Human Nutrition and Dietetics

For Churchill Livingstone

Publisher: Lucy Gardner
Copy Editor: Jennifer Bew
Indexer: Jill Halliday
Design: Design Resources Unit
Production Controller: Mark Sanderson
Sales Promotion Executive: Hilary Brown

Human Nutrition and Dietetics

Edited by

J. S. Garrow MD PhD FRCP FRCP(Edin)
Rank Professor of Human Nutrition,
St Bartholomew's Hospital Medical College,
London, UK

W. P. T. James CBE MA MD DSc FRCP(Edin) FRSE
Director of the Rowett Research Institute,
Bucksburn, Aberdeen, UK

Editorial Assistant

Ann Ralph BSc PhD
The Rowett Research Institute, Bucksburn,
Aberdeen, UK

NINTH EDITION

CHURCHILL LIVINGSTONE
EDINBURGH LONDON MADRID MELBOURNE NEW YORK AND TOKYO 1993

CHURCHILL LIVINGSTONE
Medical Division of Longman Group UK Limited

Distributed in the United States of America by Churchill
Livingstone Inc., 650 Avenue of the Americas, New York, N.Y. 10011,
and by associated companies, branches and representatives
throughout the world.

First edition 1959
Second edition 1963
Third edition 1966
Fourth edition 1969
Fifth edition 1972
Sixth edition 1975
Seventh edition 1979
Eighth edition 1986
Ninth edition 1993

ISBN 0-443-04121-0

British Library Cataloguing-in-Publication Data
A catalogue record for this book is available from the British Library.

Library of Congress Cataloging-in-Publication Data
A catalog record for this book is available from the Library of Congress.

Produced by Longman Singapore Publishers Pte Ltd
Printed in Singapore

The
publisher's
policy is to use
**paper manufactured
from sustainable forests**.

Contents

Contributors

Peter J. Aggett MSc FRCP
Head of Department of Diet, Nutrition and Health,
AFRC Institute of Food Research, Colney, Norwich;
Honorary Consultant Paediatrician, Norfolk and
Norwich Hospitals, Norwich, UK

B. Roger Allen MB FRCP
Consultant Dermatologist, University Hospital,
Nottingham, UK

Erkki Antila MD PhD
Researcher, Department of Anatomy,
University of Helsinki, Helsinki, Finland

Laurence Blendis MD FRCP(C) FRCP
Professor of Medicine, Director of Liver Diseases,
University of Toronto, Ontario, Canada

Caroline Bolton-Smith BSc PhD
Lecturer in Nutrition, University of Dundee,
Dundee, UK

Peter Boyle PhD
Director, Division of Epidemiology and
Biostatistics, European Institute of
Oncology, Milan, Italy

John Broom BSc MBChB MIBiol MRCPath
Consultant Biochemist and Senior Lecturer,
University of Aberdeen, Aberdeen Royal Hospitals,
Aberdeen, UK

Israel Chanarin BSc MD FRCPath
Consultant Haematologist, Head, Section of
Haematology, MRC Clinical Research Centre,
Harrow, Middlesex, UK

Barbara E. Clayton MD PhD FRCP FRCP(Edin) FRCPath
Honorary Research Professor in Metabolism,
University of Southampton, Southampton, UK

Bernard Crabtree (deceased) BSc PhD
The Rowett Research Institute, Bucksburn,
Aberdeen, UK

John H. Cummings FRCP
Clinical Scientific Staff, MRC Dunn
Nutrition Unit, Cambridge, UK

Garry G. Duthie BSc PhD
Senior Scientific Officer, Rowett Research
Institute, Bucksburn, Aberdeen, UK

Johanna Dwyer BSc
Tufts University Medical School and Frances
Stern Nutrition Center, New England Medical
Center Hospital, Boston, Massachusetts, USA

Hans N. Englyst PhD
Senior Scientist, MRC Dunn Clinical
Nutrition Unit, Cambridge, UK

Anne Ferguson FRCP FRCPath FRSE
Professor of Gastroenterology, University of
Edinburgh, Edinburgh, UK

Peter J. Garlick PhD
Head, Clinical Metabolism Group, Rowett
Research Institute, Greenburn Road,
Bucksburn, Aberdeen, UK

John S. Garrow MD PhD FRCP FRCPath(Edin)
Rank Professor of Human Nutrition, St
Bartholomew's Hospital Medical College,
London, UK

Cutberto Garza MD PhD
Director and Professor, Division of Nutritional
Sciences, Cornell University, Ithaca, New York, USA

Sara Gilbert BA MSc
Clinical Psychologist, Northwick Park Hospital,
Harrow, Middlesex, UK

Barbara E. Golden BSc MD DCH
Clinical Lecturer, Department of Child Health,
University of Aberdeen, Aberdeen, UK

Michael H. N. Golden FRCP
Professor of Medicine and Wellcome Senior Lecturer,
University of Aberdeen, Aberdeen, UK

Michael I. Gurr BSc PhD FIBiol
Visiting Professor, University of Reading and
Oxford Polytechnic, UK

Leif Hallberg MD PhD
Professor, Department of Medicine and Clinical
Nutrition, Gothenburg, Sweden

Charles H. Halsted MD
Professor of Internal Medicine and Chief, Division
of Clinical Nutrition and Metabolism, University
of California, Davis, California, USA

K. W. Heaton MA MD FRCP
Reader in Medicine, University of Bristol; Honorary
Consultant Physician, Bristol Royal Infirmary,
Bristol, UK

Basil S. Hetzel AC MD FRCP FRACP FFPHM FTS
Executive Director, International Council for
Control of Iodine Deficiency Disorders; Chief,
CSIRO Division of Human Nutrition,
Women's and Children's Hospital, North Adelaide,
Australia

W. Philip T. James CBE MA MD DSc FRCP FRCP(Edin)
FRSE
Director of the Rowett Research Institute,
Bucksburn, Aberdeen, UK

K. N. Jeejeebhoy MB BS PhD FRCP(C)
Professor, Department of Medicine, University of
Toronto; Staff Gastroenterologist, St Michael's
Hospital, Toronto, Ontario, Canada

I. T. Johnson PhD BSc
Head of Nutrient Absorption and Metabolism Group,
AFRC Institute of Food Research, Colney,
Norwich, UK

Izhar H. Khan MRCP
Research Fellow, Department of Medicine and
Therapeutics, University of Aberdeen,
Aberdeen, UK

Susan M. Kingman BSc PhD
Research Officer, Dunn Clinical Nutrition Centre,
Cambridge, UK

Nigel Loveridge MPhil, PhD
Bone Growth and Metabolism Unit, Rowett Research
Institute, Aberdeen, UK

Alison M. Macleod MD MRCP
Senior Lecturer in Medicine and Therapeutics,
University of Aberdeen; Honorary Consultant
Physician/Nephrologist, Aberdeen Royal
Hospitals Trust, Aberdeen, UK

Donald S. McLaren MD PhD DTMGH FRCP(Edin)
Honorary Fellow, Department of Medicine, Royal
Infirmary, Edinburgh; Honorary Head,
Nutritional Blindness Prevention Programme,
Institute of Ophthalmology, London, UK

Jim Mann MA DM PhD FRCP FFCM
Professor of Human Nutrition, University of
Otago; Head of Endocrinology, Dunedin Hospital,
Dunedin, New Zealand

Geraldine M. Neill MB ChB MSc PhD
Lecturer, Department of Medicine and Therapeutics,
University of Aberdeen, Aberdeen, UK

Donald W. M. Pearson BSc(Hons) FRCP(Glas)
FRCP(Edin)
Consultant Physician and Senior Lecturer,
Diabetic Clinic, Aberdeen Royal Hospitals
NHS Trust, Aberdeen, UK

Claude Pichard FRCP
Consultant Cardiologist, Homerton and St
Bartholomew's Hospitals, London, UK

Ann Ralph BSc PhD
The Rowett Research Institute, Bucksburn,
Aberdeen, UK

Peter Reeds MD
Department of Pediatrics, Children's Nutrition
Research Center, Baylor College of Medicine, Houston,
Texas, USA

Patricia Richmond
Senior Dietitian, Department of Nutrition and
Dietetics, Aberdeen Royal Hospitals Trust,
Aberdeen, UK

Aileen Robertson PhD
Director of Postgraduate Nutrition & Dietetic Centre,
Rowett Research Institute, Bucksburn, Aberdeen, UK

Daphne A. Roe MD
Professor, Division of Nutritional Sciences, Cornell
University, Ithaca, New York, USA

Andrew J. Rugg-Gunn PhD DSc BDS FDS
Professor of Preventive Dentistry, University of
Newcastle-upon-Tyne, Department of Child Dental
Health, The Dental School, Newcastle-upon-Tyne,
UK

Brittmarie Sandström PhD
Professor, Research Department of Human Nutrition,
The Royal Veterinary and Agricultural University,
Frederiksberg, Denmark

Roger Smith MD PhD FRCP
Consultant Physician, Metabolic Medicine, John
Radcliffe Hospital and Nuffield Orthopaedic
Centre, Oxford, UK

D. A. T. Southgate BSc PhD CBiol MJBiol
Formerly Head of Nutrition, Diet and Health
Department, AFRC Institute of Food Research
Laboratory, Colney, Norwich, UK

D. S. Tunstall Pedoe FRCP DPhil(Oxon)
Consultant Cardiologist, Homerton and
St Bartholomew's Hospitals, London, UK

R. Walker PhD CChem FRSC FIFST
Professor of Food Science, School of Biological
Sciences, University of Surrey, Guildford, UK

Thomas Westermarck MD DSc
Senior Lecturer, Vice-Chief Physician,
Helsinki Central Institute for the Mentally
Retarded, Kirkkonummi, Finland

Oliver Wrong DM FRCP
Emeritus Professor of Medicine, University
College, London; Institute of Urology and
Nephrology, The Middlesex Hospital, London, UK

Preface

Human Nutrition and Dietetics developed from A Textbook of Dietetics, which was written by Professor Stanley Davidson and Dr Ian Anderson. It was published in 1940, with a preface by Lord Boyd Orr. The first edition of Human Nutrition and Dietetics appeared in 1959, with Dr Reg Passmore as an editor, and this book, universally known as 'Davidson and Passmore', has been the leading British textbook in the field for the past three decades. Stanley Davidson died in 1981, and the continuing success of this textbook is a great tribute to the editorial skills of Reg Passmore, aided by colleagues at the Edinburgh Medical School.

Readers who are familiar with the eighth edition, which was the last to be edited by Passmore, and published in 1986, will see some changes in this ninth edition, for which explanation is needed.

First, the original format was designed for the nutrition teaching of the era in which it started, but the science and practice of human nutrition has changed radically since 1959. Classical nutrition was concerned with famine relief, wartime rationing, and the prevention of deficiency diseases in the socially disadvantaged sections of society. The older generation of people interested in nutrition (which includes past and present editors of this book) worked an apprenticeship in Third World countries, where deficiency diseases are an important cause of mortality. However, both the problems facing nutritionists, and the solutions at their disposal, have changed in many ways. These are set out in Chapter 1. It is instructive to list the main reasons why it is no longer good enough simply to supply a 'balanced diet', which includes at least the recommended amounts of all nutrients.

Nutritional epidemiology. We know that disease prevalence is significantly associated with intake of non-starch polysaccharide, different types of fat, fruit, alcohol, etc., which cannot be explained on the basis of satisfying known nutrient requirements. There is increasing evidence that many of the major diseases in developing countries are in some way related to diet, but such theories require careful and expert evaluation. Communities, and individuals, who differ markedly in diet invariably differ in other respects also, and these confounding factors must be kept in view. We have, therefore, asked the contributors to this edition to evaluate and explain the strengths and weakness of arguments linking diet to the particular disease group with which they are expert.

Changes in clinical practice. It is now necessary to provide nutritional support to people who would not have been viable in 1959; e.g. patients with extensive resection of bowel requiring total parenteral nutrition, patients with impaired immunity due to disease or suppression by drugs, and extremely premature babies. Thus, supplying normal nutrient requirements may not be enough. Also, people with inborn errors of metabolism (such as phenylketonuria) are now having children themselves, so new problems arise—for example, managing PKU in pregnancy—which would not have happened in 1959. For this reason, it is no longer possible for an individual editor to assess which are the important advances, and which are the passing fads, in the huge range of clinical conditions for which expert nutritional management is now required. For reliable advice, it is necessary to enlist the help of a clinician who has first-hand knowledge of the clinical problems, and of the efficacy and practicality of nutritional management.

Recognition of harm done by excess intake. In the days when the diet consisted essentially of tissue from plants or animals, made palatable by cooking, there was little risk of excessive intake of single nutrients. Today, for reasons given in Chapters 1 and 21, a large and ever-increasing proportion of the food we eat is processed to make it look, or taste, or keep better, or to make it easier to cook. During this processing some of the natural components of the food may be removed, or additives (which may themselves be nutrients) are added. Also, there is a flourishing 'health food' industry which offers amino acids, vitamins, minerals and other nutrients either singly or in combinations which would never normally occur in food. It is clear that excessive intake of energy, leading to obesity, is an important factor in many major diseases (see Ch. 32). Excessive intakes of a single mineral, such as zinc, may impair the metabolism of other minerals, and vitamins, especially fat-soluble ones, are toxic in excess. The new Recommended Nutrient Intakes, summarized in Appendix 2, give guidance about upper safe limits of intake. Thus, the boundary between nutrition and toxicology is no longer so clear, and new types of diet-related disorders are appearing.

These are the main reasons for asking expert clinicians to write the chapters in the second section of the book (Chs 29–50). Each chapter is supported by an up-to-date reference list which will guide the student who wishes to read more thoroughly in the topic. Of course there are also disadvantages in multi-author works: the seamless fluency of a monograph is lost, and the careful student will note some minor inconsistencies between chapters (e.g. in different chapters total body water in a 70 kg adult has been assigned values ranging from 42 to 50 kg, any of which is possible). We believe that the deeper understanding brought to the subject by these authoritative contributors more than outweighs these disadvantages.

Although the second part of the book has been radically changed, the essential structure of the eighth edition has been retained in the first part. To be competent in nutrition it is essential to have a firm grasp of the physiological and biochemical role played by nutrients, and the dietary sources from which these nutrients are derived. This is increasingly true for several reasons. Nutrition, or dieting, is now widely discussed in the popular press, and a 'diet book' is rarely absent from the best-seller list. Often the startling theories propounded in these books show that the author has no understanding of the science of nutrition. We, who claim expertise in nutrition, may be called upon to explain why the theories are unsound, and this requires a mastery of the information set out in the first part of the book.

However, confusion about nutrition in the mind of the public does not arise simply from the fictional works of ignorant authors. Nutritional science is not isolated from the economic and cultural life of society. If the public believes it should change its consumption of particular types of fat, or fruit, or meat, or sugar, this may present a serious threat to the prosperity or employment of thousands of people. Governments have a responsibility to maintain industrial activity as well as to maintain health, and there is often a conflict between these objectives. The food industry is particularly vulnerable to changes in public taste, since severe criticism of a particular food product in the media may cause virtual cessation of sales of that product in a week: no other major industry is so exposed to instant commercial disaster. By way of defence the food industry maintains a very active public relations operation which is alert to challenge and deflects any public statement which might be commercially disadvantageous.

It is also true that nutrition education of the public operates in the area where advice is given on a balance of probabilities, rather than on irrefutable evidence. It is therefore relatively easy (and profitable) for iconoclastic journalists to draw attention to the evidence that does not support the consensus view, and thus refute the experts, which is always a popular thing to do. Thus, the public is bombarded with conflicting advice, and concludes that the nutrition experts are themselves confused and incompetent. The antidote to this is to provide an accessible summary of the scientific principles on which nutrition is based, and also to make the student aware of the economic and cultural pressures which tend to distort the scientifically sound nutritional advice that should be offered to the public. We hope we have succeeded in this objective.

Editing a book of this scale is a major undertaking and we are very grateful to the many people who made it possible. The authors of chapters are identified: we thank them for their expertise, and their tolerance of the frustrations which inevitably arise in trying to achieve a balance between different contributions in a work of this size and scope. No doubt we have made errors in editing: we hope these will be identified and remedied in subsequent editions. We have relied heavily on the willingness of Mrs Elrick at the Rowett, and Mrs Churchman at Barts, to retype passages which had become too greatly altered to be legible to typesetters. Lucy Gardner at Churchill Livingstone has bolstered our morale in times of desperation, and Dr Ann Ralph has done more than we could ever have hoped or expected to check and correct both manuscripts and proofs, thereby making a very major contribution to the clarity and accuracy of the book. We thank them all most sincerely.

J.S.G.
W.P.T.J.

1993

1. Historical perspective

W. P. T. James

This chapter takes a historical perspective in looking at attitudes to food, health and nutrition in an attempt to explain the state of affairs that exists today. Some of the major landmarks are summarized in Fig. 1.1.

CHANGES IN SOCIETY

The clinician or dietitian is used to treating individual patients. Yet most of the significant changes in the patterns of disease in a population, and the causes of death, have little to do with individual therapy. Fluctuations in the patterns of health depend on environmental changes, which include social and economic conditions, the implementation of immunization programmes, women's educational status and changes in agricultural practice induced by regulations dealing with taxes, international trade, and agricultural research. All these measures operate through alterations in the provision of hygienic food with changes in its nutritional quality and through the availability of uncontaminated water. Clean housing free from overcrowding, and changes in the exposure to environmental toxicants, are also important as well as individual behaviour relating to deliberate use of toxicants, e.g. drug use, smoking and alcohol consumption. Thus the decline in deaths from infections, diseases such as scarlet fever, rheumatic fever and diphtheria, and from tuberculosis started in Europe decades before chemotherapy was available (Fig. 1.2). Immunization made a great contribution to the decline of whooping cough, poliomyelitis, measles, diphtheria and smallpox but many of these diseases were much more prevalent and serious in the poor than in the wealthy.

Measles and whooping cough continue to be scourges in the Third World with high death rates, whereas infected children in Europe or North America have much milder infections. Chapter 44 sets out the multiple mechanisms whereby nutrition can affect immunity and it is widely believed that unspecified improvements in diet have contributed to the better health of children and adults, which became apparent in affluent societies throughout the world by the 1950s. Life expectancy increased progressively with a remarkable fall in the risk of death in childhood (Fig. 1.3). This was associated with a marked reduction in the size of families as women's social and political role became more established and their education improved.

In the Third World, improvements in diet, hygiene and immunization have been less effective in reducing childhood mortality. The birth rate has fallen but women remain in general less educated, of a lower social status and less likely to control the size of their family. The resulting population explosion now threatens to outstrip food supplies, particularly in the Indian subcontinent. Studies in Kerala, one of the poorest Indian states, where paradoxically women are exceptionally well educated, show that infant mortality and the birth rate are far below that expected for such a poor society but consistent with high quality maternal care (Ratcliffe 1978). The delay between the changes in infantile mortality and contraceptive practices is variable but the longer it is the greater the population explosion. Blaxter (1993) calculated that existing agricultural practices and decreased availability of suitable land for cultivation will not be able to provide enough food for the world's population unless there are substantial and widespread decreases in population growth. As nutritionists and dietitians consider the debates about national nutritional policies, this historical perspective shows that few of the arguments are new.

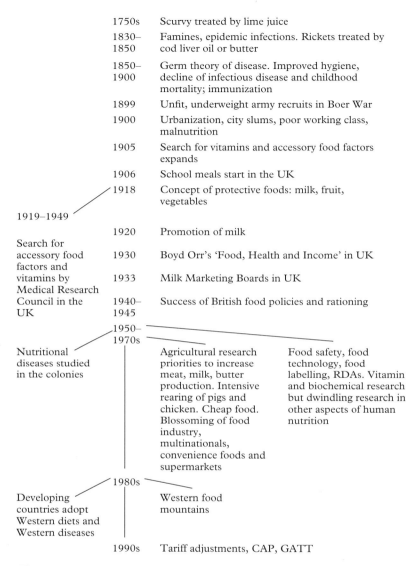

1750s	Scurvy treated by lime juice	
1830–1850	Famines, epidemic infections. Rickets treated by cod liver oil or butter	
1850–1900	Germ theory of disease. Improved hygiene, decline of infectious disease and childhood mortality; immunization	
1899	Unfit, underweight army recruits in Boer War	
1900	Urbanization, city slums, poor working class, malnutrition	
1905	Search for vitamins and accessory food factors expands	
1906	School meals start in the UK	
1918	Concept of protective foods: milk, fruit, vegetables	

1919–1949

Search for accessory food factors and vitamins by Medical Research Council in the UK

1920	Promotion of milk	
1930	Boyd Orr's 'Food, Health and Income' in UK	
1933	Milk Marketing Boards in UK	
1940–1945	Success of British food policies and rationing	

1950–1970s

Nutritional diseases studied in the colonies

Agricultural research priorities to increase meat, milk, butter production. Intensive rearing of pigs and chicken. Cheap food. Blossoming of food industry, multinationals, convenience foods and supermarkets

Food safety, food technology, food labelling, RDAs. Vitamin and biochemical research but dwindling research in other aspects of human nutrition

1980s

Developing countries adopt Western diets and Western diseases

Western food mountains

1990s   Tariff adjustments, CAP, GATT

Fig. 1.1 Landmarks in the fields of health, food and nutrition leading to the present situation.

GERM THEORY OF DISEASE AND THE NEED FOR PUBLIC HYGIENE

The Third World in the 1990s still experiences the ravages of famines, natural and man-made disasters, semi-starvation, endemic and epidemic infections and political reorganization and civil war. Similar problems, however, occurred in Western Europe only 100–150 years ago. In 1831, cholera arrived in Britain and the epidemic that followed forced the Government to take action. A Board of Health was established to issue a series of sanitary regulations. Its effectiveness led to public awareness of the need for standards of hygiene and good living conditions.

Medical science later provided a new understanding of the causes of disease, the typhoid bacillus being discovered in 1880 and the causes of leprosy and malaria in the same year. The discovery of the bacilli

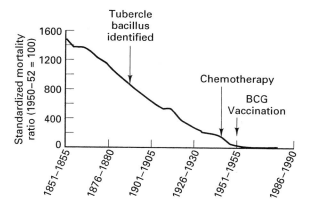

Fig. 1.2 Decline in death rate from tuberculosis in England and Wales, 1851–1990 (from Health of the Nation 1992).

causing tuberculosis, cholera, diphtheria, *Escherichia coli* diarrhoea and pneumococcal pneumonia were discovered sequentially from 1882 to 1886, so a new understanding of the importance of sanitation, hygiene and clean water reinforced the demand for major developments in water supplies, building regulations, sewerage disposal and public health education. European governments were gripped by population demands for public work based on hygienic principles and a concern for the 'evils' of uncleanliness, foul air and poor sanitation. By the beginning of this century, it was accepted that governmental action for the public's health should go hand in hand with individual care by doctors. The public health professions were strong and influential and were able to force changes in medical education to emphasize the teaching of 'sanitary science'.

POOR FOOD AND THE WORKING CLASSES

In Britain the next public health crisis came about in 1900 when the Government realized that the British had nearly been defeated in the Boer War. Recruitment proved difficult because so many young men were considered too small and sick to enter the army. The public already knew of the overcrowding and filth in the city slums and some feared that the working class, with their higher birth rates, would numerically overwhelm the upper and middle classes, thereby leading to a decline in the effectiveness and intelligence of society as 'inferior' genetic stock came to dominate Britain! However, a special committee was established and concluded that the main causes of ill health and poor physique were to be found in the homes of the poor: improper and insufficient food were claimed to be the main problem. Malnutrition was identified as a cause of ill health and poor physical and mental performance. Studies were therefore conducted throughout Britain and in many other European countries to estimate the numbers of malnourished children in different areas. High reported prevalences, e.g. of 30% in the Scottish city of Edinburgh and 60% in Manchester in Northern England, led to greater popular concern.

A subsidized School Meals Service was started in 1906 to provide needy children with food so that 'they could take advantage of the education provided'. A single meal of high quality was to include appropriate amounts of the more expensive foods such as the protein foods which the body needed for growth. A School Meals Service developed and emphasized the child's need for energy and protein. By the 1920s the dairy industry and the Government promoted the consumption of milk and in 1933 the Milk Marketing

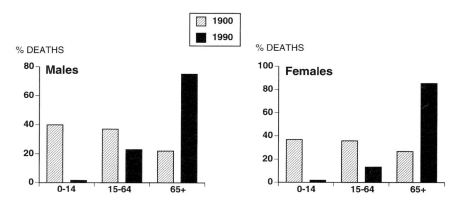

Fig. 1.3   Changes in age of death in the UK, 1900–1990 (OPCS 1990).

Boards were set up to improve the efficiency of transport and distribution of milk. School milk clubs and cheap milk were promoted incessantly, this being paid for by local authorities or charities. Cod liver oil was then added to prevent rickets. School feeding schemes increased rapidly throughout the 1930s. The poor sections of the population were specifically targeted and by the mid-1930s the use of milk was seen to be a suitable alternative to a whole meal. In practice, the switch to milk exacerbated rather than reduced the deficit in energy intake, but the growth-promoting properties of milk were by then well recognized.

IMPACT OF VITAMIN DISCOVERIES

The amazing impact on clinical medicine of the discovery of vitamins is discussed in Chapters 13 and 14. Yet the development of modern nutrition had to wait until Atwater and Benedict in the United States had set out the principles for understanding the dietary basis for meeting energy needs (Chapter 3). The modest need for protein and its constituent amino acids had also been reassessed by Chittenden. Accessory food factors were sought from 1905 onwards. Funk in Poland and Hopkins in England were then able to demonstrate that small amounts of chemicals in different foods could prevent poor growth and disease in animals fed semi-purified diets. McCollum by 1918 had already classified fruit and vegetables, as well as milk, as 'protective foods' and dietary studies on rats provided the basis for the new British Medical Research Council's report on vitamins in 1919. In the 1920s, McCarrison, head of what became India's National Institute of Nutrition, linked rat studies to human growth and deficiency disease by feeding rats on either a typical Sikh or a poor European diet. Rats fed on the Sikh diet of whole wheat, butter, milk, legumes, raw vegetables and milk grew well, whereas those fed the poor European diet grew badly on a mixture of white bread, margarine, tinned meat, boiled vegetables, jam, tea and sugar with only a little milk. Clearly the Sikh diet was better and contained more 'protective' factors. Boyd Orr in Aberdeen repeated these studies but compared a poor Scottish diet with one to which milk and green vegetables had been added. The additions promoted growth and suggested that children might also benefit from similar treatment. Thus the discovery of vitamins and the benefits to growth and the health of both experimental animals and children fed supplements of meat, milk and other protective foods re-

emphasized the importance of diet for the health of the nation.

NUTRITION IN PUBLIC HEALTH: PUBLIC ACTION OR INDIVIDUAL EDUCATION?

In Britain Fletcher and Mellanby were in charge of the British Medical Research Council from 1919–1949, and were prominent in public health. They gave preferential funding to nutrition research, a rare event in any country, so there was a flowering of research to identify food factors with unusual healthy properties. Fletcher also backed a report that showed that miners had a poor physique, low wages, a poor diet and used inappropriate cooking methods, but the Ministry of Health was unenthusiastic about nutrition education. Then poverty increased during the economic slump of 1929–1932 when 2.7 million UK adults were out of work. Soon after Mellanby (1934) outlined a programme for state action to improve the nation's diet (Table 1.1) and emphasized the importance of establishing a carefully thought out national policy.

However, a Glaswegian physiologist, Cathcart, considered that the problem of childhood malnutrition reflected poor maternal care. The potential efficiency of households to cope, the mother's cooking skills, her capacity as a general manager and household cleanliness were assessed and the father was scored on the consistency of his income and the amount of money spent on alcohol. The children's nutritional status was found not to depend on income but on the 'efficiency' of the parents. He concluded that the way to combat the problem was nutrition education with the distribution of pamphlets listing the protective foods. Nevertheless, Boyd Orr galvanized public opinion in the 1930s by emphasizing the link between poverty, a poor diet and poor health. Boyd Orr's study on Food Health and Income (1936) was one of many but the propaganda value of the report was great. United action by religious and women's groups, and by voluntary organizations, built up pressure to provide free milk to the vulnerable groups in society, i.e. to infants, school children, pregnant and lactating mothers. The Government, however, continued to resist the proposals for the widespread subsidy of milk on the grounds of cost.

WAR-TIME POLICIES

With the start of the World War II the UK Government was stimulated to act by the fear that the

Table 1.1   The changing basis of nutritional advice

1934: Mellanby's priorities for British food

Reduce	Increase	Expected benefit
Cereal and bread intake	Protective foods, i.e. milk, cheese, eggs, green vegetables	*Increase*: Stature Physical activity Mental alertness *Decrease*: Dental caries Goitre Rickets Anaemia *Probable decrease*: Middle ear infection Bronchopneumonia Tuberculosis Rheumatic endocarditis

1976–1983 Royal College of Physician's Advice on British Food

Reduce	Increase	Expected benefit
Fat, saturated fatty acid, sugar, salt intakes, i.e. eggs, milk fat (high fat cheeses)	Cereals, bread, green vegetables, fruit, polyunsaturated fatty acid intakes	*Maintain*: Stature Physical activity Mental alertness *Decrease*: Dental caries Obesity Heart disease Constipation Gallstones *Possible decrease*: Some cancers

country would be starved into submission. German submarines sank many ships bringing food from the colonies and North America and these ships provided 70% of the country's needs. British agriculture was desperately inadequate, the dairy industry had an excess of milk, which was selling poorly despite promotional campaigns, and the authorities were worried that the morale of the people would suffer if good food was not provided.

During the war there developed a coherent strategy to ensure sufficient food for all and to deal with food production, distribution, storage and sales. Prices of staple foods were fixed at below market rates, farmers were not recruited into the army and British women were mobilized for the first time to work not only in the armed forces and factories, but also on the land. Foods were rationed but everybody was allowed enough to meet their nutrient needs as calculated by a group of four medical nutritionists who based their analyses on pre-war dietary surveys. Incessant public campaigns encouraged home growing of foods and a variety of other measures, including collecting wild rose-hips to provide more vitamin C. Cooking methods and intense nutritional education left nobody in any doubt of the importance of good food. 'Protein foods' were advisable for growth and for good body repair, 'energy foods' in the form of carbohydrates and fats were good for vitality, and 'protective foods' prevented vitamin and mineral deficiencies. Eating a variety of foods from each of these three groups ensured that everybody would have a 'balanced' diet. This was the first and only time that the UK Government reorganized major economic aspects of Government as part of a coherent nutrient and food policy. By 1940 cheap milk was made available throughout the maternal and child welfare service and by 1944 free school milk was made available to all schoolchildren.

POLICIES SINCE WORLD WAR II

The UK wartime food policies were acclaimed worldwide. Throughout Europe, having enough high quality food was a recognized national priority because of the hardships of war. In the 1930s, Russia's farmers had been starved to death in their millions by Stalin for refusing to agree to collectivization, and the blockade of parts of the Netherlands in 1944 led to widespread starvation. At the end of World War II there were also 6 million refugees moving about a devastated Western Russia, Poland and Germany, searching for food, and there was a refugee problem in the Middle East. Concern for food supplies was therefore widespread and this concern has dominated agricultural and food policies worldwide ever since.

It was accepted in the 1940s that the combination of intensive nutrition education, a rationing system based on scientific principles and the development of farming and food distribution policies would ensure a balanced diet and the conquest of deficiency diseases. Massive American aid helped Europe to recover after the war. Eventually food rationing in Western Europe gave way to the enjoyment of food and the development of the food industry to ensure the widespread availability of foods with enough energy, protein and micronutrients at the cheapest possible cost. Some refinements in the understanding of human nutrition were still needed, but agricultural research and production became a priority. Meat, milk and butter production was, and continues to be, a high priority for many societies. It became accepted as a national priority that no European country should have to rely on food imports. By having enough of everything it was possible to guarantee the availability of a balanced diet. Food legislation and health policy need then only be geared to ensuring that the vulnerable groups in society had special treatment.

In the 1950s the emphasis on nutritional deficiency switched to the tropics where famine was a problem and specific deficiency diseases, such as beriberi and pellagra, were still occurring. Although the British, Dutch, French, Portuguese and Belgian Empires were coming to an end, the colonies became the obvious place for nutritional research. The British Medical Research Council promoted its nutritional research effort in Uganda, India and Jamaica. Kwashiorkor and marasmus were to be studied to establish their nutritional basis and the conquest of nutritional deficiency disease became an international priority. Platt's MRC Unit and his work at the London School of Hygiene and Tropical Medicine was seen as a back-up for tropical problems and McCance's unit in Cambridge continued to work on problems of childhood nutrition. In the UK, Nobel prize-winning biochemists, such as Krebs, were allowed to transfer from wartime nutritional research to their first love of biochemistry. By 1970 only the original Dunn Nutrition Laboratory remained as the Medical Research Council's major contribution to human nutritional research in the UK. More esoteric research into vitamins was allowed and this eventually led to the discovery by Fraser of the renal origin of 1,25 dihydroxy vitamin D.

Post-war, the Rowett Research Institute was ordered to stop doing human nutrition research, so the newly-appointed medically-qualified Director, Cuthbertson, famous for his work on patient feeding in trauma, set about boosting research into animal production. Boyd Orr, the founder of the Rowett Research Institute, was called on to establish the United Nations Food and Agriculture Organization. He soon resigned, however, because the United States and Britain were unwilling to create an Executive Food Board to control reserve stocks of world food and food prices to prevent starvation. This would have meant the transfer of power to the new United Nations, which neither the new American nor old colonial powers could accept.

THE FARMING REVOLUTION

Throughout Europe and North America it was accepted that food production must be a priority. Agricultural research institutions proliferated and Government subsidies to farmers were boosted and linked to the development of free national agricultural advisory services. Marketing boards and farming cooperatives in Europe were encouraged; tax advantages for farmers and price support schemes were developed to ensure maximum milk production from tuberculosis-free cows, and for butter and meat production. Farmers had to be supported by every conceivable means in the expectation that eventually there would be enough food for everybody to choose an enjoyable, balanced and cheap diet with sufficient energy, protein, vitamins and minerals. A diet rich in cheese, cream, meat and other dairy products was recognized as a luxury which might eventually be a regular feature of everybody's diet and not simply an occasional treat.

This policy proved spectacularly successful; the combination of agricultural science and the growth of large firms to serve the farmers led to the development of agribusinesses and a change in the whole way of farming. With new seeds, the use of fertilisers, mineral supplements, crop regulators, growth enhancers, pesticides and other management techniques, there seemed no longer to be the need to worry about crop rotation to ensure nutrient balance within the soil. Single crops could therefore be produced annually on the same soil. The needs for harvesting machinery were therefore simplified and soon monoculture systems developed throughout the Western world. Intensive livestock management with maximum productivity progressed. In the USA the barley beef system developed by Preston at the Rowett led to the use of huge feed lots where cattle stood eating barley or other cereals ad libitum instead of having to graze extensively on grass. Animal growth rates and production improved and costs fell progressively. The steady fall in food prices was seen as a major success for the farming industry.

Soon it was apparent that the conversion of cereals to animal protein was an expensive process in ruminants, e.g. cattle and sheep, but was much more efficient in a pig, so cheaper pork and bacon could be produced by controlling the environment and feeding conditions of pigs. Pigs were therefore housed in new, intensively organized, specially designed buildings where their reproductive cycle, lactation and growth rates could be monitored and manipulated by drugs, diet and a variety of management techniques. The cost of bacon and pork therefore fell rapidly and their consumption rose steadily.

Chickens then proved to be even more efficient converters of cereal to meat protein, so intensive husbandry methods were devised for egg and chicken production. Prices fell, availability improved dramatically and the wartime luxury of an occasional small piece of chicken is now changed in Europe to one where chicken is one of the commonest dishes available in any household, cafeteria or restaurant.

WESTERN FOOD MOUNTAINS

The farmers' effectiveness in responding to these policies post-war seemed to prove that they were highly responsible, public-spirited and hard-working members of the community. Government subsidies, free advice, marketing boards and new opportunities for increasing productivity meant that the European farmer began to enjoy an unprecedentedly high standard of living as food production climbed rapidly. From the low level of farm productivity in 1945, remarkable changes had occurred by 1980 when an excess production of almost every food was apparent in both Western Europe and the United States. Food mountains of unsold food had to be stored before being disposed of in some way. The financial burden of European subsidies paid on the basis of output was increasing rapidly, but in the United States huge subsidies were still not sufficient to prevent farmers being bankrupt by crop failures and falling world prices. The USA and European Economic Community then began to compete on the world market selling butter, cereals, beef and other commodities below world prices to the former Soviet Union and Eastern Europe. By maintaining high prices for Western farmers and selling cheaply abroad, Third World farmers were immediately at a disadvantage because they had little incentive to produce crops for export. In this way the affluence of European and North American farmers was preserved by the tax-payer at the expense of the rural poor in developing countries.

In the 1990s the Europeans are attempting to adjust their subsidy policies while they argue with the USA, Australasia and other countries about their need to maintain the viability of the farming community. This is part of the adjustment of the European Community's Agriculture Policy (CAP) to the General Agreement on Tariffs and Trade (GATT) as part of longstanding international trading agreements.

EMERGING PROBLEMS IN THE SECOND AND THIRD WORLDS

Dietary changes

The principal components of a country's diet tend to relate to a nation's state of affluence. The fall in the consumption of starchy foods and the rise in animal fat consumption are the most striking dietary features as societies become more affluent. Simple sugars, especially sucrose and glucose syrups, also form a much higher proportion of the total dietary carbohydrates in very affluent communities, e.g. 50% compared with the 5–10% observed in many communities with a low income. These changes are not necessarily a reflection of an intrinsic desire for meat and fat at the levels consumed in the West, although in hunter–gatherer societies on very high carbohydrate intakes fat is recognized as a flavour-rich item which is specially prized. Part of the pressure to change to Western diets comes from the widespread cultural perception that freedom and affluence is part of the enjoyable North American and European lifestyle, so any affluent subsection of an Eastern European or developing country seeks to incorporate indices of an affluent lifestyle into its behaviour. These ideas are promoted by the intense marketing of Western firms, e.g. Coca Cola, Mars, Macdonald's hamburgers and Kentucky Fried Chicken, using marketing strategies which recognize the long-term financial benefits of marketing the image, even in societies which have very different dietary patterns. Thus the Japanese, despite their complex traditions on diet with a fat content of only 13% in 1963 (Insull et al 1968), had increased their fat intake to 28% by the 1980s (FAO 1984). The marketing of American snack foods and drinks in Japan is pervasive and follows the marketing patterns seen throughout the Third World. These approaches are similar to those used in cigarette promotion (Taylor 1984). Tobacco firms increasingly deprived of their sales and lobbying in Western countries are buying up international food firms, so it is little surprise that their tactics in influencing international organizations, Government ministers, trade policies and marketing restrictions are similar.

Eastern European food policies, diets and disease

These have been based on the same nutritional principles which led to an emphasis in Western Europe on the provision of enough energy, protein and other nutrients to permit children to grow and adults to work. Agriculture and food policies were centrally organized as expected in a command economy and there was a widespread acceptance throughout the European Communist world that animal production was vital to provide plentiful supplies of meat.

With the collapse of the Communist system, policymakers throughout Eastern Europe still perceive the people's needs in old-fashioned terms with an emphasis on animal protein and fat production. Vegetables and fruit have become scarce commodities and the Eastern European countries have the most obese populations in Europe, with very high rates of diabetes, hypertension, hypercholesterolaemia, coronary heart disease and dietary-related cancers. Their rates now vie with Scotland and Northern Ireland. The nutrition and food policies of Eastern Europe are now in a state of flux with central controls abandoned, and economic rather than health issues now dominant. Surveys show that the populations of Czechoslovakia and Hungary are aware of the links between saturated fatty acid intake, elevated blood cholesterol and heart disease, but their food patterns remain imprudent with a high meat and fat consumption and with modest amounts of poor quality fruit and vegetables.

Developing country nutrition

Urbanization in the Third World has an immediate impact on the nature of the food supply because no longer is a household relying on the ready availability of home-grown produce or on its storage within the household. The cash economy is of far greater significance for the urban household's food supply, and expanding urban communities begin to place great demands on the transport and storage systems for food. Food preservation therefore becomes of even greater significance than in the rural areas, and the availability of large numbers of people within a confined area provides a ready market for development of small- and medium-sized food industries. These developments are often encouraged by Government subsidies, tax incentives or administrative support as Governments seek to solve the problems of both urban unemployment and food supply. These urban communities are then exposed to the same processes of mass production and demand convenient snack foods while being exposed to new marketing strategies by the international and local food firms.

Thus, there are social and economic pressures for urban communities to change their diet towards that of affluent societies. Dietary patterns of urban and rural dwellers in the same country usually show striking differences with higher intakes of fat, sugar and salt in urban compared with rural areas. The latter usually depend on their staple crops of cereals, tubers, vegetables and fruits.

FOOD SAFETY

With the post-war emphasis on improving food production for a balanced diet it was clearly important to ensure that the foods were safe in terms of their toxicological or compositional content. There therefore developed complex regulatory procedures, discussed in Chapters 21–24. In the UK, committees were formed based on the assumption that it was the Government's responsibility to ensure the toxicological and microbiological safety of foods. The choice of a balanced diet depended on consumer choice which in turn required general nutritional education. Food technologists and toxicologists financed by industry came to dominate the advisory processes and nutritional issues were soon considered as rather vague and unimportant in affluent societies. It was thought that food availability was based on a free market despite the huge distortion of food prices and sales by agricultural subsidies and the often unscrupulous marketing tactics of the major food firms. On an international basis, FAO and WHO established a standing committee, known as Codex Alimentarius, again composed mostly of industrial food technologists and toxicologists, to agree internationally binding regulations on analytical methods, food labelling issues and toxicological questions. Modern concepts of nutrition were either ignored or seen as a matter of persuading consumers not to indulge themselves excessively in the enjoyable foods rich in fat, sugar and salt. Thus regulatory authorities are now dominated by concepts of food toxicology and food safety and are usually unsympathetic to public health issues and remedies.

NUTRITIONAL REQUIREMENTS AND FOOD LABELLING

The emphasis on regulatory aspects of food safety combined with a wish to allow consumer choice has led the food industry and the Governments to agree on a common basis of food labelling (Chapter 24), which includes standard displays of the absolute amounts of nutrients per 100 g of food product. Additional attempts to make these labels meaningful for consumers and to justify fortification policies and health claims led industry to agree to present the confusing variety of weights and units of each nutrient in terms of the national or internationally accepted and scientifically determined values for the requirements for each nutrient. These values are traditionally set as the recommended dietary allowances (RDA). This has led to great confusion when nutritionists assess the diet of individuals (see Appendix 1). The WHO, US, UK and EC committees have produced different values and schemes for the RDA or other reference values. These are set out in Appendix 2, which also contains an explanation of some of the differences. These issues of food labelling are perceived as the basis of nutrition policies in those Western countries that emphasize health and nutrition education. In countries concerned to reduce the fat and saturated fat content of the diet, foods are increasingly labelled with their fat, carbohydrate and protein content even though it is impossible without a calculator and knowledge of one's basal metabolic rate and physical activity pattern to purchase foods according to individual need. Nevertheless, the food industry persists with labels that fail to display the real significance of the fat, sugar or salt content in terms which consumers can understand. New labelling techniques have been proposed based on a variety of new approaches, but there is understandable reluc-

tance to label food products emphasizing their undesirable nutritional qualities!

FOOD STANDARDS

Compositional standards were originally introduced as a form of consumer protection so that, for example, sausages, ice cream, butter, pies or jams could be guaranteed to have a minimum content of meat, fat or fruit (Chapter 24). The need to guarantee the quality of food stemmed from concern about having enough protein, energy or other nutrients in a food and to prevent the adulteration of good quality products. Regulations were also introduced specifying standards for production for traditional products, e.g. cheeses, and regulations were then made to protect special foods or drinks from being copied. European food regulations still allow the maintenance of many aspects of national food laws but in the EC specify that every member must allow the entry of food products from another EC country if the food is acceptable in the country of origin. There is, however, a growing belief that these standards are old-fashioned and that there should be less regulation and a greater emphasis on nutrient declaration. In practice, when food standards are relaxed, evidence is growing that many food companies compete on price by removing the more expensive ingredients, such as protein. Thus meat pies and fish fingers sold in the UK have shown a striking fall in meat and fish content since deregulation and the many firms compete with each other by producing brands at the lowest possible price and with only minor amounts of meat and fish.

THE FOOD INDUSTRY

With post-war national priorities for cheap food production, the food industries in North America and Northern Europe blossomed. Luxuries, such as confectionery, biscuits, cakes, butter, cream, meat and other more unusual foods, became readily available at a price most people could afford, so there was a huge change in eating habits once the restrictions on food supplies were overcome in the mid-1950s.

One major consequence of World War II in Western Europe and Northern America was the recognition that women could play a major role in the economic activity of a country. This new-found freedom, amplified by the widespread introduction of reliable forms of contraception, brought women into jobs before, during and after their childbearing years. The demand for a simplification of food preparation and cooking opened up a major opportunity for the sale of kitchen gadgets, refrigerators, freezers and a variety of labour-saving devices. Foods which could be bought in bulk, preserved for considerable periods of time and then easily and quickly cooked were in demand. As purchasing power increased, seasonal foods became available throughout the year as air, rail and road transport was revolutionized to move foods in chilled or frozen form across continents and halfway round the world. Food manufacturers were able to offer traditional foods in newly packaged forms: in tins, plastic containers, vacuum packs and ready cooked varieties of dishes which decades ago would have taken hours to prepare and cook, even if the ingredients had been available. The challenge for a food manufacturer was then how to establish a market niche and develop specific brands of foods which would retain consumer loyalty. Food was no longer a matter of survival and health but a pleasure, with major social connotations. As wealth increased millions from the affluent countries went abroad for their holidays, experienced new foods and cultures and thereby created new opportunities for further food products to be produced with ethnic, social or other connotations. Immigrants from Africa, Asia and the Caribbean poured into Western Europe, and from Japan, Mexico, South and Central America into the United States, bringing their own foods, cuisines, restaurants and culture.

Given these market pressures, it is no surprise to discover in Northern Europe that 70% or more of all foods now consumed are processed, preserved and/or packaged in one way or another. This 'adds value' to the product in agricultural terms, but for the consumer this means paying a higher price for the primary product in return for its preservation or modification into some 'appetizing' food produced in a form which is convenient in purchasing, preservation or serving terms.

The effect of these developments should not be underestimated. In Northern Europe the consumption of potatoes has fallen, and a large proportion of potatoes is now consumed as potato products, e.g. as chips and crisps, rather than in their fresh state. In this case the processing of potatoes had increased their monetary value very substantially but at a cost in nutritional terms of a marked increase in fat consumption.

Similar examples can be given relating to sugar and salt consumption. Sugar intakes have been declining throughout Northern Europe when expressed in terms of free sucrose bought in bags as refined sugar. However, the sugar content of food items has increased and new sugar products, e.g. soft drinks, are

an increasingly prominent component of the diet, sustained and promoted by intense advertising.

Salt has traditionally been used as a food preservative but with the advent of refrigeration and other food preservatives, the use of salt for preserving meats and vegetables for consumption in the winter has declined. Nevertheless, food manufacturers have recognized the usefulness of salt as a taste enhancer so that salt is an important ingredient of commercially produced soups and a variety of manufactured foods. The proportion of ingested salt coming from food products rather than from cooking and the use of table salt varies depending on the dominance of manufactured food products in the diet. Thus in the UK new techniques for analysis have shown that 85% of the population's salt intake comes from nonhousehold sources where the consumer cannot use his or her discretion (Sanchez-Castillo et al 1987). In Italy, by contrast, the figure is about 65% (Leclerq & Ferro-Luzzi 1991).

Thus, wherever the food industry is a major source of food products, there has been a natural tendency to develop products rich in fat, sugar and salt. New processing techniques improved the flavour of products as sugars, fats, salt and spices were added to enhance the texture, crispness and taste of products. Meat, formerly rejected as unrecoverable from carcasses, could now be removed by new grinding, washing and enzyme processes. Meats, salamis and pies were manufactured from soya or other vegetable products to resemble any meat by the judicious addition of special flavours, chemical binders, preservatives and additives. Thus food products were produced at low prices which meant that the poorer sections of the community thought they had the ideal combination of readily available, attractively packaged and cheap foods.

Major national and international food companies began to control networks of wholesale and retail outlets. The result of this intense competition is that the marketing of foods and drinks is now a major source of advertising revenue for television and radio companies, with a myriad of new products being promoted in an attempt to establish new markets.

FOOD RETAILING AND THE DEVELOPMENT OF SUPERMARKETS

Throughout Northern Europe and North America there has been a profound change in food distribution and sales, as well as in food production and processing. In Scandinavia and Northern Europe farmers traditionally sold their produce to local distributors or directly to individual village shops. Some retailers, however, prospered by buying a group of shops and converting them into highly organized purchasing and retailing businesses. This process started first in America; the improvement in the standard of living meant that most people had a car and found it convenient to shop once a week, or even once a month, rather than daily. The efficiency of supermarkets meant cheaper food, often of high quality and in a far greater variety than could be bought at a small local shop. During the 1970s and 1980s there has therefore been a revolution in the distribution and selling of food, with supermarkets taking about three-quarters

or more of all food sales in the UK. The supermarket buyers have therefore accelerated the fall in food prices and forced even more efficient ways of providing foods until, in the 1990s, supermarkets realize that they sell more profitably by concentrating on the quality of their products. Thus in the West there is at last a change from a cheap food policy based on old concerns to food being chosen as a social and enjoyable feature of life to which are now added new concerns for health. Eating for health is once more on the national agenda for almost the first time since World War II (Chapter 51).

REFERENCES

Blaxter K 1993 From hunting and gathering to agriculture. In: Leathwood P, Horisberger M, James WPT (eds) For a better nutrition in the 21st century. Nestlé Nutrition Workshop Series 27: 1–13. Nestec Ltd, Vevey

Food and Agriculture Organization 1984 Food balance sheets 1979–1981. FAO, Rome

Health of the Nation 1992 A strategy for health in England. HMSO, London

Insull W, Oiso T, Tsuchiya K 1968 The diet and nutritional status of Japanese. American Journal of Clinical Nutrition 21: 753–777

Leclercq C, Ferro-Luzzi A 1991 Total and domestic consumption of salt and their determinants in three regions of Italy. European Journal of Clinical Nutrition 45: 151–159

Mellanby E 1934 Report on the need for improved motivation of the people of Great Britain. MRC Report 2110/146, London

Office of Population Censuses and Surveys 1990 In: Annual Abstract of Statistics 1992. Central Statistical Office. HMSO, London

Orr JB 1936 Food, health and income. Macmillan, London

Ratcliffe J 1978 Social justice and the demographic transition: lessons from India's Kerala State. International Journal of Health Services 8: 123–144

Royal College of Physicians 1980 Medical aspects of dietary fibre. Pitman Medical, London

Royal College of Physicians 1983 Obesity. Journal of the Royal College of Physicians of London 17: 3–58

Royal College of Physicians and British Cardiac Society 1976 Prevention of coronary heart disease. Journal of Royal College of Physicians of London 10: 213–275

Sanchez-Castillo CP, Warrender S, Whitehead TP, James WPT 1987 An assessment of the sources of dietary salt in a British population. Clinical Science 72: 95–102

Taylor R 1984 The smoke ring. The politics of tobacco. Bodley Head, London

2. Composition of the body

J. S. Garrow

HUMAN GROWTH AND CHEMICAL MATURATION

When a human baby grows to become an adult, body weight increases about twenty-fold. Virtually all the material in the weight gained entered the body by way of food or drink (the trivial exception being oxygen, some of which will have come from inspired air), and the material gained during intrauterine growth came from the mother's diet. Therefore we are – literally – what we eat. A grossly abnormal diet may cause striking changes in body weight, configuration and composition. Fig. 2.1 shows three pigs which are littermates but are very different in size and shape because they have had different diets. The largest pig received unlimited quantities of a good diet. The smallest pig received the same diet, but in small quantities which just enabled it to remain alive, but not to grow. The third pig received the same diet as the smallest one, but also had access to unlimited amounts of sugar. This extra energy source enabled it

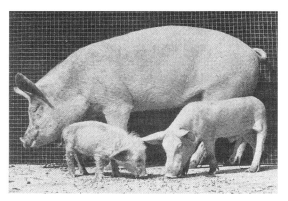

Fig. 2.1 These three pigs are littermates, about 1 year old. The largest was reared on unlimited quantities of a good diet, the smallest on very small quantities of the same diet, and the third had the same rations as the smallest pig but also had access to unlimited sugar (From McCance 1968.).

to use the small ration of protein to achieve better growth, but it is still far smaller than the well-fed pig. Apart from the differences in size it is obvious that the different diets have also altered the proportions of limbs to trunk, and the quality of the skin.

EFFECT OF PROTEIN ENERGY MALNUTRITION ON BODY COMPOSITION

Some of the earliest scientific studies on the effects of poor diets were undertaken by German paediatricians at the beginning of this century. They observed a condition in children fed only on a starchy gruel, which they called 'Mehlnahrschaden', which is roughly equivalent to what we now call kwashiorkor. They suspected that these children died of a deficiency of protein, but chemical analysis of the cadavers of malnourished children gave results which were unexpected: some of the most severely malnourished children contained the highest amount of protein in proportion to body weight (Garrow et al 1968).

In the light of subsequent research we can interpret these results. During normal growth in the uterus, and in the first year of extrauterine life, several changes in body composition occur, which are illustrated in Table 2.1. The embryo has a very high percentage of water, but with maturation the proportion of water decreases and there is a shift in the distribution of water from extracellular (with Na^+ as the chief anion) to intracellular (with K^+ as the chief anion). As the proportion of water decreases, the concentration of protein and electrolytes increases. Fat is mostly laid down during the last trimester of pregnancy, and during the first year of extrauterine life.

Severe malnutrition in children prevents normal gains in body weight, and also delays the chemical maturation of the body. A child who has starved to death will have less protein and more water than normal in its lean tissues, but because it has little fat

Table 2.1 Effect of growth, malnutrition and obesity on the composition of the body, and of fat-free tissue

	Fetus 20–25 weeks	Premature baby	Full term baby	Infant (1 yr)	Adult man	Malnourished infant	Obese man
Body wt (kg)	0.3	1.5	3.5	20	70	5	100
Water %	88	83	69	62	60	74	47
Protein %	9.5	11.5	12	14	17	14	13
Fat %	0.5	3.5	16	20	17	10	35
Remainder %	2	2	3	4	6	2	5
Fat-free wt (kg)	0.30	1.45	2.94	8.0	58	4.5	65
Water %	88	85	82	76	72	82	73
Protein %	9.4	11.9	14.4	18	21	15	21
Na (mmol/kg)	100	100	82	81	80	88	82
K (mmol/kg)	43	50	53	60	66	48	64
Ca (g/kg)	4.2	7.0	9.6	14.5	22.4	9.0	20
Mg (g/kg)	0.18	0.24	0.26	3.5	0.5	0.25	0.5
P (g/kg)	3.0	3.8	5.6	9.0	12.0	5.0	12.0

the percentage of protein *relative to body weight* may actually be higher than normal. It is therefore necessary to consider separately changes in the fat content of the body, and changes in the composition of the fat-free component. Pace & Rathbun (1945) analysed the carcases of a series of guinea-pigs ranging from lean to obese animals, and showed that the water and protein content of the fat-free body was little affected by the amount of fat.

CHEMICAL ANALYSIS OF HUMAN CADAVERS

Our understanding of the composition of the fat-free adult human body is based on chemical analyses of six cadavers which were performed between 1945 and 1956. Mitchell et al (1945) analysed a 35-year-old white male who died suddenly of a heart attack; Widdowson et al (1951) analysed two adults and a child: the adults were a man of 25 years who died of uraemia and a woman of 42 years who drowned herself; Forbes et al (1953) analysed a man of 46 who died of a fractured skull; and Forbes et al (1956) reported two more analyses: one a Negro male with bacterial endocarditis who died aged 48, and the other a man of 60 years who was found dead, presumably of a heart attack. Further data on the electrolyte composition of the last two bodies were published by Forbes & Lewis (1956). The composition of individual organs has been extensively investigated by Dickerson & Widdowson (1960) and Widdowson & Dickerson (1960).

Table 2.2 shows the water, protein and potassium concentrations of the fat-free bodies which were

Table 2.2 The contribution of water and protein to the fat-free weight of adult bodies, and in some organs (for sources of these data see text)

Age (years)	Water (g/kg)	Protein (g/kg)	Remainder (g/kg)	Potassium (mmol/kg)	K:N ratio (mmol/g)
Fat-free whole bodies					
25	728	195	77	71.5	2.29
35	775	165	60	—	—
42	733	192	75	73.0	2.38
46	674	234	92	66.5	1.78
48	730	206	64	—	—
60	704	238	58	66.6	1.75
Mean	725	205	71	69.0	2.05
Selected organs					
Skin	694	300	6	23.7	0.45
Heart	827	143	30	66.5	2.90
Liver	711	176	113	75.0	2.66
Kidneys	810	153	37	57.0	2.33
Brain	774	107	119	84.6	4.96
Muscle	792	192	16	91.2	2.99

analysed by the investigators mentioned above. It can be seen that fat-free tissue contains about 725 g of water, 205 g of protein, and 69 mmol of potassium per kg, but that there is considerable variation between the individual bodies. In the lower part of Table 2.2 the composition of various organs is shown, and it is obvious that fat-free skin, for example, has a very different water and potassium content from, say, brain or muscle.

IN VIVO MEASUREMENT OF FAT AND FAT-FREE MASS

The body composition of a hypothetical normal adult male is shown diagrammatically in Fig. 2.2. It is obviously not practicable to measure the energy stores of a patient by direct chemical analysis, so various indirect methods have been developed, which are discussed later in this chapter. These all to a greater or lesser degree rest on the assumption that the body consists of two components: fat and fat-free tissue of a fairly constant composition.

MEASUREMENT OF BODY DENSITY

The measurement of body density as an index of obesity was pioneered by Behnke et al (1942). Some national-ranking American football players had been rejected for military service because they were over-weight for height, but it was shown that their body density was high, so their excess weight was muscle and not fat, which would have caused their density to be low. The density of human tissues has been measured by Allen et al (1959).

Human fat at body temperature has a density of 0.900 g/cm^3, and a reasonable approximation for the density of the fat-free body is 1.100 g/cm^3 (Keys & Brozek 1953). Thus, a person in whom half the body weight is fat has an average density of 1.00. Obviously any mixture of fat and lean will result in an average density somewhere between 1.10 and 0.90. Making the assumptions stated above, it is possible to calculate the percentage of fat from average body density. It may be that in individuals who are very fat or very severely malnourished, the hydration of the fat-free

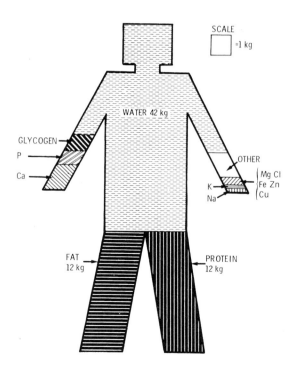

Fig. 2.2 Diagrammatic representation of the body composition of a normal adult male weighing 70 kg. The contributions of the components to body weight is represented by their area in the diagram: only fat, protein and glycogen contribute to the energy stores of the body.

body is altered (Streat et al 1985), but this causes only a small error in the estimation of body fat from density.

The practical problem is to make a very accurate estimate of the volume of the tissues of a human subject in a manner acceptable to patients. Usually this is done by asking the subject to submerge in water, so that the volume of water displaced, or the apparent weight loss of the submerged subject, can be accurately measured, but few patients are able and willing to do this. These measurements cannot be made unless the water around the subject is at rest, and in practice this means that the subject must submerge calmly and remain still under water for 30 s. An alternative method, which does not require the subject to immerse completely, is to use a tank with a plastic cover in which the subject stands up to the neck in water, and then the volume of air remaining under the cover is measured (Garrow et al 1979). Since the volume of water and of the whole tank is known, the volume of the subject can be obtained by subtraction.

MEASUREMENT OF TOTAL BODY WATER

The volume of water in the cooling system of a car can be measured by the dilution principle: if 1 litre of antifreeze is added to the radiator, and after thorough mixing of the water in the cooling system the concentration of antifreeze is found to be 5%, the total volume of water must be 20 litres. Even if there is a slow leak in the system this will not introduce much error in the estimate of volume at the time the antifreeze was added, since any leakage after complete mixing was achieved will not affect the final concentration, because the same proportion of water and antifreeze will be lost in any given time period.

Body water in living man can be similarly measured by giving a dose of water labelled with either tritium (the radioactive isotope of hydrogen) or deuterium (the stable heavy isotope of hydrogen) or ^{18}O (a stable heavy isotope of oxygen). The concentration of tritium in body water after equilibrium is reached is measured in a scintillation counter, but if either stable isotope is used it is necessary to use an isotope ratio mass spectrometer to measure the enrichment of isotope in the equilibrium sample (Halliday & Miller 1977). To obtain a measurable concentration after mixing with body water it is necessary to give a dose of about 3.7 MBq of $^{3}H_2O$ or about 1 g of D_2O. The dose of labelled water may conveniently be given orally diluted in 100 ml of tap water. The weight of water given is measured by weighing the container

before and after the subject has taken the dose through a drinking straw. It is necessary to allow about 3 hours to achieve isotopic equilibrium, and during this period no food or drink may be taken by the subject, otherwise the recently ingested water will dilute the plasma water and cause a falsely low reading, which will result in too large an apparent total body water and too low an estimate of total body fat. The loss of isotope in urine during the equilibration period of 3 hours does not contribute a significant error (<1%), so it is not necessary to measure this loss. An error of about 2% occurs because the labelled hydrogen exchanges with labile organic hydrogen atoms as well as water hydrogen (Culebras et al 1977), but this small overestimate of water can be ignored.

Having obtained an estimate of total body water (TBW, kg), fat-free mass (FFM, kg) can be obtained thus:

$$FFM = \frac{TBW}{0.73}$$

on the assumption that FFM is 73% water (Pace & Rathbun 1945). The fat content (F, kg) of a person of body weight W, kg is then:

$$F = W - FFM$$

MEASUREMENT OF TOTAL BODY POTASSIUM

All potassium, including that in the human body, is labelled with the natural radioactive isotope ^{40}K, so each gram of potassium emits about three gamma rays of high energy (1.46 MeV) each second. These rays can be detected by suitable apparatus (Burch & Spiers 1953; Boddy et al 1976; Smith et al 1979) and thus the total body potassium can be estimated.

Fig. 2.3 shows the general construction of a whole-body counter designed to measure ^{40}K. Since the radiation coming from the body is very weak, it is necessary to enclose the apparatus and subject in a massive shield made (usually) of steel and lead to reduce interference from cosmic radiation and other extraneous sources of radioactivity. The steel itself must be free from radioactivity; prewar battleship steel is a suitable material. Within the shielded volume the subject lies with detectors arrayed around him to try to catch as much as possible of the radiation: ideally the detectors should totally enclose the subject but this causes problems in getting the subject in and out of the counter, so a usual compromise is to have detectors above and below the couch on which the subject lies. Typically, the counting time for an average subject is about 1000 s, and the coefficient of variation is about

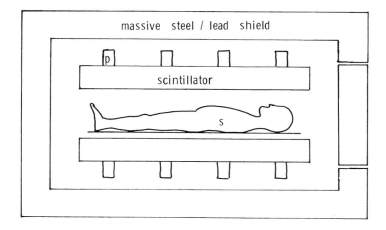

Fig. 2.3 Diagram of one type of whole-body counter designed to measure [40]K. The subject (s) lies between tanks of scintillation liquid. Gamma rays emerging from the subject pass through the scintillator and cause flashes of light which are detected by a series of photomultipliers (p). To reduce the background count rate from cosmic rays and other local radioactivity the whole instrument is enclosed in a massive shield.

3%. Longer counting times will give greater precision, but ultimately accuracy is limited by the stability of the electronics and the validity of the calibration equations.

Having obtained an estimate of total body potassium (TBK, mmol) the FFM (kg) can be calculated for women from:

$$FFM = \frac{TBK}{60}$$

and for men from:

$$FFM = \frac{TBK}{66}$$

on the assumption that fat-free tissue contains 60 mmol K/kg or 66 mmol K/kg for women and men respectively (1 g K = 25.6 mmol).

ANTHROPOMETRY

Many attempts have been made to derive equations by which the fat and the fat-free mass of the body can be estimated from the measurements of selected lengths and circumferences. The most important of these are measurements of skinfold thickness, and indices relating weight to height. These will be described in some detail.

Measurement of body fat by skinfold thickness

Most of the fat stored in the body lies immediately under the skin (Edwards 1950) and the thickness of a fold of skin picked up at strategic sites indicates the amount of subcutaneous fat. Various sites for mea-surement have been suggested; probably the best established system is that using four sites – biceps, triceps, subscapular and suprailiac. These were proposed by Durnin & Rahaman (1967) and developed by Durnin & Womersley (1974) and Womersley & Durnin (1977) to include standards based on 245 men and 324 women covering the age range from 17 to 72 years.

The measurement of skinfolds requires skill and training. Ruiz et al (1971) showed that it was important that the triceps skinfold was measured at exactly the correct site, otherwise false results were obtained. In very fat people it is impossible to obtain a true fold of skin and subcutaneous fat, and if you do so it will not fit between the jaws of the standard caliper. A theoretical limitation to the skinfold measurement is that it assumes a constant relationship between sub-cutaneous and deep fat stores, which is not confirmed by measurement at postmortem examinations (Alexander 1964), but the tables of Durnin & Womersley (1974) give different standards for percentage body fat according to age and sex, which to some extent compensates for age- and sex-related changes in the distribution of fat in the body. Jones et al (1976) found differences between the proportion of fat which was subcutaneous in Europeans, Gurkhas, Rajputs and South Indians, so there are probably also ethnic differences which should be considered when converting from skinfold thickness measurements to estimates of body fat. Despite these reservations, skinfolds are certainly the most convenient method for estimating fat in people of reasonably normal build,

The sites of measurement are biceps, triceps, subscapular and suprailiac. The position of the first two sites is on the anterior and posterior midline, respectively, of the upper arm, at the midpoint between the acromion and the olecranon processes when the elbow is flexed at 90°. The skinfold is oriented in the long axis of the limb. The subscapular site is at the lower angle of the scapula at 45° to the vertical, and the suprailiac site is a horizontal skinfold just above the iliac crest in the midaxillary line. For the measurement it is necessary to have the subject stripped to the waist or, with female subjects, wearing only a brassiere above the waist. Three measurements should be made at each site, and, if the span of readings is greater than 2 mm, more readings should be taken until a set of three consecutive readings agreeing to 2 mm is obtained. The average of the three readings is taken at each site, and the sum of these values is entered into the table given by Durnin & Womersley (1974) in the column appropriate to the age and sex of the subject. The percentage body fat related to the sum of four skinfolds is given in Table 2.3, taken from the data of Durnin & Womersley.

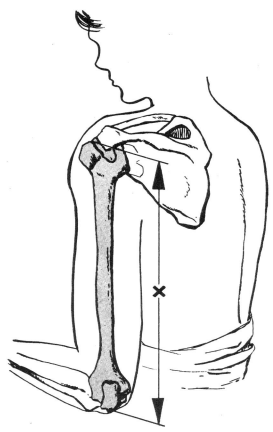

Fig. 2.4 The first step in measuring triceps skinfold, or arm circumference, is to find the midpoint (x) between the acromion and the olecranon processes.

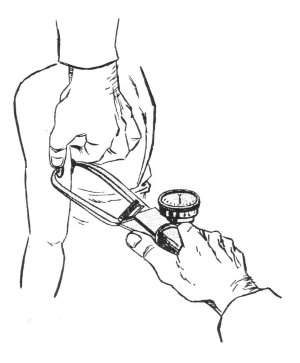

Fig. 2.5 The fold of skin and subcutaneous fat is raised as described in the text, and the thickness is measured with calipers.

provided that the measurements are made by a trained observer, and an error of about 3% of body weight (i.e. 2 kg of fat in an average subject) is acceptable. This is probably the error in skilled hands (Durnin & Womersley 1977).

The Harpenden caliper (Holtain Ltd. Bryberian, Crymmych, Pembrokeshire) is designed so the surface of the jaws applied to the skin surface remains parallel and exerts a constant pressure. To measure the triceps skinfold, first determine the midpoint between the acromion and the olecranon processes (Fig. 2.4) and mark this point. The skinfold is picked up between the forefinger and thumb of the left hand, the caliper is applied so that it closes under the spring pressure, and the reading is taken on the micrometer dial as soon as the rapid phase of compression is over, after about 5 s (Fig. 2.5), and similarly at other sites.

Table 2.3 Percentage body fat in men and women related to the sum of four skinfolds (biceps, triceps, subscapular and suprailiac) (Data of Durnin & Womersley 1974.)

Age (yrs)	Men				Women			
	17–29	30–39	40–49	50+	16–29	30–39	40–49	50+
Skinfold (mm)								
20	8.1	12.2	12.2	12.6	14.1	17.0	19.8	21.4
30	12.9	16.2	17.7	18.6	19.5	21.8	24.5	26.6
40	16.4	19.2	21.4	22.9	23.4	25.5	28.2	30.3
50	19.0	21.5	24.6	26.5	26.5	28.2	31.0	33.4
60	21.2	23.5	27.1	29.2	29.1	30.6	33.2	35.7
70	23.1	25.1	29.3	31.6	31.2	32.5	35.0	37.7
80	24.8	26.6	31.2	33.8	33.1	34.3	36.7	39.6
90	26.2	27.8	33.0	35.8	34.8	35.8	38.3	41.2
100	27.6	29.0	34.4	37.4	36.4	37.2	39.7	42.6
110	28.8	30.1	35.8	39.0	37.8	38.6	41.0	42.9
120	30.0	31.1	37.0	40.4	39.0	39.6	42.0	45.1
130	31.0	31.9	38.2	41.8	40.2	40.6	43.0	46.2
140	32.0	32.7	39.2	43.0	41.3	41.6	44.0	47.2
150	32.9	33.5	40.2	44.1	42.3	42.6	45.0	48.2
160	33.7	34.3	41.2	45.1	43.3	43.6	45.8	49.2
170	34.5	34.8	42.0	46.1	44.1	44.4	46.6	50.0

Arm muscle circumference

The mid-upper arm circumference (MUAC) can be measured as shown in Fig. 2.6. If it is assumed that the mid-arm is a cylinder of muscle covered by a layer of fat, and that the double thickness of the layer of fat is represented by the triceps skinfold (TSF), then the arm muscle circumference (AMC) can be calculated thus:

AMC=MUAC – 4.18 TSF

The combination of triceps skinfold and arm muscle circumference provides a simple field estimate of fat mass and muscle mass respectively (Heymsfield et al 1982).

Measurement of fatness by Quetelet's index

The use of Quetelet's index as a measure of fatness has been analysed by Garrow & Webster (1985). There are two ways in which fatness can be expressed: either fat as a percentage of body weight, or else fat in absolute amount (kg). When a person puts on weight the added tissue has a constant ratio of fat to FFM, with about 75% fat and 25% fat-free tissue (Webster et al 1984), so the percentage of body fat will approach 75% at infinite weight, but can never be greater than 75%. However, if fatness is expressed in absolute terms (i.e. in kg) it will increase indefinitely

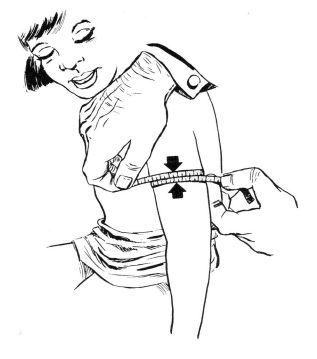

Fig. 2.6 The arm circumference is measured as shown. The arm muscle circumference can be calculated as described in the text.

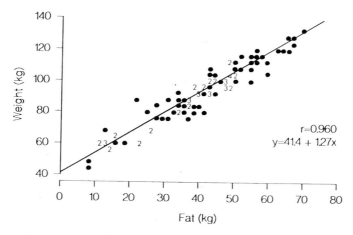

Fig. 2.7   Relation of body weight to total body fat in a series of 104 women. Body fat was calculated from the mean of estimates by density, water and potassium in each woman (Data from Webster et al 1984)

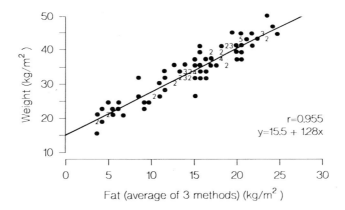

Fig. 2.8   The data shown in Fig. 2.7 corrected for differences in stature by dividing both variables by H^2. The y axis now becomes Quetelets's index.

in a linear manner with successive additions of tissue which has a constant proportion of fat. Thus the two ways of expressing the changes in fatness give different impressions of fat gain.

The data on which the argument rests are shown in Fig. 2.7. Among 104 women aged 14–60 years, who ranged from very thin to very fat, the relation of fat to body weight was well described by a straight line, with a slope of 1.27 and a correlation coefficient of 0.960 (Webster et al 1984). To correct for differences in stature, both axes may be divided by H^2: this yields the result shown in Fig. 2.8. The intercept of the regression line has changed but the slope (1.28) and the correlation coefficient (0.955) are hardly changed. The estimates of fat used to construct Figs 2.7 and 2.8 were the average values derived from measurements of

density, water and potassium in each of these 104 women, using the calculations explained above.

The data in Figs 2.7 and 2.8 suggest that as women (of a given height) increase in weight they gain 1 kg fat for every 1.27 kg weight gained: in other words 1/1.27, or 78.7%, of the excess weight is fat. For statistical reasons this is a slight overestimate of the fat content of excess weight, which, without significant error, can be rounded to 75% and 25% fat-free tissue.

Quetelet's index is not quite as accurate a method for estimating body fat as the more complex laboratory techniques described in previous sections. There is no perfectly accurate method applicable to living subjects, but under very carefully controlled conditions in a metabolic ward it is possible to estimate *change* in fat stores with considerable accuracy from measurements of energy balance or nitrogen balance. For example, measurements of body fat by density, water and potassium have been made on a series of 19 obese women, and repeated after a few weeks. The change in fat stores during the interval was estimated by energy balance and nitrogen balance, and the change estimated in this way: (2.77 + 0.71 kg fat) was assumed to be the 'true' change. By comparing the change in fat stores indicated by the change in density, water and potassium with the 'true' value for each subject, the errors of the various methods can be estimated: they are calculated to be 2.2 kg, 2.3 kg and 3.5 kg of fat by density, water and potassium respectively (Garrow et al 1979).

Measurements of 'frame size'

Despite the popular belief that skeletal size may in part explain the greater weight of some people, attempts to add measurements of 'frame size' have failed to refine the estimation of body fat from estimates based on weight and height (Himes & Bouchard 1985, Rookus et al 1985).

METHODS BASED ON ELECTRICAL CONDUCTIVITY

Two methods have been developed which depend on the difference in electrical conductivity of lean tissue (which is virtually an electrolyte solution, and hence a good conductor) and fat, which is a non-conductor. In the total body electrical conductivity (TOBEC) system the subject lies within a solenoid coil through which radiofrequency pulses are fed at a frequency of 5 MHz (Segal et al 1985). This generates an alternating magnetic field within the coil which induces a response in the subject depending on the conductivity of the tissues, and the strength of the evoked field is measured by a secondary coil. The advantage of this system is that it makes the measurement very quickly: the device was originally designed to measure the fat content of processed meat travelling on a conveyor belt. The disadvantage is that the evoked field depends on the shape of the subject as well as on his fat content; a short stout person traps more of the magnetic radiation than a tall slim person of similar body weight and composition. A new version of TOBEC consists of a coil through which the subject is passed and the evoked field is analysed by computer (van Loan & Mayclin 1987). It is not yet clear if this will provide more reliable estimates of fat and fat-free mass.

The other device which measures electrical conductivity uses a pair of electrodes attached to the left hand and left foot of the subject (Lukaski et al 1985). A current of 800 µA at a frequency of 50 MHz is passed between the outer electrodes, and the voltage drop is measured at the proximal electrodes, from which the resistance (strictly impedance, since it is an alternating current) of the tissues is calculated. In some commercial instruments the measured value for impedance is entered into a regression equation, together with anthropometric data such as weight, height, age and gender. The resultant prediction of fat-free mass and total body water agrees well with values obtained by the more complex methods described above, but much of the correlation comes from the anthropometric data, rather than from the measured impedance (Diaz et al 1989). An analysis of Danish subjects aged 35–75 years by Heitman (1990) developed a multiple regression equation using impedance measurements which had a higher correlation with fat measured by total body water and total body potassium than equivalent equations using either skinfolds or weight–height indices.

The best equation for women was:

$$F = 0.819W - 0.279H^2/R - 0.231H + 0.077A + 14.941$$

and for men:

$$F = 0.755W - 0.279H^2/R - 0.231H + 0.077A + 14.941$$

where F=fat (kg), W=weight(kg), H=height(cm), R=impedance (ohms) and A=age (years).

INFRARED INTERACTANCE

Another technique for estimating fatness is infrared interactance (Conway et al 1984). Light from a very expensive monochromator at different colours in the wavelength range 700–1100 nm is shone onto the skin surface at selected sites, and the spectrum of wavelengths reflected is analysed by computer. Fat and lean tissue have different interactive spectra, and so the lean:fat ratio at the test sites can be calculated. This technique has also been commercially developed to provide a low-cost instrument, but with very poor accuracy (Hortobagyi et al 1992).

NEUTRON ACTIVATION

The measurement of total body potassium by measuring the activity of ^{40}K in the body depends on the happy accident that all potassium, whether in the human body or elsewhere, contains this natural high-energy radioisotope, which decays very slowly indeed; it loses half its radioactivity in 1300 million years. However, if a subject is irradiated with a beam of fast neutrons the energy is captured by atoms in the body, some of which become short-lived radioactive isotopes, notably ^{49}Ca and ^{15}N. These isotopes emit radiation at characteristic energy bands, and can therefore be detected using apparatus similar to that shown in Fig. 2.3. Thus it is possible to estimate total body Ca or N, as well as K, but facilities for this investigation are available in only a few specialist centres. The apparatus is also very expensive to construct and maintain, and the radiation dose to the subject is significant, so this is unlikely to be a technique which is widely applied.

SCANNING TECHNIQUES

Computer-assisted tomography

In conventional radiography a beam of X-rays is passed through the tissues of the subject, and the pattern of absorption of the X-rays is shown by the energy recorded on a photographic film. If, instead of having a stationary wide beam forming a photographic image, the X-rays are emitted in a narrow beam from a source which travels in a semicircle around the subject, and the energy passing through the body is recorded by a detector which is mounted diametrically opposite the X-ray source, a large amount of information is gathered concerning the absorption of X-rays in the 'slice' of body which has been irradiated. A suitably programmed computer can then reconstruct the pattern of absorbing material within the slice which must have given rise to the observed changes in X-ray transmission as the instrument rotated around the subject. Since fat, water, lean tissue and bone have different absorption characteristics, the computer-assisted tomograph displays on a video screen the distribution of these tissues within the slice, as if the subject had been cut through at the level of the scan. If serial scans are performed at different levels of the body from head to feet, it is possible to build up data on the total volume of the different types of tissue, and how these tissues are distributed in different sections of the body.

This technique has provided most valuable information about the relative proportions of fat which are subcutaneous or intra-abdominal (Kvist et al 1988). The metabolic importance of intra-abdominal fat deposition is discussed in Chapter 32. However, the instrument is expensive to buy and maintain, the examination takes quite a long time, and there is a significant radiation dose to the subject, so this technique is not suitable for routine assessment of body fatness.

Nuclear magnetic resonance

Water nuclei carry an asymmetrical charge and can be made to rotate in a strong magnetic field. If radio waves at an appropriate frequency are passed through human tissue that is in a strong magnetic field, some hydrogen nuclei change their orientation in the field and flip back again when the radio waves are switched off, releasing the energy they had captured. From the emission of this released energy it is possible to construct images similar to those obtained by X-ray tomography, and also to indicate differences in the energy state, or level of hydration, of tissues. The potentialities of magnetic resonance techniques are very great, and so far it appears that the radiation involved does not damage tissues. However, it is at present a very expensive procedure whose most effective application has yet to be determined.

Photon absorptiometry

The ability of bone mineral (and other tissues) to absorb energy from a photon beam of given energy is known. Therefore, the mass of bone mineral in a limb can be estimated by scanning across the limb with a beam of photons of known energy and observing the energy which emerges at the other side, provided that the absorption from surrounding soft tissues is kept constant. The latter requirement can be achieved by immersing the limb in a tank of water. However, it is much more convenient to use a source which emits photons at two known energies (such as gadolinium-153 which emits photons at 44 and 100 keV) and to observe the attenuation of both beams as they pass through the limb. In this way it is possible to obtain information about both the bone mineral and the soft-tissue mass in the section of limb which has been scanned, and also about the lean:fat ratio in the soft tissue. The radiation dose to the subject is low, but the instrument is expensive. It is becoming an important technique for measuring changes in the bone mineral content of the body in studies of osteoporosis.

INDICES OF BODY COMPONENTS

Intracellular and extracellular water

The principal of tracer dilution to estimate total body water has been explained above. If a tracer can be found which is distributed through extracellular water, but which does not enter cells, then the volume of extracellular water can also be estimated. Some of the earliest work on the effects of nutritional status on body composition used this approach (McCance & Widdowson 1951), but it is of doubtful validity. A measure of the partitioning of body water is only required if it is suspected that it may be abnormal, but if it is abnormal it cannot be assumed that the markers which normally do not enter cells will continue to behave in this way.

Urinary creatinine excretion

Creatinine is formed by the non-enzymatic irreversible hydrolysis of creatine, and about 98% of all creatine in the body is in muscle, mainly as creatine phosphate. Thus Talbot (1938) showed that 17.9 kg of skeletal muscle contribute 1 g/day of urinary creatinine. Therefore, if an accurate 24-hour sample of urine can be collected from a subject, it is possible to estimate his muscle mass from the daily creatinine excretion, provided he has been on a meat-free diet for several days.

Urinary 3-methylhistidine excretion

During the synthesis of actin in muscle the amino acid histidine is methylated, but when the actin is broken down the methylhistidine cannot be recycled but is excreted quantitatively in the urine. Thus in subjects with normal rates of turnover of muscle protein the excretion of 3-methylhistidine in urine provides an index of muscle mass. However, in abnormal states, such as myopathies, non-muscle sources of 3-methylhistidine, such as platelets and the intestine may invalidate this method for estimating muscle mass (Rennie & Millward 1983).

Waist–hip and waist–thigh ratios

The radio of the circumference of the waist to that of the buttocks or thigh has been used as a measure of fat distribution. The technique and its interpretation is discussed in Chapter 32.

ESTIMATES OF CHANGE IN BODY COMPOSITION

For a group of people who range in body fat from 10 kg to 50 kg, many of the techniques described above will serve to rank the individuals reliably in order of fatness. However, if each of these individuals now loses 10 kg in weight, of which, say, half to three-quarters is fat, it is much more difficult to rank them in order of the proportion of fat in the weight lost. The only technique which will yield reliable information in the latter situation is either energy balance or nitrogen balance (or preferably both) done very carefully in a metabolic ward over several weeks. This is a very tedious and expensive investigation, which has therefore seldom been done (Garrow et al 1979). Therefore the reader should beware of claims that diet (or drug, or exercise) A caused a greater loss of fat than diet B, when the weight loss is <10 kg in both cases, unless the measurement of fat loss was done by careful balance techniques.

REFERENCES

Alexander MK 1964 The postmortem estimation of total body fat, muscle and bone. Clinical Science 26: 193–202

Allen TH, Krzywicki HJ, Roberts JE 1959 Density, fat water and solids in freshly isolated tissues. Journal of Applied Physiology 14: 1005–1008

Behnke AR, Feen BG, Welham WC 1942 The specific gravity of healthy men; body weight and volume as an index of obesity. Journal of the American Medical Association 118: 495–498

Boddy K, Hume R, White C et al 1976 The relation between potassium in body fluids and total body potassium in healthy and diabetic subjects. Clinical Science and Molecular Medicine 50: 455–461

Burch PRJ Spiers FW 1953. Measurement of the gamma radiation from the human body. Nature (London) 172: 519–521

Conway JM, Norris H, Bodwell CE 1984 A new approach for the estimation of body composition: infrared interactance. American Journal of Clinical Nutrition 40: 1123–1130.

Culebras JM, Fitzpatrik GF, Brennan MF, Boyden CM, Moore FD 1977 Total body water and exchangeable hydrogen. II. A review of comparative data from animals based on isotope dilution and desiccation, with a report of new data from the rat. American Journal of Physiology 232: R60–R65

Diaz EO, Villar J, Immink M, Gonzales T 1989 Bioimpedance or anthropometry? European Journal of Clinical Nutrition 43: 129–137

Dickerson JWT, Widdowson EM 1960 Chemical changes in skeletal muscle during development. Biochemical Journal 74: 247–257

Durnin JVGA, Rahaman MM 1967 The assessment of the amount of fat in the human body from measurement of skinfold thickness. British Journal of Nutrition 21: 681–689

Durnin JVGA, Womersley J 1974 Body fat assessed from

body density and its estimation from skinfold thickness: measurement on 481 men and women from 16 to 72 years. British Journal of Nutrition 32: 77–97

Edwards DAW 1950 Observations of the distribution of subcutaneous fat. Clinical Science 9: 259–270

Forbes GB, Lewis AM 1956 Total sodium, potassium and chloride in adult man. Journal of Clinical Investigation 35: 596–600

Forbes RM, Cooper AR, Mitchell HH 1953 The composition of the adult human body as determined by chemical analysis. Journal of Biological Chemistry 203: 359–366

Forbes RM, Mitchell HH, Cooper AR 1956 Further studies on the gross composition and mineral elements of the adult human body. Journal of Biological Chemistry 223: 969–975

Garrow JS, Webster J 1985 Quetelet's index (W/H^2) as a measure of fatness. International Journal of Obesity 9: 147–153

Garrow JS, Smith R, Ward EE 1968 Electrolyte metabolism in severe infantile malnutrition. Pergamon Press, Oxford, pp. 168

Garrow JS, Stalley S, Diethelm R., Pittet Ph, Hesp R, Halliday D 1979 A new method of measuring the body density of obese adults. British Journal of Nutrition 42: 173–183

Halliday D, Miller AG 1977 Precise measurement of total body water using trace quantities of deuterium oxide. Biomedical Mass Spectrometry 4: 82–87

Heitman BL 1990 Evaluation of body fat estimated from body mass index, skinfolds and impedance. A comparative study. European Journal of Clinical Nutrition 44: 831–837

Heymsfield SB, McManus C, Smith J, Stevens V, Nixon DW 1982 Anthropometric measurement of muscle mass: revised equations for calculating bone-free arm muscle area. American Journal of Clinical Nutrition 36: 680–690

Himes JH, Bouchard C 1985 Do the new Metropolitan Life insurance weight–height tables correctly assess body frame and body fat relationships? American Journal of Public Health 75: 1076–1079

Hortobagyi T, Israel RG, Houmard A, McCammon M R, O'Brien KF 1990 Comparison of body composition assessment by hydrodensitometry, skinfolds, and multiple site near-infrared spectrophotometry. European Journal of Clinical Nutrition 46: 206–211

Jones PRM, Bharadwaj H, Bhatia MR, Malhotra MS 1976 Differences between ethnic groups in the relationship of skinfold thickness to body density. In: Bhatia B, Chhina GS, Singh B (eds), Selected topics in environmental biology. Interprint Publications, New Delhi, pp. 373–376

Keys A, Brozek J 1953 Body fat in adult man. Physiological Reviews 33: 245–325

Kvist H, Chowdhury B, Tylen U, Sjostrom L 1988 Total and visceral adipose-tissue volumes derived from measurements with computed tomography in adult men and women: predictive equations. American Journal of Clinical Nutrition 48: 1351–1361

Lukaski HC, Johnson PE, Bolonchuk WW, Lykken GI 1985 Assessment of fat-free mass using bioelectrical impedance measurements of the human body. American Journal of Clinical Nutrition 41: 810–817

McCance RA 1968 The effect of calorie deficiencies and protein deficiencies on final weight and stature. In: McCance RA, Widdowson EM (eds) Calorie deficiencies and protein deficiencies. Churchill, London, pp. 319–328

McCance RA, Widdowson E M 1951 A method of breaking down the body weights of living persons into terms of extracellular fluid, cell mass and fat, and some applications of it to physiology and medicine. Proceedings of the Royal Society B, 138: 115–130

Mitchell HH, Hamilton TS, Steggerda FR, Bean HW 1945 The chemical composition of the adult human body and its bearing on the biochemistry of growth. Journal of Biological Chemistry 158: 625–637

Pace N Rathbun EN 1945 Studies of body composition: water and chemically combined nitrogen content in relation to fat content. Journal of Biological Chemistry 158:685–691

Rennie MJ, Millward DJ 1983 3-methylhistidine excretion and the urinary 3-methylhistidine/creatinine ratio are poor indicators of skeletal muscle protein breakdown. Clinical Science 65: 217–225

Rookus MA, Burema J, Deurenberg P, Van der Wiel-Wetzels WAM 1985 The impact of adjustment of a weight–height index (W/H^2) for frame size on the prediction of body fatness. British Journal of Nutrition 54: 335–342

Ruiz L, Colley JRT, Hamilton PJS 1971 Measurement of triceps skinfold thickness. An investigation of sources of variation. British Journal of Preventive and Social Medicine 25: 165–167

Segal KR, Gutin B, Presta E, Wang J, van Itallie TB 1985 Estimation of human body composition by electrical impedance methods; a comparative study. Journal of Applied Physiology 58: 1565–1571

Smith T, Hesp R, Mackenzie J 1979 Total body potassium calibrations for normal and obese subjects in two types of whole-body counter. Physics in Biology and Medicine 24: 171–175

Streat SJ, Beddoe AH, Hill GL 1985 Measurement of body fat and hydration of the fat-free body in health and disease. Metabolism 34: 509–518

Talbot NB 1938 Measurement of obesity by the creatinine coefficient. American Journal of Diseases of Children 55: 42–50

van Loan M, Mayclin P 1987 A new TOBEC instrument and procedure for the assessment of body composition: use of Fourier coefficients to predict lean body mass and total body water. American Journal of Clinical Nutrition 45: 131–137

Webster JD, Hesp R, Garrow JS 1984 The composition of excess weight in obese women estimated by body density, total body water and total body potassium. Human Nutrition: Clinical Nutrition 38C: 299–306

Widdowson EM, Dickerson JWT 1960 The effect of growth and function on the chemical composition of soft tissues. Biochemical Journal 77: 30–43

Widdowson EM, McCance RA, Spray CM 1951 The chemical composition of the human body. Clinical Science 10: 113–125

Womersley J, Durnin JVGA 1977 A comparison of the skinfold method with extent of 'overweight' and various weight–height relationships in the assessment of obesity. British Journal of Nutrition 38: 271–284

3. Energy

G. McNeill

At the end of the 18th century the French chemist Lavoisier and the physicist Laplace carried out experiments in which they placed a guinea-pig in a very small closed chamber surrounded by ice. They measured the amount of ice that melted over a 10-hour period and at the same time the amount of carbon dioxide given out by the animal. They demonstrated that there was a relationship between the heat produced by the animal and the carbon dioxide produced. Lavoisier also measured the oxygen consumption of men, and showed that it increased after food and exercise. These experiments led Lavoisier to realize that 'La vie est donc une combustion' (Life is therefore a process of combustion).

Lavoisier is generally regarded as the founder of the science of nutrition, but his life and work were cut short by the guillotine of the French revolution. The first plans to build a large human respiration chamber were made by Reynault and Reiset, who were working in Paris in the 1840s, but they were unable to obtain sufficient funds for the project. Pettenkoffer and Voit constructed a chamber in Munich in the late 19th century, in which a man could live for several days and have all his respiratory exchanges measured. After 24-hour measurements on a fasting man, the protein 'burned' was calculated from the urinary nitrogen and the fat combustion from the respiratory carbon dioxide (after deducting the carbon in the protein burned and assuming no change in the carbohydrate store of the body). A difference of only 6.2% was found between the measured oxygen absorption and that calculated as necessary for the combustion of the body materials metabolized. This accuracy indicates both their experimental skill, and the soundness of the assumptions on which their calculations were based.

It was Atwater, a student of Voit, who carried out the experiments which have established the essential quantitative physiological knowledge on which all assessments of human energy needs are based. Atwater returned to the USA from Germany in 1892 and with the help of Rosa, an engineer, constructed a human calorimeter which could measure the heat produced by a man with an accuracy of 0.1% (Fig. 3.1). At the same time the chamber incorporated the respiration apparatus of Pettenkoffer and Voit. Table 3.1 illustrates how accurately Atwater was able to measure the energy exchange of man. Since this work, our knowledge of the biochemical pathways underlying energy utilization has increased, but the understanding of the process from the whole body perspective is essentially unchanged.

The first part of this chapter gives an account of the physiology of energy exchange, and of the methods available for the measurement of energy expenditure in man. Those with an interest in the experiments which laid the foundations for our current understanding are referred to the account by Lusk (1928), which describes this classic work.

The second part of this chapter describes the factors which influence energy expenditure in man and the methods used to predict the energy requirements of individuals and groups. It is important to point out that the prediction of energy requirements involves assumptions and uncertainties which are due to the very practical nature of the task, rather than a lack of understanding of the physiological principles of energy exchange. None the less, the prediction of energy requirements is an essential part of the application of nutritional science to everyday problems.

FORMS OF ENERGY

In biological systems various forms of energy – solar, chemical, mechanical, electrical and thermal – are interchanged. Animals and plants are no exception to the first law of thermodynamics, which states that energy can only be changed between its different forms and is not created or destroyed. Animals differ from plants, in that plants can use solar energy to synthesize complex molecules such as carbohydrates,

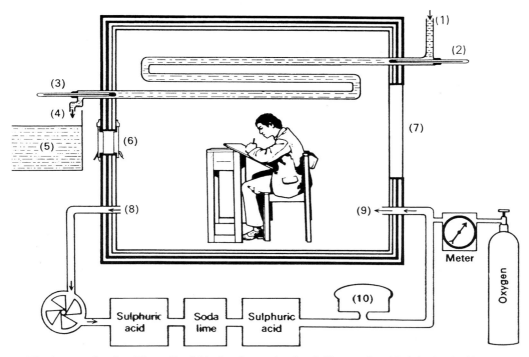

Fig. 3.1   The Atwater chamber. The walls of this chamber are insulated. Heat produced in it is absorbed by water passing in at (1) and out at (4), its temperature on entering and leaving being recorded on the thermometers (2) and (3). The volume of water that has flowed through the cooling system is measured in the vessel (5). The subject may be observed through the window (7), while food may be introduced and excreta removed through the porthole (6). Air leaves the chamber at (8) and passes through a blower and over sulphuric acid and soda-lime to absorb water and carbon dioxide. Oxygen measured by a gas meter is added to the system before the air passes into the chamber at (9). (10) is a tension equaliser. (From Bell GH, Davidson JN, Scarborough H 1968 Textbook of Physiology and Biochemistry, 7th edn. Livingstone, Edinburgh.)

Table 3.1   A 4-day experiment of Atwater and Benedict in 1899

a)	Gross energy content of food	10.31 MJ/day
b)	Gross energy of faeces	0.32 MJ/day
c)	Gross energy of urine	0.56 MJ/day
d)	Gross energy of alcohol excreted	0.09 MJ/day
e)	Energy content of net protein oxidation	0.29 MJ/day
f)	Energy content of fat stores oxidised	0.56 MJ/day
g)	Energy of nutrients oxidised [a−(b+c+d)+e+f]	10.19 MJ/day
h)	Heat produced (by direct calorimetry)	10.02 MJ/day

Difference between g) and h) = −1.6%

proteins and fats, while animals depend on the synthetic ability of plants for their source of (chemical) energy. The chemical energy which animals take in in the form of food is used to perform mechanical (muscular contraction), electrical (maintaining ionic gradients across membranes) and chemical work (synthesis of new macromolecules). However, the conversion of food energy to these other forms is not a perfectly efficient process, and around 75% of the original food energy may be dissipated as heat during these interconversions. In this respect the human body is much more efficient than most steam engines, and roughly equivalent to a good internal combustion engine. Unless the environmental temperature is very low, the heat generated as a byproduct of the essential processes will be sufficient to maintain body temperature, especially if the body is insulated by clothing. When energy utilization increases substantially, the extra heat generated is often in excess of that needed for the maintenance of body temperature, and must be dissipated by means of sweating.

UNITS OF ENERGY

The SI unit of energy is the joule (J), which is the energy used when 1 kilogram (kg) is moved 1 metre (m) by a force of 1 newton (N); 1 joule is a very small amount of energy, and in most uses in nutrition the kilojoule (kJ), i.e. 10^3J, or the megajoule (MJ), i.e. 10^6J or 10^3kJ, are more convenient. In the SI system, rates of energy use can be expressed either in J per unit time (e.g. kJ/min, MJ/24h), or in watts (W), where $1W = 1J/s$ or $1kW = 1kJ/s$. Watts can therefore be converted to kJ/min or kJ/24h by multiplying by 0.06 or 86.4, respectively.

The adoption of SI units in human nutrition has been slow, and many texts, especially those intended for non-scientists, continue to express energy in kilocalories (kcal or Cal). The calorie can be defined in a number of different ways, each of which produces a slightly different value in relation to SI units. For example, the 15°C calorie is the energy required to raise the temperature of 1 g of water from 14.5 to 15.5°C: it is equivalent to 4.1855 J, while the thermochemical calorie is the heat liberated on the total combustion of 1 g of pure benzoic acid and is equivalent to 4.184 J. The Royal Society of London recommends the use of the thermochemical calorie conversion factor, so that 1 kcal = 4.184 kJ, or 1 kJ = 0.239 kcal. For calculations which do not require great accuracy, the conversion factor of 4.2 kJ = 1 kcal is sometimes used.

To avoid duplication, the remainder of this chapter gives values in kJ or MJ, but values in kcal may be obtained by dividing by 4.184 (kJ) or 4.184 × 10^{-3}(MJ).

ENERGY CONTENT OF FOOD

The chemical energy contained in any food can be determined in a bomb calorimeter (Fig. 3.2). The food sample is placed in a small dish in a chamber filled with oxygen and surrounded by water. When the food is ignited by the passage of an electric current through a small wire, the macromolecules are completely oxidized to give water, carbon dioxide and nitrogen oxides. The energy released in this combustion is converted to heat, which causes a temperature rise in the water surrounding the central chamber. A second outer water jacket separated from the inner

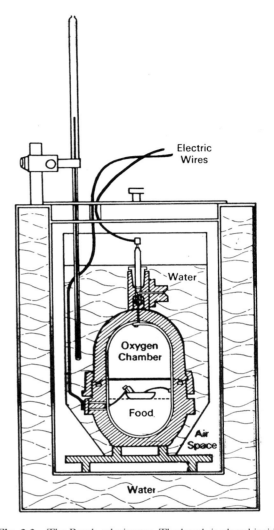

Fig. 3.2 The Bomb calorimeter. The bomb is placed inside a vessel of water, the temperature of which can be accurately measured. The foodstuff is placed in a small crucible. The bomb is filled with oxygen at high pressure and the foodstuff ignited by means of electric leads. The material in the bomb burns and the heat produced leads to a rise of temperature in the surrounding water.

chamber by a layer of air is used to insulate the inner chamber from external temperature changes.

The energy determined by bomb calorimetry is termed the gross energy (GE) of a food, and this represents the total chemical energy in the food. However, not quite all of this energy is available to the animal that eats the food, for two reasons. The first is that not all food eaten by an animal is absorbed from the digestive tract. Atwater carried out studies of young men on typical American diets of the time, and concluded that 99% of ingested carbohydrate, 95% of fat and 92% of protein are absorbed. The second reason is that in the body, nitrogen-containing compounds (notably protein) are not completely oxidized to nitrogen oxides, which would be toxic, but are converted instead to urea, which is less toxic and is excreted in the urine. The urea contains around a quarter of the chemical energy of the original protein, equivalent to 5.23 kJ/g protein.

The energy losses through faeces and urine need to be subtracted from the gross energy of a food to estimate the energy available to the body. This value is termed the metabolizable energy (ME) of the food. The ME intake of individuals on a mixed diet can be determined by performing bomb calorimetry on the food, faeces and urine over a given period of time. Table 3.2 gives an example of these calculations over 7 days for one subject on a metabolic diet.

To simplify the determination of the ME content of foods, Atwater devised a system whereby the ME content of protein, fat, carbohydrate and alcohol were estimated separately, so that the ME content of a food or diet could be predicted from knowledge of the amounts of each of these major nutrients. The ME values for the major nutrients, as calculated by Atwater, are shown in Table 3.3. The values are known as 'Atwater factors', and provide a very good approxi-

mation to the true ME content of most foods and mixed diets (Southgate & Durnin 1970). However, it should be pointed out that the exact values for ME for each major nutrient may vary with the type of the food; for example, the values assume that 6.25 g of protein contains 1 g of nitrogen, while for cereals and milk protein the values are closer to 5.7 and 6.4, respectively. A further complication is that starch has a higher energy content than the same weight of simple sugars. This problem is often solved in food composition tables by expressing the carbohydrate content of foods in terms of their constituent monosaccharides, and using the ME value of 15.7 kJ/g monosaccharide. Details of the methods used to calculate ME in each set of food composition tables should be available within the tables. Useful accounts of the history and use of the various factors used have been given by Widdowson (1955) and McCance & Widdowson (1991).

In practice, variations in the exact values used to estimate the ME content of foods are likely to introduce less error in the estimation of energy intake than differences in the energy content of different samples of the same food. Foods which are particularly variable in energy content are animal foods – especially meats – which have a very variable fat content, and foods with variable water content, since this will influence the energy content per unit weight

Table 3.2 Calculation of metabolizable energy intake. Ten women on a diet in which 55% energy was in the form of carbohydrate and which contained 30 g fibre* per 8 MJ, measured over 7 days

a)	Gross energy of diet	9279	(SD 1125)	kJ/day
b)	Faecal energy loss	647	(SD 154)	kJ/day
c)	Urinary energy loss	318	(SD 70)	kJ/day
	Metabolizable energy intake [a–(b+c)]	8314	(SD 1137)	kJ/day
	ME as a % of gross energy	89.5	(SD 1.7)	%
	ME as a % of food table ME	100.5	(SD 2.0)	%

* Southgate method

Table 3.3 Metabolizable energy of major nutrients

Nutrient	Gross energy (kJ/g)	Percentage absorbed (Atwater's values)	Digestible energy (kJ/g)	Urinary loss (kJ/g)	Metabolizable energy (kJ/g)	Atwater factor (kcal/g)
Starch	17.5	99	17.3	—	17.3	4
Glucose	15.6	99	15.4	—	15.4	4
Fat	39.1	95	37.1	—	37.1	9
Protein	22.9	92	21.1	5.2	15.9	4
Alcohol	29.8	100	29.8	Trace	29.8	7

of food. Other situations where ME values from food tables may be misleading include diets based on unusual proteins and fats, or with a high proportion of non-digestible carbohydrates such as cellulose, or in disease states where faecal and urinary losses of energy may be increased. In such situations, or when energy intake needs to be determined with a high degree of accuracy, e.g. for research purposes, there is no alternative to direct determination of ME intake by bomb calorimetry of food, faeces and urine.

MEASUREMENT OF ENERGY EXPENDITURE

Direct calorimetry

Direct calorimetry involves the measurement of the energy expended by an individual over a given period by measuring the heat emitted by the body. In principle this is simple, and a number of room-sized chambers designed to detect heat loss have been developed for human use. In practice the construction and operation of such chambers is technically difficult, as every part of the walls, floor and roof need to be sensitive to heat, and anything which produces heat other than the subject (such as the operating staff or any electrical equipment) needs to be excluded from the vicinity of the chamber. One more recent approach has been to use a water-cooled garment in which the subject can move more freely than in a calorimeter chamber. Direct calorimetry has the additional disadvantage of requiring periods of several hours or more for each measurement, since the technique assumes that no heat is stored in or lost from the body. Since direct and indirect calorimetry agree well, as can be seen from Atwater and Rosa's results, indirect calorimetry in man is usually more practical than direct calorimetry.

Indirect calorimetry

Indirect calorimetry is based on the fact that as foods are oxidized to produce heat in the body, oxygen is consumed and carbon dioxide is produced in proportion to the heat generated. This can be most simply demonstrated with a stoichiometric equation describing the oxidation of one mole of glucose:

$$C_6H_{12}O_6 + 6\,O_2 \longrightarrow 6\,CO_2 + 6\,H_2O + Heat$$
$$(180\,g)\quad(6\times22.4\,l)\quad(6\times22.4\,l)\quad(6\times18\,g)\quad2.78MJ$$

From these figures it can be seen that the energy released on oxidation of 1g of glucose is 15.4 kJ (2780/180), and that each litre of oxygen consumed is equivalent to the production of 20.7 kJ (2780/6 × 22.4) of heat. Thus from knowledge of the oxygen consumed, the heat production (more usually known as the energy expenditure) can be calculated.

Similar equations can be written for protein and fat, which show that each litre of oxygen consumed is equivalent to an energy expenditure of around 19.3 kJ, when either fat or protein is being oxidized. Table 3.4 shows these values, and the value for oxygen consumed, carbon dioxide produced, and heat produced per gram of each major nutrient. Also shown in Table 3.4 is the respiratory quotient (RQ) for each nutrient. The RQ is the ratio of the moles of carbon dioxide produced to the moles of oxygen consumed on oxidation of a given amount of each nutrient. The values are close to 0.7 for fat and 1.0 for carbohydrate, with protein having an intermediate value.

It can be seen from Table 3.4 that the energy expended per litre of oxygen consumed is very similar for all three major nutrients, so if the mixture of nutrients being oxidized is close to the mixture of nutrients in a normal diet, a value of 20.3 kJ per litre of oxygen consumed is a good approximation of the

Table 3.4 Values for oxidation of major nutrients (Brockway 1987, personal communication)

Nutrient	O_2 consumed (1/g)	CO_2 produced* (1/g)	RQ**	Energy released (kJ/g)	Energy released (kJ/l O_2)
Starch	0.829	0.824	0.994	17.49	21.10
Glucose†	0.746	0.742	0.995	15.44	20.70
Fat	1.975	1.402	0.710	39.12	19.81
Protein	0.962	0.775	0.806	18.52	19.25
Alcohol†	1.429	0.966	0.663	29.75	20.40

*CO_2 is not an ideal gas: 1 mole at STP occupies 22.26 not 22.4 litre.
**volumetric RQ
† Brockway (personal communication)

energy expenditure. For greater accuracy from indirect calorimetry, it is useful to measure the carbon dioxide production and, in experiments of sufficient duration, the urinary nitrogen excretion. The most widely used formulae in human indirect calorimetry are those developed by Weir (1949):

$$EE \ (kJ) = 16.489 \ VO_2(l) + 4.628 \ VCO_2(l) - 9.079 \ N \ (g)$$

If nitrogen excretion is not measured, but it is assumed that protein accounts for 15% of total energy expenditure, the same formula becomes:

$$EE \ (kJ) = 16.318 \ VO_2(l) + 4.602 \ VCO_2(l)$$

Similar formulae have been developed by other workers, with minor differences which arise from differences in the assumptions about the composition of carbohydrate, fat and protein. These different assumptions lead to differences between estimates of energy expenditure of less than 3% under most normal dietary conditions (Brockway 1987), although with unusual diets or in altered metabolic states these differences can increase.

If oxygen consumption, carbon dioxide production and urinary nitrogen excretion are all measured, it is possible to calculate the proportions of energy derived from the three major nutrients. The following equations are based on the values for glucose, fat and protein given in Table 3.4 and on the assumption that 6.25 g of protein contain 1 g of nitrogen:

Carbohydrate oxidation (g)
$$= 4.706 \ VCO_2 \ (l) - 3.340 \ VO_2 \ (l) - 2.714 \ N \ (g)$$
Fat oxidation (g)
$$= 1.768 \ VO_2 \ (l) - 1.778 \ VCO_2 \ (l) - 2.021 \ N \ (g)$$
Protein oxidation (g) $= 6.25 \ N \ (g)$

This approach remains valid even when there is net synthesis of lipid from carbohydrate. The results are very sensitive to the accuracy of the measurements of O_2 consumed and CO_2 produced. In unusual nutritional situations, e.g. during elemental feeding, the underlying assumptions of the stoichiometry of oxidation of the different nutrients may require alteration to avoid errors in the results (Livesey & Elia 1988).

Equipment for measuring energy expenditure by indirect calorimetry

The equipment used for the measurement of energy expenditure by indirect calorimetry ranges from the

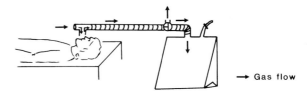

Fig. 3.3   The Douglas bag.

simple equipment designed to operate under rugged field conditions to technically sophisticated whole-body chambers. Detailed descriptions of equipment and techniques are to be found in McLean & Tobin (1987).

The most widely used system is the Douglas bag technique. In this method the subject breathes through a valve which separates inspired from expired air, and directs all the expired air into a plastic bag of capacity of up to 150 litres (Fig. 3.3). After a period in which the subject becomes accustomed to breathing through the valve, all the expired air is collected over a measured period of time. The volume of expired air is then measured and adjusted to the volume at standard temperature and pressure with no humidity. The concentration of oxygen, and sometimes of carbon dioxide, is measured in a sample of expired air from the bag, using either a chemical apparatus, such as the Haldane apparatus, or a specially designed gas analyser. The most widely used gas analysers depend on the paramagnetic properties of oxygen and the infrared absorbance of carbon dioxide, although other approaches are sometimes used. Since in well-ventilated surroundings the oxygen and carbon dioxide content of atmospheric (i.e. inspired) air can be assumed to be 20.95% and 0.03%, respectively, the amount of oxygen consumed and carbon dioxide produced, and hence the energy expenditure of the subject, can be calculated.

The Douglas bag has been used for many measurements of energy expenditure at rest and during exercise, although for the latter it is less than ideal since the bag fills quickly during heavy activity. In these situations the Kofrani–Michaelis respirometer (also known as the 'KM' or the Max Planck respirometer; Fig. 3.4) has been more widely used, since it measures expired air volume as it is collected, and therefore only a small sample of the expired air needs to be retained for subsequent gas analysis. The KM is no longer manufactured, and to take its place another portable instrument, the Oxylog, was developed. This weighs 2.2 kg and incorporates both a volume meter and oxygen sensors, so there is no need for subse-

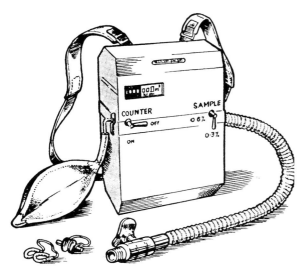

Fig. 3.4   The Kofrani–Michaelis respirometer.

quent gas analysis. Electronic components powered by rechargeable batteries calculate the oxygen consumed and provide a digital display of results on a minute-by-minute basis during the measurement. Most recently another successor to the KM, the Cosmed K2, has been produced. This weighs only 400 g and incorporates an oxygen sensor and a device for transmitting data to a radio receiver remote from the subject.

The collection of expired air with either the Douglas bag or portable respirometers introduces an element of discomfort for the subject through the necessity for a face mask or a one-way breathing valve and nose-clips. Ventilated hood systems (Fig. 3.5)

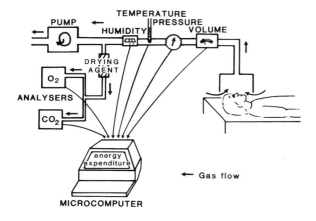

Fig. 3.5   A ventilated hood indirect calorimeter.

avoid this need by maintaining a high rate of air flow through the restricted space in which the subject breathes. More accurate gas analysers are needed, and the system is best suited to situations in which the subject is lying at rest for periods of 30 min to 6 hours.

Whole-body indirect calorimeter chambers operate on the same principle as the ventilated hood, but enclose the subject in a small room in which he or she can follow many of the activities of a normal day. A number of these chambers now exist in different countries, ranging in size from 5 to 25m^3. In the majority of these systems, both oxygen and carbon dioxide are monitored, and the subjects follow a fixed activity schedule with meals, sleep and periods of exercise. In this way a value for the 24-hour energy expenditure of subjects, and of the energy expended in standardized activities, can be obtained. The 24-hour energy expenditure may of course differ from the normal energy expenditure of the same subject under free-living conditions, due to the impossibility of simulating all forms of normal physical activity inside a calorimeter chamber.

Non-calorimetric methods As an alternative to the measurement of energy expenditure by indirect calorimetry, measurement of heart rate has been used by some workers to estimate energy expenditure over 24-hour periods. This method requires the establishment of the relationship between heart rate and energy expenditure in individual subjects by simultaneous heart-rate monitoring and indirect calorimetry. It is necessary to use a number of different activities to establish this relationship, since heart rate and energy expenditure do not follow a simple linear relationship. The method does not have the same accuracy as indirect calorimetry, but it is inexpensive and nonrestrictive to the subject, and gives information on the pattern of energy expenditure at different times of day. It can therefore be used in large numbers of subjects, and in subjects such as children, in whom 24-hour calorimetry would be difficult, to estimate energy expenditure under free-living conditions.

The most substantial recent advance in the study of energy expenditure in man has been the development of the doubly labelled water technique (Schoeller & van Santen 1982). This provides information on the total energy expenditure of a non-restricted subject over a period of up to 3 weeks, and can therefore reflect the true energy requirements of the subject. It involves the subject taking an oral dose of water containing stable (non radioactive) isotopes of both hydrogen and oxygen. The isotopes, ^2H (deuterium) and ^{18}O, mix with the normal hydrogen and oxygen in body water within a few hours. As energy is expended

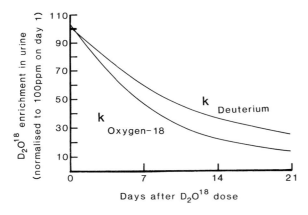

Fig. 3.6   Decline of ²H and ¹⁸O in body fluids during a doubly labelled water experiment.

in the body, carbon dioxide and water are produced. The carbon dioxide is lost from the body via the breath, while water is lost from the body through the breath, skin and urine. ¹⁸O is contained in both carbon dioxide and water and will therefore be lost from the body faster than the ²H, which is contained in water but not in carbon dioxide. The difference between the rate of loss of the two isotopes is used to calculate the carbon dioxide production of the subject, which in turn is used to calculate energy expenditure by the traditional formulae for indirect calorimetry (e.g. the Weir formula).

The rates of loss of the ¹⁸O and ²H are determined by measuring the decline in the concentration of the isotopes in any body fluid (usually urine) over the 10–21 days of the experiment (Fig. 3.6). The number of days on which samples are required varies from 2 to 21, according to the experimental protocol. Several other variables must be estimated for calculation of the results: the diet composition (to give an estimate of RQ and hence oxygen consumption), the amount of evaporative water loss, and the extent of incorporation of the isotopes into body tissue, which may be especially important during growth. Comparisons of the doubly labelled water method with whole-body indirect calorimetry suggest that the technique is capable of an accuracy of better than 5% under carefully controlled experimental conditions.

The major advantage of the doubly labelled water technique is that the subject is completely free to follow his or her normal lifestyle during the measurement. The method can therefore be used in ill, young, elderly or exceptionally active subjects, in whom other methods might be impractical. The

major disadvantage of the technique is the high cost of the doubly labelled water itself, and of the mass spectrometer required to measure the concentrations of the isotopes in the body fluid samples. A further drawback is the fact that the technique gives no information on energy expenditure at different times of the day, or on the different days of a study. However, if doubly labelled water measurements are made in combination with indirect calorimetry, a complete picture of total energy expenditure and its components can be obtained.

COMPONENTS OF ENERGY EXPENDITURE IN MAN

The energy expenditure of a man or woman over a whole day is often divided into different components which can be individually determined, as shown in Fig. 3.7. The largest single component of 24-hour energy expenditure in most individuals is the basal metabolic rate (BMR), which is the energy expenditure of an individual lying at physical and mental rest in a thermoneutral environment, at least 12 hours after the previous meal. In practice, BMR measurements are made early in the morning, before the subject has engaged in any significant physical activity, and with no ingestion of tea or coffee or inhalation of nicotine for at least 12 hours before the measurement. Heavy physical exercise on the day before the measurement may also influence the BMR (see below) and should therefore be avoided. If any of the conditions for BMR are not met, the energy expenditure should be termed the resting metabolic rate (RMR) of the subject.

The BMR of a subject is influenced by many factors, such as age, sex, body size, body composition, nutritional and physiological state, which are outlined

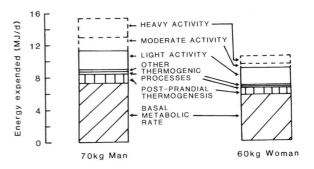

Fig. 3.7   Components of 24-hour energy expenditure in men and women.

Table 3.5 Estimates of the energy costs of selected activities (James & Schofield 1990). All values are expressed as a multiple of basal metabolic rate

Activity	Men	Activity	Women
Sitting	1.2	Sitting	1.2
Standing	1.4	Standing	1.5
Walking (normal pace)	3.2	Walking (normal pace)	3.4
Carpentry	3.5	Light cleaning	2.7
Mining with pick	6.0	Hand-threshing grain	5.0

in the following section. It is nevertheless a useful indication of the energy expenditure under standardized conditions, which can be compared within and between individuals. BMR is not necessarily the minimum metabolic rate of a subject, since estimates of sleeping metabolic rate by different workers range from 90–100% of the BMR of the same subjects.

Physical activity accounts for 20–40 % of total daily energy expenditure in most individuals. The energy expended in physical activity depends on the nature and duration of the different activities carried out in the day. Activities which involve little muscular work but which are carried out for long periods, such as sitting and standing, may contribute more to total daily energy expenditure than more strenuous activities carried out for shorter periods of time. The energy cost of any particular activity varies widely between individuals, since the size of the subject and the speed and dexterity with which he or she carries out an activity influence the energy expended (Mahadeva et al 1953). Heavy physical exercise also appears to increase the resting metabolic rate by a small amount over the following day (Maehlum et al 1986), an effect known as the 'excess post-exercise oxygen consumption (EPOC)'. Some examples of the energy cost of different activities for men and women, expressed as a multiple of BMR, are given in Table 3.5. A more comprehensive list of the energy cost of activities is given in James & Schofield (1990), although for accurate values for a particular individual or group, there is no substitute for direct measurements.

Other thermogenic processes in man include the effect of food intake, drugs, cold and hormonal state. The ingestion of food produces an increase in energy expenditure over several hours, which is usually known as postprandial thermogenesis (PPT): earlier terms include 'specific dynamic action' and 'heat increment of feeding'. The term 'diet-induced thermogenesis' (DIT) is sometimes used to describe the response to recent food ingestion, but is more usually used to describe the longer-term effects of food intake

on energy expenditure, as for example when BMR increases in over-feeding. PPT is a result of energy expended in the digestion, absorption and transport of ingested nutrients, as well as the physical activity required for ingestion and any increase in mental arousal due to the sensory stimuli from food. It is usually assumed to amount to around 10% of the energy content of a normal diet. Cold-induced thermogenesis involves shivering and non-shivering components, which increase energy expenditure to maintain body temperature when heat loss into the environment increases due to cold, air movement or lack of shelter and insulation. Other thermogenic stimuli which account for small fractions of the total daily energy expenditure are discussed below.

FACTORS INFLUENCING ENERGY EXPENDITURE IN MAN

Body size is one of the major determinants of energy expenditure in man, accounting for more than half of the variability in BMR between different individuals. Larger people have higher metabolic rates: a difference in weight of 10 kg would account for a difference in BMR of around 500 kJ/day in adult men or women, or a difference in daily energy expenditure of around 800 kJ/day in subjects with light physical activity.

Body composition is another major determinant of energy expenditure, since at rest adipose tissue has a lower metabolic rate than other ('fat-free' or 'lean') tissue. For this reason, BMR is usefully expressed per kilogram of fat-free mass. Adipose tissue, however, may contribute to the energy cost of physical activity in activities involving movement of the body.

Age affects energy expenditure in that the energy expended per unit of body weight declines rapidly from birth to old age. In children, energy expenditure is increased by the energy cost of growth, and in very young infants, by the energy required to maintain body temperature. During adulthood there is usually a decline in fat-free mass and an increase in adipose tissue, which accounts for a large part of the decline in metabolic rate after early adulthood.

Sex differences in energy expenditure are again largely accounted for by differences in body size and body composition. A 65 kg adult man will have a BMR of around 1 MJ/day higher than a woman of the same age and weight.

Diet affects energy expenditure, both immediately after a meal (see PPT above) and over longer periods (see DIT above). Postprandial thermogenesis is greater in response to protein ingestion than to the same energy intake in the form of carbohydrate or fat (Nair et al 1981). Energy intakes above or below energy requirements will lead to an increase or decrease in BMR, which is over and above that which would be expected from the change in body weight and body composition. These changes in energy expenditure are sometimes termed 'adaptive', since they act to offset the energy surplus or deficit, but they are usually around 5–15% of the difference between energy intake and expenditure, and will therefore only slightly diminish the weight change produced by the energy imbalance.

Climate affects energy expenditure due to the need to maintain body temperature, as discussed above. Air temperature, wind speed and the radiant temperature of surrounding materials are important factors. In lightly clothed adults in an indoor environment, air temperatures below 25°C may increase energy expenditure. At air temperatures above 30°C, energy expenditure may be increased by the additional work of sweating.

Genetic differences in energy expenditure have been the subject of several recent studies. Metabolic rate under standardized conditions varies by up to ±10% between subjects of the same age, sex, body weight and fat content, and there is growing evidence that some of this variation is determined by genetic factors. One recent study has shown lower RMR and energy cost of activities in Asian and African subjects than in Caucasian subjects of similar body weight and composition (Geissler & Hamoud Aldouri 1985), while other studies have detected no differences in energy expenditure between subjects of different ethnic groups.

Hormonal state can affect energy expenditure, notably in endocrine disorders such as hyper- and hypothyroidism, when energy expenditure is increased or decreased respectively. More physiological hormonal effects are seen in pregnancy and lactation. In pregnancy, BMR appears to decrease in the early stages (Durnin et al 1987), while towards the end of gestation the increase in body weight accounts for an overall increase in BMR. The early fall in BMR seems to be larger in women with low energy intakes, such as those in poor rural communities in developing countries. The net change in total daily energy expenditure in pregnancy is also determined by the change in the amount and intensity of physical activity over the gestational period, a phenomenon which is likely to vary widely between individuals and between populations. In lactation there may also be a reduction in energy expenditure in BMR, physical activity and other thermogenic processes (Illingworth et al 1986).

Psychological state may affect energy expenditure, as acute anxiety is a potent stimulant of energy expenditure. Whether chronic psychological stress influences energy expenditure is less certain.

Pharmacological agents which influence metabolic rate include everyday substances such as nicotine (Dallosso & James 1984), caffeine and theophylline (Dulloo et al 1989), all of which increase energy expenditure by small but measurable amounts, and therapeutic agents such as amphetamines and more experimental drugs used to treat obesity. Others including beta-blockers commonly used to treat high blood pressure, may reduce energy expenditure and lead to slight weight gain.

Disease processes also increase metabolic rate, especially infections with fever, tumours and burns of the skin. The mechanisms by which these processes increase energy expenditure are likely to involve intracellular signalling agents such as the cytokines, but as yet they are not fully understood.

ESTIMATION OF ENERGY REQUIREMENTS

The energy requirement of an individual is defined as 'the energy intake which will balance energy expenditure when the individual has a body size and composition and level of physical activity consistent with long-term good health; and that will allow for the maintenance of economically necessary and socially desirable physical activity. In children and pregnant or lactating women, the energy requirement includes the energy needs associated with the deposition of tissues or the secretion of milk at rates consistent with good health' (FAO/WHO/UNU 1985).

For an individual who is neither gaining or losing weight, energy intake and energy expenditure must be equal. For this reason, the energy requirements of healthy adults have frequently been estimated from estimates of energy intake. In infants and children up to 10 years of age in whom measurements of energy expenditure are difficult, current estimates of energy

Table 3.6 Estimated energy requirements of children 1–10 years (Department of Health 1991)

Age	Average weight (kg)		Energy requirement (kJ/kg/day)		Energy requirement (kJ/day)	
	Boys	Girls	Boys	Girls	Boys	Girls
1 month	4.15	4.00	480	480	1990	1920
3 month	6.12	5.70	420	420	2570	2390
6 month	8.00	7.44	400	400	6200	2980
12 month	10.04	9.50	400	400	4020	3800
2 yr	12.39	11.80	400	400	4960	4720
3 yr	14.40	13.85	400	400	5760	5540
4 yr	17.0	16.8	395	365	6730	6120
5 yr	19.3	18.9	370	345	7190	6480
6 yr	21.7	21.3	350	320	7570	6770
7 yr	24.2	23.8	325	295	7920	7050
8 yr	26.8	26.6	305	275	8240	7280
9 yr	29.7	29.7	290	255	8550	7510

Table 3.7 Equations for the prediction of basal metabolic rate (Department of Health 1991)

	Age range	Prediction equation	95% confidence limits
Men	10–17 yr	BMR (MJ/day) = 0.074(wt)* + 2.754	±0.88 MJ/day
	18–29 yr	BMR (MJ/day) = 0.063(wt)* + 2.896	±1.28 MJ/day
	30–59 yr	BMR (MJ/day) = 0.048(wt)* + 3.653	±1.40 MJ/day
	60–74 yr	BMR (MJ/day) = 0.0499(wt)* + 2.930	(N/A)
	75+ yr	BMR (MJ/day) = 0.0350(wt)* + 3.434	(N/A)
Women	10–17 yr	BMR (MJ/day) = 0.056(wt)* + 2.898	±0.94 MJ/day
	18–29 yr	BMR (MJ/day) = 0.062(wt)* + 2.036	±1.00 MJ/day
	30–59 yr	BMR (MJ/day) = 0.034 (wt)* + 3.538	±0.94 MJ/day
	60–74 yr	BMR (MJ/day) = 0.0386(wt)* + 2.875	(N/A)
	75+ yr	BMR (MJ/day) = 0.0410(wt)* + 2.610	(N/A)

*Body weight in kg

requirements are based on estimates of energy intake in subjects considered to be gaining weight at an acceptable rate. This is carried out by estimating breast milk and supplementary food intake at different ages. Unfortunately the energy content of breast milk is difficult to determine with accuracy: recent estimates of energy expenditure using deuterated water in infants suggest that the intake method may overestimate energy requirements (Prentice et al 1988). Table 3.6 lists the energy requirements of children from birth to 10 years, estimated by the Department of Health (1991).

In groups of normal-weight healthy adults, energy intake, measured over 7 days or more by the weighed food inventory technique (see Appendix 1) have been found to agree well with estimates of energy expenditure over the same period, although the agreement for each individual is usually less good than for the mean values of intake and expenditure for the combined subject in any one group. However, it should be borne in mind that even the most careful records of food intake may be subject to bias due to under-recording or changes of food habits, or due to random error if the days studied are not representative of the long-term dietary habits of the subjects. Several studies in different population groups have found that energy intake estimates are lower than energy expenditure when measured by the doubly-labelled water technique (e.g. Prentice et al 1986; Livingstone et al 1990). For this reason it is wise to assume that even the most careful estimates of energy intake in adults may not reflect habitual energy expenditure unless there is some additional evidence, such as a tendency for the mean weight of the group to remain constant over the period of recording, or reasonable agreement between the mean energy intake and the predicted energy requirements of the group.

Energy requirements can also be determined from energy expenditure, which can be estimated in a number of ways. The most common approach is the factorial method, in which the different components of energy expenditure are separately determined. BMR can be measured directly by indirect calorimetry, or can be predicted from tables based on measurements in large numbers of similar subjects. An extensive compilation of BMR data, based on a world-wide survey of some 11 000 technically acceptable measurements on individuals of all ages and both sexes, was made by FAO/WHO in the 1980s. This included all those measurements on which earlier equations for predicting BMR, such as the Harris-Benedict and Aub-du Bois formulae, were based. The data were subjected to statistical analysis, which demonstrated that simple linear equations predicting BMR from weight for different age and sex groups fitted the data as well as those including height, or based on more complex mathematical relations. More recently some additional data, notably on elderly subjects, have been added to these analyses. The resulting prediction equations for BMR are given in Table 3.7, which also shows the 95% confidence limits for the prediction of BMR in the younger age groups. This illustrates that the variation in BMR between different individuals of the same age group, weight and sex is approximately ±15%.

Once BMR has been measured or predicted, it is necessary to add on the energy required for physical activity and other thermogenic processes. The energy cost of physical activity can be measured directly by indirect calorimetry, although to do this for all the major activities of each subject is a painstaking task; the alternative is to estimate the energy cost of each activity from tables. The most comprehensive set of tables of the energy cost of activities for adults is provided by James & Schofield (1990), which is illustrated in Table 3.5. This compilation expresses the energy cost of activities as multiples of BMR for men and women, allowing one value to be given for each activity which can be applied to all individuals of any body weight and any age group. If the duration of each activity is known, its energy cost can be determined from this multiple and the measured or

Table 3.8 BMR multiples for light, moderate and heavy activity (Department of Health 1991)

Non-occupational activity level	Occupational activity level					
	Light		Moderate		Heavy	
	M	F	M	F	M	F
Non-active	1.4	1.4	1.6	1.5	1.7	1.5
Moderately active	1.5	1.5	1.7	1.6	1.8	1.6
Very active	1.6	1.6	1.8	1.7	1.9	1.7

Table 3.9 Calculation of energy requirements from activity pattern (FAO/WHO/UNU 1985)

Example a): A male office clerk aged 25 yrs; weight 65 kg; predicted BMR = 6078 kJ/day

Activity	Multiple of BMR	Hours spent in activity	kJ expended
In bed	1.0	8	2340
At work	1.7	6	2970
Discretionary			
Household tasks	3.0	2	1760
Fitness training	6.0	0.33	580
Remainder	1.4	7.67	3140
TOTAL	1.54	24	10 780

Example b): A rural woman in a developing country aged 35 yrs; weight 50 kg; predicted BMR = 5290 kJ/day

In bed	1.0	8	1780
Domestic work	2.7	3	1800
Agricultural work	2.8	4	2490
Discretionary	2.5	2	1110
Residual	1.4	7	2180
TOTAL	1.76	24	9360

predicted BMR of the subject. In this way the body weight of the subject is taken into account in the estimate of energy expenditure in activity, whereas earlier tables providing a single figure for the total energy expended in each activity, regardless of the size of the subject, did not allow for any effect of body size. Another new departure in these tables is the fact that the measurements were made in subjects without standardization of the time of meals and the influence of other thermogenic stimuli, so the value given by multiplying the BMR by the value for each activity is assumed to include the energy expended in other thermogenic processes.

The estimation of the duration of different physical activities can be made either by retrospective recall by the subject, by an activity diary kept by the subject, or by time-and-motion records kept by unobtrusive observers. If no such detailed information is available, a crude estimate may be made from knowledge of the subjects' lifestyle. To assist in this process, a recent UK report uses three activity categories for both work and leisure. The multiples of BMR for men and women in each of these categories is shown in Table 3.8. Examples of the estimation of energy requirements of a male office clerk and of a rural woman in a developing country are given in Tables 3.9 a) and b).

It is important to point out that the definition of energy requirement advanced by the WHO allows for energy expenditure in desirable physical activity (note for example the 20 minutes' daily fitness training assumed for the male office clerk in Table 3.9 a). In subjects who are below the desirable weight, or in whom the existing level of energy expenditure departs from the optimum for any reason, the correction for desirable levels can be included or omitted, according to whether the estimate of energy requirement is designed to maintain or to improve the status quo.

The energy requirements of adolescents and of pregnant and lactating women estimated by the factorial method should also include an allowance for the energy cost of tissue deposition or breast milk secretion. In normal growth, weight gain can be assumed to require 21 kJ per gram of tissue deposited (FAO/WHO/UNU 1985). By assuming appropriate rates of weight gain and standard patterns of physical activity, the energy requirements of adolescents are estimated to be around $1.65 \times$ BMR for boys or $1.57 \times$ BMR for girls.

In pregnancy, additional energy requirements have traditionally been estimated from theoretical calculations of the energy required for development of the fetus and the supporting tissues (placenta, uterus, breasts and adipose tissue depots), which suggest an additional requirement of 1200 kJ per day throughout pregnancy (Hytten & Leitch 1971). This allowance does not take into account any possible reduction in BMR or the energy expended in physical activity, and may therefore be seen as generous. Studies of women in both affluent and poor societies have rarely shown changes in energy intake of this magnitude throughout pregnancy, though there may be some increase in energy intake in the last few months. Current UK recommendations acknowledge

this by suggesting an increase of 800 kJ/day in the last trimester only (Department of Health 1991).

In lactation, some of the energy cost of breast milk secretion is met by the adipose tissue stores laid down in pregnancy (4 kg of 11 kg gained in a theoretical 'textbook' gestation). If breast milk containing 3 MJ per day is secreted for 6 months, with an estimated efficiency of production of 80%, but at the same time the adipose tissue stores laid down in pregnancy are depleted, the net increase in energy requirement will be around 2.1 MJ per day over the 6-month period. Clearly, for women who bottle-feed, or who breast-feed for periods of less than 6 months, this allowance will be too large. A recent study of the energy intake of lactating women in the UK (Goldberg et al 1991) reported an increase of energy intake of around 1.5 MJ/day as compared with non-pregnant, non-lactating values, suggesting that a reduction in physical activity and/or alterations in the thermogenic processes observed in lactation may operate to reduce the additional energy requirements of lactation in many women.

The estimation of energy requirements can therefore be seen to be an imprecise tool, but one which is necessary for indicating the food needs of individuals and populations. The final test of whether the energy requirement has been estimated correctly is whether a subject fed his or her estimated energy requirement over a period of time changes weight by the amount intended. New measurements of energy expenditure, especially those by the doubly labelled water technique, are likely to improve the process of estimating energy requirements in coming decades, but there will never be a better validation of the suitability of a subject's energy intake than the simple observation of body weight.

REFERENCES

Brockway JM 1987 Derivation of formulae used to calculate energy expenditure in man. Human Nutrition: Clinical Nutrition 41C: 463–471

Dalloso HM, James WPT 1984 The role of smoking in the regulation of energy balance. International Journal of Obesity 8: 365–375

Department of Health 1991 Dietary Reference Values for Food, Energy and Nutrients for the United Kingdom. HMSO, London

Dulloo AG, Geissler CA, Horton T, Collins A, Miller DS 1989 Normal caffeine consumption: influence on thermogenesis and daily energy expenditure in lean and post-obese human volunteers. American Journal of Clinical Nutrition 49: 44–50

Durnin JVGA et al 1987 The energy requirements of human pregnancy. Lancet: 895–900; 953–955; 1010–1012; 1072–1076; 1129–1133

FAO/WHO/UNU 1985 Energy and Protein Requirements. WHO Technical Report Series No. 724. World Health Organisation, Geneva

Geissler CA, Hamoud Aldouri MS 1985 Racial differences in the energy cost of standardised activities. Annals of Nutrition and Metabolism 29: 40–47

Goldberg GR, Prentice AM, Coward WA et al 1991 Longitudinal assessment of the components of energy balance in well-nourished lactating women. American Journal of Clinical Nutrition 54: 788–798

Hytten FE, Leitch I 1971 The Physiology of Human Pregnancy, 2nd edn. Blackwell, Oxford

Illingworth PJ, Jung RT, Howie PW, Leslie P, Isles T 1986 Diminution in energy expenditure during lactation. British Medical Journal 292: 437–441

James WPT, Schofield C 1990 Human energy requirements. Oxford University Press, Oxford

Livesey G, Elia M 1988 Estimation of energy expenditure, net carbohydrate utilization and net fat oxidation and synthesis by indirect calorimetry: evaluation of errors with special reference to the detailed composition of fuels. American Journal of Clinical Nutrition 47: 608–628

Livingstone MBE, Prentice AM, Strain JJ et al 1990 Accuracy of weighed dietary records in studies of diet and health. British Medical Journal 300: 708–712

Lusk G 1928 The elements of the science of nutrition 4th edn. Johnson Reprint Corp, New York (reprinted 1976).

Maehlum S, Grandmontagne M, Newsholme EA, Sejersted OM 1986 Magnitude and duration of excess postexercise oxygen consumption in healthy young subjects. Metabolism 35: 425–429

Mahadeva K, Passmore R, Woolf B 1953 Individual variations in the metabolic cost of standardised exercises: the effects of food, age, sex and race. Journal of Physiology 121: 225–231

McCance RA, Widdowson EM 1991 The composition of foods, 5th edn. HMSO, London

McLean JA, Tobin G 1987 Animal and human calorimetry. Cambridge University Press, Cambridge.

Nair KS, Garrow JS, Halliday D 1981 Thermic response to isoenergetic protein, carbohydrate or fat meals in lean and obese subjects. Clinical Science 62: 43P

Prentice AM, Black AE, Coward WA et al 1986 High levels of energy expenditure in obese women. British Medical Journal 292: 983–987

Prentice AM, Lucas A, Vasquez-Velasquez L, Davies PWS, Whitehead RG 1988 Are current dietary guidelines for young children a prescription for overfeeding? Lancet (ii): 1066–1069

Schoeller DA, van Santen E 1982 Measurement of energy expenditure in humans by doubly labelled water method. Journal of Applied Physiology 53(4): 955–959

Southgate DAT, Durnin JVGA 1970 Calorie conversion factors. An experimental reassessment of the factors used in the calculation of the energy value of human diets. British Journal Nutrition 24: 517

Weir JB de V 1949 New methods for calculating metabolic rate with special reference to protein metabolism. Journal of Physiology 109: 1–9

Widdowson EM 1955 Assessment of the energy value of human foods. Proceedings of the Nutrition Society 14: 142

4. Carbohydrates

H. N. Englyst and S. M. Kingman

Carbohydrates provide a great part of the energy in all human diets. In the diets of poor people, especially in the tropics, up to 85% of the energy may come from this source. On the other hand, in the diets of the rich in many countries, the proportion may be as low as 40%. Neither of these extremes is desirable.

Green plants synthesize carbohydrates from carbon dioxide and water with evolution of oxygen under the influence of sunlight. The primary products are the sugars, which are readily soluble in water and so easily transported throughout the tissue fluid of both plants and animals to provide the fuels of the cells. Sugars are polymerized to form polysaccharides, some of which are not readily soluble in water, but easily stored or incorporated into cell-wall structures.

Plant foods contain two chemically distinct types of polysaccharide, the storage polysaccharide starch, a polymer of glucose linked by α-glucosidic linkages, and the cell-wall or chemically related polysaccharides, which do not contain α-glucosidic linkages and may conveniently be called non-starch polysaccharides (NSP). Seed grains, root vegetables and plantains contain large amounts of starch and are the world's most important starchy foods. NSP is the principal and readily measurable component of what has been termed dietary fibre (see below).

Animal tissues also contain carbohydrate polymers. Glycogen is a storage polysaccharide with a structure similar to starch. Glycoproteins, found in many tissues and with diverse functions, are polypeptides containing short chains of carbohydrates. The carbohydrate-rich mucins, which are also glycoproteins, constitute a protective lining for epithelial tissues, particularly in the gut. Mucin consists of a protein core covered with carbohydrate side chains that are resistant to hydrolysis by endogenous enzymes. The amount of carbohydrate in animal tissues is small in relation to their fat and protein content, and is not important in dietary terms.

Starch and sugars are, to a large extent, broken down by digestive enzymes into monosaccharides and then absorbed in the small intestine. However, certain types of starch and sugars, and all the NSPs, escape digestion in the small intestine and become available as fermentable substrates for the colonic microflora. The main products of fermentation are carbon dioxide, hydrogen, methane and volatile fatty acids (acetic, propionic and butyric acids). The gases may be passed as flatus or absorbed and excreted through the lungs. The volatile fatty acids are absorbed and may be used as energy sources by various tissues. Thus, carbohydrates escaping digestion in the small intestine may, to a large extent, become available as a source of energy through fermentation. The widely used and long-standing nutritional term 'unavailable carbohydrates' for those components not digested in the small intestine is potentially misleading. The digestion and utilization of the various types of dietary carbohydrates is summarized in Fig. 4.1.

DIETARY SOURCES OF CARBOHYDRATE

Fig. 4.2 is a classification of the main types of food carbohydrate in the human diet. These are described in more detail below. The proportions of starch, sugar and NSPs (dietary fibre) in the diet are highly variable, as illustrated in Fig. 4.3, which gives typical nutrient profiles for three different communities from around the world (See also Chapter 16).

Monosaccharides

Glucose is found in small amounts in fruit and vegetables, particularly grapes and onions and, with fructose, is one of the main constituents of honey. Free glucose is not found abundantly in natural foods, but is manufactured from starch and sold commercially in a number of proprietary preparations. These have no

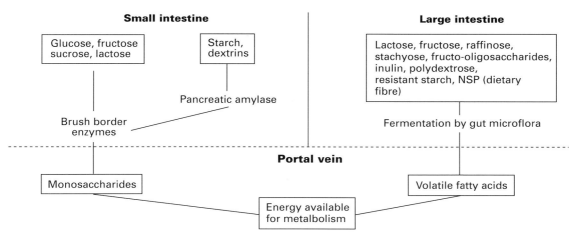

Fig. 4.1   Utilization of dietary carbohydrates

advantage over sucrose as a source of energy for healthy people, but may be useful in special high-energy diets: glucose is only half as sweet as sucrose, so more may be used to give the same sweetness.

Fructose is found in fruits, vegetables and honey. It is present also in invert sugar, a syrup made from sucrose and used extensively in the food industry.

Mannose is uncommon as a monosaccharide in foods but is present in manna, which the Israelites gathered to make bread when they were in the desert (Exodus 16: 13–35). Manna is the common name for lichens which in drought curl up into light balls that may be blown across the desert, and from which a bread may be made.

Pentoses are present as constituents of the macromolecules in the cells of all natural foodstuffs, but only in small amounts, so they are not important as a source of energy. Ribose and deoxyribose are components of nucleic acids and, as they are synthesized by all animals, are not essential nutrients.

Disaccharides

Sucrose is the sugar commonly used in the home, and is extracted commercially from sugar beet or sugar cane. Table sugar is 99% pure sucrose and is the major dietary source of this disaccharide, although it is present also in fruit and vegetables. Sucrose is readily hydrolysed by acids, and by the enzyme sucrase in the brush border of the small intestine, into glucose and fructose.

Lactose is a disaccharide of glucose and galactose that is found naturally only in milk and milk products. During childhood, lactose is hydrolysed readily by the

enzyme lactase; however, many ethnic groups lose the ability to produce lactase in adulthood, causing a condition known as lactose intolerance.

Maltose is a product of the hydrolysis of starch and comprises two molecules of glucose. It is present in malted (sprouted) wheat and barley, from which malt extract is produced commercially for use in brewing and the manufacture of malted foods.

Trehalose is a disaccharide composed of two molecules of glucose and is known as the mushroom sugar. It constitutes up to 15% of the dry matter of mushrooms and is present also in insects. The fact that we still possess the specific enzyme trehalase necessary for its hydrolysis suggests that fungi and insects were much more important foods for our ancestors than they are for us now.

Oligosaccharides

Raffinose, stachyose and verbascose are short-chain sugars composed of galactose, glucose and fructose. They are found in plant seeds – mainly legumes, such as beans and peas – and cannot be broken down by endogenous enzymes. Like NSP, these oligosaccharides are fermented in the large intestine.

Fructans is the name given to a group of oligo- and polysaccharides consisting of fructose residues attached to a single glucose molecule. The chain lengths of fructans can range from 3 to 50 residues, depending on the source. Shorter fructans predominate in cereals, whereas Jerusalem artichokes contain a larger proportion of inulin, a fructan of about 35 residues. Other sources are onions, garlic and asparagus. The hydrolysis of fructans in the stomach and the small

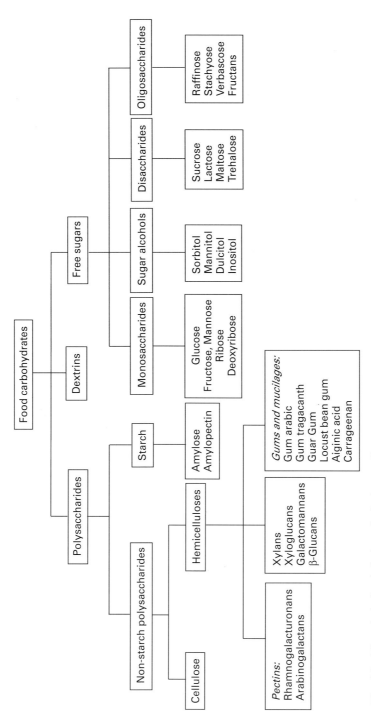

Fig. 4.2   The principal carbohydrates in the human diet

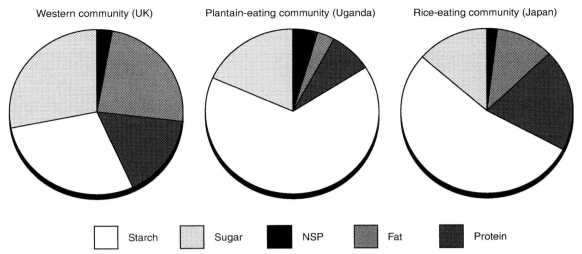

Western community (UK)   Plantain-eating community (Uganda)   Rice-eating community (Japan)

☐ Starch   ▨ Sugar   ■ NSP   ▧ Fat   ▨ Protein

Fig. 4.3 Percentage nutrient intake in three communities with different dietary intakes

intestine is negligible and any trisaccharides absorbed directly are usually excreted in the urine. The major part of fructans reaches the large intestine, where it is fermented.

Sugar alcohols

These are found in nature and are also prepared commercially. Sorbitol is found naturally in some fruit, such as cherries, but is made commercially from glucose by the use of the hydrogenating enzyme aldose reductase, which converts the aldehyde (CHO) group in the glucose molecule to the alcohol (CH$_2$OH). The manufactured product is used in 'diabetic' soft drinks, jams, chocolates and sweets. It is only 60% as sweet as sucrose, and it is absorbed from the gut more slowly and converted to fructose in the liver. It thus has less effect on blood glucose levels than sucrose, but episodic intakes above 50 g per day may lead to diarrhoea in diabetic patients consuming these products. Sorbitol is present in small amounts in nerve and other tissues, and these are increased by hyperglycaemia; this may be responsible for the impaired nerve conduction occurring in some diabetic patients.

Mannitol and dulcitol are alcohols derived from mannose and galactose, and both have a variety of uses in food manufacture. Mannitol is extracted commercially from a seaweed that grows on the coasts of Britain.

Inositol is a cyclic alcohol with six hydroxyl radicals and is allied to glucose. It is present in many foods, especially the bran of cereals. Its hexaphosphate ester

phytic acid has important nutritional effects because it impairs the absorption of calcium and iron in the small intestine (see Chapter 12).

Polysaccharides

Starch is the major carbohydrate of the human diet and is the main storage polysaccharide of dietary staples such as cereal grains, potatoes and plantains. Within the plant, starch is present in the form of granules with characteristic shapes, specific to each species. These can be seen under the microscope lying in groups inside thin-walled cells. Starch consists of two main types of polysaccharide derived from glucose. Amylose is a long, virtually unbranched chain of glucose units with $\alpha(1\rightarrow4)$ linkages. Amylopectin is a highly branched polymer with 15–30 $\alpha(1\rightarrow4)$ linked glucose units in each branch, the branches being joined by $\alpha(1\rightarrow6)$ linkages. Amylopectin predominates in most starches, but the relative amounts of amylose and amylopectin vary among different plant sources from 2% amylose in waxy corn starch to 80% amylose in high-amylose corn starch. The majority of starches contain between 15% and 35% amylose.

In starch granules the amylose and amylopectin chains are arranged in a semicrystalline structure, which makes them insoluble in water and retards their digestion by pancreatic amylase. Three crystalline forms, A, B and C, have been identified from X-ray diffraction studies (Katz 1934). When starch granules are heated in the presence of moisture, the crystalline structure is disrupted and the polysaccharide chains take up a random conformation, causing swelling of the starch and thickening of the surrounding matrix (gelatinization). The starch is then readily accessible to digestive enzymes. On cooling, the gelatinized starch begins a process of recrystallization known as retrogradation. This takes place very rapidly for amylose, while the retrogradation of amylopectin, known to be responsible for the staling of bread, takes place over several days.

Table 4.1 shows a classification of starch, based on studies in man, which has been developed for nutritional purposes. The three fractions described, which are defined in physical and chemical terms and determined in vitro, give an indication of the probable behaviour of starchy foods within the digestive tract.

The in vitro methodology involves incubating a starchy food with pancreatic amylase and amyloglucosidase under controlled conditions. The glucose released from the food within 20 minutes represents rapidly digestible starch, and that released in the following 100 minutes represents slowly digestible starch. Any starch unhydrolysed after 120 minutes is classified as resistant. Refinements to the method allow the three fractions of resistant starch to be measured separately if required.

Rapidly digestible starch (RDS) consists mainly of amorphous and dispersed starch. It is typically found in large amounts in starchy foods that have been cooked by moist heat, for instance bread and potatoes.

Slowly digestible starch (SDS), like RDS, is expected to be completely digested in the small intestine, but for one reason or another is digested more slowly. The category includes starch that is poorly accessible to enzymes, such as a portion of that in partly milled grains and seeds and in highly dense foods such as pasta. It also includes a high proportion of the granular starch in raw foods.

Resistant starch (RS) comprises the starch that may potentially resist digestion in the small intestine and therefore become available for fermentation in the large intestine. RS may be measured as a single entity or subdivided into RS_1, RS_2 and RS_3. RS_1 is physically inaccessible starch that may be found in whole or partly milled grains and seeds, and in some very dense types of processed starchy foods; RS_2 escapes digestion in the small intestine because its starch granules are intrinsically highly resistant to hydrolysis by pancreatic amylase – raw potato and banana starches are examples; RS_3 is mainly retrograded amylose formed during the cooling of gelatinized starch. Most moist-heated starchy foods will therefore contain some RS_3.

The amounts of RDS, SDS and RS in foods are highly variable. They depend partly on the source of starch, but largely on the type and extent of processing the food has undergone.

Dextrins are degradation products of starch in which the glucose chains have been broken down to smaller units by partial hydrolysis. They are the main source of carbohydrate in proprietary preparations used as oral supplements for tube feeding. 'Liquid glucose' is a mixture of dextrins, maltose, glucose and water. These products are a means of giving carbohydrates in an easily assimilated form to patients who are seriously ill. Dextrins, being larger molecules than sucrose or glucose, have less osmotic effect and so are less likely to cause osmolar diarrhoea. Dextrins should not be confused with dextran, a carbohydrate polymer obtained from bacterial cell walls. This has no place in dietary therapy, but when used intravenously is a useful plasma expander under emergency conditions. A 10% solution given intravenously causes an increase

Table 4.1   Classification of starch for nutritional purposes (from Englyst & Kingman 1990)

Type of starch	Example of occurrence	Probable digestion in small intestine
Rapidly digestible starch (RDS)	Freshly cooked starchy food	Rapid
Slowly digestible starch (SDS)	Most raw cereals	Slow but complete
Resistant starch (RS)		
Physically inaccessible starch	Partly milled grains and seeds	Resistant
Resistant starch granules	Raw potato and banana	Resistant
Retrograded amylose	Cooked potato after cooling, bread, cornflakes, etc.	Resistant

in blood volume, with a consequent rise in cardiac output and renal blood flow in patients who are in shock following haemorrhage.

Glycogen, the animal equivalent of starch, has a structure very like that of amylopectin, but is more highly branched. It is present in liver and muscle, where it is stored as a readily available energy reserve. Like starch, it is broken down by pancreatic amylase to glucose. In most foods of animal origin it is a negligible source of dietary carbohydrate, but an oyster (removed from its shell) contains about 6% of its wet weight as glycogen.

Non-starch polysaccharides (dietary fibre)

Definition

A major barrier to progress in understanding dietary fibre and its role has been the lack of an agreed chemical definition of dietary fibre. This has delayed the development of accurate methods for its measurement and resulted in the misinterpretation of studies of dietary fibre in man.

The original concept of 'dietary-fibre' (Hipsley 1953) was of material derived from the plant cell wall in foods. By 1972, dietary fibre had been defined as the skeletal remains of plant cells that are resistant to digestion by the enzymes of man (Trowell 1972), but by 1978 it was suggested by Cummings & Englyst that dietary fibre should be measured as the non-starch polysaccharides in plant foods (James & Theander 1981). In 1987, Englyst et al (1987b) proposed that dietary fibre should be defined for the purposes of food labelling as NSP, since this gives the best index of plant cell-wall polysaccharides and is in keeping with the original concept of dietary fibre.

It has been argued that dietary fibre should be defined as the food components resisting digestion in the small intestine. Such a definition would include NSP, lactose (in many ethnic groups), raffinose, stachyose and other oligosaccharides, a small amount of lignin, organic anions such as oxalate and tartrate, Maillard reaction products, some fat, hair, bone, grit and other insoluble materials, and, depending on food processing, a highly variable amount of starch and protein. In addition, lactulose, polydextrose, neosugar and similar synthetic products resistant to pancreatic amylase would be included as dietary fibre. Such a broad definition, including highly refined and synthetic products, is in clear contrast to the original concept of dietary fibre.

Resistance to the digestion of foodstuffs in the small intestine depends not only on food processing and chemical structure, but also on a number of highly variable factors not limited to the food itself. These include the extent of chewing, transit time through the stomach and small intestine, and the amount and type of other food components in the meal as a whole. The extent of digestion in the small intestine is therefore highly variable for an individual, and even larger differences in digestibility are seen between individuals or between population groups. Large differences in small-intestinal digestibility are also seen between man and animals. Defining dietary fibre as material resisting digestion in the small intestine is not analytically realistic, nor is it a scientifically meaningful alternative to defining dietary fibre, for analytical purposes, as NSP, which gives the analyst a clear task. NSP is the best index of plant cell-wall polysaccharides and is thus in keeping with the original concept of dietary fibre.

The Englyst procedure for the measurement of NSP as an index of dietary fibre has evolved from the principles laid down by Southgate (1969). Starch is completely removed enzymically and NSP is measured as the sum of its constituent sugars released by acid hydrolysis. The sugars may in turn be measured by gas–liquid chromatography (GLC, Englyst et al 1992), or high-pressure liquid chromatography (HPLC, Quigley & Englyst 1992), giving values for individual monosaccharides, or more rapidly by colorimetry (Englyst & Hudson 1992). A value is obtained for total dietary fibre and, if required, for soluble and insoluble dietary fibre. A small modification also allows cellulose to be measured separately.

Values for dietary fibre in a single food may differ considerably according to the method used for analysis, as illustrated by Table 4.2. The crude fibre technique, no longer used in human studies but still practised in the analysis of animal feedstuffs, measures only the small proportion of dietary fibre (mainly cellulose) that resists hydrolysis with acid and alkali. It therefore severely underestimates dietary fibre in foods. The neutral detergent fibre method (NDF), which measures a selective, largely insoluble fraction of dietary fibre, also tends to underestimate the total fibre present, particularly in vegetables and fruit, which are rich in soluble non-starch polysaccharides. Higher values for dietary fibre in foods are given by the Southgate method and the enzymic–gravimetric methods of Prosky et al (1985, 1988) and Mongeau & Brassard (1990), because they include substances other than the non-starch polysaccharides that are measured directly in the Englyst procedure.

The development of the two types of technique, which include different components of the diet in their measurement of dietary fibre, has led to consid-

Table 4.2   Comparison of 'dietary fibre' values obtained by different analytical methods

Sample	Crude fibre	NDF (1976)	Southgate (1969)	AOAC (Prosky) (1985)	Mongeau (1987)	Englyst (1987)
			g/100 g dry matter			
White bread	1.7	2.4	4.4	3.5	3.0	3.0
Wholemeal bread	5.1	10.6	14.2	8.8	9.2	6.6
Porridge oats, raw	2.0	6.9	7.7	10.5	11.0	8.2
Shredded wheat cereal	3.6	13.4	13.3	10.4	11.1	9.0
Sweetcorn kernels	2.2	7.9	13.5	7.7	7.8	5.9
Onion	6.1	7.6	18.0	16.9	17.3	16.7
Carrots, raw	5.7	9.2	28.7	25.4	23.4	23.4
Cabbage, raw	8.4	14.2	28.4	23.3	20.7	21.0
Apples	3.7	7.6	12.7	14.6	14.2	13.4
Oranges	2.7	3.7	12.6	12.8	13.7	13.5
Reference	1	1	2	3	3	3

1. van Soest 1978
2. Paul & Southgate 1978
3. Mongeau & Brassard 1990

erable confusion in research and the food labelling of dietary fibre. The Prosky procedure, which includes part of the starch retrograded during food processing and also 'lignin'-measuring substances as dietary fibre, leads to higher values than the Englyst procedure, but the physiological effect of the material measured by this technique is unknown and is likely to be different from that of dietary fibre measured solely as NSP. Different recommended dietary amounts (RDAs) are therefore required for dietary fibre measured by the two methods and no single conversion factor to NSP can be applied to values obtained by the Prosky procedure.

Starch included in the Prosky procedure consists mainly of retrograded amylose and it represents a proportion of the starch measured as RS. One argument advanced is that this type of starch escapes digestion in the human small intestine, as does dietary fibre. However, when the digestibility of various types of starch is tested in man it becomes clear that retrograded amylose (RS_3) represents only a small proportion of the total amount of starch escaping digestion in the small intestine.

In addition to NSP and various types of starch, other substances escape digestion in the human small intestine; for example, some protein, lactose, raffinose, stachyose and free sugars. This characteristic is therefore not unique to NSP and RS_3 and is not a rational basis for the inclusion of any type of starch with dietary fibre.

It has been suggested that retrograded amylose (RS_3) may have a faecal bulking effect and therefore should be included as dietary fibre. However, virtually all the food components that escape digestion in the small intestine, including the three types of RS (see Table 4.1), a substantial amount of protein and free sugars, are expected to have bulking effects, either directly or through fermentation and bacterial growth (Cummings & Englyst 1987). The bulking effect is therefore not unique to NSP and RS_3, and thus there is no reason to include this type of starch as dietary fibre.

The amount of RS_3 formed during the processing of starchy foods is controlled by a number of factors, including the source of starch, water content, pH, heating temperature and time, number of heating and cooling cycles, freezing and drying. The amount of RS_3 in starchy foods is therefore in the hands of those who prepare foods, either at home or in the food industry (Englyst & Cummings 1988).

The amount of RS_3 formed by normal cooking is nutritionally insignificant for most foods. However, if RS_3 were to be included as dietary fibre, the RS_3 content of some types of food could be raised substantially by food manufacturers, with the aim of boosting sales through a claim of high dietary fibre content. The inclusion of RS_3 would also cause considerable problems for food labelling. For example, different apparent 'dietary fibre' values will be obtained for the same food if it is hot, cold, frozen or dried. The apparent 'dietary fibre' content will also change if test samples are heated, cooled, frozen or dried before analysis. One or more of these treatments is always used prior to analysis by the Prosky method. Dietary fibre values obtained by the Prosky method thus do not reflect the RS content in food as eaten, but include RS produced by storage and pretreatment of the sample. For example, the RS measured in a cooled or dried potato sample will not be present in the potato when eaten hot. Thus RS, but not NSP, is affected by food processing.

In addition to the inclusion of retrograded starch, the main reason for the high values obtained for dietary fibre by the Prosky procedure is the inclusion of substances measuring as lignin. Accurately measured, lignin would be quantitatively insignificant in the diet, but the material measured as lignin may result in large overestimations of dietary fibre, especially in processed foods. Lignin is not a carbohydrate and its physiological significance (in animal studies) is very different from that of NSP. Lignin should therefore not be measured with NSP, and it is not included in the analytical definition of dietary fibre (Englyst et al 1987b). Lignin is quantitatively a minor component in the human diet and it is difficult to determine (Cummings et al 1985).

Fibre content of foods

Total, soluble and insoluble dietary fibre have been measured in 178 fruits and vegetables (Englyst et al 1988) and in 114 cereal products (Englyst et al 1989). Table 4.3 gives dietary fibre values for a selection of plant foodstuffs. When using GLC, fibre values can also be separated into cellulose and non-cellulosic polysaccharides (NCP) with values for the individual constituent sugars. These analytical fractions are of interest because of their different physiological roles.

Wheat bran has a high proportion of the total NSP in the form of insoluble NSP. In general, cereal products contain more NCP xylose than arabinose, but contain only traces of uronic acids. This is in contrast to fruit and vegetables, where arabinose, especially soluble NCP arabinose, is the predominant pentose. Fruit and vegetables generally have a high content of uronic acids originating from pectin. The main polymers making up NSP are described below.

Cellulose is the most abundant organic substance found in nature, being the principal component of cell walls in higher plants. It is a high-molecular-weight linear polymer of up to 10 000 glucose units linked by $\beta(1\rightarrow4)$ bonds. Strong inter- and intramolecular hydrogen bonding between cellulose chains leads to the formation of microfibrils and fibres, and to the development of highly stable crystalline structures. Cellulose thus shows low chemical reactivity, which explains its characteristic physical properties.

Hemicelluloses are heterogeneous, branched polymers of hexoses, pentoses and uronic acids, found in virtually all plant cell walls. They are relatively short polymers (50–2000 residues) and the constituent sugars of the polymer chains vary according to the plant source. Xylans are polymers of xylose with side chains of arabinose and glucuronic acid, found particularly in wheat, rye and barley. Galactomannans, characteristic of legumes, consist of a mannose backbone with galactose and glucose side chains. Xyloglucans, with a glucose backbone and xylose branches are found closely associated with cellulose in many plant tissues.

Pectins are branched polymers that are characteristic of immature parenchymatous tissue found in fruit and vegetables. The two main types are rhamnogalacturonans, which are polymers of rhamnose and galacturonic acid with branches of galactose and arabinose, and arabinogalactans, which are galactose chains with many short arabinose side chains. The uronic acid groups of pectins may be partially esterified with methoxyl groups. Pectin is extracted commercially from apple pomace and citrus fruit rind. It is used in food manufacture as a stabilizer and emulsifier, and as a gelling agent in jams (E440).

β-Glucans are mainly water-soluble polymers of glucose linked $\beta(1\rightarrow3)$ and $\beta(1\rightarrow4)$. Unlike cellulose, the glucose chains are branched and have a relatively low degree of polymerization. Cereals such as oats and barley are particularly good sources of these polysaccharides, and the β-glucans have been implicated in the cholesterol-reducing properties of oat bran.

Gums are water-soluble viscous polysaccharides of 10 000–30 000 units, mainly glucose, galactose, mannose, arabinose, rhamnose and their uronic acids, which may be methoxylated or acetylated. Gums are extracted commercially and used in the food industry as emulsifiers, stabilizers and thickeners. Gum arabic is obtained as an exudate from the acacia tree (*Robinia pseudacacia*); gum tragacanth, a partially soluble polysaccharide with a structure similar to pectin, is extracted from the *Sterculia* and *Khaya* species. Guar gum and locust bean gum are galactomannans. They are the storage polysaccharides of the Indian cluster bean and the locust or carob bean, respectively.

Mucilages, like exudate gums, are structurally complex, but they are generally characterized by the component D-galacturonic acid. They are found in some seeds and roots, where they are thought to prevent desiccation. Algal polysaccharides, from algae and seaweeds, are widely used as food additives. Alginic acid, extracted from brown seaweeds, is a polymer of mannuronic and guluronic acids. It is used as a

Table 4.3   Examples of the variability in the fibre composition of different foods based on detailed gas–liquid chromatographic analysis by the Englyst method

Food	Total NSP (g/100 g) Fresh weight	Dry weight	Soluble NSP (g/100 g) Dry weight	Cellulose	Rha	Fuc	Ara	Xyl	Man	Gal	Glc	UAc
Wheat bran	36.0	41.1	4.2	8.2	—	—	9.9	17.7	0.3	0.8	3.0	1.2
White bread	1.6	2.7	1.6	0.2	—	—	0.8	1.2	0.1	0.1	0.3	—
Rye bread	7.3	13.3	6.7	1.2	—	—	3.5	5.8	0.1	0.3	2.3	0.1
Oatmeal	6.6	7.4	4.1	0.4	—	—	0.9	1.3	0.1	0.2	4.2	0.3
Cornflakes	0.9	0.9	0.4	0.3	—	—	0.1	0.3	—	—	0.1	0.1
Potato	1.2	6.4	3.8	2.0	0.1	—	0.4	0.1	—	2.2	0.6	1.0
Beans, French	3.1	30.4	12.7	11.1	0.3	—	2.3	1.7	1.4	4.1	0.6	8.9
Carrots	2.4	19.5	11.4	6.4	0.7	—	2.0	0.3	0.4	3.4	0.1	6.2
Cabbage	2.9	24.4	11.8	8.0	0.7	—	4.6	1.0	0.5	2.7	0.1	6.8
Tomato	1.1	18.8	7.4	7.5	0.3	—	0.9	1.0	1.3	1.7	0.4	5.7
Apples	1.7	12.5	5.4	4.2	0.3	0.2	1.7	0.8	0.3	1.0	0.3	3.7
Oranges	2.1	15.0	9.8	3.4	0.3	—	2.2	0.6	0.4	1.8	0.1	6.2

Note: columns under "Composition of total NSP (g/100 g dry weight)" — Cellulose, then Non-cellulosic polysaccharides: Rha, Fuc, Ara, Xyl, Man, Gal, Glc, UAc.

Rha = Rhamnose   Fuc = Fucose   Ara = Arabinose
Xyl = Xylose   Man = Mannose   Gal = Galactose
Glc = Glucose   UAc = Uronic Acid

Cellulose is found in the insoluble NSP fraction but the non-cellulosic polysaccharides are present in both. Those foods with substantial uronic acid contents have these predominantly in the soluble fraction of NSP, but otherwise the monosaccharides may be found in either the soluble or insoluble polysaccharides. A dash (—) indicates only trace quantities of the monosaccharide.

thickener and stabilizer in ice cream, confectionery, beers, dairy products and other foods. Carrageenans gel strongly in the presence of Ca^{2+} or K^+ ions to give a brittle gel that is used in a large number of foods. They are sulphated galactose polymers derived from red algae.

Synthetic carbohydrates

Polydextrose is a synthetic carbohydrate that consists of randomly cross-linked glucose polymers of various sorts. It is made by thermal polymerization of glucose in the presence of citric acid and sorbitol. Two forms are available – an off-white amorphous powder and a light yellow aqueous solution, both of which are non-sweet and tasteless, but have similar functional properties to sucrose. Polydextrose is not digested in the small intestine but enters the colon, where approximately 30% is fermented by intestinal bacteria to volatile fatty acids and CO_2; the remainder is excreted in the faeces (Torres & Thomas 1981).

Neosugar is the name given to a mixture of short-chain fructo-oligosaccharides (3–5 residues) synthesized from sucrose by the action of fungal β-fructofuranosidase. It has similar characteristics to sucrose when used in cooking, but is only half as sweet and, like polydextrose, is not digested by endogenous human digestive enzymes. Neosugar is fermented to volatile fatty acids and CO_2 in the large bowel by selected bacterial strains, notably the *Bifidobacterium* spp., which increase in the faeces as a result. The energy available from neosugar through fermentation has been estimated as 1.5 kcal/g compared with 4 kcal/g from sucrose.

Dietary fibre intakes

Recent estimates suggest that the average daily intake of dietary fibre (measured as NSP) in Britain is 12 g, with little regional variation (Table 4.4). British men and women consume very similar amounts on average (Bingham et al 1985). However, there is considerable individual variation in NSP consumption, and some people have been shown to ingest up to 30 g/day on an omnivorous diet. Of the NSP in the typical British diet, approximately 48% is derived from vegetables, 10% from fruit and 38% from cereals (Bingham et al 1979).

Table 4.4 Probable intakes of NSP in different populations

Population	NSP intake (g/day)
United Kingdom (mean)	12.4
Scotland	11.9
N. England	12.4
Mid England	12.7
S. England	12.4
Wales	12.7
United States (mean)	14.6
Men	17.1
Women	12.1
Lacto-ovo vegetarian men	24.5
Lacto-ovo vegetarian women	17.1
Vegan men	44.7
Vegan women	20.9
Denmark	
Urban	13.2
Rural	18.0
Finland	
Urban	14.5
Rural	18.4
Japan	10.9
Africa	
Maize-eating area	12
Plantain-eating area	30
Millet-eating area (women)	18

Recent survey data from the USA suggest that the mean intake of NSP by the American population is slightly higher than that of the British, and that American men consume considerably more than American women. The sex difference is evident whether the population consists of omnivores, lacto-ovo vegetarians or vegans, and probably reflects a higher caloric intake by the men. Urban populations from other affluent countries, such as Denmark, Finland and Japan, have NSP intakes similar to those in Britain, although rural communities in these countries tend to consume more. Present-day intakes of dietary fibre in affluent countries are generally lower than they have been in the past, when there was a greater dependence on lightly processed carbohydrate foods.

Very few tropical or African foods have been analysed for NSP, and dietary fibre intakes in the developing world are uncertain. However, Table 4.4 gives estimates of possible NSP consumption, based on typical diets, of three African populations subsisting on different starchy staples. In areas where white rice is the staple cereal (China, India, South America), fibre intakes are thought to be similar to western intakes. However, in all these areas the amounts of starch escaping digestion may be substantial and of great importance for large-bowel physiology (see below).

DIGESTION AND ABSORPTION OF CARBOHYDRATES

The small intestine

The digestive process begins in the mouth, where chewing breaks up the structure of compact food and mixes it with saliva containing an amylase (ptyalin). The resulting bolus is swallowed. The digestion of starch begins in the bolus but this phase is relatively short, the amylase being inactivated by the gastric acid when the bolus is broken up in the stomach. Digestion occurs mainly in the small intestine through the action of amylase in the pancreatic juice. This hydrolyses the starch to short-chain dextrins and maltose. In the brush border of the intestinal epithelium there are glucosidases that further reduce the dextrin, and specific disaccharidases – maltase, sucrase and lactase – that convert maltose, sucrose and lactose into monosaccharides. The monosaccharides glucose, fructose and galactose are then transported across the epithelial cells and enter the portal vein. Free concentrations in the intestine or at the mucosal surface are likely to be high enough for passive or facilitated absorption, but as concentrations fall, active transport against a concentration gradient becomes necessary and so requires energy. The active transport system is similar to the one that absorbs glucose from the renal tubules, and involves the breakdown of ATP and the presence of Na^+. Different sugars compete for transport, and galactose and glucose are absorbed faster than fructose.

After a meal, the level of glucose in the blood rises to a maximum in about 30 min and then returns slowly to the fasting level after 90–180 min. The height of the maximum and the rate of return to normal vary with the nature of the meal, and give an indication of the rate at which starchy foods are digested in the small intestine. The glycaemic index (Jenkins et al 1981) is a physiological measurement which can be used to estimate the relative rates of glucose absorption from various foods. Subjects ingest a portion of the test food containing 50 g carbohydrate, and blood glucose levels in peripheral blood are measured every 30 min for 3 h. The area under the resultant glucose curve is compared with the area under the curve obtained when the same subject is given 50 g carbohydrate from a standard source – usually glucose or white bread. Using this technique, values, compared with an arbitrary value of 100 for white bread, range from less than 50 for legumes to over 110 for mashed potato. These values may be useful in planning diabetic diets, when the aim is to keep the level of blood glucose as low as possible. However, after a mixed meal of several foods many factors affect the rate of absorption of carbohydrate. The rate of passage through the stomach and upper small intestine is obviously important, and this depends on the amount of peristalsis and the viscosity of the bolus passing. It was believed at one time that mono- and disaccharides were absorbed much more easily than starch. However, this is not always the case. Glucose, dextrins and soluble starch are absorbed at equal rates (Wahlqvist et al 1978), indicating that luminal digestion of these soluble glucan polymers per se is not a limiting factor in glucose absorption.

The effects of food preparation on carbohydrate absorption

The gross physical form of the food, crystallinity of the starch granules and retrogradation after cooking have a major effect on the rate and extent of starch digestion in the small intestine. Thus the way food is processed and prepared in the factory and/or at home determines the proportion of dietary starch that enters the colon.

Starch contained within discrete structures such as whole grains and seeds is physically inaccessible to pancreatic amylase. Crushing, chopping and milling increase the accessibility of the starch, the rate of digestion being dependent on the final particle size (Crapo & Henry 1988, Heaton et al 1988). In foods such as pasta, starch hydrolysis is retarded by the density of the product (Hermansen et al 1986), which decreases enzyme access. Physical inaccessibility may

cause the rate of starch hydrolysis to be so slow that particles of undigested food enter the large intestine. In extreme cases, starch contained within discrete structures may be excreted in the faeces.

Cooking facilitates the hydrolysis of starch through the gelatinization of starch granules and the dispersion of the starch chains. However, foods eaten raw retain their starch within granules, which show varying degrees of resistance to digestion. Raw starch from cereals is digested slowly within the small intestine, giving a smaller glycaemic response. Raw starch from bananas shows a greater degree of resistance, up to 90% passing undigested through the small intestine (Englyst & Cummings 1986).

Retrogradation also retards digestion, and retrograded starch (mainly amylose) from processed cereal and potato products has been shown to pass through the small intestine (Englyst & Cummings 1985).

Table 4.5 shows the digestibility in vitro of starch from a selection of starchy foods. Values for the first four foods illustrate how different processing methods may affect the digestibility of starch from a single source. Raw white wheat flour, which consists mainly of ungelatinized starch granules with an 'A' type crystalline structure, is digested relatively slowly, 59% of the starch measuring as slowly digestible starch (SDS). Baking the flour into shortbread, which involves cooking in the presence of very little water, results in limited disruption of the granular structure and gives a product that is also digested slowly. On the other hand, baking the flour into bread, a process that requires a long cooking time in the presence of a moderate amount of water, leads to extensive gelatinization of the starch granules and results in a rapidly digestible product. A small amount of retrograded amylose (RS_3) is produced during baking. Wheat flour made into spaghetti is digested more slowly than bread, despite

Table 4.5   In vitro digestibility of starch in a variety of foods. The values are expressed as a percentage of the total starch present in the food.

	% RDS	% SDS	% RS$_1$	% RS$_2$	% RS$_3$
White flour	49	48	—	3	t
Shortbread	56	43	—	—	1
White bread	94	4	—	—	2
White spaghetti	52	43	3	—	3
Banana biscuits	39	23	—	38	t
Potato biscuits	47	27	—	25	1
Haricot beans	18	42	18	9	12
Pearl barley	41	41	9	—	2

RDS = rapidly digestible starch; SDS = slowly digestible starch;
RS = resistant starch; t = trace

being cooked by moist heat. This is because the dense structure of the pasta impedes its enzymic hydrolysis, as demonstrated by the 2% of starch measuring as RS_1 (physically inaccessible). Other examples of foods in which some of the starch may be physically inaccessible are haricot beans and pearl barley.

Only a small amount of raw wheat flour measures as RS_2, resistant starch granules. However, flours produced commercially from banana and potato contain starch granules which are highly resistant to digestion. Table 4.5 contains values of RS_2 in biscuits made with a 1:1 mixture of wheat flour and either banana or potato flour. Because no water is used in the formulation, the starch granules retain their crystalline structure, leading to a product in which over a third of the starch resists digestion.

The starch fractions described here are determined solely by properties inherent in the food sample (see above and Table 4.1). They therefore represent reproducible measurements by which starchy foods can be compared. However, the digestibility of starch within the small intestine depends not only on starch crystallinity and the physical form of the starchy food itself, but on a number of highly variable factors: the extent of chewing, the transit time of the food along the small intestine, the concentration of amylase available for breakdown of the starch, the amount of starch, and the presence of other food components that might retard enzymic hydrolysis. It is not possible therefore to predict accurately the digestion of starchy foods in an individual.

Undigested carbohydrate entry into the large intestine

A number of potentially fermentable substrates enter the caecum. The principal ones are NSP and starch, but a substantial amount of protein also escapes digestion in the small intestine (Table 4.6). Studies using ileostomy subjects (i.e. people who have had their large intestines removed for medical reasons) have shown that dietary NSPs are virtually completely recovered in the ileostomy effluent. Even so, for many foods more starch than NSP reaches the colon. The amount of starch escaping digestion and available for fermentation ranges from 2% for oats to 89% for bananas (Cummings & Englyst 1987).

Endogenous carbohydrates from mucin and glycoproteins that line the gut contribute a further 3–5 g of fermentable substrate per day, with normal intestine epithelial turnover in adults on a western diet. Other potential substrates for colonic fermentation include fructose, sorbitol and other poorly absorbed mono-

mers, lactose in lactase-deficient individuals, raffinose, stachyose, verbascose and fructans including inulin, and synthetic carbohydrates such as polydextrose, palatinit and neosugar. Together these provide about 5 g carbohydrate per day in a UK diet, and are of marginal significance except in some disease states.

Colonic fermentation

Once in the large intestine, carbohydrates are metabolized by the colonic microflora, which ferment them to short chain fatty acids (SCFA) with the evolution of gases (Fig. 4.4). The extent of fermentation depends on the form and solubility of the substrate. Soluble carbohydrates such as pectin are degraded almost completely, whereas the insoluble polymers in lignified material such as wheat bran are attacked to a much smaller extent.

Colonic fermentation is a complex biochemical process. Initially, large polymers are broken down into their constituent monomers, mainly glucose, galactose, arabinose, xylose and uronic acids. The sugars then enter the glycolytic pathway and are converted to pyruvate, but from there various routes may be followed depending on the microbial species present and the nature of the available substrate. The principal SCFAs produced from all substrates are acetate, propionate and butyrate, but other organic acids such as isobutyrate, valerate, isovalerate, lactate and succinate occur in small amounts. These organic acids are the major anions in the large intestine and contribute to the relatively low pH found there (5.6–6.6).

Estimates based on samples of colonic contents taken from sudden-death victims place the caecal

Table 4.6 The principal substrates available for fermentation in the human colon. The amounts estimated are based on subjects consuming a western diet (from Macfarlane & Cummings 1990)

Substrate	Amount (g/day)
Carbohydrates	
Resistant starch	8–40
Non–starch polysaccharides	8–18
Unabsorbed sugars, sugar alcohols	2–10
Oligosaccharides	2–6
Chitin and amino sugars	1–2
Nitrogenous substrates	
Dietary protein	3–9
Pancreatic enzymes and secretions	4–6
Urea and nitrate	0.5
Other substrates	
Mucin	2–3

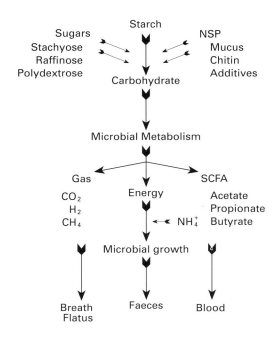

Fig. 4.4 Fermentation in the human colon (adapted from Cummings 1983)

effects – an antitumour action has been demonstrated in vitro (Kim et al 1982). Most SCFAs are cleared by the liver, with only acetate released (Pomare et al 1985) to be used as a fuel by peripheral tissues (Skutches et al 1979). Propionate is utilized within the liver, where it may modify carbohydrate and lipid metabolism.

The main gases produced during fermentation are hydrogen and carbon dioxide. Some individuals have the capacity to produce methane (CH_4) from CO_2 and H_2, thus diminishing the total volume of gas accumulating in the colon because 1 volume of CH_4 is produced from 4 volumes of H_2. In others, sulphate-reducing bacteria incorporate hydrogen into hydrogen sulphide, particularly after a high intake of dietary sulphate (Christl et al 1992).

The volume of gas resulting from carbohydrate fermentation is considerably less than would be predicted from proposed stoichiometry because of the secondary utilization of H_2 by methane, sulphate and nitrate-reducing bacteria. Using the equation of Miller & Wolin (1979) for non-methanogenic subjects

$$24.5\ C_6H_{12}O_6 \rightarrow 18\ \text{acetate} + 58\ CO_2 + 95\ H_2 + 10.5\ H_2O + 11\ \text{propionate} + 5\ \text{butyrate}$$

the fermentation of 70 g of carbohydrate would yield 24 l of H_2/day! However, flatus volume is usually about 1 l/day.

SCFA concentration in the region of 135mmol/kg. This declines as the contents progress along the colon (Fig. 4.5), SCFAs are absorbed and the availability of fermentable substrate decreases. The excretion of SCFAs in faeces is very low (10–20 mmol/day).

The efficiency of SCFA production and the molar ratios of acetate, propionate and butyrate generated from carbohydrate differ according to the substrate being utilized (Table 4.7). For example, the fermentation of starch produces SCFA with a large proportion (29%) of butyrate. In contrast, only 2% of the SCFA generated from the fermentation of pectin is in the form of butyrate. Thus the amount and type of SCFA produced in the human colon is partly dependent on the amount and type of carbohydrate entering the colon from the diet.

Acetate and propionate are rapidly absorbed from the colon and carried in the portal vein to the liver. However, butyrate is the preferred fuel for human colonocytes, particularly in the distal colon, and it is actively metabolized to ketone bodies (acetoacetate and β-hydroxybutyrate), carbon dioxide and water. The use of butyrate rather than glucose or glutamine by the colonic epithelium is thought to have beneficial

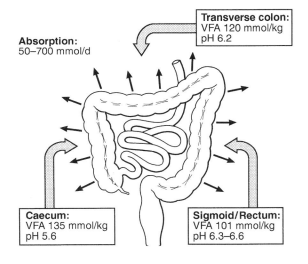

Fig. 4.5 Concentrations of volatile fatty acids in different parts of the colon

Table 4.7 Short-chain fatty acids (SCFA) produced in vitro by intestinal bacteria grown on different polysaccharide substrates. Molar ratios are given in parentheses (from Englyst et al 1987a)

| | SCFA produced(mg/mg polysaccharide) | | | |
Polysaccharide	Acetate	Propionate	Butyrate	Total
Starch	0.25 (50)	0.13 (22)	0.21 (29)	0.59
Arabinogalactan	0.19 (50)	0.20 (42)	0.04 (8)	0.43
Xylan	0.42 (82)	0.10 (15)	0.02 (3)	0.54
Pectin	0.27 (84)	0.06 (14)	0.01 (2)	0.34

The excretion of gases per rectum occurs when the production of gas exceeds the absorptive capacity of the colon, but at low levels the gases are largely absorbed and excreted through the lungs. Measurement of the hydrogen expired in breath has been used as a marker for carbohydrate fermentation (Anderson et al 1981) and may be useful in a clinical setting to detect pancreatic insufficiency. However, this technique cannot be used for reproducible assessment of the quantity of carbohydrate entering the colon (Cummings & Englyst 1991).

The energy which, through fermentation of carbohydrates to SCFA, becomes available for the tissues, represents 60–70% of the energy potentially available had the carbohydrate been hydrolysed and absorbed from the small intestine (Blaxter 1962). With such a high proportion of the energy becoming available, the old term 'unavailable carbohydrates' for those not digested in the small intestine could be misleading.

Physiological effects of carbohydrates not digested in the small intestine

Of the many carbohydrates that may escape small-intestinal digestion, the principal ones are NSP (dietary fibre) and starch. Dietary fibre has been the subject of research for several decades; however, the concept of resistant starch is relatively new and, although many assumptions have been made, the consequences of starch reaching the colon have not yet been investigated to any extent. Understanding of the physiological effects of carbohydrates that are not digested is therefore largely limited to what is known about dietary fibre from epidemiology, animal model studies and clinical investigations. For this reason this section will deal mostly with the physiological effects of dietary fibre.

Dietary fibre and disease

In the late 1940s, Dr Dennis Burkitt and Dr Hugh Trowell, surgeons working in Africa, began to notice that the pattern of diseases found in black Africans differed markedly from that seen in African or European whites. In particular they rarely encountered the diseases known as the 'diseases of civilization', a group of 17 that included constipation, appendicitis, diverticular disease, haemorrhoids, colorectal cancer, coronary heart disease and gallstones. Trowell (1960), observing that all the relatively common non-infective diseases of the large bowel were rare in sub-Saharan blacks, speculated that the protective factor might be the soft and bulky nature of their stools, which were passed easily and frequently, and which were a consequence of their high-fibre diet. Subsequently, it has been shown that lack of dietary fibre is a major factor which could be involved in several gastrointestinal diseases. A highly refined diet results in hard, dry stools that pass sluggishly through the large intestine and require a large increase in luminal pressure for their evacuation. Although such a diet, often rich in refined carbohydrates and fats, is also associated with the development of diabetes, coronary heart disease and obesity in affluent societies, it is not generally accepted that fibre deficiency is the cause of these conditions. A diet rich in dietary fibre tends to increase faecal weight, decrease intestinal transit time and may improve control of glucose and lipid metabolism. However, both the quantity and the type of dietary fibre are important in determining the effect. The division of dietary fibre into soluble and insoluble fractions and the characterization of these by GLC has been helpful in discerning the reasons for the physiological effects of fibres from different sources (see Table 4.3).

Faecal weight

People consuming a typical UK diet excrete an average of 106 g of stool per day (Cummings et al 1992) although there is wide individual variation in the weight of stool passed and the frequency of bowel movement. Dietary fibre is the only food fraction that has been shown to have a universal effect on stool weight, but recent studies suggest that starch also may be an influential factor. Increasing the dietary fibre intake of a person who is accustomed to a low-fibre diet has been shown to increase faecal weight (Table 4.8). However, there is a poor correlation between faecal weight and total dietary fibre intake per se, because the effect is highly dependent on the type of fibre given.

Table 4.9 shows the composition of faecal matter from subjects consuming a typical western diet, or the same diet supplemented with 18 g of a largely insoluble fibre (wheat bran) or a similar amount of a highly soluble fibre (cabbage fibre). On a normal diet, faeces comprise approximately 70% moisture and 30% dry matter, of which over half is derived from bacteria, a quarter is water-soluble solids and the remainder is residual fibre. Wheat bran is highly effective at increasing mean daily stool weight, principally because it is poorly degraded in the gut. The surviving fibre holds water, thus increasing the bulk of the colonic contents and encouraging faster transit. Table 4.9 shows that supplementing a western diet with bran results in faeces that are wetter and that contain more fibre, water-soluble solids and bacteria than those resulting from a normal diet.

Cabbage fibre increases mean daily stool weight and hydration to a lesser extent than wheat bran. Soluble fibre is highly fermentable by colonic bacteria and it has been estimated that, in contrast to bran, only 8% of cabbage fibre escapes degradation in the gut and contributes to stool weight. The principal change in stool composition seen with cabbage fibre is that of increased bacterial solids and water, indicating that the increase in stool weight is the result of bacterial growth, stimulated by the presence of a fermentable substrate.

Thus, two factors are involved in the faecal bulking effect of dietary fibre. Soluble fibre is readily fermented and leads to increased faecal weight through proliferation of the bacterial population. Insoluble fibre, especially if lignified like wheat bran, partially survives the fermentation process and acts directly as a bulking and water-holding agent. In general, it is the more insoluble cereal fibres that increase faecal weight the most, and that have an important laxative action.

Stool weight is closely associated with transit time. Faecal weights below 150 g/day are associated with increasing transit time, and constipation commonly occurs if the faecal output falls below 100 g/day. Epidemiological studies show that low stool weights and extended transit times are connected with increased risk from diverticular disease and bowel cancer. It has been suggested that bowel disease in the UK could be reduced if the mean faecal output could be raised to 132 g/day – a change that would require a mean NSP intake of 17.9 g/day (Cummings et al 1992).

Intestinal transit time

The intestinal transit time is the time taken for a meal to pass from the mouth to the anus. It may be measured by administering a marker by mouth and measuring the time taken for this to appear in the faeces. The marker may be a dye such as carmine red, or a capsule of tiny radio-opaque plastic shapes that may be detected in the faecal matter by X-rays. It is convenient to divide whole-gut transit time into two phases – mouth-to-caecum transit, and colonic transit. Colonic transit takes approximately ten times as long as mouth-to-caecum transit, and is the major phase affecting the whole-gut transit time.

Table 4.8   Effect of added dietary fibre on faecal weight

Fibre content of diet (g)		Source of added fibre	No. of subjects	Mean faecal weight (g/day)		Reference
Low	High			Low fibre	High fibre	
12	45	Fruit, vegetables, wholemeal cereals	46	69	185	Stass-Wolthuis et al 1979
4.1*	7.2*	+16 g of bran	8	107	174	Eastwood et al 1973
22	60	+bran	6	95	197	Cummings et al 1978
22	61	+cabbage extract	5	88	143	Cummings et al 1978
22	67	+carrot extract	6	117	189	Cummings et al 1978
22	88	+apple extract	5	141	203	Cummings et al 1978

*Crude fibre

Table 4.9 Composition of faeces from subjects consuming a normal western diet or the same diet supplemented with 18 g fibre (measured as neutral detergent fibre) from wheat bran or cabbage (from Stephen and Cummings 1980)

	Normal diet	Bran diet	Cabbage diet
Mean stool weight (g/day)	95.5	197.0	142.5
Moisture (%)	71.1	76.3	74.6
Total solids (g/day) of which:	27.0	46.0	34.6
NDF	4.6	16.2	5.7
water-soluble	6.5	9.2	8.7
bacteria	15.0	17.3	19.3

Mouth-to-caecum transit is affected by gastric emptying and small-intestinal transit, both of which may be altered by the consumption of viscous polysaccharides such as guar gum, gum tragacanth and oat bran. The viscosity of such fibres leads to prolonged gastric emptying, resulting in greater satiety and a delay in the delivery of nutrients to the small intestine (Holt et al 1979). Viscous dietary fibres also delay the absorption of low-molecular-weight nutrients such as sugars within the small intestine, particularly in the distal regions where the viscosity is increased by the absorption of water from the gut contents.

Colonic transit is influenced less by the viscosity of polysaccharides, which is rapidly reduced as fermentation proceeds. Insoluble fibres such as bran decrease colonic transit time and result in larger, softer stools. The mechanism of action of dietary fibre on colonic transit is unclear; it is not certain whether the increase in faecal bulk stimulates colonic peristalsis or whether dietary fibre has a direct effect on colonic motor activity. It is probable that a number of different factors, including the retention of fluid in the fibre matrix, the presence of poorly absorbed SCFA such as lactic acid, a low pH which inhibits salt and water absorption, an increase in bacterial cell mass and distension due to gas production, all contribute to the decrease in intestinal transit time.

Cholesterol metabolism

Crude epidemiological data suggest that the consumption of dietary fibre is inversely related to the incidence of diseases, such as coronary heart disease and gallstones, that are connected with steroid metabolism, particularly the level of cholesterol in the serum. Physiological studies also show that the addition of certain plant fibres to the diet is accompanied by significant reductions in serum cholesterol concentrations. Soluble NSP fractions (pectins, gums, etc) are the most effective; insoluble NSP fractions have very little influence on total serum cholesterol levels. The reduction in cholesterol is seen mostly in the low-density lipoprotein fraction, and is accompanied by decreases in the cholesterol content of the liver, aorta and other tissues.

The effect has been explained in terms of bile acid metabolism. Bile acids and neutral steroids are synthesized from cholesterol in the liver, secreted in the bile and normally returned to the liver via reabsorption in the small intestine (the enterohepatic cycle). Dietary fibre is supposed to interrupt this cycle by absorbing bile acids, thus preventing their reabsorption and necessitating their replacement from the cholesterol pool. In this way the serum and the bile are thought to be depleted of cholesterol.

In vitro, several NSP fractions from fruit and vegetables have been reported to bind bile acids, and in vivo, several fibre fractions have been shown to increase the daily faecal output of bile acids. However, some fibres, such as bran, which absorb bile acids do not affect serum cholesterol levels (Kay and Truswell 1977), whereas others such as beans lower serum cholesterol levels without increasing bile acid excretion (Anderson et al 1984). It is clear therefore that bile acid binding is not the sole factor involved. Chen & Anderson (1984) have suggested that hepatic cholesterol synthesis may be altered by SCFAs derived from the colonic fermentation of soluble fibres. Propionate has been shown to inhibit hydroxymethyl-glutaryl CoA reductase, the rate-limiting enzyme of cholesterol synthesis, and this may result in lower serum cholesterol levels. The overall effect of NSP on lipoprotein levels is considered in more detail in Chapter 41.

REFERENCES

Anderson IH, Levine A S, Levitt MD 1981 Incomplete absorption of the carbohydrate in all-purpose wheat flour. New England Journal of Medicine 304: 891–992

Anderson JW, Story L, Sieling B, Chen WJL, Petro M S, Story J 1984 Hypocholesterolaemic effects of oat bran or bean intake for hypercholesterolaemic men. American Journal of Clinical Nutrition 40: 1146–1155

Bingham S, Cummings JH, McNeil N I 1979 Intakes and sources of dietary fiber in the British population. American Journal of Clinical Nutrition 32: 1313–1319

Bingham SA, Williams DRR, Cummings JH 1985 Dietary fibre consumption in Britain: new estimates and their relation to large bowel cancer mortality. British Journal of Cancer 52: 399–402

Blaxter KL 1962 The energy metabolism of ruminants. Hutchinson, London

Chen WL, Anderson JW 1984 Propionate may mediate the hypocholesterolaemic effect of plant fibers in cholesterol-fed rats. Proceedings of the Society for Experimental Biology and Medicine 175: 215–218

Christl SU, Gibson GR, Cummings JH 1992 The role of dietary sulphate in the regulation of methanogenesis in the human large intestine. Gut (in press)

Crapo P.A, Henry R R 1988 Postprandial metabolic responses to the influence of food form. American Journal of Clinical Nutrition 48: 560–564

Cummings JH 1983 Fermentation in the human large intestine: evidence and implications for health. Lancet i: 1206–1209

Cummings JH, Bingham SA, Heaton KW, Eastwood MA 1992 Fecal weight, colon cancer risk and dietary intake of non-starch polysaccharides (dietary fibre). Gastroenterology 103: 1783–1789

Cummings JH, Englyst HN 1987 Fermentation in the human large intestine and the available substrates. American Journal of Clinical Nutrition 45: 1243–1255

Cummings JH, Englyst HN 1991 Measurement of starch fermentation in the human large intestine. Canadian Journal of Physiology and Pharmacology 69: 121–129

Cummings JH, Southgate DAT, Branch WJ, Houston H, Jenkins DJA, James WPT 1978 The colonic response to dietary fibre from carrot, cabbage, apple, bran and guar gum. Lancet i: 5–9

Cummings JH, Englyst HN, Wood R 1985 Determination of dietary fibre in cereals and cereal products – collaborative trials. Part 1: Initial trial. Journal of the Association of Official Analytical Chemists 23: 1–35

Eastwood MA, Kirkpatrick JR, Mitchell WD, Bone A, Hamilton T 1973 Effects of dietary supplements of wheat bran and cellulose on faeces and bowel function. British Medical Journal 4: 392–394

Englyst HN, Cummings JH 1985 Digestion of the polysaccharides of some cereal foods in the human small intestine. American Journal of Clinical Nutrition 42: 778–787

Englyst HN, Cummings JH 1986 Digestion of the carbohydrates of banana (*Musa paradisiaca sapientum*) in the human small intestine. American Journal of Clinical Nutrition 44: 42–50

Englyst HN, Cummings JH 1988 Improved method for measurement of dietary fiber as non-starch polysaccharides in plant foods. Journal of the Association of Official Analytical Chemists 71: 808–814

Englyst HN, Hudson GJ 1992 Dietary fiber and starch: classification and measurement. In: Spiller GA (ed) Dietary fiber in human nutrition. CRC Press, Boca Raton

Englyst HN, Kingman SM 1990 Dietary fiber and resistant starch. A nutritional classification of plant polysaccharides. In: Kritchevsky D, Bonfield C, Anderson JW (eds) Dietary fiber. Plenum, New York.

Englyst HN, Hay S, Macfarlane GT 1987a Polysaccharide breakdown by mixed populations of human faecal bacteria. FEMS Microbiology Ecology 95: 163–171

Englyst HN, Trowell HW, Southgate DAT, Cummings JH 1987b Dietary fiber and resistant starch. American Journal of Clinical Nutrition 46: 873–874

Englyst HN, Bingham SA, Runswick SA, Collinson E, Cummings JH 1988 Dietary fibre (non-starch polysaccharides) in fruit, vegetables and nuts. Journal of Human Nutrition and Dietetics 1: 247–286

Englyst HN, Bingham SA, Runswick SA, Collinson E, Cummings JH 1989 Dietary fibre (non-starch polysaccharides) in cereal products. Journal of Human Nutrition and Dietetics 2: 257–276

Englyst HN, Quigley ME, Hudson GJ, Cummings JH 1992 Determination of dietary fibre as non-starch polysaccharides by gas–liquid chromatography. Analyst 117: 1707–1714.

Heaton KW, Marcus SN, Emmett PM, Bilton CH 1988 Particle size of wheat, maize and oat test meals: effects on plasma glucose and insulin responses and on the rate of starch digestion in vitro. American Journal of Clinical Nutrition 47: 675–682

Hermansen K, Rasmussen O, Arnfred J, Winther E, Schnitz O 1986 Differential glycaemic effects of potato, rice and spaghetti in Type 1 (insulin-dependent) diabetic patients at constant insulinaemia. Diabetalogia 29: 358–361

Hipsley EH 1953 Dietary 'fibre' and pregnancy toxaemia. British Medical Journal 2: 420–422

Holt S, Heading RC, Carter DC, Prescott LF, Hothill P 1979 Effect of gel fibre on gastric emptying and absorption of glucose and paracetamol. Lancet ii: 636–639

James WPT, Theander O (eds) 1981 The analysis of dietary fiber in food. Marcel Dekker, New York, pp. 258–259

Jenkins DJA, Thomas DM, Wolever TMS, Taylor RH et al 1981 Glycaemic index of foods: a physiological basis for carbohydrate exchanges. American Journal of Clinical Nutrition 34: 362–366

Katz JR 1934 X-ray investigation of gelatinization and retrogradation of starch and its importance for bread research. Bakers Weekly 81: 34–37

Kay RM, Truswell A S 1977 The effect of wheat fibre on plasma lipid and faecal steroid excretion in man. British Journal of Nutrition 37: 227–235

Kim YS, Tsao D, Morita A, Bella A 1982 Effect of sodium butyrate on three human colorectal adenocarcinoma cell lines in culture. In: Malt RA, Williamson RCN (eds) Colonic carcinogenesis. Falk Symposium 31. MTP Press, Lancaster, pp. 317–323

Macfarlane GT, Cummings JH 1990 The colonic flora, fermentation and large bowel digestive function. In: Philips SE, Pemberton JH, Shorter TG (eds) The large intestine: physiology, pathophysiology and diseases. Raven Press, New York

Miller TL, Wolin M J 1979 Fermentations by saccharolytic intestinal bacteria. American Journal of Clinical Nutrition 32: 164–172

Mongeau R, Brassard R 1990 A comparison of three methods for analysing dietary fiber in 38 foods. Journal of Food Composition and Analysis 2:189–199

Paul AA, Southgate DAT 1978 The composition of foods, 4th edn. HMSO, London

Pomare EW, Branch WJ, Cummings JH 1985 Carbohydrate fermentation in the human colon and its relation to acetate concentration in venous blood. Journal of Clinical Investigation 75: 1448–1454

Prosky L, Asp N-G, Furda I, DeVries JW, Schweizer TF, Harland BF 1985 Determination of total dietary fibre in foods and food products: collaborative study. Journal of the Association of Official Analytical Chemists 68: 677–679

Prosky L, Asp N-G, Schweizer TF, DeVries JW, Furda I 1988 Determination of insoluble, soluble, and total dietary fiber in foods and food products: interlaboratory study. Journal of the Association of Official Analytical Chemists 71: 1071–1023

Quigley ME, Englyst HN 1992 Determination of neutral sugars and hexosamines by high-performance liquid chromatography with pulsed amperometric detection. Analyst 117: 1715–1718

Skutches GL, Holroyde CP, Myers RN, Paul P, Reichard G A 1979 Plasma acetate turnover and oxidation. Journal of Clinical Investigation 64: 708–713

Southgate DAT 1969 Determination of carbohydrates in foods. II. Unavailable carbohydrates. Journal of the Science of Food and Agriculture 20: 331–335

Stass-Wolthuis M, Hautvast JGAJ, Hermus RJ et al 1979 The effect of a natural high-fiber diet on serum lipids, fecal lipids and colonic function. American Journal of Clinical Nutrition 32: 1881–1888

Stephen AM, Cummings J H 1980 Mechanism of action of dietary fibre in the human colon. Nature 284: 283–284

Torres A, Thomas RD 1981 Polydextrose and its application in foods. Food Technology July: 44–49

Trowell H 1960 Non-infective disease in Africa. Edward Arnold, London, pp. 217–222

Trowell H 1972 Ischaemic heart disease and dietary fiber. American Journal of Clinical Nutrition 25: 926–932

Van Soest P 1978 Fiber analysis tables. American Journal of Clinical Nutrition 31: S281–S284

Wahlqvist ML, Wilmshurst EG, Murton CR, Richardson EN 1978 The effect of chain length on glucose absorption and the related metabolic response. American Journal of Clinical Nutrition 31: 1998–2001

5. Proteins

P. J. Garlick and P. J. Reeds

Protein generally comprises about 10–15% of dietary energy, but its significance is more than simply as a source of energy. It is the major functional and structural component of all the cells of the body, and it is ubiquitous throughout life forms. All the enzymes, membrane carriers, blood transport molecules, intracellular matrix, hair, fingernails, etc. are proteins, as are many hormones and a large proportion of membranes. Moreover, their constituent amino acids act as precursors of many coenzymes, hormones, nucleic acids and other molecules essential for life. Thus an adequate supply of dietary protein is essential to maintain cellular integrity and function, and for health and reproduction.

Protein molecules in both the diet and the body are even more complex and variable than carbohydrates and fats, and contain a greater variety of elements. The characteristic element of protein is nitrogen, which constitutes about 16% of its weight, so that nitrogen metabolism is often considered to be synonymous with protein metabolism. Carbon, oxygen and hydrogen are also abundant elements, and there are smaller proportions of sulphur and phosphorus.

This chapter briefly describes the most relevant aspects of protein metabolism in healthy and diseased states. Additional material will be found in the references given under specific topics, and in the series of books entitled *Mammalian Protein Metabolism*, which although dated, still represent the best comprehensive account of the subject and its relation to nutrition (Munro & Allison 1964a,b, Munro 1969, 1970).

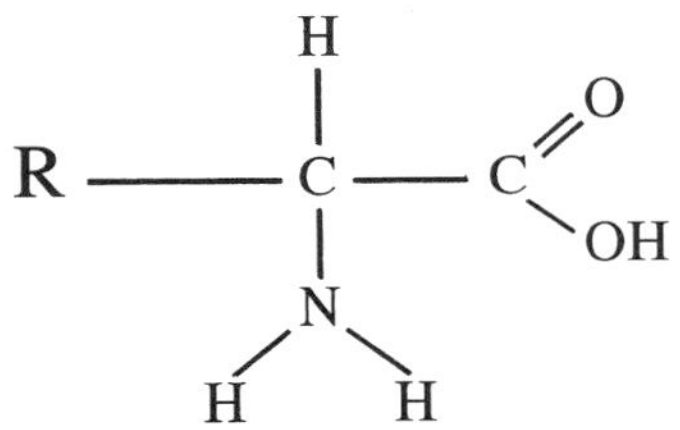

CHEMISTRY OF PROTEINS AND AMINO ACIDS

Proteins

Proteins are macromolecules consisting of long chains of amino acid subunits. The general formula for an amino acid is shown in Fig. 5.1, and the properties of the 20 or so different amino acids found in protein are discussed in the next section. In the protein molecule, the amino acids are joined together by 'peptide' bonds, which result from the elimination of water between the carboxyl group of one amino acid and the amino group of the next in line. In biological systems the chains so formed might be anything from two amino acid units (dipeptide) to thousands of units long, corresponding to molecular weights ranging from hundreds to hundreds of thousands of Daltons. Fig. 5.2 is an example showing the amino acid sequence of a small polypeptide chain, the hormone insulin. Many hormones are even smaller than this, some having fewer than ten amino acids.

The polypeptide chains do not exist as long straight chains, nor do they curl up into random shapes, but instead fold into a definite three-dimensional structure. Some proteins might be globular in shape and some might be rigid rods. Their exact shape depends on their function and their interaction with other molecules. Many proteins are composed of several separate peptide chains held together by ionic or covalent links. An example is haemoglobin of the erythrocyte, each active unit of

Fig. 5.1 The general formula of an amino acid. R represents the side chain, which determines the specific characteristics of each individual amino acid.

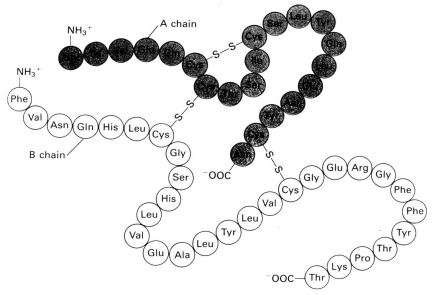

Fig. 5.2   The primary structure of the human insulin molecule. (Reproduced with permission from Darnell et al 1986)

which consists of two pairs of dissimilar subunits (the α and β chains). Many enzymes alter their shape in response to the presence of either their substrates or of other small molecules which modify their activity.

As will be seen below, the most important aspect of proteins from a nutritional point of view is their amino acid composition, but the protein's structure might also influence its nutritional availability. Some proteins, such as hair, are highly insoluble and are resistant to digestion: others are resistant to attack by the hydrolytic enzymes of the intestine (e.g. the mucins secreted by the intestine).

Amino acids

The structures of the twenty or so amino acids found in protein are shown in Table 5.1. The difference between them lies in the structure of the side chain (designated R in Fig. 5.1). As well as differences in size, these side groups carry different charges at physiological pH (e.g. ⊕ for diamino acids and ⊖ for dicarboxylic amino acids); some groups are hydrophobic (branched chain and aromatic amino acids) and some hydrophilic (most others).

These side chains have an important bearing on the ways in which the higher orders of protein structure are stabilized, and are intimate parts of many other aspects of protein function. Attractions between posi-

tive and negative charges pull different parts of the molecule together. Hydrophobic groups tend to cluster together in the centre of globular proteins, while hydrophilic groups remain in contact with water on the periphery. The ease with which the thiol groups in cysteine form sulphur–sulphur bonds is an important factor in the stabilization of folded structures within a polypeptide, and is a crucial element in the formation of interpolypeptide bonds (e.g. insulin, Fig. 5.2). The hydroxyl and amide groups of amino acids provide the sites for the attachment of the complex oligosaccharide side chains that are a feature of many mammalian proteins. Histidine and the dicarboxylic acids are critical features in ion-binding proteins, such as the calcium-binding proteins (e.g. troponin C), critical for muscular contraction, and the iron-binding proteins responsible for oxygen transport.

Some amino acids in protein only achieve their final structure after their precursors have been incorporated into the polypeptide. Notable examples of such post-translational modifications are the hydroxyproline and hydroxylysine residues found in the collagens, and the methylated histidines and lysines found in actin and myosin (not shown in Table 5.1). The former amino acids are critical parts of the cross-linking of collagen chains that lead to rigid and stable structures. The role of the methylated amino acids in contractile protein function is unknown.

Table 5.1   L-amino acids of nutritional significance

Name	Abbreviation	Formula
Aliphatic side chains		
Glycine	Gly	H—CH—COOH / NH$_2$
Alanine	Ala	CH$_3$—CH—COOH / NH$_2$
Valine★	Val	(CH$_3$)$_2$CH—CH—COOH / NH$_2$
Leucine★	Leu	(CH$_3$)$_2$CH—CH$_2$—CH—COOH / NH$_2$
Isoleucine★	Ile	CH$_3$—CH$_2$(CH$_3$)CH—CH—COOH / NH$_2$
Aromatic side chains		
Phenylalanine	Phe	C$_6$H$_5$—CH$_2$—CH—COOH / NH$_2$
Tyrosine	Tyr	HO—C$_6$H$_4$—CH$_2$—CH—COOH / NH$_2$
Tryptophan	Trp	indole—CH$_2$—CH—COOH / NH$_2$
Hydroxyl groups in side chains		
Serine	Ser	CH$_2$—CH—COOH / OH NH$_2$
Threonine	Thr	CH$_3$—CH—CH—COOH / OH NH$_2$
Sulphur-containing side chains		
Cysteine★★	Cys	HS—CH$_2$—CH—COOH / NH$_2$
Methionine	Met	CH$_3$—S—CH$_2$—CH$_2$—CH—COOH / NH$_2$
Imino acids		
Proline†	Pro	CH$_2$—CH$_2$ / CH$_2$—N(H)—CH—COOH
Acidic side chains and their amides		
Glutamic acid	Glu	HOOC—CH$_2$—CH$_2$—CH—COOH / NH$_2$
Glutamine	Gln	H$_2$N—CO—CH$_2$—CH$_2$—CH—COOH / NH$_2$
Aspartic acid	Asp	HOOC—CH$_2$—CH—COOH / NH$_2$
Asparagine	Asn	H$_2$N—CO—CH$_2$—CH—COOH / NH$_2$

Table 5.1   (*Cont'd*)

Name	Abbreviation	Formula
Basic side chains		
Lysine	Lys	$H_2N-CH_2-CH_2-CH_2-CH_2-CH-COOH$, NH_2
Arginine	Arg	$H_2N-C(=NH)-NH-CH_2-CH_2-CH_2-CH-COOH$, NH_2
Histidine	His	imidazole ring $-CH_2-CH-COOH$, NH_2
Ornithine††	Orn	$H_2N-CH_2-CH_2-CH_2-CH-COOH$, NH_2

Amino acids in italics are classed as nutritionally essential for humans
* Leucine, valine and isoleucine are known as the branched-chain amino acids
** Cysteine is often found as a dimer (cystine), linked through the sulphur atoms (–S–S–) by oxidation
† Proline is strictly speaking an imino acid rather than an amino acid
†† Ornithine is not found in protein but is an important intermediate in urea synthesis

In Table 5.1, eight of the amino acids are marked as 'nutritionally essential'. The carbon skeletons of these amino acids cannot be synthesized from simpler molecules in animals, and therefore must be provided in the diet. Their significance will be discussed further later in the chapter.

PROTEIN DIGESTION AND ABSORPTION

The processes by which ingested proteins are degraded in the intestine and absorbed as free amino acids into the circulation are dealt with in many other texts (e.g. Alpers 1987, Hopfer 1987) and brief details only will be given here.

After ingestion, proteins are denatured by the acid in the stomach and then pass into the small intestine, where the peptide bonds are hydrolysed by a variety of proteolytic enzymes. These bond-specific enzymes originate in the pancreas and include trypsin, chymotrypsin, elastin and carboxypeptidase. The resultant mixture of free amino acids and small peptides is then transported into the gut cells by a series of carrier systems, each specific for a limited range of substrates. After hydrolysis of the peptides, the free amino acids are then secreted into the bloodstream or are further metabolized within the gut itself.

For a number of reasons, protein absorption might be incomplete. Some of the proteins, because of their physical or chemical structure, are resistant to proteolytic attack and therefore pass through the small intestine relatively unmodified. Furthermore, the absorption of free amino acids and peptides may be less than 100%, particularly if gut function is impaired. This occurs in a number of clinical conditions, such as intestinal infection or injury, and when certain 'antinutritional' factors such as lectins or trypsin inhibitor proteins are present in the diet. This unabsorbed protein or amino acid then passes through into the colon. Metabolism by the colonic microflora then occurs, but the amino acids are no longer available to the body and are excreted in the faeces, mainly in the form of bacterial protein.

Absorbed amino acids pass into the portal vein and then on to the liver, where a proportion of the amino acids is taken up and used: the remainder pass through into the systemic circulation and are then transported into the tissue's cells.

PATHWAYS OF METABOLISM OF AMINO ACIDS

The major cellular pathways of metabolism are illustrated in Fig. 5.3.

Protein synthesis and degradation

The biochemical mechanism by which free amino acids are linked together by peptide bonds to form proteins can be found in any biochemistry textbook. From a nutritional and metabolic point of view, it is important to recognize that protein synthesis is a continuing process that takes place in almost all cells of the body. In a steady state, when neither growth nor protein loss is occurring, protein synthesis is

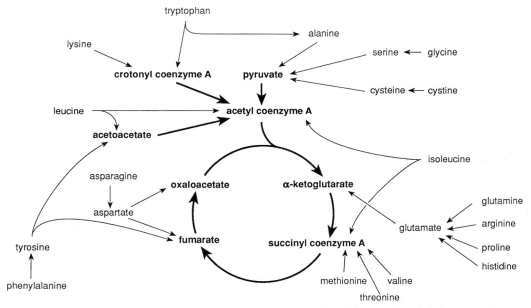

Fig. 5.3   Metabolism of the carbon skeletons of the amino acid chains (light arrows) and their points of entry into the general pathways of metabolism of glucose and fat (bold arrows).

balanced by an equal amount of protein degradation. The mechanism of intracellular protein degradation, by which the protein is hydrolysed to free amino acids, is more complex and is not as well characterized as that of synthesis. The details, as presently understood, can be found in Bond & Butler (1987) and Mortimore et al (1989).

These processes, by which all proteins are being continuously broken down and resynthesized, are known as 'protein turnover'. In the adult human body, more than 250 g of protein are synthesized and degraded daily. This compares with a dietary intake of only 70 g. The amount of protein turned over is greater in infants and less in the elderly, when compared with young adults on a bodyweight basis (Table 5.2). This relationship between protein turnover and age is similar to that between protein requirement and basal metabolic rate (BMR; see Chapter 3) and age. Some tissues are more active in protein turnover than others. Thus the liver and intestine, despite their rather small contribution to the total protein content of the body (see below), are together believed to contribute as much as 50% of whole body protein turnover. Conversely, skeletal muscle is the largest single component of body protein mass (about 50%), but contributes only about 25% of body protein turnover.

At the tissue level proteins are continually being synthesized and degraded as a sensitive means of regulating the amount of each separate enzyme or structural component. Other proteins might be secreted from the cell after synthesis, and are subsequently degraded at a distant site. Examples of such proteins are serum albumin, synthesized in the liver, antibodies in the B-lymphocytes, digestive enzymes in the pancreas, and peptide hormones in the endocrine glands.

Amino acid nitrogen metabolism

About 10–15 g of nitrogen are excreted each day in the urine of a healthy adult, mostly in the form of urea, with smaller contributions from ammonia, uric

Table 5.2   Whole-body protein synthesis in humans at different ages

	Protein synthesis		
	g/kg/day	g/g Protein requirement	g/kcal BMR
Newborn (premature)	17.4	5.4	0.15
Infants (~ 1 year)	6.9	4.1	0.13
Young adults	3.0	5.2	0.11
Elderly	1.9	4.5	0.11

Original data of Young et al (1975), as modified by Waterlow et al (1978)

Table 5.3 Approximate distribution of nitrogen in urinary constituents in human subjects receiving a normal balanced diet

Compound	g Nitrogen/24h
Urea	12.9
Ammonia	0.7
Amino acids	0.7
Creatinine	0.65
Uric acid	0.3
Hippuric acid	0.05
Total	15.30

From Diem (1962)

acid, creatinine and some free amino acids (Table 5.3). These are the end products of body nitrogen metabolism, with the major part – that in urea and ammonia – arising from the oxidation of amino acids. Uric acid and creatinine are indirectly derived from amino acids and will be considered later. Additional material on these processes can be found in biochemistry textbooks.

The separation of the nitrogen from the individual amino acids and its conversion to a form that can be excreted by the kidney, mainly as urea, can be considered as a two-part process. The first steps are usually one of two types of enzymic reaction, transamination or deamination. Transamination is a reversible reaction which uses the keto acid products of glucose metabolism (pyruvate, oxaloacetate and α-ketoglutarate) as recipients for the nitrogen. Most amino acids can take part in these reactions, with the result that their nitrogen is concentrated into just three amino acids: alanine from pyruvate, aspartate from oxaloacetate and glutamate from α-ketoglutarate. For the majority of amino acids this process takes place largely in the liver, but for the three branched-chain amino acids – leucine, isoleucine and valine – transamination occurs mainly peripherally, particularly in skeletal muscle. Here the main products are alanine and glutamine, which then pass into the circulation. These are very important carriers of nitrogen from the periphery to the intestine and liver. In the small intestine the glutamine is extracted and metabolized to ammonia, alanine and citrulline, which are then conveyed to the liver.

Nitrogen is also removed from amino acids by deamination reactions, which result in the formation of ammonia. A number of amino acids can be deaminated, either directly (histidine), by dehydration (serine, threonine), by way of the purine nucleotide cycle (aspartate) or by oxidative deamination (glutamate). These latter two processes are important because glutamate and aspartate are recipients of nitrogen by transamination from other amino acids, including alanine. Glutamate is also formed in the specific pathways for the degradation of arginine and lysine. Thus, nitrogen from any amino acid can be funnelled into the two precursors of urea synthesis, ammonia and aspartate.

Urea synthesis takes place in the liver by the cyclic pathway known as the Krebs–Henseleit cycle. The essential reaction in this process is the hydrolysis of the amino acid arginine by the enzyme arginase to urea and another amino acid, ornithine, which is not found in protein. The remaining part of the cycle involves the resynthesis of arginine using ammonia and aspartate. Thus, although the arginine is the direct precursor of urea, it is not consumed, as the nitrogen is all derived from the ammonia and aspartate.

After synthesis, the urea passes from the liver to the kidney, where it is excreted into the urine. Although the excretion of urea dominates nitrogen excretion as a whole, significant quantities of ammonium ions are also excreted. As pointed out above, there are some metabolic pathways, notably the purine nucleotide cycle, whereby purine nitrogen is converted to ammonium ions. Much of the ammonia produced by this cycle in skeletal muscle is transported into the blood as glutamine. Some of this glutamine is metabolized in the kidneys, where the enzyme glutaminase leads to the release of ammonium ions and glutamate. This glutamate is then utilized in the synthesis of glucose in the kidney. The generation of ammonium ions from glutamine has a specific role in acid–base homeostasis, as ammonium ion excretion serves as the main vehicle for the excretion of excess hydrogen ions during acidosis.

Amino acid carbon metabolism

For most amino acids, removal of the nitrogen generates their keto acid analogues. Many of these are already in a form suitable for entry into the pathways of oxidative metabolism (see Fig. 5.3). For example, α-ketoglutarate from glutamate, and pyruvate from alanine, are intermediates of the glycolysis/tricarboxylic acid pathway of glucose oxidation. All the others have specific degradative systems that give rise to intermediates that can be metabolized in these oxidative pathways. Thus, protein can make a significant contribution to the body's energy supply. This is particularly true in non-growing adults, who on average consume, and therefore oxidize, about 10–15% of their dietary energy as protein. Protein will form a much smaller contribution to energy supply during chronic starvation, or in protein-restricted diets. Conversely, protein oxidation may rise considerably in highly traumatized or septic individuals, when large amounts of body protein are lost: this loss can compromise recovery or even lead to death (see below).

Once the amino acid deamination products enter the tricarboxylic acid cycle or the glycolysis pathway, their carbon is also available for use in biosynthetic pathways, particularly for glucose and fat. Which of these two can be formed depends on its point of entry into the general metabolism (see Fig. 5.3). If they enter as acetyl-CoA, then only fat or ketone bodies can be formed. Other amino acids can, however, enter metabolism in such a way that their carbons can be used for gluconeogenesis. This is the basis for the classical nutritional description of amino acids as either ketogenic or glucogenic (i.e. able to give rise to either ketones or glucose). Many amino acids can give both products and so are both ketogenic and glucogenic (see Fig. 5.3).

The synthesis of glucose from amino acids is quantitatively dominated by alanine, glutamate and aspartate. However, as substantial amounts of these three amino acids are derived from the amination of intermediates of glucose metabolism (by transamination from other amino acids), a significant proportion of glucose synthesis by this route really represents recapture and recycling via the liver of 3-carbon units derived from glucose. This occurs by way of the so-called glucose–alanine cycle (which is a direct parallel of the Cori cycle, see Chapter 8) and the glucose–glutamine cycle. Since the donors of nitrogen may be either glucogenic or ketogenic amino acids, these cycles function as much as a mechanism for transporting nitrogen from the periphery to the liver, as for glucose production. The cycle involving glutamine transport from the periphery to the gastro-intestinal tract is also vital to the synthesis of arginine and proline, and is critical to the prevention of the build-up of excessive ammonia in the circulation.

Non-protein pathways of amino acid nitrogen utilization

Although in general the utilization of dietary amino acids is dominated by their incorporation into protein, amino acids are also involved in the synthesis of other nitrogenous compounds important to physiological viability (Table 5.4). In general, it seems unlikely that amino acid utilization in these pathways has a major influence on the availability of

amino acids for protein synthesis. Some pathways, however, have the potential to exert a substantial impact on the utilization of certain amino acids. This is particularly true for glycine which, as Table 5.4 shows, is involved in at least five quantitatively significant synthetic pathways. Its utilization in the synthesis of creatine (muscle function), haem (oxygen transport and oxidative phosphorylation) and glutathione (protective reactions) is not only of great potential physiological importance, but also can involve substantial quantities of the amino acid. For example, in the absence of a dietary source of creatine, an adult man requires the daily provision of at least 1.2 g of glycine in order to sustain adequate rates of creatine and haem synthesis. In milk-fed premature infants, glycine supply may well be a primary nutritional limitation to growth (Jackson 1989). This so-called non-essential amino acid is then needed in the diet for optimum growth, and may be termed 'conditionally essential'. Similarly, the synthesis of carnitine (involved in intracellular fatty acid transport) could under some circumstances become of quantitative significance to lysine requirements. These may be important nutritional considerations in individuals consuming marginal amounts of proteins of plant origin, and undoubtedly have an impact on overall amino acid utilization when protein intake is very low (Reeds 1990).

MAINTENANCE OF BODY PROTEIN

Protein and amino acid reserves

Protein

The body of a 70 kg man contains about 11 kg of protein and the approximate distribution of this

Table 5.4 Non-protein pathways of amino acid utilization

End product	Precursor amino acids
Serotonin	Tryptophan
Nicotinic acid	Tryptophan
Catecholamines	Tyrosine
Thyroid hormones	Tyrosine
Melanin	Tyrosine
Carnitine	Lysine
Taurine	Cysteine
Glutathione	Glutamate, cysteine, glycine
Nucleic acid bases	Glutamine, asparatate, glycine
Haem	Glycine
Creatine	Glycine, arginine, methionine
'Methyl group metabolism'	Methionine, glycine, serine
Bile acids	Glycine, taurine

Table 5.5 Body content of protein in adults and newborn babies, indicating the approximate distribution of protein among the tissues (from Lentner 1981)

	Newborn	Adult
Whole body (kg)		
Body weight	3.5	70
Total protein	0.41	11
Tissue protein (% total)		
Muscle	29	43
Skin	21	15
Blood	19	16
Liver	5	1.8
Brain	6	1.5
Kidney	1	0.3

among the various tissues is illustrated in Table 5.5. Nearly half this protein is present as skeletal muscle, while the other structural tissues (e.g. skin) and blood are large contributors. The metabolically active visceral tissues (e.g. liver and kidney) contain comparatively small amounts of protein (together about 10% of the total). The distribution among the organs varies with developmental age. As can be seen from Table 5.5, the newborn infant has proportionately less muscle and much more of brain and visceral tissues. It is also notable that, despite the very wide variety of different enzymes and proteins within a single organism, almost one-half of the total protein content of the body is present in just four proteins (myosin, actin, collagen and haemoglobin). Collagen in particular might comprise 25% of the total. Moreover, in malnutrition, this proportion can rise to 50% because of the substantial loss of non-collagen proteins, whereas collagen itself is retained (James 1977).

Even in the adult, when the protein mass of the body has reached a plateau, it can be influenced by a variety of nutritional and pathological factors. Thus, when diets high or low in protein are given, there is a gain or loss of body protein over the first few days, before re-equilibration of protein intake with oxidation/excretion occurs. This phenomenon has led to the concept of a 'labile protein reserve', which can be gained or lost from the body as a short-term store for use in emergencies, or to take account of day-to-day variations in dietary intake. Studies in animals have suggested that this immediate labile store might be contained in the liver and visceral tissues, as they lose protein very rapidly during starvation or protein depletion, by as much as 40%, while skeletal muscle loses protein much more slowly. This concept has been discussed in detail by Munro & Allison (1964a). The reserve in man is unlikely to account for more

than 300–400 g of protein, a mere 3% of the total body content. Thus, the immediately accessible stores of protein cannot be considered in the same light as the huge stores of fat: the labile protein reserve is similar in weight to the glycogen store. However, it should be recognized that this protein reserve is unlike the fat and glycogen stores, whose primary roles are for energy use. The protein lost during fasting is functional body protein and there is no evidence for a protein pool serving only as a store.

There is a wide range of variation in dietary intake to which the body is able to adapt over a period of days, after which no further change in protein content occurs. However, pathological conditions such as starvation, injury, infection, cancer and diabetes can cause substantial rates of protein loss. If these conditions go unchecked for more than a few days there may be a serious depletion of the body protein mass, which might eventually become life-threatening. Although the evidence from short-term changes in diet suggests that the main loss of protein is from the viscera, in chronic illness the largest single contributor to protein loss is from skeletal muscle, which, as noted above, comprises nearly 50% of the protein mass of the healthy subject. A considerable amount of research effort has therefore gone into understanding the mechanism of protein loss from the whole body and from muscle in these pathological states, and into possible nutritional and other means of minimizing or reversing it. This will be described in later chapters.

Free amino acids

Although the free amino acids dissolved in the body fluids are only a very small proportion of the body's total mass of amino acids, they are very important for the nutritional and metabolic control of the body's proteins.

The content of free and protein-bound amino acids in rat muscle is shown in Table 5.6. It can be seen that there is a considerable range, and that their concentration in the free pool is in no way related to their concentration in body proteins. In the human body, free phenylalanine comprises less than 0.2% of its total body pool, and corresponds to only about 1.5 hours worth of protein synthesis, or one-quarter of the day's intake of protein. Free glutamate and alanine comprise a much larger proportion of their respective body pools, but they could not be considered as reserves for more than a very short time. In human muscle, glutamine has an exceptionally large free pool, containing about 10–15 g

Table 5.6 Comparison of the pool sizes of free and protein bound amino acids in rat muscle

	μmol/g wet weight		
	Protein	Free	Ratio
Essential amino acids			
Isoleucine	50	0.16	306
Leucine	109	0.20	556
Lysine	58	1.86	31
Methionine	36	0.16	225
Phenylalanine	45	0.07	646
Threonine	60	1.94	31
Valine	83	0.31	272
Non-essential amino acids			
Alanine	111	2.77	40
Arginine	67	0.25	269
Aspartic acid (+ amide)	110	1.13	97
Glutamic acid (+ amide)	148	9.91	15
Glycine	117	1.94	60
Histidine	26	0.39	67
Serine	74	1.96	38
Tyrosine	36	0.14	266

Data of E B Fern, quoted in Waterlow et al (1978)

nitrogen. After trauma, this pool can become depleted by as much as 50% and its loss might then make a significant contribution to the total loss of nitrogen.

Although the plasma compartment is the most easily sampled, the concentration of most amino acids is higher in the intracellular pool of tissues. Typically, large neutral amino acids, such as leucine and phenylalanine, are 1–2-fold more concentrated in muscle than plasma, while others – notably glutamine, glutamic acid and glycine – are 10–50-fold more concentrated. Dietary variations or pathological conditions can result in substantial changes in the concentrations of the individual free amino acids in both the plasma and tissue pools. These have been widely studied with a view to understanding the mechanisms regulating the protein content of tissues. More detailed discussions of free amino acids are reported by Fürst (1985) and Waterlow et al (1978, Chapter 4).

Protein turnover

The exchange between the body protein and the free amino acid pool is illustrated by the highly simplified scheme shown in Fig. 5.4. Here, all the proteins in the tissues and circulation are lumped together into a single pool. Similarly, there is a second pool, consisting of the free amino acids dissolved in the body fluids. The arrows into and out of the protein pool show the continual degradation and resynthesis of these macromolecules (i.e. protein turnover). The other major pathways which involve the free amino acid pool are the supply of amino acids by the gut from the absorbed dietary proteins, the de novo synthesis (non-essential amino acids, see below) and their loss by oxidation, excretion or conversion to other metabolites. Although this scheme represents protein metabolism in the body as a whole, with

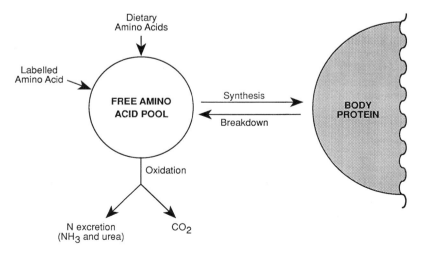

Fig. 5.4 Simple representation of whole-body protein and amino acid metabolism. This two-pool model has been found useful for calculating rates of protein turnover from data obtained with isotopic tracers.

minor modifications it can also be used to represent protein metabolism in individual organs, or indeed the metabolism of a single protein.

Regulation of the protein content of the body is achieved by modulation of the rates of any or all of the transfer processes. Because the body protein mass is continually being degraded to free amino acids and resynthesized, the net loss or gain depends on the net balance between these two processes. This is illustrated in Fig. 5.5, which shows that when the protein is in balance, the rates of synthesis and degradation are equal (A in the figure). When protein is lost, this must result from an excess of degradation over synthesis, but there are several alternative mechanisms: protein degradation might be stimulated (B), protein synthesis inhibited (C), or some combination of these (D, E, F). This mechanism would apply equally well for the protein of the whole body, a single organ or a single enzyme. In each case the amount of protein is regulated by alterations in the rates of these biochemically distinct processes of synthesis and degradation.

Over the last century a great deal of knowledge has been gained on how protein metabolism is controlled by nutrients and hormones, and how it is altered in pathological states. This understanding has gone hand in hand with the development of a variety of techniques for assessing the control and integration of protein metabolism in the whole organism. These range from methods for evaluating the net gains and losses of protein from body tissues, to techniques for assessing amino acid fluxes and protein turnover rates. An appreciation of the principles underlying these techniques, and of their accuracy, advantages and limitations, will be helpful when reading the literature on the nutritional control of protein metabolism.

Methods for assessing protein and amino acid metabolism

Body composition

Assessment of the protein status of the individual can be achieved by the sequential measurement of certain aspects of body composition and the comparison of these values to population estimates. This subject is discussed in much greater detail in Chapter 2 but some points merit emphasis here.

Most methods of assessing protein status attempt to measure some index of cellular mass, and usually attempt to partition the body weight between its lipid and non-lipid components. Four characteristics of the lean tissue or fat-free mass are generally used in indirect estimations of cellular or protein mass:

1. The densities of lean tissues and fat stores are different. Thus the measurement of the specific gravity of the body (by measuring the apparent loss in weight when the body is totally immersed in water), when combined with a knowledge of the specific gravity of lean (>1.0) and fat (<1.0) tissue, allows the proportion of fat and lean to be calculated.

2. The concentration of water in the lipid stores is much less than that in lean tissues. Thus measurements of body water give valuable information on lean–fat relationships. Developments in the mass spectrometric measurement of deuterium have led to an expansion of investigations of body water and its relationship to growth.

3. Cells contain high concentrations of potassium. Thus measurements of whole-body potassium content are also indices of cellular, and hence protein, mass. Potassium has a long-lived radioisotope (^{40}K) that is present in all potassium, so that measurements of the natural radiation emitted by the body allow the measurement of body potassium, and hence lean body mass.

4. The electrical properties of lean and fat tissues are different. This is exploited in two methods that measure either the conductivity (the TOBEC technique) or impedance (the BIA techniques), and derive values of the conductive volume of the body. This is also a measure of the fat-free body mass.

These techniques are being used with increasing frequency and provide a valuable addition to the classical balance techniques.

Synthesis or
degradation

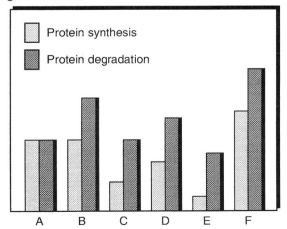

Fig 5.5 Illustration of the various different ways in which changes in protein synthesis and degradation can contribute to body protein loss. For description, see text.

Nitrogen balance

Because the nitrogen economy is dominated by that of protein, and because there are available highly sensitive methods (e.g. the Kjeldahl method) for measuring nitrogen, an individual's handling of dietary protein is classically defined from measurements of nitrogen balance. This is the algebraic sum of nitrogen intake and nitrogen loss via the urine, faeces and skin. At nitrogen equilibrium the sum is zero; positive nitrogen balance is taken as a sign that body protein is being deposited and negative balance indicates body protein loss. The state of nitrogen balance does not, of course, tell us anything about the mass of the body's proteins, nor their distribution, concentration or function.

At the practical level it must be recognized that because we do not eat continuously, nitrogen excretion in both the urine and faeces is not constant throughout the day, or even between days. Furthermore, because the urea pool in the body is large and turns over with a half-life of approximately 12 hours, it may take 2 days for a change in urea synthesis (i.e. nitrogen balance) to be fully reflected in the urine. The combination of the delay in the urea pool and the inevitable day-to-day variations in nitrogen excretion mean that the proper assessment of protein gain or loss by this method must involve prolonged collections (of at least 72 hours). Ideally the start and end of the balance measurements should be defined by the appearance of some external marker (such as a dye) in the faeces.

There are other potential sources of error in this method. For example, it is extremely difficult to measure accurately the quantities of nitrogen lost in sweat and by desquamation, and most reports rely on the limited number of reports in which these losses have been quantified. Values as high as 1 g N and as low as 90 mg have been reported for adults. These estimates represent 8% and 1% respectively of current estimates for the amount of protein-nitrogen needed by adults for achieving nitrogen balance. For this reason alone, measured nitrogen balance tends to overestimate the true balance, that is, it overestimates protein deposition and underestimates protein loss.

Many diets, for example human milk, contain significant quantities of non-protein nitrogen, so that the simple assumption that dietary nitrogen is all in dietary protein may be wrong. Furthermore, the utilization of nitrogen in the non-protein pathways listed above can lead to nitrogen retention but not protein retention. Therefore, nitrogen balance is only a crude method of examining protein balance in the body.

Whole-body protein and amino acid kinetics

Much biochemical information on the regulation of protein metabolism has been obtained by studying isolated organs or tissue homogenates in vitro. However, studying the influence of nutrition on the integrated metabolism of protein requires techniques that can be used in the intact animal or human. In animals, the radioactive isotopes ^{14}C, tritium and ^{35}S have been used, but in man it is more acceptable to label with stable (non-radioactive) isotopes such as ^{13}C, deuterium and ^{15}N. The principles are the same whether radioactive or stable isotopes are chosen: only the method of detection differs, radioactive isotopes being measured by their radiation and stable isotopes by mass spectrometry.

Rates of protein turnover in the whole body were first studied by Schoenheimer's group, using the then newly available isotope ^{15}N (Waterlow et al 1978). The techniques that have evolved from these early studies have been based on the concept that body protein metabolism can be represented by a simplified model such as that shown in Fig. 5.4. One such technique is the continuous infusion of a carbon-labelled amino acid, e.g. [1-^{13}C]leucine. The infusion is given intravenously over a period of hours, during which the isotopic enrichment (i.e. the ratio of labelled to total molecules, usually expressed as atom per cent excess over the natural abundance) rises to a plateau value. This plateau value (A_{max}) is used to calculate the total rate of turnover (Q) of the free leucine in the body from the expression

$$Q = i / A_{max}$$

The term i is the rate of infusion of the isotope. This equation is derived on the assumption that at plateau the rates of entry and exit from the free leucine pool are equal for both labelled and unlabelled molecules (i.e. there is a steady state). Thus, Q is also known as the flux rate, appearance rate or irreversible loss rate. As shown in Fig. 5.4, the appearance of leucine can be partitioned into intake from the diet (I) and entry from the degradation of body protein (D), de novo synthesis being zero for an essential amino acid such as leucine (see below). Similarly, loss from the free leucine pool can be partitioned into protein synthesis (S) and other pathways of metabolism (O), of which only oxidation to CO_2 and urinary N is taken to be significant. Since entry and exit are equal in the steady state:

$$Q = I + D = S + O$$

Having determined the flux (Q), it is possible to calculate the rate of whole body protein degradation

(D), since the dietary intake (I) of leucine is known. By assessing the production of labelled CO_2 in the breath it is also possible to measure the rate of leucine oxidation (O), thus allowing the rate of whole-body protein synthesis to be calculated.

By this means the rates of metabolism of an individual amino acid by oxidation and by the synthesis and degradation of body protein can be determined. A very similar approach is used with ^{15}N, which is usually given as [^{15}N]glycine. The difference is that because of transamination, this label acts as a tracer for total free amino nitrogen, rather than for an individual amino acid. Also, estimates of the plateau enrichment in the free amino acid pool are not usually made on the plasma, but instead on two end products of nitrogen metabolism in the urine, urea and ammonia.

The choice of which isotopic label to use depends on the type of experiment which is planned. Carbon (^{13}C or ^{14}C) labelling is more suited to short-term (e.g. 4 hours) measurements in a controlled environment where frequent blood and breath sampling is possible. ^{15}N methods are more suitable for free-living subjects and patients, when urine sampling is possible but regular blood and breath sampling are inconvenient. The application of the method can be made even simpler when the ^{15}N label is given orally as a single dose. Both methods involve many assumptions (Waterlow et al 1978), but in practice the two approaches have been shown to give very similar results, thus adding confidence to the data obtained with either.

Protein turnover in individual tissues

The techniques for this are more invasive than for the whole body, in general requiring measurements on samples of tissue. Although studies involving tissue sampling in man are becoming more common, the bulk of the data on tissues have been obtained in experimental animals. The procedure for measuring tissue protein synthesis is to give an isotopically labelled amino acid and to assess its incorporation into the protein of the tissue under study. However, the calculation also requires that the isotopic enrichment of the free amino acid at the site of protein synthesis be monitored throughout the incorporation period. This can present difficulties because of the compartmentation of free amino acid pools within cells, so that this measurement cannot reliably be made on plasma or tissue free amino acids. Special techniques can be used to minimize the problem (e.g. by giving the label as a large, non-tracer dose, or by

measurements on the amino acid bound to transfer RNA; Waterlow et al 1978; Garlick et al 1991).

It is also possible to obtain information on the state of protein synthesis in tissues in vivo non-isotopically, by measurements on ribosomes. By extracting the ribosomes from a tissue biopsy and centrifuging at high speed, they can be separated into those which are aggregated into polyribosomes (polysomes, i.e. those that are actively synthesizing protein) and those which are free. Decreases in both the ratio of polysomal to non-polysomal RNA and the total amount of ribosomes in the tissue have been taken as indicative of a decrease in the rate of protein synthesis in traumatized patients (Wernerman 1991).

Protein degradation is more difficult to assess in individual tissues in man, but in animals it can be estimated from values for the rates of synthesis and growth of tissue protein. In man, rates of degradation in certain tissues can be estimated by performing balance techniques across limbs or organs (see below), and in muscle by measuring the urinary excretion of 3-methylhistidine. This amino acid is found only in the actin and myosin of muscle, where it is synthesized by methylation of specific histidine residues of the proteins. After degradation of the proteins the 3-methylhistidine is not reincorporated into protein, but is instead excreted quantitatively in the urine, thus supplying a direct measure of the rate of degradation of actin plus myosin. Although the results cannot be equated solely with the degradation of skeletal muscle, because there is 3-methylhistidine in smooth muscle (e.g. in the gut), this method has proved very useful for studies in patients because of its totally non-invasive nature (Sjölin et al 1989).

Limb or organ amino acid balance techniques

In addition to the amino acid fluxes into and out of protein, there are exchanges of amino acids between tissues. When a tissue has a discrete blood supply which allows all the blood entering and leaving to be sampled, it is then possible to measure the total uptake or output of amino acids and other nutrients. The forearm or leg can be used to represent the metabolism of skeletal muscle (or with special cannulation, fat), and arterial and hepatic vein catheters can be used to study the splanchnic bed (i.e. liver and intestine). This approach has been used, for example, to demonstrate the role of the liver in the metabolism of amino acids absorbed from the diet (Abumrad et al 1989).

The organ balance technique measures only the net balance of an amino acid in a tissue, but with the addition of an isotopically labelled amino acid, the synthesis and degradation of tissue protein can also be estimated simultaneously. The technical and theoretical problems of such studies need careful attention, however (Wernerman & Vinnars 1987; Garlick et al 1991).

Amino acid oxidation

Measuring nitrogen excretion provides no information on the rates of catabolism of individual amino acids. However, since ^{13}C-labelled amino acids have become available, increasing use has been made of breath $^{13}CO_2$ measurements (see above) as indices of the oxidation of individual amino acids (Waterlow et al 1978; Young 1987). When the labelled amino acid is not limiting in the diet, the rate of $^{13}CO_2$ production can be used as an index of total amino acid catabolism. The principal advantage of labelling the amino acid is that there is little delay between a change in amino acid catabolism and a change in labelling of breath carbon dioxide, so the method is not as time-consuming as classical nitrogen balance. Furthermore, this approach can be used to examine more dynamic aspects of the regulation of amino acid catabolism.

The technique can also be used to investigate specifically the metabolism of a single amino acid, and thereby estimate the requirement for this amino acid under suitable dietary conditions. This technique has been used as part of a new but controversial approach to the re-evaluation of essential amino acid requirements in adults (See below and Chapter 52).

PHYSIOLOGICAL CONTROL OF PROTEIN METABOLISM

The following gives a brief summary of some of the physiological and pathological modulators of protein metabolism which are of particular relevance to nutrition, together with a description of some possible hormonal mediators. Because direct studies in man are limited by ethical considerations, our knowledge in this area also comes from laboratory measurements of tissue metabolism and extensive studies in experimental animals. More detailed analyses can be found in Waterlow et al (1978), Garlick (1980), Waterlow & Jackson (1981), Reeds & Garlick (1984), Waterlow (1984), Garlick et al (1988), and a collection of articles in *Diabetes/ Metabolism Reviews* (volume 5, 1989).

Age and growth

The whole-body rate of protein turnover of 200–300 g/day in adult man corresponds to about 3–4 g/day/kg body weight. In babies and children, however, the rate expressed in this way is far higher. Table 5.2 gives examples of turnover at ages ranging from premature infants to elderly adults, showing a gradual decrease in turnover with increasing age. Similar changes with age have been demonstrated for both dietary protein requirements and metabolic rate. Although a relationship between protein turnover rate and mature body weight has been well documented in mammals ranging widely in body size, the changes from birth to senescence shown in Table 5.2 result more from differences in the stage of maturity. Thus, immature animals in general have higher rates of both synthesis and degradation of protein than do adults.

One property of immaturity is the high capacity for growth, which in itself is strongly related to the synthesis and degradation of cellular and structural proteins. Rates of whole-body protein synthesis have been shown to correlate positively with rates of growth or protein retention, both in preterm infants and in children recovering from malnutrition. Although rates of degradation also increase somewhat at higher growth rates, the difference between synthesis and degradation increases, thus giving rise to greater protein retention.

Studies in animals have shown that protein turnover in individual tissues is also higher in the newborn than in adults. Changes in muscle are particularly pronounced. During the first few weeks of life in rats, there is an approximately tenfold decline in protein synthesis. There is a slower fall in degradation as the rate of growth declines, so that at maturity synthesis and degradation are equal, with zero growth. Measurements on tissues have not been made in humans during growth, but the changes are likely to be much less pronounced because of man's very prolonged period of development and very slow growth compared with most other species.

Dietary intake

Responses to meals

Dietary factors should be separated into acute responses, such as those occurring after individual meals, and chronic effects, such as might accompany a prolonged change in diet. For most of us, dietary intake is not continuous but is taken as discrete meals, interspersed with periods of fasting. The normal state might therefore be divided into two phases: absorptive, which is the period during which the nutrients are actively absorbed from the gut, and post-absorptive, which occurs after absorption has finished and before the next meal. In the post-absorptive state the body is using its stores of nutrients and is in a state of catabolism. The oxidation of amino acids continues, despite the absence of intake, and this results in the loss of tissue protein, notably from skeletal muscle and the splanchnic area. This continued drain of amino acids occurs despite the ability of the body to recycle most of the amino acids from protein degradation back into the synthesis of new proteins. The loss occurs because there is a need for the precursors of gluconeogenesis, and to continue the synthesis of some of the many compounds for which amino acids act as precursors. Feeding later replenishes the proteins lost during fasting.

The anabolism which accompanies feeding in the adult is brought about mostly by a decrease in the rate of whole-body protein degradation, rather than by an increase in protein synthesis. This contrasts with the pronounced increases in synthesis when food is given to infants or animals during rapid growth. There is also an increase in the rate of amino acid oxidation if the meal contains a plentiful supply of protein. After absorption by the intestine, some of the dietary amino acids are removed by the intestinal cells for protein synthesis and some are selectively oxidized, e.g. glutamine. Most of the amino acids are then passed to the liver, where they are extracted. Thus the peak in amino acid concentrations in the portal blood after protein ingestion is much higher than those measured routinely in venous blood samples. The extracted hepatic amino acids serve to increase the protein content of the liver by inhibiting protein degradation while maintaining protein synthesis. There also seems to be an increase in the production rate of secretory proteins, such as serum albumin. Amino acids escaping extraction by the liver are mostly taken up by muscle for synthesis into protein as part of the largest protein reserve in the body. The three branched-chain amino acids – leucine, isoleucine and valine – which are not extracted by the liver to the same extent as the others, are also extensively oxidized in peripheral tissues such as muscle.

As the rate of amino acid absorption declines, protein turnover changes and a net flow of amino acids from protein begins. Many of the amino acids from net protein degradation in the muscle pass directly to the liver to be converted to glucose precursors. The glycogen reserve is limited to about one day's supply, so the post-absorptive supply of glucose by gluconeogenesis from amino acids is important. The branched-chain amino acids, which are normally very abundant in protein, are trans-aminated in muscle, giving rise to large amounts of alanine and glutamine, which are then transported to the liver to act as precursors for glucose and urea. On the way, glutamine is largely extracted by the small intestine and converted to alanine.

Starvation

If another meal is not forthcoming, the post-absorptive state progresses into starvation. Here the priority is to restrict the loss of protein by minimizing the need for glucose. Thus, over a period of a week or so the brain adapts to using ketone bodies as its main oxidative substrate in place of glucose, and there is a concomitant reduction in the oxidation of amino acids and in urinary nitrogen excretion. Typically, the rate of nitrogen excretion is about 12 g/day in well-nourished subjects, and falls to only about 3 g/day in the fully adapted starved state. Starvation is accompanied by a fall in protein synthesis in most tissues, particularly in skeletal muscle, where degradation is also depressed. This fall in both synthesis and degradation limits both the loss of protein and the expenditure of energy which would be needed to maintain these processes. Only during the terminal phase, when other supplies of energy have become exhausted, is there an increase in degradation, resulting in a very rapid loss of protein.

Injury and disease

This is dealt with in more detail in Chapter 31. Injury, infection, burns and cancer all result in a loss of body protein. The ensuing negative nitrogen balance is proportional to the degree of trauma, ranging from a few grams of nitrogen per day after minor or moderate surgery, to more than 30 g N/day with severe burns. The latter value corresponds to a loss of about 1 kg of lean tissue per day. Thus it is clear that if this condition persists for more than a few days, survival is threatened and recovery impaired. This metabolic response is aggravated by the starvation which frequently accompanies trauma. However, metabolically trauma and starvation are rather different. The loss of protein in starvation affects most tissues to a similar extent, whereas with trauma there is a pronounced loss of skeletal muscle, with preservation of the visceral protein mass. Also, the adaptation which limits glucose utilization, and hence protein loss, during starvation does not occur in severe trauma.

In general there is an increase in whole-body rates of both protein synthesis and degradation, with the increase in degradation predominating, thus resulting in the net loss of total body protein. The site of the increased synthesis is thought to be the liver and the cells of the immune system, whereas synthesis in skeletal muscle is depressed. Hence this loss of protein from the relatively non-essential organs such as muscle will provide the substrates necessary for the repair of injured tissue (e.g. wound healing) and for activating the host defence mechanisms. The latter include the 'acute phase response', in which there is an increase in the synthesis of a series of plasma proteins by the liver (e.g. fibrinogen, C-reactive protein, α1-acid glycoprotein).

Clinicians have attempted to reverse the loss of body protein by nutritional means. As oral intake is generally not possible in very sick patients, intravenous infusions of artificial nutrient mixtures are given. Although this procedure has been shown to reduce the nitrogen losses substantially, it is only partially effective and patients do not regain muscle mass until the underlying pathology is treated successfully. For this reason there has been much research aimed at redesigning the composition of the nutrients given, and tailoring them for particular disease states (see Chapter 31). Because of chemical instability or insolubility in water, several amino acids (e.g. glutamine, tyrosine, cysteine) cannot easily be given in the free form, and alternative forms, for example dipeptides, are being tested. Mixtures enriched with certain amino acids are also being assessed. For example, branched-chain amino acids have been used for reversing the amino acid imbalance experienced during liver failure (Chapter 34), and, furthermore, are considered by some to enhance muscle anabolism. There are also mixtures designed to minimize nitrogen excretion for use in kidney failure, by replacing some of the essential amino acids with their keto acid analogues (Chapter 40).

Hormonal and other mediators

Anabolic factors

Hormones can be broadly separated into anabolic factors, which are responsible for modulating the disposition of nutrients after feeding and for growth, and catabolic factors, which mediate tissue loss during starvation and trauma. The most notable anabolic hormone is insulin. This is a peptide hormone produced by the ß-cells of the pancreas, and secreted predominantly in response to the increasing plasma glucose concentration after meals. The rise in circulating insulin is thought to be a major factor in controlling the retention of absorbed protein. In vitro studies on animal tissues have shown that insulin can stimulate protein synthesis in skeletal muscle and inhibit degradation in both muscle and liver. The effects of this hormone are very rapid: infusion of insulin into growing rats stimulates muscle protein synthesis within minutes. Increases in amino acid concentrations, particularly of the branched-chain amino acids leucine, isoleucine and valine, induce similar effects to those of insulin in vitro. In the intact animal these two factors appear to act synergistically to initiate the response to feeding. During starvation and malnutrition the levels of insulin are much reduced, thus in part mediating the loss of body protein.

Growth hormone (GH), a peptide hormone produced by the pituitary gland, also stimulates protein deposition in muscle and other tissues. GH acts indirectly, by stimulating the secretion of insulin-like growth factor-1 (IGF-1, somatomedin-C) by the liver. The polypeptide IGF-1 has a more prolonged effect than insulin, which is consistent with its role in a continuous process such as growth.

Catabolic factors

During fasting there is a rise in the plasma concentration of glucagon, a peptide hormone produced by the pancreatic α-cells. It promotes gluconeogenesis in the liver from free amino acids and lactate. This effect is rapid (i.e. within minutes of a rise in glucagon level), so glucagon balances insulin in the acute control of the responses to feeding and fasting. The ratio of insulin to glucagon concentrations seems to be more important than the absolute level of either. Although glucagon has also been shown to inhibit muscle protein synthesis at high concentrations, it is not clear at present whether it has a direct action on the periphery in vivo at normal physiological levels.

Cortisol is a steroid hormone produced by the adrenal cortex, which has rather similar, but slower (2–4h), effects to those of glucagon. It also has direct effects on muscle, decreasing protein synthesis and increasing protein degradation. In the liver it modifies the activities of a number of enzymes by altering the rate of production of their specific messenger RNAs, and hence the rate of enzyme synthesis. Cortisol secretion is much increased after trauma and injury, a characteristic it shares with glucagon and adrenaline, the three together being known as the 'stress hormones'. These are thought to be responsible for mediating many, but not all, of the metabolic responses to trauma, such as the high rate of gluconeogenesis and the mobilization of muscle protein.

In the last 10 years a new group of hormonal mediators, known as the cytokines, has been identified. These peptides are produced by activated macrophages, particularly in response to local injury, and are involved in organizing the metabolic and immunological events following trauma. Of those influencing protein metabolism the most studied are tumour necrosis factor (TNF, cachectin), interleukin-1 (IL-1, endogenous pyrogen) and interleukin-6 (IL-6). When injected, they bring about fever and negative nitrogen balance. Injections of TNF or IL-1 stimulate liver protein synthesis and inhibit muscle protein synthesis in rats, and IL-6 is believed to be involved in the initiation of the acute-phase response in the liver. Their mode of action, whether their effects are direct or mediated by some other cytokine or hormone, and their role in relation to the stress hormones is not currently clear.

PROTEIN AND AMINO ACID REQUIREMENTS

Much of the quantitative research on protein and amino acid metabolism is directed towards identiying the amounts of amino acids that should be supplied in the diet in order to support optimum health. The dietary recommendations emerging have important implications both for public health and also for food policy and the agricultural economy.

Requirements and allowances

The subject of human essential amino acid requirements is under debate and the current recommendations are being reappraised (Beaton & Chery 1988, Millward & Rivers 1988, Young et al 1989). When reading the literature on human protein 'requirements' it is important to be aware that this term is often used in an ill-defined fashion. The way in which it is applied to protein nutrition by various authors is very dependent on the way in which they approach the issue of how to assess the adequacy of the diet. Those investigating the relationship between protein intake and body protein status (e.g. nitrogen retention, weight gain, linear growth) tend to describe requirements in terms of dietary protein supply. Those who adopt a more direct biological approach define requirements in terms of the rates of the pathways (tissue growth, amino acid catabolism, protein turnover) discussed above. The first group defines requirements in practical terms, i.e. as dietary allowances, whereas the second group defines them in biological terms, i.e. as amino acid needs. Both groups recognize explicitly that amino acid needs are primarily a function of physiological and reproductive status, but the first approach gives a higher requirement than the second. Dietary protein is not absorbed with 100% efficiency, and there is inevitably some extra amino acid catabolism associated with the surge in plasma and tissue amino acid concentrations after a protein meal. So it is not surprising that the two approaches to assessing requirements give different answers.

Components of protein and amino acid requirements

Nutritional and metabolic classification of amino acids

Older views of the nutritional classification of amino acids categorized them into two groups, essential (indispensable) and non-essential (dispensable). Essential amino acids were those that man could not synthesize and therefore had to have in the diet. Although the classification of the essential amino acids has been maintained, the definition of non-essential amino acids has become blurred as more information on the intermediary metabolism of these compounds becomes available. Recent authors (Laidlaw & Kopple 1987) now divide non-essential amino acids into two classes: truly non-essential and conditionally essential. Non-essential amino acids are now more rigidly defined as those synthesized either by reductive amination of a keto acid by ammonium ions, or by transamination of a carbon chain synthesized in the central pathways of carbon metabolism, i.e. the glycolytic pathway or the Kreb's cycle. According to this definition only glutamate, aspartate and alanine should be regarded as truly non-essential.

Conditionally essential amino acids (Table 5.7) are now defined as those that derive from the metabolism of either other amino acids or other complex nitrogenous metabolites. A key point is that the synthesis of these amino acids does not involve the simple transamination. It has, of course, been known for many years that there is a close metabolic and nutritional interrelationship between methionine and cysteine, and between phenylalanine and tyrosine, so

Table 5.7   Precursors of conditionally essential amino acids

Amino acid	Precursors
Cysteine	Methionine, serine
Tyrosine	Phenylalanine
Arginine	Glutamine/glutamate, asparatate
Proline	Glutamate
Histidine	Adenine, glutamine
Glycine	Serine, choline

Table 5.8   Comparison of the composition of body protein and the amino acid pattern for optimum protein utilization for growth in the pig (g amino acid/16 g N)

	Body protein	Growth pattern
Leucine	6.9	7.8
Threonine	4.2	4.7
Lysine	7.8	6.8
Methionine	2.1	1.9
Cysteine	1.9	1.7
NEAA/EAA	52/48	54/46

From Reeds (1990) and Fuller et al (1989)
NEAA/EAA is the ratio of non-essential to essential amino acids

many formulations of recommended dietary amino acid allowances (see below) consider these amino acids as pairs. However, only the thiol group of cysteine is derived from methionine, while its carbon and nitrogen are derived from serine. Similarly, arginine and proline require the provision of excess glutamate and aspartate, while histidine is derived from adenine and glutamine. Finally, although known for many years, it has only recently been generally accepted that amino nitrogen is not freely interchanged between all amino acids. Serine, lysine and threonine nitrogen, for example, is not readily transferred to glutamate, aspartate or alanine.

The term 'conditionally essential', then, recognizes that in principle these amino acids may be needed in the diet unless abundant amounts of their precursors are available for their synthesis at nutritionally significant rates. There may be physiological circumstances (for example in the newborn) in which the enzymes involved in what are quite complex synthetic pathways may be present in inadequate amounts, so that there is then a dietary requirement for this amino acid.

Amino acid utilization in growth

Dietary protein is not only needed for maintaining protein turnover and the variety of products of amino acid metabolism, but also for laying down as new tissue during growth. The extra amino acids needed approximate to the amino acid composition of the new protein being laid down (Table 5.8).

Maintenance protein requirements

Even when mammals consume no protein, nitrogen losses continue. Provided the dietary energy supply is adequate, these so-called 'endogenous' losses are closely related to body weight, and even more to basal metabolism. Thus, although immature individuals excrete more nitrogen per unit body weight than

adults when consuming a low-protein diet, there is little age-related difference when nitrogen excretion is related to (body weight)$^{0.75}$ or to body surface area. This suggests that amino acid catabolism is linked to fundamental body metabolism.

In man, because normal growth is very slow and because man is a long-lived species, the maintenance needs (i.e. the replacement of endogenous losses in order to maintain nitrogen and/or body protein equilibrium) are of crucial nutritional importance and account for well over 90% of lifetime needs for dietary protein. Unfortunately, although it has proved relatively easy to formulate approximate recommendations based on nitrogen balance and expressed in terms of dietary protein, it has proved difficult to define these protein needs exactly. It is much more difficult to define them in terms of amino acid intake. There are four reasons for this. First, nitrogen equilibrium in adults is difficult to measure precisely, whereas it is very clear when an infant is not growing because of an inadequate protein intake. Secondly, dietary requirements defined in terms of maintaining nitrogen equilibrium are potentially very sensitive to the preceding diet and other issues of the nutritional design (Millward et al 1990). Thirdly, the choice of the method for assessing needs, e.g. amino acid nitrogen balance versus amino acid carbon balance and turnover (Young 1987), may influence the final recommendation (Reeds 1990). Finally, the maintenance needs for individual amino acids will reflect amino acid utilization in a number of pathways unrelated to protein metabolism, so measuring nitrogen balance may be inappropriate without assuming the effectiveness of production of these other products of amino acid metabolism. It is therefore not surprising that the dietary protein and amino acid requirements of adults in particular, remain controversial.

Potential contributors to maintenance needs

In considering the basis of maintenance protein needs it is important to remember that the metabolic pool of amino acids derives both from the diet and from body protein degradation. It has been assumed for decades that the body's capacity to conserve individual amino acids varies, so the pattern of amino acids needed in the diet to match their individual catabolic rates does not correspond with the composition of body protein. For example, the essential amino acid requirements of adults have been assumed to be equivalent to about one-eighth of the minimum need for amino acid nitrogen, compared with the usual composition of non-collagen body protein, in which approximately half the amino acids are essential. This implies that there is very effective recycling of the essential amino acids released from protein degradation back into protein synthesis. Under conditions where the diet is protein-free, the efficiency of amino acid recycling is over 90%. The difference between the proportion of essential amino acids needed to maintain constant body tissue function and protein stores, and the proportions of individual amino acids needed for depositing new protein, can be expected to be very different. Studies in growing animals vividly display the higher requirements for essential amino acids during growth. Several differences become apparent. First, the proportion of non-essential amino acids in the total protein needed appears to be much higher than the proportion in body protein. Secondly, the ratio of cysteine to methionine requirement is higher close to maintenance than during growth, and thirdly, the proportion of threonine in the optimum dietary amino acid pattern appears to be similar for both nitrogen equilibrium and growth. Two pathways of amino acid loss are important contributors to these requirements.

1. The non-protein pathways of amino acid metabolism were described above. Some non-essential (e.g. glutamate) and conditionally essential (e.g. cysteine, glycine, arginine), rather than essential, amino acids are the major substrates for those pathways that produce products other than urea, CO_2 and water. These pathways place an obligatory requirement on specific amino acids. The products of these pathways, for example creatine, may themselves be converted to metabolites which are lost, such as creatinine; the haem of haemoglobin also enters the red cells, which, when broken down, yield the haem for metabolism and excretion through the bile. The demand for end products such as creatine and haemoglobin is of sufficient magnitude to have a significant impact on the needs for their amino acid precursors under conditions of inadequate protein supply. For example, the daily creatinine losses in an adult require the utilization of quantities of glycine and arginine that are equivalent to 80% and 250% of the amounts of these amino acids released by the net loss of body protein under protein-free feeding conditions. The end products of these pathways of amino acid metabolism (e.g. haem, creatine and glutathione) are of great functional importance. Therefore it is not surprising that animals and man maintain body protein turnover and the catabolism of some amino acids, in order to ensure that these products can be resynthesized so that the child or adult is not placed at risk.

2. Intestinal protein losses continue even under conditions of protein-free feeding, and faecal nitrogen loss (i.e. bacterial protein) may account for 50% of the basal loss of nitrogen. Obviously under this dietary circumstance the only source of amino acids for the accretion of bacterial biomass is the body amino acids. In those studies in which highly digestible protein-containing diets have been given to subjects previously ingesting protein-free diets, faecal nitrogen excretion changed by only a small extent. Thus, it seems likely that when humans consume diets that do not provide an excessive quantity of protein, a high proportion of the faecal nitrogen loss originates from a combination of gastrointestinal secretions and the partial capture of the significant quantities of urea hydrolysed by the microbes adhering to the wall in the large intestine (Jackson 1989).

The following points support the view that the intestinal route of protein (amino acid) loss is of quantitative significance to maintenance protein needs. First, continued cell turnover, enzyme and mucin secretion are necessary for maintaining the integrity of the gastrointestinal tract and its normal digestive physiology. Secondly, animal studies show that the amino acid composition of the proteins leaving the ileum for bacterial fermentation in the colon is quite different from that of body protein. In particular, the secretions are relatively rich in non-essential amino acids. Probably because mucin secretions make a substantial contribution to the endogenous outflow, the proteins that exit the terminal ileum are rich in threonine and cysteine, two amino acids that appear to be of special significance to amino acid needs close to nitrogen equilibrium.

Estimates of protein and amino acid requirements

These are dealt with in detail in the report produced by the FAO/WHO/UNU Expert Consultation (FAO 1985), which met in Rome in 1981. A further meeting in Washington, formally sponsored by FAO and WHO, was held in 1990 and resulted in a modification to the policy on the essential amino acid requirements of adults (see below). Tables of requirements as set out by this UN group are given in Appendix 2. Where the latest UK dietary reference value (DRV) report differs from the UN figures, both values are given. As will be explained in Chapter 52, the UN figures relate to the upper values of the requirement range, so the UK reference nutrient intake (RNI) corresponds in practice to the UN values. The estimated average requirement is also provided in the UK report, and so is included in the tables in Appendix 2. Issues relating to pregnancy and lactation are dealt with in Chapter 25. Table 5.9 gives examples of the process used in calculating the protein requirements in children. Specific details of these calculations are discussed below.

Measurements in children

The protein requirements for babies are based on complex calculations of the total intake and nitrogen content of breast milk fed directly or by bottle to babies in the first 4–6 months of life. Yet 20% of the total nitrogen in breast milk is in the form of non-amino acid nitrogen, such as urea. Because babies grow well on this milk, provided they have enough, the total nitrogen is assumed to be utilized and figures are calculated as though the nitrogen were all protein. From 6–12 months, the breast-fed child is still growing rapidly, but now has to rely on other sources of food, i.e. supplementary feeds. For these requirement values, reliance is placed on short-term nitrogen balance studies using milk or egg protein. Additional studies were carried out on children aged 1–5 years using soya milk or mixed sources of protein as well as nitrogen-balance measurements conducted with milk. Different nitrogen intakes were chosen, allowances were made for skin losses and a slope of nitrogen retention in relation to intake was calculated to obtain the maintenance requirement. Adjustments had to be made for the different digestibility of the different proteins: mixed feeding leads to additional faecal nitrogen loss compared with the faecal losses on a milk diet, so the true maintenance needs of absorbed amino acids are less than the protein intake. Conversely, once the maintenance and growth requirements of children are estimated, the true needs for dietary proteins have to be increased to make allowance for incomplete digestibility or

Table 5.9   Calculating the safe level of milk protein and other dietary proteins for children

Age (years)	Maintenance needs	Growth needs	Estimated average requirement	CV%	Add 2SD	Reference nutrient intake	Type of diet	Digestibility (%)	RNI with allowance for digestibility	Amino acid score (%)	RNI with allowance for both digestibility and protein quality
	(mg N/kg/day)					(g Protein/ kg/day)			(g Protein/ kg/day)		(g Protein/ kg/day)
0.5–0.75	120	80	200	16	264	1.65	Wheat and veg	66	2.5	76	3.3
2–3	118	28	146	12	181	1.13	Rice 70% Fish 30%	73	1.5	81	1.9
5–6	115	17	132	12	164	1.02	Beans and corn 95% Veg 5%	59	1.7	89	1.9
9–10	111	17	128	12	155	0.99	Mixed; animal 45%	80	1.2	100	1.2

Data taken from WHO/FAO/UNO (1985) with each digestibility value specified for each individual diet.
Digestibility D% = $100 \times (I-F)/I$, where, I = N intake and F = faecal N on the diet.
CV% is the coefficient of variation, which combines a CV for maintenance of 12.5% and a growth CV of 35%. The diets and corresponding digestibility values are taken from individual studies cited in the report to illustrate the varying values. In general, adults can be considered to have an 85% digestibility of nitrogen on unrefined diets and a value of 95% on refined diets. The amino acid scores take account of the limiting amino acids of the mixed diet.

additional endogenous nitrogen excreted from the intestine in response to the particular diet. To obtain an estimate of the recommended daily allowance (RDA) or RNI, allowance must also be made for the individual variability in requirements which, for healthy children, amounted to about 12.5% as a coefficient of variation (CV).

Requirements for growth

The variability of weight gain has to be considered when assessing the protein needs of children in every-day life. If energy intakes are high, but the quality or amount of protein or micronutrients is inadequate, then children, particularly when recovering from mal-nutrition, can put on weight as fat, with only modest increases in body protein. Different amounts of protein are also laid down from day to day, so in order to maintain an adequate average growth rate, the child must be provided with enough protein for the days when growth is rapid. The effect of the intermittent growth rate is therefore to increase requirements. In addition, children from developing countries are frequently ill with respiratory or gastrointestinal infections which arrest growth, impair absorption and reduce body weight. Additional protein (and energy) therefore needs to be available for catch-up growth. If allowance is made for the variability between individual children in their main-tenance requirement (CV 15%) and for the greater natural variation in growth rate (CV 35%), then RNI (see Chapter 49), which takes both of these into account, is likely to meet the needs of many children for catch-up growth. Under the scheme illustrated in Table 5.9, the higher the growth rate, the greater the need for total protein and for protein with a high amino acid score.

Amino acid scores

Traditionally, the amino acid composition of a protein was compared with that of milk or egg protein to assess whether it had sufficient essential amino acids to match those of milk or eggs, which have a composition similar to that found in total body protein. Rat growth studies showed the importance of having the correct complement of amino acids to allow growth to occur, so emphasis came to be laid on the importance of animal proteins in supporting growth. If a diet is based almost completely on cereals, then lysine, methionine plus cysteine, threonine and tryptophan are the most limiting amino acids. If, however, a diet is mixed, for example with additional beans or a mixture of different cereals, then the composition of one food will balance the other and compensate for deficiencies. If a small amount of animal protein is included in the diet, then it is unusual to find one of the amino acids to be limiting. If the lysine score of a food – for example, wheat – is 0.73, this means that 37% (i.e. (1–0.73)/0.73) more wheat would in theory be needed to make up the deficiency. Alternatively, adding an animal protein to the diet will improve the score and enhance the ability of a child to grow.

Digestibility

This will vary with the diet and tends to be less in children than in adults. Details can be found in the FAO/WHO/UNU report (FAO 1985). The digestibility figures provided in Table 5.9 only refer to the output of faecal nitrogen in excess of that observed on a milk diet, since the maintenance requirements were calculated assuming some faecal nitrogen loss.

In adults, the process of calculating requirements is a little simpler because no allowance for growth is needed. However, the same principles of adding the need for high-quality protein to dietary estimates will apply to people gaining weight as they recover from illness.

There are many outstanding issues in relation to amino acid and protein requirements. The contro-versy over the level of essential amino acids noted above is discussed more extensively in Chapter 51 because of its major policy issues.

REFERENCES

Abumrad NN, Williams P, Frexes-Steed M et al 1989 Inter-organ metabolism of amino acids in vivo. Diabetes/Metabolism Reviews 5: 213–226

Alpers DH 1987 Digestion and absorption of carbohydrates and proteins. In: Johnson LR (ed) Physiology of the gastrointestinal tract, 2nd edn, Volume 2. Raven Press, New York, pp. 1469–1487

Beaton GH, Chery A 1988 Protein requirements of infants: a reexamination of concepts and approaches. American Journal of Clinical Nutrition 48: 1403–1412

Bond JS, Butler PE 1987 Intracellular proteases. Annual Review of Biochemistry 56: 333–364

Darnell J, Lodish H, Baltimore D 1986 Molecular cell biology. Scientific American Books, New York, p. 59

Diem K 1962 Documenta Geigy Scientific Tables, 6th edn. Geigy UK, Macclesfield, p. 528

FAO/WHO/UNU 1985 Energy and protein requirements. Report of a joint expert consultation. WHO Technical Report Series no 724. Geneva, WHO

Fuller MF, McWilliam R, Wang TC, Giles LR 1989 The optimum dietary amino acid pattern for growing pigs. 2. Requirements for maintenance and for tissue protein accretion. British Journal of Nutrition 62: 255–267

Fürst P 1985 Regulation of intracellular metabolism of amino acids. In: Bozzetto F, Dionigi R (eds) Nutrition in cancer and trauma sepsis. (Proceedings of the Sixth Congress of ESPEN). Karger, Basle, pp. 21–53

Garlick PJ 1980 Protein turnover in the whole animal and specific tissues. In: Neuberger A (ed) Comprehensive biochemistry, Volume 19B. Elsevier, Amsterdam, pp. 77–210

Garlick PJ, Burns HJG, Palmer RM 1988 Regulation of muscle protein turnover: possible implications for modifying the responses to trauma and nutrient intake. Baillière's Clinical Gastroenterology 2: 915–940

Garlick PJ, Wernerman J, McNurlan MA, Heys SD 1991 Organ-specific measurements of protein turnover in man. Proceedings of the Nutrition Society 50: 217–225

Hopfer U 1987 Membrane transport mechanisms for hexoses and amino acids in the small intestine. In: Johnson LR (ed) Physiology of the gastrointestinal tract, 2nd edn, Volume 2. Raven Press, New York, pp. 1499–1526

Jackson AA 1989 Optimizing amino acid and protein supply and utilization in the newborn. Proceedings of the Nutrition Society 48: 293–301

James WPT 1977 Research in malnutrition and its application to parenteral feeding. In: Johnston IDA (ed) Advances in parenteral nutrition. (Proceedings of an International Symposium, Bermuda), pp. 521–531

Laidlaw SA, Kopple JD 1987 Newer concepts of the indispensable amino acids. American Journal of Clinical Nutrition 46: 593–605

Lentner C 1981 Geigy Scientific Tables, 8th edn. Volume 1: Units of measurement, body fluids, composition of the body, nutrition. Ciba-Geigy, Basle

Millward DJ, Rivers J 1988 The nutritional role of indispensable amino acids and the metabolic basis for their requirements. European Journal of Clinical Nutrition 42: 367–393

Millward DJ, Price GM, Pacy PH, Halliday D 1990 Maintenance protein requirements: the need for conceptual re-evaluation. Proceedings of the Nutrition Society 49: 473–487

Mortimore GE, Pösö AR, Lardeux BR 1989 Mechanism and regulation of protein degradation in liver. Diabetes/Metabolism Reviews 5: 49–70

Munro HL 1969 Mammalian protein metabolism, Volume III. Academic Press, New York

Munro HL 1970 Mammalian protein metabolism, Volume IV. Academic Press, New York

Munro HL, Allison JB 1964a Mammalian protein metabolism, Volume I. Academic Press, New York

Munro HL, Allison JB 1964b Mammalian protein metabolism, Volume II. Academic Press, New York

Reeds PJ 1990 Amino acid needs and protein scoring patterns. Proceedings of the Nutrition Society 49: 489–497

Reeds PJ, Garlick PJ 1984 Nutrition and protein turnover in man. In: Draper HH (ed) Advances in nutritional research, Volume 6. Plenum Press, New York, pp. 93–138

Sjölin J, Stjernström H, Henneberg S et al 1989 Splanchnic and peripheral release of 3-methylhistidine in relation to its urinary excretion in human infection. Metabolism 38: 23–29

Waterlow JC 1984 Protein turnover with special reference to man. Quarterly Journal of Experimental Physiology 69: 409–438

Waterlow JC, Jackson AA 1981 Nutrition and protein turnover in man. British Medical Bulletin 37: 5–10

Waterlow JC, Garlick PJ, Millward DJ 1978 Protein turnover in mammalian tissues and in the whole body. North Holland, Amsterdam

Wernerman J 1991 Ribosome profiles from human skeletal muscle as a measure of protein synthesis. Clinical Nutrition 10, Suppl: 6–11

Wernerman J, Vinnars E 1987 The effect of trauma and surgery on interorgan fluxes of amino acids in man. Clinical Science 73: 129–133

Young VR 1987 Kinetics of human amino acid metabolism, nutritional implications and some lessons. American Journal of Clinical Nutrition 46: 709–725

Young VR, Steffee WP, Pencharz PB, Winterer JC, Scrimshaw N S 1975 Total human body protein synthesis in relation to protein requirements at various ages. Nature 253: 192–194

Young VR, Bier DM, Pellet PL 1989 A theoretical basis for increasing current estimates of the amino acid requirements in adult man with experimental support. American Journal of Clinical Nutrition 50: 80–92

6. Fats

M. Gurr

SOME DEFINITIONS

Surprisingly, there is no precise definition of the word 'fat'. The term is generally applied to those foods that are obviously fatty in nature, greasy in texture and immiscible with water. Familiar everyday examples are butter and other spreads, cooking oils and the fatty parts of meats. We think of fats as solid in texture, as distinct from oils, which are liquid at ambient temperatures. Chemically, however, there is little distinction between a fat and an oil, since the substances that the layman regards as fats are all composed predominantly of esters of glycerol with fatty acids.

Edible fats are triacylglycerols (Fig. 6.1a) and are chemically quite distinct from the oils used in the petroleum industry, which are hydrocarbons. The melting points of the triacylglycerols (and, therefore, the degree of 'hardness' of the fat) increase with the chain lengths of the constituent fatty acids and their degree of saturation (Table 6.1 and see Fig. 6.2). Thus, the 'hard fats', such as lard, contain a relatively high proportion of saturated long-chain fatty acids.

Chemists and biochemists use the term 'lipid' to describe a chemically varied group of substances that have in common the property of being insoluble in water but soluble in solvents such as chloroform, hydrocarbons, alcohols or ethers (Gunstone & Norris 1983, Gurr & Harwood 1991, Gurr 1992). This definition includes a far wider range of chemical substances than simply the triacylglycerols; for example the phospholipids (Fig. 6.1b), glycolipids (Fig. 6.1c), sterols (Fig. 6.1d) and the fat-soluble vitamins (Chapter 13). In this chapter, we will tend to reserve the word fats for the fatty components of foods and diets and use the word lipid when discussing the metabolism of fats in the body.

In nutrition and dietetics, a distinction is often made between 'visible' and 'invisible fats'. Visible fats are those clearly apparent to the consumer: the spreads, the cooking oils and the fat on meats. In contrast, a great deal of the fat in many of our foods is

Table 6.1 Some important fatty acids in foods

Common name	Chemical name	Shorthand nomenclature
Saturated		
Short chain		
Butyric	Butanoic	4:0
Caproic	Hexanoic	6:0
Medium chain		
Caprylic	Octanoic	8:0
Capric	Decanoic	10:0
Long chain		
Lauric	Dodecanoic	12:0
Myristic	Tetradecanoic	14:0
Palmitic	Hexadecanoic	16:0
Stearic	Octadecanoic	18:0
Monounsaturated		
Oleic	*cis*-9-Octadecenoic	18:1 (*n*-9)
Elaidic	*trans*-9-Octadecenoic	
Erucic	*cis*-13-Docosenoic	22:1 (*n*-9)
Polyunsaturated		
Linoleic	*cis*, *cis*-9,12-Octadecadienoic	18:2 (*n*-6)
α-Linolenic	all-*cis*-9,12,15-Octadecatrienoic	18:3 (*n*-3)
Arachidonic	all-*cis*-5,8,11,14-20:4 Eicosatetraenoic	20:4 (*n*-6)
EPA	all-*cis*-5,8,11,14,17-Eicosapentaenoic	20:5 (*n*-3)
DHA	all-*cis*-4,7,10,13,16,19-docosahexaenoic	22:6 (*n*-3)

In the shorthand system, the number before the colon denotes the number of carbon atoms in the fatty acid hydrocarbon chain and the number after the colon, the number of double bonds. The number in parenthesis denotes the unsaturated fatty acid 'family' according to the positional distribution of the double bonds. When the double bond furthest from the carboxyl group is three carbons from the methyl end of the chain, the acid belongs to the *n*-3 family; similarly, the *n*-6 and *n*-9 families have the terminal double bond 6 and 9 carbons from the methyl terminal respectively. If it is required to specify the position from the carboxyl end (as in the official chemical naming system), the shorthand can be written: *c*9-18:1, *c*9, *c*12-18:2 etc (*c* and *t* are the shorthand forms for *cis* and *trans* respectively).

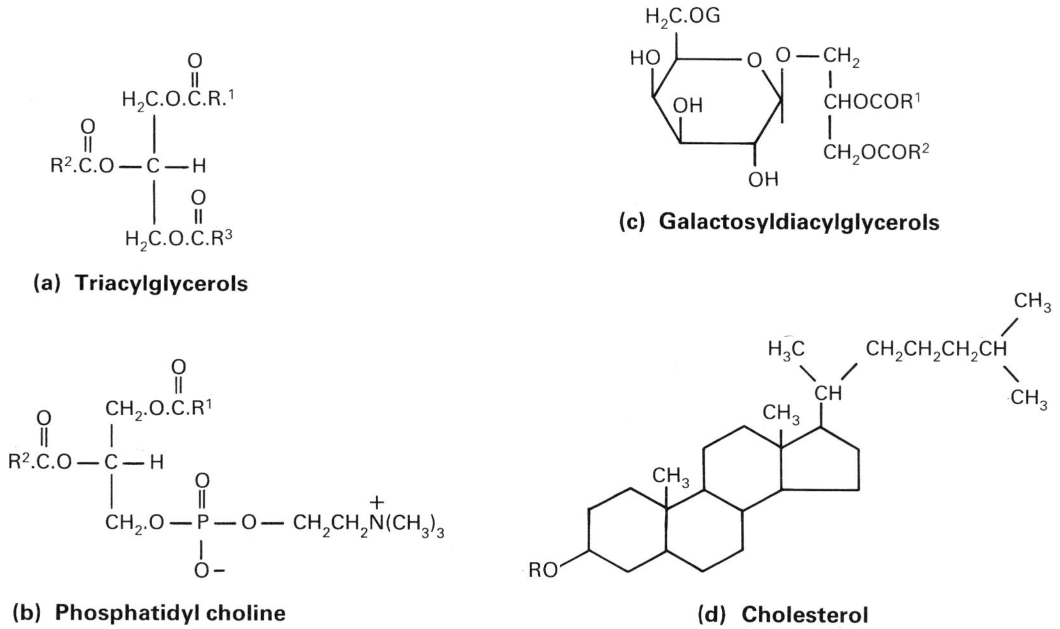

(a) Triacylglycerols

(c) Galactosyldiacylglycerols

(b) Phosphatidyl choline

(d) Cholesterol

Fig. 6.1 Structures of some important food and body lipids. (a) Triacylglycerols (sometimes called triglycerides) are the major storage lipids; R represents the hydrocarbon chain of the fatty acids; (b) Phosphoglycerides: a subclass of a broader group of lipids that contain phosphorus; generally called phospholipids. R represents the hydrocarbon chain of the fatty acids; several low-molecular-weight bases can be esterified with the phosphate; the commonest is choline ($OH.CH_2.CH_2.N^+(CH_3)_3$) in which case the phospholipid is phosphatidylcholine, sometimes called by its trivial name lecithin. Other bases present in naturally occurring phospholipids are ethanolamine, serine, inositol and glycerol; the positions occupied by fatty acids are numbered 1 and 2; the phosphate is at position 3. When the hydroxyl at position 2 is free and not esterified with a fatty acid, the compound is known as known as a lysophospholipid (e.g. lysophosphatidylcholine); (c) Galactosyldiacylglycerols: here a sugar replaces the phosphate ester; R again represents fatty acid hydrocarbon chains; G may be hydrogen, in which case the lipid is monogalactosyldiacylglycerol or another galactose molecule, in which case the lipid is digalactosyldiacylglycerol; (d) Cholesterol: cholesterol is the main sterol of animal tissues and is present as the free alcohol (in which group R is a hydrogen atom) or as cholesteryl esters (in which group R is a fatty acid).

hidden by incorporation during preparation and cooking, for example in cakes, biscuits and potato crisps, or in the formulation of processed meats and sausages and in emulsions such as mayonnaises. Like the visible fats, these hidden fats will be mainly triacylglycerols, but hidden fats may also be present in the membranes of plant and animal tissues, and these will be mainly the phospholipids, glycolipids and cholesterol. Hence, the total fat in the diet is hard to measure, because different samples of the same food may vary widely in fat content as well as in fat type, especially in the case of meat. Only approximate figures for total fat content are provided by food tables or nutritional labelling.

TYPES OF FATS IN THE BODY AND THEIR FUNCTIONS

The pioneering work on the chemistry of the natural fats was by the Liverpool chemist T. P. Hilditch and his classic book *The chemical composition of natural fats* (Hilditch & Williams 1964) makes fascinating reading, although the painstaking chemical techniques that he had to use have been supplanted by modern chromatographic methods.

Lipid molecules of various types are important constituents of all cells in the body. It is convenient to divide them into three categories: 1) structural, 2) storage, and 3) metabolic fats. It should be emphasized, however, that there is considerable overlap between these types. Structural fats may also perform a storage function; metabolic fats are derived from both storage and structural fats and sometimes the same molecules may fulfil all three roles (Gurr 1992).

Structural fats

Structural fats are those that contribute to the architecture of cells, mainly as constituents of cell membranes. In animal membranes the phosphoglycerides are the major lipids, while in plant cells the glycosyl-glycerides predominate (Fig. 6.1c). Phosphoglycerides are mixed acid esters of glycerol with two fatty acid and one phosphoric acid residues (Fig. 6.1b). (The general term to describe lipids containing phosphorus is 'phospholipid'. Some phospholipids are derivatives of the base sphingosine rather than glycerol, but for practical dietetic purposes only the phosphoglycerides need be considered.) The student interested in the chemistry of food phosphoglycerides should consult Gunstone & Norris (1983), Mead et al (1986), Gurr & Harwood (1991), Ansell et al (1973), Vance & Vance (1985) and Gurr et al (1992) for the more detailed chemistry and biochemistry of lipids and their constituent fatty acids. Phospholipids are called 'polar' lipids or, more technically 'amphiphilic' lipids (from the Greek: 'liking both', because they possess chemical groupings that associate with water (hydrophilic groups) in juxtaposition with hydrophobic moieties that are lipid-soluble. For example, the most abundant animal phospholipid, phosphatidylcholine (Fig. 6.1b) contains a polar moiety consisting of the negatively charged phosphate residue and the positively charged choline group. The fatty acids are responsible for the fat-like properties.

Fatty acids consist of hydrocarbon chains with a terminal carboxyl group, and it is the latter that forms the ester linkage with glycerol in the phosphoglycerides and triacylglycerols. Naturally occurring fatty acids normally have even-numbered carbon chains ranging from 4 to 22 carbon atoms in length, although chains with an odd number of carbon atoms do occur and it is possible to find chain lengths longer than 22. Sometimes the chains may be branched or contain various constituents such as hydroxyl groups. Despite the bewildering variety of fatty acids found in nature, those of quantitative significance in human nutrition are limited in number and are shown in Table 6.1. The carbon chains may be completely saturated or contain one (monounsaturated) or several (polyunsaturated) ethylenic double bonds. The most important structures are illustrated in Fig. 6.2.

In biological membranes, the phospholipid molecules associate together to form a bilayer that forms a continuum throughout the membrane, with the fatty acid chains pointing inwards towards each other and the polar headgroups on the surfaces (Singer & Nicolson 1972). In the membranes of nervous tissue and in most plant membranes, glycolipids (those in which the polar moiety is a sugar rather than a phosphodiester) are important constituents of the bilayer. Protein molecules, which may have a mainly structural function or serve as enzymes or receptor molecules, are inserted into the phospholipid bilayer, interacting by non-covalent forces with both the polar and non-polar regions of the lipids (Fig. 6.3). They may be located at external or internal faces or project through from one side to the other. Lipid molecules are quite mobile along the plane of the membrane, and there may be limited movement across the membrane. Indeed the patterns of lipid molecules on each side of some membranes are quite different, a phenomenon known as 'membrane asymmetry' (Rothman & Lenard 1977). The fatty acid chains are in constant motion, and the degree of molecular motion within the membrane (often referred to as 'fluidity') is influenced by the nature of the fatty acid chains, interactions between the fatty acid chains and cholesterol, and interactions between proteins and lipids.

The chemistry of the individual fatty acids influences their shape (Fig. 6.4), which in turn determines the space they occupy in the bilayer. Straight-chain saturated fatty acids can pack together in an almost crystalline array, and molecular motion tends to be minimized compared with unsaturated or branched acids, which occupy more space (Fig. 6.3) and are more mobile. A relatively high proportion of unsaturated fatty acids, and especially polyunsaturated fatty acids, seems to be an essential requisite for the proper functioning of cell membranes. Dietary fat is able to influence membrane composition, but only within certain limits. Storage fats, by contrast, are far more variable in composition (see below). Foods containing membranes are, therefore, important sources of certain polyunsaturated fatty acids in the diet.

Cholesterol plays an important role in stabilizing the hydrophobic interactions within animal membranes by inserting itself between the fatty chains in the bilayer (Fig. 6.3). Animals consuming diets relatively rich in polyunsaturated fatty acids tend to accumulate a higher proportion of these acids in the membrane bilayer. Under these circumstances the proportion of cholesterol to phospholipids increases, maintaining the fluidity of the membrane constant (Edwards-Webb & Gurr 1988). The metabolic functions of the membrane require that fluidity be maintained within certain limits (Wahle 1983). For reasons that are not completely understood, cholesterol seems to be the only sterol that will allow the proper functioning of animal membranes. Plant membranes, in contrast, have little or no cholesterol and contain mainly β-sitosterol. Dietary cholesterol, therefore, comes almost entirely from animal foods.

Membranes can be thought of as barriers between

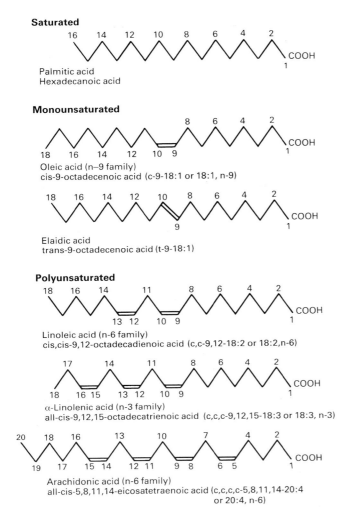

Saturated

Palmitic acid
Hexadecanoic acid

Monounsaturated

Oleic acid (n–9 family)
cis-9-octadecenoic acid (c-9-18:1 or 18:1, n-9)

Elaidic acid
trans-9-octadecenoic acid (t-9-18:1)

Polyunsaturated

Linoleic acid (n-6 family)
cis,cis-9,12-octadecadienoic acid (c,c-9,12-18:2 or 18:2,n-6)

α-Linolenic acid (n-3 family)
all-cis-9,12,15-octadecatrienoic acid (c,c,c-9,12,15-18:3 or 18:3, n-3)

Arachidonic acid (n-6 family)
all-cis-5,8,11,14-eicosatetraenoic acid (c,c,c,c-5,8,11,14-20:4
or 20:4, n-6)

Fig. 6.2 Some fatty acids occurring in food and body lipids. The zig-zag lines represent hydrocarbon chains, with a carbon atom at the intersection of lines: thus, ⌇⌇⌇ represents CH_2-CH_2-CH_2-CH=CH-CH_2 etc. According to a biochemical convention, the numbering of the carbon chain is from the carboxyl group (-COOH). Thus a substituent such as a methyl group on the 4th carbon from the carboxyl group of a 16-carbon saturated fatty acid would be 4-methyl-hexadec*a*noic acid, etc. If a double bond occurs between carbon atoms 9 and 10 of an 18-carbon acid, the fatty acid is called 9-octadec*e*noic acid. The nomenclature *n-3*, *n-6*, *n-9* describes families of fatty acids in which the last double bond in the chain is 3, 6, or 9 carbon atoms from the methyl end of the molecule. The suffixes *c* and *t* below double bonds in the formulae denote the geometrical configuration of the double bond, *cis* or *trans*. The terms 'monounsaturated' and 'monoenoic' etc. are interchangeable. In subsequent figures and tables in this chapter, a common shorthand notation for fatty acids will be used. In this system, the fatty acid is identified by a number denoting the number of carbon atoms in its hydrocarbon chain, followed by a colon, followed by a number denoting the number of double bonds. Thus, stearic acid (18 carbon atoms with no double bonds) is represented as 18:0 and octadecenoic acids (18 carbon atoms with 1 double bond in an unspecified position and with an unspecified geometrical configuration) as 18:1, etc. If the unsaturated acid needs to be identified more precisely, it can be done by indicating the position(s) and configuration(s) of the double bonds, thus: oleic acid, *c*9-18:1; linoleic acid, *c*9, *c*12-18:2, etc. In some cases, it is useful to specify the family to which the fatty acid belongs; thus, 18:3 may be either 18:3*n*-3 (α-linolenic acid, all-*cis*-9,12,15-18:3) or 18:3*n*-6 (γ-linolenic acid, all-*cis*-6,9,12-18:3).

the cell and its environment, or between one part of a cell and another. Another sort of barrier in which structural lipids are important is the surface of the skin, or fur in animals, or the leaf surface of plants. These 'surface lipids' are not very important in nutrition, but are interesting in that their composition is quite different from other lipids in comprising significant quantities of odd-chain and branched-chain fatty acids, acids with double bonds in unusual positions, and sterols of different structures. The skin is an important source of vitamin D (see Chapter 13).

Storage fats

Storage fats are those that provide a long-term reserve of metabolic fuel for the organism. Triacylglycerols are

by far the most important storage form of lipids (see Fig. 6.1a). (In older biochemical literature and in current literature for the more general reader, you will normally find these compounds referred to as triglycerides. The term 'triacylglycerol' is the officially approved nomenclature and will be used throughout this chapter. It is entirely synonymous with triglyceride.)

There tends to be a distinction between the types of fatty acids fulfilling a storage role (and, therefore, esterified in triacylglycerols) and those playing a structural role (and, therefore, found mainly in amphiphilic lipids). Storage fats tend to contain a higher proportion of saturated or monounsaturated fatty acids, although this is only a general guideline, since the composition of storage lipids is influenced strongly by the fatty acid composition of the diet in simple-stomached animals,

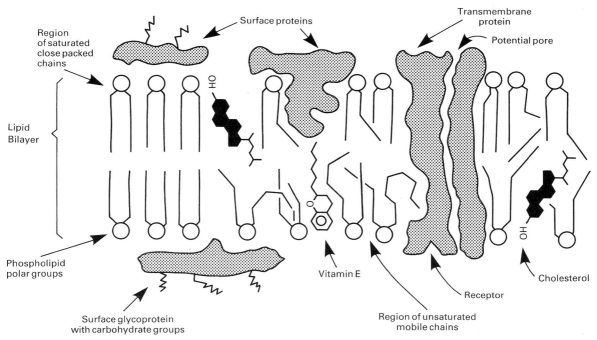

Fig. 6.3 Lipids in biological membranes. A schematic representation of what a biological membrane might look like. The small spheres are the polar head groups of phospholipid molecules which form a double layer (lipid bilayer) throughout the membrane with fatty acid chains (represented by the tails) pointing inwards towards each other. Cholesterol and vitamin E are inserted between the fatty acid chains. Protein molecules (represented by large stippled shapes) are inserted at intervals into the bilayer, sometimes mainly at one face or the other, sometimes extending right through. Sugar groups are attached to the surface proteins.

or by the fermentative activities of the rumen micro-organisms in ruminants.

In man and the animals that provide man's food, the biggest reservoir of fatty acids to supply the long-term needs for energy is the adipose tissue (see section on metabolism, below). Other tissues, such as the liver of mammals, can accommodate fat in the form of small globules, but only in the short term. The excessive accumulation of fat in mammalian liver is a pathological condition. Many species of fish that contribute to the human diet, however, normally store fat in the liver or flesh rather than in the adipose tissue (Wiseman 1984).

Milk fat is also a form of energy store, for the benefit of the newborn and, like adipose tissue fat, is composed mainly of triacylglycerols (Christie 1983). Egg-yolk lipids likewise provide a store of fuel for the developing embryo. In western countries, where the amount of fat in the diet is generally high, human adipose tissue normally stores fatty acids derived from the diet. When the diet is rich in carbohydrates, as occurs in some countries, or in commercially impor-

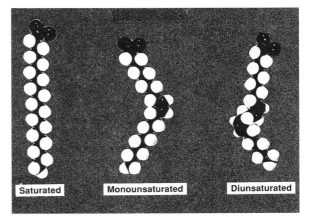

Fig. 6.4 Space-filling molecular models indicating the shapes of fatty acids.

tant animals such as pigs, cattle and poultry, the adipose tissue is able to synthesize fatty acids, mainly palmitic, stearic (saturated) and oleic (monounsaturated). The mammary gland is unique in making short- and medium-chain fatty acids (chain lengths up to 10 or 12 carbon atoms), whereas all other tissues produce long-chain fatty acids (mainly 16 and 18 carbon atoms). The pattern of milk fatty acids is characteristic of each species. In ruminants, the composition is markedly influenced by the activities of the rumen microorganisms, while in simple-stomached animals, the composition is influenced by the amount and type of fat in the diet (Wiseman 1984).

Metabolic fats

Storage fats and structural fats are present in bulk. They fulfil their specialized functions as a result of their chemical and physical properties. Thus, triacylglycerols are ideal for storage since they have an energy density over twice that of carbohydrates, and they take up less space than, say, glycogen, as they are not hydrated. The amphiphilic properties of phospholipids are ideal for membrane structure: they can interact with both proteins and non-polar lipids, and the lipid in the bilayer provides an insulating environment for the metabolic activities of the membrane.

Metabolic fats is a term that refers to those lipids that as individual molecules undergo metabolic transformations to produce a specific substance of physiological and nutritional importance. The molecules in question are no different from those classified earlier as storage or structural lipids, and indeed, metabolic lipids are derived from these other compartments.

Thus, fatty acids make a major contribution to the production of cellular energy, but must first be released from storage fats and directed into metabolic pathways in the mitochondria of cells to generate usable chemical energy. Specific types of unsaturated fatty acids that are stored in the membrane phospholipids can be released and transformed into hormone-like substances called 'eicosanoids'.

Cholesterol is metabolized in the adrenal gland to a variety of steroid hormones, and in the liver to a variety of bile acids that are secreted in the bile and are subsequently involved in the digestion and absorption of dietary fats in the alimentary tract.

Fat-soluble vitamins also participate in metabolic processes of diverse kinds, many of them incompletely understood. They may be stored in the adipose tissue or liver for some time before being involved in these processes. Vitamin E is stored in the membrane lipid bilayers, where it serves to prevent the oxidation of the highly unsaturated membrane fatty acids.

These various metabolic functions will be discussed in more detail in a later section on lipid metabolism.

FATS IN TRANSPORT

Body fats, even when they are part of structural or storage pools, are in a dynamic state. There is a continuous exchange of fatty acids in membranes or in adipose tissue with fatty acids in the blood. Fats have to be transported from tissues where they are synthesized, into storage, or from storage pools to sites of metabolism. Fats absorbed from the alimentary tract after the digestion of fats in the diet have to be transported to sites of storage or metabolism, depending on the animal's current energy state. The mode of transport of lipids in the blood is by means of large particles that are aggregates of many lipid molecules stabilized by a surface amphiphilic coat of proteins and polar lipids. These are the lipoproteins (see Fig. 6.9, Table 6.6). They play a key role in lipid metabolism, and defects in lipoprotein transport are reflected in a number of common metabolic diseases.

FATS IN FOODS

Food fats from adipose tissue

These are not only the visible fats attached to meats, but also cooking fats processed from adipose tissue, such as lard and suet. Although predominantly composed of triacylglycerols, the fat also contains some cholesterol, the fat-soluble vitamins A, D, E and K, and also small traces of fat-soluble substances from the environment, such as pesticides and antioxidants added to the animal feed.

Although palmitic and oleic acids are likely to be the major components whatever the source of the fat, the proportions of the different fatty acids are markedly affected by the diet of simple-stomached animals, of which pigs and poultry are economically the most important (Wiseman 1984). Thus, the inclusion of vegetable oils in pig and poultry diets results in a higher proportion of linoleic acid and a lower proportion of palmitic and oleic acids than the inclusion of tallow, which tends to give a body fat similar to that of animals fed on cereals alone (Table 6.2). Feeding supplements that contain high proportions of lipids with unsaturated fatty acids, or including appreciable amounts of copper in pig diets, result in a soft back fat (Wiseman 1984). This may be useful to encourage a higher polyunsaturated to saturated fatty acid (P/S) ratio in the human diet, but

Table 6.2 Fatty acid composition of some animal storage fats important in foods

Food fat	4:0–12:0	14:0	16:0	16:1	18:0	18:1	18:2	20:1 22:1	LC PUFA	Others
				g/100 g total fatty acids						
Lard (1)	0	1	29	3	15	43	9	0	0	0
Lard (2)	0	1	21	3	12	46	16	0	0	1
Poultry	0	1	27	9	7	45	11	0	0	1
Beef suet	0	3	26	9	8	45	2	0	0	7
Lamb	0	3	21	4	20	41	5	0	0	6
Milk (cow)	13	12	26	3	11	29	2	0	0	4
Milk (goat)	21	11	27	3	10	26	2	0	0	0
Egg yolk	0	0	29	4	9	43	11	0	0	4
Cod-liver oil	0	6	13	13	3	20	2	18	20	5

LC PUFA = long-chain polyunsaturated fatty acids

may be counterproductive if the purchaser is averse to the texture of the fat, as some surveys show.

Ruminant adipose tissue fat (mainly beef and mutton fat in the UK) is less variable than that of pigs and poultry because 90% of the unsaturated fatty acids in the animals' diets are hydrogenated (i.e. converted into relatively more saturated fatty acids by the reduction of double bonds) by microorganisms in the rumen (Table 6.2). The fat, therefore, contains a higher proportion of saturated and monounsaturated fatty acids and a lower proportion of polyunsaturated fatty acids than pig fat (i.e. lard) and poultry fat. It also contains more *trans*unsaturated and branched-chain fatty acids. *Trans* double bonds are formed by isomerization of the more common *cis* double bonds during the hydrogenation process catalysed by enzymes in certain of the anaerobic rumen micro-organisms (Gurr & Harwood 1991).

In traditional farming practice, ruminants feed on pasture or on cereal-based concentrates that have a low fat content. Variations in adipose tissue fatty acid composition can occur, depending on the species of animal and the type of feed. For example, feeding sheep a diet rich in barley leads to much higher proportions of branched-chain fatty acids and results in a softer carcase fat. A more recent trend, to improve the efficiency of animal production, is to feed ruminants, especially dairy cows, fat supplements or crushed oilseeds (Wiseman 1984). In this way, modest changes in adipose tissue composition can be effected, although not so extensive as by feeding so-called 'protected' fat, in which the fat particles are treated in such a way as to prevent hydrogenation in the rumen (McDonald & Scott 1977). It was thought that these products would be useful for people on lipid-lowering diets (see Chapter 41), but they have not been successful in the marketplace because of their cost and their susceptibility to oxidative deterioration,

contributing to poor taste and a short shelf-life. It is more effective to approach the problem of lipid lowering by using lean meat, which provides mainly structural fat with a high P/S ratio (Watts et al 1988).

Milk fat

Cows' milk and the dairy products derived from it currently contribute 24% of the fat in the UK diet, although this figure is slowly decreasing as the sales of lower-fat milks increase at the expense of full-fat milk. In 1983 only 3% of liquid milk sold in the UK was of the lower-fat varieties, whereas in 1991 the figure was 42%. Cow's milk is the only milk of quantitative importance in the UK, but in some countries goat's and sheep's milk are of considerable importance, and there is increasing interest in these milks in the UK.

Milk fat (Christie 1983) is composed mainly of triacylglycerols, which are present as an emulsion in which the fat globules are stabilized by a surrounding membrane composed of proteins, phospholipids and cholesterol. The fat globules also contain small amounts of cholesterol esters and fat-soluble vitamins, mainly A, D and β-carotene. The fatty acid composition of ruminant milk fat is characterized by a high proportion of short- and medium-chain saturated fatty acids, long-chain saturated and monounsaturated fatty acids, and very small proportions of polyunsaturated fatty acids (see Table 6.2). They also contain small quantities of a wide variety of branched- and odd-chain fatty acids.

Butter is a common food fat, containing 15% water as an emulsion in oil. The fat is derived entirely from cow's milk fat and its composition does not normally vary greatly, compared with margarines which do. Experimentally it has been shown that feeding cattle supplements of varieties of oats with a high fat content or feeding crushed oilseeds can elevate the proportion of oleic acid (see Table 6.5). Commercial exploitation of this finding could have two advantages, first in providing a product that is more spreadable from the refrigerator, and therefore more convenient, and secondly in providing a product with a higher unsaturated to saturated fatty acid ratio.

Cream is an example of an emulsion of milk fat in water whose textural properties and quantitative contribution of fat to the diet depend on the total concentration of fat in the emulsion. Fat emulsions markedly influence the palatability of food.

Eggs

Eggs provide a significant source of fat in many human diets. One egg on average provides 6–7 g triacylglycerols and phospholipids and 250–300 mg cholesterol. The fatty acid composition is shown in Table 6.2. The importance of eggs in food lies not only in the nutritive value of the fats, but in the contribution made by the egg-yolk lipoproteins to the structure of food, particularly to the textural quality of cake after baking.

Fish oils

Fish are classified broadly into 'lean' fish that store their reserve fats as triacylglycerols in the liver (e.g. cod), or 'fatty' fish (e.g. mackerel, herring) where the fat is located in the flesh. In either case, the oils have a high content of fatty acids with 20 or more carbon atoms, a high proportion of which contain five or six double bonds and belong to the 'n-3' family (see Tables 6.1, 6.2). These are broad generalizations; wide variations in fatty acid composition occur depending on the species of fish, its diet and the season of the year.

Muscle meats

The fats eaten in muscle meats comprise mainly phospholipids and free cholesterol, although in many meat animals the muscles are infiltrated with storage triacylglycerols (marbling). Five fatty acids account for over 85% of the total muscle fatty acids: palmitic, stearic, oleic, linoleic and arachidonic acids (Table 6.3). The composition of the marble fat tends to resemble more the composition of the adipose tissue.

Vegetable oils

Most oil-bearing plants store their fat as triacylglcerols in the seed endosperm (e.g. rape, sunflower, soybean) or the fleshy fruit exocarp (e.g. avocado). Some, like the palm, store the oil in both the exocarp (palm oil) and the endosperm (palm kernel oil). Seed oils vary widely in their fatty acid compositions (see Table 6.4) (Gunstone et al 1986). One fatty acid usually predominates, is frequently of unusual structure and is characteristic of the particular plant family. Seed oils that are of dietary importance, however, are generally those in which the predominant fatty acids are the common ones: palmitic, stearic, oleic and linoleic acids. The exceptions are coconut and palm kernel oils, which are unusual in containing saturated fatty acids of medium chain length (C8–C14). Elsewhere in nature, only milk fat contains these acids.

Seed oils are also important dietary sources of phospholipids, chlorophylls, carotenoids, tocopherols and plant sterols, such as β-sitosterol, although the latter is not absorbed from the human gut. Some may contain unusual fatty acids which, if ingested in large amounts, may have toxic or otherwise undesirable metabolic effects. A good example is the old variety of

Table 6.3 Fatty acid composition of some structural fats important in foods

Food	16:0	16:1	18:0	18:1	18:2	18:3	20:4	LC PUFA	Others
			g/100 g total fatty acids						
Beef (muscle)	16	2	11	20	26	1	13	0	11
Lamb (muscle)	22	2	13	30	18	4	7	0	4
Lamb (brain)	22	1	18	28	1	0	4	14	12
Chicken (muscle)	23	6	12	33	18	1	6	0	1
Chicken (liver)	25	3	17	26	15	1	6	6	1
Pork (muscle)	19	2	12	19	26	0	8	0	14
Cod (flesh)	22	2	4	11	1	trace	4	52	4
Green leaves	13	3	trace	7	16	56	0	0	5

LC PUFA = long-chain polyunsaturated fatty acids
Source: Gurr (1992)

Table 6.4 The fatty acid compositions of some vegetable oils important in foods

Oil	8:0	10:0	12:0	14:0	16:0	18:0	18:1	18:2	18:3	20:1 +22:1	Others
					g/100 g total fatty acids						
Avocado	0	0	0	0	20	1	60	18	0	0	1
Coconut	8	7	48	16	9	2	7	2	0	0	1
Corn	0	0	0	1	14	2	30	50	2	0	1
Olive	0	0	0	trace	12	2	72	11	1	0	2
Palm	0	0	trace	1	42	4	43	8	trace	0	2
Palm kernel	4	4	45	18	9	3	15	2	0	0	0
Peanut	0	0	trace	1	11	3	49	29	1	0	6
Rape (high erucic)	0	0	0	trace	4	1	24	16	11	43	1
Rape (low erucic)	0	0	0	trace	4	1	54	23	10	trace	8
Safflower (high oleic)	0	0	0	0	5	2	73	17	1	0	2
Safflower (high linoleic)	0	0	0	0	6	3	15	73	1	0	2
Soyabean	0	0	trace	trace	10	4	25	52	7	0	2
Sunflower	0	0	trace	trace	6	6	33	52	trace	0	3

Adapted from Gurr (1992) and Mattson & Grundy (1985)

rapeseed, which contained the 22-carbon monoenoic fatty acid erucic acid (see Table 6.4). When toxicity studies with experimental animals indicated that high dietary concentrations of rapeseed oil could cause lipid infiltration into heart muscle followed by necrosis of the tissue, the plant breeders embarked on a breeding programme to eliminate the erucic acid, thought to be the toxic constituent. Most varieties now grown are of the 'zero erucic' type. It was never demonstrated scientifically, however, that toxic effects would occur in man.

Plant leaves

The structural lipids of plant leaves, provided by such foods as lettuce, cabbage and other green vegetables, provide most of the α-linolenic acid in the diet. The fatty acid composition is very simple and varies little between different types of leaves. Five fatty acids account for over 90% of the total: palmitic, hexadecenoic, oleic, linoleic and α-linolenic (see Table 6.3) (Gunstone et al 1986).

MODIFICATION OF FATS DURING FOOD PROCESSING

Margarine is the oldest example of a fat manufactured to simulate a natural product – butter – although there are now many more fat spreads available with different compositions and physical characteristics (Table 6.5).

Modern margarine, like butter, is an emulsion of

Table 6.5 The fatty acid compositions of some familiar spreading fats

Spread	Average fat content of product (g/100 g product)	4:0– 12:0	14:0	16:0	18:0	20:0	22:0	16:1	18:1	20:1	22:1	18:2	18:3	20:4 +20:5	22:5 +22:6	Others
							(g/100 g total fatty acids)									
Butter*	85	13	12	26	11	0	0	3	28	0	0	2	trace	0	0	5
Butter†	85	9	7	20	14	0	0	2	35	0	0	5	1	0	0	7
Hard margarine	85	trace	6	20	8	2	2	6	22	9	9	5	trace	7	4	0
Soft margarine	85	1	5	16	5	2	3	6	25	7	9	9	trace	7	5	0
Polyunsaturated margarine	85	3	1	11	9	1	1	trace	18	1	1	53	1	trace	trace	0
Blended low-fat spread	50	12	9	24	9	0	0	2	21	0	0	14	trace	0	0	9

Compiled from Gurr (1992)
*Normal butter from cows grazed on pasture
†Butter from cows grazed on pasture with supplement of crushed soybeans

water in fat. The aqueous component is skimmed milk (or sometimes an artificial 'milk' made by adding dried protein to water) which has been incubated briefly with lactic acid bacteria. These organisms break down the lactose, proteins and fats in the milk to a very small extent, and in the process low-molecular-weight fermentation products are formed, which contribute to the flavour. This is not unlike the process used for making yoghurt, but is not continued long enough for the milk to curdle. All margarines are made by blending fats and oils from different animal and vegetable sources, the blend depending on the supply and cost of oils at a given time, and the physical and nutritional properties desired for a particular branded product (e.g. hard, soft, polyunsaturated, etc). Some natural oils (e.g. fish, soybean), because of their degree of unsaturation, have melting points that are too low for successful product formulation. They would also oxidize readily and so have too short a shelf-life before becoming inedible. This problem is normally overcome by catalytic hydrogenation (Gunstone & Norris 1983, Perkins & Visek 1983), which results in a decrease in the number of double bonds, an increase in the proportion of *trans* fatty acids and a randomization of double-bond positions along the chain. Other processing techniques include inter-esterification (which randomizes the positions of the fatty acids on the triacylglycerol molecules; in natural oils they are specifically distributed) or fractionation (which separates out fats of different melting points).

As explained above, seed oils rich in polyunsaturated fatty acids are liquid at room temperature, and in the earlier days of margarine making, the only way to achieve a solid margarine was to hydrogenate the oil. The solid physical characteristics of the 'high polyunsaturates' margarines which are now widely available are achieved not by hydrogenation but by clever use of emulsifier technology. Margarine and butter are known technically as 'water-in-oil emulsions', i.e. the predominant phase is oil with water droplets dispersed in it. Cream, by contrast, is an 'oil-in-water emulsion'. So that the oil and water phases do not separate (such as, for instance, when French dressing is left standing), the emulsion must be stabilized, and this is achieved by the use of an emulsifier, i.e. a chemical that has both hydrophilic (water-attracting) and lipophilic (fat-attracting) parts of the molecule. The molecules form a coat around the droplets of oil or water and keep them in suspension. Examples of natural emulsifiers are the bile salts (see Figs 6.7, 6.8) and the apolipoproteins.

Emulsifiers used in the food industry include phospholipids and lysophospholipids, monoglycerides and a number of approved synthetic emulsifiers. By choosing appropriate emulsifiers and blending with carefully selected oils, even highly polyunsaturated oils can be incorporated into a solid (albeit soft) margarine. Nevertheless, even soft margarines need to incorporate some 'hardstock' (i.e. a small amount of a hard fat) to achieve the required physical properties. Examples of margarine compositions are given in Table 6.5. Even within a particular margarine brand, the composition may change within defined limits from batch to batch because fats and oils are blended to give a least-cost formulation. Therefore, these compositions should be regarded as rough guides only.

With the skilful use of modern emulsifier technology, the aqueous phase can be increased from about 15% in margarines to around 70% to give low-fat spreads that may have applications in energy-reduced diets. Other manufactured fats, such as shortenings, whose role is to 'shorten' or tenderize baked foods by preventing the cohesion of wheat gluten strands, do not contain an aqueous phase. They are made from mixtures of partially hydrogenated vegetable oils with or without animal fats, and are found in biscuits, cakes, doughnuts, pastries, breads and many fried foods.

HOW DO WE DETERMINE FOOD FAT CONTENT AND COMPOSITION?

Nutritionists need to be able to quantify, easily and accurately, the total fat content of a food or of a whole diet, and to determine the amount of different types of fat present. Moreover, to be able to make the appropriate food choices, consumers need education in the nature and distribution of food fats. An important aid to food selection is the sensible labelling of products, and to supply this information the food manufacturer needs at his command an appropriate analytical facility. It is important to decide precisely what information is required, because although modern technology is capable of providing extremely detailed analytical data for individual lipid components, the consumer seldom requires this amount of detail. The provision of extensive analytical data would certainly add to the cost of the product, so that it is important to distinguish between the basic information that is useful to consumers, and the more detailed data required by the research nutritionist or the hospital dietitian.

Extraction of fat (Osborne & Voogt 1978, Christie 1982, Gunstone & Norris 1983)

A commonly used method is to extract the finely divided dried food by continuous refluxing with light petroleum. This method determines only the readily extractable storage fats and is limited in its application. In the Weibull method, wet proteinaceous foods with a low carbohydrate content are treated first by boiling with dilute hydrochloric acid to break the chemical bonds that bind the lipids into the structure of the food, before extraction with light petroleum. Alternatively, the Roese-Gottlieb method employs an initial treatment with an alcoholic solution of ammonia to disrupt the lipid-protein bonds without breaking down heat and acid-sensitive carbohydrates, which would interfere with the extraction. These methods extract mainly the hydrophobic lipids. Extraction with a mixture of two volumes chloroform and one of methanol is the method of choice when the analyst wishes to determine all the individual lipid components in the food.

Determination of individual fat components (Christie 1982, Gurr 1992)

Phospholipids and cholesterol can be determined in the mixture by specific colorimetric reactions, while triacylglycerols and cholesterol can be determined by enzymic methods for which there are readily available commercial kits. More detailed information on individual lipids in the extracted mixture and on their fatty acid components is best obtained by chromatographic procedures such as thin-layer, gas–liquid or high-performance liquid chromatography. These methods can now be highly automated for rapid, specific and highly reproducible quantitative and qualitative analysis.

Measurement of energy value

The energy value of a food or fat can be measured by bomb calorimetry. The sample is burned in an atmosphere of oxygen, and the heat generated by this process is measured and used to calculate the gross energy value of the sample (Osborne & Voogt 1978; see also Chapter 15).

The research worker investigating dietary fats will need to have all the above-mentioned techniques at his command, but the practical nutritionist or dietitian may find all the compositional data required in food tables, such as those found in *McCance and Widdowson's The composition of foods* (Holland et al

1991). Versions of these tables are now available on computer tapes, and software programs are available that allow the dietitian to use these data for the formulation or analysis of practical diets. It has to be remembered that the foods analysed by the compilers of the tables were not precisely the same as those that you will be dealing with, so that the limitations have to be recognized. The tables are convenient, but there is no substitute for direct analysis.

CONSUMPTION OF FATS IN THE DIET

There are enormous differences between different cultures in the part that fat plays in the diet. The Ho tribe in India make little or no use of fat in their food preparation, and their fat intake has been estimated to be no more than 2–4 g/day, or 2% of their dietary energy intake. Certain Eskimo communities, however, may consume as much as 80% of their energy intake as fat. In the UK, people eat on average about 100 g of fat a day, and this contributes about 42% of dietary energy intake. It is difficult to obtain an accurate figure for two main reasons. First, the most reliable figures for UK food consumption, the Annual Reports of the National Food Survey Committee (Ministry of Agriculture, Fisheries and Food 1990) deal only with food eaten in the home. We do not really know how the nutrient profile of food eaten in restaurants and canteens compares with that eaten at home, but the fat intake estimates of the National Food Survey are likely to be a little lower. Secondly, there are enormous differences between individuals in the average amounts of fat they eat, and one individual may consume very different quantities from day to day. Marr (1981) has calculated that one needs to record food intakes over a period of 10 days to get a reliable estimate of an individual's fat intake. Many studies rely on a 24-hour recall, and even the best normally only record weighed intakes over 7 days (see Marr 1981, Bingham 1987 and Appendix 1).

WHY DO WE EAT FAT?

Palatability

For most people, foods are more palatable if they have a substantial fat content. For the nutritionist or dietitian, this is not an unimportant matter, since whatever its nutrient composition may be, food has no nutritive value if it is not eaten. In countries where the choice of food is abundant, palatability is a major factor in determining food choice and, therefore, nutrient intakes. Indeed, there is evidence that price and the appearance and taste of food are more influential in determining food choice than interest in its nutritive value or 'healthiness', although the latter is now beginning to assume more importance for consumers than hitherto.

Fats contribute to palatability principally in two ways: by the response to their texture in the mouth ('mouthfeel') and by the olfactory responses of taste in the mouth and aroma in the nose ('flavour'). Mouthfeel has much to do with the way in which fat is associated with other food components, particularly in the form of emulsions. Thus, butter, cream and milk are all different types of emulsions of milk fat, but they each cause a different sensation in the mouth that is more pleasant than that which comes from consuming a pure fat. Aroma is due to low-molecular-weight volatile compounds derived from the decomposition of lipids by lipolysis, oxidation and microbial or thermal degradation. These processes may generate free short-chain fatty acids, aldehydes, ketones, lactones and other volatile compounds.

An energy source

Most people think primarily of fats as sources of metabolic energy. Triacylglycerols represent a very concentrated form of fuel with a gross energy value of 38 kJ/g. A brief description of how fats are metabolized to yield this energy in usable form is given below.

A source of essential nutrients

Dietary lipids provide two types of essential nutrients: the essential fatty acids and the fat-soluble vitamins. The latter are discussed in detail in Chapter 13.

Essential fatty acids

In a classic paper in 1929, two American nutritionists, Burr and Burr, described how acute deficiency states could be produced in rats by feeding fat-free diets, and that these deficiencies could be eliminated or prevented by adding only certain specific fatty acids to the diet. It was shown that fatty acids related to linoleic acid were the most effective, and the term 'vitamin F' was coined for them, although they are now always referred to as essential fatty acids, (EFA). EFA deficiency can be produced in a variety of animals, including man, but the condition is best documented in the laboratory rat. The disease is characterized by skin symptoms such as dermatosis and the skin becomes 'leaky' to water. Growth is retarded, reproduction is impaired and there is

degeneration or impairment of function in many organs of the body. Biochemically, EFA deficiency is characterized by changes in the fatty acid composition of many tissues, especially the biological membranes, whose function is impaired, and in the mitochondria, the efficiency of production of metabolic energy by the oxidation of fatty acids is reduced. Well documented EFA deficiency in man is rare, but was first seen in children fed virtually fat-free diets (Hansen et al 1958, Soderhjelm et al 1970). Four hundred infants were fed milk formulae containing different amounts of linoleic acid. When the formulae contained less than 0.1% of the dietary energy as linoleic acid, clinical and chemical signs of EFA deficiency ensued. The skin abnormalities were very similar to those seen in rats, and these and other signs of EFA deficiency disappeared when more linoleic acid was added to the diet. Hansen and his colleagues, who described this work, argued for substantial requirements, but the controversy in this field is highlighted by Cuthbertson (1976), who argued that the requirements had been overstated.

Earlier, in 1938, one volunteer male lived for 6 months on an experimental low-fat diet, containing only about 2 g butter fat daily (Brown et al 1938). He remained in good health throughout and no skin lesions developed, but he lost a little weight and the proportions of linoleic and arachidonic acids in his plasma lipids fell. It can be concluded that his requirement for EFA was very small in relation to the stores of linoleic acid in his adipose tissue fat. In contrast, the infants described above were of very low birthweight and were subsequently fed on skimmed milk, then the orthodox treatment for such infants. Thus, they had not been able to lay down a normal store of EFA before birth, and after birth were given an EFA-deficient diet. Today, great care is taken to see that the feeds of all babies, but especially those of very low birthweight, contain all the essential nutrients, and EFA deficiency in infants is apparently rare and usually the result of inadequate care.

However, at least two important uncertainties remain. First, until recently attention has been devoted almost entirely to linoleic acid ($18:2n-6$). The importance of α-linolenic acid ($18:3n-3$, see below) has now been recognized and some infant formulae are being supplemented with α-linolenic acid to give a ratio of $18:2n-6$ to $18:3n-3$ of approximately 5:1. Secondly, human milk (but not infant formulae) contains small amounts of long-chain polyunsaturated fatty acids, principally arachidonic ($20:4n-6$) and docosahexaenoic ($22:6n-3$, DHA) acids. These are derived from linoleic and α-linolenic acids respectively, by further chain elongation and desaturation (see later section on Fatty acid metabolism). These are necessary for the very active brain development that is occurring at this time, since about 50% of the dry weight of brain is composed of lipids, of which up to 50% are the long-chain polyunsaturated fatty acids. Whereas many body tissues, including brain, contain the enzymes necessary for converting linoleic and α-linolenic acids into long-chain polyunsaturated fatty acids, it is uncertain whether they are able to convert as much as is required. It is likely that premature babies will need to be supplied with dietary long-chain polyunsaturated fatty acids, but it remains uncertain whether full-term babies given formula feeds need these fatty acids in the diet.

In 1971, the first unequivocal case of EFA deficiency in an adult was reported (Collins et al 1971). The patient, a man of 44, had had all but 60 cm of his bowel surgically removed. He was then given intravenous feeding only, with preparations containing no fat, and after 100 days he developed a scaly dermatitis. A biochemical test that allows early diagnosis of EFA deficiency before the appearance of skin lesions depends on the failure of tissues to produce arachidonic acid (all-cis-5,8,11,14–20:4) and at the same time, to produce an excess of all-cis-5,8,11–20:3 (Fig. 6.5). The metabolic basis for these changes is described below. The ratio of 20:3/20:4 (the triene/tetraene ratio) measured in plasma phospholipids is used as a biochemical index of EFA status. In health, the ratio is about 0.1 or less, rising to 1.0 in severe EFA deficiency. Using this ratio as a diagnostic criterion, three patients with chronic disease of the small bowel who had been treated with low-fat diets but not given intravenous feeding, were found in a London hospital (Press et al 1974). They responded successfully to the application to the skin of lipids containing a high proportion of linoleic acid. Holman (1983) has used a more sophisticated method of serum fatty acid profiling to pinpoint subtle defects in polyunsaturated fatty acid metabolism. A whole spectrum of unsaturated fatty acids, including positional and geometric isomers, is analysed instead of simply the two mentioned above.

There is no question that linoleic acid is essential for man. Overt EFA deficiency is seen only when it provides less than 1–2% of dietary energy, or 2–5 g daily for an adult. Rather more may be needed in pregnancy or lactation, although we cannot be precise because the body contains considerable stores in the adipose tissue and little is known about its ability to adapt to lower intakes. The argument that an even higher intake – say 10% of energy – is desirable in view of its effects in lowering the concentration of cholesterol in the blood, has nothing to do with the essentiality of linoleic acid in its strictest sense.

The essentiality of linolenic acid for man has remained in doubt. A case has been described of a young girl displaying neurological symptoms 4–5 months after being on total parenteral nutrition, in which the fat component contained mainly linoleic acid and only a minute quantity of α-linolenic acid

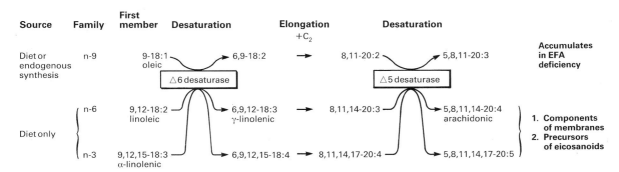

Fig. 6.5 The metabolism of three different families of unsaturated fatty acids. The first member of the *n*-9 family, oleic acid, can be taken in from the diet or can be formed in body tissues, whereas linoleic and α-linolenic acids, the first members of the *n*-6 and *n*-3 families respectively, can only come from the diet. The first step in their metabolism is the introduction of a new double bond at position 6 by an enzyme called 6-desaturase. All three fatty acids compete for this enzyme. There follows a series of alternate competitive elongation and desaturation steps. The products formed from oleic acid accumulate only when linoleic acid is absent from, or present in only very small amounts in, the diet. They are therefore markers of essential fatty acid deficiency. Arachidonic acid (*n*-6 family) is the major long-chain polyunsaturated fatty acid in human membranes of most tissues; DHA (*n*-3 family), is a characteristic component of nervous tissue.

(Holman et al 1982). When safflower oil was replaced by soybean oil, containing much more α-linolenic acid, the neurological symptoms disappeared. More recently, a Norwegian group (Bjerve et al 1987) provided evidence for α-linolenic acid deficiency in elderly patients fed by gastric tube. Like linoleic acid, α-linolenic acid cannot be made by the human body and must come from the diet. Since a large proportion of the lipids of the brain, and of specialized tissues such as the retina, are composed of polyunsaturated fatty acids of the n-3 family derived from dietary α-linolenic acid, it is reasonable to assume its essentiality. It seems quite certain, however, that only small amounts of this nutrient are required in human diets, as reviewed by Zollner (1986) and the British Nutrition Foundation (1992).

As discussed above, there may be circumstances when the enzymes catalysing the conversion of 18:3n-3 into long-chain polyunsaturated fatty acids are working at less than optimal activity, in which case the long-chain polyunsaturated fatty acids may be regarded as essential nutrients, rather than simply as essential metabolites. The resolution of this question awaits further research. The question of requirements for EFA has recently been addressed by a publication of the UK Department of Health (1991) which states that 18:2n-6 should provide at least 1% of dietary energy, and 18:3n-3 at least 0.2%, for infants, children and adults.

Why are some fatty acids essential?

Two distinct roles to account for the essentiality of linoleic and α-linolenic acids have been discussed. These are as membrane components and as precursors for a group of physiologically active metabolites, the eicosanoids (British Nutrition Foundation 1992).

Membranes

During EFA deficiency, changes occur in the properties of membranes, for example, the permeability to water and small molecules, which can be correlated with changes in the fatty acid composition of the membrane. Membranes of liver mitochondria isolated from EFA-deficient animals have smaller proportions of linoleic and arachidonic acids, and larger proportions of oleic and 5,8,11-eicosatrienoic acid than those of healthy animals. β-oxidation and oxidative phosphorylation are less efficient. These changes at the molecular level are reflected in the animal's poorer performance in converting food energy into metabolic energy for growth and maintenance of body function (Holman 1970). It seems that the stability and integrity of the membrane and its ability to provide an environment for the efficient functioning of the enzymes, receptors and other proteins embedded into the lipid bilayer, can only be supported by the presence of lipids with a certain pattern of polyunsaturated fatty acids, in ways that are as yet incompletely understood.

Eicosanoids

Arachidonic acid and other C20 and C22 polyunsaturated fatty acids of the n-3 and n-6 families can be metabolized to a range of compounds that exert a multitude of physiological activities at concentrations down to 10^{-9} g per gram of tissue (Needleman et al 1986, Sanders 1988). These include the ability to contract smooth muscle, to inhibit or stimulate the adhesion of blood platelets, and to cause the constriction or dilation of blood vessels with related influence on blood pressure. As early as the 1930s, physiologists were discovering that fatty acid-like substances in seminal plasma could cause a strong contraction or relaxation of smooth muscle, and the active factor was called prostaglandin. Further work in Sweden and the Netherlands demonstrated that the activity was associated with oxygenated unsaturated fatty acids that could be shown by radiotracer techniques to be derived directly from arachidonic acid (Samuelsson et al 1978). In the intervening years, several more classes of compounds have been discovered: prostacyclins, thromboxanes and leukotrienes. These are now collectively referred to as eicosanoids, because they are derived from 20-carbon precursor fatty acids, the eicosenoic acids, as illustrated in Fig. 6.6.

Two groups of these metabolites, the prostacyclins and the thromboxanes have essentially opposite physiological effects. Prostacyclins, formed in arterial walls, are among the most powerful known inhibitors of platelet aggregation. They relax the arterial walls and promote a lowering of blood pressure. Thromboxanes, found in platelets, stimulate platelets to aggregate (an important mechanism in wound healing), contract the arterial wall and promote an increase in blood pressure. The balance between these activities is important in maintaining normal vascular function. Several studies have demonstrated that altering the amounts and types of n-6 and n-3 fatty acids in the diet can influence the spectrum of eicosanoids produced. For example, the substitution of fish oils in which n-3 fatty acids predominate for diets in which linoleic acid (n-6) is the main

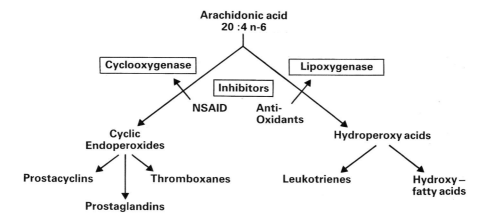

Fig. 6.6 The two major pathways of arachidonic acid metabolism to eicosanoids. NSAID = non-steroidal anti-inflammatory drugs (e.g. aspirin).

polyunsaturated fatty acid (as typified by the average UK diet) results in changes in plasma and platelet fatty acid profiles from arachidonic acid to eicosapentaenoic acid as the predominant polyunsaturated fatty acid, and a reduction in the formation of thromboxane A_2 and an increase in the formation of thromboxane A_3 by platelets (Weber et al 1986; Sanders 1988). In general, the potency of eicosanoids derived from n-3 polyunsaturated fatty acids is less than that of those derived from n-6 polyunsaturated fatty acids. Thus, blood platelets are stimulated to aggregate less strongly by the 3-series thromboxanes than those of the 2-series, and thrombotic tendency is reduced. Moreover, the n-3 polyunsaturated fatty acids also tend directly to inhibit the cyclooxygenase enzyme responsible for eicosanoid biosynthesis.

Polyunsaturated fatty acids are also metabolized to another type of eicosanoid known as leukotrienes. Arachidonic acid (n-6) is metabolized to leukotriene B_4, which has considerable inflammatory potential, while eicosapentaenoic acid (n-3) is metabolized to leukotriene B_5, which is one to two orders of magnitude less inflammatory. Dietary n-3 fatty acids may inhibit the formation of leukotriene B_4, thus reducing inflammatory responses.

The physiological effects of the eicosanoids are so powerful that they are generated locally and destroyed immediately they have produced their effect. The excretion of eicosanoid breakdown products in urine has been used as a method for estimating daily eicosanoid production and requirements. The essential fatty acid precursors of the eicosanoids are released from the membrane phospholipids, which can therefore be regarded as a vast body store of EFAs that are immediately available for eicosanoid biosynthesis. As they are depleted, they must be replaced by new polyunsaturated fatty acids biosynthesized by the pathways illustrated in Fig. 6.5. The mechanisms by which the relative proportions of the different eicosanoids are regulated, particularly how diet influences this regulation, and the quantitative relationship between the requirements for essential fatty acids, which are measured in grams, and the daily production of eicosanoids, which is measured in micrograms, are subjects for further research.

BASICS OF FAT METABOLISM

Digestion

Triacylglycerols, which form the bulk of the fats in the diet, must be broken down into partial glycerides and fatty acids by a pancreatic lipase in the small intestine before they can be absorbed efficiently. This is the process of digestion. In most adults, the processes of fat digestion and absorption are very efficient and over 95% of the 100 g or so a day consumed in the UK are probably digested and absorbed. Much larger quantities, up to 250 g/day or even more, can sometimes be absorbed if the body is short of energy. Arctic explorers and lumberjacks frequently consume such large amounts.

The newborn baby has to adapt to the relatively high fat content in breast milk after relying mainly on glucose as an energy substrate in fetal life. He can digest fat, but not as efficiently as the older child or adult, because his pancreatic and biliary secretions are not fully developed (Hamosh 1979a). Neonatal fat digestion is aided by the activity of a lipase secreted from the lingual serous glands and carried into the stomach, where hydrolysis occurs, without the need for bile salts, at a pH of around 4.5–5.5 (Hamosh 1979b). The activity is probably stimulated by the action of sucking and the presence of fat in the mouth. The products of hydrolysis are mainly 2-monoacylglycerols, diacylglycerols and non-esterified fatty acids, the latter being richer in medium chain length acids than the original glycerides. There is also evidence that a lipase in human breast milk contributes to fat digestion in the newborn (Fredrikzon et al 1978). Later in life, the process of fat digestion also begins in the stomach, where a churning action helps to form a coarse fat emulsion. This is not hydrolysed, but enters the small intestine and is modified by mixing with bile and pancreatic juice (Carey et al 1983). The biliary secretion, which is enhanced as the amount of dietary fat increases (Hill 1974), contains bile acids that are formed in the liver from cholesterol (Fig. 6.7). The first and rate-limiting step is hydroxylation at C7, followed by oxidation of the side chain with the formation of a carboxyl group to produce chenodeoxycholic acid. Further hydroxylation at C12 yields cholic acid. These two primary bile acids are excreted in the bile as conjugates with taurine or glycine. The polar groups and the shape of the molecules make the bile acids effective detergents and enable them to solubilize the fats present in the small intestine.

Digestion takes place in the duodenum, catalysed by a pancreatic lipase. The main products of triacyl-glycerol digestion are 2-monoacylglycerols and non-esterified fatty acids. Phospholipid digestion yields lysophosphoglycerides and a fatty acid released from position 2 of the phosphoglycerides by pancreatic phospholipase. Cholesterol esters in the dietary fat must be hydrolysed by a pancreatic cholesterol esterase before absorption can occur.

As digestion progresses, the oil phase decreases in volume as the lipolytic products pass into 'mixed micelles': large molecular aggregates consisting of monoacylglycerols, fatty acids longer than C12, bile salts and phospholipids (Fig. 6.8). The mixed micelles are able to draw into the hydrophobic core the less water-soluble molecules such as cholesterol, the carotenoids, tocopherols and some undigested triacylglycerols.

Absorption

Lipid absorption occurs mainly in the jejunum. The digestion products pass from the mixed micelles into the enterocyte membrane by passive diffusion (Carey et al 1983). A diffusion gradient is maintained by 1) the presence of a fatty acid binding protein which immediately binds to fatty acids entering the cell, and 2) the rapid re-esterification of fatty acids to the monoacylglycerols, which are the main digestion products crossing the intestinal mucosa (Carey et al 1983) (Fig. 6.8). Cholesterol absorption is completed by re-esterification catalysed by acyl-CoA: cholesterol acyltransferase, or by the reversal of cholesterol esterase. The former enzyme is induced by high concentrations of dietary cholesterol. Triacylglycerols and cholesterol esters resynthesized in the enterocytes are esterified with fatty acids having chain lengths greater than 12 carbon atoms.

Short (C4–C6) and medium (C8–C10) chain fatty acids are absorbed directly into the portal blood and carried to the liver, where they are rapidly oxidized (Fig. 6.8). They do not, therefore, contribute to plasma lipids, nor are they deposited in adipose tissue in significant quantities. About 4 g/day are absorbed

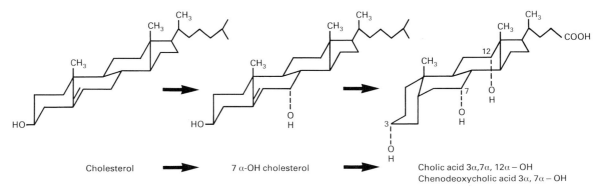

Fig. 6.7 Metabolic conversion of cholesterol into bile acids. Note the preponderance of hydrophobic groups on one side of the planar molecule, hydrophilic on the other.

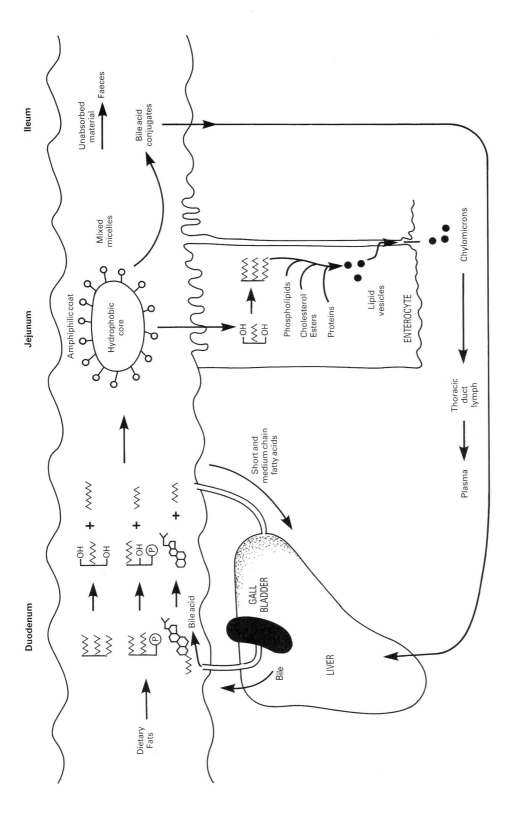

Fig. 6.8 Digestion and absorption of lipids in the small intestine. The enzyme pancreatic lipase catalyses the breaking of ester bonds in positions 1 and 3 of triacylglycerols, releasing 2 moles of fatty acid per mole of triacylglycerol, with 1 mole of 2-monoacylglycerol remaining. Bile salts aid in the emulsification of the fat droplets, while co-lipase anchors the enzyme to the surface of the fat droplets. Phospholipids are split by a pancreatic phospholipase A_2, releasing the fatty acid in position 2 and leaving a lysophospholipid. A cholesterol ester hydrolase splits the fatty acid from cholesterol esters. Lipolysis products are stabilized in mixed micelles comprising surface-active components: monoacylglycerols, long-chain fatty acids and bile salts with unhydrolysed triacylglycerols, cholesterol and fat-soluble vitamins in the hydrophobic interior. Short-chain fatty acids are absorbed as free acids into the portal blood. Monoacylglycerols and long-chain fatty acids from mixed micelles are transported across the brush border and re-esterified in the enterocytes. Reformed triacylglycerols are stabilized with phospholipids and apoproteins and exported into plasma as chylomicrons.

from dairy products; further smaller amounts may be derived from food products that incorporate coconut and palm kernel oils.

Defects in fat digestion and absorption

Failure to assimilate lipids of dietary origin into the body may arise from defects in digestion (maldigestion) or absorption (malabsorption) (Sickinger 1975). Maldigestion can occur because of incomplete lipolysis. Thus pancreatic insufficiency, from pancreatitis, a pancreatic tumour or in diseases of malnutrition such as kwashiorkor, can lead to a failure to secrete enough lipase. Alternatively there may be enough functional lipase but a failure to produce bile because of biliary disease, with obstruction of the bile duct, or chronic liver disease. The commonest cause of biliary insufficiency in affluent societies, however, arises from bile-salt deficiency induced by surgical resection of the ileum, where active transport of bile salts occurs (see Chapter 34). Bile-salt deficiency results in an inability to effect micellar solubilization of lipolysis products. Gastric disturbances also affect digestive efficiency; thus, maldigestion seems to arise from defects in a variety of organs contributing to different aspects of the digestive process.

Malabsorption may occur even when digestion is functioning normally, due to defects in the absorptive surfaces of the small intestine. There may be a variety of causes, some common ones being bacterial invasion or sensitization of the gut to dietary components such as gluten, as in coeliac disease. Malabsorption syndromes (often called 'sprue') are characterized by dramatic changes in the morphology of the intestinal mucosa. The epithelium is flattened and irregular, and atrophy of the villi reduces the absorbing surface. A common feature of all fat malabsorption syndromes is a massively increased excretion of fat in the faeces (steatorrhoea), which arises not only from unabsorbed dietary material but also from the bacterial population that proliferates in the gut. Patients with poor fat absorption are at increased risk of deficiencies of energy, fat-soluble vitamins and essential fatty acids. The clinical management of fat malassimilation is facilitated by replacing normal dietary fats by medium-chain triacylglycerols (MCT) (Sickinger 1975). This product is refined from coconut oil and consists of the fraction containing mainly C8 and C10 saturated fatty acids, which are more efficiently digested and absorbed directly into the portal blood, bypassing the normal absorptive route. For other dietetic approaches to steatorrhoea and diarrhoea, see Chapter 33.

Lipid Transport (Fig. 6.9)

During active fat absorption, the triacylglycerols synthesized in the enterocyte acquire a stabilizing coat of phospholipids and apolipoproteins (apoA and apoB). These chylomicrons, large spherical particles 75–600 nm in diameter, are secreted into the lymphatic vessels (see Fig. 6.8) and pass via the thoracic duct to the jugular vein. In the bloodstream they acquire apolipoproteins C and E (Table 6.6).

The first tissues encountered by the chylomicrons are the lungs, but they pass through the lungs and the ventricles of the heart with little modification, and then rapidly enter the capillaries of the skeletal muscles, heart, mammary glands and adipose tissues, where they interact with the enzyme lipoprotein lipase (LPL). This enzyme catalyses the hydrolytic breakdown (lipolysis) of triacylglycerols by the release of fatty acids, which are then taken up into the cells of the target tissue. After a meal, an elevated insulin concentration directs most of the chylomicron breakdown to adipose tissue by activating the adipose tissue LPL. The hormonal balance during a fast activates muscle LPL, while during lactation, the LPL of the mammary glands is elevated under the stimulation of prolactin, to ensure a supply of substrates for milk-fat synthesis. About half the chylomicron triacylglycerols are hydrolysed in 2–3 minutes, but the particles are not completely degraded. Remnant particles, containing proportionately less triacylglycerol and more cholesterol are poor substrates for the LPL and are taken up by the liver, where the cholesterol is used for membrane or new lipoprotein biosynthesis, or converted into bile acids.

If the diet contains an appreciable amount of fat, endogenous fatty acid and triacylglycerol biosynthesis are suppressed, although, since the process of lipid turnover is occurring continually in all tissues, a low level of biosynthetic activity is always present. (The biochemistry of lipid synthesis cannot be covered in this chapter and the student is referred to Gurr & Harwood (1991) and Vance & Vance (1985) for a fuller account). Fatty acid synthesis in human adipose tissue (measured in isolated adipocytes and subcellular fractions) increases up to elevenfold when subjects change from a high-fat to a high-carbohydrate diet (Sjöström 1973). Under these conditions, the liver is probably the dominant human organ for lipid synthesis, and the newly synthesized fat is exported as very low-density lipoproteins (VLDL), similar to chylomicrons but smaller, less dense and containing relatively more phospholipids, cholesterol and proteins. Nevertheless, Sjöström (1973) found that fatty acid synthesis de novo was of little quantitative importance in human beings,

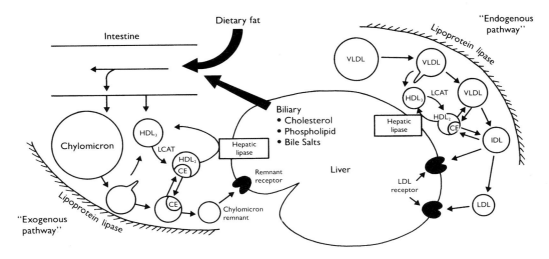

Fig. 6.9 The metabolism of lipoproteins. The 'exogenous pathway' is concerned with the transport and metabolism of fat coming from the diet. The fats are packaged as chylomicrons, which circulate and are removed from the plasma by the enzyme lipoprotein lipase, mainly in the adipose tissue. The chylomicrons are not entirely consumed by this enzyme but are degraded to smaller particles called remnants, which are removed by the liver. Parts of the chylomicrons also go into making HDL which, in conjunction with the enzyme LCAT, remove excess cholesterol from membranes and other lipoprotein particles, converting it into cholesteryl esters. This process involves the interconversion of two forms of HDL: HDL_2 and HDL_3 and cholesteryl esters are taken to the liver for further processing. The endogenous pathway is concerned with the transport and metabolism of fats made in the body itself. The products are the VLDL which are metabolized in a manner analogous to the chylomicrons. Their remnants are usually called intermediate-density lipoproteins (IDL) and are further metabolized to LDL which are taken up by the specific LDL receptor.

even when carbohydrates were the main source of dietary energy.

High rates of fatty acid synthesis can occur in the mammary gland during lactation. The medium-chain fatty acids, caprylic (octanoic) and capric (decanoic) acids, are produced specifically by the mammary gland and in no other tissue. They can, therefore, act as a marker of endogenous fatty acid synthesis. When the amount of fat in the human diet is very low, there is a marked elevation of milk medium-chain fatty acids compared with the concentrations in the milk of women on a high-fat diet (Read et al 1965a). The proportion is highest after the main meal, and falls within a few hours (Read et al 1965b).

Chylomicrons and VLDL are types of molecular aggregates of lipids and proteins called lipoproteins (Table 6.6) (Segrest & Albers 1986), whose function is to transport lipids in the plasma to tissues where they are needed as sources of energy, components of membranes or precursors of biologically active metabolites. Nature has solved the problem of how to stabilize lipids in an aqueous environment by coating the lipid particles with a layer of amphiphilic lipids and proteins. The protein components (called apolipoproteins) have another function. They confer specificity on the lipoproteins and determine the way in which they are metabolized, and, to a large extent, the tissues in which they are metabolized. The apoproteins recognize and interact with specific receptors on cell surfaces, following which the receptor–lipoprotein complex is taken into the cell by a process of endocytosis. There are several apolipoprotein peptides, identified by a series of letters A–E, but as research continues, more and more subclasses are being discovered. Thus apolipoprotein C is now divided into apoC-I, II and III. While many of these peptides are involved in receptor recognition, some are also involved in the functioning of enzymes of lipoprotein metabolism; thus apoC-II is needed for the activation of lipoprotein lipase and apoA-I for an enzyme involved in cholesterol esterification (Table 6.7). An individual's apolipoprotein profile is genetically determined, and variants are now recognized that result in specific metabolic disorders.

Table 6.6 Composition and characteristics of the human plasma lipoproteins

	Chylomicrons	VLDL	LDL	HDL
Protein (% particle mass)	2	7	20	50
Triacylglycerols (% particle mass)	83	50	10	8
Cholesterol (% particle mass) (free + esterified)	8	22	48	20
Phospholipids (% particle mass)	7	20	22	22
Particle mass (daltons)	$0.4–30 \times 10$	$10–100 \times 10$	$2–3.5 \times 10$	$1.75–3.6 \times 10$
Density range (g/ml)	> 0.95	0.95–1.006	1.019–1.063	1.063–1.210
Diameter (nm)	> 70	30–90	18–22	5–12
Apolipoproteins	A_1, B-48 C_1, C_2, C_3	B-100, E	B-100	A_1, A_2

Source: Gurr & Harwood (1991)

Table 6.7 Characteristics of the human apolipoproteins

Shorthand name	Molecular weight (Daltons)	Amino acid residues	Function	Major sites of synthesis
A_1	28 000	243	Activates LCAT*	Liver Intestine
A_2	17 000	154	Inhibits LCAT? Activates hepatic lipase	Liver
B-48			Cholesterol clearance	Intestine
B-100	350–550 000		Cholesterol clearance	Liver
C_1	6 605	57	Activates LCAT?	Liver
C_2	8 824	79	Activates LPL**	Liver
C_3	8 750	79	Inhibits LPL? Activates LCAT?	Liver
E	34 000	279	Cholesterol clearance	Liver

*LCAT   Lecithin-cholesterol acyltransferase
**LPL   Lipoprotein lipase
Source: Gurr & Harwood (1991)

Whereas chylomicrons are the major carriers of fat from the diet, VLDLs are involved in transporting endogenously synthesized lipids. They are degraded by a mechanism similar to that described for chylomicrons. The VLDL remnant is normally called an 'intermediate-density lipoprotein' (IDL). The name arises because further degradation yields a particle called a low-density lipoprotein (LDL). This class of lipoprotein is the major carrier of cholesterol in human beings, so that in a person with a plasma cholesterol of 5 mmol/l, about 70% is carried on LDL. The particles are 18–22 nm in diameter and comprise 20% protein and 80% lipid, of which cholesterol contributes 50%, 80% of which is cholesterol ester, mainly 18:2, 18:1 and 16:0. Their role is to deliver cholesterol to tissues for the vital functions of membrane synthesis and repair. The discharge of cholesterol can occur by passive endocytosis or by a specific receptor-mediated uptake process (Brown et al 1981) in which the receptor recognizes the apoB component of LDL and binds to it. The LDL-receptor complex is taken into the cell and the LDL degraded by lysosomal enzymes. The resulting free cholesterol interacts with the endoplasmic reticulum membranes in which are located the enzymes of cholesterol biosynthesis, and inhibits hydroxymethyglutaryl-CoA (HMGCoA) reductase, the rate-limiting enzyme in the sequence. In this way, endogenous cholesterol biosynthesis is regulated by the amount available from the diet. Familial hypercholesterolaemia, an inherited disorder characterized by high circulating concentrations of LDL, results from the absence of the LDL receptor (Brown et al 1981).

The remaining important class of lipoproteins is the type known as high-density lipoproteins (HDL). Their role is to carry cholesterol from peripheral cells to the liver, where it is degraded or repackaged, a process known as 'reverse cholesterol transport'. HDLs have attracted a great deal of research attention recently, since it was realized that a low plasma concentration may be indicative of increased risk of cardiovascular disease, and it has been proposed that they may have a protective role. Nevertheless, it has yet to be shown that procedures that lead to an elevation of HDL do indeed reduce the risk of this disease. Protein (mainly ApoA-I and II, with some C, D and E peptides) constitutes 50% of the mass of HDL, while approximately 22% is phospholipid, 20% cholesterol ester and only 8% triacylglycerol. A key step in reverse cholesterol transport is catalysed by the enzyme lecithin cholesterol acyltransferase (LCAT). A fatty acid is transferred from phosphatidylcholine to cholesterol to form a cholesterol ester, as illustrated in Fig. 6.10. In human plasma, LCAT is associated with HDL and the phospholipid substrate is also present in HDL, having been transferred from chylomicron remnants or IDL during the degradation of chylomicrons or VLDL. The cholesterol substrate is derived from the surfaces of plasma lipoproteins or the plasma membranes of cells. LCAT, by consuming cholesterol, promotes its net transport from cells into plasma. Molecules of cholesterol ester transferred to lipoproteins containing apoB or apoE are taken up by the liver, thereby completing the process of reverse cholesterol transport. The integration of lipoprotein metabolism is illustrated in Fig. 6.9.

The amounts and proportions of lipoproteins in the plasma, especially the chylomicrons and VLDL,

respond to the influx of digestion products from lipids and carbohydrates after the consumption of a meal. The average long-term concentrations of VLDL, LDL and HDL may also to some extent be determined by habitual intakes of fats and carbohydrates.

1. Increasing the dietary intake of cholesterol increases plasma cholesterol by only a small extent (about 0.5 mmol/l or 2 mg/dl) for every 100 mg cholesterol consumed daily, and this is mainly in the LDL fraction.
2. The substitution of saturated fatty acids by monounsaturated or n-6 polyunsaturated fatty acids leads to a reduction of the concentration of LDL-cholesterol. HDL cholesterol is not reduced unless linoleic acid provides more than about 12% of dietary energy.
3. The addition of long-chain n-3 PUFA (mainly 20:5 and 22:6) to diets leads to a reduction in the concentration of VLDL, but not LDL or HDL.
4. The replacement of dietary saturated fatty acids with carbohydrates leads to decreased concentrations of LDL and HDL and, in some people, increased concentrations of VLDL.
5. The replacement of dietary n-6 PUFA with carbohydrates leads to increased LDL-cholesterol concentrations, with little change in HDL, and, in some people, increased concentrations of VLDL.

The mechanisms by which these changes occur are poorly understood. In part, they may result from reductions in the rate at which the apoB receptors in the liver remove LDL, brought about by some saturated fatty acids (specifically 12:0 and 14:0) and reversal of this effect by some unsaturated fatty acids. Alternatively, different types of fatty acids and carbohydrates may influence rates of biosynthesis of LDL from VLDL (Grundy & Denke 1990).

Fatty acid metabolism

Most body tissues contain enzymes for the biosynthesis of fatty acids and their esterification in triacylglycerols, phospholipids and other body lipids (Vance & Vance 1985; Gurr & Harwood 1991). This is known from experiments with samples of biopsied tissue, limited tracer studies in vivo, or by inference from studies in other species. When the fat content of the diet is low, rates of fatty acid synthesis are high, particularly in the liver, to supply the needs of the body in respect of structural and storage fat, the main products being palmitic and oleic acids. However, this hardly ever occurs in western man, whose diet generally contains a high proportion of its energy as

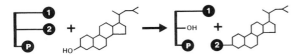

Fig. 6.10 The lecithin–cholesterol acyltransferase reaction (LCAT). The reaction is responsible for the formation of cholesteryl esters in plasma and involves the participation of HDL particles (see also Fig. 6.9).

fat. At most times, the enzymes of fat synthesis are 'switched off' and the needs for storage and structural fats are satisfied from dietary intake.

Diet may control fatty acid synthesis by influencing the synthesis or activities of biosynthetic enzymes through the availability of cofactors, such as pantothenic acid or biotin, or by influencing the concentrations of circulating hormones which induce or suppress the synthesis of some enzymes of lipid metabolism. Although many hormones are involved, the dominant role is undoubtedly played by insulin, which suppresses glucose synthesis in the liver, encourages glycogen and fatty acid synthesis, stimulates the uptake of glucose into adipose tissue, and inhibits the breakdown of fat in that tissue.

To achieve the desired physical properties of lipids in cells, a high degree of unsaturation is required. Virtually all tissues contain enzymes (desaturases) that insert double bonds into saturated fatty acids, normally at position 9. Thus, palmitic and stearic acids, arising either from the diet or biosynthesis in the tissues, are desaturated to palmitoleic (cis-9-hexadecenoic) and oleic (cis-9-octadecenoic) acids respectively. Human tissues also contain desaturases that catalyse the introduction of further double bonds to produce polyunsaturated fatty acids. These desaturations, alternating with elongations of the chain, give rise to several families of polyunsaturated fatty acids, depending on the structure of the precursor fatty acid, as illustrated in Fig. 6.5. The most important families are termed n-3, n-6 and n-9. In the course of evolution, human beings lost the ability to make the enzymes that catalyse the introduction of double bonds between positions 12–13 and 15–16, as present in linoleic and α-linolenic acids, which are formed in plants. Yet these fatty acids and higher fatty acids derived from them are essential to life, for reasons explained earlier; they must therefore be present in the diet.

Because the same desaturases are involved in the metabolism of the different polyunsaturated fatty acid families (Fig. 6.5), it can be demonstrated that substrates on the different pathways compete with each other for desaturases, thus influencing the proportions of the end products formed. The affinity of the 6-desaturase for its substrates is in the order 18:3 > 18:2 > 18:1. Normally, conditions are such that the pathway beginning with linoleic acid (the n-6 series) predominates, and arachidonic acid is the major end product. If the amount of linoleic acid in the diet is very small compared with oleic acid, the n-9 pathway will begin to predominate, giving rise to an excessive production of 5, 8, 11–20:3. This explains why the ratio of 20:3(n-9) to 20:4(n-6) is an indicator of essential fatty acid deficiency, as described earlier. Other acids, such as the isomeric fatty acids formed during hydrogenation, can also compete with linoleic acid, and diets with excessive amounts of these isomers and limiting amounts of linoleic acid could also give rise to EFA deficiency, as defined by these biochemical criteria. For most individuals this rarely occurs, but some individuals eating strange diets in which hardened fats provide much of the energy could be at risk.

If the diet contains a large contribution from fish oils rich in n-3 fatty acids, the balance of polyunsaturated fatty acid metabolism can be tipped towards the n-3 family, causing the stimulation of production of eicosanoids derived from these precursors. There is good evidence that these eicosanoids reduce the ability of platelets to aggregate, and this may explain why the Eskimos, whose diets are rich in n-3 fatty acids, are little troubled by thrombosis despite their extremely high total fat intakes. We cannot assume, however, that indiscriminate use of these highly unsaturated fatty acids is entirely without risk. The conversion of polyunsaturated fatty acids into eicosanoids is an example of enzymically controlled oxidation. Uncontrolled oxidation of PUFA by free radical chain reactions can occur in the presence of oxygen and a catalyst such as iron. The living body is protected against such uncontrolled peroxidation by two main mechanisms: the organization of lipids in membrane bilayers in juxtaposition with lipid-soluble antioxidants such as vitamin E, and the presence of enzyme systems such as superoxide dismutase, which destroy initiating radicals. There is growing evidence that diets deficient in natural antioxidants such as vitamins C and E, and environmental factors producing free radicals (e.g. smoking) can cause oxidative stress, which if it overtaxes an individual's capacity to scavenge free radicals, can lead to degenerative changes over long periods (Gey 1986).

Storage of fat in the body: white adipose tissue

There are two types of adipose tissue, white and brown, which perform entirely different functions. White adipose tissue is concerned with fat storage, while brown adipose tissue is an organ that has evolved to provide body heat.

White adipose tissue, which in man provides a reserve of fuel, consists mainly of mesenchymal connective tissue cells called adipocytes (Hausman 1985). Fat is stored in these cells as a single droplet which pushes the nucleus and cytoplasm to the periphery of the cell. Adipocytes have an enormous potential to expand as more fat needs to be accommodated. The cells are supplied by a capillary network and receive nerves from the autonomic nervous system, the fibres of which appear to terminate in close relation to both cells and blood vessels. The amount of cellular material in adipose tissue is not generally appreciated. Thus, if a healthy man carries 10 kg of adipose tissue (about 15% of his body weight) of which 85% is fat, he has 1.5 kg of fat-free adipose tissue. This is about the weight of his liver and contains about 200 g protein. A healthy woman has more fat in relation to her body weight than a man: usually about 25%, which would amount to 15 kg or so. In a very emaciated person this is reduced to about 1 kg, while some very obese people can carry around 100 kg or even more. The health problems associated with excessive adipose tissue mass are described in Chapter 32. The adipose tissue is not evenly distributed. In man, about two-thirds is located under the skin (subcutaneous) and one-third internally (visceral). As well as storing fuel, visceral fat provides a protective cushion for the internal organs and external fat acts as insulator, as well as providing a cushioning effect. Men tend to deposit more adipose tissue around the abdomen and this is accentuated with age, while women tend to deposit more in the upper and lower body, particularly over the hips and thighs. An abdominal distribution seems to be more associated with health problems such as raised blood pressure, diabetes and an increased risk of cardiovascular disease than the female distribution, for reasons that are still obscure (Stern and Haffner 1986, and Chapter 32).

The development of white adipose tissue begins in fetal life (Hausman 1985) and the newborn baby weighing 3.5 kg has about 560 g adipose tissue. Fetal adipose tissue has to synthesize most of its fat from glucose; fat cells therefore possess all the pathways for the biosynthesis of lipids de novo. These enzymes are largely suppressed by high fat intakes later in life. Adipose tissue is, however, anything but an inert mass of fat, and the lipids contained in it are undergoing continuous turnover, even when the total mass of fat is neither increasing or decreasing. The time taken for half the linoleic acid in adult adipose tissue to be replaced has been estimated to be somewhere between 350 and 750 days (Hirsch et al 1960). The activity of lipoprotein lipase (controlled by insulin) determines the rate of entry of fatty acids from circulating lipids into the fat cell, and the activity of a hormone-sensitive triacylglycerol lipase (stimulated by

catecholamines) controls the lipolysis of stored fat prior to the export of fatty acids into the blood, where they are carried on serum albumin before further metabolism by ß-oxidation (Vance & Vance 1985, Gurr & Harwood 1991) in muscle, liver or other tissues needing fuel.

Because of this slow turnover of fatty acids, the composition of the adipose tissue tends to reflect the fat composition of the diet for some time in the past. This was graphically illustrated in human babies by Widdowson et al (1975) as a result of a 'natural' experiment. It had become customary for Dutch mothers to feed their babies a formula in which the manufacturers had replaced cow's milk fat by vegetable oil rich in linoleic acid. The concentration of linoleic acid in the Dutch babies' adipose tissue rose steadily, reaching nearly 50% of total fatty acids in some children by 40 weeks of age, whereas in the British babies it remained at between 2% and 4%, reflecting the intake of formulae based on cow's milk fat (Table 6.8). There was even a slight difference at birth, suggesting that the Dutch mothers' diets also contained more linoleic acid than their British counterparts', and that this had influenced the composition of the fetal fat, since the human placenta is quite permeable to fatty acids.

Because it is a compound derived entirely from the diet and not from body synthesis, linoleic acid in adipose tissue makes an ideal marker for the type of dietary fat consumed. Small pieces of fat tissue are taken by needle biopsy and analysed for fatty acids by gas–liquid chromatography. The method is a more reliable measure of habitual fatty acid intake than dietary surveys, which have a large random error (Katan et al 1986; Berry et al 1986). It can also be used as a good estimate of *trans* fatty acid intake (Katan et al 1986), but a simple relationship between dietary intake and adipose tissue composition does not hold true for all fatty acids. For example, the adipose tissue concentrations of α-linolenic and arachidonic acids tend to be lower than predicted from amounts in the diet. Recently, there has been interest in the composition of adipose tissue in relation to mortality and morbidity from cardiovascular disease. A lower content of linolenic acid has been found in the adipose tissue of men living in Edinburgh (where the incidence of cardiovascular disease is relatively high) compared with those in Stockholm (where it is lower), and in healthy Scottish men compared with patients prone to coronary heart disease (Wood et al 1987) (Table 6.8). The association of dietary fats and cardiovascular disease is discussed in more detail in Chapter 41.

Table 6.8 Some examples of adipose tissue fatty acid compositions

| Fatty acid | British babies given formulae with a cow's milk fat component[*] | Dutch babies given formulae with a vegetable fat component[*] (g/100 g total fatty acids) | Healthy adult men in the Stockholm–Edinburgh heart study | | |
| | | | Edinburgh | | Stockholm |
			1976[†]	1988[†]	1976[†]
14:0	9	4	4.1	3.3	4.3
16:0	32	30	24.9	24.7	23.7
16:1	7	14	8.1	8.1	6.4
18:0	6	3	5.7	4.8	5.9
18:1	43	41	46.4	44.5	44.5
18:2	3	8	7.3	11.3	11.8
18:3	0	0	2.5	2.8	2.4
Others	0	0	1.0	0.5	1.0

[*]Adapted from Widdowson et al 1975
[†]From data supplied by Dr. R. Riemersma from the Edinburgh–Stockholm study (see also Wood et al 1987)

Thermogenesis: brown adipose tissue

Mammals can react to cold by muscular activity – typically by shivering – which produces heat. Heat is also produced in chemical reactions, which are thermodynamically inefficient, for example those that release energy as heat rather than storing it in ATP. Normally, the oxidation of substrates in the electron transport chain of the mitochondria is coupled to the synthesis of ATP. In brown adipose tissue mitochondria, this process is bypassed, producing heat. The high concentration of cytochromes in the mitochondria which pack the cells and surround the lipid droplets they use as fuel gives the tissue its brown appearance.

In newborn babies, brown adipose tissue is conspicuous, especially in the thorax around the thymus gland and in the dorsal subcutaneous fat in the neck and between the scapulae (Hull & Hardman 1970). At birth, heat production by shivering in response to cold is ineffective, and the activation of brown adipose tissue is the chief mechanism for controlling body temperature in a cold environment. In adults, brown adipose tissue is not conspicuous and it is difficult to know whether this is because it atrophies or simply becomes obscured by the greater mass of white adipose tissue that develops around it. The activation of brown adipose tissue as a means of disposal of excess dietary energy and for controlling body weight occurs in some species, but its significance in man remains controversial (Chapter 9).

REFERENCES

Ansell GB, Hawthorne JN (eds) 1982 Phospholipids. Elsevier, Amsterdam

Berry EM, Hirsch J, Most J, McNamara DJ, Thornton J 1986 The relationship of dietary fat to plasma lipid levels by factor analysis of adipose tissue fatty acid composition in a free-living population of middle-aged American men. American Journal of Clinical Nutrition 44: 220–231

Bingham A 1987 The dietary assessment of individuals: methods, accuracy, new techniques and recommendations. Nutrition Abstracts and Reviews Series A 57: 705–742

Bjerve KS, Mostad, IL, Thoresen L 1987 α-Linolenic acid deficiency in patients on long-term gastric tube feeding: estimation of linolenic acid and long-chain unsaturated n–3 fatty acid requirements in man. American Journal of Clinical Nutrition 45: 66–77

British Nutrition Foundation 1992 Unsaturated fatty acids: nutritional and physiological significance. Report of the British Nutrition Foundation's Task Force. Chapman and Hall, London

Brown WR, Hansen AE, Burr GO, McQuarrie I 1938 Effects of prolonged use of an extremely low-fat diet on an adult human subject. Journal of Nutrition 16: 511–524

Brown MS, Kovanen PT, Goldstein JL 1981 Regulation of plasma cholesterol by lipoprotein receptors. Science 212: 628–635

Burr GO, Burr MM 1929 A new deficiency disease produced by rigid exclusion of fat from the diet. Journal of Biological Chemistry. 82: 345–367

Carey MC, Small DM, Bliss CM 1983 Lipid digestion and absorption. Annual Review of Physiology 45: 651–677

Christie WW 1982 Lipid analysis, Pergamon Press, Oxford

Christie WW 1983 The composition and structure of milk lipids. In: Fox PF (ed) Developments in dairy chemistry 2. Lipids. Applied Science Publishers, London

Collins FD, Sinclair AJ, Royle JP, Coats DA, Maynard AT, Leonard RF 1971 Plasma lipids in human linoleic acid deficiency. Nutrition and Metabolism 13: 150

Cuthbertson WFJ 1976 Essential fatty acid requirements in infancy. American Journal of Clinical Nutrition 26: 559–568

Department of Health 1991 Dietary reference values for food energy and nutrients for the United Kingdom. Report on Health and Social Subjects 41. HMSO, London

Edwards-Webb JD, Gurr MI 1988 The influence of dietary fats on the chemical composition and physical properties of biological membranes. Nutrition Research 8: 1297–1305

Fredrikzon B, Hernell O, Bläckberg L, Olivecrona T 1978 Bile salt-stimulated lipase in human milk: evidence of activity in vivo and of a role in the digestion of milk retinol esters. Pediatric Research 12: 1048–1052

Gey KF 1986 On the antioxidant hypothesis with regard to arteriosclerosis. Bibliotheca Nutritia Dieta 37: 53–91

Grundy SM, Denke MA 1990 Dietary influences on serum lipids and lipoproteins. Journal of Lipid Research 31: 1149–1172

Gunstone FD, Norris FA 1983 Lipids in foods. Pergamon Press, Oxford

Gunstone FD, Harwood JL, Padley FB 1986 The lipid handbook. Chapman and Hall, London

Gurr MI 1992 Role of fats in food and nutrition. Elsevier Applied Science Publishers, London

Gurr MI, Harwood JL 1991 Lipid biochemistry: an introduction. Chapman & Hall, London

Hamosh M 1979a The role of lingual lipase in neonatal fat digestion. In: Development of mammalian absorptive processes. CIBA Foundation Symposium No. 70, Excerpta Medica, Amsterdam pp. 92–98

Hamosh M, 1979b Fat digestion in the newborn: role of lingual lipase and preduodenal digestion. Pediatric Research 13: 615–622

Hansen AE, Haggard ME, Boelsche AN, Adam DJD, Wiese HF 1958 Essential fatty acids in infant nutrition: clinical manifestations of human linoleic acid deficiency. Journal of Nutrition 66: 565–576

Hausman GJ 1985 The comparative anatomy of adipose tissue In: Cryer A, Van R L R (eds) New perspectives in adipose tissue: structure, function and development. Butterworths, London, pp. 1–21

Hilditch TP, Williams, PN 1964 The chemical composition of natural fats, 4th edn. Chapman & Hall, London.

Hill MJ 1974 Colon cancer: a disease of fibre depletion or of dietary excess? Digestion 11: 289–306

Hirsch J, Farquar JW, Ahrens EH, Peterson ML, Stoffel W 1960 Studies of adipose tissue in man: a microtechnique for sampling and analysis. American Journal of Clinical Nutrition 8: 499–511

Holland B, Welch AA, Unwin ID, Buss DH, Paul AA, Southgate D A T 1991 McCance and Widdowson's The composition of foods, Royal Society of Chemistry, Cambridge and MAFF

Holman RT 1970 Biochemical activities of and requirements for polyunsaturated fatty acids. Progress in the Chemistry of Fats and other Lipids 9: 607–682

Holman RT, Johnson SB 1983 Essential fatty acid deficiencies in man. In: Perkins EG, Visek WJ (eds) Dietary fats and health. American Oil Chemists' Society, Champaign, Illinois, USA

Holman RT, Johnson SB, Hatch TF 1982 A case of human linolenic acid deficiency involving neurological abnormalities. American Journal of Clinical Nutrition 35: 617–623

Hull D, Hardman MJ 1970 Brown adipose tissue in newborn mammals In: Lindberg O (ed) Brown adipose tissue. Elsevier, New York, pp. 97–115

Katan MB, Van Staveren WA, Deurenberg P et al 1986 Linoleic and trans-unsaturated fatty acid content of adipose tissue biopsies as objective indicators of the dietary habits of individuals. Progress in Lipid Research 25: 193–195

McDonald IW, Scott TW 1977 Foods of ruminant origin with elevated content of polyunsaturated fatty acids. World Review of Nutrition and Dietetics 26: 144–207

Marr JW 1981 Individual variation in dietary intake. In: Turner MR (ed) Preventive nutrition and society. Academic Press, London, pp. 77–83

Mattson FH, Grundy SM 1985 Comparison of dietary saturated, monounsaturated and polyunsaturated fatty acids on plasma lipids and lipoproteins in man. Journal of Lipid Research 26: 194–204

Mead JF, Alfin-Slater RB, Howton D, Popjak G. 1986 Lipids: chemistry, biochemistry and nutrition. Plenum Press, New York

Ministry of Agriculture, Fisheries and Food 1990 Household Food Consumption and Expenditure: Annual Report of the National Food Survey Committee. HMSO, London

Needleman P, Turk J, Jakschik BA, Morrison A R, Lefkowith J B 1986 Arachidonic acid metabolism. Annual Review of Biochemistry 55: 69–102

Osborne DR, Voogt P 1978 The analysis of nutrients in foods. Academic Press, London

Perkins EG, Visek WJ (eds) 1983 Dietary fats and health. American Oil Chemists' Society, Champaign, Illinois, USA

Press M, Kikuchi H, Shimoyama T, Thompson GR 1974 Diagnosis and treatment of essential fatty acid deficiency in man. British Medical Journal 2: 247–250

Read WWC, Lutz PG, Tashjian A 1965a Human milk lipids. II. The influence of dietary carbohydrates and fat on the fatty acids of mature milk. A study in four ethnic groups. American Journal of Clinical Nutrition 17: 180–183

Read WWC, Lutz PG, Tashjian A 1965b Human milk lipids. III. Shortterm effects of dietary carbohydrates and fat. American Journal of Clinical Nutrition 17: 184–187

Rothman J E, Lenard J 1977 Membrane asymmetry. Science 195: 743 and 752

Samuelsson B, Goldyne M, Granstrom E, Hamberg M, Hammarstrom B, Malmsten C 1978 Prostaglandins and thromboxanes. Annual Review of Biochemistry 47: 997–1029

Sanders TAB 1988 Essential and trans fatty acids in nutrition. Nutrition Research Reviews 1: 57–78

Segrest JP, Albers JJ (eds) 1986 The lipoproteins: Volume 128, Preparation, structure and molecular biology; Volume 129, Characterization, cell biology and metabolism. In: Methods in enzymology. Academic Press, New York

Sickinger K 1975 Clinical aspects and therapy of fat malassimilation with particular reference to the use of medium-chain triglycerides. In: Vergroesen A J (ed) The role of fats in human nutrition. Academic Press, London, pp. 116–209

Singer SJ, Nicolson GL 1972 The fluid mosaic model of the structure of cell membranes. Science 175: 720–731

Sjöström L 1973 Carbohydrate-stimulated fatty acid synthesis de novo in human adipose tissue of different cellular types. Acta Medica Scandinavica 194: 387–404

Soderhjelm L, Wiese HF, Holman RT 1970 The role of polyunsaturated fatty acids in human nutrition and metabolism. Progress in the Chemistry of Fats and Other Lipids 9: 555–585

Stern MP, Haffner SM 1986 Body fat distribution and hyperinsulinaemia as risk factors for diabetes and cardiovascular disease. Arteriosclerosis 6: 123–130

Vance DE, Vance JE (eds) 1985 Biochemistry of lipids and membranes. Benjamin Cummings Publishing Co., Menlo Park, California, USA

Wahle KWJ 1983 Fatty acid modification and membrane lipids. Proceedings of the Nutrition Society 42: 273–287

Watts GF, Ahmed W, Quiney J et al 1988 Effective lipid-lowering diets including lean meat. British Medical Journal 296: 235–237

Weber PCV, Fischer S, Schacky CV, Lorenz R, Strasser T 1986 Conversion of dietary eicosapentaenoic acid to prostanoids and leukotrienes in man. Progress in Lipid Research 25: 273–276

Widdowson EM, Dauncy MJ, Gairdner DMT, Jonxis JHP, Pelikan-Filipkova M 1975 Body fat of British and Dutch infants. British Medical Journal 1: 653–655

Wiseman J (ed) 1984 Fats in animal nutrition. Butterworths, London

Wood DA, Riemersma RA, Butler S et al 1987 Linoleic acid and eicosapentaenoic acid in adipose tissue and platelets and risk of coronary heart disease. Lancet 1: 177–183

Zöllner N 1986 Dietary linolenic acid in man – an overview. Progress in Lipid Research 25: 177–180

7. Alcohol: its metabolism and effects

W. P. T. James

Ethyl alcohol (ethanol, C_2H_5OH) is the principal alcohol of nutritional significance in nature. Methyl alcohol (methanol, CH_3OH) is only ingested as a cheap alternative to alcohol by misguided individuals seeking intoxication, despite the high risk of retinal damage and permanent blindness induced by the formaldehyde formed by methanol metabolism. Ethyl alcohol has been produced by most civilizations by fermenting carbohydrate, particularly sugars. It is bactericidal at a concentration of about 70%, and is therefore used as a simple disinfectant for skin preparations or for sterilizing instruments. Its bactericidal properties have also served as a preservative; fruits may be preserved for long periods in distilled spirits. On an industrial basis, alcohol produced by the fermentation of starches is used in some countries as a cheap additional component of petrol for cars.

Alcohol consumption is a feature of many societies, but its effects are so striking and abuse so common that several religions have banned its consumption or counselled against its use; these include Muslims, devout adherents of Buddhism, members of the Hindu Brahmin caste, Mormons and some Christian Presbyterian sects such as Methodists and Quakers. Strict codes of conduct relating to alcohol consumption have often been imposed, and some of the oldest known codes of laws regulate drinking houses, for example in Babylonia around 1770 BC. Alcohol has assumed considerable cultural significance, and secret recipes were developed, often in monasteries, to produce liqueurs and other spirits. In religious rites and festivals alcohol is often used both as a vehicle for participants to attain a 'divine' state of drunkenness, and as a symbol, as when red wine takes the place of sacrificial blood; in the Christian religion, the wine represents the blood of Christ.

The Aztecs of Mexico used alcohol in preparing their victims for sacrifice, and ethanol was also recognized as useful for dulling pain and limiting the stress of surgery before anaesthetics became available.

Different societies have different drinking habits, with beer and spirits dominating in the colder regions where cereals and tubers are ready sources of carbohydrate for fermentation; in warmer climates grapes are grown for wine, sherry and port production, and fruits for the manufacture of liqueurs (Table 7.1).

ALCOHOL INTAKE

This is difficult to estimate because of the social stigma of excess drinking in many societies, and the cerebral effects of alcohol also induce forgetfulness. Many epidemiological analyses record only 40–60% of the intake expected from alcohol sales. Anonymous questionnaires are more reliable than individual records or interviews. Independent estimates of consumption are crude and depend on direct biochemical monitoring of alcohol levels in urine, blood or breath. Excess consumption leads to altered liver metabolism, e.g. elevated α-amino-n-butyric acid, or liver damage with leakage of cytoplasmic liver enzymes into the blood (e.g. γ-glutamyl transpeptidase).

Figure 7.1 shows the changing pattern of drinking in a predominantly beer-drinking country, Britain. These statistics ignore home-brewing, but this contributes less than 2% of total alcohol intake, which currently provides about 6% of the average energy intake of adults. The fluctuations in the amount and type of drink reflect the reduction in availability of alcohol during the 1939–1945 war, and a combination of rising incomes and changing tastes as more northern Europeans holiday in the wine-growing regions of Europe. Drinking habits vary widely worldwide, with declining wine-drinking in France and Italy, but persisting high intakes with episodic drinking are found in Sweden, where taxation is high and sales are restricted in an effort to limit consumption. During the era of prohibition in the USA, illicit alcohol production was widespread and substantial, with an estimated 3 billion litres being produced in

Table 7.1   Typical measures of a variety of alcoholic drinks

Beverage	Origin	Volume (ml)	Alcohol content (%)	Alcohol (g)	Sugar (g)	Energy (kJ)
Beer, lager		280	3.5–5.5	7.5–12.3	8–15	335–502
'Diet'lager		280	4.0–6.0	9.0–13.4	2–10	377–544
Wine	Grapes	120	10–13	9.5	1–3	293–544
Dry sherry		60	18	8.5	1.5	272
Port		45	21	7.0	5.0	293
Whisky	Barley, rye	24	40	7.5	0	209
Gin		24	40	7.5	0	209
Rum	Sugar cane	24	40	7.5	0	209
Mixers:						
Regular		120	0	0	6–12	100–167
Sugar-free		120	0	0	0	0
Liqueurs		30	15–30	5–10	8–10	320–390

Note: 1 unit of alcohol = 8 g or $\frac{1}{2}$ pint beer, 1 small glass table wine, 1 glass sherry or a single measure of spirits
Adapted from Wright & Marks (1985)

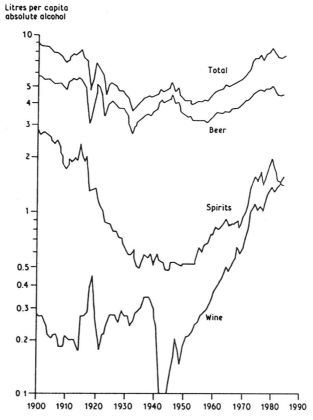

Fig. 7.1   Changes in alcohol consumption in Britain. Reproduced with permission from the Royal College of Physicians (1987)

1930, 3 years before prohibition was repealed. There seems to be a perceived need for alcohol and other drugs in most societies.

Drinking habits also vary within a population, and reflect the interaction of personal and environmental factors. In the UK, men drink twice as much as women and the young more than the old; married adults drink less than single men and women. Usually poor people drink more than the affluent sector of society, and permitted drinking hours influence the pattern of drinking and its consequences. Thus in Scotland in the past, and currently in Australia, shorter hours for licensed drinking has led to heavy, rapid and episodic drinking. Changes in consumption can be assessed from tax-collecting statistics, as shown in Fig. 7.1, but can also be revealed by monitoring the death rates from cirrhosis. A man of average size, e.g. 65 kg, who drinks 170 g ethanol daily for 25 years has a 50% chance of developing liver cirrhosis, and women are equally susceptible at only half that intake (see below). Additional factors, such as hepatic or other nutritional factors, may influence death rates from cirrhosis, which are particularly high in North America, France and Italy. Cirrhosis is causing an increasing mortality in eastern Europe.

ALCOHOL ABSORPTION AND METABOLISM

Some of the alcohol in the stomach is immediately metabolized by the substantial amounts of alcohol dehydrogenase enzyme found in the gastric mucosa. This in part explains the marked discrepancy in the response in blood alcohol levels when alcohol is given orally rather than intravenously. This 'first-pass' metabolism of alcohol is reduced in chronic drinking, because the amount of enzyme falls as gastritis develops with heavy drinking; blood levels then increase after a standard dose. The H_2-antagonist drugs used to reduce gastric acidity in patients with duodenal ulceration, also suppress gastric dehydrogenase, so these patients will have higher blood alcohol levels. Women have less gastric alcohol dehydrogenase activity than men, so they show a greater rise in blood alcohol. This may explain their greater susceptibility to the toxic effects of alcohol. Chinese and North American Indians also absorb ethanol more rapidly than Caucasians. Absorption can be delayed if alcohol is taken slowly throughout the course of a meal, when presumably the gastric mucosal enzyme can metabolize a portion of the ingested dose. Slowed absorption and increased

gastric metabolism may also explain the reduced effects of alcohol when it is preceded by a drink of cream or oil before a party. Once absorbed, the alcohol spreads rapidly into the body-water space, so the smaller size and greater fat content in women amplify the rise. A 65 kg man, on drinking 1 unit of alcohol, can expect to increase his blood alcohol level within the first hour by 150 mg/l, whereas a 55 kg woman shows a rise of about 200 mg/l. In a healthy person alcohol is cleared from the blood by the liver at a constant rate of 15 mg/100 ml blood per hour, i.e. about 6 g alcohol per hour in absolute terms. This rate of metabolism differs markedly from person to person and is noticeably affected by drugs (see below). Alcohol metabolism adapts to heavy intakes by showing an accelerated clearance for reasons which are now becoming clear, but the metabolic and medical consequences of high intake are varied and serious. A higher rate of ethanol metabolism is reported in Chinese, Eskimos, some Mexican and Canadian native Americans, and in the Japanese. Caucasians metabolize on average 90–110 mg ethanol/kg body weight/h, whereas Mongoloids including the Chinese and Japanese, oxidize 120–140 mg ethanol/kg/h. Nevertheless, given the variety of factors which influence ethanol metabolism, for example differences in lean body mass, dietary habits and variable previous alcohol intake (see below), it is by no means certain that these differences are genetic in origin.

ALCOHOL METABOLISM

The liver is the principal site of ethanol metabolism, and four routes of metabolism have been described (Table 7.2). The principal route is via alcohol dehydrogenase in the cytoplasm of the liver cell, with the generation of acetaldehyde and NADPH. Acetaldehyde is toxic and is normally rapidly removed by entering the mitochondria for conversion to acetylCoA prior to oxidation in the tricarboxylic cycle. In many tissues alcohol stimulates the proliferation of microsomal membranes, where a specific cytochrome P-450 fraction IIE1 is induced, but other P-450 isozymes are also capable of metabolizing alcohol, in what is collectively known as the microsomal ethanol-oxidizing system (MEOS). This system, by using rather than generating NADPH, alters the energy coupling of alcohol oxidation to oxidative phosphorylation. Thus heat is generated. Alcoholics have an induced MEOS system, and when

Table 7.2   The metabolism of alcohol

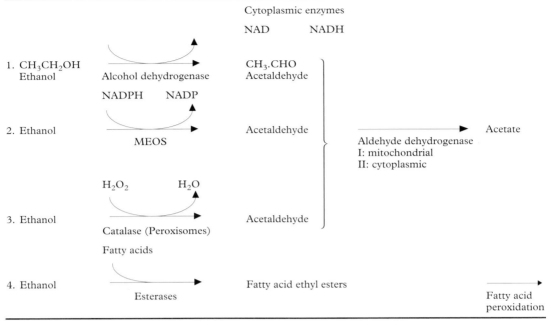

MEOS = microsomal enzyme oxidizing system, particularly the cytochrome P-450 IIE1 enzyme. The alcohol dehydrogenase is present in liver and gastric mucosa; the MEOS is induced in the liver and other tissues by repeated ingestion of ethanol and catalase is also present in several tissues. Esterases are widespread, e.g. in brain, heart and pancreas, and produce little or no acetaldehyde from alcohol. The esterases may contribute to the cell damage by producing non-oxidative esterases, which can be metabolized by fatty acid peroxidation to produce abnormal free radical activity.

given a weight maintenance diet plus extra alcohol fail to gain weight, whereas normal people do (Fig. 7.2). When alcoholics receive 50% of their energy as alcohol instead of carbohydrate, they lose weight. However, modest drinkers, without an induced MEOS, maintain weight (Lieber 1991).

ALCOHOL–DRUG INTERACTIONS

At higher alcohol intakes the MEOS plays a major part in ethanol metabolism, but it also has a profound effect in stimulating drug metabolism (Fig. 7.3). It also serves to activate xenobiotics, e.g. carbon tetrachloride, thereby enhancing their toxicity. The cytochrome P-450 dependent generation of carcinogens is also increased. This may explain why alcohol consumption is a major risk in the development of oesophageal cancer and seems to increase the risk of a variety of cancers, for example breast and lung cancers (see Chapter 45). For the same reason, heavy drinkers are also more susceptible to the hepatotoxicity of industrial

solvents, anaesthetics, chemical carcinogens, many commonly-used drugs and even such readily available analgesics as phenacetin.

The interactions between alcohol and drug metabolism are complex. Once the MEOS is induced, alcohol competes with a variety of drugs for the MEOS, thereby reducing drug clearance and metabolism if alcohol is taken at the same time. However, when the drug is taken without alcohol a marked acceleration in the metabolism of some commonly used drugs is observed (Table 7.3 and Fig. 7.3). Thus the short- and long-term effects of alcohol have opposite effects on drug metabolism. Doctors and dietitians frequently fail to forewarn patients of these dangers. Ethanol enhances the metabolism of endogenous and exogenous steroids, e.g. vitamin D, and increases the catabolism of testosterone and its conversion to oestrogens, producing a fall in blood testosterone levels. This effect is amplified by alcohol's inhibition of the testicular synthesis of testoterone.

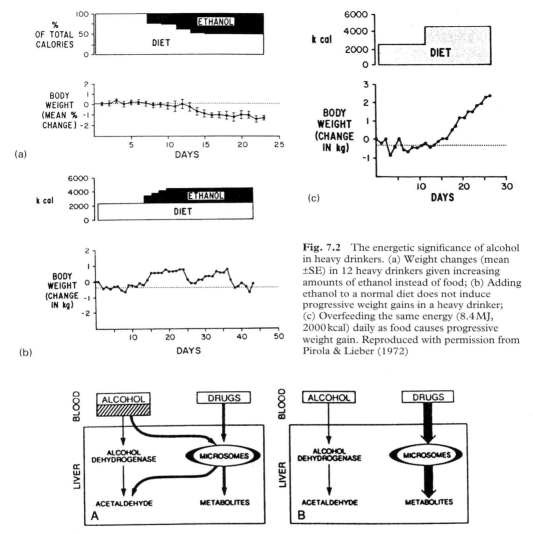

Fig. 7.2 The energetic significance of alcohol in heavy drinkers. (a) Weight changes (mean ±SE) in 12 heavy drinkers given increasing amounts of ethanol instead of food; (b) Adding ethanol to a normal diet does not induce progressive weight gains in a heavy drinker; (c) Overfeeding the same energy (8.4 MJ, 2000 kcal) daily as food causes progressive weight gain. Reproduced with permission from Pirola & Lieber (1972)

Fig. 7.3 The effects of high alcohol intakes on drug metabolism. (a) Alcohol induces the microsomal ethanol-oxidizing system (MEOS) but competes with drugs as a substrate. When alcohol is drunk, drug metabolism is therefore inhibited; (b) when the chronic drinker fails to drink alcohol on the day a drug is taken, then the persisting MEOS accelerates normal drug metabolism. (Adapted from Lieber 1988)

Alcohol dehydrogenase

This enzyme (ADH) oxidizes many alcohols to their corresponding aldehydes and is an enzyme widely found in nature – in animals, plants and micro-organisms. Alcohols arising in foodstuffs and fruits are readily metabolized by these ADHs to acetaldehyde. ADH may also play a part in retinol–retinal inter-conversion in the eye (see Chapter 13), in the metabolism of steroids and bile acids, and the catabolism of short-chain alcohols responsible for food flavours. The enzyme also seems to play a key role in the metabolism of dopamine, so its physio-logical function is extensive. ADH also metabolizes methanol and the ethylene glycol used as antifreeze, both of which are toxic. Digitalis compounds given to treat cardiac failure are also metabolized. ADH therefore has a fundamental physiological role.

ADH is a protein with two subunits (molecular weight 40 000 each). Its activity differs between

Table 7.3 Acute and chronic effects of alcohol on drug metabolism

Acute effects with decreased metabolism of:	Chronic effects of high alcohol intakes with increased metabolism of:
Benzodiazepines	Benzodiazepines
Barbiturates	Barbiturates
Phenothiazines	-
Tricyclic antidepressants	-
Chlormethiazole	Chlormethiazole
Dextropropoxyphene	-
Monoamine oxidase inhibitors	-
Oral hypoglycaemic agents	Tolbutamide
Phenytoin	Phenytoin
Warfarin	Warfarin
Metronidazole	-
	Paracetamol
	Alkylating agents
	Anitipyrine
	Meprobamate

From the Royal College of Physicians (1987) with permission

people for genetic reasons, there being at least five different gene loci controlling its activity, with eight known types of subunit. During development, different forms – isozymes – of ADH appear at different stages. Different isozymes also occur in different tissues and in different locations within the cell, and have variable abilities to metabolize ethanol. The pattern of isozyme varies according to race, because of the varying gene influences. Thus one variant (ADH Indianapolis) is found in 25% of American blacks but is absent from white Americans, Germans and Japanese. Only about 5–10% of the English, 9–14% of Germans, and 20% of Swiss have an atypical type (ADH$_2$), but this variant occurs in over 85% of the Japanese, Chinese and Mongoloid races. The atypical ADH has several times the catalytic activity of other ADHs. This enzyme form may explain the more rapid conversion of alcohol to acetaldehyde in the Japanese and Mongoloids, who have a higher blood acetaldehyde level after alcohol than do whites. This may also explain the greater prevalence of alcohol intolerance in these races, but there is no link between the presence of this atypical ADH type and alcohol intolerance on an individual basis.

Normally acetaldehyde concentrations increase only in the liver, because acetaldehyde is usually rapidly metabolized to acetate by acetaldehyde dehydrogenase (ALDH). This enzyme acts via an NAD-dependent step which converts acetaldehyde and many other aldehydes in the body to acetylCoA or the corresponding keto acids. ALDH also exists in a number of isomeric forms, controlled by different gene loci.

ALDH I isoenzyme has a low Km in the mitochondria, so rapid metabolism at low concentrations of acetaldehyde is likely in those with this isoenzyme. The isoenzymes are inhibited by the drug disulfiram (Antabuse) which is used to deter alcoholics from drinking because it limits the metabolism of acetaldehyde, thereby producing extremely unpleasant 'hangovers' as well as toxic effects as acetaldehyde accumulates. Oriental populations of Mongoloid origin have a deficiency of ALDH I isoenzyme, as do 40% of South Americans, but not North American Indians. Caucasian and Negroid populations rarely show an absence of ALDH I. ALDH I-deficient Japanese have a 15-fold increase in plasma acetaldehyde compared with Japanese with normal ALDH I levels (Table 7.4) and ^{13}C ethanol given orally is converted to $^{13}CO_2$ more slowly (Lehmann et al 1986).

THE ACUTE RESPONSE TO ETHANOL

These are listed in Table 7.5. The range of reactions are many and individuals differ markedly in their responses, which are determined by the extent to which alcohol stimulates the sympathetic nervous system and by the rate of production of acetaldehyde and acetate. The most frequent responses are an increase in heart rate and peripheral vasodilation. This explains the great sense of warmth, which can be hazardous in cold environments when individuals remove clothes and rapidly lose body heat while believing themselves to be overheated. In some individuals a moderate amount of alcohol exerts a very marked effect, with facial flushing, palpitation, tachycardia and muscle weakness. This 'alcohol intolerance' is found in only 5–10% of Europeans compared with 60–85% of orientals and American Indians, who often develop a marked aversion to alcohol. Adults of mixed oriental–Caucasian blood have a flushing response after drinking alcohol similar to that of orientals. In Caucasians alcohol intolerance runs in families, with fast-flush (after only one drink)

Table 7.4 The metabolic response to ethanol in Japanese with alcohol intolerance

	Peak blood levels	
	Ethanol (mmol/1)	Acetaldehyde (μmol/1)
Normal	10.3±1.9	2.1±1.7
ALDH-1-deficient	10.9±2.3	35.4±12.8

From Harada et al (1981)

Table 7.5   Acute psychophysiological responses to ethanol

Objective symptoms	Subjective symptoms
Disturbed left ventricular performance	Cutaneous erythema and facial flushing
Cardiac depression	Blotching of the trunk and arms
Hypotension	Hot feeling in the stomach/nausea
Tachycardia	Dizziness/hangover
Bradycardia	Numbness in hands or feet
Peripheral vasodilation	Abdominal discomfort
Increased skin temperature	Muscle weakness
Augmented flow in arteries	Shakes
Increase in heart rate	Chest distress/palpitation

From Agarwal & Goedde (1990), with permission

and slow-flush (two or more drinks induce flushing) family groups; autosomal dominance is, however, not yet clear.

This flushing response may depend on aldehyde effects and not on alcohols, with acetaldehyde being a greater stimulator of catecholamine release from the adrenal medulla and sympathetic nervous system than ethanol. Plasma acetaldehyde and catecholamines, as well as urinary catecholamines, rise after ethanol ingestion in those who flush. Other metabolites are involved, however, including the vasodilators histamine and the prostaglandins. When aspirin, an inhibitor of the cyclo-oxygenase enzyme needed for prostaglandin synthesis, is given to subjects with alcohol intolerance, then alcohol-induced flushing of the face is blocked (Truitt et al 1987). Other mediators, for example endorphins, have also been implicated in studies with opioid antagonists (Ho et al 1988).

If flushing depends on acetaldehyde concentrations, then its rate of metabolism as well as production is important. This flushing is so unpleasant that it is not surprising that the drinking habits of orientals with ALDH I deficiency are in general more modest than those observed in Caucasians. Japanese who experience flushing after drinking ethanol also consume less than their normal compatriots.

Ethanol also promotes water loss by the kidney. This diuresis can lead to dehydration in spirit drinkers who consume high amounts of concentrated alcohol without additional water. The water loss occurs because alcohol inhibits the normal response of the hypothalamic osmoreceptors; the rate of arginine vasopressin release therefore falls below what it should be for the plasma osmolality. With the fall in the output of this antidiuretic hormone, the distal tubule no longer concentrates the urine and substantial losses of body water occur.

ALCOHOLISM

In general the prevalence of alcoholism is much lower in the Japanese, Chinese and other ethnic groups within the Mongolian race than among Caucasians, and this may relate to the rate and routes of alcohol metabolism. Whereas normally over 40% of Japanese have ALDH I deficiency, in Japanese alcoholics the isoenzyme is deficient in only 2–5%, implying that having an ALDH I deficiency is a great deterrent to drinking. Similar findings are seen in Taiwan.

North American and Mexican Indians have several times the prevalence of alcoholism seen in white US citizens. These groups also metabolize alcohol faster, rarely have ALDH I deficiency, and can therefore be expected to metabolize acetaldehyde satisfactorily. When deficiency occurs, the Indians drink less than normal and alcoholism is rare in this group, as in the Japanese and Taiwanese with a similar deficiency.

Despite the expected rapid ethanol and acetaldehyde metabolism of the American Indians, flushing is common. Although this has been linked with acetaldehyde accumulation in orientals, histamine or prostaglandin effects may dominate in the Indians, who probably originated as a subgroup of the Mongolian race.

It seems clear that there are several metabolic factors which influence the immediate behavioural and physiological responses to a drink containing ethanol. Genetic–environmental interactions determine the alcohol-drinking behaviour not only of different racial groups, but also that of individuals within any one society. Alcoholism is a familial condition, with sons and brothers of alcoholic men having a 25–50% risk of alcoholism themselves. There is also over a 55% concordance of alcoholism in identical twins, compared with a rate of 28% in non-identical twins of the same sex (see Schuckit & Rayses 1979).

These differences must still reflect important environmental pressures, because otherwise the identical twins would have a 100% concordance for alcoholism. Genetic factors play an important role: adoption studies in Scandinavia clearly show a more than fourfold increase in the children of alcoholics, even when the children were separated from the parents at birth and raised without knowing their biological parent's drinking problems. Conversely, children adopted into alcoholic families have relatively low rates of alcoholism (Goodwin 1987; Dinwiddie & Cloninger 1989). Alcohol preferences can also be bred into strains of animals.

In view of the low rate of alcoholism in Japanese and Taiwanese with ALDH I deficiency who exhibit elevated acetaldehyde concentrations and flushing after small doses of ethanol, it is surprising that Caucasian children of alcoholics with a concomitant high risk of alcoholism tend to have high levels of acetaldehyde after a standard dose of ethanol (Schuckit & Rayses 1979). This implies that the acute aversion induced by acetaldehyde can be overcome in some way. One possible explanation is that acetaldehyde can condense directly with biogenic amines (e.g. dopamine, serotonin) to form isoquinoline derivatives such as salsolinol, and acetaldehyde also competes with the aldehyde metabolites of amines for the aldehyde dehydrogenase pathway. One aldehyde, dopamine aldehyde (DOPAL), can therefore accumulate and condense with dopamine itself to form the addictive opiate-like compound tetrahydropapaveroline (THP). THP is formed in the brain after alcohol drinking, particularly in the amine-rich regions of the cerebral cortex, and acts as a false transmitter (Fig. 7.4). Salsolinol infused into the brain ventricles of the rat at low doses produces morphine-like behaviour, with a remarkable increase in the preference for ethanol drinking. At high doses salsolinol induces stimulatory effects which make the symptoms of alcohol withdrawal in the chronically drinking animal worse. Experimentally, an inhibitor of ALDH I given either into the blood or directly into the rat brain, leads to an increase in the voluntary consumption of alcohol as the endogenous formation of biogenic aldehydes increases (Critcher & Myers 1987). Biogenic amines are also found in the urine of alcoholics, but the evidence that these quinoline derivatives are the key to alcohol addiction is still lacking.

BIOCHEMICAL ASPECTS OF ALCOHOLISM

The changes seen in individuals drinking too much alcohol are influenced not only by the amount drunk

but by the individual's genetic predisposition, nutritional state, the diet eaten with the alcohol drinking, and the sex and hormonal status of the individual. Pre-existing organ damage will also alter the spectrum of changes and disease.

The direct toxic effects of ethanol and local acetaldehyde produced in the epithelium probably account for the inflammatory changes in the oesophagus and stomach found in heavy drinkers. As the damage progresses, gastric secretion falls and intestinal damage, with reduced enzyme activities, including disaccharidases, becomes common. The importance of alcohol in reducing folate absorption is dealt with in Chapter 14, but other nutrients can also be malabsorbed. The diarrhoea which follows heavy drinking may depend on fluid overload, which produces a cholera-like effect as the alcohol passes

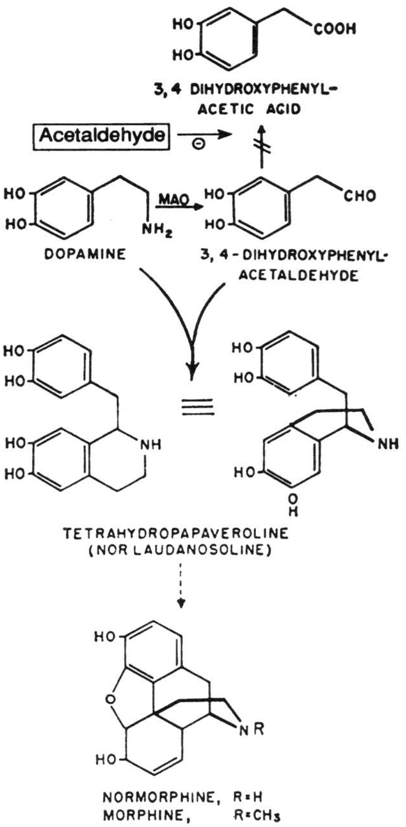

Fig. 7.4 An example of one route whereby ethanol ingestion could induce the production of addictive metabolites in the brain. (Modified from Davis & Walsh 1970)

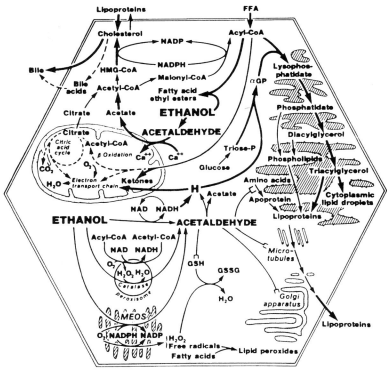

Fig. 7.5 The metabolic effects of alcohol on lipid metabolism in the liver.
(Reproduced with permission from Lieber 1985)

rapidly into the colon. It may also be metabolized by microorganisms to induce an acetaldehyde-stimulated colonic response.

Liver changes

Chronic alcoholism produces liver changes which progress from fatty infiltration to hepatitis, fibrosis and cirrhosis. The biochemical basis of liver damage has been covered by Lieber (1985, 1988a) who has summarized the metabolic effects of ethanol in a diagram (Fig. 7.5). Lieber points out that many toxic effects and disturbances in intermediary metabolism can be linked to the generation of NADPH by alcohol. The induction of the MEOS system in the cytoplasm is also important (see Metabolism above) and acetaldehyde itself is toxic, with effects on collagen metabolism. The catalase enzyme system in the cytoplasm peroxisomes uses the hydrogen peroxide generated by fatty acid oxidation and other oxidative reactions (see Table 7.2) but the formation of fatty acid ether esterases, when these are metabolized, induces free radical activity which is increas-

ingly recognized as an important contributor to hepatic disease. The concentrations of glutathione (a free radical scavenger) tend to be reduced in alcoholic liver disease, particularly when iron levels are raised, with conjugated diene formation (Situnayake et al 1990). Experimentally, therapy with vitamin E helps to prevent alcoholic liver damage, but the reduced vitamin A content of the alcoholic liver, despite adequate intakes and plasma vitamin A concentrations, probably reflects the effect of alcohol on the recently discovered stellate cells in the liver, which selectively store vitamin A (Blomhoff et al 1991). Providing vitamin A to patients with alcoholic liver disease seems to exacerbate rather than help the problem (Lieber 1988a). Lipids also accumulate, because of the increased direct channelling of ethanol as a substrate to acetate via acetaldehyde, with the subsequent conversion of acetylCoA to fatty acids. The changed redox state contributes to this conversion. About half the increase in liver size in heavy drinkers is explained by the excess fat. Export protein secretion is inhibited, probably by the effect of acetaldehyde on the cytoplasmic microtubules, which are responsible for the secretion of proteins such as transferrin, so that export proteins accumulate in the liver, as do fatty acid-binding proteins. As alcohol ingestion continues, mitochondrial damage becomes obvious and fatty acid oxidation becomes impaired, as may alcohol metabolism in the mitochondria. Fatty acids must therefore be oxidized by the peroxisomes. The increase in ethanol metabolism in the cytoplasm accelerates free radical generation and a further fall in the protective concentrations of glutathione. Clearly, if the dietary provision of the precursors for glutathione – cysteine, glycine and glutamate – are not provided, and a poor-quality diet lacking in vitamin A, β-carotene and vitamins E and C, is also eaten by heavy drinkers, it is little wonder that the liver disease is exacerbated. Microsomal oxidases induced by alcohol accentuate superoxide and H_2O_2 production, and the P-450 IIE 1 enzyme in the cytochrome P-450 system (see Metabolism above) is also induced and generates hydroxyl radicals. Indices of lipid peroxidation in the phospholipid portion of the blood lipids return to normal within 2–4 days when alcoholics stop drinking and return to a normal diet (Fink et al 1985).

Acetaldehyde itself promotes fibrinogenesis by stimulating collagen synthesis, as well as directly interacting with proteins within the membranes of the liver cell. With cellular damage developing, the liver becomes inflamed and this will exacerbate the development of fibrosis and eventually the full picture of cirrhosis develops, with progressive loss of actively functioning liver tissue. Autoimmune responses are also important and may be triggered by the development of an abnormal cytokeratin, which seems to develop in vitamin A deficiency.

Nutritional factors

The influence of alcohol on nutritional status is reviewed by Lieber (1988b) and the nutritional management of alcohol-related disease is dealt with in Chapter 48. The role of nutrition in the development of cirrhosis was debated for years, because many patients are malnourished and it was not clear whether the poor diet of alcoholics was primarily responsible for the liver damage, or whether sick patients with liver disease becoming anorexic became secondarily malnourished.

Pancreatitis

Alcohol directly inhibits the secretion of pancreatic enzymes, but how this relates to the development of chronic relapsing pancreatitis in alcoholics is uncertain. Hyperlipidaemia, especially hypertriglyceridaemia, seems particularly liable to cause pancreatitis, and alcohol is known to induce high plasma triglycerides in susceptible subjects, presumably both by stimulating triacylglycerol synthesis and by inducing insulin resistance. How elevated plasma VLDLs are linked to pancreatitis remains unclear. Women are more sensitive to pancreatitis than men, presumably because of the speed and extent of the rise in plasma ethanol on drinking.

Cardiac and muscle effects

The cardiac effects of alcoholism can progress from cellular swelling, fatty infiltration and inflammation to fibrosis and progressive weakness of the muscle, with the development of an alcoholic cardiomyopathy and congestive heart failure. Most patients with this problem are drinking over 80 g of alcohol daily, the alcohol damaging the muscle proteins themselves, presumably through the action of acetaldehyde. Ethanol also inhibits the binding of actin and myosin, thus interfering with muscular contractility. This is made worse by the mitochondrial damage.

Not only is cardiac muscle affected, but so too are the arteriolar muscles. High blood pressure is common in heavy alcohol drinkers and should be one of the first issues to be assessed and dealt with. The hypertension may also reflect the effects of alcohol on the sympathetic nervous system (see Hypertension and cerebrovascular disease below). This hypertension and the high cardiac output of patients with alcoholic liver disease (see Chapter 48) may induce cardiac hypertrophy, which is another feature of alcoholism, before the direct effects of ethanol on the heart induce congestive cardiac failure.

Given the alcohol-induced increase in blood pressure it is not surprising that there is a link between alcohol drinking and strokes (Altura & Altura 1989).

Ethanol drinking also affects skeletal muscle function; muscle weakness is common in heavy drinkers, and myopathy develops in alcoholics. Alcohol is toxic to striated muscle in a dose-dependent manner (Urbano-Marquez et al 1989). Damage to skeletal muscle is evident on electron microscopic study in volunteers given 225 g ethanol daily for a month (Rubin et al 1976). What determines the progression from the membrane damage seen in many patients to the loss of myofibrils and fibrosis is unknown. The myopathy tends to be of the proximal type, presumably because the larger muscles take up the greatest amounts of ethanol. Patients may become seriously incapacitated and unable to walk.

Brain

The immediate depressive and euphoric effects of ethanol on mental function are well recognized and are summarized in relation to blood alcohol level in Table 7.6. In some societies episodic heavy drinking is the rule, and this can lead to much more serious problems than those encountered in individuals consuming the same amount of alcohol but on a regular basis. Brainstem and cerebellar functions are affected before the cerebral cortex, and the behavioural response may depend on the social environment: in congenial company the drinker often feels excited, whereas solitary drinking may lead to feelings of isolation and depression. As blood levels rise, individuals often feel that they have greater ability when in fact their motor and intellectual performance is clearly deteriorating. Emotional restraint is then lost before drowsiness and coma, with depressed tendon responses, and a low blood pressure and low body temperature develop as alcohol levels rise. Death usually results from respiratory depression or the inhalation of vomit.

DELETERIOUS CONSEQUENCES OF ALCOHOL INTAKE

Different types of drinker can be classified on the basis of their consumption of alcohol and their ability to cope. A 'social drinker' may take two to three units of alcohol a day, and does not become intoxicated. A 'heavy drinker' usually drinks six units a day without apparent immediate harm, whereas a 'problem drinker' has physical, psychological, social, family, legal or occupational problems attributable to drink. A 'dependent drinker' is usually a consistent drinker with a tolerance to alcohol, which is increased early but reduced later. Withdrawal symptoms are relieved by further alcohol. In all types of drinker, individual variation in the susceptibility to alcohol is great. These are summarized in Table 7.7 and dealt with in detail in an excellent report from the British Royal College of Physicians (1987).

Alcohol withdrawal symptoms

When a regular heavy drinker stops consuming alcohol he can experience a variety of responses, ranging from tremor and hallucinations to epileptic fits and delirium tremens. Tremor is common

Table 7.6   Effects of specific quantities of alcohol intake on blood ethanol concentrations and mental function

Number of drinks	Blood alcohol level (mg/100 ml)	Effects
1 pint of beer or 2 glass of wine or a double whisky	30	Increasing likelihood of having an accident
1.5 pints of beer or 3 whiskies or half a (75 cl) bottle of wine	50	Increasing cheerfulness, impaired judgement and loosening of inhibitions
2.5 pints of beer or 5 whiskies or 5 glasses of wine	80	Loss of driving licence if caught
5 pints of beer or 10 whiskies or 1 litre of wine	150	Loss of self-control; exuberance; quarrelsomeness slurred speech
6 pints of beer or half a bottle of spirits or 2 (75 cl) bottles of wine	200	Stagger; double vision; loss of memory
0.75 bottle of spirits	400	Oblivion; sleepiness; coma
1 bottle of spirits	500	Death possible
	600	Death certain

From the Royal College of Physicians (1987), with permission

Table 7.7   Summary of physical health hazards associated with alcohol abuse

Nervous system
Acute intoxication; 'blackouts'
Persistent brain damage:
   Wernicke's encephalopathy
   Korsakoff's syndrome
   Cerebellar degeneration
   Dementia

Cerebrovascular disease
   Strokes, especially in young people
   Subarachnoid haemorrhage
   Subdural haematoma after head injury
Withdrawal symptoms:
   Tremor, hallucinations, fits
Nerve and muscle damage:
   Weakness, paralysis, burning sensation in hands and feet

Liver
Infiltration of liver with fat
Alcoholic hepatitis
Cirrhosis and eventual liver failure
Liver cancer

Gastrointestinal system
Reflux of acid into the oesophagus
Tearing and occasionally rupture of the oesophagus
Cancer of the oesophagus
Gastritis
Aggravation and impaired healing of peptic ulcers
Diarrhoea and impaired absorption of food
Chronic inflammation of the pancreas leading in some to diabetes and malabsorption of food

Nutrition
Malnutrition from reduced intake of food, toxic effects of alcohol on intestine, and impaired metabolism, leading to weight loss
Obesity, particularly in early stages of heavy drinking

Heart and circulatory system
Abnormal rhythms
High blood pressure
Chronic heart muscle damage leading to heart failure

Respiratory system
Fractured ribs
Pneumonia from inhalation of vomit

Endocrine system
Overproduction of cortisol leading to obesity, acne, increased facial hair, and high blood pressure
Condition mimicking overactivity of the thyroid, with loss of weight, anxiety, palpitations, sweating and tremor
Severe fall in blood sugar, sometimes leading to coma
Intense facial flushing in many diabetics taking the antidiabetic drug chlorpropamide

Reproductive system
In men, loss of libido, reduced potency, shrinkage in size of testes and penis, reduced or absent sperm formation and hence infertility, and loss of sexual hair
In women, sexual difficulties, menstrual irregularities, and shrinkage of breasts and genitalia.

Occupation and accidents
Impaired work performance and decision making
Increased risk and severity of accidents

The fetus, the child, and the family
Damage to the fetus and the fetal alcohol syndrome
Acute intoxication in young children:
   hypothermia, low blood sugar levels, depressed respiration
Effect on physical development and behaviour of the child through heavy drinking by parents

Interaction of alcohol with medicinal substances
Increased likelihood of unwanted effects of drugs
Reduced effectiveness of medicines

affecting a third of patients with alcoholic neurological problems. It appears 12–24 hours after the last drink, with restlessness and insomnia. The tremor subsides within hours or days unless suppressed with further alcohol. Isolated or generalized epileptic fits occur 12–48 hours after withdrawal, and may precede delirium tremens. This develops 2–5 days after alcohol withdrawal with an abrupt onset, often at night, of nightmares and disorientation. Agitated subjects tremble with hallucinations, sweat, and may become feverish. This phase subsides after 2–3 days but dehydration, circulatory collapse, hypothermia, pneumonia and injury may be lethal.

Prolonged alcohol abuse: Wernicke's encephalopathy

Thiamin deficiency associated with alcoholism is the cause of this frequently undiagnosed condition. Mental changes, abnormal eye movements and unsteadiness can be arrested by the intravenous injection of thiamin (see Chapter 14). The confused state tends to recover first, with abnormal eye movements persisting for days or weeks, and nystagmus sometimes for months. Some alcoholics present with an isolated progressive cerebellar defect. Only 14% of cases of Wernicke's encephalopathy had been diagnosed before death in one study from Australia (Harper 1979), and there is little evidence that diagnosis is better elsewhere. The brain has characteristic lesions in the brain stem and close to the cerebral ventricles. Korsakoff's syndrome may follow Wernicke's encephalopathy, which is why the two names are frequently linked.

Korsakoff's syndrome is characterized by extreme loss of memory, and this is associated anatomically with more chronic lesions which may not respond so readily to thiamin. With chronic abuse there is clear evidence of cerebral ventricular enlargement, this being found in young male heavy drinkers with no symptoms. Surprisingly, there can be substantial improvement in the ventricular enlargement shown on computerized tomographic scanning if the drinking stops, but the improvement depends on the degree of cerebral atrophy, particularly of the white matter, which is prominent in those with Wernicke's encephalopathy and alcoholic liver disease.

Peripheral nerve damage

Functional loss of the peripheral sensory and motor nerves is a frequent complication of chronic alcohol abuse, and is more common in alcoholic women. Burning discomfort, extreme skin sensitivity and weakness of the hip and thigh muscles are not unusual. Tendon reflexes are lost and evidence of neuropathy of the autonomic nervous system may be found.

Fetal alcohol syndrome

There is a clear correlation between maternal alcohol abuse during pregnancy and fetal abnormalities. Intakes of more than 10 units (80 g) alcohol per day is linked with the fetal alcohol syndrome. This has four features: intrauterine growth retardation, typical facial features (e.g. poor formation of the mid-face (maxillary) area, a small fissure between the eye lids), neurodevelopmental abnormalities including microcephaly, and a variety of other congenital abnormalities, e.g. of the joints and heart. There is considerable variability in the development of this syndrome in women who drink heavily. The basis for this variability is unknown, but babies may have only one or more of the syndrome's features and be less severely affected than in the extreme form. About 1 in 1 000 live babies worldwide are affected with the full syndrome, whereas some fetal alcohol effects are more frequent, at 3 per 1 000.

These observations question whether it is safe for pregnant women to drink any alcohol. Currently there is little evidence that modest drinking, i.e. less than 10 units/80 g alcohol *per week* has a harmful effect (Royal College of Physicians 1987). Effects on the fetus are much more clearly documented with smoking and the use of illegal drugs rather than with alcohol use (Plant 1985). Nevertheless, maternal and, curiously, paternal drinking may reduce birthweight, so it is probably sensible for women to abstain from alcohol or to have only the occasional drink, especially in early pregnancy when fetal development is occurring. Alcohol does appear in breast milk at the same concentration as in plasma, but this level of input to the baby will be harmless.

SOCIAL–ECONOMIC ASPECTS OF ALCOHOL USE

These are well set out in the Royal College of Physicians' report. Table 7.8 lists the cost of alcohol abuse to a nation. The costs to a country where alcohol use is substantial are immense in both economic and social terms. There is a loss of production from workers who fail to turn up for work (typically at the beginning of the working week), or who have accidents or illness at work. Other obvious

Table 7.8   Cost of alcohol abuse to the nation

Cost to industry
   Sickness absence
   Unexplained absence from the job and lateness to work
   Reduced efficiency and decision making at work
   Higher accident rates
   Impaired industrial relations
   Early retirement and premature death
   Higher labour turnover and retraining
Cost to the NHS
   Psychiatric care
   Non-psychiatric care
   GP care
Social response costs
   Expenditure by national alcohol bodies
   Research
Cost of material damage
   Road traffic accidents
   Home accidents, industrial accidents and fire damage
Cost of criminal activities
   Police costs associated with traffic offences (excluding
      cost of accidents)
   Other criminal offences
   Drink-related court cases
   Probation, judiciary and prison service

From the Royal College of Physicians (1987), with
permission

contributors to cost include motor car accidents and
injuries at home arising from carelessness. Physical
abuse by angry intoxicated men is another contributor
to the economic costs. About a third of home
accidents in Britain are related to alcohol.

Figure 7.6 shows the risk of road accidents in
relation to the blood alcohol level. The British legal
limit is currently set at 80 mg per 100 ml of blood, but
a slowness to respond to emergencies is already evident at lower concentrations in the susceptible, so it is
little surprising that an excess number of accidents
occur after very small amounts of alcohol. The risk is
greater in the young adult and elderly person, and in
those who are not habitual drinkers. Pedestrians as
well as drivers are also injured or killed, because they
too misjudge distances and the speed of cars when
crossing roads.

For children brought up in homes with alcoholic
parents there is a sixfold increase in risk of behavioural problems (Nylander 1960) and these emotional
problems persist into adult life, with alcohol and drug
abuse as common disorders. Whether this is a
reflection of social or genetic influences is uncertain.
Hyperactive and delinquent children are more likely
to have alcoholic parents. Young, heavy drinkers may
have lost one or more parents in early life, or have
spent part of their time in institutional care.

METABOLIC EFFECTS OF ALCOHOL: CARBOHYDRATE CHANGES: GLUCOSE CHANGES

Both hyperglycaemia and hypoglycaemia may be
encountered after alcohol ingestion. Acute hypoglycaemia may result from drug–alcohol interactions
and reflect an inhibition of gluconeogenesis. A fall in
blood glucose also occurs 6–36 hours after an

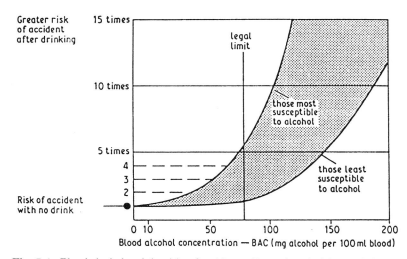

Fig. 7.6   Blood alcohol and the risks of accidents. (Reproduced with permission
from the Royal College of Physicians 1987)

alcoholic binge, especially if the alcohol is taken on an empty stomach. Young children are also susceptible to alcohol and can display unusual behaviour when given quite small amounts by their parents. Glucose intolerance sometimes leading to diabetes is also encountered in chronic heavy drinking, but the diabetes is usually mild.

Alcohol induces an increase in high-density lipoproteins especially in HDL_2. VLDL synthesis increases as alcohol increases the hepatic triglyceride secretion responsible for the hypertriglyceridaemia. An increase in VLDL catabolism to HDL_2 may explain the response to alcohol, but the feminizing action of alcohol may also be responsible (see below).

Sex hormone metabolism

Ethanol affects mainly the liver and gonads, with little effect on the control of sex steroid metabolism at the pituitary level. Within minutes of taking a drink of alcohol there are changes in the plasma sex hormones. In young male volunteers the plasma concentrations of the oestrogens conjugated in the liver to glucuronides and monosulphates increased in parallel with the concentrations of blood alcohol (Andersson et al 1987), and this is presumed to reflect the change in the redox state of the liver as ethanol is oxidized. The rise in oestradiol monosulphate will then increase the availability of the oestrogenic hormone to the peripheral tissues. Alcohol is also known to directly inhibit testosterone synthesis in the testis, so testosterone levels commonly fall in habitual drinkers. In addition, there is now evidence that some drinks, e.g. whisky, contain congeners which have high oestrogenic activity, as one might expect if they contain phyto-oestrogens (Gavaler et al 1987) derived from the barley or other cereal used for fermenting the alcoholic drinks. Alcoholic women also lose their libido and suffer from ovarian atrophy, with menstrual disturbances and sterility. There is premenopausal shrinking of their breasts and external genitalia. Heavily drinking men show many signs of feminization, with testicular atrophy, gynaecomastia, loss of libido and changes in skin and hair growth. These changes may depend not only on the direct effects of alcohol but also on the effects of liver disease in altering sex steroid breakdown.

CARCINOGENIC EFFECTS OF ALCOHOL

The role of alcohol in enhancing the risk of cancer is dealt with in Chapter 45.

ALCOHOL AND ITS LINKS WITH CHRONIC ADULT DISEASE

Alcohol provides a ready source of energy, but the effects on energy expenditure will depend on the chronicity and intensity of alcohol intake (see Alcohol metabolism above). The acute effect of alcohol on energy expenditure is also variable, with a post-prandial thermogenic response over a few hours amounting to 0–8% of the alcohol energy ingested. How alcohol intake interacts with the physiological control of food intakes is unclear, but weight gain in young men in the 20–30-year-old group has been linked with the onset of frequent drinking. There is also some suggestion that alcohol drinking (and smoking) are particularly conducive to fat deposition in the omental area, thus producing a selective increase in the waist–hip ratio (Seidell, personal communication) with all its associated hazards (see Chapter 32).

Hypertension and cerebrovascular disease

Alcohol stimulates the development of high blood pressure in previously normotensive adults (Puddey et al 1985) and seems to play an important part in the early stages of hypertension. The effect seems to be mediated independently of obesity, and occurs at very modest alcohol intakes. Given this effect on blood pressure, it is perhaps surprising that alcohol consumption is linked to a lower incidence of cardiovascular disease. At modest intakes, e.g. 35–100 g alcohol per week, the risk of ischaemic strokes (in both men and women) seems to be 40–60% less, and any enhanced risk of stroke with heavier drinking in both sexes seems to be linked with subarachnoid haemorrhages (Stampfer et al 1988). Subdural and extradural haematomas are frequent in heavy drinkers because they often fall and injure their heads. Acute bouts of drinking may also lead to cerebral infarcts in young adults, perhaps by altering clotting and/or by inducing acute rises in blood pressure. In heavy drinkers, i.e. >300 g/week, the selective extra risk of stroke in men is four times greater than in non-drinkers (Gill et al 1986), even after adjusting for the hypertension and smoking observed so frequently in these men.

Coronary heart disease

Recent studies (Shaper 1990; Rimm et al 1991) show a clear inverse relationship between the degree of alcohol intake and the incidence of coronary heart disease, with a progressive fall to 40% below the rate of non-drinkers in those consuming more than 30 g per day. Originally there was a concern that the higher mortality rate of non-drinkers simply reflected the inclusion in this group of sick individuals who had given up heavy drinking. The new data, however, suggest that the effect is genuine but the mechanism for the protective effect remains obscure. A metabolic effect on lipid metabolism with an increase in HDL_2 cholesterol levels is a plausible explanation, but the feminization effects of alcohol may also indicate a protective effect which is sex-hormone mediated.

REFERENCES

Altura BM, Altura BT 1989 Cardiovascular functions in alcoholism and after acute administration of alcohol: heart and blood vessels. In: Agarwal DP, Goedde HW (eds) 1990 Alcohol metabolism, alcohol intolerance and alcoholism. Springer-Verlag, Berlin.

Andersson SHG, Cronholm T, Sjovall J 1987 Effects of ethanol on conjugated gonadal hormones in plasma of men. Alcohol and Alcoholism Suppl 1: 529–531

Blomhoff R, Green MH, Green JB, Berg T, Norman KR 1991 Vitamin A metabolism: new perspectives on absorption, transport and storage. Physiological Reviews 71: 952–990

Critcher EC, Myers RD 1987 Cyanamide given ICV or systemically to the rat alters subsequent alcohol drinking. Alcohol 4: 347–353

Davis VE, Walsh MJ 1970 Alcohol amines and alkaloids: a possible biochemical basis for alcohol addiction. Science 167: 1005–1006

Dinwiddie SH, Cloninger CR 1989 Family and adoption studies of alcoholism. In: Goedde HW, Agarwal DP (eds) Alcoholism: biomedical and genetic aspects. Pergamon, New York, pp. 259–276

Fink R, Clemens MR, Marjot DH et al 1985 Increased free-radical activity in alcoholics. Lancet ii: 291–294

Gavaler JS, Imhoff AF, Pohl CR, Rosenblum ER, Van Thiel DH 1987 Alcoholic beverages: a source of estrogenic substances. Alcohol and Alcoholism Supp 1: pp. 545–549

Gill JS, Zezulka AV, Shipley MJ, Gill SK, Beevers DG 1986 Stroke and alcohol consumption. New England Journal of Medicine 315:1041–1046

Goodwin DW 1987 Adoption studies of alcoholism. In: Goedde HW, Agarwal DP (eds) Alcoholism: biomedical and genetic aspects. Pergamon, New York, pp. 259–276

Harada S, Agarwal DP, Goedde HW 1981 Aldehyde dehydrogenase deficiency as a cause of facial flushing reaction to alcohol in Japanese. Lancet ii: 982

Harper C 1979 Wernicke's encephalopathy: a more common disease than realized. A neuropathological study of 51 cases. Journal of Neurology, Neurosurgery and Psychiatry 42: 226–231

Ho SB, DeMaster EG, Shafer RB et al 1988 Opiate antagonist nalmefene inhibits ethanol-induced flushing in Asians: a preliminary study. Alcoholism (NY) 12: 705–712

Lehmann WD, Heinrich HC, Leonhart R et al 1986 ^{13}C-ethanol and ^{13}C-acetate breath tests in normal and aldehyde dehydrogenase deficient individuals. Alcohol 3: 227–231

Lieber CS 1985 Alcohol and liver: metabolism of ethanol, metabolic effects and pathogenesis of injury. Acta Medica Scandinavica (Suppl) 703: 11–55

Lieber CS 1988a Biochemical and molecular basis of alcohol-induced injury to liver and other tissues. New England Journal of Medicine 319: 1639–1650

Lieber CS 1988b The influence of alcohol on nutritional status. Nutrition Reviews 46: 241–254

Lieber CS 1991 Perspectives: do alcohol calories count? American Journal of Clinical Nutrition 54: 976–982

Nylander I 1960 Children of alcoholic fathers. Acta Paediatrica Scandinavica 49: 1–134

Pirola RC, Lieber CS 1972 The energy cost of the metabolism of drugs including ethanol. Pharmacology 7: 185–196

Plant M 1985 Women, drinking and pregnancy. Tavistock Publications, London

Puddey IB, Beilin LJ, Vandongen R, Rouse I , Rogers P 1985 Evidence for a direct effect of alcohol consumption on blood pressure in normotensive men in a randomized controlled trial. Hypertension 7: 707–773

Rimm EB, Giovannucci EL, Willett WC et al 1991 Prospective study of alcohol consumption and risk of coronary disease in man. Lancet 338: 464–468

Royal College of Physicians 1987 A great and growing evil. The medical consequences of alcohol abuse. Tavistock, London

Rubin E, Katz AM, Lieber CS, Stein EP, Puskin S 1976 Muscle damage produced by chronic alcohol ingestion. American Journal of Pathology 83: 499–515

Schuckit MA, Rayses V 1979 Ethanol ingestion: differences in blood acetaldehyde concentrations in relatives of alcoholics and controls. Science 203: 54–55

Shaper AG 1990 Alcohol and mortality: a review of prospective studies. British Journal of Addiction 85: 837–847

Situnayake RD, Crump BJ, Thurnham DI, Davies JA, Gearty J, Davis M 1990 Lipid peroxidation and hepatic antioxidants in alcoholic liver disease. Gut 31: 1311–1317

Stampfer MJ, Colditz GA, Willett WC, Speizer FE, Hennekens CH 1988 A prospective study of moderate alcohol consumption and the risk of coronary heart disease and strokes in women. New England Journal of Medicine 319: 267–273

Truitt EB, Gaynor CR, Mehl DL 1987 Aspirin attenuation of alcohol-induced flushing and intoxication in oriental and occidental subjects. Alcohol and Alcoholism Suppl 1: 595–600

Urbano-Marquez A, Estruch R, Navarro-Lopez F, Grau JM, Mont L, Rubin E 1989 The effects of alcoholism on skeletal muscle and cardiac muscle. New England Journal of Medicine 320: 409–415

Wright J, Marks V 1985 The effect of alcohol on carbohydrate metabolism. In: Rosalki SB (ed) Clinical biochemistry of alcoholism. Churchill Livingstone, Edinburgh, pp. 135–148

8. Fuels of tissues

B. Crabtree[†] and P.J. Garlick

The energy supplied by the diet is mostly in the form of complex macromolecules of carbohydrate, protein and fat. This energy cannot be used by the tissues until these have been broken down into smaller molecules such as monosaccharides, free fatty acids (FFA) and amino acids (AA). An account of the energy present in different foods and of the small losses that occur in making it available to the tissues has been given in Chapter 3. The digestive processes break down the large molecules into smaller ones, which are then transported in the blood to be either used directly, or stored mainly as glycogen (for glucose residues), protein (for amino acids) and triglycerides (for FFA). These stores enable the tissues to be supplied with fuel even when supply via the digestive tract is limited (e.g. during fasting). Ethanol is also a source of energy, as described in Chapter 7. Table 8.1 lists the major fuels that circulate in the blood and which serve as fuels for the tissues under different conditions. The relative importance of each fuel is determined by the amounts stored in the tissues and by the dietary and/or metabolic state of the individual. It is regulated by a complex series of feedback interactions ultimately controlled by hormones, particularly glucagon, insulin and the thyroid hormones.

The immediate source of energy for cell metabolism is nucleoside triphosphate (NTP), usually in the form of adenosine triphosphate (ATP), and all fuels are used to generate this by phosphorylating the corresponding diphosphate. We will therefore consider the metabolism and role of ATP before discussing fuel utilization generally.

METABOLIC ROLE OF ATP AND OTHER NUCLEOSIDE TRIPHOSPHATES

Although ATP is the major nucleoside triphosphate involved in cellular energy metabolism, it is not the only one. Guanosine triphosphate (GTP) is produced

Table 8.1 Substances which circulate in the blood and are used to supply energy

Fuel	Source
Glucose	Dietary carbohydrate Glycogen stores Gluconeogenesis in liver and kidney from lactate, amino acids and glycerol
Free fatty acids	Dietary fats Triglyceride stores (especially in adipose tissue) Synthesized from carbohydrate in liver and adipose tissue, especially after feeding low-fat diets
Amino acids	Dietary protein Tissue protein stores Synthesized from carbohydrates
Ketone bodies (acetoacetate, 3-hydroxybutyrate)	Produced from FFA and some amino acids in liver
Glycerol	Produced from triglyceride breakdown
Lactate	Anaerobic glycolysis
Acetate	Gut fermentation of carbohydrates Produced from FFA in liver and muscle, and from ethanol in liver
Ethanol	Dietary intake Gut fermentations
Fructose	Dietary sucrose
Galactose	Dietary intake, especially as milk lactose

in the Krebs cycle (Fig. 8.1) and is hydrolysed to GDP during protein synthesis, during ribosome movement and in the cellular response to hormones which involves cyclic AMP. Cytosine triphosphate (CTP) hydrolysis occurs during the synthesis of phospholipids, and uridine triphosphate (UTP) hydrolysis occurs during the synthesis of glycogen and lactose from hexose phosphate. Details of the metabolic pathways referred to in this chapter may be found in any general biochemical text, such as

[†] Bernard Crabtree sadly died on 16 July 1992, aged 48.

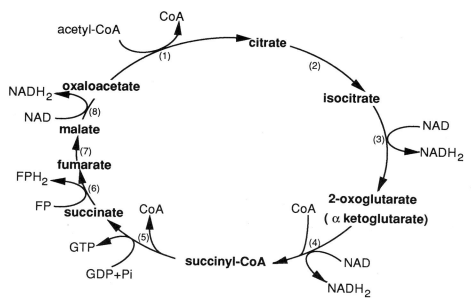

Fig. 8.1 The Krebs tricarboxylic acid cycle. FP and FPH$_2$ denote oxidized and reduced flavoprotein, respectively. P$_i$ denotes inorganic phosphate. Reactions: (1) citrate synthase; (2) aconitase; (3) isocitrate dehydrogenase; (4) 2-oxoglutarate (or α-ketoglutarate) dehydrogenase; (5) succinyl-CoA synthetase; (6) succinate dehydrogenase; (7) fumarase; (8) malate dehydrogenase. In contrast with glycolysis, this cycle occurs in the mitochondrial matrix; for further details see Stryer (1988).

McGilvery & Goldstein (1983), Newsholme & Leech (1983) or Stryer (1988).

All the nucleoside triphosphates (NTP) and diphosphates (NDP) equilibrate with ATP and ADP, via the activity of nucleoside diphosphate kinase

$$ATP + NDP \rightleftharpoons ADP + NTP$$

so effectively there is one pool of nucleoside triphosphate which we will consider as 'ATP'.

ATP HYDROLYSIS AND METABOLIC CYCLING

ATP hydrolysis supplies the chemical energy for muscular contraction to produce mechanical work and heat. When ATP hydrolysis is used for metabolic processes such as biosynthesis, for example, the synthesis of fatty acids from carbohydrates or the synthesis of glucose from lactate, the situation is somewhat more complex. Although ATP has, under these conditions, been regarded as transferring 'free energy' between reactions, this concept is flawed (see Crabtree & Nicholson 1988). It is better to regard the coupling of reactions, and whole biosynthetic pathways, to ATP hydrolysis as a means of enabling them to proceed at physiologically acceptable substrate concentrations. Indeed, this is the main reason why

ATP hydrolysis is so important for the maintenance of life. Its role in the active transport of ions, e.g. Na$^+$ and K$^+$ (Fig. 8.2), is an example of such a facilitation by ATP, allowing a net movement of these ions in a direction which would otherwise be impossible at the concentrations observed in living cells. Moreover, this coupling enables reactions and systems to proceed simultaneously in opposing directions to produce cycles, for example the PFK/FBPase substrate cycle that occurs on the glycolytic pathway in many tissues

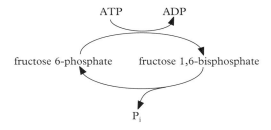

Here the conversion of fructose 6-phosphate (F6P) into fructose 1,6-bisphosphate (FBP) (catalysed by 6-phosphofructokinase, or PFK) is facilitated by coupling it to ATP hydrolysis, and proceeds at the same time as the dephosphorylation of FBP (catalysed by fructose bisphosphatase, or FBPase) to produce a cycle which results in the net hydrolysis of ATP to ADP and P$_i$ (inorganic phosphate). All such cycles

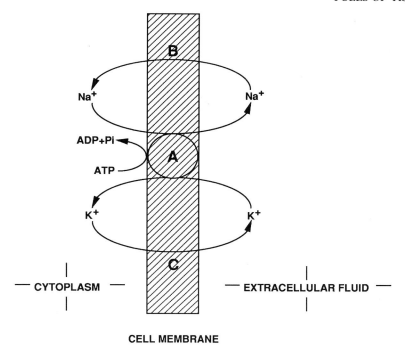

Fig. 8.2 The cell membrane Na⁺/K⁺ pump. A: Na⁺/K⁺ ATPase; B and C: 'passive' re-entry or escape of Na⁺ and K⁺, respectively. This diagram is not stoichiometric, since 3 mol of Na⁺ and 2 mol of K⁺ are transported per mol of ATP hydrolysed, but is designed to illustrate the cyclic nature of this process, once again at the expense of ATP hydrolysis. For further details see Harold (1986).

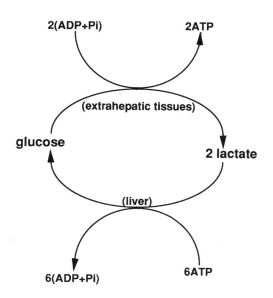

Fig. 8.3 The Cori cycle. Only the net yield or consumption of ATP by the components of the cycle are shown: for details of the gluconeogenic pathway see Stryer (1988). Note that there is a net consumption of 4 mol of ATP per revolution of this cycle, illustrating the need for ATP consumption if such cycles are to exist (see text).

must result in a net hydrolysis of ATP. For this reason they are sometimes referred to as 'futile cycles', since they appear to waste ATP. However, this apparent wastage of ATP is a price worth paying for an increased flexibility of metabolic response (see below). Another cycle, encompassing the whole body, is the Cori cycle which cycles carbohydrate reserves between glucose and lactate (Fig. 8.3) (see overleaf).

PRODUCTION OF ATP

ATP is produced by two main processes, often referred to as 'substrate-level' and 'oxidative' phosphorylation. The most familiar examples of substrate-level phosphorylation occur during glycolysis, at the reactions catalysed by diphosphoglycerate kinase and pyruvate kinase: the reactions producing or consuming ATP by this pathway are outlined in Fig. 8.4. Another example of substrate-level phosphorylation occurs in the Krebs cycle, when GTP is formed during the conversion of succinyl-CoA into succinate: an outline of this pathway is given in Fig. 8.1.

However, most tissues obtain most of their ATP by oxidative phosphorylation, which occurs in the mitochondria and, unlike substrate-level phosphorylation,

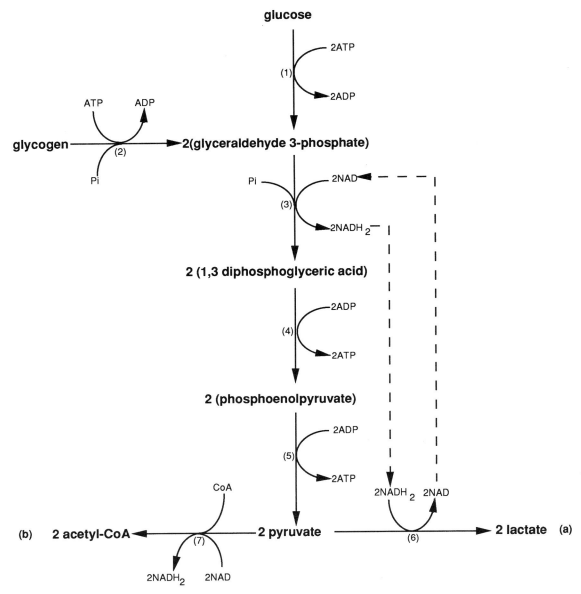

Fig. 8.4 The ATP-consuming and producing reactions of glycolysis. (a) Anaerobic glycolysis; (b) Aerobic glycolysis, in which pyruvate is oxidized to acetyl-CoA. Reactions: (1) span from hexokinase to aldolase, in which ATP is used at hexokinase and phosphofructokinase (PFK); (2) span from phosphorylase to aldolase, in which ATP is used at PFK; (3) glyceraldehyde 3-phosphate dehydrogenase; (4) span from diphosphoglycerate kinase to enolase, in which ATP is produced at diphosphoglycerate kinase; (5) pyruvate kinase; (6) lactate dehydrogenase; (7) pyruvate dehydrogenase. All the reactions except (7) are cytoplasmic. Only the principal intermediates and steps involving ATP and NAD are shown: for further details see Stryer (1988).

requires an intact membrane. The basic principles of this mechanism (often referred to as the chemiosmotic theory), involve the cyclic extrusion and re-entry of H^+ across the mitochondrial inner membrane, as outlined in Fig. 8.5. For calculations of the yields of ATP it should be noted that up to 3 mol of ATP are formed per mol of NADH (i.e. reduced nicotinamide–adenine dinucleotide), whereas only 2 mol are formed per mol of FPH_2 (reduced flavoprotein), oxidized by the mitochondrial respiratory chain.

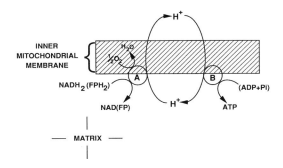

Fig. 8.5 The production of ATP by oxidative phosphorylation. A: the respiratory chain; B: ATP synthetase (F_2 ATPase). This diagram is a highly condensed illustration of the principle involved, i.e. the extrusion of H^+ by the respiratory (electron-transport) chain followed by their subsequent re-entry via ATP synthetase, and does not show the stoichiometries involved. For these and further details see Nicholls (1982) or Harold (1986). This system allows the production of up to 3 or 2 mol of ATP per mol of $NADH_2$ or FPH_2 oxidized, respectively.

Anaerobic glycolysis

Anaerobic glycolysis (Fig. 8.4) proceeds in the absence of oxygen, and this property is important for many tissues. Figure 8.4 shows that there is a net yield of 2 mol of ATP when 1 mol of glucose is converted into 2 mol of lactate, and this ATP is all derived from substrate-level phosphorylation. There are also no problems with disposing of the cytoplasmic $NADH_2$ (generated at the glyceraldehyde 3-phosphate dehydrogenase reaction) because this is recycled to NAD when pyruvate is converted into lactate.

The major source for anaerobic glycolysis is often glycogen. Since only 1 mol of ATP is needed for the conversion of glycogen into glyceraldehyde 3-phosphate (Fig. 8.4), the net yield from glycogen-derived glucose is 3 molecules of ATP when lactate is the end product.

These yields of ATP from anaerobic glycolysis are small compared with those resulting from complete oxidation to CO_2, so the process is energetically inefficient. However, it is the only ATP-producing system that can operate in the absence of oxygen, and it is therefore essential for tissues which have little, if any, oxidative capacity. For example, red cells do not contain mitochondria and are therefore totally dependent on anaerobic glycolysis to provide the ATP for ion transport; this is also the case for eye tissues, which need to be as transparent as possible and which therefore cannot tolerate the presence of mito-chondrial pigments. Other tissues that rely heavily, if

not exclusively, on anaerobic glycolysis are the renal medulla cells and also many malignant tumours (Newsholme & Leech 1983). Their intrinsic demand for carbohydrate means that glucose must be conserved as much as possible during fasting. The body's carbohydrate reserves of glycogen are limited: their associated 3 g of water per g of glycogen makes it a heavy storage form of energy compared with fat, which can be stored almost endlessly.

All these glucose-dependent tissues produce lactate from glucose continuously under all conditions. The lactate may either be oxidized (e.g. in heart and other muscles) or be recycled to glucose in the liver, via the process referred to as gluconeogenesis. This recycling spans the whole body (unlike the PFK/FBPase substrate cycle which occurs in individual cells), and is termed the Cori cycle after its discoverer (see Fig. 8.3). It becomes very important when body carbohydrate reserves are limited (e.g. during fasting), since under such conditions carbohydrate must be spared for those tissues which rely heavily or exclusively on this substance as a fuel (especially the brain). The effects of fasting will be discussed in more detail in a later section, but essentially pyruvate (and hence carbohydrate and lactate) oxidation is strongly inhibited by a reduction in the activity of pyruvate dehydrogenase (see Fig. 8.4), so that nearly all the carbohydrate used by the brain, red cells, etc. is returned to the liver and recycled by the Cori cycle. The ATP deficit of 4 mol per revolution of the Cori cycle is supplied by the oxidation of other fuels, especially fat, in the liver.

Another situation where anaerobic glycolysis becomes important is when a tissue becomes transiently short of oxygen, for example in many muscles at the onset of, or during, exercise (Newsholme & Leech 1983). The blood supply to muscles is regulated to increase only during exercise. This may take several minutes, during which the exercising muscle becomes short of oxygen. During this period the ATP demands are met by anaerobic glycolysis from the muscle glycogen stores. However, the rate of glycolysis is quite high under these conditions (because of the relative inefficiency of anaerobic glycolysis in producing ATP) and the glycogen stores can only last for a few minutes. Therefore, if the muscle does not receive an adequate blood supply by then, it will rapidly become fatigued as glycogen is depleted and lactate and H^+ ions build up.

This also explains why sprinters can maintain their level of exercise for only a short time, and why techniques to increase glycogen storage are important in pre-race training. The high ATP demands associated with sprinting cannot be met by any physiological rate of blood supply and are therefore limited by the initial stores of glycogen and the tolerance of the muscle fibres to lactic acid. Dietary regimens have therefore been developed to increase the initial glycogen stores in the muscles of sprinters to improve their performance as well as improving their blood supply (see Chapter 28). However, in most people, only a small fraction of the muscles' ATP demands during the day are met anaerobically.

Anaerobic glycolysis is also important when oxygen supplies are limited by pathological situations, for example, after a heart attack, a severe haemorrhage or severe burns. The tissues around severe burns depend on anaerobic glycolysis because the regenerating cells which form the granulomatous mass in a healing wound have a large demand for ATP, but their blood supply is restricted due to vascular damage.

Oxidative formation of ATP: aerobic metabolism

When oxygen is available to a tissue with many mitochondria, glycolytically produced pyruvate may enter the mitochondria and be converted into acetyl-CoA (see Fig. 8.4). This is a 'point of no return' because mammalian tissues have no significant pathway for converting acetyl-CoA back into carbohydrate (in contrast with many other organisms). The reaction producing acetyl-CoA (catalysed by pyruvate dehydrogenase) is strongly inhibited when carbohydrate supplies are scarce. For details of the biochemical mechanisms involved see Randle (1986).

When pyruvate is oxidized to acetyl-CoA, the NADH produced in the cytoplasm during glycolysis (Fig. 8.4) must now be reoxidized by the mitochondria. However, since NAD and NADH cannot cross the mitochondrial inner membrane, their reoxidation is carried out indirectly using several shuttles, of which the most important are the malate/aspartate and glycerophosphate shuttles. Details of these can be found in any biochemical texts (e.g. Newsholme & Leech 1983). With the malate shuttle, the cytoplasmic reducing equivalents appear as mitochondrial NADH, so that 3 mol of ATP are formed during their subsequent reoxidation. However, with the glycerophosphate shuttle, the cytoplasmic reducing equivalents appear as mitochondrial reduced flavoprotein (FPH_2) and therefore only 2 mol of ATP are formed during their subsequent reoxidation. Hence the yield of ATP under aerobic conditions depends on the shuttle used in vivo, and this information is not always available. Therefore we shall here assume the upper limit of 3 mol of ATP per mol of cytoplasmic NADH reoxidized.

From the pathways summarized in Fig. 8.2 and 8.4 it can be seen that, using the appropriate ATP equivalents, the oxidation of 1 mol of pyruvate yields $(5 \times 3) + 1 + (1 \times 2) = 18$ mol of ATP. Since 2 mol of pyruvate are produced per mol of glucose oxidized, and there is a net production of 2 mol of ATP between glucose and pyruvate, the total yield is 38 mol of ATP per mol of glucose oxidized to CO_2. If glycolytic NADH is reoxidized by the glycerophosphate shuttle, the yield of ATP would only be 36 mol.

The ATP yield of aerobic glycolysis is therefore more than ten times that of anaerobic glycolysis. Under conditions of oxygen and glucose availability, aerobic glycolysis predominates. This is the case for heart muscle in the normal fed state, when anaerobic glycolysis serves only to supply extra ATP during short-lasting increases in cardiac output (Goodale et al 1959). Aerobic glycolysis is also of great importance for sustained exercise (as opposed to sprinting). Thus, in marathon runners as much as 50% of the power output may be derived from aerobic glycolysis, and if the muscle glycogen reserves become depleted, performance is severely diminished.

Under aerobic conditions other fuels can also supply ATP, notably free fatty acids (FFA) and ketone bodies, both of which become especially important during fasting. Lactate is also an important fuel in the normal fed state, especially for heart muscle during exercise (Harris et al 1964). The metabolic significance of acetate is unclear. Among the amino acids, glutamine is an important fuel for the kidney (especially in late starvation), small intestine, lymphocytes and some tumour cells. In addition to regenerating ATP, glutamine also supplies nitrogen for purine and pyrimidine synthesis, which is essential for rapidly dividing cells such as lymphocytes and intestinal cells; in the kidney, glutamine also supplies NH_3 which is excreted in the urine as NH_4^+, thereby helping to dispose of H^+ during acidotic states (Newsholme & Leech 1983).

A list of ATP yields and heat changes associated with each of the main fuels is given in Table 8.2.

OVERALL PRODUCTION OF ATP IN THE HUMAN BODY

Table 8.3 shows how the carbohydrate, fat, protein, and ethanol in a diet providing 10.8 MJ might generate approximately 145 mol of ATP per 24 hours. The amount of ATP produced varies a little with the exact fatty acid composition of the diet, and also slightly with the nature of the carbohydrate. The energy conversion of protein hydrolysis and oxidation depends on the amino acid composition of the

Table 8.2 ATP yields of the main fuels and the heat associated with ATP turnover. ATP yields can be calculated by assuming the conventional pathways of oxidation (Newsholme & Leech 1983; Stryer 1988), but numerous assumptions are necessary. The final column represents the energy released (as heat) when 1 mol of ATP is hydrolysed and then regenerated by the corresponding fuel in vivo (Krebs 1964; Newsholme & Crabtree 1976).

Fuels	End product(s)	ATP yield (mol per mol of fuel oxidized)	Energy value of fuel (kJ/mol)	Energy released per mol ATP regenerated in vivo (kJ/mol ATP)
Glucose	CO_2	38	2800	74
Glycogen	CO_2	39	2800	72
Palmitic acid (C16 saturated)	CO_2	129	10 000	78
Lactate	CO_2	21	1370	65
Acetate	CO_2	10	878	88
Glutamine	$CO_2 + NH_3$	27	2570	95

Table 8.3 Estimated daily production of ATP from the energy ingested by a subject on a Western diet

Food eaten	Amount (g)	Energy content (mmol)	Energy content (kJ/g)	Energy content (total kJ)	ATP generated in mol per mol substrate	ATP generated in mol total
Carbohydrate as glucose (mol wt 180)	300	1667	16	4800	38	63.4
Fat as triglyceride (mol wt av. 861.5) yielding on hydrolysis	100	116	37	3700		
Glycerol (mol wt 92)	10.7	116			20	2.3
Fatty acids saturated, e.g. palmitic acid (mol wt 254)	22.1	87			129	11.2
monounsaturated, e.g. oleic acid (mol wt 282)	49.1	174			144	25.2 } 51.0
polyunsaturated, e.g. linoleic acid (mol wt 280)	24.4	87			142	12.4
Protein as amino acid (mol wt av. 110)	80	727	17	1360		
Oxidation in deamination to urea						1.4
as glucose		288				10.4
as 3-hydroxybutyric acid		145				3.7 } 16.9
as acetoacetate		61				1.4
Alcohol as ethyl alcohol (mol wt 46)	35	761	29	1020	18	13.7
Total kJ and mol of ATP generated/day				10 800		145

protein, and approximately 30% of the protein energy is excreted as urea.

The production of ATP does not proceed at a fixed rate, however, but must vary rapidly in response to changed cellular demands for ATP. Since an adult's body may contain only 200 mmol of ATP, despite a production of approximately 140 mol per day, ATP is turned over extremely rapidly and, were its supply to stop, would be exhausted within about 1 minute. Muscle contraction may increase ATP demand by several hundred-fold, so ATP production must adjust rapidly. In muscle (and other tissues) there are therefore some very sensitive feedback mechanisms which can increase the rates of glycolysis and fatty acid oxidation very rapidly, with only a small change in the concentration of ATP. Details of these mechanisms may be found in Newsholme & Leech (1983).

The dependence on a continuous supply of fuel and oxygen to maintain the ATP pool in the brain accounts for the almost immediate loss of consciousness when the blood supply to the brain stops, and the rapid irreversible damage that results after

2 minutes, when the small amounts of fuel and oxygen remaining in the cerebral bloodstream have been exhausted. These examples show that although ATP can function as an 'energy currency', it does not serve as a significant store of energy in the body.

SYSTEMS USING ATP: ENERGY COSTS OF STORAGE AND FACTORS DETERMINING THE EFFICIENCY OF STORING FUELS

As stated previously, ATP hydrolysis generates the chemical energy for mechanical work (notably muscle contraction), and also supplies the facilitation needed for such processes as ion pumping. Indeed, the Na^+/K^+ system operates as a continuous cycling of ions across the cell membrane (see Fig. 8.2), which results in a continuous hydrolysis of ATP, perhaps equivalent to 20% of the basal metabolic rate in some animals (e.g. sheep and guinea pig) (Kelly & McBride 1990).

The most widespread use of ATP is in biosynthesis, either to store fuels for later use or to provide new cellular structures (especially proteins and phospholipids). Calculations of ATP usage can be made for each storage system, but these are usually only approximate. As there may be alternative pathways using different amounts of ATP, the ATP may not always be regenerated by the fuel being stored, and the yields of ATP may vary according to the metabolic state of the individual. Storage processes may also increase the rate of operation of substrate cycles and use more ATP than

predicted by the overall storage pathway. Thus the true energy costs are not always predictable.

Regeneration of ATP by alternative pathways

Recent work strongly suggests that, after a fast, little if any glucose is taken up by the liver (after refeeding with carbohydrates) because the glucose is metabolized to lactate in the extrahepatic tissues and then returned via the Cori cycle to the liver, where it is converted into glycogen by gluconeogenesis (Fig. 8.6b). The total cost of this process of glycogen synthesis is 5 mol of ATP per mol of glucose stored, compared with 2 mol for the direct pathway (Fig. 8.6a). At present the reason why glucose is stored as glycogen in such a roundabout way is not clear, but it may allow glucose to be taken immediately to the brain instead of being diverted to glycogen synthesis in the liver. Similarly, the ATP used by, and hence the efficiency of, the conversion of glucose into fatty acids (for subsequent storage as triglycerides in adipose tissue) depends on the relative importance of the pentose phosphate pathway and the pyruvate/malate cycle as suppliers of the $NADPH_2$ required for fat synthesis de novo (Newsholme & Leech 1983; Smith et al 1983).

Regeneration of ATP from different fuels

From Table 8.2 it can be seen that the energy released per mol of ATP cycled between ATP and ADP is very similar – approximately 75 kJ/mol – whether ATP

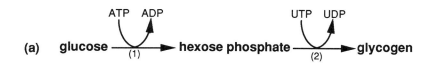

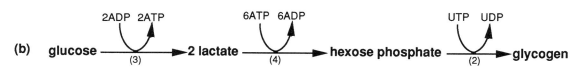

Fig. 8.6 Storage of glucose as glycogen in the liver. (a) Direct pathway; (b) Indirect pathway. Reactions: (1) glucokinase (liver); (2) glycogen synthesis (liver); (3) anaerobic glycolysis (extrahepatic tissues); (4) gluconeogenesis (liver). The reactions refer to the net fluxes, since several steps involve substrate cycling (see Fig. 8.7). For further details see McGarry et al (1987).

synthesis is supported by glucose or long-chain fatty acids (FFA); so that this value can be used to calculate efficiencies under most normal conditions. Thus, the energy cost associated with the direct storage of 1 mol of glucose as glycogen is approximately $2 \times 75 = 150\,kJ$, which is approximately 5% of the total energy of that amount of glucose. Similar calculations, using the ATP demands associated with the storage of fatty acids as triglycerides (Fig. 8.7b), show that this can be achieved with an efficiency of approximately 97% and the storage of amino acids as protein can be calculated to have an efficiency of approximately 80%. From these values it can be seen that the cost of

storing amino acids as proteins is a much greater percentage of their energy content than that of storing glucose as glycogen, or fatty acids as triglycerides.

Variations in the yield of ATP: uncoupling of oxidative phosphorylation

The above efficiencies are only valid if the ATP yields of the fuel are those given in Table 8.2. However, this may not always be the case, and ATP yields should not therefore be regarded as being constant under all conditions. For the oxidation of all major fuels, a large proportion of the ATP is synthesized by mitochondrial oxidative phosphorylation. This process involves the pumping of H^+ out of the mitochondrial matrix by the enzyme systems oxidizing NADH and FPH_2, followed by the synthesis of ATP during H^+ re-entry (see Fig. 8.2). However, H^+ may re-enter via other pathways (e.g. the transfer of ATP out of the mitochondria, the pumping of other ions such as Ca^{2+} across the membrane). The operation of these alternative re-entry systems for H^+ reduces the yield of ATP (Nicholls 1982; Harold 1986). In brown adipose tissue the mitochondrial membrane contains a protein (thermogenin) which permits most, if not all, the H^+ to re-enter without any ATP synthesis at all. The mitochondria are then completely uncoupled and the ATP yields are only those of the associated substrate-level phosphorylations of the fuels (see Figs 8.1 and 8.4): much lower than the fully coupled yields. This low ATP yield requires a high rate of fuel oxidation to supply the demands for ATP, and this produces much more heat. This uncoupling therefore enables brown adipose tissue to provide sufficient heat to warm essential organs immediately after birth, and in animals waking from hibernation (Cannon & Nedergaard 1985).

Although other mammalian tissues are unlikely to operate such a near-total uncoupling of oxidative phosphorylation under normal conditions, there may be a partial and variable uncoupling depending on the metabolic and nutritional state of the animal. Consequently, the yields of ATP per mol of fuel oxidized must be regarded as upper limits and not constants.

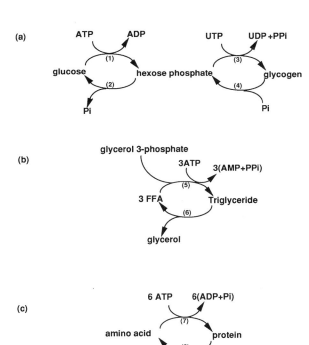

Fig. 8.7. Substrate cycles associated with fuel storage. (a) Storage of glucose (direct pathway) in liver; (b) Storage of FFA in adipose tissue, liver and muscle; (c) Storage of amino acids in muscle and liver. PP_i denotes pyrophosphate. Reactions: (1) glucokinase; (2) glucose 6-phosphatase; (3) glycogen synthetase; (4) glycogen phosphorylase; (5) FFA esterification pathway; (6) 'hormone sensitive' lipase; (7) protein synthesis; (8) protein degradation. Since the formation of AMP is equivalent to the hydrolysis of 2 ATP mol, the ATP costs (mol) of these cycles are as follows: glucose/hexose phosphate and hexose phosphate/glycogen, 1 each: FFA/triglyceride, 7 (6 for the formation of 3 mol of fatty acyl-CoA plus 1 required for glycerol 3-phosphate synthesis): amino acid/protein, 6 (although this value is conjectural) (see Newsholme & Leech 1983).

Increased ATP utilization by substrate cycling

The potential for substrate cycling is present at each storage site (Newsholme & Crabtree 1976, and Fig. 8.7). If some of the glucose molecules cycle between glycogen and glucose before being deposited as glycogen by the direct pathway (Fig. 8.7a), the amount of extra ATP used will depend on the rate of cycling. Therefore the cost in vivo will be greater and the efficiency of storage less. Similar conclusions apply to the storage of fatty acids as triglycerides and the storage of amino acids as protein (Fig. 8.7). The extra utilization of ATP due to an increased rate of operation of these and other substrate cycles may be one reason for the increased heat production which follows the ingestion of food (i.e. the thermic effect or 'specific dynamic action' of food).

Substrate cycles may have several physiological roles (Newsholme & Crabtree 1976; Newsholme et al 1984). As with the uncoupling of mitochondrial oxidative phosphorylation in brown adipose tissue, they may be involved in heat production and the dissipation of excess fuels. In addition, high rates of cycling can provide a high sensitivity and/or speed of response of fuel storage or mobilization to changes in the supply of, or demand for, the fuel (Crabtree & Newsholme 1985). Unfortunately, although these cycles are known to operate in humans (Schulman et al 1985; Elia et al 1987; Myoshi et al 1988), it is quite difficult to measure their rates of operation accurately (Crabtree & Lobley 1988), so that their actual energy costs cannot yet be calculated precisely. Current evidence suggests that the amino acid protein cycles, i.e. protein turnover, accounts for 10–15% of the basal metabolic rate (Waterlow & Jackson 1981). Other cycles (except for the Na^+/K^+ cycle, Fig. 8.2) are energetically less important, with each one accounting for no more than approximately 1% of the basal metabolic rate. However, in the condition of malignant hyperpyrexia induced in genetically susceptible people and pigs, exposure to the anaesthetic halothane leads to a large increase in the rate of substrate cycling at PFK/FBPase in pig muscle in vivo (Clark et al 1973). The catecholamines, insulin, glucagon and the thyroid hormones can all increase substrate cycling, and these hormones are all known to be important regulators of energy metabolism.

Unlike most substrate cycles, the protein/amino acid cycles (protein turnover) and the Na^+/K^+ cycle (see Fig. 8.2) operate at a high activity most of the time. This is probably because the Na^+/K^+ cycle is important in maintaining cell volume as well as the membrane potential, and must therefore operate continuously to counteract any potentially harmful changes. Likewise, protein turnover has to be continuously active to enable a rapid and sensitive control of enzyme and protein concentrations. The extra consumption of ATP by substrate cycles and the ability to vary the yields of ATP by using different pathways and uncoupling oxidative phosphorylation, enables the body to respond to both anticipated and actual energy demands in a very flexible manner; the importance of this flexibility outweighs the extra energy costs involved.

ASSIMILATION OF FUELS

Carbohydrates

A normal meal containing about 100 g of carbohydrate is absorbed over a 2–4-hour period. During this time the liver stores approximately 50 g as glycogen, only 10 g of which is produced directly from glucose (see Fig. 8.6a). The rest is synthesized indirectly from lactate produced by the extrahepatic tissues (McGarry et al 1987). Glucose is also stored as glycogen in muscle, probably via the direct conversion of glucose to hexose phosphate and thence to glycogen (see Fig. 8.6a).

These processes are helped by the secretion of insulin, which promotes the conversion of liver hexose phosphates into glycogen and also the transport of glucose across the cell membrane of extrahepatic tissues, especially muscle. Insulin also reduces the rate of lipolysis and increases the rate of FFA esterification in adipose tissue (Fig. 8.7b). This lowers the blood FFA concentration, which in turn lowers the rate of FFA uptake and metabolism by both liver and muscle. The fall in FFA levels relieves the inhibition of glucose metabolism (including oxidation) caused by FFA metabolism.

If a diet high in carbohydrates is ingested, excess glucose can be converted into FFA and stored as triglycerides, but in humans there is little evidence for this being an important pathway. In the typical high-fat western diet, most of the triglyceride store is derived from dietary fat, with little if any glucose being converted into FFA. When this conversion does occur the most important tissue seems to be the liver, although some conversion can occur in adipose tissue and is stimulated by insulin (Sims & Danforth 1987).

Fats

The digestion and absorption of fats is much slower than that of starch or protein because fat delays gastric emptying and enters the circulation mainly through the lymphatic channels, as chylomicrons. These are particles in which FFA are present as triglycerides (TG) and their production may give the plasma an opalescent appearance after a fatty meal; they also enable fat absorption to bypass the liver. Although the half-life of chylomicrons in blood is quite short (less than 1 hour in man) (Eisenberg & Levy 1975), their synthesis takes several hours. This, together with the relatively slow rates of fat digestion and absorption, means that a patient usually has to fast for as long as 12 hours before the basal blood triglyceride concentration can be measured.

Chylomicron triglycerides are hydrolysed to glycerol and FFA in several tissues – notably liver and adipose tissue – by the enzyme lipoprotein lipase (often termed 'clearing-factor lipase'). This enzyme is synthesized intracellularly and is then transported across the cell membrane into the capillary bed, where it hydrolyses chylomicron TG to produce a locally high concentration of FFA. These then diffuse (or are transported on 'fatty acid-binding' proteins) into the tissue, where they are either oxidized, or re-esterified and stored as endogenous TG (especially in adipose tissue). In the liver, FFA are re-esterified and resecreted as very low-density lipoprotein, VLDL (Robinson 1970; Cryer 1985). Very low-density lipoprotein triglycerides are hydrolysed by lipoprotein lipase in adipose and other extrahepatic tissues (notably muscle), so there is a whole-body cycling of fat (as VLDL-TG and FFA) between the liver and extrahepatic tissues. This cycle, which is similar to the Cori and glucose/alanine cycles (Figs 8.3 and 8.8), is involved in fat storage, rather than oxidation (see Newsholme & Crabtree 1976).

Chylomicron- and VLDL-triglyceride serve to transport FFA for storage, or for the synthesis of milk fats during lactation, whereas FFA serve mainly as a transport form for oxidation (Newsholme & Leech 1983). A rise in FFA concentration above 2 mM (the normal blood concentraton is 0.3–0.6 mM in fed individuals) can damage platelets and produce cardiac arrythmias (Newsholme & Leech 1983). In contrast, the transport of relatively large amounts of FFA as triglycerides in the blood for storage does not upset the body's capacity for metabolizing glucose or damage essential functions.

Lipoprotein lipase is under hormonal control (Robinson & Wing 1970; Cryer 1985) which allows triglyceride fatty acids to be targeted according to metabolic requirements. For example, the enzyme activity in adipose tissue decreases on fasting, whereas that in muscle increases, allowing blood triglyceride to be diverted from storage towards oxidation. During lactation the activity of lipoprotein lipase in the lactating mammary glands increases, whereas that in adipose tissue decreases, thereby diverting triglycerides towards the mammary gland for the synthesis of milk fat. These effects are long term and probably involve changes in the synthesis and/or degradation of the enzyme (under the control of hormones such as insulin and, in lactation, prolactin). However, there are also short-term changes in activity which may result from the enzyme being interconverted between an active and a less active form. This could explain the cyclical variation of lipoprotein lipase activity during the day. It increases in adipose tissue after a meal but then decreases again until the next meal. In muscle, however, it decreases after a meal and then increases again, until the next meal. Insulin, and possibly the catecholamines, may be responsible for these changes.

Water-soluble short- or medium-chain fatty acids (MCT) are not transported as chylomicrons but are carried in solution to the liver via the portal blood for oxidation. Consequently MCT seldom, if ever, reach the fat stores of the body.

Amino acids

Proteins are rapidly digested in the duodenum and jejunum and, after a meal, amino acid concentrations in the blood rise at the same time as glucose. Once absorbed, the amino acids are transported to the liver in both the plasma and the red cells. (Approximately 25% of the alanine and an appreciable proportion of serine, threonine, methionine, leucine, isoleucine and tyrosine are carried between tissues in the red cells.) The greatest increases are in the branched-chain amino acids leucine, isoleucine and valine, because the liver extracts relatively small amounts of these (Wahren et al 1976). Consequently, within 30 minutes of ingesting a protein-rich meal, there is an increase in the uptake of the branched-chain amino acids in muscle for storage or oxidation. In rats there is then a substantial flow of keto acids, derived from

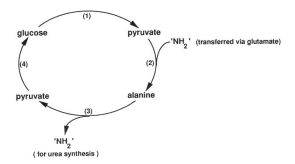

Fig. 8.8 The glucose/alanine cycle. Reactions: (1) glycolysis (muscle); (2) alanine aminotransferase (muscle); (3) alanine aminotransferase (liver); (4) gluconeogenesis (liver).

the transamination of branched-chain amino acids, from the muscles to the liver, but this does not occur to any extent in humans (Palmer et al 1985).

However, the rate of delivery of amino acids to the systemic circulation is actually quite slow. For example, after a meal containing 47 g of beef protein, containing approximately 10 g of branched-chain amino acids, only 1 g of these pass into the systemic circulation per hour and plasma amino acid concentrations are raised by 50–100% for up to 8 hours (Wahren et al 1976). This prolonged output into the systemic circulation is the result of a moderation or 'buffering' of ingested amino acids by the intestine and, to a lesser extent, the liver. As the amino acid supply to the liver increases, the breakdown of hepatic proteins is reduced. The result is that the rise in blood amino acids is buffered by an increased mass of liver (and gut) protein, and the subsequent turnover of this maintains the outflow of amino acids to the peripheral tissues for several hours.

Although glutamate and aspartate represent approximately 20% of the ingested protein, they do not appear to any sizable extent in the portal blood, because, with asparagine and glutamine, they are used as fuels for the small intestine, where they are converted to alanine. Amino groups removed during amino acid oxidation in muscle are also transported to the liver as alanine, via the glucose/alanine cycle (Fig. 8.8). In this cycle, alanine is formed from glucose taken up by the muscle and is then transported to the liver where it is reconverted into glucose, with the amino group being converted into urea. The cycle serves to transfer amino groups from muscle to liver, whereas the Cori cycle transfers energy from liver to muscle (and other extrahepatic tissues). Even after feeding, there is a substantial release of alanine by resting muscle, and hence glucose/alanine cycling.

After their entry into the liver, several amino acids, most notably alanine, are either metabolized to glucose or oxidized to produce ATP. Over a 24-hour period the rate of amino acid oxidation approximately equals the amount ingested, but there is a surge in oxidation after each meal.

The sequence of changes of amino acid metabolism is closely regulated by insulin, which stimulates amino acid uptake and the synthesis of protein. Studies in growing animals show quite clearly that insulin stimulates both protein synthesis and inhibits protein degradation in muscle. However, in adult man the situation is less clear and only the inhibition of degradation has been demonstrated. In addition, after a meal rich in protein but low in carbohydrates, glucagon levels are also elevated and serve to maintain liver gluconeogenesis, which would otherwise be inhibited by the raised concentration of insulin (Felig et al 1976).

USE OF FUELS DURING FASTING

Stores of carbohydrate are relatively small and exist mostly as glycogen in muscle and liver (Table 8.4). However, since muscle does not possess glucose 6-phosphatase activity, it cannot release glucose into the blood, although it can and does release lactate for glucose synthesis in the liver (via the Cori cycle). In contrast, the liver releases glycogen-derived glucose directly into the blood in response to a fall in plasma insulin and a rise in glucagon concentrations. This process is the most immediate and important supplier of glucose for the brain and other tissues during the overnight fast. However, these glycogen reserves can only supply the body's glucose needs for approximately 12 hours, so that if fasting is prolonged beyond this time, for example by missing breakfast, or during a religious fast (Malhotra et al 1989), other sources of glucose must take over (Cahill 1976; Newsholme & Leech 1983).

Table 8.4 Available fuel reserves in an adult man (modified from Cahill 1976)

Tissue (Weight in kg)	Glucose and glycogen		Mobilizable proteins		Triglycerides	
	(g)	(kJ)	(g)	(kJ)	(g)	(kJ)
Blood (10)	15	255	100	1700	5	185
Liver (1)	100	1700	100	1700	50	1850
Intestines (1)	0	0	100	1020	0	0
Brain (1.4)	2	34	40	680	0	0
Muscle (30)	300	5100	4000	68 000	600	22 200
Adipose tissue (15)	20	340	300	5100	12 000	444 000
Skin, lung, spleen (4)	13	220	240	4080	40	1480
Total	450	7649	5000	82 280	12 695	469 715

Table 8.5 The pattern of release of some amino acids from the human forearm and their contribution to muscle protein (data from Ruderman 1975)

Amino acid	Amino acids released (%)	Muscle protein (%)
Alanine	28.0	6.4
Glutamine	23.0	6.6
Lysine	8.7	12.6
Glycine	7.9	4.0
Histidine	2.8	3.1
Valine	2.8	3.5
Leucine	2.0	6.2
Isoleucine	2.0	3.9
Aspartate	0	7.0
Glutamate	−7.9 (net uptake)	11.7

A further decrease of insulin results in the mobilization of muscle amino acids, mostly in the form of glutamine and alanine (Table 8.5). Alanine passes to the liver for conversion to glucose, whereas glutamine serves as an energy source for both the intestine and the kidney. In early fasting, much of the glutamine is converted into alanine by the intestine, and this alanine is then further metabolized by the liver. However, as fasting becomes more prolonged, the metabolism of glutamine to glucose by the kidney increases, to provide NH_3 for the excretion of H^+ associated with the high concentrations of ketone bodies (see below). In late starvation, a significant proportion of the body's glucose may derive from the kidneys.

Muscle protein cannot continue to provide glucose substrates if fasting is prolonged for more than a few days, because the body would soon be depleted of essential proteins. Muscle protein supplies no more than approximately 4 kg of protein for gluconeogenesis under extreme conditions with another 1 kg of protein coming from other tissues.

In the initial stages of fasting, the fall in insulin and rise in glucagon concentrations increase the mobilization of FFA from adipose tissue (see Fig. 8.7b). This leads to a progressive rise in the blood concentration of FFA (Fig. 8.9) and to an increasing use of this fuel by muscle and liver. In these latter tissues, FFA utilization is not as tightly controlled by the feedback effects of ATP and related metabolites as that of glucose (Newsholme & Leech 1983; Crabtree & Newsholme 1985). Therefore, an increased blood concentration of FFA increases the rate of FFA oxidation, which in turn inhibits both glucose oxidation, by inhibiting pyruvate dehydrogenase (see Fig. 8.4), and glycolysis, by inhibiting phosphofructokinase (Newsholme & Leech 1983). The net result

is that these tissues virtually stop taking up and oxidizing glucose and meet nearly all their ATP demands by oxidizing FFA. Consequently, the limited amount of glucose in the body is spared for those tissues which are absolutely dependent on it, especially the brain. (FFA cannot be transported across the blood–brain barrier). The glycerol released by lipolysis in adipose tissue (see Fig. 8.7b) is also transported to the liver and converted into glucose.

In the initial stages of fasting, most of the FFA used by the liver is oxidized or re-exported as VLDL. However, as fasting progresses, liver FFA oxidation is increasingly switched (as a result of the increasing glucagon/insulin ratio) from complete oxidation or VLDL production to the production of the partially oxidized end products acetoacetate and 3-hydroxybutyrate, known as ketone bodies. (Acetone may also be formed by the spontaneous decarboxylation of acetoacetate, and is responsible for the characteristically sweet odour of a ketotic subject, but its metabolic significance is negligible.) The production of ketone bodies by the liver becomes so great that, after several days' starvation, they become the fuel with the highest concentration in the blood (Fig. 8.9). Moreover, the predominant ketone body produced by liver during fasting is 3-hydroxybutyrate, which yields three more ATP molecules than acetoacetate on complete oxidation.

Ketone bodies are oxidized by muscle and spare glucose by essentially the same mechanisms as those

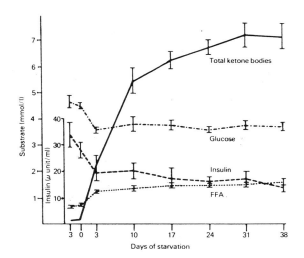

Fig. 8.9. Concentrations of blood total ketone bodies and glucose, insulin and FFA in 37 obese subjects during prolonged starvation (means ± SEM) (data from Owen & Reichard 1975).

operating with FFA oxidation; moreover, they are used in preference to FFA, and their contribution to muscle energy production consequently rises from approximately 10% after an overnight fast to 50–80% after 3–7 days' starvation (Owen & Reichard 1975). Furthermore, unlike FFA (which are transported bound to plasma albumin), ketone bodies are water-soluble and can therefore cross the blood–brain barrier and be used to supply ATP for the brain. Thus, after a few days of starvation, ketone bodies supply 10–20% of the energy requirements of the brain, and if starvation is prolonged for several weeks, this proportion is increased even further. As a consequence of the increased oxidation of ketone bodies by the brain, its requirements for glucose are reduced from approximately 100g/day in fed conditions or early fasting to approximately 40g/day after several weeks' starvation (Table 8.6). For unknown reasons, the brain requires some glucose at all times.

In very late starvation (after 6 weeks in obese subjects) the pattern of ketone body utilization changes, so that they now contribute only approximately 10% of muscle energy requirements, with the deficit being made up by FFA. This tends to conserve ketone bodies for the brain and kidney, which are by now heavily dependent on them. Moreover, the increased concentration of ketone bodies inhibits muscle proteolysis, possibly by inhibiting muscle leucine oxidation.

The endocrinological control of fuel metabolism in the late stages of starvation is quite complicated (Newsholme & Leech 1983). Although glucagon and insulin are still important, several other hormones come into prominence. The thyroid hormone, T_3, stimulates protein degradation, and its lowered blood concentration during long-term starvation may help to reduce proteolysis. Fig. 8.10 summarizes the main endocrinological factors involved in fasting.

A summary of fuel requirements and utilization during a short fast and long-term starvation is given in Table 8.6, from which the importance of the ketone bodies is clear. Far from being pathological, as was once believed, ketone bodies are important fuels for human and other mammalian tissues because they spare glucose for the brain and conserve muscle protein. By serving as an alternative fuel, they also help to prevent dangerously large increases in blood FFA. In addition, they serve as important sources of energy for the tissues of newborn infants: because milk is a high-fat/low-carbohydrate diet, the relatively limited amounts of carbohydrate that are ingested must be spared for the brain and other tissues which are absolutely dependent on glucose (Robinson & Williamson 1980; Newsholme & Leech 1983).

Acetate is another fuel (derived from gut fermentations and from the partial oxidation of FFA in the liver) which is oxidized by muscle and other tissues in preference to glucose, FFA and perhaps even ketone bodies (Karlsson et al 1977; Akanji et al 1988). Therefore, acetate oxidation may also help to spare glucose during periods when carbohydrates are in short supply. However, in contrast to ketone bodies,

Table 8.6 Fuel supplies and utilization during a short fast and prolonged starvation (adapted from Cahill 1976)

Tissue	Fuel	Fasting 3 days (g/day)	Starvation 6 weeks (g/day)
Energy supplies from:			
Adipose tissue	FFA	180	180
Liver	Ketone bodies	150	150
	Glucose	150	80
	Glycerol	20	20
	Lactate + pyruvate	40	40
	Amino acids	70	20
Muscle	Glycogen	20	0
	Amino acids	75	20
Energy utilized by:			
Brain	Glucose	100	40
	Ketone bodies	50	100
Liver	Amino acids	70	20
Muscle	Amino acids	75	20
Other tissues	Glucose	50	40
	FFA	30	30
	Ketone bodies	100	50

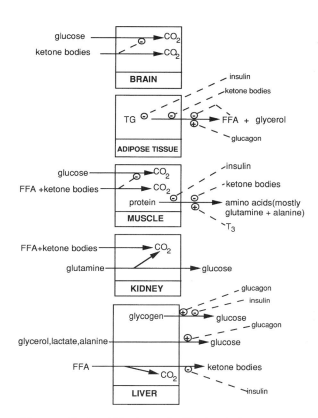

Fig. 8.10 Fuel mobilization and utilization during starvation. The relative importance of each fuel depends on the duration of fasting (see text). Net fluxes are represented by solid lines: broken lines represent regulatory interactions, with + and - denoting activation and inhibition, respectively.

significant amounts of acetate are absorbed from the gut fermentation of dietary carbohydrates, especially those associated with diets rich in non-starch polysaccharides and resistant starch diets (Scheppach et al 1988). Acetate is also produced by tissues other than the liver (e.g. muscle) and is the main end product of ethanol metabolism in the liver (Newsholme & Leech 1983). Consequently, the turnover of blood acetate is quite high even after feeding.

FUEL SUPPLY DURING EXERCISE

Measurements of the uptake of glucose by arteriovenous differences in concentration across the tissue show that, even in normal fed subjects, resting skeletal muscle uses very little glucose. The total glucose consumption of all the skeletal muscles of an adult male is 20–25 mg/min, which is approximately 25% of that by the brain: moreover, the respiratory quotient (see

Chapter 3) of resting muscle is close to 0.7, reflecting the dominance of fat as a fuel (Andres et al 1956).

This situation changes dramatically when exercise begins and carbohydrates, in the form of endogenous glycogen stores and blood glucose, become major fuels. Anaerobic glycolysis of glycogen into lactate is the major source of ATP during the initial stages of exercise and for short-lasting sprints of 100–200 metres (Newsholme & Leech 1983). More sustained exercise requires a continuous supply of blood-borne fuels, such as glucose and FFA, as well as oxygen.

The contribution of FFA increases as exercise is prolonged (Fig. 8.11). Nevertheless, glucose still supplies approximately 40% of the fuel in many subjects, even if heavy exercise continues for nearly 3 hours (Table 8.7). Since blood glucose and muscle glycogen reserves are being continuously oxidized during sustained exercise, glucose carbon is being continuously removed from the body pool of carbohydrates and must therefore be replaced. As in fasting, this glucose is derived firstly from liver glycogen and, when this becomes depleted, by gluconeogenesis in the liver. Since the Cori cycle only

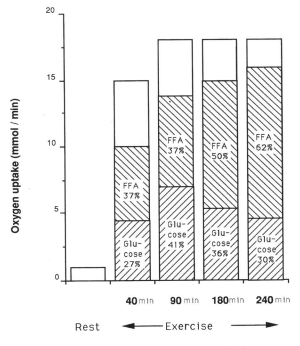

Fig. 8.11 Uptake of oxygen and substrates by the legs during prolonged exercise. Hatched areas represent the proportion of total oxygen uptake contributed by the oxidation of blood FFA and glucose. Open portions indicate the oxidation of non-blood borne fuels, such as muscle glycogen and intramuscular lipids (data from Ahlborg et al 1974).

Table 8.7 Relative proportions of carbohydrate and fat in the fuel mixture during prolonged heavy work with energy expenditure at 900–1000 W (Christensen & Hansen 1939)

Time (min)	Respiratory quotient	Percentage of energy from	
		Carbohydrate	Fat
0–30	0.910	69	31
30–60	0.890	63	37
60–90	0.875	57	43
90–120	0.855	50	50
120–150	0.840	45	55
150–162	0.825	40	60

recycles glucose carbon and does not replenish glucose lost by oxidation (see Fig. 8.3), this glucose must be derived from amino acids and glycerol (as in fasting). Indeed, muscle output of alanine increases during sustained exercise in proportion to the intensity of the work. At the same time, there is an increased oxidation of branched-chain amino acids by muscle, which may also supply some of the energy. During exercise the brain continues to require its usual supply of glucose (approximately 100 g/day), so that there is a heavy and continuous demand for liver gluconeogenesis in sustained exercise.

All the above changes are associated with a lowered blood insulin and, if exercise is prolonged, a raised blood glucagon concentration (as in fasting). The blood concentrations of the catecholamines are also elevated, and at least one of their roles may be to increase the rate of substrate cycling in muscle and other tissues, thereby providing extra sensitivity for the control systems involved in ATP production. As exercise is prolonged, many other hormones, for example growth hormone and the steroid hormones, become involved. However, there is usually (but not always) little change in the blood concentrations of the thyroid hormones, or in the basal metabolic rate. Further details of the hormonal changes during exercise can be found in the reviews by Galbo (1985) and Terblanche (1989).

Why heavy sustained exercise should require carbohydrate oxidation and not be supported exclusively by FFA (or ketone body) oxidation, is as yet unclear. In many individuals the power output is seriously reduced if the carbohydrate reserves are consumed. Moreover, this requirement for carbohydrate during sustained exercise seems to vary with the individual. For example, two medical students offered to walk 28 miles in 7 hours with no breakfast. After 23 miles, one of them suddenly collapsed, but recovered within 30 minutes after being given oral glucose: measurements of his respiratory exchanges showed that he had used 150 g of carbohydrate during the walk and the proportion of carbohydrate in his metabolic mixture had fallen from 65% to 35%. However, the other student, who completed the walk with little difficulty, used only 125 g of carbohydrate for the entire walk, at the end of which the proportion of carbohydrate in his 'metabolic mixture' was 10% (Fonseka et al 1965). The highly trained Scandinavian athletes who provided the data for Table 8.7 used approximately 325 g of carbohydrate during their prolonged exercise, but they had probably eaten breakfast.

Recovery from exercise

Once exercise has stopped, muscles continue to take up blood glucose at three to four times the resting rate for some time, and thereby replenish their reserves of glycogen. However, since the demand for ATP is now very much lower, the uptake of glucose by the muscles falls after the cessation of exercise, resulting in a rise in blood glucose concentration (Maehlum et al 1986). Blood FFA concentrations also increase and, as in fasting, inhibit glucose oxidation by muscles. Thus muscle glucose is directed towards the resynthesis of glycogen which occurs before the resynthesis of glycogen in the liver (Maehlum et al 1978).

Blood ketone bodies also rise immediately after exercise, particularly in those subjects who use FFA to supply most of their fuel for sustained exercise, for example trained athletes who have eaten a low-carbohydrate diet before a race (Koeslag et al 1980). This phenomenon, referred to as a post-exercise ketosis, results from an increased blood (and thus FFA) supply to the liver after exercise. Since ketone bodies inhibit FFA mobilization from adipose tissue (see Fig. 8.9), post-exercise ketosis may represent a safety mechanism to prevent a sudden and dangerously large rise in blood FFA concentrations after exercise (Newsholme & Leech 1983).

After short-lasting exercise, these metabolic changes are often accompanied by a rapid increase in the concentration of blood insulin, especially in the portal blood; however, if the exercise was prolonged, insulin concentrations may remain low for some time. Catecholamine and glucagon concentrations may also remain elevated, possibly serving to maintain the rates of some substrate cycles after exercise. The elevated glucagon concentration may also ensure the continuation of liver gluconeogenesis (from glycerol and lactate). Indeed, gluconeogenesis in the liver continues after exercise at approximately twice the resting (i.e. the pre-exercise) rate: presumably this supplies glucose for the resynthesis of glycogen.

The changes in amino acid metabolism are equally rapid after exercise. During heavy prolonged exercise in trained athletes, the production of urea (derived from the nitrogen of the amino acids used for liver gluconeogenesis) can rise by 60%. However, after exercise, the much lower demands for muscle ATP lead to a reversal of the output of amino acids from muscle, so athletes usually remain in a net nitrogen balance over the entire day of an event.

After a period of appreciable exercise, the uptake of oxygen by the body remains elevated, sometimes for as long as 72 hours. This effect, which used to be known as the 'oxygen debt', is now termed 'excess post-exercise oxygen consumption' (EPOC) (Gaesser & Brooks 1984) and shows a great deal of individual variation. It reflects an increased oxidation of body fuels (mostly fat) during this period and, although some of the EPOC represents the energy costs involved in the resynthesis of liver and muscle glycogen (and protein) stores, a significant part results from the several substrate cycles (see earlier) (Newsholme 1978, Maehlum et al 1986). Regular exercise, as well as helping with weight maintenance, also improves glucose tolerance, hyperinsulinaemia and other hormonal changes that may predispose to obesity (Terblanche 1989).

REFERENCES

Ahlborg G, Felig P, Hagenfeldt L, Hendler R, Wahren J 1974 Substrate turnover during prolonged exercise in man. Journal of Clinical Investigation 53: 1080–1090

Akanji AO, Ng L, Humphreys S 1988 Plasma acetate levels in response to intravenous fat or glucose/insulin infusions in diabetic and non-diabetic subjects. Clinica Chimica Acta 178: 85–94

Andres R, Cader G, Zierler KL 1956 The quantitatively minor role of carbohydrate in oxidative metabolism by skeletal muscle in intact man in the basal state. Journal of Clinical Investigation 35: 671–682

Cahill GF 1976 Starvation in man. Clinical Endocrinology and Metabolism 5 (2): 397–415

Cannon B, Nedergaard J 1985 The biochemistry of an inefficient tissue: brown adipose tissue. Essays in Biochemistry 20: 110–164

Christensen EH, Hansen O 1939 Untersuchunger uber die Verbrennungsborgange bei langdauernder, schewer Muskelarbeit. Skandinavisches Archiv fur Physiologie 81: 152–159

Clark MG, Williams CH, Pfeifer WF et al 1973 Accelerated substrate cycling of fructose 6-phosphate in the muscles of malignant hyperthermic pigs. Nature 245: 99–101

Crabtree B, Newsholme EA 1985 A quantitative approach to metabolic control. Current Topics in Cellular Regulation 25: 21–76

Crabtree B, Lobley GE 1988 Measuring metabolic fluxes in organs and tissues with single and multiple tracers. Proceedings of the Nutrition Society 47: 353–364

Crabtree B, Nicholson BA 1988 Thermodynamics and metabolism. In: Jones MN (ed) Biochemical thermodynamics, 2nd edn. Elsevier, Amsterdam, pp. 347–394

Cryer A 1985 Lipoproteins and adipose tissue. In: Cryer A, Van RLR (eds) New perspectives in adipose tissue. Butterworths, London, pp. 183–198

Eisenberg S, Levy RI 1975 Lipoprotein metabolism. Advances in Lipid Research 13: 1–89

Elia M, Zed C, Neale G, Livesey G 1987 The energy cost of triglyceride fatty acid recycling in non-obese subjects after an overnight fast and four days of starvation. Metabolism 36: 251–255

Felig P, Wahren J, Sherwin R, Hendler R 1976 Insulin, glucagon and somastatin in normal physiology and diabetes mellitus. Diabetes 25: 1091–1099

Fonseka CC, Hunter WM, Passmore R 1965 The effect of long-continued exercise on plasma growth hormone levels in human adults. Journal of Physiology (London) 182: 26P–27P

Gaesser GA, Brooks GA 1984 Metabolic bases of excess post-exercise oxygen consumption: a review. Medicine and Science in Sports and Exercise 16: 29–43

Galbo H 1985 The hormonal response to exercise. Proceedings of the Nutrition Society 44: 257–266

Goodale WT, Olson RE, Hackel DB 1959 The effects of fasting and diabetes mellitus on myocardial metabolism in man. American Journal of Medicine 27: 212–220

Harold FM 1986 The vital force: a study of bioenergetics. Freeman, New York

Harris P, Howel Jones J, Bateman M, Clouverakis C, Gloster J 1964 Metabolism of the myocardium at rest and during exercise in patients with rheumatic heart disease. Clinical Science 26: 145–156

Karlsson N, Fellenium E, Kiessling K-H 1977 Influence of acetate on the metabolism of hydroxybutyrate in the perfused hindquarter of the rat. Acta Physiologica Scandinavica 99: 113–122

Kelly JM, McBride BW 1990 The sodium pump and other mechanisms of thermogenesis in selected tissues. Proceedings of the Nutrition Society 49: 185–202

Koeslag JH, Noakes TD, Sloan AW 1980 Post-exercise ketosis. Journal of Physiology (London) 301: 79–90

Krebs HA 1964 The metabolic fate of amino acids. In: Munro H N, Allison J B (eds) Mammalian protein metabolism, vol. 1, Academic Press, New York, pp. 125–177

McGarry JD, Kuwajima M, Newgard CB, Foster DW 1987 From dietary glucose to liver glycogen: the full circle round. Annual Review of Nutrition 7: 51–73

McGilvery RW, Goldstein G 1983 Biochemistry, a functional approach. Saunders, Philadelphia

Maehlum S, Felig P, Wahren J 1978 Splanchnic glucose and muscle glycogen metabolism after glucose feeding during postexercise recovery. American Journal of Physiology 235: E255–E260

Maehlum S, Grandmontagne M, Newsholme EA, Sejersted OM 1986 Magnitude and duration of excess post-exercise oxygen consumption in healthy young subjects. Metabolism 35: 425–429

Malhotra A, Scott PH, Scott J, Gee H, Wharton BA 1989 Metabolic changes in Asian Muslim pregnant mothers observing the Ramadan fast in Britain. British Journal of Nutrition 61: 663–672

Myoshi H, Schulman GI, Peters EJ, Wolfe MH, Elahi D, Wolfe RR 1988 Hormonal control of substrate cycling in humans. Journal of Clinical Investigation 81: 1545–1555

Newsholme EA 1978 Substrate cycles: their metabolic, energetic and thermic consequences in man. Biochemical Society Symposia 43: 183–205

Newsholme EA, Crabtree B 1976 Substrate cycles in metabolic regulation and in heat generation. Biochemical Society Symposia 41: 61–109

Newsholme EA, Leech AR 1983 Biochemistry for the medical sciences. Wiley, Chichester

Newsholme EA, Challiss RAJ, Crabtree B 1984 Substrate cycles: their role in improving sensitivity in metabolic control. Trends in Biochemical Sciences 9: 277–280

Nicholls DG 1982 Bioenergetics: an introduction to the chemiosmotic theory. Academic Press, New York

Owen OE, Reichard GA 1975 Ketone body metabolism in normal, obese and diabetic subjects. Israel Journal of Medical Science 11: 560–570

Palmer TN, Caldecourt MA, Snell K, Sugden MC 1985 Alanine and inter-organ relationships in branched-chain amino and 2-oxo acid metabolism. Bioscience Reports 5: 1015–1033

Randle PJ 1986 Fuel selection in animals. Biochemical Society Transactions 14: 799–806

Robinson AM, Williamson DH 1980 Physiological roles of ketone bodies as substrates and signals in mammalian tissues. Physiological Reviews 60: 143–187

Robinson DS 1970 The function of the plasma triglycerides in fatty acid transport. Comprehensive Biochemistry 18: 51–116

Robinson DS, Wing DR 1970 Regulation of adipose tissue clearing factor lipase activity. In: Jeanrenaud B, Hepp D (eds) Adipose tissue: regulation and metabolic function. Academic Press, New York, pp. 41–46

Ruderman NB 1975 Muscle amino acid metabolism and gluconeogenesis. Annual Review of Medicine 26: 245–258

Scheppach W, Cummings JH, Branch WJ, Schrezenmeir J 1988 Effect of gut-derived acetate on oral glucose tolerance in man. Clinical Science 75: 355–361

Schulman GI, Ladenson PW, Wolfe MH, Ridgeway EC, Wolfe RR 1985 Substrate cycling between gluconeogenesis and glycolysis in euthyroid, hypothyroid and hyperthyroid man. Journal of Clinical Investigation 76: 757–764

Sims EAH, Danforth E 1987 Expenditure and storage of energy in man. Journal of Clinical Investigation 79: 1019–1025

Smith GH, Crabtree B, Smith RA 1983 Energy metabolism in the mammary gland. In: Mepham TB (ed) Biochemistry of lactation. Elsevier, Amsterdam, pp. 121–140

Stryer L 1988 Biochemistry, 3rd edn. Freeman, San Francisco

Terblanche SE 1989 Recent advances in hormonal response to exercise. Comparative Biochemistry and Physiology 93B: 727–739

Wahren J, Felig P, Hagenfeldt L 1976 Effect of protein ingestion on splanchnic and leg metabolism in normal man and in patients with diabetes mellitus. Journal of Clinical Investigation 57: 987–999

Waterlow JC, Jackson AA 1981 Nutrition and protein turnover in man. British Medical Bulletin 37: 5–10

9. Energy balance and weight regulation

J. S. Garrow

WEIGHT REGULATION IN LABORATORY RODENTS

The field of energy balance and weight regulation provides good examples of the problems which arise when results obtained by observing small laboratory animals are extrapolated to man. A pure-bred strain of laboratory rat or mouse is a convenient model in which to study the influences of various factors on body weight: for example, lesions of the hypothalamic nuclei will cause operated animals to alter their feeding behaviour and body weight, compared with unoperated control animals. For experimental purposes it is essential that the animals should behave in a uniform and predictable manner under controlled conditions, so that small changes in body weight or composition can be shown to be statistically significant. However, the human species is not genetically pure, so uniformity of feeding behaviour is not to be expected in human subjects.

The mechanisms which control body weight, as revealed by results obtained by classic neurophysiological studies in laboratory rodents, can be briefly summarized. Up to about 1972 (for example in the 5th edition of this textbook), it was accepted that energy intake was controlled by the activity in two groups of nerve cells at the base of the brain: a 'hunger centre' in the lateral hypothalamus, and a 'satiety centre' in the ventral hypothalamus. If the nucleus of the former was damaged the animals became indifferent to food, and would starve to death unless artificially fed, while lesions of the latter nucleus caused the animals to eat ravenously and become obese (Kennedy 1950). However Gold (1973) showed by very precise knifecut lesions that it was not the ventromedial nucleus which controlled satiety, but nearby noradrenergic tracts, and that lesions of the lateral hypothalamus did not specifically affect hunger, but caused general apathy. If rats with a lateral hypothalamic lesion were nursed through their initial period of apathy they would again regulate body weight, and if given amphetamine – which is both a central nervous system stimulant and an appetite suppressant in normal animals – they would increase their food intake. In the light of this information the 'dual centre' explanation of regulation of food intake had to be abandoned.

It became evident that the control of food intake in the laboratory rat depended on a large number of variables. Russek (1976) devised a mathematical model which would predict food intake if the following were known: the concentrations in the blood of glucose, insulin, glucagon and adrenalin; the amount of glycogen stored in the liver; the rate of utilization of glucose by the lateral hypothalamus; body weight and osmolarity, and air temperature. No doubt all these factors (and perhaps others) would also affect human food intake if we lived in wire cages and were offered only laboratory chow and water. In fact there are both physiological and social differences between humans and the laboratory rat which bring into play a set of important influences which may override the physiological control mechanisms which have been described in the rat.

NORMAL VARIATION IN BODY WEIGHT IN MAN

A rat is liable to die after a week of total starvation, whereas a normal person will probably survive for 10 weeks: this is because man has a large store of energy in the form of fat. Fig. 9.1 shows the relative magnitude of daily energy intake, faecal energy losses, energy output and energy stores in a normal adult. (For a description of methods for measuring energy stores see Chapter 2, and for the processes by which energy is transformed within the body see Chapter 3.)

It is obvious that man does not need to balance energy input against output each day as accurately as a rat does, since the energy stores will be mobilized if

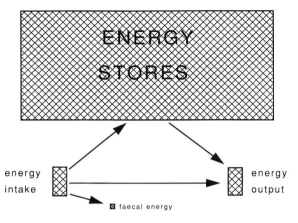

Fig. 9.1 In normal man the energy stores (mainly fat) contain about 70 times as much energy as daily intake or expenditure. Energy losses in faeces are about 5% of daily intake.

energy intake is lower than requirements, or replenished if intake is higher than requirements, provided that a balance is maintained over a period of several months. Large fluctuations in fat stores will be reflected by fluctuations in body weight: the energy value of adipose tissue is about 7000 kcal/kg. The fluctuations in body weight that occur in a normal population are shown in Fig. 9.2. In the town of Framingham, virtually everyone undergoes a routine examination every 2 years, at which (among other things) weight is measured (Gordon & Kannel 1973). These histograms show the difference between maximum and minimum weights observed after 10 examinations, spanning 18 years. Among both men and women the average peak-to-peak fluctuation was 10 kg, so we can calculate that energy stores varied by some 70 000 kcal in the average person. These facts

are not in dispute, but there is still fierce controversy between those who consider that energy balance in man is, or is not, precisely regulated. The facts can be used to support either view. We can say that a system which allows an error in energy balance of 70 000 kcal – the equivalent of about 1 month's energy intake – is not very precise. On the other hand, we can say that over 18 years the average person in Framingham had an energy intake of about 15 000 000 kcal, so an error of 70 000 kcal is less than 0.5% of turnover, which is precise regulation. Furthermore, the 10 kg variation was not the average difference between the start and end of the 18-year period, but a maximum deviation at some time in between: most individuals finished with a body weight within 5 kg of their initial weight, so long-term regulation is still more precise.

In this chapter we review the mechanisms which tend to maintain stability of body weight, both in the short term and over the whole adult lifetime.

CONTROL OF ENERGY INTAKE IN MAN

The physiological mechanisms which control energy intake in the rat certainly also exist in man. If a person is deprived of food he becomes hungry, and if he has eaten a lot he becomes satiated. Hunger can be suppressed by drugs, such as amphetamine which acts on adrenergic neuroreceptors in the brain, or by fenfluramine, which increases the concentration of brain serotonin, probably by inhibiting its reuptake. People who suffer damage to the hypothalamus, either from trauma or tumour, may display abnormalities of weight regulation (Bray 1982). Therefore there are good reasons to believe that areas in the hypothalamus process signals coming from sensors of many types, and relay to the cerebral cortex signals

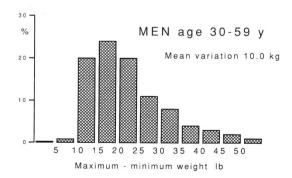

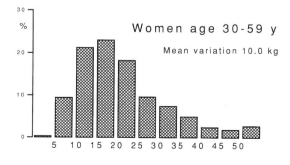

Fig. 9.2 Variations in body weight among the male and female adult population of Framingham (Gordon & Kannel 1973). Individuals were measured every 2 years for 18 years, and the difference between highest and lowest weight (in lbs) is shown.

which we interpret as hunger or satiety. The input to the hypothalamus probably includes all those used in the predictive equation of Russek, but if this was the whole story, we should be able reliably to sense the energy content of a meal, and to regulate energy intake when the energy density of the meal was altered. Some experiments show that this is not done very accurately by most people, and in this respect there seems to be a difference between man and the lower animals.

Perception of the energy content of a meal

Wooley et al (1972) supplied volunteers with one liquid meal per day, in which they could alter the energy content without altering the volume, taste or appearance. For a baseline period of 5–10 days the meal provided the same amount of energy as that normally consumed by the volunteers, but for the next 14–21 days the meal provided either 50% less or more than the usual amount of energy, the average difference being 230 kcal (960 kJ). At 15, 30, 60 and 120 minutes after the test meal, the subjects were asked to guess if the meal they had just consumed provided more or less energy than usual. Of the 262 estimates 55% were correct and 45% incorrect, which is not much better than the result which would be expected by chance. Thus human subjects are not good at recognizing the energy content of the meal they have just eaten. There was also no difference between normal and obese subjects in their ability to guess the energy load they had just consumed.

Satiety is a conditioned reflex

When we eat, the food is absorbed from the gut and there are many potential signals which might cause satiety: it has been suggested that the important messengers might be metabolites of food (such as glucose) entering the bloodstream or nerve signals arising from the gut as food is absorbed, or hormones released from the gut wall in response to the presence of food in the gut lumen. The problem with all these suggestions is that they do not explain how the last mouthful of a meal is determined; the signals listed above require that food should already be in the intestine, if not actually absorbed, before the signals can be generated, but while this is happening there is time for many more mouthfuls to be ingested before the meal is terminated.

A solution to this problem is offered in a study by Booth et al (1976). They gave normal volunteers meals consisting of a lemon-flavoured drink, sand-wiches and a dessert of yoghurt. The lemon-flavoured drink had on some days 65 g of starch, and on other days 5 g of starch, but these were indistinguishable by taste or appearance. The dessert yoghurt was in two flavours, of which one was given on the days when there was a large starch preload, and the other when there was a small starch preload. After some days the volunteers unconsciously but reliably ate fewer sand-wiches and less yoghurt after the high than after the low preload. This phase of the experiment showed that the volunteers were able to respond to a covert alteration in the starch preload by altering voluntary food intake thereafter.

In the second phase of the experiment the volunteers were given a 35 g of starch preload at all meals, but it was observed that for a few days they ate less on the days when they were served the yoghurt flavour previously associated with the high preload, than when they were served the yoghurt previously associated with the low preload. This result showed that satiety in these circumstances is to some extent *conditioned*: the subjects felt full after less food because the yoghurt flavour was associated with an experience of earlier satiety in the previous phase of the experiment.

Sensory specific satiety

Another insight into the nature of satiety was pro-vided by Rolls et al (1984). They offered normal volunteers a four-course meal consisting of sausages, then bread and butter, then a chocolate dessert, and lastly bananas, and recorded the weight of food consumed at each course and its energy value. On other occasions the volunteers were offered meals of four courses with each course the same: thus there would be a meal of sausage, followed by sausage, followed by sausage, and then sausage, and similarly for each of the other items on the above menu. The total weight of food was 44% greater, and energy intake was 60% greater, when the meal had four different types of food than when it had only one. This is a formal demonstration of a principle which underlines gastronomy: that an appetizing meal should provide variety and contrasts in taste, colour and texture. It is a common experience that, having partaken of a banquet which provided much more nourishment than we need, we may believe ourselves to be incapable of eating any more. However, if a particularly attractive item is produced – perhaps the first strawberries of the season – we find the ability to eat is miraculously restored.

These findings show us that novelty and variety in food makes it more difficult to regulate intake by physiological mechanisms. If, like the laboratory rat, we were fed chow of constant composition, we would no doubt regulate our food intake accurately according to our requirements. We would do this because at each meal we would acquire experience about the quantity of food which fulfilled our needs, and having ingested that amount we would feel satiated by the conditioning effect demonstrated by Booth et al. However, this mechanism works only for meals of which we have had previous experience. If each meal is novel, we have no experience of that meal with which conditioning of satiety can occur. If our cuisine is varied as well as novel, the task of regulation is made still more difficult, because satiety is 'sensory-specific': we may be satiated to sausages but not yet satiated to bananas. The application of this theory to diet in affluent countries is obvious: food technologists are constantly inventing new flavours and textures which may not exist in any natural food, with the laudable intention of stimulating our appetite and their sales. It is not surprising that the physiological mechanism which evolved to regulate intake of the monotonous diet of our forefathers is no match for such sophistication.

Sensory-specific satiety must have urged our forefathers to eat a variety of foods, and not just the large animal which they had recently killed, or the stem of bananas which had recently become ripe. In this way the quality of the diet is improved, because the more different foods there are in a diet the less likely it is that there will be an overall deficiency of specific nutrients, such as vitamins or essential amino acids. It is therefore a great advantage to the poor peasant whose food supply is limited, monotonous and intermittent, and for whom the main nutritional danger is undernutrition. However, in affluent countries the greater danger is overnutrition and obesity, which is discussed further in Chapter 32.

LONGER-TERM CONTROL OF APPETITE

These studies relate to the immediate impact of sensory stimulus on the intake of energy on the same day, although in Booth's conditioning study the full responsiveness of individuals required several days to become fully effective. Slower adjustments in food intake to changes in energy balance are evident over a 2–6 day period in infants, children and adults. Thus Fomon et al (1969) showed that newborn babies fed a dilute milk formula would compensate by taking a much greater volume of formula so that their total energy intake was close to those fed a concentrated formula. The adjustment was surprisingly good, so

that within a month of birth the two groups of babies had almost exactly the same energy intake. Further evidence of the importance of the physiological appetite drive is the response of children recovering from malnutrition. Ashworth (1969) in Jamaica showed that, once the first few days of treatment had allowed for recovery from the acute metabolic problems of protein–energy malnutrition, the children became extremely hungry and could eat twice the energy requirement for their age and size. Growth rates accelerated to 15 times the normal rate, until the children reached their expected weight for height. At this point almost all the children dramatically reduced their food intake within 1–2 days, and returned their growth rates to a much slower one expected for healthy children of their age and size. This suggests that powerful signals relating to body size or composition must be involved.

In adult women it is recognized that food intake shows an unconscious cyclical decrease during the follicular phase, with a rise in the luteal phase (Dalvit 1981). This fluctuation is compatible with the supposed depressive effects of some oestrogens on food intake in animals and a rise in intake when progesterone secretion dominates, e.g. during the luteal phase (Czaja 1978). The cyclical changes in intake exceed the similar cycle in energy expenditure which can occur independently of intake (Bisdee et al 1989), so premenopausal women appear to be in a shifting state of energy balance over the whole of a menstrual cycle. In lactation women also experience hunger and show a rise in food intake which compensates to a large extent for the cost of milk synthesis and production (Thomson et al 1970). Without this compensation weight loss would amount to about 450–600 g per week during normal lactation. Studies in adults fed liquid diets, camouflaged to allow changes in the energy density of the diets, also clearly show that within 1–3 days both men and women unconsciously begin to drink more if an energy-dilute mixture is fed. Similarly, in studies on lean and obese adults, Porikos claimed that all subjects began to compensate within about 3–6 days for surreptitious changes in the energy density of a variety of normal-looking meals, whether the dietary manipulations involved a switch in carbohydrate or fat content (Porikos & Pi-Sunyer 1984). Studies on sledging expeditions in polar regions (Masterton et al 1957) show that exercise does induce a compensatory change in intake, unless the food is very unpalatable or the subjects are conscious of their weight; psychological factors then seem to override their physiological mechanisms.

Cross-sectional studies of the energy intake of western adults of different ages imply that intake steadily declines with age, as physical exercise and general activity diminish. Without this decline the population would become even more overweight and obese than currently observed, and it seems likely that an appreciable part of this fall in intake is a physiological response to the reduced demand for energy. The problem is in assessing the relative importance of conscious social conditioning and physiological mechanisms in determining the control of food intake.

DIETARY PATTERNS AND QUALITY IN RELATION TO APPETITE CONTROL

Short-term studies suggest that a small carbohydrate-rich snack taken 30–60 minutes before a meal reduces food intake, but that a similar load taken 2 hours before the meal does not. This led Booth to suggest that the widespread practice of snacking or 'grazing' helps to delude the normal control system without taking account of the constant bombardment of novel tastes (Booth et al 1970). There is also increasing interest in the proposition that a diet rich in fat is particularly conducive to energy imbalance, since a number of studies find that individuals on a high-fat diet are more overweight (Dreon et al 1988). Flatt et al (1985) suggest that this depends on an appetite drive for carbohydrate rather than fat, and that fat is not particularly good at suppressing food intake. This theory relates to earlier animal experiments, where rats were shown to regulate independently their carbohydrate and protein intakes (Ashley & Anderson 1975). On this basis, dietary fat is conducive to weight gain, not because of its energy density or poor induction of energy expenditure, but because it is not involved as much as the other macronutrients in the mechanisms controlling food intake. Other aspects of diet which have been invoked in explaining the imperfect energy imbalance of adults in affluent societies include the use of foods low in dietary fibre (non-starch polysaccharides) and the widespread consumption of alcohol. Fibre-rich foods are proposed as limiting food intake because they induce gastric distension (Heaton 1973), and alcohol because it either suppresses or eludes the normal control mechanisms. Assessing the validity of each of these claims is difficult, but there seems little doubt that conscious signals, e.g. of overweight, clothes or social factors relating to body shape, can induce many people to alter their food intake irrespective of any physiological control mechanisms.

ABSORPTION OF ENERGY FROM THE GUT

It is sometimes suggested that the regulation of energy balance depends in part on the proportion of ingested energy which is absorbed from the gut (Macnair 1979). There is no evidence for this view: about $95 \pm 2\%$ is absorbed, in both thin and obese people, and this ratio alters little during overfeeding or underfeeding.

CONTROL OF ENERGY OUTPUT

The components of energy output, and the techniques by which they can be measured, have been described in Chapter 3. We here consider the extent to which alterations in energy output contribute to the regulation of energy balance and stability of body weight.

Adaptation to underfeeding

Much of our understanding about the effects of undernutrition on energy output comes from two classic experiments conducted in the USA in the aftermath of the world wars. Benedict et al (1919) recruited 34 volunteers at the International Young Men's Christian Association College in Springfield, Mass, and underfed them for about 3 months, so as to reduce their body weight by 10% of the starting value. They comment: 'Investigators who work entirely with small animals and domestic fowl can have little conception of the perplexities which arise in working with a considerable number of adults'. One of these perplexities was that the national festivals of Thanksgiving and Christmas interrupted the experiment: the subjects went home, pledged to maintain their experimental restricted diet. The chief results of the study are shown graphically in Fig. 9.3. The striking findings are that resting metabolic rate (RMR, or basal heat production, as Benedict called it) decreased rapidly at first, and then more slowly, with continuing weight loss. After the breaks at Thanksgiving and Christmas there was a sharp but transient increase in RMR which quickly settled to a low level when the diet was again administered under strict supervision.

The other great study of experimental undernutrition was undertaken by Keys et al (1950), who restricted the diet of volunteers over a period of 24 weeks to achieve a loss of 25% of body weight. They confirmed the decrease in metabolic rate, and calculated that 65% of the decrease could be accounted for by the metabolic activity of the tissue which had been lost. Analysis of many underfeeding experiments shows that the decrease in energy expenditure has three components

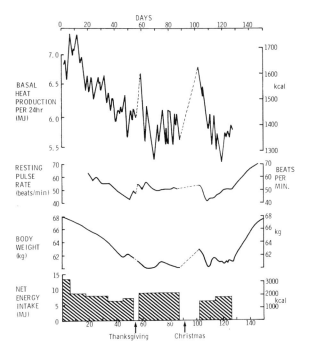

Fig. 9.3 The effect of a restricted diet on the basal metabolic rate, resting pulse rate and body weight of normal young men (data of Benedict et al 1919). The experiment was interrupted for holidays at Thanksgiving and Christmas, and after 126 days the subjects ate ad libitum.

(Garrow & Webster 1989). First, if energy intake is decreased the thermic effect of feeding (which is about 10% of energy intake) is similarly decreased. Secondly, there is an adaptive decrease in metabolic rate which occurs during the first week, related in part to a decrease in sympathetic activity. The magnitude of this decrease is significantly related to the initial metabolic rate – usually about 5–8%. Thirdly, there is the decrease in metabolic rate which can be explained by the weight lost: most investigators find a decrease of 10–12 kcal/day per kg weight loss. The effect of all three processes is that a person who lost weight from, say, 100 kg to 70 kg (a 30% reduction in weight) would experience about a 15% reduction in energy requirements for weight maintenance. Thus a decrease in energy intake causes a reduction in body weight but, provided the decrease is not too great, a new equilibrium will be reached at which the reduced requirement will be satisfied by the reduced intake, and body weight will again stabilize.

Adaptation to overfeeding

If a normal subject is supplied with dietary energy in excess of expenditure, this excess will be stored, mainly in adipose tissue. However, it is not true that a normal person in energy balance who increases his energy intake by 1000 kcal/day will increase his energy stores by 1000 kcal/day. The reverse of the adaptation to undernutrition will apply: there will be increased thermic effect from feeding of about 100 kcal/day in response to the extra 1000 kcal intake, and RMR will increase by about 10–12 kcal/day per kg increase in body weight. In addition there is a metabolic cost associated with the synthesis of glycogen, protein and fat in the extra tissue; the magnitude of this cost depends on the substrates from which these tissues are made. On top of all these costs there seems to be an additional type of thermogenesis, mediated in part by hormonal changes, e.g. in thyroid metabolism, and by increased sympathetic activity, which disposes of some of the excess energy intake and limits weight gain. The magnitude of this adaptive thermogenesis is in dispute: it differs between different strains of experimental animals, and between young and old animals of the same strain.

The only experiment of overfeeding normal subjects which approaches the magnitude of the underfeeding experiments of Benedict et al (1919) and of Keys et al (1950) is a study in Vermont by Sims et al (1973). This experiment was designed primarily to test the hypothesis that obesity caused the insulin insensitivity which is a characteristic of non-insulin-sensitive diabetes mellitus, so unfortunately data on energy metabolism were not systematically collected. Nineteen normal young men, with no family history of diabetes or obesity, were overfed and increased in weight by 21%, of which 73% was fat. Since the weight gain was about 16 kg, this represents an increase in energy stores of about 110 Mcal over 250 days, or about 440 kcal/day. The estimated energy requirement of the men at baseline was about 4000 kcal/day and during overfeeding their intake was about 7000 kcal/day, so on this calculation the energy stored was only about 15% of the excess intake. Even though there were no rigorous measurements made of energy balance in this study, these figures suggest that there was a large adaptive thermogenesis in the men in response to overfeeding.

However, more recent studies of more minor degrees of overfeeding have failed to find the expected large increases in energy expenditure. Metabolic rate increased significantly with overfeeding, but only about 14% of the excess energy intake was dissipated in measured increased metabolic rate, which implies that the remainder of the excess went into energy stores (Norgan 1990, Diaz et al 1991). The relative ability of lean and obese people to burn off excess energy intake, and whether this is a factor in the aetiology of obesity, is considered in Chapter 32.

PHYSICAL ACTIVITY AND ENERGY BALANCE

The nutritional implications of competitive sports are discussed in Chapter 28. We consider here the effects on energy balance of varying the level of physical activity within the range which can be achieved by the ordinary non-athlete: for example, increasing the metabolic rate to seven times the resting level for 1 hour. Assuming a metabolic rate of about 1.3 kcal/min at rest and 10 kcal/min during exercise, this means that exercise involves the expenditure of about 500 kcal/h. However, to calculate the effect of this on overall energy balance it is necessary to consider the effect of the exercise on subsequent RMR, and also on food intake.

It is claimed that exercise causes a prolonged increase in metabolic rate after the exercise ceases, and this is true of the high levels of work achieved by elite athletes, but there is no detectable effect after exercise of the intensity considered here (Freedman-Akabas et al 1985, Pacy et al 1985).

It has also been claimed that exercise causes a reduction in food intake, and again this is true for some hours after exhausting exercise. Mayer et al (1954) reported a strange relationship between physical activity and food intake in rats. If the rats were made to run at 1 km/h for 1, 2, 3 or 4 hours a day, the higher rates of work were associated (as expected) with greater food intake. However, rats which were exercised for 40 minutes, 20 minutes, or not at all, ate more than the rats exercised for 1 hour per day. Mayer et al (1954) suggested that moderate exercise had the effect of reducing food intake compared with a totally sedentary condition. This conclusion was apparently supported by another study on workers in a jute mill in west Bengal (Mayer et al 1956), but that study was seriously flawed (Garrow 1988). Carefully controlled experiments by Woo & Pi-Sunyer (1985) showed that among both normal and obese subjects exercise is associated with an increase in food intake, but the increase tends not to match the increased energy expenditure, so there is a net energy deficit.

INTEGRATING INTAKE AND EXPENDITURE

The independent studies on adaptations in intake or expenditure are interesting physiological experiments, but when attempting to explain the actual responses in energy balance and weight regulation in real life we need to recognize that several factors may be operating at once on both sides of the energy balance equation. Compensatory adjustments occur in both intake and output, so that unravelling the importance of one or other adjustment is not easy. Models have been constructed which show that small increases in daily intake, e.g. of 100–200 kcal, will induce small increases in body weight with an associated rise in energy expenditure as the mass of lean tissue increases. If these changes occur on a daily basis, month by month, then after 3–5 years the adult is still eating 200 kcal/day more, but is now heavier and has come into energy balance. Thus, body fat buffers short-term energy imbalance, and changes in lean tissue mass and the cost of moving a smaller or greater body weight also buffers small changes in intake over a period of several years.

FACTORS PREDISPOSING TO WEIGHT VARIABILITY IN MAN

Since so many factors may affect energy balance, and hence weight stability, it is of interest to know the characteristics of people who do, or do not, maintain a constant body weight. Rissanen et al (1991) analysed the weight change of over 12 000 adults aged 25–64 years in Finland over an interval of 5 years. The average weight of 6504 men increased by 0.60 kg, and that of 6165 women increased by only 0.06 kg. However, among men and women 17.5% and 15.1% respectively gained more than 5 kg, and 10.5% and 13.8% lost more than 5 kg. These investigators considered many factors, but the ones which were most significantly associated with a risk of significant weight gain were a low level of education, chronic disease, little physical activity, heavy alcohol consumption, getting married or stopping smoking. It is possible to think of plausible metabolic mechanisms by which these features might predispose to a positive energy balance, but another observation was that, while parity increased the risk of weight gain in the women of the lower educational level, it was associated with a decreased risk of weight gain among women of a higher educational level. The only plausible explanation of these findings is that control of body weight in the long term is achieved by a conscious limitation of energy intake (or possibly increase in energy expenditure) when an unacceptable increase in body weight is noticed. The socioeconomic factors which predict weight gain presumably do so by altering the level of weight gain which is considered unacceptable.

HEALTH CONSEQUENCES OF WEIGHT VARIATION

If people maintain a reasonable weight by cycling gains and losses, does it matter? We do not know, but there is some evidence that people whose weight is stable have less liability to die young, particularly of heart disease, than those who show large weight changes during adult life (Wannameethe & Shaper 1990, Lissner et al 1991). It may be that people who vary in weight are anxious people who are always going on diets and coming off them, so the increased mortality reflects the type of person rather than the actual fluctuation in weight. However, from what we know of the metabolic consequences of overfeeding and starvation, it is likely that weight fluctuation is itself harmful to health. Thus from a public health viewpoint it is desirable that people should maintain a body weight which is within the desirable range for height, and also that they should remain at a reasonably stable weight throughout adult life.

REFERENCES

Ashley DVM, Anderson GH 1975 Food intake regulation in the weanling rat: effects of the most limiting essential amino acids of gluten, casein and zein on the self selection of protein and energy. Journal of Nutrition 105: 1405–1411

Ashworth A 1969 Growth rates in children recovering from protein–calorie malnutrition. British Journal of Nutrition 23: 835–845

Benedict FG, Miles WR, Roth P, Smith M 1919 Human vitality and efficiency under prolonged restricted diet. Carnegie Institution, Washington, DC, p. 83

Bisdee JT, James WPT, Shaw MA 1989 Changes in energy expenditure during the menstrual cycle. British Journal of Nutrition 61: 187–199

Booth DA, Campbell HT, Chase A 1970 Temporal bounds of post-ingestive glucose-induced satiety in man. Nature 228: 1104

Booth DA, Lee M, McAleavey C 1976 Acquired sensory control of satiation in man. British Journal of Psychology 67: 137–147

Bray GA 1982 Regulation of energy balance. Proceedings of the Nutrition Society 41: 95–108

Czaja JA 1978 Ovarian influences on primate food intake: assessment of progesterone actions. Physiology & Behaviour 21: 923–928

Dalvit SP 1981 The effect of the menstrual cycle on patterns of food intake. American Journal of Clinical Nutrition 34: 1811–1815

Diaz E, Prentice AM, Goldberg GR, Murgatroyd PR, Coward WA 1991 Metabolic and behavioural aspects to altered energy intake in man. 1. Experimental overfeeding. Proceedings of the Nutrition Society 50: 110A

Dreon DM, Frey-Hewitt B, Ellsworth N, Williams PT, Terry RB, Wood PD 1988 Dietary fat: carbohydrate ratio and obesity in middle-aged men. American Journal of Clinical Nutrition 47: 995–1000

Flatt JP, Ravussin E, Acheson KJ, Jequier E 1985 Effects of dietary fat on postprandial substrate oxidation and on carbohydrate and fat balances. Journal of Clinical Investigation 76: 1019–1024

Fomon SJ, Filer LJ, Thomas LN, Roger RR, Proksch AM 1969 Relationship between formula concentration and rate of growth of normal children. Journal of Nutrition 198: 241–254

Freedman-Akabas S, Colt E, Kissilef HR, Pi-Sunyer FX 1985 Lack of sustained increase in metabolic rate following exercise in fit and unfit subjects. American Journal of Clinical Nutrition 41: 545–549

Garrow JS 1988 Obesity and related diseases. Churchill Livingstone, Edinburgh

Garrow JS, Webster JD 1989 Effects on weight and metabolic rate of obese women of a 3.4 MJ (800 kcal) diet. Lancet i: 1429–1431

Gold RM 1973 Hypothalamic obesity: the myth of the ventromedial nucleus. Science 182: 488–490

Gordon T, Kannel WB 1973 The effects of overweight on cardiovascular disease. Geriatrics 28: 80–88

Heaton KW 1973 Food fibre as an obstacle to energy intake. Lancet 2: 1418–1421

Kennedy GC 1950 The hypothalamic control of food intake in rats. Proceedings of the Royal Society B 1137: 535–549

Keys A, Brozek J, Henschel A, Mickelson O, Taylor HL 1950 The biology of human starvation. University of Minnesota Press, Minneapolis, p. 1385

Lissner L, Odell PM, D'Agostino RB et al 1991 Variability of body weight and health outcomes in the Framingham population. New England Journal of Medicine 324: 1839–1844

Macnair AL 1979 Burning off unwanted energy. Lancet ii: 1300

Masterton JP, Lewis HE, Widdowson EM 1957 Food intakes, energy expenditure and faecal excretion of men on a polar expedition. British Journal of Nutrition 11: 346

Mayer J, Marshall NB, Vitale JJ, Christensen JH, Mashayekhi MB, Stare FJ 1954 Exercise, food intake and body weight in normal rats and genetically obese adult mice. American Journal of Physiology 177: 544–548

Mayer J, Roy P, Mitra KP 1956 Relation between caloric intake, body weight and physical work. American Journal of Clinical Nutrition 4: 169–175

Norgan NG 1990 Thermogenesis above maintenance in humans. Proceedings of the Nutrition Society 49: 217–226

Pacy PJ, Barton N, Webster JD, Garrow JS 1985 The energy cost of aerobic exercise in fed and fasted normal subjects. American Journal of Clinical Nutrition 42: 764–768

Porikos KP, Pi-Sunyer FX 1984 Regulation of food intake in human obesity: studies with caloric dilution and exercise. Clinics in Endocrinology and Metabolism 13: 547–561

Rissanen AM, Heliovaara M, Knekt P, Reunanen A, Aromaa A 1991 Determinants of weight gain and overweight in adult Finns. European Journal of Clinical Nutrition 45: 419–430

Rolls BJ, Van Duijvenvoorde PM, Rolls ET 1984 Pleasantness changes and food intake in a varied four-course meal. Appetite 5: 337–348

Russek M 1976 A conceptual equation of intake control. In: Novin D, Wyrwicka W, Bray GA (eds) Hunger: basic mechanisms and clinical implications. Raven Press, New York, pp. 327–347

Sims EAH, Danforth E, Horton ES, Bray GA, Glennon JA, Salans LB 1973 Endocrine and metabolic effects of experimental obesity in man. Recent Progress in Hormone Research 29: 457–496

Thomson AM, Hytten FE, Billewicz WZ 1970 The energy cost of human lactation. British Journal of Nutrition 24: 565–572

Wannamethee G, Shaper AG 1990 Weight change in middle-aged British men: implications for health. European Journal of Clinical Nutrition 44: 133–142

Woo R, Pi-Sunyer FX 1985 Effect of increased physical activity on voluntary intake in lean women. Metabolism 34: 836–841

Wooley SC, Wooley OW, Dunham RB 1972 Can calories be perceived, and do they affect hunger in obese and non-obese humans? Journal of Comparative and Physiological Psychology 80: 250–258

10. Water and monovalent electrolytes

O. Wrong

BODY COMPOSITION

Water is the main constituent of the body, comprising 72% of fat-free weight – about 45 litres in the average 70 kg man, and slightly less in the average woman of this weight because of the greater proportion of body fat. Of this 45 litres, about 30 are intracellular fluid (ICF), and 15 are extracellular fluid (ECF), and of the latter volume about one-fifth, or 3 litres, is plasma water within the intravascular space. Transcellular fluids (e.g. cerebrospinal fluid, fluids in the eye and the ear, and intestinal secretions) comprise further small parts of the ECF compartment, but usually have slightly different ionic structures owing to the selective properties of the organs secreting them.

The monovalent electrolytes sodium (Na^+), potassium (K^+) and chloride (Cl^-) are conveniently considered at the same time as body water, for these ions are responsible for almost the entire osmolality of body fluids, and their disposition within the body determines the volume of ICF and ECF, K^+ being predominantly confined intracellularly with accompanying magnesium, phosphate (largely organically combined) and proteinate anion, whereas Na^+ and Cl^- are sequestered mainly in the ECF. The amounts of these ions in the body have been measured by whole-carcase analysis, by isotope dilution studies, and by neutron activation analysis. Values obtained by the last method are shown in Table 10.1.

Figure 10.1 shows the ionic composition of ECF and ICF by the 'ionogram' method of display popularized by Gamble (1947). Concentrations are expressed per kilogram of water, not per litre of fluid, in order to avoid problems caused by the high solid content of plasma and ICF; in addition, the unit of concentration is not the familiar millimole, but the more old-fashioned milliequivalent (mEq), a unit of electrical equivalence or charge which is equal to the millimole multiplied by the valency, and is therefore identical to the millimole for the monovalent ions

Table 10.1 Total body Na^+, K^+ and Cl^- by neutron activation analysis (From Cohn et al 1976, and Ellis et al 1976.)

		average (mmol)	average (mmol/kg)
Na^+	Men	3540	47
	Women	2620	43
K^+	Men	3190	26
	Women	2030	25
Cl^-	Men	2110	28
	Women	1720	28

considered here. The use of mEq makes it clear that the electrical charge of anions and cations is equal in each compartment. The total concentration of ions in mEq is greater in ICF than in ECF because of the greater electrical charge of the polyvalent intracellular ions, particularly proteinate, but the osmolality (a measure of the number of molecules in solution per kg of water) of the two fluids is identical. Plasma, because of the Donnan effect of its higher protein content, has slightly lower concentrations of Cl^- and bicarbonate than the ECF ionogram shown, and a slightly higher Na^+ concentrations by about 5%.

Active cellular extrusion of Na^+ at the cell membrane, which involves the enzyme Na^+/K^+-linked ATPase, is responsible for the predominantly extracellular position of Na^+ and the intracellular position of K^+. The exact ionic composition of ICF varies a little between different cell types and in many tissues is still largely conjectural because of analytical problems; the 13 mEq/kg of ICF Na^+ shown in Fig. 10.1 is an estimate for muscle cells, the predominant cell type in the body, but Na^+ concentrations are higher in cells actively involved in secreting or absorbing Na^+, including the renal tubules, sweat and lacrimal glands, and the secreting and absorbing cells in the alimentary tract. About half of total body Na^+ is immobilized in bone, apparently

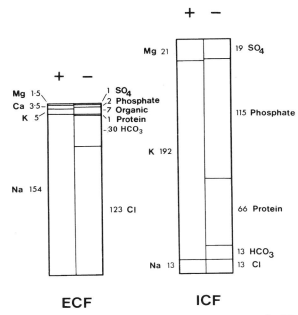

Fig. 10.1 Electrolyte composition (mEq/kg water) of ECF and ICF.

an integral part of the mineral lattice. Tracer experiments have shown that this bone Na^+ is not fully exchangeable with the Na^+ in ECF, and it appears to be unavailable to support ECF volume or osmolality in clinical states of Na^+ depletion or hyponatraemia.

The asymmetric distribution of diffusible ions between ECF and cell fluid produces an electric charge across the cell membrane averaging about 80 mV, negative on the cell interior. This membrane potential is important for many cell functions, and most obviously for the normal excitable behaviour of muscle and nerve. The *ratio* of ECF to ICF concentrations determines the contribution of each ion to this membrane potential, and in clinical practice the ECF concentration of K^+ appears to be particularly important, probably because the concentration is normally so low that quite small changes have a much more marked effect on the ECF/ICF ratio than do much larger changes in ICF concentration.

Like Na^+, Cl^- is predominantly an extracellular ion, but it is not sequestered in bone. Cl^- concentrations in ICF vary from about 3 mmol/1 in skeletal muscle to 90 mmol/1 in red cells and neuroglia, with intermediate levels in the ICF of the secreting and absorbing cells of the renal tubule and alimentary tract. In red cells, Cl^- has a particular function in

relation to the transport of carbon dioxide, as plasma Cl^- exchanges with erythrocyte bicarbonate when blood is deoxygenated in the peripheral capillary bed (the 'chloride shift'), and so assists the venous carriage of carbon dioxide to the lungs, where the process is reversed. Cl^- also has a special role in the stomach, for gastric juice at its most acid has a pH of 0.9 and contains 140 mmol/1 each of Cl^- and hydrogen ion.

Water and monovalent ions are unlike some other nutrients in that there are no storage depots in the body. The amounts present in the body are controlled at a very constant level by a precise balance between intake and output, and in particular by control of urinary losses, which form the main avenue of output.

WATER BALANCE

The intake of water comprises water drunk, water present in the food eaten, and metabolic water, which is derived from the metabolism of foodstuffs, including the metabolism of body tissues. Output consists of water lost as urine, the water lost in faeces, and water lost from the skin and to a lesser extent from the lungs.

Table 10.2 shows the water balance of a healthy young man leading a sedentary life in a temperate climate. It should be noted that the volume of water drunk as fluid is roughly equal to the urine volume, but that these figures represent only one-half of the total water input and output. In clinical practice it is seldom useful to obtain a precise figure for water balance, as this procedure entails more trouble and patience for medical staff and subject than can usually

Table 10.2 The daily water balance of a young man leading a sedentary life on a diet providing 8.8 MJ (2110 kcal) daily. Mean of five daily measurements. (From Passmore et al 1955.)

	Water (ml/day)
Intake:	
Water content of solid food	1115
Liquid drunk	1180
Metabolic water	279
	2574
Output:	
Urine	1294
Faecal water	56
Evaporative water loss	1214
	2565
Water balance	+9

be justified by the usefulness of the information obtained. The serial measurement of body weight is the simplest way of determining changes in body water, and has a degree of accuracy (a clinical beam-balance has a precision of 0.1% or better) which cannot be matched by measurements of fluid intake and output. Daily weight measurements are particularly useful in following the response of fluid-overloaded or depleted subjects to treatment; for example, a grossly oedematous subject may lose 10–20 kg in weight within 10 days after the initiation of effective diuretic therapy. Although changes in body solids – as with malnutrition or re-feeding – can of course lead to profound alterations in body weight, the changes are not as rapid as the day-to-day changes which are often seen with fluctuations in total body water.

Of the six components of water balance listed in Table 10.2, only two – fluid intake and urine volume – are controlled by homoeostatic mechanisms responsive to the state of body water. A water deficit produces increased osmolality of all body fluids, and this increase, working through the increased osmolality of the plasma circulating through the brain, stimulates the thirst centre and the osmoreceptor, two hypothalamic centres which are intimately connected both functionally and structurally, to cause thirst and the release of the antidiuretic hormone vasopressin. This hormone acts on receptors in the renal collecting tubule to cause increased water absorption and reduced urinary volume. When the body contains an excess of water the reverse processes occur: reduced plasma osmolality inhibits thirst and the osmoreceptor centre, drinking ceases and in the absence of vasopressin water absorption in the renal tubules is reduced, with a consequent water diuresis. These mechanisms are exquisitely sensitive and precise, coming into action with deficits and excesses of only 200–300 ml, so that total body water in a healthy 70 kg man, drinking fluids as dictated by thirst alone, varies by no more than 500 ml, and the changes in plasma osmolality which produce these effects are so small that they can only be detected in the laboratory with difficulty.

Because water balance is controlled by thirst and the release of vasopressin, and these two mechanisms respond to ECF osmolality – which is in osmotic equilibrium with ICF osmolality – it follows that the total amount of water in the body is ultimately determined by the amount of osmotically active solute present, i.e. by the quantities of Na^+ and K^+ and their accompanying anions in the body. The mechanisms by which the body controls these amounts are considered below.

Individual components of water balance

Thirst

Although everyone experiences thirst from time to time, it plays little day-to-day role in the control of water intake of most healthy subjects living in a temperate climate, in whom fluid intake is determined by many other considerations, such as water taken as a vehicle for nutrients (e.g. soups, milk), in tea and coffee as mild stimulants, and in alcoholic beverages drunk on social occasions or for the purpose of intoxication. Urine losses, which reflect water intake, are therefore often much greater than they would be if dictated by thirst alone, and urinary osmolality is lower. In a hot arid environment, as in Arabia, insensible water losses may increase many fold and be accompanied by copious visible sweating. The resultant thirst that develops ensures that fluid intake keeps up with body losses. Although body fluid osmolality is the chief stimulus to thirst, local drying of the mouth and throat also causes a sensation of thirst, for example when a well-hydrated speaker pauses in a lecture to take a drink in order to moisten his tongue and lips before continuing.

Urine excretion

The quantity of urine is not determined solely by the amount of surplus body water available, for the kidney also rids the body of solute, which requires the passage of urine for its excretion. Urine osmolality can vary from a minimum value of about 50 mosmol/kg to a maximum of 900–1200 mosmol/kg. This last figure, 1200 mosmol/kg, is close to the osmolality of seawater, and is more than four times that of body water, at 285 mosmol/kg. The chief solutes requiring excretion in the urine are the urea produced from the metabolism of protein, and Na^+ and K^+ derived from food, with their accompanying anions. Table 10.3 shows that the average urinary excretion of solute is approximately 1000 mosmol/day, an amount which requires about 1 litre of urine daily for its excretion. However, daily excretion of solute, and hence the obligatory urine volume, varies greatly between subjects, depending on the amount of food eaten. Consumers of large amounts of meat may excrete almost double this amount of solute, for meat is the major source of urinary urea, K^+ and phosphate, and is usually consumed with large amounts of sodium chloride. Vegetarians and eaters of small amounts of meat derive most of their energy from carbohydrate, and so produce not only small amounts of urea but also small amounts of other urinary solutes. Some years ago the

Table 10.3 Contribution of main urinary solutes to urinary osmolality. Urinary cations are assumed to be accompanied by equivalent anion (Cl⁻ bicarbonate, phosphate, sulphate, urate, etc)

	Daily adult excretion		Contribution to urinary mosmol	
	Mean	Range	Mean	Range
Urea (g)	25	14–35	417	233–583
Creatinine (g)	1.6	1.0–2.0	14	8–18
Na^+ (mmol)	180	75–350	360	150–700
K^+ (mmol)	65	30–100	130	60–200
Ca^{2+} (mmol)	5.8	1.1–10.0	12	2–20
Mg^{2+} (mmol)	3.9	1.2–7.0	8	2–14
Total mmol			941	455–1535

author found that healthy subjects living on a 20 g protein diet (as was then advocated for chronic renal failure) and drinking water as dictated by thirst, might have a urinary volume under 600 ml/day owing to their very low excretion of solute.

Faecal water

Although 7–8 litres of fluid are secreted daily into the alimentary tract, in health this volume is almost all reabsorbed. Normal subjects pass 50–400 g of faeces each day, the amount being largely determined by the dietary content of undigestible fibre. On the international scale, Europeans eat little fibre and have a small faecal mass, averaging about 100 g/day. The water content of faeces averages 75% by weight, with an extreme range of 60–90%. Faecal water is slightly hypertonic, owing to bacterial generation of fresh solute in the large intestine, with an average pH of 7.0, range 5.0–8.0. The main faecal ions in solution in faecal water are short-chain fatty acid anions, K^+ and bicarbonate, but faeces also contain large amounts of calcium, magnesium and phosphate, precipitated in insoluble forms.

Fluid loss from the skin

Sweat glands occur in all parts of the external skin. Some water evaporates from the skin surface even in the absence of sweating. In a temperate climate, subjects at rest are not aware of the small amounts of sweat secreted by their skin, which evaporates and contributes to 'insensible' fluid loss. The normal function of sweat is to cool the body by its evaporation, so that sweat secretion increases and becomes obvious as liquid sweat on the skin when body temperature is increased by a high ambient temperature or by heavy muscular exertion. In extreme cases, losses of sweat of 2500 ml/hour have been recorded; losses of 10–12 litres/day are not uncommon.

Fluid loss from the lungs

Air leaving the lungs is saturated with water vapour at 37°C, i.e. at a pressure of one atmosphere it contains 44 mg water/l. This amount of water is lost from the body during mouth-breathing, and represents an increment of 32 mg/l over the 12 mg/l present in inspired air at an ambient temperature of 20°C and fairly average humidity of 70%, or a net loss of 320 ml/day at a normal resting pulmonary ventilation of 10 000 l/day.

The amount of water vapour carried by air at complete saturation (100% humidity) is markedly dependent on temperature, e.g. 5 mg/l at 0°C, increasing to 17 mg/l at 20°C, and 52 mg/l at 40°C. An obvious example both of the water lost from the body in expired air, and of the effect of temperature in determining how much water vapour can be carried in air, is seen in subjects in a very cold environment, whose exhaled breath becomes visible when water picked up in the lungs condenses as a fine mist. The dog takes advantage of the relationship between air temperature and its water-carrying capacity in reducing respiratory water loss, by means of a heat exchanger in the nasal mucosa. Inspired air is warmed as it passes over the turbinates and expired air is cooled when it passes in the reverse direction, so giving up much of its water content. Whether this mechanism is of any importance in man is unknown, and man certainly lacks the cold moist nose of dogs; in any event, this effect would be lost during mouth-breathing, which usually accompanies increased respiratory excursion. Water loss from the lungs is increased by fever, and by a reduced water content of inspired air, such as results from a reduced ambient temperature or relative humidity. An example is the increased respiratory loss of water during mountain climbing (Hunt 1953), which arises partly from the increased ventilation caused by muscular exertion and a reduced ambient oxygen content, and partly from the reduced water content of inspired air caused by reduced relative humidity, temperature and atmospheric pressure.

SODIUM, CHLORIDE AND POTASSIUM

Na^+, Cl^- and K^+ balances can be measured as they are for water, but with greater ease as these ions do not volatilize appreciably, and are neither created nor destroyed in the body, so no allowances need to be made for metabolic production or insensible losses. For a complete balance it is necessary only to determine dietary intake, either by the use of food tables or with greater accuracy by analysis of a duplicate diet, and measure what is lost in urine, faeces or any abnormal body secretions (e.g. vomit, intestinal secretion and fistulae). Sweat losses are usually negligible, especially in a temperate climate, and are habitually disregarded. The construction of such an electrolyte balance has little clinical value, except occasionally when investigating electrolyte deficiencies of obscure origin.

Correction by the body of abnormal Na^+, Cl^- and K^+ balances takes much longer to complete than do corrections in water balance. When total body water is altered by an extra water load or deficit, the excess is excreted in the urine, or the deficit is made up by increased drinking and reduced urine volume, within 2–4 hours. Control of Na^+, Cl^- and K^+ balance is no less precise, but takes 2–5 days to be complete, or even longer when the initial disturbance is marked. At the same time there are usually changes in the volume of body water which are secondary responses to changes in its osmolality. Thus, after a generous helping of salted fish many people are conscious of increased thirst, which is a response of their thirst centre to increased ECF osmolality caused by the extra load of sodium chloride. As a result, more water is drunk, while increased vasopressin release causes urine flow initially to be reduced. ECF osmolality is thus returned to normal by the newly conserved water, but at the expense of an increase in ECF volume. Over the next 2–4 days the extra water, Na^+ and Cl^- are slowly excreted in the urine, and ECF volume is restored to normal.

Electrolyte intake

Dietary intakes of Na^+ and K^+ are very similar to the urinary outputs shown in Table 10.3. The amounts of dietary Na^+ and Cl^- vary to a greater extent than those of K^+, owing to the large but variable amounts of common salt, NaCl, consumed by healthy subjects. Small amounts of both Na^+ and Cl^- are ingested in other forms (e.g. sodium bicarbonate in baking powder, citrate and tartrate in effervescent drinks, sulphite as a preservative, monosodium glutamate as a flavour-enhancer), but these amounts are small in comparison to the intake of Na^+ and Cl^- together in common salt. Evidence for this conclusion comes from recent observations (Sanchez-Castillo et al 1987), showing that the ratio of urinary Na^+ to Cl^- in the inhabitants of a Cambridgeshire market town, consuming their usual intake, was 1.03 (standard error 0.008), i.e. the excretion of the two ions was almost identical; as excretion of either ion by routes other than the urine is negligible, it follows that the *intake* of the two ions was nearly identical. This study also established that 85% of the dietary salt intake, which averaged 9 g or 155 mmol/day, was from foodstuffs brought into the household, and the remaining 15% was added during domestic cooking or at the table.

Table 10.4 shows the Na^+, Cl^- and K^+ content of some common foods. Most natural foods, particularly cereals, vegetables and fruits, contain little Na^+ and Cl^-. Meats and fish contain larger amounts, due to the presence of Na^+ and Cl^- in the ECF of the animal from which the food was obtained. Cows' milk

Table 10.4 Electrolyte content of some common foods. Values, from Paul & Southgate (1978), expressed as mmol/100 g.

	Na^+	K^+	Cl^-
Natural foods:			
Wholemeal wheat flour	0.1	9	1
Beef, lean	3	9	2
Cod, frozen steaks	3	8	3
Eggs, boiled	4	4	5
Cows' milk, fresh	2	4	3
Lettuce, raw	0.4	6	1
Cabbage, raw	0.3	7	1
Carrots, raw	4	6	2
Potatoes, raw	0.3	15	2
Oranges	0.1	5	0.1
Bananas	0.1	10	0.2
Apples, eating	0.1	0.3	0.03
Processed foods:			
White bread	23	3	25
Bacon, raw lean	81	9	79
Kippers, baked	23	7	23
Cheese, cheddar	27	3	30
Salted butter	38	0.5	38
Beans, canned in tomato sauce	21	7	23
Tomato ketchup	49	15	51

contains about 22 mmol/1 of Na^+ and Cl^-, essential for the development of the ECF of the growing calf, but most of this is lost in the whey when cheese is made, and most commercial cheeses contain large amounts of salt added during preparation. During manufacture large amounts of salt are added to almost all forms of processed foods, particularly preserved meat and fish, pickles, spices, soups and sauces, with the dual purpose of enhancing flavour and increasing shelf life by retarding bacterial spoilage. Even bread, the biblical staff of life, has salt added during manufacture. Extreme examples of the use of salt as a preservative are its addition to bacon, salami, various forms of salted fish, and exotic foods such as olives.

The K^+ contained in foods is present in their unprocessed form, as K^+ is an essential element of all forms of life, both animal and plant, whereas Na^+ and Cl^- are essential constituents of animals but not of most plants. Furthermore, K^+ is not added to foods because it does not enhance their flavour, the taste of the potassium ion being generally considered unpleasant, and described as 'metallic' or 'fishy'. K^+ is an intracellular ion, so highly cellular tissues such as animal meat contain large amounts, but it also has a high concentration in certain fruits, particularly banana, tomato and citrus fruits. Because K^+ is found in all forms of natural food, it is difficult to construct a diet from which it is absent, and those who have tried to produce potassium depletion experimentally have had recourse to various purified extracts of natural foods, such as sucrose, butter and vegetable oils, or milk from which K^+ has been removed by passage through an ion-exchange resin. When subjects are found to be spontaneously consuming very little K^+, it is almost invariably the case that they are eating extremely little of any foodstuff, as for example in anorexia nervosa.

Salt appetite

Na^+ and Cl^- are essential constituents of all forms of animal life, yet are virtually absent from vast areas of the land surface of the earth. Both ions form practically no insoluble compounds and so over millions of years have been leached out of the earth's surface by rainwater, being now confined to the oceans except for a few landlocked collections of water such as the Dead Sea and the lakes of the Rift Valley in East Africa, and scanty salt deposits and subterranean collections representing former ocean beds. As a consequence, many animals have developed very efficient mechanisms for the conservation of their body Na^+ and Cl^-, and these include an appetite for salt. This is most marked in herbivorous animals, which consume plants that usually contain negligible Na^+ and Cl^-, whereas carnivorous animals can benefit from the salt content of their animal prey. Salt appetite, particularly its nervous and humoral control, has been discussed in detail by Denton (1982), and it is clear from his work that the salt appetite is primarily for Na^+ rather than for Cl^-, as some salts of Na^+ other than the chloride are as avidly sought as sodium chloride, and chloride salts are not sought unless presented as sodium chloride. The term 'salt appetite' has usually been understood to mean both a craving to consume salt, and an increased ability to detect traces of salt by taste. Both aspects are increased by the physiological stimulus of Na^+ deficiency, whatever its primary cause. An example is the ability of sheep and cattle, Na^+-depleted by prolonged lactation and subsistence on fresh pasture containing no Na^+, to track down the location of a 'salt-lick' over a distance, apparently by detecting minute traces of volatilized salt in the air.

It is likely that primitive man had a well-developed salt appetite, for many primitive communities subsisted on agriculture and lived hundreds or thousands of miles from the nearest supply of salt. Salt depletion caused by faecal losses during gastroenteritis, or resulting from injury with loss of blood, must in the past have increased the need for salt and the advantage for survival of an efficient salt appetite. Depletion of body K^+ was, by contrast, a rare event, owing to the abundance of K^+ in all natural foods, so that a 'potassium appetite' would have little survival value and has not developed. Not surprisingly, salt has been used as a commodity for barter by many primitive peoples, and with the more modern advent of rapacious governments has frequently been subject to an excise tax.

Nowadays salt is cheap and easily transported; it can be stored indefinitely, and so is readily available in civilized communities. Salt appetite as a biological urge has largely disappeared, to be replaced by a hedonistic use of salt as a general enhancer of flavour when added to other foods. The normal physiological requirement for salt has not been definitely established, but is probably less than 10 mmol/day, though liable to be increased by physiological losses such as lactation, menstruation, parturition or heavy sweating. The average salt intake is about 20 times this minimal figure. In these circumstances, the retention of an efficient salt appetite becomes a biological irrelevance, but it is still very occasionally seen in subjects at lifelong risk of Na^+ depletion, such as those with Na^+-losing renal disease, adrenal insufficiency or a sodium-losing form of adrenal hyperplasia, where the salt appetite may have been imprinted in childhood as a result of chronic Na^+ depletion (Denton 1982). It can be argued that the modern appreciation of salt as a food additive is a manifestation of salt appetite, but there appears to be an important difference in that salt appetite is increased by the appropriate physiological stimulus of Na^+ deficiency, whereas the classic studies of McCance (1936) indicated that contemporary man does not experience an increased desire for salt even when experimentally salt-depleted.

Electrolyte output

Urine

Because dietary intake of Na^+, Cl^- and K^+ is usually greatly in excess of the needs of the body, and intestinal absorption is virtually complete, it falls to the kidney to excrete excesses of these ions, and so indirectly to control the volumes of ECF and ICF.

Renal capacity to excrete Na^+ and Cl^- has a range of at least 2000-fold, from 0.5 mmol/day or less (seen, for example, after completion of a successful course of intense diuretic therapy in a patient with cardiac failure or nephrotic syndrome who is avidly conserving Na^+), to more than 1000 mmol/day, depending on the real or perceived needs of the body. In most situations Na^+ appears to be the prime mover, Cl^- accompanying it, and so preserving acid–base equilibrium; but urinary Cl^- can be conserved to values of under 1 mmol/day in selective Cl^- deficiency, which is seen most typically after prolonged loss of gastric hydrochloric acid.

Urinary Na^+ excretion represents a balance between the amount of Na^+ filtered by the renal glomeruli – of the order of 25 000 mmol/day in normal subjects – and the almost equally large amount reabsorbed by the renal tubules. The control of Na^+ excretion is achieved by mechanisms that are still incompletely understood, but which are responsive to changes in ECF volume, or some critical component of ECF volume (e.g. renal afferent arteriolar pressure, or atrial filling pressure), rather than to changes in ECF Na^+ concentration. Of these, the best established are glomerular filtration rate and two humoral factors – the renin/angiotensin/aldosterone system and atrial natriuretic peptide – which modify the renal tubular reabsorption of Na^+.

Renal control of K^+ excretion has a less extensive range than that of Na^+ and Cl^-. During experimental K^+ deficiency in man, urinary excretion has fallen to 7–12 mmol/day, with total K^+ deficits of 700–

1200 mmol, at which time plasma K^+ has fallen to below 3.5 mmol/l and definite symptoms of K^+ deficiency have developed. Whether more profound K^+ deficiency would have led to a lower urinary K^+ is not known, nor have the upper limits of urinary K^+ excretion been determined. Urinary K^+ excretion is less influenced by glomerular filtration rate than is that of Na^+, and experimental evidence suggests that much of the K^+ that appears in the urine is secreted by the distal nephron, filtered K^+ being almost entirely absorbed more proximally in the tubule. In chronic renal failure, when glomerular filtration rate is markedly reduced, urinary K^+ may exceed the small amount filtered; an important factor here is increased aldosterone secretion, a physiological response to hyperkalaemia, which enhances the distal tubular absorption of Na^+ and the secretion of K^+.

Alimentary losses

Saliva is not normally lost from the body in significant amounts, except rarely in patients with dysphagia. Unlike other alimentary secretions, it is normally hypotonic, with Na^+, K^+ and Cl^- concentrations averaging 10, 21 and 16 mmol/l respectively. The secretion of gastric oxyntic cells consists of almost pure isotonic hydrochloric acid, with Cl^- and hydrogen ion concentrations of 140–150 mmol/l each; selective loss of this secretion can cause Cl^- deficiency, with an accompanying hypochloraemic alkalosis. Bile, pancreatic and small-intestinal fluids are isotonic, with Na^+ concentrations of 120–140 mmol/l, K^+ 10–30 mmol/l. Pancreatic juice contains large amounts of bicarbonate (HCO_3^-), and throughout the small intestine Cl^- is actively reabsorbed and partly replaced by HCO_3^-.

In the large intestine, which determines ionic losses from the alimentary tract, the Na^+ contained in fluid delivered by the small intestine is largely reabsorbed and replaced by secreted K^+, and Cl^- is simultaneously replaced by HCO_3^- and short-chain fatty acid anions, the latter generated by the anaerobic bacterial metabolism of carbohydrate residues. The mucosal reabsorption of Na^+ and Cl^-, and the secretion of K^+ and HCO_3^-, are all active movements. Faecal losses of Na^+, normally only a fraction of those of K^+ and negligible in relation to urinary Na^+ losses, are under the influence of aldosterone, which enhances the mucosal absorption of Na^+ and increases further secretion of K^+, just as it does in the distal renal tubule.

Sweat

Sweat is hypotonic to plasma, but does contain low concentrations of electrolytes, averaging Na^+ 45, K^+ 10 and Cl^- 30 mmol/l. Na^+ and Cl^- concentrations fall at high rates of sweating, or when heavy sweating continues for several days. Increased aldosterone secretion may be partly responsible, for it is known that aldosterone reduces the Na^+ concentration in sweat. (When Conn in 1955 described the first recorded patient with 'primary aldosteronism', caused by an adrenal cortical adenoma, his initial suspicion that the patient had an excess of circulating Na^+-retaining hormone was due to the finding of abnormally low sweat Na^+ and Cl^- concentrations.)

BODY DEFICITS

Water depletion

The term 'dehydration' strictly means deficiency of water, but is usually applied to states of combined Na^+ and water deficiency, with reduced ECF volume. Because of this misleading usage it is best to avoid the term altogether, referring to pure water losses as 'water depletion' and the more common loss of isotonic salt and water as 'saline depletion' or 'ECF depletion'.

The existence of a water deficit always implies a defect of either the thirst/drinking mechanism or of the osmoreceptor/antidiuretic mechanism, or of both. The thirst mechanism may be defective because subjects do not experience thirst (e.g. a hypothalamic lesion damaging the thirst centre, or coma from any cause) or they cannot respond appropriately to thirst (infancy, debilitated subjects, dysphagia or those shipwrecked at sea or lost in the desert). The osmoreceptor/antidiuretic mechanism may be defective because a pituitary lesion prevents the production of vasopressin (cranial diabetes insipidus), or the renal tubules respond inadequately to the hormone (nephrogenic diabetes insipidus, osmotic diuresis). Whatever the underlying defect, the resultant water deficiency is more severe when insensible water loss is increased by a high ambient temperature, fever or increased respiratory excursion.

The symptoms of a water deficit depend on the defect giving rise to that deficit. Severe thirst develops provided the hypothalamic thirst centre is functioning. Urine becomes scanty and highly concentrated, as long as vasopressin production is unimpaired and the renal tubules are capable of responding to it. Clouding of consciousness, muscle twitching and coma eventually develop as the water deficit becomes more severe. Cerebral venous thrombosis is a recognized complication. Neurological deficits may persist after the water deficit has been made good: these are seen particularly tragically in familial nephrogenic diabetes insipidus, an X-linked recessive condition which is often not diagnosed until several weeks after birth, when it is at last realized that a male infant who fails to thrive and is excessively wet and miserable is suffering from a severe renal water-losing state, by which time irreversible brain damage has often developed.

Physical signs, particularly the classic signs of 'dehydration' (hypotension, reduced tissue turgor, cold extremities), are conspicuously absent. The diagnosis can most readily be made by the demonstration of increased plasma concentrations of Na^+, Cl^- and osmolality. Values of plasma Na^+ over 148 mmol/l and osmolalities of over 315 mmol/kg are diagnostic. Plasma urea and creatinine concentrations are normal. Despite the high plasma Na^+, urinary Na^+ is usually low – a seeming paradox unless it is realized that ECF volume, which is reduced though not markedly so, rather than ECF Na^+ concentration, is the factor controlling renal Na^+ excretion. The most severe cases of water deficit have been recorded in patients with combined destruction of the thirst centre and of vasopressin release caused by hypothalamic disease, a double lesion occasionally seen in eosinophil granuloma, in which a plasma Na^+ of over 200 mmol/l has been encountered.

The nature of the underlying disturbance in body fluid volumes and concentrations is easily understood by reference to first principles, as shown in the top panel of Fig. 10.2. Because ECF and ICF are in osmotic equilibrium, a deficit in total body water, although usually initially sustained by the ECF, is rapidly distributed over total body water, and only one-third of the deficiency is then sustained by the ECF; consequently, signs of reduced ECF volume are late to appear, by which time total body osmolality is dangerously increased and the neurological features of a raised plasma osmolality dominate the clinical picture.

Treatment depends on the cause. Mild defects can be treated by oral water, with desmopressin (DDAVP) when the osmoreceptor/vasopressin mechanism is disturbed. When intravenous therapy is required, the appropriate fluid is 2.5–5.0% dextrose intravenously, *not* pure water as this causes haemolysis. The total body water deficit can readily be calculated from the degree of elevation of plasma

Loss of water

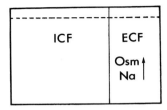

Loss of saline

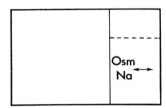

Fig. 10.2 Effect of a 10% contraction in body fluid volume. Loss of water alone (top panel) is distributed over total body water (as shown by interrupted line) with increased solute concentrations in both ECF and ICF. Loss of the same volume in isotonic saline (lower panel) is sustained entirely by the ECF compartment, with no change in ICF volume and initially no change in solute concentrations.

Na^+, assuming that the defect is distributed over total body water, but in some cases the clinical condition has appeared to worsen after a rapid correction of the hyperosmolar state, and it is generally recommended that in severe cases the plasma Na^+ concentration should be lowered only slowly to the normal range over the first 48 hours of treatment, or longer.

Combined Na^+, Cl^- and water deficit (saline deficiency)

A general reduction in ECF volume, with isotonic loss of Na^+, Cl^- and water, is much more frequently seen in clinical practice than a pure water deficit. This is the state traditionally described as 'dehydration' because the subject looks dry, a term which is misleading as it obscures the fact that the primary loss is usually of Na^+ and never of water.

The causes of saline deficiency are shown in Table 10.5. In some cases isotonic fluid has been lost as such from the ECF compartment, as when fluid is lost

Table 10.5 Causes of saline deficiency (combined depletion of water, Na^+ and Cl^-)

Gastrointestinal losses
  Vomiting
  Gastric or small bowel drainage
  Diarrhoea
  Intestinal fistulas (ileostomy, colostomy)
Renal losses
  Adrenal (especially mineralocorticoid) deficiency
  Chronic renal failure
  Renal tubular disease (e.g. Fanconi and Bartter
    syndromes, renal tubular acidosis)
  Postobstructive nephropathy
  Osmotic diuresis (e.g. uncontrolled diabetes)
  Diuretic drugs
Skin losses
  Sweating
  Burns
Deliberate parenteral removal of saline
  Paracentesis
  Haemodialysis, peritoneal dialysis
  Haemofiltration

from the intestine by suction or in the profuse diarrhoea of cholera, but in others (e.g. adrenal insufficiency, sodium-losing renal disease) the primary loss is more clearly of Na^+, with a secondary commensurate loss of water owing to the effect of a low ECF osmolality in suppressing thirst and vasopressin release. The experiments of McCance, in which Na^+ and Cl^- depletion was caused by forced sweating and water replacement, showed that body water losses (as shown by body weight) paralleled those of Na^+ until a deficit of 300 mmol of Na^+ had been reached; beyond this point weight fell little further, despite continuing Na^+ loss. This late stabilization of body water is the result of increased vasopressin secretion, stimulated by hypovolaemia; with further Na^+ losses plasma Na^+ concentration falls progressively, though not usually to such a severe degree as may be seen in pure water excess (see below).

Saline-depleted subjects feel physically exhausted and apathetic. Blood pressure is reduced, particularly in the erect position, and the pulse is rapid. Subcutaneous turgor is reduced, but this sign is difficult to assess as it can be mimicked by the loss of subcutaneous fat from wasting disease, and by old age which leads to atrophy of the elastic fibres. Eyeball tension is reduced, peripheral veins are collapsed and the extremities may be cold. The mouth is usually dry due to a reduction in salivary flow, but this sign is unreliable as it occurs in many mouth-breathing patients, even in the absence of saline depletion.

Reduced renal blood flow leads to oliguria and diminished renal function, and in severe cases to total renal failure, a form of 'prerenal uraemia', which can mimic closely the clinical picture of renal failure caused by intrinsic renal disease.

Provided the renin/angiotensin/aldosterone mechanism is intact, urinary Na^+ and Cl^- excretion is markedly lowered due to hyperaldosteronism secondary to ECF contraction. The blood shows increased haematocrit, haemoglobin and protein concentrations due to shrinkage of the plasma volume, with increased concentrations of urea, creatinine and urate caused by reduced renal function, and plasma Na^+ and Cl^- concentrations which are normal or moderately reduced.

The bottom half of Fig. 10.2 shows graphically the nature of the change in body fluid compartments. Primary loss of Na^+ reduces the osmolality of body water, leading to suppression of thirst and a water diuresis, which restores body fluid osmolality to normal at the expense of a reduced ECF volume. The reduction in body water is sustained entirely by the extracellular fluid; ICF volume is not reduced because there is no loss of intracellular electrolyte and no increase in ECF osmolality, as in pure water depletion, tending to draw water from the intracellular compartment.

In mild cases treatment is best achieved by the oral administration of Na^+ salts (Table 10.6), especially sodium chloride. Subjects usually retain water in parallel, so that the deficit of both Na^+ and water is replaced. However, the amount of Na^+ required may be more than subjects can tolerate by mouth, or intake may be impaired by gastrointestinal disease, in which case physiological saline intravenously is the treatment of choice. When very large deficits are being replaced, it is sensible to provide some of the Na^+ in the form of an anion which is metabolized to bicarbonate (e.g. lactate, acetate, citrate), and imitate the composition of ECF (Fig. 10.1) by adding K^+ and calcium, which can be done with Hartmann's solution containing Na^+ 131, K^+ 5, calcium 2, Cl^- 111 and lactate 29 mmol/l.

Chloride depletion

Body Cl^- usually follows body Na^+, both ions being depleted together, but occasionally body Cl^- is markedly reduced, with a relative preservation of Na^+. Selective depletion of Cl^- is most often seen in patients who have lost large amounts of gastric hydrochloric acid from pyloric stenosis or self-induced vomiting, and less often in patients who have received excessive diuretics combined with salts of potassium other than the chloride (usually bicarbonate or tartrate) to prevent potassium depletion. Usually patients show signs of saline depletion caused by an accompanying Na^+ deficit, and have a low plasma K^+, but their disproportionate Cl^- deficiency is shown by the existence of a hypochloraemic alkalosis and urinary Cl^- concentrations and Cl^-:Na^+ ratios which are close to zero. When provided with sodium or potassium chloride (and it is best to provide both salts) these patients avidly retain Cl^- and excrete an alkaline bicarbonate-rich urine, thus correcting their Cl^- deficiency and alkalosis while simultaneously restoring body Na^+ and K^+.

Potassium depletion

The causes of K^+ depletion are shown in Table 10.7. K^+ depletion is always associated with abnormal losses of K^+ from the body, and has not been reliably reported from reduced K^+ intake alone. Certainly anorexia nervosa is often associated with K^+ depletion, but on close examination there have always turned out to be increased K^+ losses – often concealed by the patient – such as self-induced vomiting or purgation, or diuretic abuse. In any K^+-depleted patient the decision as to whether increased losses are occurring through the kidney or the alimentary tract can be made by measurement of urinary K^+, which is below 20 mmol/day when the kidneys are conserving K^+ normally.

In clinical practice plasma K^+ reduced below 3.4 mmol/l is usually accepted as evidence of a total

Table 10.6 Content of some common electrolyte supplements

	Molecular weight	Cation content (mmol/g)	Availability in UK
Sodium chloride	58.5	17	300 mg tablets and 600 mg slow-release ('Slow- Na') preparation
Sodium bicarbonate	84	12	500 mg and 1000 mg gelatin capsules
Potassium chloride	74.5	13.5	600 mg slow-release ('Slow-K') and many other proprietary preparations
Potassium bicarbonate	100	10	Effervescent potassium tablets, 6.5 mmol K^+/tablet
Potassium citrate	324	9	Various mixtures

Table 10.7 Causes of K^+ depletion

Gastrointestinal
Vomiting
Gastric or small bowel drainage
Diarrhoea (especially purgation, villous tumours of large
  intestine)
Intestinal fistulas
Ureterocolic anastomosis
Urinary losses
Steroid excess (Cushing's syndrome, primary and secondary
  hyperaldosteronism, juxtaglomerular tumour)
Renal tubular disease
Osmotic diuresis (especially uncontrolled diabetes)
Diuretic drugs
Chronic metabolic acidosis or alkalosis

body deficit. However, only 2% of the total body K^+ is in the extracellular compartment, so that it is theoretically possible for abnormal plasma values to result from shifts of K^+ between the cells and the ECF, whatever the state of total body K^+. Net shifts of K^+ from cells to ECF occur when tissues are rapidly destroyed, as with massive haemolysis or soft-tissue trauma, when glycogen is broken down as in uncontrolled diabetes, in systemic acidosis, and in adrenergic blockade. Conversely, there is a net shift from ECF to ICF during glycogen synthesis (e.g. after glucose and insulin administration), when acidosis is corrected, and during catecholamine release. In familial hypokalaemic periodic paralysis, the normal relationship between ECF and ICF potassium is disturbed and attacks of paralysis are associated with sharp reductions in plasma K^+, caused by an intracellular shift, though total body K^+ is normal. Provided these factors can be excluded, it is reasonable to assume that the level of plasma K^+ gives an approximate indication of total body K^+.

Symptoms of potassium deficiency include lethargy, constipation and muscular weakness, which can proceed to generalized flaccid paralysis. Renal function is reduced, frequently with thirst and polyuria caused by the reduced urinary concentrating power. Cardiac excitability is increased and the heart becomes more sensitive to digitalis; changes in the electrocardiogram include lengthening and flattening of the T wave and the appearance of a U wave, but these findings are not specific. Plasma changes include a plasma K^+ below 3.4, and often a metabolic alkalosis with a high plasma HCO_3^-, caused by an intracellular shift of hydrogen ion from the ECF, unless the cause of K^+ depletion also predisposes to acidosis as in diabetic ketoacidosis, renal tubular disease, or from loss of alkaline intestinal secretions.

Plasma levels below 1.5 mmol/l are rarely seen, and have been associated with deaths from respiratory paralysis or cardiac arrhythmia.

Treatment is best achieved by oral K^+ supplements, preferably the chloride. Intravenous K^+ is seldom required and should not exceed 20 mmol/h or 300 mmol in all, in view of the dangerous direct effects of a high plasma K^+ on the myocardium.

Oral electrolyte supplements

The most commonly used supplements are detailed in Table 10.6. Na^+ is usually given as the chloride, except where metabolic acidosis needs to be treated, when the bicarbonate is used. Both Na^+ salts may cause ECF expansion with cardiac embarrassment in those with reduced cardiac reserve, or when Na^+ excretion is impaired by renal failure. Na^+ salts are gastric irritants, and should be taken with food. This advice applies even more to potassium salts: all solid forms of K^+ have, on occasion, led to intestinal ulceration and stricture formation, probably the direct result of a high K^+ concentration at the site of dissolution, which has even been reported, although less frequently, with the waxed slow-release preparation 'Slow-K'. For this reason liquid forms of K^+ are preferable, and for patients are most conveniently obtained by the use of effervescent tablets. Potassium citrate is traditionally used for symptomatic relief in urinary infections, and is appropriate in acidosis associated with K^+ deficiency. Otherwise potassium is best given as the chloride, in view of the frequency of an associated Cl^- deficiency. Many diuretic preparations contain potassium, added to prevent diuretic-induced K^+ deficiency, but their K^+ content is usually inadequate for this purpose, which can be better achieved by the addition of a potassium-sparing diuretic such as amiloride or triamterene.

BODY EXCESSES

Water excess

The word 'overhydration' is usually applied to oedematous states in which Na^+ and water have been retained in isotonic proportions (saline excess or ECF excess), water retention in most cases being secondary to Na^+ retention. An excess of body water alone is much less common, and is often described as water 'intoxication', particularly when it develops rapidly.

The presence of a pure water excess implies either an excessive intake of water, or the failure of water diuresis. Frequently both factors are present, for maximum urine output by healthy kidneys is in the range 600–1200 ml/h, so either water must be consumed at an even faster rate than this if the capacity of the kidneys to excrete the water load is to be exceeded, or water excretion must be impaired. Excess water intake can arise from an abnormal thirst, as described in 'beer-drinkers hyponatraemia', and in obsessional polydipsia. Very occasionally it has been reported as deliberately self-induced by a subject who mistakenly thought that water 'intoxication' might be as pleasant as alcoholic intoxication, but at much less cost! The postoperative patient is at particular risk because he is often given large volumes of water (as 5% glucose) intravenously, or fluid may have been absorbed from the prostatic venous bed at prostate surgery, at a time when surgical trauma has led to an increased release of endogenous vasopressin. In other patients the water diuresis which normally corrects water excess may be absent because of renal failure, or from the increased release of ADH caused by drugs such as barbiturates or anaesthetics. The syndrome of inappropriate secretion of antidiuretic hormone (SIADH) is a chronic hyponatraemic state which may complicate several malignant conditions and a miscellany of drugs, metabolic and other diseases, as shown in Table 10.8.

Clinical features depend on the speed of onset, being most marked when the water excess develops rapidly. Nausea and vomiting are usually the first symptoms, progressing to confusion, muscle cramps, convulsions and coma. In very chronic cases these symptoms may be absent, but subjects may be apathetic or show behavioural changes which are only apparent to those who know them well. Generalized oedema and hypertension, the physical signs of ECF expansion, are absent. The most useful and reliable sign is a depression of plasma Na^+, Cl^- and osmolality values. In chronic cases plasma Na^+ may be as low as 105 mmol/l in the virtual absence of symptoms, but in acute water excess neurological features usually develop when plasma Na^+ drops as low as 120 mmol/l. Despite hyponatraemia, urine Na^+ excretion is usually raised, a physiological response to increased ECF volume.

The accompanying changes in body fluid volumes are shown in the top panel of Fig. 10.3. Water excess initially expands and dilutes the extracellular compartment, but the reduction in its osmolality causes a net shift of water into the ICF until ECF and ICF osmolality become equal and the water load has been distributed evenly across the total body water, with equal dilution of ECF and ICF ionic concentrations and osmolality. Because total body water is three times as large as the ECF volume, only one-third of the water excess remains in the ECF, and the signs of ECF expansion, such as oedema, are late to appear, by which time neurological features have developed, believed to be caused by the passive entry of water into the cerebral cells, and the resultant cell swelling.

The treatment of severely ill patients is aimed at increasing plasma Na^+ and osmolality to normal by withholding dilute fluids and administering hypertonic saline (2–5%) intravenously, coupled with a high-ceiling diuretic such as frusemide to increase sodium excretion in a dilute urine. It has been claimed that permanent neurological damage, associated in particular with central pontine myelinosis, may result from too rapid a correction of hyponatraemia, and that the plasma Na^+ should not be raised at a rate faster than 0.7 mmol/l/h or elevated to completely normal values, although there is some evidence that this dangerous complication develops during the initial water excess rather than during its treatment. In the chronic syndrome of inappropriate ADH release, therapy is aimed more at discovering and correcting the underlying cause, if possible. The correction of

---

Table 10.8   Causes of the syndrome of inappropriate ADH secretion (SIADH)

Malignant disease
Carcinoma, especially bronchus, pancreas, prostate, colon, lymphoma

Neurological
Meningitis, encephalitis, stroke, peripheral neuritis

Respiratory
Pulmonary tuberculosis, lung abscess

Psychiatric
Schizophrenia, acute mania

Metabolic
Adrenal or thyroid deficiency, acute porphyria

Drugs
Chlorpropamide, carbamazepine, vincristine, cyclophosphamide

Expansion with water

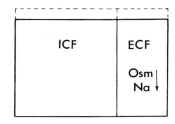

Expansion with saline

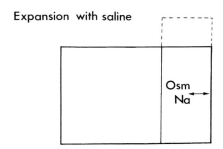

Fig. 10.3 Effect of a 10% expansion in body fluid volume. Gain in water alone (top panel) is distributed over total body water (as shown by interrupted line) with equal dilution of ECF and ICF solute. A gain of the same volume of isotonic saline (lower panel) is sustained entirely by the ECF compartment, with no change in solute concentrations.

water excess by withholding fluids is frequently attempted, but is often difficult because there may be an associated abnormal thirst; in these cases the renal loss of excess water may be achieved by the use of demeclocycline, lithium or a high-ceiling diuretic.

Saline excess

Isotonic retention of Na^+, Cl^- and water with consequent ECF expansion leading to generalized oedema is the commonest abnormality of electrolyte and water metabolism in western communities. Usually the primary cause is the failure of some critical part of the circulation, leading to compensatory renal conservation of salt and water; less often the retention is caused by renal failure. The nature of the signal by which an inadequate circulation triggers the kidney to conserve Na^+ and water is not usually clear, but in various circumstances it may include reduced glomerular perfusion, a reduced release of atrial natriuretic factor, and stimulation of the renin/angiotensin/aldosterone system. The many clinical conditions in which this sequence occurs

include primary cardiac disease; hypoalbuminaemia from any cause, including protein starvation and nephrotic syndrome, in which net transudation of plasma fluid into interstitial spaces is increased; portal hypertension in which ECF is sequestered into the portal venous bed; and the 'idiopathic' oedema of otherwise healthy women in whom the capillary permeability to plasma albumin is increased. When the defect primarily responsible for saline retention lies in the left side of the heart, as in cases of ischaemic and hypertensive heart disease, the attendant increase in pulmonary venous pressure usually causes the retained saline to settle in the lungs, causing pulmonary oedema. In this confined space, the accumulation of no more than 1 litre of saline can cause death through asphyxia. In most other oedematous conditions the retained saline collects in the more capacious systemic circulation, which can accommodate very much larger volumes; a 70 kg man has usually accumulated more than 5 litres of saline by the time bilateral ankle oedema is first noted, more than 10 litres when it extends to the sacrum, and excesses of 20–30 litres are not uncommon.

Symptoms of the underlying disease are usually present. Pulmonary oedema usually causes severe exertional and nocturnal breathlessness. When systemic oedema appears, its site is largely determined by gravity – swelling of the ankles at the end of the day, and of the face, particularly around the eyes, on first rising in the morning in those who are not prevented by breathlessness from sleeping horizontally at night. Systemic blood pressure is usually increased when saline retention is the result of renal failure rather than circulatory inadequacy, and correction of the saline excess corrects this hypertension. Plasma Na^+, Cl^- and osmolality are usually normal, with a scanty urine containing little Na^+ and Cl^- while saline is being actively retained.

The lower panel of Fig. 10.3 shows graphically the attendant disturbances of body fluids. The retention of Na^+ leads to retention of an isosmotic volume of water through the thirst and antidiuretic mechanisms. ECF volume is consequently expanded, but its electrolyte composition and osmolality are not altered, so that the ICF is unchanged and the ECF sustains the whole increase in volume.

Treatment is by dietary Na^+ restriction, by diuretics which increase urinary Na^+ excretion, and occasionally by invasive procedures causing the loss of isotonic saline – aspiration of ascites and pleural effusions, ultrafiltration during peritoneal or haemodialysis, or haemofiltration. It is possible to construct a nutritionally adequate diet containing as little as 20 mmol of Na^+ daily, but this requires specially prepared food (particularly salt-free bread) and it is more practical to restrict salt intake less severely and combine a more liberal diet with an effective diuretic regime. A 40-mmol Na^+ diet can be achieved by eating ordinary foodstuffs and avoiding all preserved meats, relishes, soups, pickles and cheeses, and adding no salt during cooking or at the table. The thiazide diuretics are the standby of treatment, but in those with resistant oedema, particularly the oedema of renal failure, high-ceiling diuretics such as frusemide or bumetamide are usually required. When diuretic therapy is prolonged, it may need to be accompanied by a potassium-sparer (e.g. amiloride) to prevent diuretic-induced K^+ deficiency. It can be argued that the treatment of oedema by diuretics and Na^+ restriction is unphysiological when Na^+ retention is part of a compensatory mechanism to preserve circulatory integrity, as is usually the case. However, man's ability to conserve Na^+ avidly developed in his primitive ancestors, in whom the threat to the circulation arose much more frequently from lack of dietary Na^+, or from Na^+ losses in diarrhoea, than from primary heart disease or the circulatory problems created by liver disease or hypoalbuminaemia. Na^+ retention is an inappropriate response to the latter conditions, in which body Na^+ is not reduced, and frequently exacerbates the primary circulatory problem. Obvious circulatory inadequacy, with hypotension and poor peripheral perfusion, is occasionally precipitated when intensive diuretic therapy is pursued excessively, or in those with a very grave circulatory defect, but in most patients oedema can be greatly improved by diuretic therapy without this problem arising.

Na+ excess

A true excess of Na^+ and Cl^- without accompanying water is very rarely seen, and arises only in bizarre and usually iatrogenic circumstances, as when a patient on haemodialysis is mistakenly dialysed against a concentrated salt solution, or infants are given a high Na^+ feed.

Salt intake and arterial blood pressure

Hypertension is one of the commonest diseases of western man, and currently there is much controversy regarding the role of dietary salt in the condition. Experimental work on animals and epidemiological studies of primitive communities in Polynesia and Amazonia have suggested a close direct relationship between Na^+ intake and blood pressure, but the relevance of these observations to western man is uncertain. Significant reductions in the blood pressure of hypertensive subjects were obtained by the use of the Kempner rice diet in the 1930s, before the advent of effective drug treatment for hypertension, but this diet entailed Na^+ restriction to under 10 mmol/day, which many subjects found intolerable, and the effects of more modest reductions in dietary Na^+ have not been consistent. Certainly most people consume much more Na^+ than they need, and reductions in Na^+ intake of the order of 50% have significantly reduced the blood pressure of a few patients with 'essential' (i.e. idiopathic) hypertension. Advice that salt intake should be reduced by the population as a whole was not considered warranted by Swales (1980) and Denton (1982). However, new analyses (Law et al 1991) back current national and international policies which suggest that the average sodium intakes of Western diets should be reduced (Chapter 51).

Potassium excess

The dissociation of total body K^+ and plasma K^+ has already been discussed under potassium deficiency. Hyperkalaemia is usually associated with an increase in total body K^+, but plasma K^+ can also increase due to the transfer of cellular K^+ to the ECF, without any increase in total body K^+, as arises in massive cell destruction (e.g. septic shock, rhabdomyolysis, intravascular haemolysis), during treatment with β-adrenergic blockers and the muscle depolarizer succinylcholine, in acidosis and digitalis poisoning, and in the very rare form of familial periodic paralysis associated with hyperkalaemia. Increased total body K^+ may be associated with increased K^+ intake (and suicide from potassium intoxication has been recorded in a patient who deliberately took a massive oral overdose of the K^+ supplement which had been prescribed to prevent diuretic-induced hypokalaemia) but is usually caused by reduced renal excretion of K^+. In acute renal failure, reduced excretion of K^+ may be associated with one or other of the conditions in which K^+ transfer from cells to the ECF occurs (e.g. acidosis or muscle trauma), and the combined effects of reduced excretion and the increased cellular release of K^+ may give rise to a hyperkalaemic emergency requiring urgent treatment. Chronic hyperkalaemia is most common in chronic renal failure, particularly when the effect of aldosterone on the mineralocorticoid receptor in the distal renal tubule is inhibited. This structure normally triggers the reabsorption of Na^+ from the tubular lumen in exchange for secreted K^+ and hydrogen ion, and is the final effector in a complex sequence involving the juxtaglomerular apparatus, renin, angiotensin I and II, aldosterone and the receptor itself. Failure of any part of this sequence can cause chronic hyperkalaemia, as for example in hyporeninaemic hypoaldosteronism, in primary adrenal disease, in the various renal defects of hyperkalaemic renal tubular acidosis, or when potassium-sparing diuretics interfere with K^+ secretion by the distal tubule.

Although rarer than K^+ depletion, potassium intoxication is more dangerous because of the risk that it will lead to cardiac arrest. Patients may experience premonitory paraesthesiae around the mouth, or muscle weakness, but usually there is no warning and the heart once stopped cannot be restarted, probably because the ischaemic tissues release more K^+. Cardiac arrest may occur when the plasma K^+ is over 7 mmol/l, but even values of over 10 mmol/l have been survived. The electrocardiogram provides a useful monitor of the early cardiac effects: increasing hyperkalaemia progressively causes peaked T waves, broadening of the QRS complex, absent P waves due to atrial paralysis, slurring of the ST segments into the T waves, and most ominously of all a sinewave pattern immediately preceding cardiac arrest.

Detailed studies of body fluid volumes in K^+ intoxication do not appear to have been made, but because of the predominantly intracellular position of K^+ an increase in ICF cation content and osmolality is to be expected, with secondary transfer of water from the ECF and the expansion of ICF at the expense of ECF. However, patients with hyperkalaemia usually have renal insufficiency, which tends to cause Na^+ retention, which would obscure some of these changes.

Treatment of K^+ intoxication entails the removal of all sources of K^+ intake and drugs which cause hyperkalaemia, particularly K^+-sparing diuretics and β-adrenergic blockers. Acidosis should be treated, mineralocorticoid deficiency corrected and steps taken to improve renal function. In chronic cases oral cation exchange resins in the sodium or calcium form (Resonium®) are effective in removing K^+ from the body because of their effect in binding K^+ in the large intestine, and have an efficiency of about 1 mmol K^+/g. In the acute hyperkalaemic emergency insulin and glucose may be given to promote the cellular uptake of K^+, and intravenous calcium gluconate is valuable in opposing the effect of hyperkalaemia on the heart, although it does not lower plasma K^+. Peritoneal dialysis and haemodialysis are both effective in lowering plasma K^+, and may be required by these patients anyway because of their attendant renal failure.

WATER AND ELECTROLYTE METABOLISM OF INFANTS

Infants have some important water and electrolyte differences from adults. They have a larger proportion of body water – about 80% by weight at full-term birth – which is partly but not entirely explicable by their lower fat content. ECF and ICF at birth average 55% and 45% of body water respectively, a reversal of the normal adult relationship. Electrolyte concentrations in ECF are similar to those of adults, except that Cl^- concentrations are 3–4 mmol/l higher, bicarbonate concentrations are lower by the same amount, and plasma phosphate is about double the adult value. Glomerular filtration rate is about half the adult value when expressed per unit of surface area, but very similar in relation to body mass. Urinary diluting and acidification processes are similar to adults, but maximum urinary concentration at 600 mosmol/kg is only half that of the adult kidney, largely because the excretion of urea (which normally assists the concentrating mechanism) is much lower owing to the intense protein anabolism associated with growth.

Saline depletion is common in infants, most often as a result of diarrhoea, which may be infective in origin or the result of high-carbohydrate feeds, but because of their greater surface area in relation to body mass, their high respiratory rate and their lower urinary concentrating power, infants are at greater risk than adults of developing a water deficit, a danger which is increased by their inability to communicate a sensation of thirst. Saline depletion and water depletion are often combined, a state known as 'hypertonic dehydration', in which the infant is depleted of both water and Na^+, but the water depletion is proportionately greater, so that plasma Na^+ and osmolality are increased.

Infants are also at risk because their fluid intake may not be ideal, yet they have virtually no choice in the matter. Cows' milk contains too much salt and protein, which gives rise to urea, and both these substances require excretion through kidneys with a reduced concentrating power, hence causing water depletion by creating an osmotic diuresis. Because of their low glomerular filtration, maximum solute excretion by infants is reduced, partly explaining the ease with which they develop saline excess and oedema – commonly seen after neonates with birth asphyxia have been resuscitated with the aid of intravenous sodium bicarbonate, or in infants at 1 month of age ('30-day oedema') who have been given feeds with too high an Na^+ content.

The hunger of growing infants, combined with their obligatory fluid intake, may also give rise to problems. Gross salt excess with hypernatraemia has caused death in infants fed on cows' milk to which salt has been added in mistake for sugar, a feed which would be rejected by older children. On the other hand, acute water intoxication can develop when infants continue to drink their usual dilute feed if there is any reason for an antidiuresis (such as excess vasopressin activity); this is not a danger in adults because their food is not in fluid form, and even a mild excess of body water inhibits further drinking.

REFERENCES

Cohn SH, Vaswani A, Zanzi I, Aloia JF, Roginsky MS, Ellis KJ 1976 Changes in body chemical composition with age measured by total-body neutron activation. Metabolism 25: 85–95

Conn JW 1955 Primary aldosteronism, a new clinical syndrome. Journal of Laboratory and Clinical Medicine 45: 6–17

Denton D 1982 The hunger for salt. Springer Verlag, Berlin.

Ellis KJ, Vaswani A, Zanzi I, Cohn S H 1976 Total body sodium and chlorine in normal adults. Metabolism 25: 645–654

Gamble JL 1947 Chemical anatomy, physiology and pathology of extracellular fluid. Harvard University Press, Cambridge, Mass.

Hunt J 1953 The ascent of Everest. Hodder & Stoughton, London, p. 275

Law MR, Frost CD, Wald NJ 1991 By how much does dietary salt restriction lower pressure? British Medical Journal 302: 811–824

McCance RA 1936 Medical problems in mineral metabolism. III Experimental human salt deficiency. Lancet i: 823–830

Passmore R, Meiklejohn AP, Dewar AD, Thow RK 1955 Energy utilization in overfed thin young men. British Journal of Nutrition 9: 20–27

Paul AA, Southgate DAT 1978 Mc Cance and Widdowson's The composition of foods, 4th edn. HMSO, London; Elsevier, Amsterdam

Sanchez-Castillo CP, Warrender S, Whitehead TP, James WPT 1987 An assessment of the sources of dietary salt in a British population. Clinical Science 72: 95–102.

Swales JD 1980 Dietary salt and hypertension. Lancet i: 1177–1179.

11. Bone mineral

R. Smith

This chapter deals with the minerals normally found in the skeleton and gives an outline of the normal physiology and metabolism of bone. The reader needs to be aware that the skeleton itself is not inert, and should not be analysed and dealt with as such. In addition to the mineral component, it is important to note first that there is an important organic component to bone; secondly, that the skeleton is continually being removed and replaced by the action of the bone cells within it; thirdly, that these cells are themselves controlled by mechanical and hormonal factors which are often in opposition; and fourthly, the skeleton has a mechanical as well as a biochemical function, and thus is not just a repository for calcium (Smith 1984). Understanding the physiology of bone is important to a knowledge of its diseases, and this chapter should be read in conjunction with Chapter 37. Both include a consideration of osteoporosis, the most common and important of the metabolic bone diseases. The physiology of bone is described in detail by Vaughan (1981) and particular aspects are discussed in the book by Tam et al (1989) and in a Ciba Foundation Symposium (Evered & Harnett 1988).

COMPOSITION AND PHYSIOLOGY

The important minerals within bone are calcium, phosphate and magnesium. There is about 1 kg of calcium in the adult skeleton, as a complex crystalline material with phosphate in the form of hydroxyapatite. This mineral is laid down in an organized manner on an organic matrix, the main constituent of which is collagen. There are also important non-collagen proteins within the skeleton.

Bone mineral

Although calcium in fully mineralized bone is present as hydroxyapatite, this is preceded by other crystal forms and during mineralization there is always a small fraction of mineral in an amorphous form. Mineralization appears to occur in two separate ways (Smith 1984), and there is controversy about how much these overlap. The first involves the formation of crystals within matrix or mineralizing vesicles, themselves derived from osteoblasts. This system is widespread throughout the skeleton, occurring in calcifying cartilage, in normal and in ectopic ossification. In the second process, mineral appears to be laid down in a very orderly fashion, beginning in the hole zones of organized fibrils of collagen (see below). This process was described many years ago and the initial stages are seen well in the calcification of the turkey leg tendon. The complexity of this process is illustrated in Fig. 11.1 (Arsenault 1988). The way in which mineralization occurs in vesicles is now largely understood, but there are unsolved problems concerning in vivo calcification. These concern the local control of calcification, and the possible presence of inhibitors to prevent mineralization. One theory, for which there is considerable support, relates to the presence of alkaline phosphatase, which is also a pyrophosphatase, in the matrix vesicles (and the osteoblast). This enzyme could locally degrade pyrophosphate, which normally inhibits mineralization, and also locally increase inorganic phosphate concentration, thus promoting mineralization.

Organic matrix

Collagen

It is often forgotten that the skeleton contains more than half of the body's collagen. There are numerous genetic types of collagen, but the major component of this extracellular protein is the fibrillar collagens, of which adult bone contains only Type I (Prockop & Kivirikko 1984; Smith 1986). This is a heteropolymer containing two similar chains (α1) and one different (α2) wound in a helical fashion around each other.

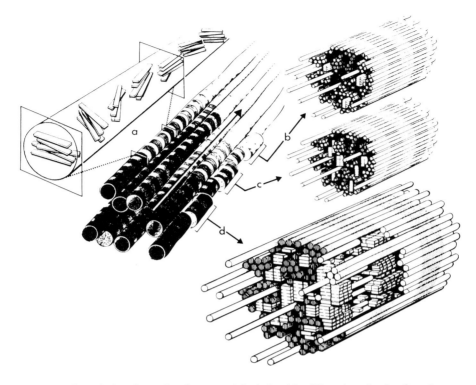

Fig. 11.1   Complexity of crystal–collagen spatial relationships. The mineralization front is extending in the direction of the main arrow. The increased periodic banding along the fibrils is due to the deposition of hydroxyapatite within the gap zones (dark bands). In Fig **a** the crystals have been drawn as exaggerated rods. In Figs **b, c** and **d** the apatite crystals gradually increase in number and change orientation from one figure to the next. At advanced stages of mineralization, apatite is shown to extend from the gap zone into the overlap, as observed in dark-field images. (From Arsenault 1988, with permission.)

Each chain has a glycine in every third position and may be expressed as a repeat of $(Gly\ X\ Y)_{338}$, where X is often proline and Y is hydroxyproline. The exact and precisely repetitive nature of this structure is essential for helix formation, for cross-linking, and for structurally sound fibre formation. One particular feature relevant to mineralization is the three-dimensional overlap structure, referred to as a quarter stagger array, which provides gaps or hole zones in which mineralization first begins (Fig. 11.1).

Non-collagen proteins

There is a wide variety of non-collagen substances within the organic matrix whose function is largely unknown. In addition there are factors apparently capable of promoting cartilage formation (and possibly that of bone; Wozney et al 1988). The non-collagen components of bone have recently been reviewed (Triffitt 1987), and may be classified into sialoproteins, proteins which contain carboxyglutamic acid (Gla-proteins), phosphoproteins including osteonectin, and bone proteoglycans. In addition there are components of the proteins of plasma which may be selectively concentrated in bone, such as $\alpha 2$ HS glycoprotein. Finally, bone contains its own specific proteoglycans.

The present state of knowledge and classification of the types and functions of non-collagen substances is provisional. One important point that determines the apparent forms and distribution of the non-collagen components is the starting tissue (for instance, fetal or adult bone); another is the method of extraction used.

Cells

The turnover of bone is controlled by the activities of its bone cells – osteoblasts, osteoclasts and osteocytes (Owen & Friedenstein 1988). The osteoblasts and osteoclasts appear to act in remodelling units whose activities are closely coupled by locally acting cell messages, only some of which have been identified. Osteoclasts are derived from haemopoietic cells, and are responsible for the resorption of bone. Osteoblasts belong to the stromal cell system and are responsible for bone formation. Osteocytes derived from osteoblasts lie within the mineralized bone matrix, communicating with each other through the canaliculi of bone. At any given time only a minor percentage of bone cells are active. The apparently inactive cells on the surface have been labelled 'bone lining' cells; they may or may not be inactive osteoblasts.

The ways in which bone cells 'talk' to each other are very complex and have been reviewed elsewhere (Krane et al 1988). It is particularly important to realize that the skeleton is constantly being resorbed and replaced, and also to recognize the central position of the osteoblast in this process. The osteoblast responds to a large number of endocrine and mechanical signals; further, it appears to control mineralization and to modify the activity of the major bone-resorbing cell, the osteoclast (Chambers 1988).

CALCIUM

The most important mineral constituent of the skeleton is calcium. This is vital for a large number of functions within the body, including the muscular, neurological and endocrine systems (Evered & Harnett 1986). The adult skeleton contains about 1 kg of calcium and is in equilibrium with the plasma calcium at a concentration of about 2.25–2.60 mmol/l (9–10.4 mg/100 ml). A large number of factors control calcium balance (Fig. 11.2). The amount of calcium within the skeleton changes with age, according to its size and composition, increasing during growth and declining in parallel with the bone loss of later years (Kanis & Passmore 1989).

Calcium balance and its control

The external balance of calcium, i.e. the difference between intake and output, is determined by exchange between the skeleton, the intestine and the kidney (Fig. 11.2). These fluxes are controlled by the action of the calciotrophic hormones, parathyroid hormone, 1,25-dihydroxycholecalciferol, and calcitonin

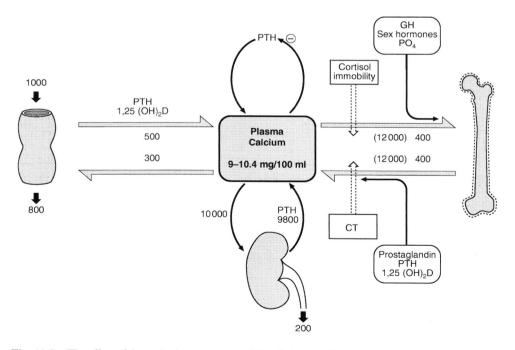

Fig. 11.2   The effect of the major hormones on calcium balance in the normal adult. The figures in brackets are an estimate of the possible exchange of calcium through the cellular barrier of bone. Units are in mg/day (to convert to mmol divide by 40). CT = Calcitonin, GH = Growth hormone. Note that PTH (parathyroid hormone) is suppressed by an increase in plasma calcium. (From Smith 1984.)

(MacIntyre 1986). They are also influenced by sex hormones, growth hormones, corticosteroids and a variety of locally acting hormones. Physiological changes in calcium balance occur during growth, pregnancy, lactation and with increasing years. These subjects have been reviewed elsewhere (Smith 1984), but it is important to summarize the control mechanisms and effects of the calciotrophic hormones, so called because of their major effects on calcium metabolism. They are vitamin D (via its most active metabolite 1,25(OH)$_2$D$_3$), parathyroid hormone (PTH) and calcitonin (CT). There are two main reasons not to be too rigid about this classification, namely that it is now recognized that the effect of these hormones is not limited to those on calcium metabolism, and that there are many other locally active hormones which have effects on calcium metabolism. A number of these have been identified as the result of continuing investigation into the hypercalcaemia of malignant disease (Mundy 1988).

The actions of the classic calciotrophic hormones, the locally acting hormones (cytokines) (Krane et al 1988) and the hormones controlling hypercalcaemia of malignancy have been extensively reviewed. The summary that follows is intended to provide a brief update.

Vitamin D

All the actions of vitamin D are mediated through its active metabolite 1,25(OH)$_2$D$_3$, except that there is some evidence in animals that the dihydroxylated metabolite 24,25(OH)$_2$D$_3$ is not entirely inert (Haussler et al 1988; Reichel et al 1989). Vitamin D is synthesized in the skin (Fig. 11.3) under the action of ultraviolet light; it is only when ultraviolet exposure of the skin is limited that vitamin D becomes an essential nutrient. The term vitamin for vitamin D is now considered as a misnomer, and it is more appropriate to call it a hormone. Advances in our understanding of vitamin D include the mechanisms of its formation in the skin, the metabolic steps it undergoes, and the action of 1,25(OH)$_2$D$_3$. Although the actions of 1,25(OH)$_2$D$_3$ concern calcium transport and are important in the control of plasma calcium (particularly by controlling the intestinal absorption of calcium and the osteoclastic resorption of bone, probably via osteoblasts) it has been shown that the calciotrophic function is only one aspect of 1,25(OH)$_2$D$_3$ metabolism. The identification of the specific cell receptor for this metabolite has led to its discovery in a wide range of tissues (Haussler et al 1988). Important among the non-calciotrophic effects of

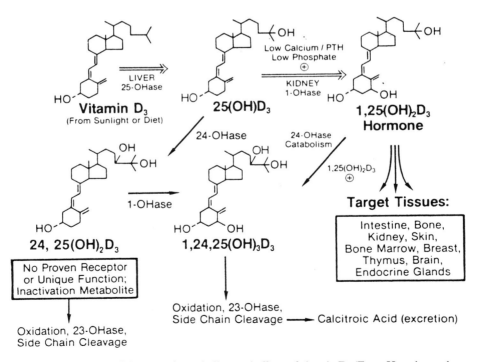

Fig. 11.3 An outline of the normal metabolism and effects of vitamin D. (From Haussler et al 1988, with permission.)

$1,25(OH)_2D_3$ are those on cell differentiation and on the immune system (Reichel & Norman 1989).

In practice, the elucidation of vitamin D metabolism has led to the logical treatment of the many causes of rickets and osteomalacia (Chapter 37), and explained the cause of such variable conditions as renal glomerular osteodystrophy and vitamin D-dependent rickets. Since the major circulating vitamin D metabolite is 25-hydroxy vitamin D, its concentration gives a reliable measure of whole-body vitamin status. Thus it is low in elderly people, in Asian immigrants, in late winter, and in people with nutritional osteomalacia (Stamp et al 1980). It has been suggested that impaired production of $1,25(OH)_2D_3$ contributes to postmenopausal osteoporosis (Tsai et al 1984; Prince et al 1988).

Parathyroid hormone (PTH) and PTH-related peptide (PTHrP)

PTH controls plasma calcium by its indirect action on intestinal calcium absorption (by controlling 1α hydroxylation of 25(OH)D), and its direct effect on the renal reabsorption of calcium, and on bone resorption. This last effect is thought to take place via the osteoblast, which contains PTH receptors whereas the osteoclast does not. The direct action of PTH on the cells of the renal tubule and bone is mediated by the classic activation of adenyl cyclase; there is also increasing evidence of action via the phosphokinase C and inositol triphosphate pathway (Farndale et al 1988).

The secretion and synthesis of PTH is controlled at various stages in its metabolism by the plasma calcium concentration. The parathyroids are unique among endocrine systems in being stimulated by a decline rather than an increase in calcium concentration. In disease states the activity of these glands (as well as their size) may be increased by hyperplasia secondary to prolonged hypocalcaemia (Table 11.1). Hyper-

Table 11.1   Causes of abnormal plasma calcium

Hypercalcaemia
Malignant disease
Primary hyperparathyroidism
Sarcoidosis (and other granulomas)
Vitamin D overdosage
Milk alkali syndrome
Immobilization
Thyrotoxicosis
Hypercalcaemia of infancy
Familial hypocalciuric hypercalcaemia

Hypocalcaemia
Vitamin D deficiency (and disturbances of its metabolism)
Hypoparathyroidism (and pseudohypoparathyroidism)

plasia may also be primary (without obvious cause), as may parathyroid adenomata, some of which appear to be monoclonal.

Recent studies on the humoral hypercalcaemia of malignancy have identified a hormone whose amino terminal sequence and biological actions are very similar to those of PTH (Fukuyama et al 1988). Hence the hormone has been labelled PTHrP (parathyroid hormone-related peptide or protein). Interestingly, there is some evidence that this is a physiological fetal hormone (Care & Abbas 1987).

Calcitonin

The physiological role of calcitonin remains a mystery (MacIntyre 1986). Measurements of its concentration in elderly people with or without femoral neck fracture or osteoporosis have been controversial. There is some evidence that it has a role in protecting the skeleton during times of stress, such as growth and pregnancy. It is known that CT and CT gene-related peptide (CGRP) are produced by alternative splicing from a common gene. CGRP is a very active vasopeptide but has negligible effects on calcium metabolism.

The effects of other hormones on the skeleton

The skeleton is affected by growth hormone, sex hormones, thyroxine, corticosteroids and less so by insulin (Raisz 1988). An excess of growth hormone during childhood and before the epiphyses close will cause gigantism, and after epiphyseal closure, acromegaly. In contrast, lack of growth hormone is a well recognized cause of proportionate short stature, and hypopituitarism will lead to osteoporosis. Oestrogen lack, after oophorectomy or a naturally occurring menopause, is an important cause of accelerated bone loss. Lack of testosterone, associated for instance with cryptorchidism, is a predictable but less well recognized cause of osteoporosis in men. An excess of corticosteroids may be the result of Cushing's syndrome and produces severe osteoporosis with excessive callus; more commonly it is iatrogenic due to the high-dose glucocorticoid treatment of asthma, or, for instance, temporal arteritis. Finally, thyrotoxicosis produces excessive bone turnover, with an increase in resorption disproportionate to the increase in bone formation, and eventual osteoporosis. It may be associated with hypercalcaemia (Table 11.1).

Locally acting agents

Changes in calcium metabolism are also brought about by locally acting hormones. These have been particularly studied in the hypercalcaemia associated with malignancy (Mundy 1988) (Table 11.1). In addition to the importance of PTHrP in the hypercalcaemia of malignant solid tumours, immune-cell products such as lymphotoxin, tumour necrosis factor (TNF) and interleukin promote bone resorption, and a variety of osteotrophic cytokines may have a central role in normal bone remodelling. The many factors capable of stimulating bone resorption include tumour necrosis factors α and β, transforming growth factors α and β, epidermal growth factor, platelet-derived growth factor and arachidonic acid metabolites such as prostaglandins and leukotrienes. Recent advances show that many cytokines with different names which have been studied in different systems are, in fact, identical (see Chapter 31).

Abnormal plasma calcium

The changes in plasma calcium in disease states (Table 11.1) illustrate different ways in which its homoeostatic mechanisms may be disturbed. Hyperparathyroidism and malignant disease are the two main causes of hypercalcaemia, in both of which there are increases in bone resorption and the renal reabsorption of calcium.

In the hypercalcaemia of sarcoidosis (and related granulomata) there is uncontrolled $1,25(OH)_2D_3$ production from 25-hydroxy vitamin D. In the previously common milk alkali syndrome, the administration of large amounts of oral calcium and alkali produced a systemic alkalosis associated with hypercalcaemia and progressively reduced renal glomerular function; however, with the decline in such regimens for peptic ulceration, a more common form of presentation is the slow onset of hypercalcaemia and uraemia due to the excessive consumption of calcium-containing 'indigestion' tablets. Therapeutic vitamin D overdosage may result from inappropriately large doses of native vitamin D or its metabolites. The cause of hypercalcaemia of infancy (the elfin face syndrome) is not yet fully elucidated. Familial hypocalciuric hypercalcaemia appears to be related to minimal hyperplasia of the parathyroid glands (Marx 1982).

THE SKELETON AND GROWTH

It must be clear that during growth the skeleton increases in size, in calcium content and in calcium requirements (Kanis & Passmore 1989) (Fig. 11.4). After growth stops, there is probably also a phase during which the amount of bone and its calcium content together (referred to as bone mass) continue to increase. The time of peak bone mass is debated, though the age of about 30 years is often quoted.

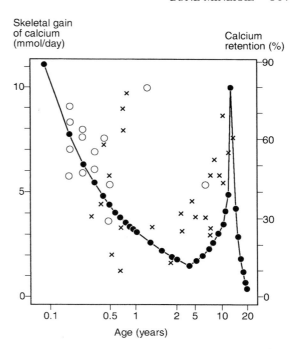

Fig. 11.4   Demonstration of estimated requirements of calcium in females during growth (●–●). Right ordinate shows the percentage of dietary intake of 500 mg that must be retained. Data points show observations from healthy children with high (x) or low (O) intakes of calcium.

Before this time, osteoblastic new bone formation exceeds osteoclastic new bone resorption (the reverse of osteoporosis). Peak bone mass is greater in men than women and has important determinants (see below). Since the amount of bone in later years is determined by the starting amount (the peak bone mass) and its subsequent loss, both are directly relevant to the subsequent development of osteoporosis.

After the age of peak bone mass, the amount of bone declines. This is brought about by an imbalance between resorption and formation, in favour of resorption. In the long bones there is endosteal bone resorption and periosteal new bone formation. The trabeculae become thin and may be perforated, and the cortex becomes porous (Fig. 11.5).

OSTEOPOROSIS

This is defined as a condition in which the amount of bone per unit volume is decreased but the composition remains unchanged (Riggs & Melton 1986; Smith 1987). The bone becomes porous, due to the imbalanced action of the forming and resorbing cells just described. In addition to the main definition there

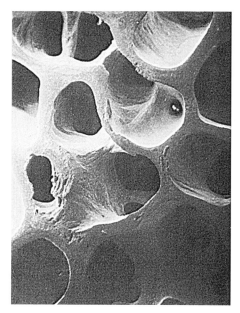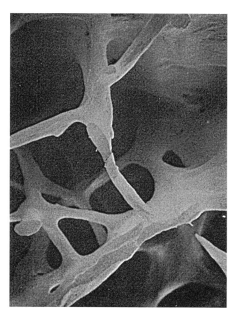

Fig. 11.5   Scanning electron microscopy to show the trabecular bone structure in (left) normal, and (right) osteoporotic, bone. (From Dempster et al 1986, with permission.)

are two qualifying points which are clinical and statistical. These are that the loss of bone is sufficient to predispose to fracture (the symptoms of osteoporosis are related to the structural failure it causes), and that the reduction in the amount of bone is more than 2SD from the mean for the young adult. There are many causes of osteoporosis (see Chapter 37) (Riggs & Melton 1986; Raisz 1988; Raisz & Smith 1989). However, if the definition of no change in composition is strictly adhered to, this excludes such bone diseases as those associated with malignant disease or parathyroid bone disease (osteitis fibrosa cystica).

Importance of osteoporosis

Osteoporosis is important because it predisposes to fractures, of which the common ones are vertebral, the forearm and the femoral neck (Riggs & Melton 1986). Vertebral compression fractures occur at an earlier age than femoral neck fractures, and in trabecular rather than cortical bone. The most important fracture associated with osteoporosis is the femoral neck fracture (proximal femoral fracture), because of its high frequency and because it leads to immediate disability, early and late mortality, and considerable morbidity; the incidence, and therefore cost, of femoral neck fracture is increasing out of proportion to the age of the population (Riggs & Melton 1986).

Whether or not a fracture occurs depends on the force of the injury – most often a fall – and the strength of the bone; the causes of fractures, especially in the elderly, are often multiple. Nevertheless, osteoporosis must be an important contributor to fracture, and its prevention and treatment are therefore of considerable clinical and economic importance. The most important determinants of osteoporosis are the peak bone mass and its subsequent rate of loss.

Factors determining peak bone mass

The amount of bone present in the young adult (when bone mass is at its peak) is determined by genetic factors, gender, the use of the skeleton, the nutritional intake, which includes calcium (Heaney 1986), and endocrine factors. It is, however, difficult to distinguish the effect of calcium intake on peak bone mass from that of energy and protein, since in any diet they tend to be associated. Less important factors tending to decrease bone mass are cigarette smoking, excessive alcohol consumption and self-imposed starvation, as in anorexia nervosa (Stevenson et al 1989) (Table 11.2).

Bone mass differs from one race to another, being at a maximum in Negroes and least in Caucasians and Orientals. Within races peak bone mass appears to be familial. Reviews on bone density at various sites in twins show that the correlation is closer in monozygotic

Table 11.2 Factors determining peak bone mass

Genetic
Race
Family
Gender

Nutritional
Calcium
Protein energy

Endocrine
Growth hormone
Sex hormones
Calciotropic hormones

Mechanical

Table 11.3 Risk factors for bone loss

Immobility
Early menopause
Positive family history
Low calcium intake
Underweight
Alcohol
Smoking

and dizygotic pairs (Pocock et al 1987); from the difference in correlation between these two groups it is possible to determine a factor called heritability, and it has been suggested that bone mass is controlled by single genes (or a set of them). Other observations demonstrate that the daughters (and siblings) of osteoporotic mothers have a bone mass – when corrected for age – which is intermediate between normal and that of the osteoporotic mothers. Such data are not easy to interpret, but they do emphasize the genetic importance of bone mass (Evans et al 1988; Seeman et al 1989). This is seen in its most obvious form in the inherited disorders of collagen which lead to osteogenesis imperfecta (Cole et al 1989).

It is common knowledge that failure to use the skeleton during growth leads to overall bone loss, with bizarre changes in the limbs: this is most clearly demonstrated in limbs which cannot be used in conditions such as poliomyelitis, muscular dystrophy and osteogenesis imperfecta. The evidence that continual use of the growing skeleton increases bone mass in experimental animals has been provided by Lanyon & Rubin (1983).

Again, the effect of proper nutrition on peak bone mass is commonly assumed but less easy to prove (Angus & Eisman 1988; Picard et al 1988). Starvation in childhood associated with protein energy malnutrition leads to temporary cessation of growth and eventual short stature. Such reduced intakes include a reduction in calcium, but the effect of an isolated low calcium intake on the growing human skeleton is not well defined. Deprivation of calcium in growing animals may lead to a form of osteoporosis; in man it is virtually impossible to produce bone disease by calcium restriction alone, and in children any bone disease produced resembles rickets (Kanis & Passmore 1989).

Loss of bone

Peak bone mass is lower in women than in men, and subsequent bone loss is greater, largely because of the accelerated loss of bone in the menopausal and post-menopausal periods. Thus bone density falls below the so-called fracture threshold many years earlier in women than in men. Against this background of bone loss, which occurs in all subjects, there are other factors which are thought to increase the rate of loss. On the whole, these are thought to be the same factors which decrease peak bone mass – namely, immobility and lack of exercise, low calcium intake, smoking and alcoholism (Table 11.3). The possible relationship of bone loss to calcium deficiency has been vigorously discussed (Nordin 1988, 1989; Kanis & Passmore 1989; Barrett-Connor 1989). Important factors to consider are the form of calcium given, the efficiency of its absorption and the recommended requirements (Blanchard 1989). Cross-sectional studies of the population show no relation between calcium intake and bone mass at cortical and trabecular sites. Likewise, the rate of bone loss appears to be unrelated to prevailing calcium intake (Riggs et al 1987; Stevenson et al 1988). Further, the addition of calcium alone to the diet does not reduce the rate of postmenopausal bone loss (the evidence for this is convincing but not unanimous) (Stevenson et al 1988; Selby et al 1988). However, increasing calcium intakes may have different effects on different types of bone, and any beneficial effect occurs in cortical bone (Riis et al 1987). There is some evidence that dietary calcium can help to reduce bone loss in association with increased physical exercise or hormone replacement therapy (HRT) (Ettinger et al 1987). Also, maximal peak bone density appears to be related to a high lifetime calcium intake plus adequate serum oestrogen levels (Cauley et al 1988). Finally, the most effective treatment to prevent postmenopausal bone loss is recognized to be combined oestrogen plus progesterone (oestrogen alone in hysterectomized women). Current work has stressed the therapeutic usefulness of naturally occurring hormones and their lack of side effects. It also emphasizes the importance of physical activity, calcium intake and oestrogen therapy in the prevention of proximal femoral fractures (Cooper et al 1988; Holbrook et al 1988, Lau et al 1988).

PHOSPHORUS

The distribution, function and control of phosphorus within the body is different from that of calcium, and for those interested in bone phosphorus has often taken a secondary role. Nevertheless, the effects of phosphorus deficiency are widespread and there are important bone diseases related to disorders of phosphorus metabolism.

Distribution and function

Phosphorus, in both its organic and its inorganic forms, is widely distributed throughout the body; nevertheless, 85% is contained within the skeleton. A deficiency of phosphate may produce osteomalacia, myopathy, growth failure and defects in leucocyte function. Phosphate is necessary for the innumerable biochemical reactions involving organic phosphates such as adenose triphosphate, and is an integral part of phospholipids, phosphoproteins and phosphosugars.

Phosphorus balance

In the normal person, many factors control phosphorus balance (Fig. 11.6), of which the most important is the amount reabsorbed by the renal tubules. The effect of hormones on phosphate balance is not fully elucidated. When vitamin D is given to a D-deficient subject, intestinal phosphate absorption increases. PTH reduces the renal reabsorption of phosphate, leading to hypophosphataemia; and calcitonin increases phosphate excretion by the

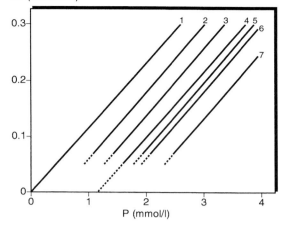

Fig. 11.7   Changes in TmP in various disorders. 1 and 4 are the lines for GFR (inulin clearance) and normal phosphate clearance respectively; 2 and 3 represent the reduced phosphate reabsorption (TmP) in hyperparathyroidism and inherited hypophosphataemia. TmP is increased by treatment with the diphosphonate EHDP (5), in hypoparathyroidism (6) and in tumoral calcinosis (inherited hyperphosphataemia) (7).

kidney. Plasma phosphate is normally higher in children than in adults. The renal handling of phosphate is expressed in terms of the maximum tubular reabsorption of phosphate (TmP) in relation to the glomerular filtration rate (GFR).

In hyperparathyroidism TmP is reduced, whereas in tumoral calcinosis with hyperphosphataemia it is increased above normal (Fig. 11.7).

Abnormal plasma phosphate (see also Chapter 37)

The main causes of hypo- and hyperphosphataemia may be renal or dietary, and inherited or acquired (Table 11.4). In vitamin D-resistant rickets (inherited

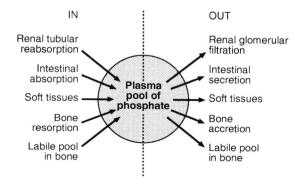

Fig. 11.6   Factors determining plasma phosphate concentration. (From Smith 1980, with permission.)

Table 11.4   Causes of abnormal plasma phosphate

Hypophosphataemia
Inherited: Vitamin D-resistant rickets
Acquired: Hyperparathyroidism
 Aludrox overdosage
 Vitamin D deficiency
 Prolonged parenteral nutrition

Hyperphosphataemia
Inherited: Tumoral calcinosis
 Pseudohypoparathyroidism
Acquired: Hypoparathyroidism
 Renal glomerular failure

hypophosphataemia), tumoral calcinosis (inherited hyperphosphataemia), hyper- and hypoparathyroidism, there is a shift in the TmP/GFR. In contrast, the main determinants of hypophosphataemia in vitamin D deficiency and aluminium hydroxide overdosage is a reduction in intestinal phosphate absorption. Hyperphosphataemia in renal glomerular failure results from the continuing intestinal absorption of phosphate with declining renal clearance.

MAGNESIUM

Magnesium, like potassium, is widely distributed in the soft tissues and in the skeleton, which contains up to 70% of the total body content. It is the most abundant divalent intracellular action and is involved in a large number of metabolic processes. The plasma magnesium level is remarkably constant and depends on rapid adaptation by the kidney; thus a fall in magnesium intake is rapidly followed by a fall in urinary output, and only later by hypomagnesaemia. Homoeostatic mechanisms, such as those described for calcium, for the selective mobilization of magnesium from the tissues do not appear to exist. The way in which the body protects against magnesium loss is by a reduction in urinary excretion, and only if the intake is very low for a long time or intestinal losses are high do the tissues lose magnesium significantly.

There are, however, inherited disorders in which selective magnesium malabsorption results in hypomagnesaemia and hypocalcaemia.

Like plasma calcium, the total plasma magnesium (1.7–2.3 mg/100 ml) is composed of an ionized fraction (1.3 mg%), a small complexed fraction (0.3 mg%), and a protein-bound fraction which is measured by the difference between total and ultrafiltrable magnesium.

Net intestinal magnesium absorption appears to be linearly related to intake (like phosphorus), but at very low intakes a negative magnesium balance can occur. Absorption in man appears to be predominantly through the small intestine and is influenced by many factors. Clinical studies suggest that it is increased by both vitamin D and parathyroid hormone, although the mechanisms for this are obscure.

Hypomagnesaemia and hypermagnesaemia

Hypomagnesaemia occurs in association with hypocalcaemia, but may also occur on its own. Probably its most common cause is malabsorption, especially where this results from small-bowel resection. Other causes include dietary deficiency: protein calorie malnutrition and prolonged intravenous feeding; excessive renal loss, as with diuretics and alcohol; and diabetes, in which there is both an increase in the renal loss of magnesium and increased transport of magnesium (as well as potassium) into the soft tissues when insulin is given.

The effect of magnesium on the parathyroid glands themselves is uncertain; in hyperparathyroidism the situation is complex. Hypomagnesaemia has been described, but this also occurs after parathyroidectomy.

Hypermagnesaemia is most commonly seen in patients with renal glomerular failure, and the bone of patients with renal failure shows an increase in magnesium content. It has been suggested that this delays the transition of bone mineral from amorphous to crystalline, and affects the normal formation of bone matrix collagen.

OTHER BONE MINERALS

There are a number of other minerals normally present in bone, whose deficiency or excess can lead to skeletal disease. These include copper, aluminium and fluorine (see Chapter 37); strontium, which is present in those foods which are rich in calcium, but in much smaller amounts than calcium and has attracted interest only because of its radioactive form ^{90}Sr which is produced in nuclear explosions and incorporated into the skeleton.

REFERENCES

Angus RM, Eisman JA 1988 Osteoporosis: the role of calcium intake and supplementation. Medical Journal of Australia 148: 630–633

Arsenault AL 1988 Crystal–collagen relationships in calcified turkey leg tendons visualised by selected-area dark-field electron microscopy. Calcified Tissue International 43: 202–212

Barrett-Connor E 1989 The RDA for calcium in the elderly: too little, too late. Calcified Tissue International 44: 303–307

Blanchard J 1989 Calcium and osteoporosis: some caveats and pleas. Calcified Tissue International 44: 67–68

Care AD, Abbas SK 1987 Calcium homeostasis in the adult and foetus. Frontiers in Hormone Research 17: 203–210

Cauley JA, Gutai JP, Kuller LH et al 1988 Endogenous oestrogen levels and calcium intakes in postmenopausal women: relationships with cortical bone measures. Journal of the American Medical Association 260: 3150–3155

Chambers TJ 1988 The regulation of osteoclastic development and function. In: Cell and molecular biology of vertebrate hard tissues. Ciba Foundation Symposium 136: 92–107

Cole WG, Jaenisch R, Bateman KF 1989 New insights into the molecular pathology of osteogenesis imperfecta. Quarterly Journal of Medicine 70: 1–4

Cooper C, Barker DJP, Wickham C 1988 Physical activity, muscle strength and calcium intake in fractures of the proximal femur in Britain. British Medical Journal 297: 1443-1446

Ettinger B, Genant HK, Cann CE 1987 Postmenopausal bone loss is prevented by low-dose oestrogen with calcium. Annals of Internal Medicine 106: 40–45

Evans RA, Marel GM, Lancaster EK, Kos S, Evans M, Wong SYP 1988 Bone mass is low in relatives of osteoporotic patients. Annals of Internal Medicine 109: 870–873

Evered D, Harnett S 1986 Calcium and the cell. Ciba Foundation Symposium 122. Wiley, Chichester

Evered D, Harnett S 1988 Cell and molecular biology of vertebrate hard tissues. Ciba Foundation Symposium 136. Wiley, Chichester

Farndale RW, Sandy JR, Atkinson SJ, Pennington SR, Meghji S, Meikle MC 1988 Parathyroid hormone and prostaglandin E_2 stimulate both inosotol phosphates and cyclic AMP accumulation in mouse osteoblast cultures. Biochemical Journal 252: 263–268

Fukuyama S, Bosma TJ, Goad DL, Voelkel EF, Tashjian AH 1988 Human parathyroid hormone (PTH)-related protein and human PTH: comparative biological activities on human bone cells and bone resorption. Endocrinology 123: 2841–2848

Haussler MR, Mangelsdorf DJ, Komm BS et al 1988 Molecular biology of the vitamin D hormone. Recent Progress in Hormone Research 44: 263–305

Heaney RP 1986 Calcium, bone health and osteoporosis. In: Peck WA (ed) Bone and mineral research, Volume 4. Elsevier Science Publishers, pp. 255–301

Holbrook TL, Barrett-Connor E, Wingard D 1988 Dietary calcium and the risk of hip fracture: 14-year prospective population study. Lancet ii: 1046–1049

Kanis JA, Passmore R 1989 Calcium supplementation of the diet. British Medical Journal 298: 137–140, 205–208

Krane SM, Goldring MB, Goldring SR 1988 Cytokines. In: Cell and molecular biology of vertebrate hard tissues. Ciba Foundation Symposium 136 Wiley, Chichester, pp. 239–256

Lanyon LE, Rubin CT 1983 Regulation of bone mass in response to physical activity. In: Dixon A St J, Russell RGG, Stamp TCB (eds) Osteoporosis, a multidisciplinary problem. London, Royal Society of Medicine, pp. 51–61 (International Congress Series 55)

Lau E, Donnan S, Barker DJP, Cooper C 1988 Physical activity and calcium intake in fracture of the proximal femur in Hong Kong. British Medical Journal 297: 1441–1443

MacIntyre I 1986 The hormonal regulation of extracellular calcium. British Medical Bulletin 42: 343–352

Marx SJ 1982 Familial hypocalciuric hypercalcaemia. In: Heath D, Marx SJ, Clinical Endocrinology 2. Butterworths International Medical Reviews, London, Butterworths, pp. 217–232

Mundy GR 1988 Hypercalcaemia of malignancy revisited. Journal of Clinical Investigation 82: 1–6

Nordin BEC 1976 Calcium, phosphate and magnesium metabolism. Churchill Livingstone, Edinburgh

Nordin BEC 1988 The calcium debate. Medical Journal of Australia 148: 608

Nordin BEC 1989 The calcium deficiency model for osteoporosis. Nutrition Reviews 47: 65–72

Owen M, Friedenstein AJ 1988 Stromal stem cells: marrow-derived osteogenic precursors. In: Cell and molecular biology of vertebrate hard tissues. Ciba Foundation Symposium 136, Wiley, Chichester, pp. 42–60

Picard D, Ste-Marie LG, Coutu D et al 1988 Premenopausal bone mineral content relates to height, weight and calcium intake during early childhood. Bone and Mineral 4: 299–309

Pocock NA, Eisman JA, Hopper JL, Yeates MG, Sambrook P N, Eberl S 1987 Genetic determinants of bone mass in adults. A twin study. Journal of Clinical Investigation 80: 706–710

Prince R, Dick I, Boyd F, Kent N, Garcia-Webb P 1988 The effects of dietary calcium deprivation on serum calcitriol levels in premenopausal and postmenopausal women. Metabolism 37: 727–731

Prockop DJ, Kivirikko KI 1984 Heritable diseases of collagen. New England Journal of Medicine 311: 376–386

Raisz LG 1988 Local and systemic factors in the pathogenesis of osteoporosis. New England Journal of Medicine 318: 818–828

Raisz LG, Smith J 1989 Pathogenesis, prevention and treatment of osteoporosis. Annual Review of Medicine 40: 251–267

Reichel H, Norman AW 1989 Systemic effects of vitamin D. Annual Review of Medicine 40: 71–78

Reichel H, Koeffler P, Norman AW 1989 The role of the vitamin D endocrine system in health and disease. New England Journal of Medicine 320: 980–991

Riggs BL, Melton LJ 1986 Involutional osteoporosis. New England Journal of Medicine 314: 1671–1686

Riggs BL, Wahler HW, Melton LJ, Richelson LS, Judd HL, O'Fallon WM 1987 Dietary calcium intake and the rate of bone loss in women. Journal of Clinical Investigation 80: 979–982

Riis B, Thomsen K, Christiansen C 1987 Does calcium supplementation prevent postmenopausal bone loss. New England Journal of Medicine 316: 173–177

Seeman E, Hopper JL, Bach LA et al 1989 Reduced bone mass in daughters of women with osteoporosis. New England Journal of Medicine 320: 554–558

Selby PL, Davidson CE, Francis RM, Robinson CG 1988 Calcium and postmenopausal bone loss. British Medical Journal 297: 481–482

Smith R 1980 Calcium, phosphorus and magnesium metabolism. In: Owen R, Goodfellow J, Bullough P (eds) Scientific foundations in orthopaedics and traumatology. Heinemann, London, pp. 213–223

Smith R 1984 Recent advances in the metabolism and physiology of bone. In: Baker P F (ed) Recent advances in physiology Vol 10. Churchill Livingstone, Edinburgh, pp. 317–348

Smith R 1986 The molecular genetics of collagen disorders. Clinical Science 71: 129–135

Smith R 1987 Osteoporosis: cause and management. British Medical Journal 294: 329–332

Stamp TCB, Walker PG, Berry W, Jenkins MV 1980 Nutritional osteomalacia and late rickets in Greater London,

1974–1979. Clinical and metabolic studies in 45 patients. Clinics in Endocrinology and Metabolism 9: 81–105

Stevenson JL, Whitehead MI, Padwick M et al 1988 Dietary intake of calcium and postmenopausal bone loss. British Medical Journal 297: 15–17

Stevenson JC, Lees B, Devenport M, Cust MP, Ganger KF 1989 Determinants of bone density in normal women: risk factors for future osteoporosis. British Medical Journal 298: 924–928

Tam CS, Heersche JNM, Murray TM 1989 Metabolic bone disease: cellular and tissue mechanisms. CRC Press

Triffitt JT 1987 The special proteins of bone tissue. Clinical Science 72: 399–408

Tsai K-S, Heath III H, Kumar R, Riggs BL 1984 Impaired vitamin D metabolism with ageing in women. Journal of Clinical Investigation 73: 1668–1672

Vaughan J 1981 The physiology of bone, 3rd edn. Clarendon Press, Oxford

Wozney JM, Rosen V, Celeste AJ 1988 Novel regulations of bone formation; molecular clones and activities. Science 242: 1528–1534

12. Iron, zinc and other trace elements

L. Hallberg, B. Sandström and P. J. Aggett

IRON

L. Hallberg

IRON IN THE BODY

Amounts and physiological roles

Iron has several vital functions in the body: as a carrier of oxygen to the tissues from the lungs, as a transport medium for electrons within cells, and as an integrated part of important enzyme reactions in various tissues (Bothwell et al 1979, Hallberg 1982, 1984, Dallman 1986).

The main part of the iron in the body is present in the red cells as haemoglobin (Table 12.1), which is a molecule composed of four units, each containing one haem group and one protein chain. The ingenious structure of haemoglobin allows it to be fully loaded with oxygen in the lungs and partially unloaded in tissues, e.g in the muscles. The extent of unloading is determined by several factors, such as the local partial pressure of oxygen and carbon dioxide, the concentration of protons (lactic acid), and the local temperature in, for example, the working muscle. Myo-globin is the oxygen reserve in the muscles and is built like haemoglobin, but with only one haem unit and one globin chain. Several enzymes, such as the cytochromes, also have one haem group and a protein chain. Their structures do not permit a reversible loading and unloading of oxygen but act as electron carriers within the cell. Their role in the oxidative metabolism is thus to transfer energy within the cell and the mitochondria. A very great number of iron-containing enzymes have been described, and they play key roles not only in oxygen and electron transport but as signal-controlling substances in some neurotransmitter systems in the brain, for example, the dopamine and serotonin systems. Other key functions for the iron-containing enzymes (e.g. cytochrome P-450) is in the synthesis of steroid hormones and bile acids (hydroxylation) and the detoxification of various foreign substances in the liver.

Ferritin and haemosiderin are specially designed for the reversible storage of iron. Ferritin is a ball-shaped protein which, in its interior, can store about 4500 iron atoms. Very small amounts of ferritin (apoferritin) are present in plasma and reflect the amounts of iron present in the iron stores. Haemosiderin is a kind of polymer of ferritin micelles, which is metabolically less active but serves the same purpose as ferritin in the storage of iron.

Transferrin is a protein with the single function of transporting iron between different compartments in the body. It carries the iron from the intestinal mucosal cells to the red-cell precursors in the bone marrow and to other cells in the body during growth and development. It also carries iron from iron stores in the liver and other organs and from macrophages in the reticular–endothelial system, where the red cells are mainly destroyed.

Iron metabolism

The metabolism of iron can be described as two loops, one internal and one external (Fig. 12.1). The

Table 12.1 Iron compounds in the body

	75 kg man (mg)	55 kg woman (mg)
Functional iron		
Haemoglobin	2400	1600
Myoglobin	350	230
Haem enzymes } Non-haem enzymes	150	110
Transferrin-bound iron	3	2
Total functional iron	~2900	~1940
Storage iron		
Ferritin } Haemosiderin	500–1500	0–300
Total iron	~4000	~2100

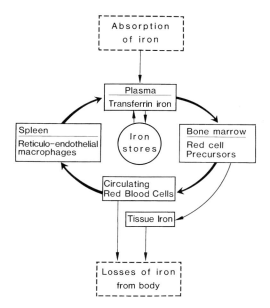

Fig. 12.1 Schematic representation of the metabolism of iron. A main internal loop with a continuous reutilization of iron and an external loop represented by iron losses from the body and absorption of iron from the diet.

internal loop is represented mainly by the formation and destruction of red cells. When a red cell dies, after about 120 days, it is usually taken care of by the macrophages of the reticular–endothelial system of the body. The iron is released and delivered to the transferrin molecules in the plasma. Transferrin, a protein specially designed for iron transport in plasma, brings the iron back to the red-cell precursors in the bone marrow, or to other cells in different tissues under growth and development. There is thus a continuous reutilization of the iron from haemoglobin in the red cells back to new red cells or other tissues. The internal iron metabolism can be studied by labelling the

transferrin-bound iron with a radioactive iron tracer. The total turnover of iron can be measured in plasma, and its appearance in the red cells can be used to quantify the erythropoiesis. Monitoring the radioactivity over different organs has also been used to study further the metabolism of iron in man. The external loop is represented by the losses of iron from the body from cell losses, including bleeding and the absorption of dietary iron. Special methods are available to study the losses and the absorption of iron (see below).

Mechanisms for the maintenance of iron balance

The body has three mechanisms for maintaining iron balance and preventing iron deficiency:
  1. The continuous reutilization of iron from catabolized red cells in the body, as mentioned above.
  2. The regulation of the absorption of iron from the intestines, with an increased iron absorption in the presence of iron deficiency and a decreased absorption in states of iron overload.
  3. The access of the specific storage protein ferritin, which can store and release iron to meet excessive iron demands, such as in the last trimester of pregnancy, and thus serve as a 'bank account' for iron in the body.

IRON REQUIREMENTS

Basal iron losses

Iron is not actively excreted from the body in the urine or in the intestines. Iron is only lost with cells from the skin and the interior surfaces of the body – intestines, urinary tract and airways. The total amount lost is estimated at 14 mg/kg body weight/day. For children, it is probably more correct to relate these losses to body surface (Table 12.2).

These losses have been calculated in the following way: after intravenous administration of the long-lived

Table 12.2 Basis for calculation of absorbed iron requirements for growth

Age (years) and sex	Weight gain (kg)	mg iron/kg body weight				Mean iron required for growth (mg/day)
		Haemoglobin	Myoglobin	Enzymes	Total	
0.25–1.0	4.2	32	3	2	37	0.65
1–2	2.4	32	3	2	37	0.24
2–6	7.9	32	6	2	40	0.22
6–12	20.2	33	6	2	41	0.38
Boys 12–16	26.2	37	7	2	46	0.66
Girls 12–16	15.2	34	7	2	43	0.36
Adult men	–	39	7	2	48	–
Adult women	–	34	7	2	43	–

radioisotope, ^{55}Fe, the rate of decrease of the specific activity of iron in haemoglobin is followed for several years. Iron is continuously lost from the body and replaced by absorbed non-radioactive iron. The rate of 'dilution' of radioiron by this absorption of iron then gives a measure of iron losses, assuming a steady state. A 55 kg woman thus loses about 0.8 mg of Fe/day and a 70 kg man about 1 mg. The range of individual variation has been estimated at ±15% (Green et al 1968).

Earlier studies suggested that sweat iron losses could be considerable, especially in a hot, humid climate. However, new studies which took extensive precautions to avoid the interference of contamination of iron from the skin during the collection of total body sweat, have shown that these sweat iron losses are negligible (Brune et al 1986).

Growth

The newborn term infant has an iron content of about 250–300 mg (75 mg/kg body weight). During the first 2 months of life, there is a decrease in the haemoglobin concentration due to the improved oxygen supply for the newborn infant, compared with the intrauterine situation of the fetus. This will lead to a considerable redistribution of iron from catabolized red cells to iron stores. This iron will cover the needs during the first 4–6 months of life, and this is the reason why the iron requirements during this period can be covered from breast milk alone, which contains very little iron. Due to the marked supply of iron to the fetus during the last trimester of pregnancy, the iron status is much less favourable in the premature and low birthweight infant than in the full-term infant. An extra supply of iron is therefore needed in these infants even during the first 6 months.

Calculations of iron requirements for growth were recently reviewed by an expert group for an FAO/WHO publication on iron requirements, and these are given in Table 12.2 (FAO/WHO 1988). For the full-term infant, iron requirements will rise markedly after the age of 4–6 months and amount to about 0.5–0.8 mg/day during the remaining part of the first year. These requirements are thus very high, especially in relation to body size and energy intake.

Within the first year of life the full-term infant must almost double its total iron content and triple its body weight. The change in body iron during this period occurs mainly between 6 and 12 months of age. Between 1 and 6 years of age, the body iron content is again doubled. The iron requirements of the infant and child are of the same magnitude as in adult man. The absorbed iron requirements in infants and children are very high in relation to their energy requirements. For example, in infants 6–12 months of age, about 1.5 mg of iron needs to be absorbed per 1000 kcal, and about half this amount up to the age of 4 years.

In the weaning period, the iron requirements in relation to energy intake are the highest during the lifespan of man, disregarding the last trimester of pregnancy, when iron requirements to a large extent have to be covered from the iron stores of the mother – see section on iron and pregnancy. The rapidly growing, weanling infant has no iron stores and has to rely on dietary iron. It is possible to meet these high requirements if the diet consistently has a high content of meat and ascorbic-acid rich foods. In developed countries today, infant cereal products are the staple foods in this period of life. Commercial products are regularly fortified with iron and ascorbic acid, and they are usually given together with fruit juices and solid foods containing meat, fish and vegetables. The fortification of cereal products with iron and ascorbic acid is important in meeting the high dietary needs, especially considering the importance of an optimal iron nutrition during this phase of brain development. It is possible that in primitive societies and among our ancestors the weanling infant might have covered some of its excessive iron needs during this period by eating iron-rich soil. Even if the fraction of iron absorbed from soil is low, the amount expected to be absorbed might still be considerable. One parallel is the importance of soil iron for the rapidly growing piglet.

Iron requirements are also very high in adolescents, particularly during the period of rapid growth. There is a marked individual variation in growth rate and the requirements may be considerably higher than the calculated mean values given in Table 12.2. Girls usually have their growth spurt before the menarche, but growth does not stop at that time. Their total iron requirements are therefore considerable.

Menstrual iron losses

Menstrual blood losses are very constant from month to month for an individual but vary markedly from one woman to another (Hallberg et al 1966). The main part of this variation is genetically controlled. Menstrual losses have been observed to be the same in populations which are geographically widely separated (Burma, Canada, China, Egypt, England and Sweden). These findings thus strongly suggest that the main source of variation in iron status in different populations is not related to varying iron requirements but to a variation in the absorption of iron from the diet. In this statement infestations with hookworm in different populations are disregarded. The mean menstrual iron loss, averaged over the entire menstrual cycle of 28 days, is about 0.56 mg/day. The frequency distribution of physiological menstrual blood losses is highly skewed. Adding the average basal iron losses (0.8 mg), the distribution of the total iron requirements in adult women can be calculated (Fig. 12.2). The mean daily total iron requirement is 1.36 mg. In 10% of women it exceeds 2.27 mg and in 5%, 2.84 mg. In 10% of menstruating, still-growing teenagers, the corresponding daily total iron requirements exceed 2.65 mg, and in 5% of these girls they will exceed 3.21 mg / day. The FAO/WHO publication has incorrectly used slightly lower figures for girls, due to incomplete sampling of menstrual blood and not to truly lower losses. The methods of calculating iron requirements in women, and their variations, have been re-examined (Hallberg & Rossander-Hultén 1991).

In postmenopausal women and in physically active elderly people, the iron requirements are the same as in men. When physical activity decreases due to ageing, the blood volume and haemoglobin mass will also diminish, leading to a shift of iron from the haemoglobin mass and thus to a reduction of the daily iron

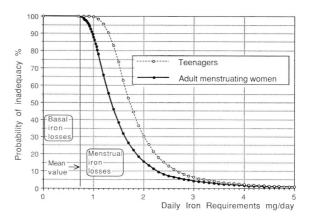

Fig. 12.2   Distribution of daily iron requirements in adult menstruating women and in menstruating teenagers. The graph illustrates the probability of inadequacy at different amounts of iron absorbed. The left part is basal obligatory losses (0.8 mg) and the right part the varying menstrual iron losses.

requirements. The absorbed iron requirements for different groups are given in Table 12.3. Pregnancy and lactation are dealt with separately below.

Table 12.3   Absorbed and dietary iron requirements. Partly based on FAO/WHO report (1988) and partly on new calculations of the distribution of iron requirements in menstruating women. Due to the very skewed distribution of iron requirements in these women, dietary iron requirements are calculated for two levels of coverage, 90% and 95%, in these groups

Group	Age (years)	Mean body weight (kg)	Growth require-ments (mg/day)	Basal losses Median (mg/day)	Menstrual losses Median (mg/day)	Menstrual losses 95th per. (mg/day)	Total requirements Median (mg/day)	Total requirements 95th per. (mg/day)	Dietary iron requirements Bioavailability 15% (mg/day) 90th percentile	Dietary iron requirements Bioavailability 15% (mg/day) 95th percentile
Children	0.25–1	8	0.56	0.21			0.77	0.96		#
	1–2	11	0.24	0.25			0.49	0.61		#
	2–6	16	0.22	0.34			0.56	0.70		4.7
	6–12	29	0.38	0.56			0.94	1.17		7.8
Boys	12–16	53	0.66	0.80			1.46	1.82		12.1
Girls	12–16	51	0.36	0.79	0.48*	1.90*	1.73	3.21	17.7	21.4
Adult men		70		0.98			0.98	1.27		8.5
Adult women										
Menstruating		55		0.77	0.48*	1.90*	1.36	2.84	15.1	18.9
Post-menopausal		55		0.77			0.77	1.00		6.7
Lactating		55		1.05			1.05	1.31		8.7

* Effect of the normal variation in Hb concentration not included in this figure
# Bioavailability of food during this period varies greatly

DIETARY IRON ABSORPTION

There are two kinds of iron in the diet, with respect to the mechanism of absorption – haem iron and non-haem iron – utilizing two separate receptors on the mucosal cells (Hallberg 1981, Baynes & Bothwell 1990, Table 12.4). After the uptake of haem iron into the mucosal cells, the porphyrin ring is split by a special enzyme (haemoxygenase) within the cells and its iron is released. Non-haem and haem iron then have a common pathway and leave the mucosal cells in the same chemical form, utilizing the same transfer system to the serosal side of the mucosal cells. As far as non-haem iron is concerned, receptors on the luminal side probably compete with complexing luminal ligands for the iron ions. It is probable that iron can only be absorbed into the cells and pass the mucosal membrane in its ferrous form. Reducing substances, especially ascorbic acid, must therefore be present in the mucin layer of the mucosal cells for iron to be absorbed. Ascorbic acid thus seems to have a physiological role in iron absorption. As man cannot synthesize ascorbic acid, it must come from the diet.

Haem iron absorption

Haem iron in meat and meat products constitutes about 1–2 mg, or 5–10%, of the daily iron intake in most industrialized countries. In developing countries, the haem content of diets is usually negligible. The average absorption of haem iron in meat is about 25% (Hallberg et al 1979). In contrast to non-haem iron, the absorption of haem iron is very little influenced by the iron status of the subject. For unknown reasons, haem iron which is not given together with meat is less well absorbed. For example, the iron absorption from a portion of blood sausage, providing about 40–50 mg of haem iron, is only about 2–3%. Considering the great amount of iron in blood products, however, the amount of iron absorbed from such foods is still high.

The absorption of haem iron from a meal can be measured using biosynthetically radioiron-labelled haemoglobin, which is mixed into the haem-containing food, e.g. a hamburger. Haem iron can be degraded and converted to non-haem iron if foods are cooked at a high temperature for too long. Calcium (see below) is the only other dietary factor that influences the absorption of haem iron.

Non-haem iron absorption

Non-haem iron is the main form of dietary iron. The main sources are cereals, vegetables, pulses, beans, fruits, etc. In contrast to haem iron, the absorption of non-haem iron is very much influenced by the individual iron status: more iron is absorbed by iron-deficient subjects and less by iron-replete subjects. Moreover, the absorption of non-haem iron is much influenced by several factors in the diet (see below).

Early studies with the chemical balance technique, employing long balance periods due to the small fraction of iron absorbed, gave important information about the magnitude of iron absorption from the whole diet. Early studies on individual food items biosynthetically labelled with radioiron also provided valuable information. Nothing was known, however, about the absorption of iron from meals and the marked variation in absorption from different meals, or about the influence of various dietary factors on the absorption of iron.

The observation that a radioiron tracer added as an inorganic iron salt to a food or a meal uniformly labelled almost all non-haem iron present in the food/meal, probably by isotopic exchange, suddenly made it possible to measure iron absorption from different meals with this 'extrinsic tag technique'. Employing two different radioiron isotopes (^{55}Fe and ^{59}Fe), the absorption from two meals could be compared in the same subject and factors influencing the absorption could be identified and their effects quantified.

There was still a considerable problem in interpreting the results of iron absorption measurements due to the markedly varying absorption in subjects with different iron status. This was overcome, however, by relating in each subject the absorption from a

Table 12.4   Factors influencing dietary iron absorption

Haem iron absorption
    Amount of haem iron present in meat
    Content of calcium in meal
    Food preparation (time, temperature)

Non-haem iron absorption
    Iron status of subjects
    Amount of bioavailable non-haem iron
    (adjustment for fortification iron and contamination iron)
    Balance between dietary factors enhancing and inhibiting iron absorption

Factors enhancing iron absorption
    Ascorbic acid
    Meat, fish, seafood
    Certain organic acids

Factors inhibiting iron absorption
    Phytates
    Iron-binding phenolic compounds
    Calcium
    Soy protein

certain meal to the absorption from a physiological dose (3 mg Fe^{2+}) of an iron salt given in a fasting state. The absorption from this reference dose thus serves as an 'internal standard'. Recent studies indicate that a 60% absorption from this reference iron dose corresponds to the absorption in non-anaemic subjects with no iron stores (Hallberg & Rossander-Hultén 1991). In this way, the iron absorption from a certain meal or diet can be expressed as a single figure by adjusting all absorption values to this 60% reference absorption, i.e. to the absorption in borderline iron-deficient subjects. Another possibility is to use serum ferritin for the same purpose. It is thus possible to compare iron absorption from different meals, to compare groups of subjects, and to quantify the influence of various dietary or other factors on iron absorption (Hallberg 1980).

Factors influencing non-haem iron absorption

Foods may contain factors (ligands) which strongly bind iron ions, thus inhibiting absorption. Examples are phytates and certain phenolic compounds. Other dietary factors may enhance iron absorption, e.g. ascorbic acid, meat and fish (Table 12.4).

Phytates

Phytates are salts of inositol hexaphosphates, which are a storage form of phosphates and minerals in all kind of grains, seeds, nuts, vegetables and fruits. In western-type diets about 90% of phytates originate from cereals. Phytates strongly inhibit iron absorption in a dose-dependent fashion and even rather small amounts of phytate have a marked effect. Ascorbic acid in sufficient amounts can partly counteract this inhibition (Hallberg et al 1989).

Bran has a very high content of phytate. High-extraction-rate flour has thus a much higher content of phytates than white wheat flour. In bread, part of the phytate in bran is degraded to inositol phosphates during the fermentation of the dough by the phytase present in flour. These inositol phosphates also inhibit iron absorption. Prolonged fermentation for a couple of days (sourdough fermentation) can almost completely degrade the phytate and will thus increase iron absorption (Brune et al 1992). Oats strongly inhibit iron absorption because of their high phytate content, due to the fact that the native phytase in oats is destroyed by heat treatment.

Fibre components as such in the diet have almost no influence on iron absorption. Fibre-rich foods, however, especially those present in cereals, are rich in phytates. An increased intake of fibre through a higher consumption of bran products, high-extraction flour and oats will lead to a reduction of the total iron absorption. The very low fractional absorption is not compensated by the higher iron content of most of these foods. Any advantages to a higher intake of this kind of fibre, which mainly influences faecal bulk and counteracts constipation, must be carefully balanced against the disadvantage of the markedly reduced absorption of iron, and probably also other minerals such as calcium and zinc.

Phenolic compounds

Almost all plants contain some phenolic compounds as part of their defence system against insects, animals and man. Thousands of such compounds are known, but only some of them – and actually only some molecular structures in these compounds – seem to be responsible for the inhibition of iron absorption. It is mainly the galloyl group in these phenolic compounds that specifically binds iron (Brune et al 1989). Well known foods containing much iron-binding polyphenols are tea, coffee and cocoa. Many vegetables (e.g. spinach) and several herbs and spices (e.g. oregano) contain appreciable amounts of galloyl groups and thus inhibit iron absorption. This inhibition can also be partly counteracted by, for example, ascorbic acid and meat.

Calcium

Given as a salt or in the form of dairy products, e.g. milk or cheese, calcium markedly interferes with the absorption of iron (Hallberg et al 1991, 1992). The inhibition is equally strong for haem and non-haem iron. As little as one glass of milk (about 165 mg of calcium) reduces iron absorption by more than half. The mechanism of action is unknown, but the balance of evidence strongly suggests that the inhibition is not localized to the gastrointestinal lumen but to the mucosal cell itself and to the common final transfer step for haem and non-haem iron. Calcium and iron are both essential nutrients and calcium thus cannot be considered as an inhibitor in the same sense as phytates or phenolic compounds. The calcium content of a meal has a marked inhibitory effect on the bioavailability of iron, however. These findings may either lead to an avoidance of excess dietary calcium or increased dietary iron intake in groups with a high calcium intake. Epidemiological studies show an association between the intake of milk and the prevalence of iron deficiency.

Soy protein

The addition of soy protein to a meal reduces the fraction of iron absorbed. This inhibition is probably explained by its high content of phytates. Due to the high content of iron in soy proteins, the net effect on iron absorption of an addition of soy products to a meal is usually positive. In infant foods containing soy proteins, their inhibiting effect can be overcome by the addition of ascorbic acid.

Ascorbic acid

This is the most potent enhancer of non-haem iron absorption. Native ascorbic acids in fruits, vegetables and juices increases iron absorption to the same extent as synthetic vitamin C.

There is a strong exponential dose-related effect of ascorbic acid on non-haem iron absorption (Hallberg et al 1986). The main mechanism for the action of ascorbic acid is probably a reduction of ferric to ferrous iron. Ferric ions bind more strongly to various ligands than does ferrous iron. Even at the normal pH range in the duodenum, dietary iron can be converted into ferric hydroxide and be precipitated in an unabsorbable form. Moreover, as mentioned above, iron can probably only pass the mucosal membrane in its ferrous form, which implies that ascorbic acid also seems to play a role in the mucin layer.

Ascorbic acid may also facilitate iron absorption by the formation of soluble iron–ascorbate complexes. The effect of ascorbic acid on iron absorption is so marked and essential that its effect on iron absorption should be considered as one of the physiological roles of ascorbic acid in the body. Each meal should preferably contain at least 25 mg of ascorbic acid. Therefore, these requirements of ascorbic acid for iron absorption should be taken into account when calculating the requirements for vitamin C.

Meat, fish, seafood

All these foods promote the absorption of non-haem iron, but the mechanism for this effect has not been established. It should be pointed out that meat also enhances the absorption of haem iron to about the same extent (see above). Meat thus promotes iron nutrition in two ways. It stimulates the absorption of non-haem iron and it provides the well-absorbed haem iron. Epidemiologically, the intake of meat has been found to be associated with a lower prevalence of iron deficiency.

Organic acids

Organic acids, such as citric acid, have been found in some studies to enhance the absorption of non-haem iron. This effect is not so consistently observed as that for ascorbic acid. Sauerkraut, as well as other fermented vegetables, and even some fermented soy sauces, have an enhancing effect on iron absorption. The nature of this effect is not yet established.

Iron absorption from meals

The pool concept (see above) in iron absorption implies that there are two main pools in the gastrointestinal lumen: one pool of haem iron and another pool of non-haem iron, and that iron absorption takes place independently from these two pools. The pool concept also implies that the absorption of iron from the non-haem pool is a resultant of all ligands present in the mixture of foods included in a meal. If the iron in one food item is well absorbed when given alone, and if other foods in the same meal contain an excess of ligands inhibiting iron absorption, e.g. phytates, the absorption will be poor from all iron compounds present in that meal. The non-haem iron absorption from a certain meal is thus not only dependent on its iron content but also, and to a marked degree, on the composition of the meal, i.e. the balance between all factors enhancing and inhibiting the absorption of iron. The bioavailability can vary more than tenfold from meals with a similar content of iron, energy, protein and fat. Just the addition of certain spices, e.g. oregano, or a cup of tea, may reduce the bioavailability by half or more. On the other hand, the addition of certain vegetables or fruits containing ascorbic acid may double or even triple the iron absorption, depending on the other properties of the meal and the amounts of ascorbic acid present.

Much is known today about the amount of iron needed to be absorbed by different groups of subjects and about the variations of iron requirements in these groups. The new knowledge about the variation in iron absorption from different meals and types of diets with, for example, different amounts of ascorbic acid, meat, phytates, etc., must be carefully considered in translating 'absorbed iron requirements' into dietary iron requirements (see below) and into recommended intakes. It is obvious that different intake figures are needed for different types of diet with a different bioavailability of iron. As energy expenditure and thus energy intake sets the limit for the amount of food eaten and thus for meal size, it is practical to relate the bioavailability of iron in different meals to its energy content. This has been named 'bioavailable nutrient density' and is a feasible measure in comparing different meals, in the construction of menus and in the calculation of recommended intakes.

IRON BALANCE

Iron balance means that a steady state is present, when the absorption of iron from the diet covers both the actual losses of iron from the body and the requirements for growth and/or pregnancy (a kind of growth). The absorption of non-haem iron is markedly influenced by the iron status. The more iron that is present in the stores, the less iron is absorbed. An increased erythropoiesis (e.g. after an acute blood loss) also increases iron absorption.

The amount of iron lost with menstruation is influenced by the haemoglobin level. During the development of an iron-deficiency anaemia, menstrual iron losses will thus successively decrease when the haemoglobin level diminishes. Skin iron losses will also decrease in a state of iron deficiency, and increase if a subject develops iron overload. Sooner or later a point is reached when iron losses are equal to the amount of iron absorbed from the diet. These facts imply that there are an infinite number of iron balance states when absorption equals loss. Take a hypothetical example: in a population of menstruating women with varying menstrual iron requirements, consuming exactly the same diet, the iron status may vary from anaemia of different degrees to iron stores of different magnitudes. This variation in iron status occurs in spite of the fact that iron absorption is higher in women with anaemia and lower in women with iron stores. In an unknown way, iron status influences the 'setting' of the ability of the mucosal cells to absorb iron. Thus, the regulation of the iron absorption in relation to iron status tries to maintain iron balance. This regulation, however, can only partially counteract the variation in iron requirements.

Any measures taken to change the iron losses or the absorption of iron in a population will move the existing point of balance, and will thus affect the prevalence and severity of iron deficiency in that population. For example, iron fortification of foods will increase absorption and lead to a reduction in prevalence of iron deficiency in the population, and an increase of iron stores. The more iron that accumulates in the stores, however, the less iron will be absorbed. This feedback system means that new states of iron balance will be obtained if more iron is available for absorption. It also means that, in a state of positive iron balance, the amount of iron in stores will at certain new balance levels flatten out to new steady states. There is thus no risk of a development of iron overload in otherwise healthy subjects. In healthy men aged about 30 years, iron stores are usually between 500 and 1000 mg in western countries, and in older men the stores may have reached a level of 1500 mg if the diet has had a high iron content and good bioavailability. The iron stores in women seldom reach 500 mg; 20–30% usually have no iron stores at all. The average amount of iron in the stores can be estimated to be around 150 mg (see section on pregnancy).

IRON DEFICIENCY AND IRON-DEFICIENCY ANAEMIA

These two concepts are often incorrectly used synonymously. A definiton of the concepts may clarify some confusion about the very varying prevalence figures given in the literature. A hypothetical example is used to explain the concepts: assume that a negative iron balance is induced in an iron-replete woman by the insertion of an intrauterine contraceptive device. Her menstrual iron losses will then be doubled. Iron absorption progressively increases but cannot fully balance the higher iron losses. Her iron stores will then be successively emptied. During this phase of negative iron balance, less and less stainable iron is seen in bone marrow smears and serum ferritin is also successively reduced. Iron stores are defined as empty when no more iron is seen in smears made with an adequate technique. At the same time, the serum ferritin in the plasma has reached the level of about 15 µg/l.

When iron can no longer be mobilized from the iron stores, insufficient amounts of iron will be delivered to transferrin, the circulating transport protein for iron. The binding sites for iron on transferrin will thus contain less and less iron. This is usually described as a reduction of the transferrin saturation (TS). When the transferrin saturation drops to a certain critical level (usually considered to be 16%) the red-cell precursors, which continuously need iron for the formation of haemoglobin, will get an insufficient supply of iron. At the same time, the supply of iron to other tissues by transferrin will also be impaired. Cells with a high turnover rate, e.g. intestinal mucosal cells with a short lifespan, are the first to be affected. An iron deficiency can thus be expected, especially in growing tissues. Using special transferrin receptors, the iron–transferrin complex is taken up by the various tissues in the body. There are marked diurnal variations in the saturation of transferrin, since the turnover rate of iron in plasma is very high. This fact makes it difficult to evaluate the iron status from single determinations of transferrin saturation. The uptake of iron by different cells seems to be related both to transferrin saturation and the number of transferrin receptors on the cell surface.

The haemoglobin production will be impaired rather early in the development of iron deficiency, and the haemoglobin level starts to fall below the individual woman's own normal (optimal) value. If the negative iron balance is sufficiently severe and longstanding, the impaired haemoglobin formation will sooner or later lead to the individual haemoglobin value passing below the 2.5th percentile value of the population. When that occurs, anaemia is considered to be present according to current definitions. This implies that the prevalence of iron-deficiency anaemia (a haemoglobin level below the 2.5th percentile value of the population) is less frequent than iron deficiency defined as an absence of iron stores, and thus the beginning of an insufficient supply of iron to various tissues.

Diagnosis of iron deficiency

The absence of iron stores (iron deficiency) can be diagnosed by showing that there is no stainable iron in the reticular-endothelial cells in bone marrow smears, or a low concentration of ferritin in the serum (15 µg/l or less). Even if an absence of iron stores may not necessarily be associated with any immediate negative effects, it is a reliable and good indicator of an increased risk of compromised supply of iron to different tissues.

A diagnosis of iron deficiency anaemia can be suspected if anaemia is present in subjects who are iron deficient, as described above. Preferably, to establish fully the diagnosis, the subjects should respond adequately to iron treatment.

An iron-deficient erythropoiesis can be suspected using several methods (e.g. besides the criteria above for iron deficiency). Examples are low transferrin saturation and a high content of transferrin receptors in the plasma, high red-cell protoporphyrin in the red cells, and a microcytic hypochromic anaemia.

Causes of iron deficiency

Nutritional iron deficiency implies that the diet cannot cover physiological iron requirements. Worldwide, this is the most common cause of iron deficiency.

Pathological causes

In many tropical countries, infestation with hook-worms leads to intestinal blood losses that may be considerable. Usually the diet is also poor in these populations. The severity of infestation with hook-worms varies considerably between subjects and regions. The average blood loss can be well estimated by egg-counts in the stools.

In clinical practice, a diagnosis of iron deficiency must always lead to a search for the pathological causes of blood loss, e.g. tumours in the gastro-intestinal tract or uterus, especially if uterine bleedings have increased or changed in regularity. Patients with achlorhydria absorb dietary iron less well (a reduction of about 50%) and patients who have undergone gastric surgery, especially if the operation has been extensive, may sooner or later develop iron deficiency due to an impaired absorption of iron.

In communities which are largely vegetarian, purely nutritional factors are of great importance, often as the only factor causing iron deficiency. Thus 63% of 138 Hindu Indian vegetarians in an affluent community in London who presented with cobalamin deficiency, showed overt iron deficiency as well (53 women and 38 men). Marrow iron stores were absent in 71% (Chanarin et al 1983).

Prevalence of iron deficiency

Iron deficiency is probably the most frequent nutritional deficiency disorder in the world. A recent estimate, using WHO criteria, indicated that around 600–700 milion of the world's population have iron deficiency anaemia (De Maeyer & Adiels-Tegman 1985). In industrialized countries, the prevalence of iron deficiency anaemia is much lower, and usually varies between 2% and 8%. However, the prevalence of iron deficiency, including both anaemic and non-anaemic subjects (see definitions above), is much higher. In western industrialized countries, for example, the abscence of iron stores or subnormal serum ferritin values are found in about 20–30% of women of childbearing age.

Worldwide, the highest prevalence figures for iron deficiency are found in infants, children, teenagers and women of childbearing age. Thanks to better information and access to fortified cereals for infants and children, the iron situation has markedly improved in these groups in industrialized countries, where the highest prevalences today are observed in menstruating women and teenagers of both sexes.

Deleterious effect of iron deficiency

Studies in animals have clearly shown that iron deficiency has several negative effects on important functions in the body (Dallman 1986). Physical working capacity in rats has been shown to be significantly reduced in iron deficiency; this is especially valid for endurance activities. This negative effect seems to be less related to the degree of anaemia and more to an impaired oxidative metabolism in the muscles, with an increased formation of lactic acid, in turn due to a lack of iron-containing enzymes, which are rate limiting for the oxidative metabolism (Scrimshaw 1984).

The fairly recently observed, and now well established, relationship between iron deficiency and brain function is of great importance for the choice of strategy in combating iron deficiency (Lozoff 1988, Youdim 1988). Several structures in the brain have a high iron content, of the same magnitude as that observed in the liver. There is an active transferrin-receptor mediated transport of iron into the brain. In man, the iron content in the brain increases continuously during development and up through the teenage period. About 10% of brain iron is present at birth, at the age of 10 the brain has reached only half its normal iron content, and optimal amounts are first reached at the age of 20–30 years. Of great importance is the observation that the lower iron content of the brain in iron-deficient growing rats cannot be restituted by giving iron later on. This fact strongly suggests that the supply of iron to the brain cells mainly takes place during an early phase of their development, and thus that early iron deficiency may lead to irreparable damage.

Several brain functions have been shown to be negatively influenced by iron deficiency, especially functions related to the neurotransmitter systems (Youdim 1988). The dopamine system, for example, has several important roles in the brain: iron deficiency leads to a reduced sensitivity of the dopamine-D2 receptor, possibly leading to a loss of receptors. This is associated with an impaired catabolism of biogenic amines, such as serotonin, as well as with the catabolism of endogenous opiopeptides. It has been shown, for example, that there is an impairment in memory and learning, an increase in the pain threshold, a reduction in the release of the thyrotropin release hormone (TRH), and hence a reduction of thyroid function and thermoregulation in the body. It was observed early on that spontaneous physical activity was reduced in rats. Another finding was the reversal of the circadian rhythm of the body in iron deficiency. Some of the functional changes that have been observed may be normalized by iron therapy, whereas others, such as learning, seem to be unaffected.

Iron deficiency also negatively influences the normal defence systems against infection. The cell-mediated immunological response by the action of T-lymphocytes is impaired due to a reduced formation of these cells, due in turn to a reduced DNA synthesis depending on the function of ribonucleotide reductase, which requires a continuous supply of iron for its function.

The phagocytosis and killing of bacteria by the neutrophil leucocytes is an important component of the defence against infection. These functions are impaired in iron deficiency. The killing function is based on the formation of free hydroxyl radicals, the respiratory burst, and results from the activation of the iron-sulphur enzyme NADPH oxidase and probably also cytochrome B (a haem enzyme). Myeloperoxidase is another important, much-studied enzyme involved in this defence system which is also impaired in iron deficiency. The functional impairments observed in several experimental studies and in animals correspond to similar observations in man.

In populations with long-standing iron deficiency, a reduction in physical working capacity has been demonstrated by several groups. An improvement has also been reported after iron administration, using placebo administration as a control.

The impairment of the immunological defence against infection which was found in animals is also regularly found in man. The administration of iron normalizes these changes within 4–7 days. It has been difficult to demonstrate, however, that the prevalence of infection is higher, or their severity more marked, in iron-deficient subjects than in controls. This may well be ascribed to the difficulty in studying this problem using a good experimental design and controlling for other potential factors.

A relationship between iron deficiency and behaviour, such as attention, memory and learning, has been demonstrated in infants and small children. In most recent well controlled studies no effect of the administration of iron has been noted. This finding is thus consistent with the observations in animals. The therapy-resistant behavioural impairments and the fact that there is an accumulation of iron during the whole period of brain growth should be considered as a strong argument for the more active and effective combating of iron deficiency in women, especially during pregnancy, in infants and children, and up through the period of adolescence into early adulthood.

DIETARY IRON REQUIREMENTS

To translate the absorbed iron requirements given in Table 12.3 into dietary iron requirements, two main facts must be considered:

1. The iron status of the body desired to be maintained in a certain fraction of a certain population group (e.g. presence of iron stores in 95% of menstruating women).
2. The bioavailability of iron in different diets.

The body iron status markedly affects iron absorption. About twice as much iron is absorbed from a certain diet in borderline iron-deficient subjects with no iron stores compared to subjects having about 300 mg of storage iron. This implies that, in order to maintain such an amount of storage iron, since the absorption is halved, twice as much iron is needed in the diet to cover the physiological demands, other conditions being the same. The figures for bioavailability in Table 12.3 are estimated for subjects with no iron stores.

The bioavailability of iron varies markedly between typical diets in different populations. The reason is variation of the various factors mainly influencing the absorption of iron from different meals. Examples are the intake of meat, ascorbic-acid rich vegetables, milk products and phytates. There is no doubt that the bioavailability of dietary iron in diets in many developing countries is very low, due to an excess of inhibitors of iron absorption and a low intake of absorption promotors such as meat and fish. Among industrialized countries there is probably also a variation in bioavailability in different segments of the population (e.g. lower in most vegetarians). Recently, however, attempts were made to estimate the bioavailability of dietary iron in western populations using indirect methods (e.g. calculation of the coverage of iron requirements in population groups with known dietary intake). Several such studies gave remarkably consistent results, suggesting that in borderline iron-deficient subjects the bioavailability may reach a level around 14–16% (Hallberg & Rossander-Hultén 1991). The average figure of 15% used in Table 12.3 does not consider that only a minor fraction of presently used fortification iron joins the non-haem iron pool.

IRON AND PREGNANCY

The iron requirements during pregnancy are well established (Table 12.5). Most iron is required to increase the haemoglobin mass of the mother: this increase occurs in all healthy pregnant women who

Table 12.5   Iron requirements in pregnancy

	Gross loss Fe (mg)
Fetus	300
Placenta	50
Expansion of maternal red cell mass	450
Basal iron losses	240
Total	1040
At delivery:	
Contraction of maternal red cell mass	+450
Maternal blood loss	−250
Net gain	+200
Net total losses	840

have sufficiently large iron stores or who are adequately supplemented with iron. The increase is directly proportional to the increased need for oxygen transport during pregnancy and is one of the important physiological adaptations that occurs in pregnancy (Hallberg 1988).

A main problem for iron balance in pregnancy is the fact that iron requirements are not equally distributed over its duration. The exponential growth of the fetus implies that iron need is almost negligible in the first trimester and that more than 80% relates to the last trimester. The total daily iron requirements, including the basal iron losses (0.8 mg), increase during pregnancy to about 10 mg during the last 6 weeks.

Iron absorption during pregnancy is determined by 1) the amount of iron in the diet, 2) its bioavailability (meal composition), and 3) the changes in iron absorption that occur during pregnancy. Several studies have found that the composition of the diet is almost unchanged during pregnancy in spite of the extra energy requirements related to the pregnancy per se. These are mainly balanced, however, by a simultaneous reduction in physical activity. There are fairly marked changes in the fraction of iron absorbed during pregnancy. In the first trimester, there is a marked decrease in the absorption of iron, which is closely related to the reduction in iron requirements during this period compared with the non-pregnant state (see below). In the second trimester, iron absorption is increased by about 50%, and in the last trimester it may increase by up to about four times.

Even considering the marked increase in iron absorption, it is impossible for the mother to cover her very high iron requirements from the diet alone. It can be calculated that, with diets prevailing in most industrialized countries, there will be a deficit of about 400–500 mg of iron between total iron requirements and the amounts of iron absorbed during pregnancy (Fig. 12.3)

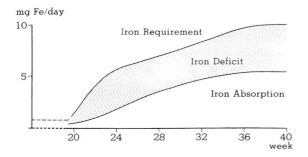

Fig. 12.3 Daily iron requirements and daily dietary iron absorption in pregnancy. The hatched area represents the deficit of iron that has to be covered by iron stores or iron supplementation.

An adequate iron balance can be achieved if iron stores of this magnitude are available. However, it is uncommon for women to have iron stores of this magnitude and a great proportion of women have no stores at all. It is therefore recommended that iron supplements in tablet form, preferably together with folic acid, are given to all pregnant women, due to the difficulty of correctly evaluating iron status in pregnancy with routine laboratory methods.

At delivery, the average blood loss corresponds to about 250 mg of iron. At the same time, however, the haemoglobin mass of the mother is gradually normalized, which implies that about 200 mg of iron from the expanded haemoglobin mass (450–250 mg) is returned to the mother. To cover the needs in a following pregnancy, a further 300 mg of iron must be accumulated in the iron stores in order for the woman to start her next pregnancy with 500 mg of stored iron. The time required for this restitution depends on the type of diet, the length of lactation and the magnitude of her menstrual iron losses. In lactating women, the daily iron loss in breast milk is about 0.3 mg. Together with the basal iron losses of 0.8 mg, the total iron requirements during the lactation period amount to 1.1 mg/day. This is therefore less than the average losses in the menstruating woman. Still, it can be estimated that a restoration of iron stores up to 500 mg probably takes years with present diets.

It is possible to estimate the distribution of iron stores in women from the distribution of serum ferritin. Very consistent results are obtained in population samples in Sweden and the USA. About 25–30% have no iron stores and median iron stores are about 150 mg. Only 20% achieve iron stores of about 250 mg and only 5% reach 400 mg.

In early man, dietary iron absorption and the magnitude of iron stores were probably considerably high-er than in present-day women, due to a much higher intake of animal protein (meat in various forms), and a probable very high intake of ascorbic acid. The balance calculations thus looked quite different in early women, and there was probably no difficulty in rebuilding iron stores up to 500 mg during a lactation period of about 6 months between pregnancies. This perspective is necessary in order to accept the paradoxical recommendation today that iron tablets and folate should be given in a physiological state such as pregnancy.

Early in pregnancy there are marked hormonal, haemodynamic and haematological changes. There is, for example, a very early increase in the plasma volume, which has been used to explain the 'physiological anaemia of pregnancy', observed also in iron-replete women. The primary cause of this phenomenon, however, is more probably an increased ability of the haemoglobin to deliver oxygen to the tissues (fetus). This change is induced early in pregnancy by increasing the content of 2-3-DPG in the red cells, which shifts the haemoglobin–oxygen dissociation curve to the right. The 'anaemia' is thus a consequence of this important adaptation and is not primarily a desirable change, for example to improve placental blood flow by reducing blood viscosity.

Another observation has likewise caused some confusion about the rationale of giving extra iron routinely in pregnancy. In more extensive studies of pregnant women there is a U-shaped relationship between various pregnancy complications and the haemoglobin level – i.e. with more complications both at low and at high levels. There is nothing to indicate, however, that high haemoglobin levels (within the normal non-pregnant range) per se have any negative effects.

There is a clear association, however, between low haemoglobin values and prematurity. A recent extensive study (Liebermann et al 1988) showed that a woman with a haematocrit of 37% had twice the risk of having a premature birth as a woman whose haematocrit was between 41% and 44% (p <0.01). A similar observation was reported in another extensive study in the USA (Garn et al 1981). These materials were examined retrospectively and the cause of the lower haematocrit was not examined.

In summary, the marked physiological adjustments occurring in pregnancy are not sufficient to balance its very marked iron requirements, and the pregnant woman has to rely on her iron stores, if present. The composition of the diet has not been adjusted to the present low-energy demanding lifestyle in industrialized countries. This is probably the main cause of the critical iron balance situation in pregnancy today, due to absent or insufficient iron stores in women before they become pregnant. The 'unnatural' need to give extra nutrients such as iron and folate to otherwise healthy pregnant women should be considered in this perspective.

PREVENTION OF IRON DEFICIENCY

The prevention of iron deficiency has become even more urgent in recent years, with the accumulation of evidence strongly suggesting a relationship between even mild iron deficiency and brain development, and especially with the observation that functional defects affecting learning and behaviour cannot be reversed by giving iron later on. As mentioned, iron deficiency is common both in developed and in developing countries.

Great efforts have been made by WHO to develop methods to combat iron deficiency. Generally this can be achieved by selecting one or more of the following strategies:

1. Iron supplementation – i.e. giving iron tablets to certain target groups such as pregnant women and preschool children.
2. Iron fortification of certain foods.
3. Food education to improve iron absorption from the diet.

Several factors determine the feasibility and effectiveness of different strategies, such as the health infrastructure of a society, the economy, access to suitable vehicles for iron fortification, etc. The solutions are therefore often quite different in developing and in developed countries.

In developing countries the choice of strategies is more limited. Iron supplementation is usually only given to pregnant women, sometimes to school children. The efficacy depends on several factors such as cost, the pharmaceutical properties of the iron tablets used, the delivery system of tablets and, not least, the methods used to motivate the women to take the tablets. Iron supplementation has proved to be effective if there is an adequate infrastructure at the village level.

The use of iron fortification is also limited by several factors besides cost. It is often difficult to find vehicles for the iron fortificant that are centrally produced and that reach the target groups to a sufficient degree. A main disadvantage of iron fortification in developing countries is its potentially low efficacy. The bioavailability of the dietary iron is often very low and the iron intake quite high. The increase of the iron content of the diet by the addition of fortification iron is therefore less rational. It should be emphasized that the absorption of the added fortification iron, the soluble part of which joins the common non-haem pool, will be as poor as the absorption from the native dietary iron.

Food education is another main alternative for improving iron nutrition, with attempts to increase the bioavailability of the dietary iron by modifying meal composition. The bioavailability of dietary iron is a balance between dietary factors enhancing and inhibiting iron absorption; iron absorption may thus be improved by, for example, increasing the content of ascorbic-acid rich foods (e.g. certain vegetables and fruits). Another main possibility is to reduce the content of foods or drinks that inhibit iron absorption, e.g. to avoid tea with main meals and to reduce the intake of foods containing iron-binding phenolic compounds, such as certain vegetables or spices. Similarly, a reduction in intake of foods with a high phytate content, or the application of improved techniques in the milling of cereals, would increase iron absorption. Considering the marked effects on the bioavailability of dietary iron even by minor components in the diet, it is reasonable to predict that feasible and effective methods could be developed to improve the diet. Systematic research in this area is required, and more effective nutritional information and education are then needed. Food education combined with agricultural and other information programmes will probably be the main basis for the long-term improvement of iron nutrition in developing countries. In some countries, this may be the only strategy available at present.

The situation is quite different in developed countries. Iron supplementation is nowadays given mainly to pregnant women. The distribution of iron requirements in menstruating women is very skewed. It would therefore seem reasonable to give iron tablets to women with the highest requirements, rather than trying to improve the diet for the whole population. The problem, however, is that women with heavier menstrual losses and greater iron requirements are not aware of this fact and cannot be identified by simple methods.

Iron fortification is an adequate method to combat iron deficiency in developed countries. Important reasons are that the main problem is the lack of dietary iron and that the bioavailability of the dietary iron is usually rather good. This means that the bioavailability of the added fortification iron will also be good, provided that an iron compound is chosen that has a good potential bioavailability (solubility). Moreover, in developed countries adequate vehicles are available to carry the iron fortificant to the target groups in the population in suitable amounts. In western countries, iron fortification is mainly used for flour (bread, pasta products), other cereal products and infant foods. In this situation iron fortification will be the action of choice. A remaining problem is the rather poor bioavailability of most iron fortificants used today.

The improvement of nutritional information is paradoxically more urgent today than ever before. The nutritional requirements for iron, for example, are the same today as in earlier generations, but the energy requirements are much lower with our present lifestyle. More iron thus needs to be absorbed per unit energy, and several strategies need to be considered and used in parallel. Besides iron fortification, more information should be given about the importance of a suitable meal composition for iron nutrition. There are certainly arguments for a higher intake of dietary fibre but it is advisable to choose fibre components with a low phytate content such as fruits and vegetables. Dairy products are needed as a source of calcium, but should preferably not be included in the main meals providing most of the dietary iron. Tea and coffee should be limited to snacks, but should preferably not be taken with main meals. It is important to examine critically what dietary modifications are feasible and effective. It is a challenge for the scientific nutritional society to formulate simple, understandable and uniform messages about diet to the general public.

TREATMENT OF IRON DEFICIENCY

The cause of iron-deficiency anaemia may be purely nutritional, in that the diet cannot cover the physiological losses of the subject. In the individual patient, however, the possibility that there is a pathological cause, such as a tumour in the uterus or the gastrointestinal tract, must always be considered. Thus, in clinical practice the treatment of iron-deficiency anaemia usually has two components: treatment of the cause of iron deficiency and treatment of the deficiency.

To treat a patient with moderate iron-deficiency anaemia only by improving the diet would take a very long time – probably several years. A good diet is important for the prevention of iron deficiency, but is not sufficient to treat existing iron deficiency anaemia. Oral iron therapy is usually very effective if well absorbed iron tablets are given at a sufficient dose for a sufficiently long time. Motivation of the patient by explaining why and how the tablets should be taken is essential for effective treatment. Sometimes a

therapeutic failure is due to the poor properties of the iron tablet: the coating must be sufficiently good to prevent oxidation of the ferrous iron to ferric, but at the same time not too resistant to allow the tablets to disintegrate and be dissolved in the gastrointestinal tract.

Parenteral iron preparations can also be used. Because of their potentially more severe side effects and risks they should only be used in patients who cannot absorb iron due to a malabsorptive disease, in patients with inflammatory intestinal disorders and in patients with more marked side effects to oral iron, e.g. consistent nausea and epigastric pain which cannot be ameliorated by reducing the dose of oral iron. (Pregnancy, see separate section above.)

IRON OVERLOAD

The amount of storage iron in the body seldom exceeds 2000 mg – in fact, in women it seldom exceeds 400–500 mg and in men, 1500 mg. Increased amounts may occur by increased absorption from the intestines or by increased parenteral administration of iron given as parenteral iron preparations or as blood transfusions.

A higher intake of dietary iron will lead to increased absorption. However, as the amount of iron in store increases, the fraction of dietary iron absorbed will successively decrease. Moreover, the losses of iron from the body will increase due to the higher iron content of the desquamated cells. Therefore, in otherwise healthy subjects, a high dietary intake of iron will not lead to any organ damage due to a pathological accumulation of iron. The only 'nutritional' iron overload condition described in healthy people are in Bantu populations consuming large amounts of a special beer with a very high iron content, brewed in iron containers. Iron overload has also been observed in alcoholics consuming large amounts of wine with a high iron content.

Iron overload may also occur in patients who have certain chronic anaemias with an increased, ineffective erythropoiesis which induces an increased absorption of dietary iron. The best known condition of this type is thalassaemia major.

In idiopathic hereditary haemochromatosis, the absorption of dietary iron is increased, resulting in serious organ damage. For example, in the liver the iron overload may cause cirrhosis, in the pancreas diabetes, in the testis hypogonadism, and in the heart serious cardiac disturbances. The iron overload can be prevented by early prophylactic phlebotomy. It is therefore important to recognize this disorder at an early stage of its development before organ damage becomes clinically manifest. The prevalence of this recessively inherited disorder probably varies considerably between different geographical regions. A recent estimate based on analyses of random population samples in Sweden is about 1 in 1000 population (Hallberg et al 1989). Differences in the bioavailability or amount of dietary iron will probably only affect the prevalence of this disorder to a limited extent, but may influence the age at which the disease reaches such a state that it becomes clinically manifest and is detected.

ZINC

B. Sandström

The essentiality of zinc has been known for more than 100 years and its role in the normal growth of animals was demonstrated in rats and mice in the 1930s. Two of the pioneers in human zinc research, as in so many other nutrition research areas, were McCance and Widdowson. In the late 1930s and early 1940s they undertook a number of studies of zinc metabolism in man, of the fate of injected zinc and of the effects of white and brown bread on zinc absorption and balance (McCance & Widdowson 1942a, 1942b). For many years human nutritionists paid relatively little attention to zinc, assuming, in the absence of known signs of zinc deficiency, that present intakes were sufficient. In the late 1960s and early 1970s came the first reports of zinc-responsive growth failure in adolescent boys in the Nile Delta of Egypt and in rural Iran (Sandstead et al 1967, Halstead et al 1972). At the same time, advances in analytical techniques made the measurement of zinc in foods and tissues a routine procedure at many laboratories. The intense research of the last 15 years has led to a more extensive understanding of the biochemical roles of zinc than for any other of the trace elements, and to the identification of the clinical manifestations of severe zinc deficiency in man. However, despite this, we still do not understand the metabolic origin of the pathological changes in zinc deficiency, we lack diagnostic criteria for marginal deficiency, and we have a meagre scientific basis for setting recommendations for the dietary intake of zinc.

THE ROLES OF ZINC

The major biochemical roles of zinc are as a constituent of metalloenzymes and in stabilizing the structure of organic components and membranes. The first described zinc-containing enzyme was carbonic anhydrase, in 1940, and since then more than 200 different zinc enzymes have been identified in plant and animal tissue (Vallee & Galdes 1984). Alcohol dehydrogenase, superoxide dismutase, DNA-polymerase, RNA-polymerase, alkaline phosphatase and carboxypeptidase are all zinc metalloenzymes and examples can be found in each of the six IUB classes of enzymes. This means that zinc is involved in, for example, nucleic acid synthesis, protein digestion, protein synthesis, carbohydrate metabolism, dark adaptation, bone metabolism, oxygen transport and protection against free radical damage. In some of these enzymes zinc is present at the active site, e.g. acting as an electron acceptor; in others and in non-enzyme proteins the function of zinc is structural, as S-S bridges or cross-links between thiolates and imidazoles.

Bound zinc stabilizes the structures of RNA, DNA and ribosomes, and recent studies suggest that zinc affects normal chromatin restructuring and gene expression (Chesters 1989). Zinc also seems to have an important role in the structure and function of membranes (Bettger & O'Dell 1981).

Zinc is essential for the immune defence systems. A suboptimal zinc intake in experimental animals causes marked atrophy of the thymus, a reduction in leucocytes and in antibody-mediated, cell-mediated and delayed-type hypersensitivity responses (Fraker et al 1987).

ZINC METABOLISM

Absorption

The mechanisms for zinc absorption and the factors controlling it are poorly understood. Under the influence of enzymes and gastric juices, zinc is most likely released from the food matrix during digestion and associated with low-molecular weight ligands such as amino acids, peptides, organic acids and phosphates. The fate of these substances is probably of great importance for the degree of zinc absorption, as indicated by the observation that the absorption of zinc from aqueous solutions of zinc taken in the fasting state is 60–80% (Sandström et al 1985, Sandström & Cederblad 1987), while in the presence of food it can vary from 5% to 40% (Sandström 1989). Animal studies suggest that the mucosal uptake of zinc is carrier-mediated and occurs via several processes which can be both saturable and non-saturable (Coppen & Davis 1987).

Distribution of zinc in the body

Zinc is present in all the tissues and fluids of the body. Figure 12.4 gives a schematic presentation of the

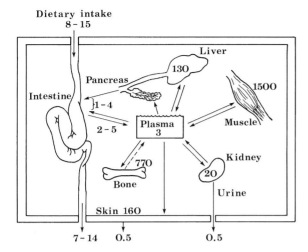

Fig. 12.4 Zinc metabolism in adult man. Intake, absorption, intestinal endogenous excretion and zinc losses via faeces, urine and skin are given in mg/day. Estimates of total zinc content (mg) of organs and tissues are indicated.

distribution and turnover of zinc. The total body content has been calculated as 2–3 g in an adult man, of which skeletal muscle accounts for approximately 60% and bone for about 30%. Zinc is a primarily intracellular ion and the concentrations in extracellular fluids are relatively low. Plasma zinc represents only about 0.1% of total body content, it has a rapid turnover and the levels appear to be under close homoeostatic control. The majority of zinc in plasma is bound to albumin acting as the transport vehicle. High concentrations of zinc are found in the choroid of the eye and in prostatic fluids.

The distribution of zinc between extracellular fluids, tissues and organs is affected by hormonal balance and stress situations. The liver probably plays an important role in this redistribution. The body seems to be dependent on a small pool of 'active' zinc and there is no 'store' in a conventional sense. Zinc in bone, which normally has a low turnover rate, can be mobilized in extreme cases, such as zinc deficiency during pregnancy (Hurley & Tao 1972). High intakes of zinc induce synthesis of metallothioneine, a small sulphur-containing protein that binds zinc and could represent an intracellular storage form (Richards & Cousins 1976). It has been suggested that metallothioneine is involved in the 'fine-tuning' of the intracellular levels of 'active' zinc.

Excretion of zinc

Zinc is lost from the body via the kidneys, the skin and the intestine (see Fig. 12.4). The intestine is the

major route of zinc excretion and zinc is lost via the digestive juices and in shed intestinal cells. Endogenous intestinal losses can be as high as 2–4 mg/day (Jackson et al 1984, Turnlund et al 1984, 1986, 1987, Wada et al 1985).

Approximately 0.5 mg of zinc/day is lost in the urine in healthy subjects. The majority of the primarily filtered zinc in the kidneys is reabsorbed and urinary excretion is unaffected by normal day-to-day variations in zinc intake. Starvation and muscle catabolism increase zinc losses in the urine and faeces (Jackson & Edwards 1982). Daily losses of zinc through the desquamation of skin, the outgrowth of hair and sweat are difficult to measure but have been estimated as 0.5 mg.

The prostatic fluids have a high concentration of zinc and an ejaculation of semen can contain up to 1 mg of zinc (Baer & King 1984). Zinc losses with menstruation are small (0.01 mg/day) (Greger & Buckley 1977).

Losses of zinc can be substantially increased in many diseases, for example, in inflammatory bowel disease intestinal losses can be large (Wolman et al 1979) and in kidney diseases and alcoholism large urinary losses have been reported (Lindeman et al 1978).

Homoeostasis

The tissue content of zinc is maintained over a wide range of dietary zinc intakes. This is made possible by changes in absorption as well as excretion. Figure 12.5 shows how the fractional absorption decreases and intestinal secretion increases when zinc intake is increased (Jackson et al 1984, Wada et al 1985). At a chronically low zinc intake, zinc absorption seems to be very efficient (59%–84%) (Jackson et al 1988). Urinary losses and losses via the skin also decrease at a low zinc intake (Hess et al 1977, Milne et al 1983).

INDICES OF ZINC STATUS

The homoeostatic regulation of zinc distribution and tissue concentration and the intracellular location of zinc make the assessment of zinc status difficult. So far, the only way to prove a poor zinc status is to give a zinc supplement and find a resulting biochemical or functional improvement, or the disappearance of clinical signs.

Circulating levels of zinc in plasma or serum are the most widely used indices of zinc status. Although plasma zinc is decreased in severe zinc deficiency, the levels can be affected by a number of conditions that are unrelated to zinc status. Infection, fever, or the intake of a protein-rich meal lower plasma zinc,

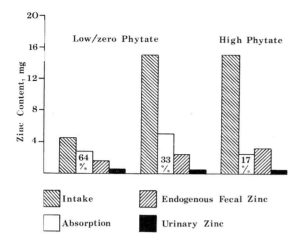

Fig. 12.5 Absorption, endogenous and urinary excretion of zinc at two levels of zinc intake and at a high (2.34 g) phytate intake. Data from Wada et al (1985) and Turnlund et al (1984).

whereas long-term fasting, contaminated test tubes and haemolysis give an analysed value that is higher than normal. Other biochemical indices used are the zinc levels in white blood cells, erythrocytes and hair, and the urinary excretion of zinc. Of the functional indices, the zinc tolerance test (Fickel et al 1986), taste acuity (Bales et al 1986) and dark adaptation (Sandström et al 1987) have been tested. None of these biochemical and functional measures has so far proven useful in identifying marginal zinc deficiency in man. The reason for this could be the notable feature of zinc deficiency that overt symptoms can occur with almost no reduction in the tissue concentration of zinc (Aggett et al 1983), and that the addition of zinc very rapidly improves the symptoms before any change in the tissue content. The detection of mild zinc deficiency is therefore at present not possible, as no reliable, sensitive index of zinc status is available.

A promising analytical development is a sensitive and rapid method to measure metallothioneine. In experimental animals the circulating levels of metallothioneine in plasma and the erythrocytes are correlated to tissue levels and to zinc status (Bremner et al 1987). Circulating metallothioneine levels are less sensitive than plasma zinc to infection and trauma, and might be useful for population surveys of zinc status.

ZINC DEFICIENCY

Severe zinc deficiency in man has been observed in an inborn error of zinc metabolism, acrodermatitis enteropathica (Moynahan 1974), in patients fed incomplete parenteral solutions (Kay et al 1976, Tucker et al 1976), in patients with Crohn's disease (McClain et al 1980) and occasionally in infants (Kuramoto et al 1986). The clinical features of zinc deficiency are circumoral and acral dermatitis, diarrhoea, alopecia and neuropsychiatric manifestations. Zinc-responsive night blindness has been observed in alcoholism and in patients with Crohn's disease (Morrison et al 1978). Failure to thrive, growth retardation, immune defects and delayed sexual maturation are also regarded as clinical manifestations of zinc deficiency.

Zinc deficiency is also a part of malnutrition. Skin ulcerations, reduced resistance to infection and growth failure are indications of zinc deficiency. Studies of Jamaican children recovering from malnutrition have shown that zinc status affects not only rate of growth but also the composition of synthesized tissue. Lean tissue synthesis is closely and positively related to dietary zinc intake (Golden & Golden 1985).

Long-term studies of marginal zinc intakes in Rhesus monkeys have provided important information about the possible consequences of zinc deficiency during pregnancy, infancy and early adolescence. These studies indicate that vitamin A metabolism, immune defence and skeletal maturation are especially sensitive to an insufficient zinc intake (Golub et al 1984a, Baly et al 1984, Leek et al 1988). An early sign of zinc deficiency in animals is a reduced feed intake leading to a reduced growth rate. This could be viewed as a useful adaptation to an inadequate zinc supply.

In experimental zinc depletion, healthy subjects with intake of an almost zinc-free diet for 5 weeks have shown signs of dermatitis, sore throat and immune defects (Baer & King 1984, Baer et al 1985). Changes in energy metabolism and decreased circulating levels of blood proteins have also been noted in studies of experimental diets with a low zinc content (5.5 mg/day) (Wada & King 1986). However, the values were still within the normal range and these observations and measurements can hardly be used for the evaluation of zinc status in an individual or a population.

A reduced growth rate is so far the only clearly demonstrated sign of mild zinc deficiency in man. Controlled zinc supplementation studies in infants and children in Colorado have shown a significantly greater weight increment in male infants after zinc supplementation (Walravens & Hambidge 1976, Walravens et al 1983). Supplementation was associated with an increase in energy and protein intake (Krebs et al 1984).

In the studies of Rhesus monkeys the zinc-deprived group had more complications of pregnancy than controls (Golub et al 1984b). Low maternal serum zinc levels in pregnant women have in some studies been associated with pregnancy complications (Jameson 1976, Simmer et al 1987, Lazebnik et al 1988). It has also been suggested that maternal leucocyte zinc at the start of third trimester could be used as a predictor of fetal growth retardation (Wells et al 1987). The association between indications of a low zinc status and pregnancy outcome is poorly understood, and it has not been possible to relate it to dietary zinc intake. Partly because of plasma expansion, plasma zinc levels are decreased in pregnancy and it is not clear when the levels are to be considered too low for a normal pregnancy. Zinc supplementation of 15–45 mg/day has so far failed to improve pregnancy outcome, except for a possible reduction in the incidence of a dysfunctional labour pattern (Kynast & Saling 1986) (for review see Swanson & King 1987).

ZINC IN FOOD SOURCES

Large variations in zinc content can be found between otherwise nutritionally similar food sources. Some examples of the relation between zinc and energy and protein contents are given in Table 12.6. These data indicate the variations in zinc intake that can arise from the selection of foods to cover energy needs. Other energy sources such as fats, oils, sugar and alcohol have a low zinc content.

In animal food sources, the fat content becomes one of the major determinants of the zinc content, as fat tissue contains much less zinc than muscle tissue. In general, dark red meat has a higher zinc content than white meat and fish muscle tissue has a lower zinc content than meat.

Cereals are the major source of energy and also of zinc in large parts of the world. The supply of zinc from cereals is dependent on the degree of refinement of the grain. Zinc is mainly located in the outer layer of the grain, and a low extraction rate means that the majority of the content of zinc as well as of other minerals is removed (Schroeder et al 1967). The content of zinc in vegetable foods is also dependent on variety, class and growing location. Up to ten fold variations in the zinc content of wheat has been reported, depending on the botanical variety (Davis et al 1984). Because of their high water contents, green leafy vegetables and fruits are only modest sources of zinc.

Food processing and preparation could also affect the zinc content of foods. Zinc from galvanized cook-

Table 12.6 Zinc contents of selected foods expressed on a raw wet weight basis and in relation to their protein and energy contents. Reproduced with permission from Sandström (1989)

	mg/g raw wet weight	mg/g protein	mg/MJ
Beef			
lean	43	0.21	8.3
fat	10	0.11	0.4
Pork			
lean	24	0.12	3.9
fat	4	0.06	0.1
Chicken			
light meat	7	0.03	1.4
dark meat	16	0.08	3.0
Fish, cod	4	0.02	1.2
Milk	3.5	0.11	1.3
Cheese, Cheddar type	40	0.15	2.4
Butter	1.5	–	0.05
Lentils	31	0.13	2.4
Wheat			
wholemeal	30	0.23	2.2
white	9	0.08	0.6
Maize (sweetcorn)	12	0.29	2.2
Rice (polished)	13	0.20	0.8
Potatoes	3	0.14	0.8
Yam	4	0.20	0.7
Coconut	5	0.16	0.3

ing utensils and water pipes was probably in former days an important additional source of zinc. On the other hand, leakages of up to 20% of the zinc content of food into cooking water or canning media have been observed (Meiners et al 1976, Schmitt & Weaver 1982).

ZINC INTAKE

The daily intake of zinc from diets typical of industrialized countries that are characteristically associated with high intakes of fat, refined sugar and animal protein, is approximately 10–12 mg or 1.0–1.4 mg/MJ (Spring et al 1979, Gibson & Schythes 1982, Sandstead et al 1982, Welsh & Marston 1982, Murphy & Calloway 1986). In the British Household Survey 1979 (Spring et al 1979), animal protein sources accounted for about two-thirds of the average intake of 9.1 mg of zinc (Fig. 12.6). A lower zinc intake 7 mg/day – is reported for a fish-based diet in areas around the Amazon (Shrimpton 1984), where signs of zinc deficiency in the population have also been observed.

Similar low intakes are also found for a population in Papau New Guinea (Ross et al 1986). A cereal-based unrefined diet can have a higher zinc intake.

Analyses of Indian foods have shown a zinc intake of 16 mg (1.4 mg/MJ) (Soman et al 1969) and calculations of rural Iranian diets give intakes of 19–22 mg/day (Maleki 1973).

DIETARY FACTORS AFFECTING ZINC ABSORPTION

No study has so far been able to find a correlation between dietary zinc intake and the indices of zinc status. This could be largely due to the insensitivity of zinc status indices, but could also be due to the fact that no attempt has been made to estimate the amount of zinc available in the diet. In contrast to the major components of the diet – fat, carbohydrates and protein – where 90–97% is absorbed, only a fraction of the total zinc content of the diet is taken up. Organic substances acting as ligands facilitating uptake, or as complexing agents reducing the solubility and absorption of zinc, and other trace elements competing with zinc for uptake sites and carriers, can lead to a large variation in fractional zinc absorption.

The way zinc is metabolized complicates studies of dietary zinc absorption in man. As indicated in Fig.12.4, unabsorbed endogenous intestinal excretion can account for a substantial part of what is found in faeces. Conventional approaches such as the metabolic balance technique require long periods on a constant diet before equilibrium is achieved (Schwartz et al 1986) and are not sensitive enough to identify factors affecting absorption, or to compare different diets. This technique can be improved by the use of stable zinc isotopes, and a limited number of such studies have been performed. With radioactive zinc isotopes it is possible to determine zinc absorption with a high degree of precision, and this technique also allows that systematic study of individual dietary factors. However, all isotope techniques require expensive analytical equipment and the knowledge about dietary zinc absorption is still limited.

A dietary factor known to impair zinc absorption in man is myoinositol hexaphosphate, alias phytic acid, in wholegrain cereals, legumes and other vegetables. At the pH values encountered in foods, phytic acid will be strongly negatively charged and will have a strong potential to bind positively charged molecules such as zinc. The presence of phytic acid is the most likely reason for the low absorption of zinc observed from wholemeal bread and soy formula (Sandström et al 1980, Sandström et al 1983, Nävert et al 1985, Lönnerdal et al 1984). The reduction of the phytic acid content of bread by long-term fermentation and the removal of phytic acid in soy formula increase zinc absorption (Nävert et al 1985, Lönnerdal et al 1988).

The absorption of zinc from a phytic-acid containing meal can also be improved by increasing the animal protein content of the diet (Sandström et al 1980, 1989). Protein seems to act as an 'antiphytate' agent, which could be through a protein–phytic acid interaction not including zinc, or through an increased solubility and facilitation of zinc absorption by peptides and amino acids liberated during digestion. In the typical modern diet, with a high degree of refinement of vegetable foods and a reasonable intake of animal protein, the phytic acid content is low and not likely to have significant effects on zinc absorption. The early studies by McCance & Widdowson (1942a) showed that zinc balance can be maintained on a mixed diet with as much as 50% of the energy as brown bread.

A diet almost entirely based on unleavened wholemeal bread with a high phytic acid content and low intake of animal proteins has been suggested as a major factor in the growth failure of adolescent boys in Egypt and Iran (Sandstead et al 1967, Halstead et al 1972). This type of diet can be assumed to give a low zinc absorption, and probably also increases endogenous losses of zinc, as shown in Fig. 12.5. Contributing factors were geophagia, which can be assumed further to reduce zinc absorption, and large zinc losses due to intestinal parasitic infections.

Elements with similar physicochemical properties may compete for binding sites and transport mechanisms. The zinc ion, with its 10 outer electrons in d

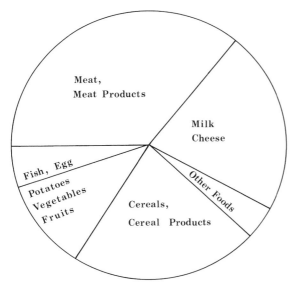

Fig. 12.6   Contribution of food groups to zinc intake in the British Household Survey 1979 (Spring et al 1979)

orbital forms a tetrahedral sp^3 chelate configuration and prefers a coordination number of four. These parameters are identical to those for Cu^+ and Cd^{2+}, and interactions between these elements have been shown in model experiments. In the human diet, the level of zinc is always higher than that of copper and cadmium, and in practice these elements are not likely to affect zinc absorption. Radio-zinc studies have shown that tin reduces zinc absorption (Valberg et al 1984). The level of tin normally found in the human diet is low and unlikely to interfere with zinc absorption. Food in unlacquered cans, however, can contain appreciable amounts of tin.

In aqueous solutions of iron and zinc, iron decreases zinc absorption (Valberg et al 1984, Sandström et al 1985). Iron added to a meal had no effect on zinc absorption, indicating that iron enrichment, to the extent that it is used in food, has no deleterious effects on zinc absorption. However, pharmacological doses of iron during pregnancy could adversely affect zinc status (Hambidge et al 1983).

A number of other nutrients or substances found in food have, in model experiments, been shown to affect zinc absorption (for review, see Sandström Lönnerdal 1989). The nutritional significance of most of these substances when occurring in human diets is, however, uncertain.

The zinc content of the diet is an important factor for the amount of zinc that is absorbed. The decrease in fractional absorption with increasing intake is not proportional to the increase, and a larger amount is absorbed from a higher intake (see Fig. 12.5).

In Fig. 12.7 some examples of fractional and total zinc absorption from single meals are given, illustrating the effect of zinc content and of the composition of the meal. For animal-protein based meals the total zinc content is a good indicator of the amount of absorbable zinc. The knowledge about zinc availability in entirely or mainly vegetarian meals is limited. Diets based on legumes seem comparable to animal protein diets, with similar zinc and protein contents despite the presence of inositol phosphates (Sandström et al 1989). Unrefined cereal-based diets present the largest risk for low zinc absorption. For the evaluation of these diets it is important to know not only the amount of inositol hexaphosphate, but also of lower inositol phosphates which can be formed during the preparation of the diet. It has been shown that the inositol pentaphosphate form has a zinc-depressing effect similar to the hexa form, while lower inositol phosphates do not affect zinc absorption (Sandström & Sandberg 1992).

ZINC REQUIREMENT

The 'true' physiological requirement of zinc, i.e. the amount that has to be absorbed to replace endogenous losses, to provide zinc for tissue synthesis and during growth and for milk secretion, is dependent on the age and physiological status of the subject. This requirement differs from the dietary requirement of

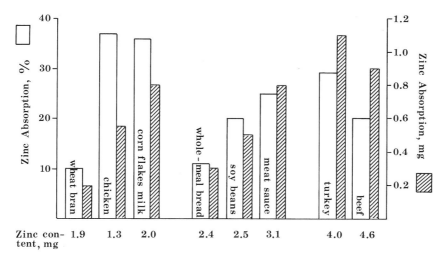

Fig. 12.7 Examples of fractional and total zinc absorption from composite meals. The major components are indicated in the bars. Data from Sandström & Cederblad (1980), Nävert et al (1985), Valberg et al (1984), Lykken et al (1986), Sandström et al (1987), Gallaher et al (1988).

zinc, that has to take into account the composition of the diet, which influences absorption and utilization.

Physiological requirement

Adults

The endogenous losses of zinc have been measured in studies using zinc-free diets, and on a normal zinc intake by the use of stable zinc isotopes (Hess et al 1977, Turnlund et al 1982, 1984, 1986, Swanson et al 1983, Wada et al 1985). In healthy adults consuming a typical industrial refined diet providing 10–12 mg of zinc, the endogenous losses of zinc are approximately 2.5 mg/day. Elderly people over 65 years of age consuming a similar diet require about 1.5 mg/day. The intake of phytic acid increases intestinal losses of zinc (see Fig. 12.5) and it has been estimated that individuals consuming vegetarian diets need as much as 4 mg of absorbed zinc per day.

Pregnancy

The total zinc requirement for gestation, for the fetus, placental tissue, amniotic fluid, uterine and mammary tissue and maternal blood have been estiamted at 100 mg (Swanson & King 1987). The rate of tissue gain thus gives a daily requirement of zinc during the last part of pregnancy of approximately 0.7 mg. If the same endogenous losses are assumed during pregnancy, the total requirement for tissue growth and replacement of losses is 3.2 mg/day towards the end of pregnancy.

Lactation

The concentration of zinc in human milk drops during lactation from 2.5 µg/ml in the first month to approximately 1 µg/ml after 3 months. Assuming a total milk volume of 750 ml/day, this gives an additional zinc requirement of 2 mg/day in early lactation and approximately 0.7mg/day after 3 months (Krebs et al 1985). Larger milk volumes and higher zinc concentrations have been reported which, especially in early lactation, could give a much higher requirement of zinc.

Infants

The estimated zinc requirement for growth is about 175 µg/kg body weight/day in the first month and decreases to about 30 µg/kg/day at 9–12 months (Krebs & Hambidge 1986). The endogenous losses of zinc are related to body size and the total requirement of zinc in infants has been estimated at 1–1.2 mg/day in males and 0.9–1.05 mg/day in females.

Dietary zinc requirement and recommended allowances

Knowledge about the dietary factors affecting the absorption and utilization of zinc and the net effect of these factors is still limited. However, from the available studies in adults using stable or radioactive zinc isotopes, it can be estimated that from a refined diet typical for industrialized countries 20–40% is absorbed depending on zinc content. From wholegrain-cereal based diets 10–15% absorption has been reported. The absorption of zinc in periods of increased zinc requirement such as infancy, adolescence, pregnancy and lactation is essentially unknown.

Earlier dietary recommendations for zinc intake in adults have varied from 8 mg/day in Czechoslovakia to 12–16 mg in Australia (IUNS 1983). Many countries have adopted the 15 mg recommendation of the USA (NRC 1980); this figure was based on results from zinc balance studies and on a calculated turnover rate of body zinc at 6 mg/day allowing for 40% absorption. The USA recommendations published in 1989 use the factorial approach and assume an average requirement for absorbed zinc of 2.5 mg/day and an absorptive efficiency of 20%, resulting in a recommended intake of 15 mg for men and 12 mg for women. The UK panel of 1991 assumed slightly lower obligatory endogenous losses – 2.2 mg for men and 1.6 mg for women – but a higher absorptive efficiency of 30%. These estimates give RNIs of 9.5 mg for men and 7.0 mg for women.

Further studies of zinc utilization from and zinc metabolism at different diets and intake levels are essential before the zinc requirement can be adequately defined. It is, however, obvious that dietary zinc recommendations have to take into consideration the composition of the diet and not only the total zinc content.

ZINC TOXICITY

Zinc has a relatively low order of toxicity compared to most other trace elements. Only a few occasions of acute zinc poisoning have been reported. Nausea, vomiting, diarrhoea and fever were observed after intake of food and beverages contaminated with zinc from galvanized containers, and lethargy was observed after the ingestion of 4–8 g of zinc (Brown et al 1964, Murphy 1970, Gallery et al 1972). Long-term zinc intakes higher than requirement could, however, interact with the metabolism of other trace elements. Copper seems to be especially sensitive to high zinc doses. Low copper and ceruloplasmin levels and anaemia have been observed after high doses of zinc (Porter et al 1977, Patterson et al 1985) and at an intake of 50 mg/day effects on both iron and copper status indices have been reported (Yadrick et al 1989). Excessive zinc intake also impairs immune responses (Chandra 1984). These observations indicate that there is reason to be concerned about the safety of consuming zinc supplements over long periods.

SUMMARY

The role of zinc in cell replication and growth and its stabilizing function in organic compounds, including membranes, makes it a key nutrient for optimal function and health. In severe deficiency a number of organs and functions are affected, whereas the functional consequences of a marginal zinc deficiency is less well understood. Growth impairment in male infants is so far the only clearly demonstrated sign of mild zinc deficiency in an otherwise 'healthy' population. The body has efficient mechanisms for maintaining tissue zinc content constant over a large range of intakes, and it seems possible to adapt to relatively low zinc intakes without loss of function. In modern society the typical refined diet with a high content of fat and sugar gives a low zinc intake, especially in subjects with a low energy requirement. In other parts of the world the diet can contain larger amounts of zinc but, due to the presence of complexing agents and a reduced availability of zinc, the intake can be insufficient for periods of high requirement, such as during adolescent growth.

OTHER TRACE ELEMENTS

P. J. Aggett

There is a wide range of trace elements which have become recognized as essential when careful animal growth studies are performed with very purified diets. These experiments are difficult to design and even more difficult to do, because the environment is so easily contaminated with dust or metal objects which provide enough of the trace element to avoid the deficiency. This means that in practice some of these deficiencies are rare, and only arise in humans if children or adult patients are on a very odd diet or fed intravenously with purified nutrients from which the trace element has been omitted. Rarely deficiency also occurs because of genetic disorders involving the

metabolism or function of the mineral. Table 12.7 lists the essential trace elements and those where possible deficiencies may occur.

Mammals have evolved complex and often poorly understood methods for controlling the uptake and/or excretion of the principal trace elements (see this chapter on iron and zinc, and Chapter 36 on Thyroid diseases and iodine.). This problem differs from that of vitamins, which are either readily stored (e.g. the fat-soluble forms) or metabolized and excreted (e.g. the water-soluble forms).

COPPER

Copper (Cu) is widely distributed in the body, and is incorporated into organic complexes, e.g. metalloprotein enzymes which are involved in such fundamental functions as the cytochrome chain of mitochondrial oxidation, the synthesis of the complex proteins of collagenous tissues in the skeleton and blood vessels, and in the synthesis of neurotransmitters (e.g. noradrenaline) and neuropeptides (e.g. encephalins). Table 12.8 lists some of the principal cuproenzymes in the body. The adult contains only 80 mg of Cu (range 50–120 mg); 40% is located in muscle, 15% in the liver, 10% in the brain and 6% in the blood. Most of the red cell Cu is in the metalloenzyme superoxide dismutase, which is involved in free radical scavenging. In plasma, 60% of Cu is bound to caeruloplasmin, 30% to transcuprein and the rest to albumin and amino acids.

Adults consume 1–2 mg of Cu daily. Good dietary sources are shellfish, legumes, wholegrain cereals, nuts and liver. Particularly high Cu concentrations are found in pig's liver because of the current practice of adding high concentrations of Cu to pig feed to alter the intestinal microflora and perhaps improve the growth of the animal. Copper piping used for water distribution can add 0.1 µg/day to intakes in hard water areas, but 10 times this amount in acid and soft water conditions. Cu is absorbed in the small intestine, probably by two transport systems which extract between 35% and 70% of dietary Cu from low-molecular weight organic complexes in the lumen (Cousins 1985); the sulphate and nitrate forms of Cu are readily absorbed, uptake from Cu carbonate depends on its being solubilized by gastric acid but Cu sulphide and porphyrin are unavailable. The body controls the circulating Cu concentration by altering the biliary secretion of a Cu complex: 0.5–1.5 mg of Cu is lost by this route daily (Brewer et al 1991) since the biliary complex is poorly reabsorbed. Caeruloplasmin and transcuprein transport Cu around the body .

Table 12.7 Trace elements: essential and possible essential minerals

Element	Function	Deficiency features
Essential		
Copper	Metalloenzymes (see Table 12.8)	See Table 12.9
Selenium	In glutathione peroxidase and type I deiodinase	Cardiomyopathy: possible involvement in iodine deficiency disorders
Manganese	Metalloenzymes and enzyme activated	Uncertain human effects
Molybdenum	Cofactor in three oxidases	Abnormal sulphur metabolism, developmental and neurological abnormalities
Chromium	Insulin sensitivity	Glucose intolerance
Possibly essential		
Fluoride	Involved in bone mineralization	Exacerbates dental caries
Arsenic	Methionine and polyamine metabolism	Growth retardation and reproductive failure. Perinatal mortality increased
Boron	Membrane signal transduction	Growth retardation, fragile bones, interaction with systemic metabolism of Mg, Ca and P
Bromine	Can substitute for chloride and iodide	Insomnia in renal dialysis patients
Lithium		Depressed growth and fertility
Nickel	Metabolism of branched chain amino acids and propionic acid	Depressed growth and reproduction, defective haematopoiesis, altered metabolism of vitamin B_{12}, iron, zinc and copper
Silicon	Cross-linking of glycoproteins and induction of calcification	Impaired collagen formation and endochrondrial ossification
Vanadium	Regulation of phosphoryl transfer enzymes and receptor phosphorylation	Neurological, skeletal and thyroid defects

The importance of caeruloplasmin is uncertain despite its many oxidase and free radical scavenging properties, because people with a genetically low concentration of caeruloplasmin appear to suffer no defects. High intakes of Cu induce the protein metallothionein in the intestinal epithelium; this binds Cu and blocks its further uptake. Zinc and iron block

Cu absorption and can induce Cu deficiency; excessive mineral supplements can therefore be dangerous and can lead to deficiencies. The intestinal uptake of Cu increases, however, when Cu intakes fall.

Copper deficiency

The symptoms and signs of deficiency are summarized in Table 12.9 (Danks 1988). Experimentally, reduced metabolic activity has been found in the brain and heart; cardiac slowing and altered conduction of the neuromuscular control of the heart's rhythms has been defined together with heart muscular hypertrophy; other effects, not necessarily found in humans, include degeneration of the exocrine pancreas, and a defective secretion of thyroxine in response to TSH stimulation.

Copper deficiency is seen most frequently in preterm infants, in term infants who have been inappropriately fed on unmodified cow's milk, and in children with protracted diarrhoea (Castillo-Duran et al 1988). Children recovering from malnutrition are also often deficient: Cu supplementation (1.25 μmol (80 μg)/kg body weight daily) reduces the rate of infections and maintains plasma concentrations of Cu (Castillo-Duran 1983). Parenteral nutrition, with solutions

Table 12.8 The principal mammalian cuproenzyme activities (see O'Dell 1990)

Cytochrome C oxidase	Mitochondrial; requires iron; oxidative phosphorylation
Superoxide dismutase	Cytosolic antioxidant: $2O_2 + H_2O \rightarrow H_2O_2 + O_2$
Dopamine-β-hydroxylase	Synthesis of adrenaline and noradrenaline
Tyrosinase	Tyrosine → dopa → dopaquinone in pigment production in choroid and epidermis
Uricase	Renal and hepatic metabolism of uric acid
Lysyl oxidase (and related enzymes)	Condensation of amino acids → cross-links of elastin and collagen
Amine oxidases	Plasma and connective tissues
Caeruloplasmin	Multiple oxidase activities
Thiol oxidase	Formation of disulphide linkages

Table 12.9 Clinical features of copper deficiency (Danks 1988)

Babies fail to thrive; feed poorly
Oedema with low serum albumin
Anaemia with altered iron metabolism and bone marrow changes
Impaired immunity with low neutrophil count
Skeletal changes numerous with fractures and generalized osteoporosis
Herniae and tortuous dilated blood vessels from collagen and elastin cross-linking defects
Hair and skin depigmentation, with steely, uncrimped hair

which provide inadequate amounts of Cu, can also be a risk for both children and adults (Shike et al 1981). Menkes' syndrome is an X-linked autosomal defect in the intracellular metabolism of copper which is manifested by features of Cu deficiency despite there being a systemic excess of the metal. The principal features of Menkes' syndrome are abnormal hair, failure to thrive, progressive cerebral degeneration, loss of skin and hair pigmentation, thrombosis and arterial rupture, and hypothermia. Hypothermia is evident soon after birth, and growth retardation, with poor mental development and convulsions, occurs from 3 months of age onwards (Chapter 42).

The occurrence of dietary Cu deficiency in adults is less well documented, but it has been proposed that low intakes may be atherogenic, impair cardiac function and cause abnormal heart rhythms, perhaps secondary to the defective metabolism of catecholamines and encephalins. Copper-responsive increases in plasma LDL cholesterol, decreases in HDL cholesterol, electrocardiographic and rhythmic changes have been seen in adults on experimental intakes of 0.7–1.0 mg/day for 4 weeks or more, but some of these abnormalities may have arisen from the diets used, which were often very unusual in composition (Reiser et al 1985). On more customary diets there were no observed changes in plasma lipids, cardiac rhythm or electrical conductivity, or caeruloplasma changes in men on intakes of 0.79 mg/day for 42 days (Turnlund et al 1989). For adults on parenteral nutrition, 0.3 mg/day is probably adequate (Shike et al 1981).

Copper excess

Copper toxicity arises from the deliberate ingestion of copper salts, or accidentally from contamination of water and drinks. In acute toxicity the gastrointestinal tract is affected with vomitting and diarrhoea. Variable degrees of intravascular haemolysis occur, hepato-cellular necrosis and renal tubular failure result, and death may ensue.

With chronic exposure, Cu accumulates in the liver and toxicity is insidious. Eventually hepatic necrosis or cirrhosis with liver failure develops. Some infants and young children, at least, are particularly vulnerable. Indian childhood cirrhosis, which presents at 1–3 years of age, possibly results from the ingestion of milks which have been stored or heated in copper or brass utensils (Bhave et al 1992). A similar syndrome in western infants may arise from the consumption of feeds which have been prepared from acidic well water which has leached copper from pipes (Spitalny et al 1984, Müller-Hocker et al 1988).

Wilson's disease (hepatolenticular degeneration) is an autosomal recessive defect in Cu metabolism with excessive accumulation of hepatic Cu. Despite substantial increases in tissue Cu concentrations, the biliary excretion of Cu is reduced in Wilson's disease. Copper accumulating in the liver, eye, brain and kidneys accounts for most of the pathological changes. Acute or chronic liver failure may occur with cirrhosis in children and adolescents, and gallstones may also occur at this age. Cerebellar changes begin between 12 and 30 years, with deteriorating mental function and spasticity. Behavioural changes and psychosis are also common. The Cu deposited in the eyes produces the characteristic Kayser–Fleischer rings of greenish or golden-brown pigment in the cornea; this is found in the neurological but not necessarily in the liver-affected cases. Chronic haemolysis is common, probably because of the increased oxidative stress induced in the erythrocytes by the excess Cu. Proximal renal tubular abnormalities occur, with excess excretion of amino acids, glucose, uric acid, phosphate, calcium and proteins. Almost all patients develop bone abnormalities with osteoporosis, fractures, bone cysts and rickets in children being the commonest features.

Assessing copper status

This is usually assessed by measuring plasma Cu concentrations. Plasma or serum Cu ranges from 0.8 to 1.2 µg/ml, and female levels are 10% higher than males. Plasma Cu is increased threefold in late pregnancy and in women taking oestrogen-based oral contraceptives. It also raises during the acute-phase response to stress as caeruloplasmin concentrations increase. A Cu level of <0.8 µg/ml is abnormal and low levels of caeruloplasmin (180–400 mg/l), urinary Cu (32–64 µg/24 h) and hair Cu (10–20 µg/g) are also found in very deficient subjects. A fall in the concentration of erythrocte superoxide dismutase (0.47 ± 0.067 mg/mg haemoglobin) seems a more sensitive test of mild Cu deficiency, and fall in the neutrophil count may also be indicative of a marginally low Cu status. In chronic Cu toxicity, plasma levels of Cu and caeruloplasma may exceed the reference levels indicated.

Copper requirements

This has been considered in some detail by Mills (1991). The adult band requirement is probably about 0.6 mg/day for women and 0.7 mg/day (13 mg/kg) for men. The recommended nutritional intake (RNI) on this basis has been set at 17 µg/kg/day (see Appendix 2). The USA considered the requirements so uncertain that they simply considered 1.5–3.0 mg Cu/day as a likely safe and adequate range of Cu intakes in adults. In the full-term baby, liver Cu stores are, at 8 mg, probably adequate for the first 1–2 months of life. Estimates based on the need to maintain these levels at 1.3 µg/kg during growth allow for some potential endogenous loss of Cu, and assuming a 50% efficiency of absorption led the UK Panel to set RNIs at different levels during the first year of life depending on the growth rate. Since by 1 year of age the RNI for Cu had fallen from 47 to 36 µg/kg/day, the RNI for children was then interpolated to take account of declining growth needs up to the adult values (see Appendix 2). Adaptive changes in Cu homoeostasis were presumed to be capable of accommodating the needs of pregnancy, but 0.38 mg/day was added for lactating mothers, who secrete about 0.22 mg of Cu/day in their milk.

SELENIUM

Selenium (Se), as a selenocysteine residue, is essential for at least two mammalian oxidase enzymes. The cytosolic antioxidant enzyme glutathione peroxidase uses glutathione to reduce a variety of organic hydroperoxides (hydrogen peroxide, hydroperoxides of sterol, steroids, prostaglandins, free fatty acids, proteins and nucleic acids) to the corresponding alcohol (Levander 1987, Sunde 1990). Once reduced glutathione has provided the H (protons) to convert hydrogen peroxide to water with the help of glutathione peroxidase, then the reduced glutathione is regenerated in the cell by glutathione reductase and NADPH produced by the glucose monophosphate shunt. Glutathione peroxidase is found throughout the body but its concentration is readily monitored in the erythrocytes. Without glutathione peroxidase the

ability of cells to cope with oxidative stress is impaired, although a variety of other antioxidants is also available to the cell. Hepatic microsomal type 1 iodothyronine 5'-deiodinase (Arthur et al 1990, Behne et al 1990) has been found in rats, and raises the possibility that Se deprivation may influence systemic responses to marginal iodine intakes in humans. Another selenoprotein may be essential for normal sperm morphology and viability (Watanabe & Endo 1991).

In the plasma, most Se is associated with α-2 and β-globulins, and with glycoproteins, amongst which selenoprotein P may be involved specifically with Se transport (Motchnik & Tappel 1990); less than 2% exists as glutathionine peroxidase (GSHpx).

The total body content of Se (3–30 mg) varies according to the geochemical environment and dietary intakes. Customary adult daily intakes of Se vary between 20 and 300 µg according to the Se content of the soil from which the foods are derived. Good sources of Se are cereal grains, meat and fish (Levander 1987). In the People's Republic of China, dietary intakes range from 11 to 5000 µg/day, at which extremes deficiency and toxicity syndromes occur (Yang et al 1988). However, in New Zealand and Finland intakes of 15–40 µg/day have not been associated with disease although Se-responsive biochemical alterations, such as suboptimal whole-blood GSHpx activity, are found: peak GSHpx activity occurs with whole-blood Se concentrations of about 100 µg/1 (Robinson 1988, Casey 1988).

Se is present in foods mainly as selenomethionine and selenocysteine. Selenoamino acids are probably absorbed by similar energy-dependent and sodium co-transport mechanisms to their sulphur analogues. Although the bioavailability of inorganic Se is less than that of organic forms, this is probably of little practical significance because all the usual dietary forms of Se are absorbed efficiently.

Two Se pools exist in tissues. The biologically active pool of Se depends on selenocysteine, which can be synthesized endogenously from inorganic Se and serine. The other pool is selenomethionine in protein. This pool is subject to factors influencing methionine metabolism, and its constituent Se is not necessarily available for Se-dependent processes. For example, when methionine intake is limited, selenomethionine is used as methionine even if there is a concomitant Se deficiency. However, if methionine supply is adequate, Se released from degraded selenomethionine is then available to contribute to the active Se pool.

Systemically selenoamino acids can be degraded to yield amino acid residues and selenite. Inorganic Se anions are sequentially reduced from selenate via selenite to selenide by glutathione reductase systems, possibly including those in erythrocytes. The homoeostasis of Se is mediated usually by adjustments in Se catabolism, with the excretion of various reduced and methylated derivatives (e.g. trimethylselonium) in the urine. At excessive intakes dimethylselenide is produced which, when exhaled, has a characteristic garlic odour (Sunde 1990, Levander 1987).

Selenium deficiency

In man, the most striking Se-responsive syndrome is that of Keshan's desease, which is an Se-responsive cardiomyopathy that predominantly affects children, young adolescents and young women in the People's Republic of China: populations with intakes of less than 12 µg/day are at risk, whereas those with intakes of 19 µg are not (Chen et al 1980, Yang et al 1988).

Keshan's disease is found particualrly in areas where geochemical analyses show low Se levels in the soil: this leads to low Se levels in staple cereals and in samples of blood, hair and other tissues taken from populations living in these areas. Nevertheless, other factors, e.g. the seasonal swings in the development of heart failure, are unexplained.

A virus infection may promote the deficiency syndrome, as may low intakes of vitamin E, proteins, methionine and other trace elements. Excess toxin intake may also be involved. Clinically, Keshan's disease is classified into four types based on the severity, i.e. acute, subacute, chronic and insidious. The heart muscle shows extensive damage, particularly to the mitochondria, and with enzyme leakage there is clear evidence of cardiac and skeletal muscular damage as the plasma creatine kinase increases. Congestive cardiomyopathy, with low Se levels, has also been reported in patients receiving total parenteral nutrition. In such patients, less severe deficiencies involving skeletal myopathy with increased plasma creatinine kinase activities, macrocytosis and lightening of the skin and hair pigmentation, have also been documented, as has an increased degree of haemolytic sensitivity to peroxide of the red cells in vitro. The latter is the only clear evidence of the metabolic effects of significantly reduced GSHpx activity; similar changes have been reported in a child with undernutrition (Mathias & Jackson 1982). Se deficiency (in animal models) has been associated with defective microsomal oxidation of xenobiotics and with disturbed cellular immune funtion (Dhur et al 1990).

Kashin–Beck disease is an osteoarthritic condition involving severe joint deformity which afflicts children 5–13 years of age living in different areas of the (former) Soviet Union and China. Cartilaginous degeneration is prominent, and it has been suggested as another form of Se deficiency (Yang et al 1988). The involvement of Se in this syndrome and its mechanism of action still has to be established.

Selenium status and chronic diseases

States of mild to moderate Se deficiency have been proposed as contributing to a large number of diseases, e.g. cardiovascular disease, infertility, ageing, eye disease (e.g. cataract formation) and macular degeneration, diabetic retinopathy and cancer. In none of these has a firm link been established, although the potential involvement of a mild impairment in antioxidant activity with reduced glutathione peroxidase levels cannot be discounted. Thus, low Se states have been associated with platelet aggregability and prospective studies have also suggested an increased risk of stroke and coronary heart disease in subjects with low serum Se (Virtamo et al 1985). Although substantial evidence suggests that Se supplementation can decrease cancer incidence, in a variety of rodent studies of carcinogenesis the human studies provide conflicting evidence. It seems clear that Se status does not play a significant role in the development of breast cancer, but Se's potential role in modulating the risk of alcohol and smoking-related tumours of the oesophagus and lung is unclear (Willett et al 1991).

Assessing selenium status

Selenium concentrations in plasma and red cells fall as Se intake is lowered, but plasma concentrations, which change more rapidly, do not necessarily reflect tissue Se concentrations (Levander 1987). The enzymatic activity of red-cell glutathione peroxidase (GSHpx) is a valid index of Se in populations or individuals with a low Se intake, and is easier to measure than Se itself. At higher Se intakes, 55–65% of dietary Se continues to be absorbed, but urinary Se output rises and blood and tissue Se levels, as well as GSHpx activities, reach a plateau (Diplock & Chaudhry 1988).

Selenium requirements

Balance studies are of little value in assessing Se requirements because of the metabolic adaptation to changing intakes (Levander 1987). Graded supplementation studies of Chinese men on low Se intakes have been used in conjuction with GSHpx measurements to assess the intake at which plateau activities are achieved. Adjustments for body weight and individual variation led the USA to recommend 70 and 55 µg/day for adults. British RNI values are little different (see Appendix 2). The USA recommends an extra 10 µg of Se/day during pregnancy, but the UK does not because of the adaptive changes in pregnancy. Recommendations for children are extrapolated from adult data, with infant RNI being set to take account of a growth requirement of 0.2 µg of Se/kg weight gain.

Selenium excess

Severe selenosis at dietary intakes of 3.2–6.7 mg/day (Yang et al 1988) presents with malodorous breath, an erythematous bullous and intensely itchy dermatitis, dystrophic nails, dry brittle hair, alopecia and neurological abnormalities involving neuropathies with paraesthesia, paralysis and hemiplegia. Mottled tooth enamel and caries are endemic in affected areas.

MANGANESE

Manganese (Mn) was shown to be essential for the growth reproduction of rodents in 1931 and Mn deficiency was later found to be a practical problem in the poultry and pig industries. Only occasional individuals have been found with Mn deficiency. The average human contains 10–20 mg, a quarter of which is found in bone. Manganese cannot be stored, but functions as a key constituent of metalloenzymes and as an enzyme activator IV. Mn is a component of arginase, pyruvate carboxylase and mitochondrial superoxide dismutase. It is also needed for various hydrolase, kinase, decarboxylase and phosphotransferase activities, and for glutamine synthetase activity. Phosphoenol pyruvate carboxylase, prolidase and glycosyl transferases specifically require Mn, otherwise in-vivo activating roles may be more dependent on magnesium (Hurley & Keen 1987).

Mn is particularly abundant in vegetable-based diets and beverages such as tea, and it would seem that current population intake is adequate even for non-drinkers of tea. Most daily intakes are 2.0–3.0 mg/day but some achieve intakes of 8.3 mg daily. Mn absorption occurs throughout the small intestine but only about 10% of dietary Mn is absorbed. This fractional absorption rate increases at low intakes and renal conservation of the metal also occurs. High levels of dietary calcium, phosphorus and phytate impair the intestinal uptake of the element, but this is probably insignificant because as yet no well documented case of human Mn deficiency has been reported. Neonatal absorption rates are higher than adults and there may be special transport mechanisms controlling uptake. The overall control of body Mn seems to be by variations in the biliary excretion of Mn. Mn is also found in intestinal and pancreatic secretions.

Manganese deficiency

Mn-deprived animals produce numerous abnormalities in their offspring, with congenital irreversible ataxia as a prominent feature. This arises from the improved development of the calcified otoliths in the inner ear, which are responsible for maintaining balance. Growth retardation and impaired skeletal development are also prominent features, with bowed shorter long bones and many cartilaginous problems leading to joint abnormalities and displaced tendons. Pancreatic damage may explain the impaired insulin secretion and glucose intolerance. Fat accumulation in the liver and kidneys may also occur with a low serum cholesterol, particularly a low HDL cholesterol (Hurley & Keen 1987).

One possible human case of Mn deficiency has been described. This was a man who was being fed an experimental diet designed to induce vitamin K deficiency. The volunteer lost weight, his serum concentrations of cholesterol, triglycerides and phospholipids fell and his prolonged prothrombin time did not respond to vitamin K supplements. All these features responded rapidly when a normal diet was supplied. Only retrospectively was it realized that Mn had been omitted from the experimental diet (Doisey 1972). In a systematic study, men fed a low-Mn diet (0.01 mg/day) developed an evanescent skin rash and hypocholesterolaemia; however, neither feature responded unequivocally to Mn repletion (Friedman et al 1987).

Interest in possible Mn deprivation in humans has been stimulated by reports of Mn-responsive carbohydrate intolerance, and either reduced Mn concentrations in the hair of some mothers whose babies had congenital abnormalities or in the blood or hair, or both, of children with skeletal abnormalities, osteoporosis and non-traumatic epilepsy, and in those on synthetic diets (Hurley & Keen 1987, Anonymous 1988).

Manganese excess

Mineworkers in Chile exposed to Mn ore dust developed – possibly as a result of inhalation rather than ingestion – 'manganic madness', manifested by psychosis, hallucinations and extrapyramidal damage with features of Parkinsonism. Mn toxicity of dietary origin has not been well documented. However, an increased incidence of a Parkinsonian syndrome has been described in an area in Greece where the well water supplies have a high Mn content (Kondakis et al 1989).

MOLYBDENUM

Molybdenum (Mo) occurs as a cofactor bound to a pterin in three major enzymes in human and animal tissues: xanthine oxidase, sulphite oxidase and aldehyde oxidase activities. The element is therefore needed for the metabolism of purines, pyrimidines, quinolines, sulphite and bisulphite (Mills & Davis 1986, Rajagopalan 1988).

An autosomal defect in the hepatic synthesis of this factor is responsible for a distinctive fatal syndrome of infants involving severe developmental retardation, neurological abnormalities, ectopic eye lenses and an impaired metabolism of sulphur amino acids and nucleotides (Wadman et al 1983). An analogous metabolic syndrome has been reported in a patient on prolonged intravenous feeding who developed hypermethionaemia, low urinary excretion of sulphate but increased thiosulphaturia, an intolerance of intravenous sulphur amino acids manifest as an encephalopathy, and low urinary and plasma uric acid concentrations; all of these features responded to Mo supplementation (Abumrad et al 1981).

Intestinal absorption of dietary Mo is highly efficient (approximately 80%) The element is metabolized as an anion (molybdate) and renal excretion is altered in response to changes in Mo absorption.

Reported daily intakes in adults range between 44 and 460 µg; as with other dietary anions, there is considerable geographic variation in intakes. Moresponsive defects have been observed in adults experimentally fed 25 µg daily. The tissue concentrations of Mo vary markedly depending on geographical area: populations living in regions with a high Mo soil content tend to have higher tissue concentrations.

The possibility that disturbed copper metabolism may occur in populations subsisting in a Mo-rich geochemical environment (Kovalsky et al 1961) has been emphasized by the success of tetrathiomolybdate in the management of Wilson's disease (Brewer et al 1991). Hitherto such a problem was thought to be relevant only to ruminants, in which sulphur and Mo interact to interfere with the absorption of copper (Mills & Davis 1986). Given the rare evidence of Mo deficiency and the limited studies on Mo metabolism, only provisional RDAs and requirement figures have been set (see Appendix 2).

FLUORIDE

Fluoride has a role in bone mineralization and in the hardening of tooth enamel, but its essentiality is not proven unequivocally. None the less, low intakes are associated with an increased incidence of dental caries, and the addition of fluoride, at 1 mg/kg, to water supplies reduces this. The body burden is regulated by renal excretion.

Children with fluoride intakes in excess of 0.1 mg/kg body weight daily have mottled teeth indicative of mild fluorosis (Leverett 1982). Chronic high intakes of fluoride cause bone disease and joint abnormalities (Krishnamachari 1986). This fluorosis is particularly common in Tanzania, South Africa, the Indian subcontinent, China and, possibly, Senegal, where a high fluoride content in the subsoil water enters the food chain either directly or via plants. This problem is exacerbated in some areas by increases in the water table after dams have been built. It may also arise from the need to drill deeper wells as the water table recedes. In arid regions, large intakes of fluorine may also arise from drinking large volumes of water, the fluorine content of which may be within the acceptable range of advisory authorities (Brouwer et al 1988). Fluorosis is more common in populations subsisting on sorghum, since this cereal retains the element.

Severe fluorosis may present as early as 6 years of age, and affects men more than women. The earliest evidence is dark mottling of the tooth enamel. In otherwise asymptomatic individuals, radiological evidence of focal areas of osteosclerosis and osteoporosis, with calcification of ligaments and tendons, may be present. This advances and patients develop stiffness, joint pains and deformities of the spine, and of the legs (genu varum and genu valgum) – bent tibiae and fibulae. Occasionally the arms are similarly affected. Low calcium intakes and high intakes of molybdenum may exacerbate the syndrome. High fluoride intakes may also interfere with iodine metabolism, causing hypothyroidism.

CHROMIUM

Trivalent chromium (Cr(III)) is thought to potentiate the action of insulin, possibly by optimizing the number of membrane insulin receptors or their interaction with insulin, or both (Stoecker 1990, Offenbacher &

Pi-Sunyer 1988). It is reported to have been beneficial in the management of both hyperglycaemic and hypo-glycaemic responses to glucose loads. A proposed 'glucose tolerance factor' comprising chromium with nicotinic acid, cysteine and glycine has not been characterized, but patients in whom chromium-responsive defects have been described (see below) benefited from parenteral supplements of inorganic chromium. However, experience with Cr(III) in the management of diabetes mellitus has produced inconsistent results, generating scepticism about the element's essentiality; some of the effects of chromium may arise from a non-specific effect on phosphoglucomutase (Anonymous 1988). Additionally, the element may have a direct or indirect role in the metabolism of lipids, perhaps via insulin action. Chromium may participate in RNA synthesis from the DNA template (Okada et al 1981).

Chromium (III) absorption is low at 0.5 to 2.0% of dietary intake. Organic chromium is absorbed efficiently but is also excreted rapidly in the urine. Foods with a high chromium content are meat, whole grains, nuts, legumes and brewer's yeast. Refined products have a low chromium content.

Chromium deficiency has been described in adults and a child on prolonged parenteral nutrition (Anonymous 1988, Brown et al 1986). The features included an insulin-resistant hyperglycaemia, elevated serum lipids, weight loss, ataxia, peripheral neuro-pathy and encephalopathy. The adult patients responded to intravenous chromium chloride (CrCl3), but the response in the child was less conclusive.

Trivalent chromium has a low level of toxicity but hexavalent chromium is more toxic in animal models in which, at intakes of 50 µg/g diet, chromium causes renal and hepatic necrosis and growth retardation.

Assessing chromium status

Tissue chromium stores do not readily equilibrate with blood chromium and measurements of blood Cr concentrations are poor indices of Cr status. High urinary Cr levels may be a good indication of excessive intakes. There is at present no good measure of Cr status.

Chromium requirements

Only tentative recommendations have been developed by the UK, USA and WHO bodies who have considered the evidence recently.

OTHER TRACE ELEMENTS

Some other elements may be essential, but it is difficult to establish this and many of the proposed roles are awaiting confirmation (Nielsen 1990, 1984). Current concepts are abstracted in Table 12.7.

REFERENCES

Abumrud NN, Schneider AJ, Steel D, Rogers LS 1981 Amino acid intolerance during prolonged total parenteral nutrition reversed by molybdate therapy. American Journal of Clinical Nutrition 34: 2551–2559

Aggett PJ, Crofton RW, Chapman M, Humphries WR, Mills CF 1983 Plasma leucocyte and tissue zinc concentrations in young zinc deficient pigs. Pediatric Research 17: 433

Anonymous 1988 Is chromium essential for humans? Nutrition Reviews 46: 17–20

Anonymous 1988 Manganese deficiency in humans: fact or fiction? Nutrition Reviews 46: 348–352

Arthur JR, Nicol F, Beckett GJ 1990 Hepatic iodothyronine 5-deiodinase: the role of selemium. Biochemical Journal 272: 537–540

Baer MJ, King JC 1984 Tissue zinc levels and zinc excretion during experimental zinc depletion in young men. American Journal of Clinical Nutrition 39: 556–570

Baer MT, King JC, Tamura T et al 1985 Nitrogen utilization, enzyme activity, glucose intolerance and leucocyte chemotaxis in human experimental zinc depletion. American Journal of Clinical Nutrition 41: 1220–1235

Bales CW, Steinman LC, Freeland-Graves JH, Stone JM, Young RK 1986 The effect of age on plasma zinc uptake and taste acuity. American Journal of Clinical Nutrition 44: 664–669

Baly DL, Golub MS, Gershwin ME, Hurley LS 1984 Studies on marginal zinc deprivation in rhesus monkeys. III. Effects on vitamin A metabolism. American Journal of Clinical Nutrition 40: 199–207

Baynes RD, Bothwell TH 1990 Iron deficiency. Annual Review of Nutrition 10: 133–148

Behne D, Kyriakopoulos A, Meinhold H, Köhrle J 1990 Identification of Type I iodothyronine 5'-deiodinase as a selenoenzyme. Biochemical and Biophysical Research Communications 173: 1143–1149

Bettger WJ, O'Dell BL 1981 A critical physiological role of zinc in the structure and function of biomembranes. Life Sciences 28: 1425–1438

Bhave SA, Pandit AN, Singh S, Walia BNS, Tanner MS 1992 The prevention of Indian childhood cirrhosis. Annals of Tropical Paediatrics (in press)

Bothwell TH, Charlton RW, Cook JD, Finch CA 1979 Iron metabolism in man. Oxford, Blackwell Scientific Publications

Bremner I, Morrison JN, Wood AM, Arthur JR 1987 Effects of changes in dietary zinc, copper and selenium supply and of endotoxin administration on metallothionein I concentrations in blood cells and urine in the rat. Journal of Nutrition 117: 1595–1602

Brewer GJ, Dick RD, Yuzbasiyan Gurkin V, Tankanow R, Young AB, Kluin KJ 1991 Initial therapy of patients with Wilson's disease with tetrathiomolybdate. Archives of Neurology 48: 42–47

Brouwer ID, De Bruin A, Backer Dirks O, Hautvast JGAJ 1988 Unsuitability of World Health Organization guidelines for fluoride concentrations in drinking water in Senegal. Lancet i: 223–225

Brown MA, Thom JV, Orth GL, Cova P, Juarez J 1964 Food poisoning involving zinc contamination. Archives of Environmental Health 8: 657–660

Brown RO, Forloines-Lynn S, Cross RE, Heizer WD 1986 Chromium deficiency after long-term total parenteral nutrition. Digestive Diseases and Sciences 31: 661–664

Brune M, Magnusson B, Persson H, Hallberg L 1986 Iron losses in sweat. American Journal of Clinical Nutrition 43: 438–443

Brune M, Rossander-Hultén L, Hallberg L 1989 Iron absorption and phenolic compounds: importance of different phenolic structures. European Journal of Clinical Nutrition 43: 547–558

Brune M, Rossander-Hultén L, Hallberg L, Erlandsson M, Sandberg A-S 1992 Iron absorption from bread. Inhibiting effect of cereal fiber, phytate and inositol phosphates with different number of phosphate groups. Journal of Nutrition 122: 442–449

Casey CE 1988 Selenophilia. Proceedings of the Nutrition Society 47: 55–62

Castillo-Duran C, Fisberg M, Valenzuela A, Egana JI, Uauy R 1983 Controlled trial of copper supplementation during the recovery from marasmus. American Journal of Clinical Nutrition 37: 898–903

Castillo-Duran C, Vial P, Uauy R 1988 Trace mineral balance during acute diarrhea in infants. Journal of Pediatrics 113: 452–457

Chanarin I, Malkouska V, O'Hea A-M, Rinsler MG, Price AB 1983 Megaloblastic anaemia in a vegetarian Hindu community. Lancet ii: 1168–1172

Chandra RK 1984 Excessive intake of zinc impairs immune responses. Journal of the American Medical Association 252: 1443–1446

Chen X, Yang G, Chen J, Wen Z, Ge K 1980 Studies on the relations of selenium and Keshan disease. Biological Trace Element Research 2: 91–107

Chesters JK 1989 Biochemistry of zinc in cell division and tissue growth. In: Mills CF (ed) Zinc in human biology. Springer-Verlag, Berlin, pp. 109–118

Cook JD, Layrisse M, Martinez-Torres C, Walker R, Monsen E, Finch CA 1972 Food iron absorption measured by an extrinsic tag. Journal of Clinical Investigations 51: 805–815

Coppen DE, Davies NT 1987 Studies on the effects of dietary dose on ^{65}Zn absorption in vivo and on the effects of zinc status on ^{65}Zn absorption and body loss in young rats. British Journal of Nutrition 57: 35–44

Cousins RJ 1985 Absorption, transport, and hepatic metabolism of copper and zinc: special reference to metallothionein and ceruloplasmin. Physiological Reviews 65: 238–309

Dallman PR 1986 Biochemical basis for the manifestations of iron deficiency. Annual Review of Nutrition 6: 13–40

Danks DM 1988 Copper deficiency in humans. Annual Review of Nutrition 8: 235–257

Davis KR, Peters LJ, Cain RF, LeTourneau D, McGinnis J 1984 Evaluation of the nutrient composition of wheat. III. Minerals. Cereal Foods World 29: 246–248

DeMaeyer E, Adiels-Tegman M 1985 The prevalence of anaemia in the world. World Health Statistics Quarterly 38: 302–316

Dhur A, Galan P, Hercberg S 1990 Relationship between selenium, immunity and resistance against infection. Comparative Biochemistry and Physiology 96: 271–280

Diplock AT, Chaudhry FA 1988 The relationship of selenium biochemistry to selenium responsive disease in man. In: Prasad A (ed) Essential and toxic trace elements in human health and disease. Alan R Liss, New York, pp 211–226

Doisy EA 1972 Micronutrient controls on biosynthesis of clotting proteins and cholesterol. In: Hemphill DD (ed) Trace substances in environmental health VI. University of Missouri, Columbia, p. 193

FAO/WHO 1988 Report of a joint Expert Group: Requirments of vitamin A, iron, folate and vitamin B_{12}. FAO Food and nutrition series No 23. Food and Agricultural Organization of United Nations Rome

Fickel JJ, Freeland-Graves JH, Roby MJ 1986 Zinc tolerance tests in zinc-deficient and zinc-supplemented diets. American Journal of Clinical Nutrition 43: 47–58

Fraker PJ , Jardieu P , Cook J 1987 Zinc deficiency and immune function. Archives of Dermatology 123: 1699–1701

Friedman BJ, Freeland-Graves JH, Bales CW et al 1987 Manganese balance and clinical observations in young men fed a manganese-deficient diet. Journal of Nutrition 117: 133–143

Gallaher DD, Johnson PE, Hunt JR, Lykken GI, Marchello MJ 1988 Bioavailability in humans of zinc from beef: intrinsic vs extrinsic labels. American Journal of Clinical Nutrition 48: 350–354

Gallery EDM, Bloomfield J, Dixon SR 1972 Acute zinc toxicity in haemodialysis. British Medical Journal 4: 331–333

Garn SM, Ridella SA, Petzold AS, Falkner F 1981 Maternal hematological levels and pregnancy outcomes. Seminars in Perinatology 5: 155–162

Gibson RS, Scythes CA 1982 Trace element intakes of women. British Journal of Nutrition 48: 241–248

Golden BE, Golden MHN 1985 Effect of zinc supplementation on the composition of newly synthesized tissue in children recovering from malnutrition. Proceeedings of the Nutrition Society 44: 110A

Golub MS, Gershwin ME, Hurley L, Baly DL, Hendrickx AG 1984a Studies of marginal zinc deprivation in rhesus monkeys. II. Pregnancy outcome. American Journal of Clinical Nutrition 39: 879–887

Golub MS, Gershwin ME, Hurley LS, Baly DL, Hendrickx AG 1984b Studies of marginal zinc deprivation in rhesus monkeys. I. Influence on pregnant dams. American Journal of Clinical Nutrition 39: 265–280

Green R, Charlton R, Seftel H et al 1968 Body iron excretion in man. A collaborative study. American Journal Medicine 45: 336–353

Greger JL, Buckley S 1977 Menstrual blood loss of zinc, copper, magnesium and iron by adolescent girls. Nutrition Reports International 16: 639–647

Hallberg L 1980 Food iron absorption. In: Cook J D (ed) Iron. Churchill Livingstone, Edinburgh, pp.116–133

Hallberg L 1981 Bioavailability of dietary iron in man. Annual Review of Nutrition 1: 123–147

Hallberg L 1982 Iron absorption and iron deficiency. Human Nutrition: Clinical Nutrition 36C: 259–278

Hallberg L 1984 Iron. In: Brown ML (ed) Present knowledge in nutrition, 5th edn. The Nutrition Foundation Inc., Washington DC, pp 459–478

Hallberg L 1988 Iron balance in pregnancy. In: Berger H (ed) Vitamins and minerals in pregnancy and lactation Nestlé Nutrition Workshop Series, Vol 16, Nestec Ltd., Vevey / Raven Press Ltd. New York, pp 115–127

Hallberg L, Björn-Rasmussen E 1972 Determination of iron absorption from whole diet. A new two-pool model using two radioiron isotopes given as haem and non-haem iron. Scandinavian Journal of Haematology 9: 193–197

Hallberg L, Rossander-Hultén L 1991 Iron requirements in menstruating women. American Journal of Clinical Nutrition 54: 1047–1058

Hallberg L, Högdahl A-M, Nilsson L, Rybo G 1966 Menstrual blood loss: a population study. Variations at different ages and attempts to define normality. Acta Obstet Gynecologica Scandinavica 45: 320–351

Hallberg L, Björn-Rasmussen E, Howard L, Rossander L 1979 Dietary haem iron absorption. A discussion of possible mechanisms for the absorption-promoting effect of meat and for the regulation of iron absorption. Scandinavian Journal of Gastroenterology 14: 769–779

Hallberg L, Brune M, Rossander L 1986 Effect of ascorbic acid on iron absorption from different types of meals. Human Nutrition Applied Nutrition 40A: 97–113

Hallberg L, Brune M, Rossander L 1989 Iron absorption in man: ascorbic acid and dose-dependent inhibition by phytate. American Journal of Clinical Nutrition 49: 140–144

Hallberg L, Björn-Rasmussen E, Jungner I 1989 Prevalence of hereditary haemochromatosis in two Swedish urban areas. Journal of Internal Medicine 225: 249–255

Hallberg L, Brune M, Erlandsson M, Sandberg A-S, Rossander-Hultén L 1991 Calcium: effect of different amounts on non-heme and heme iron absorption in man. American Journal of Clinical Nutrition 53: 112–119

Hallberg L, Rossander-Hultén L, Brune M, Gleerup A 1992 Calcium and iron absorption – mechanism of action and nutritional importance. European Journal of Clinical Nutrition 46: 317–327

Halstead JA, Ronaghy HA, Abadi P et al 1972 Zinc deficiency in man: the Shiraz experiment. American Journal of Medicine 53: 277–284

Hambidge KM, Krebs NF, Jacobs MA, Favier A, Guyette L, Ikle DN 1983 Zinc nutritional status during pregnancy: a longitudinal study. American Journal of Clinical Nutrition 37: 429–442

Hess FM, King JC, Margen S 1977 Zinc excretion in young women on low zinc intakes and oral contraceptive agents. Journal of Nutrition 107: 1610–1620

Hurley LS, Keen CL 1987 Manganese. In: Mertz W (ed) Trace elements in human and animal nutrition, Vol. 1. Academic Press, San Diego, pp 185–223

Hurley LS, Tao S 1972 Alleviation of teratogenic effects of zinc deficiency by simultaneous lack of calcium. American Journal of Physiology 222: 322–325

IUNS 1983 Recommended dietary intakes around the world, part 2. Nutrition Abstracts and Reviews 53: 1076–1119

Jackson MJ, Edwards RHT 1982 Zinc excretion in patients with muscle disorders. Muscle Nerve 5: 661–663

Jackson MJ, Jones DA, Edwards RHT, Swainbank IG, Coleman ML 1984 Zinc homoeostasis in man: studies using a new stable isotope-dilution technique. British Journal of Nutrition 51: 199–208

Jackson MJ, Giugliano R, Giugliano LG, Oliveira EF, Shrimpton R, Swainbank IG 1988 Stable isotope metabolic studies of zinc nutrition in slum-dwelling lactating women in the Amazon valley. British Journal of Nutrition 59: 193–203

Jameson S 1976 Effects of zinc deficiency in human reproduction. Acta Medica Scandinavica 593 (Suppl): 1–89

Kay RG, Tasman-Jones C, Pybus J, Whiting R, Black H 1976 A syndrome of acute zinc deficiency during total parenteral alimentation in man. Annals of Surgery 183: 331–340

Kondakis XG, Makris N, Leotsinidis M, Prinou M, Papapetropoulos T 1989 Possible health effects of high manganese concentration in drinking water. Archives of Environmental Health 44: 175–178

Kovalsky VV, Jaravaja GA, Smavonjan DM 1961 Changes in purine metabolism in man and animals in various molybdenum-rich biogeochemical provinces. Zhurnal Obshcheiviologii 22: 179–191

Krebs NF, Hambidge KM 1986 Zinc requirements and zinc intakes of breast-fed infants. American Journal of Clinical Nutrition 43: 288–292

Krebs F, Hambidge KM, Walravens PA 1984 Increased food intake of young children receiving a zinc supplement. American Journal of Diseases of Children 138: 270–273

Krebs NF, Hambidge KM, Jacobs MA, Rasbach JO 1985 The effects of a dietary zinc supplement during lactation on longitudinal changes in maternal zinc status and milk zinc concentrations. American Journal of Clinical Nutrition 41: 560–570

Krishnamachari KAVR 1986 Skeletal fluorosis in humans: a review of recent progress in the understanding of the disease. Progress in Food and Nutrition Science 10: 279–314

Kuramoto Y, Igarashi Y, Kato S, Tagami H 1986 Acquired zinc deficiency in two breast-fed mature infants. Acta Dermato-Venereologica (Stockh) 66: 359–361

Kynast G, Saling E 1986 Effect of oral zinc application during pregnancy. Gynecologic and Obstetric Investigation 21: 117–123

Lazebnik N, Kuhnert BR, Kuhnert PM, Thompson KL 1988 Zinc status, pregnancy complications, and labor abnormalities. Americal Journal of Obstetrics and Gynecology 158: 161–166

Leek JC, Keen CL, Vogler JB et al 1988 Long-term marginal zinc deprivation in Rhesus monkeys. IV Effects on skeletal growth and mineralization. American Journal of Clinical Nutrition 47: 889–895

Levander OA 1987 A global view of human selenium nutrition. Annual Review of Nutrition 7: 227–250

Leverett DH 1982 Fluorides and the changing prevalance of dental caries. Science 217: 26–30

Lieberman E, Ryan KJ, Monsen RR, Schoenbaum SC 1988 Association of maternal hematocrit with premature labor. American Journal of Obstetrics and Gynecology 159: 107–114

Lindeman RD, Baxter DJ, Yunice AA, Kraikitpanitch S 1978 Serum concentrations and urinary excretions of zinc in cirrhosis, nephrotic syndrome and renal insufficiency. American Journal of the Medical Sciences 275: 17–31

Lönnerdal B, Cederblad Å, Davidsson L, Sandström B 1984 The effect of individual components of soy formula and cow's milk formula on zinc bioavailability. American Journal of Clinical Nutrition 40: 1064–1070

Lönnerdal B, Bell JG, Hendrickx JG, Burns RA, Keen CL 1988 Effect of phytate removal on zinc absorption from soy formula. American Journal of Clinical Nutrition 48: 1301–1306

Lozoff B 1988 Behavioral alterations in iron deficiency. Advances in Pediatrics 35: 331–360

Lykken GI, Mahalko J, Johnson PE et al 1986 Effect of browned and unbrowned corn products intrinsically labeled with ^{65}Zn on absorption of ^{65}Zn in humans. Journal of Nutrition 116: 795–801

McCance RA, Widdowson EM 1942a Mineral metabolism of healthy adults on white and brown bread dietaries. Journal of Physiology 101: 44–85

McCance RA, Widdowson EM 1942b The absorption and excretion of zinc. Biochemical Journal 36: 692–696

McClain G, Soutor C, Zieve L 1980 Zinc deficiency: a complication of Crohn's disease. Gastroenterology 78: 272–279

Maleki M 1973 Food consumption and nutritional status of 13-year-old village and city schoolboys in Fars province, Iran. Ecology of Food and Nutrition 2: 39–42

Mathias PM, Jackson AA 1982 Selenium deficiency in kwashiorkor. Lancet i: 1312–1313

Meiners CR, Derise NL, Lau HC, Crews MG, Ritchey SJ, Murphy EW 1976 The content of nine mineral elements in raw and cooked mature dry legumes. Journal of Agriculture and Food Chemistry 24: 1126–1127

Mills CF 1991 The significance of copper deficiency in human nutrition and health. In: Momcilovic B (ed) Trace elements in man and animals 7. IMI, Zagreb, Ch. 5, pp 1–4

Mills CF, Davis GK 1986 Molybdenum. In: Mertz W (ed) Trace elements in human and animal nutrition, 5th edn, Vol. I. Academic Press, New York, pp 429–463

Milne DB, Canfield WK, Mahalko JR, Sandstead HH 1983 Effect of dietary zinc on whole-body surface loss of zinc: impact on estimation of zinc retention by balance method. American Journal of Clinical Nutrition 38: 181–186

Morrison SA, Russell RM, Carney EA, Oaks EV 1978 Zinc deficiency: a case of abnormal dark adaptation in cirrhosis. American Journal of Clinical Nutrition 31: 276–281

Motchnik PA, Tappel AL 1990 Multiple selenocysteine content of selenoprotein P in rats. Journal of Inorganic Biochemistry 40: 265–269

Moynahan EJ 1974 Acrodermatitis enteropathica; a lethal inherited human zinc deficiency disorder. Lancet ii: 399–400

Muller-Hocker J, Meyer U, Wiebecke B et al 1988 Copper storage disease of the liver and chronic dietary copper intoxication in two further German infants mimicking Indian childhood cirrhosis. Pathology Research and Practice 183: 39–45

Murphy JV 1970 Intoxication following ingestion of elemental zinc. Journal of American Medicine Association 212: 2119–2120

Murphy SP, Calloway DK 1986 Nutrient intakes of women in NHANES II, emphasizing trace minerals, fiber and phytate. Journal of the American Dietetic Association 86: 1366–1371

National Research Council (Committee on Dietary Allowances, Food and Nutrition Board) 1980 Zinc. In: Recommended Dietary allowances, 9th edn. National Academy of Sciences, Washington DC, pp. 144–147

Nävert B, Sandström B, Cederblad Å 1985 Reduction of the phytate content of bran by leavening in bread and its effect on absorption of zinc in man. British Journal of Nutrition 53: 47–53

Neilsen FH 1984 Ultratrace elements in nutrition. Annual Review of Nutrition 4: 21–41

Neilsen FH 1990 Other trace elements. In: Brown ML (ed) Present knowledge in nutrition, 6th edn. International Life Sciences Institute Nutrition Foundation, Washington DC, pp 294–307

O'Dell BL 1990 Copper. In: Brown ML (ed) Present knowledge in nutrition, 6th edn. International Life Sciences Institute Nutrition Foundation, Washington DC, pp 261–267

Offenbacher EG, Pi-Sunyer FX 1988 Chromium in human nutrition. Annual Review of Nutrition 8: 543–563

Okada S, Ohba H, Taniyama M 1981 Alterations in ribonucleic acid synthesis by chromium (III). Journal of Inorganic Biochemistry 15: 223–331

Patterson WP, Winkelmann M, Perry MC 1985 Zinc-induced copper deficiency: megamineral sideroblastic anemia. Annals of Internal Medicine 103: 385–386

Porter KG, McMaster D, Elmes ME, Love AHG 1977 Anemia and low serum copper during zinc therapy. Lancet ii: 774

Prohaska JR, Wittmers LE, Haller EW 1988 Influence of genetic obesity, food intake and adrenalectomy in mice on selected trace element-dependent protective enzymes. Journal of Nutrition 118: 739–746

Rajagopalan KV 1988 Molybdenum: an essential trace element in human nutrition. Annual Review of Nutrition 8: 401-427

Reiser S, Smith JC, Mertz W et al 1985 Indices of copper status in humans consuming a typical American diet containing either fructose or starch. American Journal of Clinical Nutrition 42: 242–251

Richards MP, Cousins RJ 1976 Metallothionein and its relationship to the metabolism of dietary zinc in rats. Journal of Nutrition 106: 1591–1599

Robinson MF 1988 The New Zealand selenium experience. American Journal of Clinical Nutrition 48: 521–534

Ross J, Gibson RS, Sabry JH 1986 A study of seasonal trace element intakes and hair trace element concentrations in selected households from the Wosera, Papua New Guinea. Tropical and Geographical Medicine 38: 246–254

Sandstead HH, Prasad AS, Schulert AR et al 1967 Human zinc deficiency, endocrine manifestations and response to treatment. American Journal of Clinical Nutrition 20: 422–442

Sandstead HH, Henriksen LK, Greger JL, Prasad AS, Good RA 1982 Zinc nutriture in the elderly in relation to taste acuity, immune response, and wound healing. American Journal of Clinical Nutrition 36: 1046–1059

Sandström B 1989 Dietary pattern and zinc supply. In: Mills C F (ed) Zinc in human biology. Springer-Verlag, Berlin, pp. 351–363

Sandström B, Cederblad Å 1980 Zinc absorption from composite meals II. Influence of the main protein source. American Journal of Clinical Nutrition 33: 1778–1783

Sandström B, Cederblad Å 1987 Effect of ascorbic acid on the absorption of zinc and calcium in man. International Journal of Vitamin and Nutrition Research 57: 87–90

Sandström B, Lönnerdal B 1989 Promoters and antagonists of zinc absorption. In: Mills CF (ed) Zinc in human biology. Springer-Verlag, Berlin, pp. 57–78

Sandström B, Sandberg A-S 1992 Inhibitory effects of isolated inositol phosphates on zinc absorption. Journal of Trace Elements and Electrolytes in Health and Disease 6: 99–103

Sandström B, Arvidsson B, Cederblad Å, Björn-Rasmussen E 1980 Zinc absorption from composite meals. I. The significance of wheat extraction rate, zinc, calcium and protein content in meals based on bread. American Journal of Clinical Nutrition 33: 739–745

Sandström B, Cederblad Å, Lönnerdal B 1983 Zinc absorption from human milk, cow's milk and infant formulas. American Journal of Diseases of Children 137: 726–729

Sandström B, Davidsson L, Cederblad Å, Lönnerdal B 1985 Oral iron, dietary ligands and zinc absorption. Journal of Nutrition 115: 411–414

Sandström B, Davidsson L, Lundell L, Olbe L 1987 Zinc status and dark adaptation in patients subjected to total gastrectomy: Effect of zinc supplementation. Human Nutrition. Clinical Nutrition 41C: 235–242

Sandström B, Kivistö B, Cederblad Å 1987 Absorption of zinc from soy protein meals in humans. Journal of Nutrition 117: 321–327

Sandström B, Almgren A, Kivistö B, Cederblad Å 1989 Effect of protein level and protein source on zinc absorption in humans. Journal of Nutrition 119: 48–53

Schmitt HA, Weaver CM 1982 Effects of laboratory-scale processing on chromium and zinc in vegetables. Journal of Food Science 47: 1693–1695

Schroeder HA, Nason AP, Tipton IH, Balassa JJ 1967 Essential trace metals in man: zinc. Relation to environmental cadmium. Journal of Chronic Diseases 20: 179–210

Schwartz R, Apgar BJ, Wien EM 1986 Apparent absorption and retention of Ca, Cu, Mg, Mn and Zn from a diet containing bran. American Journal of Clinical Nutrition 43: 444–455

Scrimshaw NS 1984 Functional consequences of iron deficiency in human populations. Journal of Nutritional Science and Vitaminology 30: 47–63

Shaw JCL 1988 Copper deficiency and non-accidental injury. Archives of Diseases in Childhood 63: 448–455

Shike M, Roulet M, Kurian R, Whitewell J, Stewart S, Jeejeebhoy KN 1981 Copper metabolism and requirements in total parenteral nutrition. Gastroenterology 81: 290–297

Shrimpton R 1984 Food consumption and dietary adequacy according to income in 1200 families, Manaus, Amazonas, Brazil. Archivos Latinoamericanos de Nutricion 34: 615–629

Simmer K, Iles CA, Slavin B, Keeling PWN, Thompson RPH 1987 Maternal nutrition and intrauterine growth retardation. Human Nutrition. Clinical Nutrition 41C: 193–197

Soman SD, Panday VK, Joseph KT, Raut SJ 1969 Daily intake of some major and trace elements. Health Physics 17: 35–40

Spitalny KC, Brondum J, Vogt RL, Sargent HE, Kappel S 1984 Drinking-water-induced copper intoxication in a Vermont family. Pediatrics 74: 1103–1106

Spring JA, Robertson J, Buss DH 1979 Trace nutrients. 3. Magnesium, copper, zinc, vitamin B_6, vitamin B_{12} and folic acid in the British household food supply. British Journal of Nutrition 41: 487–493

Stoecker BH 1990 Chromium. In: Brown ML (ed) Present knowledge in nutrition, 6th edn. International Life Sciences Institute Nutrition Foundation, Washington DC, pp 287–293

Sunde RA 1990 Molecular biology of selenoproteins. Annual Review of Nutrition 10: 451–474

Swanson CA, King JC 1987 Zinc and pregnancy outcome. American Journal of Clinical Nutrition 46: 763–771

Swanson CA, Turnlund JR, King JC 1983 Effect of dietary zinc sources and pregnancy on zinc utilization in adult women fed controlled diets. Journal of Nutrition 113: 2557–2567

Tucker SB, Schroeter AL, Brown Jr PW, McCall JT 1976 Acquired zinc deficiency. Journal of the American Medical Association 235: 2399–2402

Turnlund JR, Michel MC, Keyes WR, King JC, Margen S 1982 Use of enriched stable isotopes to determine zinc and iron absorption in elderly men. American Journal of Clinical Nutrition 35: 1033–1040

Turnlund JR, King JC, Keyes WR, Gong B, Michel MC 1984 A stable isotope study of zinc absorption in young men: effects of phytate and α-cellulose. American Journal of Clinical Nutrition 40: 1071–1077

Turnlund JR, Durkin N, Costa F, Margen S 1986 Stable isotope studies of zinc absorption and retention in young and elderly men. Journal of Nutrition 116: 1239–1247

Turnlund JR, Betschart AA, Keyes WR, Acord LL 1987 A stable isotope study of zinc bioavailability in young men from diets with white vs wholewheat bread or beef vs soy. Federation Proceedings 46: 879

Turnlund JR, Keys WR, Anderson HL, Acord LL 1989 Copper absorption and retention in young men at three levels of dietary copper by use of the stable isotope ^{65}Cu. American Journal of Clinical Nutrition 49: 870–878

Valberg LS, Flanagan PR, Chamberlain MJ 1984 Effects of iron, tin, and copper on zinc absorption in humans. American Journal of Clinical Nutrition 40: 536–541

Vallee B, Galdes A 1984 The metallobiochemistry of zinc enzymes. In: Meister A (ed) Advances in enzymology, Vol 56. John Wiley, New York, pp. 283–430

Virtamo H, Valkeila E, Alfthan G et al 1985 Serum selenium and the risk of coronary heart disease and stroke. American Journal of Epidemiology 122:276–282

Wada L, King C 1986 Effect of low zinc intakes on basal metabolic rate, thyroid hormones and protein utilization in adult men. Journal of Nutrition 116: 1045–1053

Wada L, Turnlund JR, King JC 1985 Zinc utilization in young men fed adequate and low zinc intakes. Journal of Nutrition 115: 1345–1354

Wadman SK, Duran M, Beemer FA et al 1983 Absence of hepatic molybdenum cofactor: an inborn error of metabolism leading to a combined deficiency of sulphite oxidase and xanthine dehydrogenase. Journal of Inherited Metabolic Disease 6 (Suppl 1): 78–83

Walravens PA, Hambidge KM 1976 Growth of infants fed a zinc supplemented formula. American Journal of Clinical Nutrition 29: 1114–1121

Walravens PA, Krebs NF, Hambidge KM 1983 Linear growth of low-income preschool children receiving a zinc supplement. American Journal of Clinical Nutrition 38: 195–201

Watanabe T, Endo A 1991 Effects of selenium deficiency on sperm morphology and spermatocyte chromosomes in mice. Mutation Research 262: 93–99

Wells JL, James DK, Luxton R, Pennock CA 1987 Maternal leucocyte zinc deficiency at start of third trimester as a predictor of fetal growth retardation. British Medical Journal 294: 1054–1056

Welsh SO, Marston RM 1982 Zinc levels of the US food supply 1909–1980. Food Technology 36: 70–76

Willett WC, Stampfer MJ, Hunter D, Colditz GA 1991 The epidemiology of selenium and human cancer. In: Aitio A,

Avo A, Järvisalo J, Vainio H (eds) The Royal Society of Chemistry, Cambridge, pp 141–155

Wolman SL, Anderson GH, Marliss EB, Jeejeebhoy KN 1979 Zinc in total parenteral nutrition: requirements and metabolic effects. Gastroenterology 76: 458–467

Yadrick MK, Kenney MA, Winterfeldt EA 1989 Iron, copper and zinc status: response to supplementation with zinc or zinc and iron in adult females. American Journal of Clinical Nutrition 49: 145–250

Yang G, Ge K, Chen J, Chen X 1988 Selenium-related endemic diseases and the daily selenium requirement of humans. World Review of Nutrition and Dietetics 3: 98–152

Youdim MBH (ed) 1988 Brain iron: neurochemical and behavioural aspects. Taylor & Francis, London

13. Fat-soluble vitamins

D. S. McLaren, N. Loveridge, G. Duthie and C. Bolton-Smith

VITAMIN A (RETINOL)

D.S. McLaren

More than 100 years before Christ, physicians in China and Egypt were prescribing the application of ox liver to the eyes for a disease that appears to have been night blindness (on the evidence that later on the Greeks borrowed the Egyptian prescriptions found in the Ebers Papyrus to treat what they called 'nuktalo'pia'). The Roman physician Celsus (25 BC–AD 50) first used the term xerophthalmia. It was a not uncommon cause of blindness in children in 19th century Europe and some parts of the tropics, and it was the first sign of a dietary deficiency induced in an experimental animal, described by Magendie in 1816 in dogs restricted to a diet of wheat gluten, starch, sugar and olive oil. McCollum and Davies isolated fat-soluble vitamin A in 1913, but it was not until 1930 that its structure was fully elucidated and the biological conversion of β-carotene to vitamin A was demonstrated (McLaren 1980).

CHEMISTRY AND NOMENCLATURE

Vitamin A (all-*trans*-retinol, vitamin A1 alcohol) is the parent of a class of chemical compounds called retinoids, both natural and synthetic, which have many of the structural features of vitamin A, including the extensive system of conjugated double bonds. Approximately 2500 retinoids have been synthesized in a search for more effective and safer compounds to be used therapeutically against neoplasms of epithelial origin and some skin disorders. Also included in the vitamin A family are the provitamin A carotenoids, chief among which is β-carotene. The majority of carotenoids in nature are not converted to vitamin A, but those commonly found in human diets, such as lycopene and lutein, are absorbed from the intestine unchanged and are found in the circulation. Their metabolism and ultimate fate in the body are unknown. Most carotenoids can serve as singlet oxygen quenchers and as antioxidants, properties not shared by retinol, and this may be important in relation to the prevention of cancer (see Chapter 45). The structural formulae of a selection of retinoids and carotenoids are shown in Figure 13.1.

FOOD SOURCES

Preformed vitamin A is chiefly found in dairy products such as milk, butter, cheese and egg yolk, in some fatty fish, and in the liver of farm animals and fish. Liver oils (cod, halibut, shark) are the richest natural sources of the vitamin and are used as dietary supplements. Carotenes in the chloroplasts of plants act as catalysts of photosynthesis by chlorophyll, and so are most abundant in the darker green leaves of such widely distributed vegetables as spinach, pumpkin, sweet potato, turnip tops and watercress. Generally, starchy roots contain little carotene, with the exception of carrots. Yellow fruits such as papaya, mango, apricots and peaches are good seasonal sources. Most of the carotenoid in tomatoes is the non-provitamin lycopene. The oils of some palms are the richest provitamin A sources known (Table 13.1).

Vitamin A and the carotenes are stable to the temperatures of ordinary cooking methods. Some loss will occur when foods are fried in butter or palm oil. Prolonged exposure to the open air in the sun-drying of fruits causes considerable destruction. Cod liver oil should be packaged in darkened glass bottles and gelatin capsules. The latter are also used for dispensing retinyl palmitate for prophylaxis (see p. 215); even so, in the tropics protection from direct sunlight and high temperatures is necessary.

REQUIREMENTS

For any nutrient these will vary according to age and some other factors and are also determined by

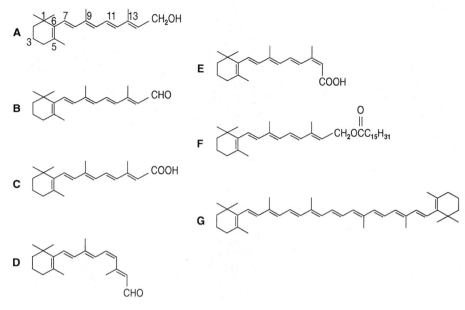

Fig. 13.1   Formulae of vitamin A and related compounds. A all-*trans*-retinol, approved numbering system; B all-*trans*-retinal; C all-*trans*-retinoic acid; D 11-*cis*-retinal; E 13-*cis*-retinoic acid; F retinyl palmitate; G all-*trans*-β-carotene.

whatever level of protection against deficiency is chosen. For vitamin A an additional complication is the need to express requirements or recommended dietary allowances (RDAs) in units that allow for the differing potency of retinol and the provitamin carotenoids. This unit is the retinol equivalent (RE) and the following relationships apply:

$$
\begin{aligned}
1.0\,\mu g\ RE = &\quad 1.0\,\mu g\ retinol \\
= &\quad 6.0\,\mu g\ \beta\text{-carotene} \\
= &\quad 12.0\,\mu g\ other\ provitamin\ carotenoids \\
= &\quad 3.3\ (IU)\ international\ units\ retinol \\
= &\quad 9.9\ (IU)\ international\ units\ \beta\text{-carotene}
\end{aligned}
$$

One IU of retinol equals $0.3\,\mu g$ of retinol, whereas one IU of β-carotene equals $0.6\,\mu g$ of β-carotene. This non-equivalence of the IU values for retinol and β-carotene causes confusion and is one of the reasons that IU values are being superseded.

Several national and international bodies have recently published their recommendations for vitamin A intakes (Olson 1990). Most of the differences can be accounted for by the different body weights used for reference adults. The figures in Appendix 2 include those for the healthy British population and others that are similar.

The mean intake of vitamin A in the form of provitamin carotenoids and of preformed vitamin A differs considerably in different parts of the world (FAO 1989). In Europe the daily intake is 666 RE carotenoids and 531 RE preformed vitamin (comparable figures are Africa 725 and 170; Asia 564 and 103; and the Americas 437 and 483 respectively). Care has to be exercised in the use of food composition tables for the estimation of the vitamin A value of foodstuffs. Units other than RE are frequently used and the conversion equivalents given above should be employed. In addition, the method of analysis of the food material used for determining the carotenoid content is important. In the past this usually resulted in a figure that overestimated the provitamin carotenoid content, as inactive carotenoids were also included. High-pressure liquid chromatography (HPLC, see p. 211) estimates individual carotenoids and retinoids separately and is being increasingly used in dietary analysis.

PHYSIOLOGY

Retinol and retinoic acid play fundamental roles in the economy of the body that are only recently beginning to be unravelled. In foods, preformed vitamin A is

Table 13.1 Dietary sources of provitamin and preformed vitamin A (typical values) (µg retinol/100 g edible portion)

Vegetable/fruit sources	
Mango (golden)	307
Papaya (solo)	124
Cucurbita (mature pulp)	862
Buriti palm (pulp)	3000
Red palm oil	30 000
Carrot	2000
Dark green leafy vegetables	685
Tomato	100
Apricot	250
Sweet potato, red and yellow	670
Animal sources	
Fatty fish liver oils:	
Halibut	900 000
Cod	18 000
Shark	180 000
Herring and mackerel	50
Dairy produce	
Butter	830
Margarine, vitaminized	900
Eggs	140
Milk	40
Cheese, fatty type	320
Meats	
Liver: sheep and ox	15 000
Beef, mutton, pork	0–4

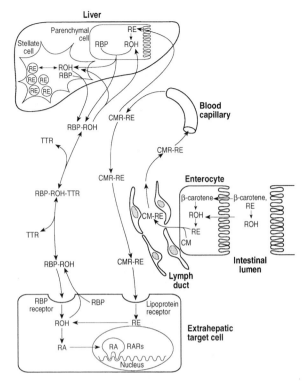

Fig. 13.2 Major pathways for retinoid transport in the body. Dietary retinyl esters (REs) are hydrolysed to retinol (ROH) in the intestinal lumen before absorption by enterocytes, and carotenoids are absorbed and then partially converted to retinol in the enterocytes. In the enterocytes, retinol reacts with fatty acids to form esters before incorporation into chylomicrons (CMs). Chylomicrons then reach the general circulation by way of the intestinal lymph, and chylomicron remnants (CMRs) are formed in blood capillaries. Chylomicron remnants, which contain almost all the absorbed retinol, are mainly cleared by the liver parenchymal cells, and to some extent also by cells in other organs. In liver parenchymal cells, retinyl esters are rapidly hydrolysed to retinol, which then binds to RBP. Retinol-RBP is secreted and transported to hepatic stellate cells. Stellate cells may then secrete retinol-RBP directly into plasma. Most retinol-RBP in plasma is reversibly complexed with transthyretin (TTR). The uncomplexed retinol-RBP is presumably taken up in a variety of cells by cell surface receptors specific for RBP. Most of the retinol taken up will then recycle to plasma, either on the 'old' RBP or bound to a newly synthesized RBP. (RA, retinoic acid; RAR, retinoic acid receptor.) Reproduced with permission from Blomhoff et al (1990).

present mainly as retinyl ester and this together with the provitamin carotenoids aggregates with other lipids during proteolytic digestion in the stomach. In the upper part of the small intestine hydrolysis occurs under the action of pancreatic esterases, and bile facilitates micelle formation and transfer across the intestinal villus cells. Absorption of vitamin A is about 80% in the presence of adequate fat intake. Carotenoid absorption is very bile-salt dependent and is only about half that of vitamin A. Conversion of β-carotene and other carotenoids into vitamin A occurs mainly in the intestinal mucosal cells and the major pathway is by the oxidative cleavage of the central 15,15′ double bond (Olson 1989). Figure 13.2 illustrates the major pathways of retinoid transport from the intestine to the liver and to target cells (Blomhoff et al 1990).

The major form of circulating vitamin A, holo-retinol-binding protein (holoRBP), consists of a 1:1 complex of all-*trans*-retinol with RBP (molecular weight 21 000) and its release from the liver and up-take by the target cells is under homoeostatic control which is little understood. In contrast, circulating carotenoids, about 15–30% of which are β-carotene and the rest mostly non-provitamin carotenoids, are carried by various classes of lipoproteins and the concentrations are directly related to dietary intake.

METABOLISM

Vitamin A is depleted from the liver at the relatively low net rate of about 0.5%/day (Sauberlich et al 1974), but within the body it is in a highly dynamic state. The half-life value for holo-RBP bound to transthyretin is about 11 hours (Goodman 1984), so it is one of the more rapidly turned over transport proteins.

Vitamin A undergoes many enzymatic transformations in the body. In addition to those already mentioned, retinal is reversibly reduced to retinol and irreversibly converted to retinoic acid in many tissues (Bhat et al 1988). Retinol is also conjugated in a number of ways, most notably in forming Schiff bases with e-amino groups of proteins, as in the important interaction between 11-*cis*-retinal and opsin and the opsin proteins (rhodopsin in the rods for night vision and porphyropsins in the cones for day and colour vision) in the eye. Isomerizations of carotenoids and vitamin A take place, for example the conversion of all-*trans*- to 11-*cis*-retinol in the eye (Bernstein et al 1987). Retinol, retinal and retinoic acid are bound to specific retinoid-binding proteins which are involved in their transport, biological transformation, protection from oxidation, and in the protection of lipid structures like membranes from the surface action of vitamin A.

FUNCTIONS

Cellular differentiation

Changes that are characteristic of vitamin A deficiency have been extensively studied in the bulbar conjunctiva and in most epithelial structures, including those of the respiratory, gastrointestinal and genitourinary tracts. It has been demonstrated (Petkovich et al 1987, Giguere et al 1987) that cell nuclei contain four receptors for retinoic acid, termed RAR-α to γ. It is hypothesized that retinoic acid is transported to the nucleus on cellular retinoic acid binding protein (CRABP), where it interacts with one or more of the RARs. The activated RAR interacts with the different hormone response elements of appropriate genes to influence transcription. Retinoic acid is a powerful morphogen in embryonic development. A nuclear receptor for retinol has not yet been identified.

Vision

The role of vitamin A in vision was the subject of classic studies, especially of George Wald, for which he was awarded the Nobel prize (Wald 1943). In both phototopic (day and colour) and scotopic (night) vision the aldehyde form of vitamin A, retinal, in its *cis* configuration, 11-*cis*-retinal, binds to the rod or cone opsins to form rhodopsin or porphyropsins respectively. Light causes retinal to change to the *trans* configuration and this initiates a complex series of reactions that cause a decrease in sodium ion entry to sodium channels, leading to a change in membrane potential that is transmitted to the brain. Not all of the energy contained in the light is dissipated in the nerve impulse and the remainder is used to release opsin and regenerate *cis*-retinal from *trans*-retinal for further participation in the visual cycle. The rod system is much more sensitive to a lack of vitamin A than that of the cones, resulting in night blindness. The role of retinoids in vision has been reviewed in much greater detail (Olson 1990).

Other processes in which vitamin A is known to be involved include fetal development, the immune response (especially cell-mediated immunity), haematopoiesis (possibly through interactions with iron) (Mejia et al 1979), spermatogenesis, appetite, hearing and physical growth. It is now thought that its fundamental role in cellular development may be implicated in most of these (Underwood 1984).

ANALYSIS

The choice of analytical technique will be determined largely by cost and availability. For the accurate separation and determination of vitamin A compounds and individual carotenoids in low concentrations in tissues and foodstuffs, HPLC is the preferred method. Straight-phase, reverse-phase, isocratic and gradient HPLC systems are available, depending upon special needs (Bhat & Sundaresan 1988). For routine hospital use or field studies in which analysis is to be carried out on the spot, and when retinol determination in serum is of primary concern, spectrophotometric or fluorometric methods are adequate and inexpensive (International Vitamin A Consultative Group 1982).

ASSESSMENT OF VITAMIN A STATUS

In the case of vitamin A the capacity of the body to store large amounts, especially in the liver, means that the state of these stores and other components that are influenced by them can be used to categorize status. As is the case for all nutritional indices, individual values must be interpreted with caution unless grossly deviant from normal, and they are primarily of use in assessing the vitamin A status of population groups.

Liver reserves

On the basis of experimental animal and human studies the lower limit of a satisfactory liver vitamin A concentration is considered to be 0.07 µmol/g (20 mg/g) in both sexes (Olson 1987). Direct measurement in postmortem samples has been advocated as a rough indication (WHO 1982). Of considerable promise are two tests, the RDR (relative dose response) and the MRDR (modified relative dose response) in which the indirect assessment of liver reserves is made from a plasma assay (Flores et al 1984, Tanumihardjo et al 1990). The basis for such tests is the finding that in the presence of vitamin A deficiency with diminished liver stores, apoRBP accumulates in the liver to several times its normal concentration. In the RDR, after baseline serum retinol has been measured, 450 µg retinyl palmitate is given orally. Some of this is taken up by the liver, combines with some of the excess apoRBP there and, as holoRBP is released into the circulation and in proportion to the pre-existing deficiency, causes a rise in serum retinol, which is sampled again after about 5 hours. The result of the test is expressed as the difference between the two serum retinol values divided by the final value, expressed as a percentage. Results of 50–20% indicate marginal liver stores, >50% indicates a deficiency.

Serum retinol

The large capacity of the liver to store vitamin A means that in both progressive deficiency and toxicity the serum fails to reflect vitamin A status. It does so only in the later stages of these processes, when clinical signs are also present. Even so, because it is readily measured and standards are available (Pilch 1987) it is part of the criteria for a public health problem for WHO and standards have been set for certain population groups (Table 13.2).

Conjunctival impression cytology

This non-invasive test for subclinical vitamin A deficiency is based on the detection by simple staining techniques of early histological changes in the bulbar conjunctiva, such as loss of goblet cells, the appearance of mucin lakes and xerotic changes in epithelial cells (Natadisastra et al 1987). At present it is unclear how specific to vitamin A deficiency the changes are. In many places where widespread deficiency is suspected, chronic eye infections and local trauma from dust, smoke and ultraviolet light may lead to similar changes (Carlier et al 1991).

Table 13.2 Plasma vitamin A levels and vitamin A status

Status	Plasma vitamin A µmol/l	(µg/dl)
Deficient	<0.35	(<10)
Marginal	0.35–0.70	(10–20)
Satisfactory	0.70–1.75	(20–50)
Excessive	1.75–3.5	(50–100)
Toxic	>3.5	(>100)

Ocular manifestations (xerophthalmia)

These show a progression, with an increasing severity of deficiency which is broadly indicated in the Xerophthalmia Classification of WHO (Table 13.3). By the time the subject is exhibiting evidence of night blindness, the serum retinol level will be depressed. Before this stage, in cooperative subjects, dark adaptometry may be performed to reveal objective evidence of the impairment of dark adaptation in positive cases (McLaren 1980). Details of the various eye signs are given below.

VITAMIN A DEFICIENCY AND XEROPHTHALMIA

Prevalence

Xerophthalmia is still the major cause of blindness in young children despite intensive prevention programmes over the past 20 years or so (see p. 216). The parts of the world most seriously affected include south and east Asia, and some countries of Africa, Latin America and the Near East.

It has been estimated (WHO 1991) that about 6–7 million new cases of xerophthalmia occur every year, with about one in ten suffering corneal damage. Of these 60% are dead within 1 year, and of the survivors

Table 13.3 Xerophthalmia classification by ocular signs

Night blindness (XN)
Conjunctival xerosis (X1A)
Bitot's spot (X1B)
Corneal xerosis (X2)
Corneal ulceration/keratomalacia $<\frac{1}{3}$ corneal surface (X3A)
Corneal ulceration/keratomalacia $\geq\frac{1}{3}$ corneal surface (X3B)
Corneal scar (XS)
Xerophthalmic fundus (XF)

Reproduced with permission from WHO/UNICEF/IVACG 1988

25% remain totally blind and 50–60% are partially blind. As a result about 3 million children under the age of 10 years are blind from this cause at any one time. An additional 20–40 million suffer from mild deficiency, which may have serious consequences for their survival (see p. 216).

Experimental deficiency

Two deprivation experiments on adult volunteers showed that body reserves are sufficient to last for many months before early signs of deficiency appear, and that about 600 µg of retinol was necessary to reverse the changes (Hume & Krebs 1949, Sauberlich et al 1974).

Secondary deficiency

Although malabsorptive states and chronic liver disease are the most common causes of xerophthalmia occurring in the presence of adequate dietary intake, there are several other mechanisms that have been described (Table 13.4).

Ocular manifestations

Posterior segment

Impaired dark adaptation is the first sign of xerophthalmia, most usually measured by dark adaptometry but also by rod scotometry (Hume & Krebs 1949). Other causes of rod dysfunction must be ruled out. For field studies in young children, careful history taking and observation make night blindness a useful tool (Sommer et al 1980). Since the 1920s reports have been made from the Far East of the occasional occurrence of changes in the fundus, consisting of yellowish spots in the peripheral fundus, visible on ophthalmoscopy. The subjects have usually been adolescents and response to vitamin A has been slow (McLaren 1980).

Anterior segment

The loss of goblet cells and early keratinizing changes in the bulbar conjunctiva, known as conjunctival xerosis (X1A), and the more advanced stage of the same process called Bitot's spot, usually precede changes in the cornea. However, in very young children advanced corneal damage known as keratomalacia may supervene without any obvious alteration to the conjunctiva. Bitot's spot consists of a heaping up of keratinized epithelial cells, most commonly occurring

Table 13.4 Secondary or endogenous causes of vitamin A deficiency

Diseases	Mechanisms
Coeliac disease, sprue, obstructive jaundice, ascariasis, giardiasis, partial or total gastrectomy	Impaired absorption of lipids including vitamin A
Chronic pancreatitis	Lack of enzymes (lipases), in some cases secondary to zinc deficiency
Cystic fibrosis	Excessive fecal loss, unrelated to amount of fat in stools★
Enzyme defect	Failure to cleave β-carotene in small intestine★★
Chronic liver disease, especially cirrhosis	Impaired storage, mostly in stellate cells which are involved in collagen formation+ Zinc deficiency may predispose
Heterozygotic reduction of plasma RBP	One case reported of keratomalacia due to reduced transport++

★Ahmed et al 1990
★★McLaren & Zekian 1971
+Blomhoff et al 1990
++Matsuo et al 1988

on the temporal aspect of the bulbar conjunctiva in the interpalpebral fissure near the limbus (Fig. 13.3). It usually takes the form of a small plaque of a silvery-grey hue with a foamy surface. Exceptionally, the material may be scattered widely over the conjunctiva. When associated with generalized conjunctival xerosis it is usually part of the vitamin A deficiency eye

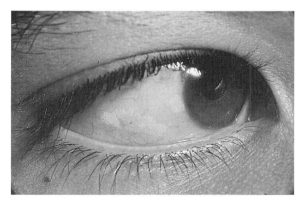

Fig. 13.3 Vitamin A-deficient eye showing Bitot's spots.

syndrome. The subjects are preschool age children, and there is a prompt response to vitamin A. In older children and adults Bitot's spots are often isolated lesions with no accompanying evidence of vitamin A deficiency, and in these circumstances they may be stigmata from earlier deficiency or caused by local irritation. Consequently it is of great importance that studies designed to estimate the prevalence of vitamin A deficiency and xerophthalmia should concentrate on preschool-age children, and wherever possible complement eye examination with biochemical tests (WHO 1982). As deficiency progresses the cornea becomes hazy (X2), but this stage appears to be of short duration as the corneal stroma rapidly becomes infiltrated with round cells, giving the cornea a milky bluish hue. The final stage consists of a unique pathological process known as colliquative necrosis, in which the cornea virtually melts away to a varying degree in extent and depth (X3a and b) (Fig. 13.4).

Some degree of visual impairment is inevitable and frequently there is total destruction of the eye with superadded infection. Fortunately the process is sometimes less advanced in one eye and some sight may be salvaged with prompt treatment (Fig. 13.5). Subsequent keratoplasty has restored sight to the privileged very few, but health provision in most circumstances is quite incapable of this.

Epidemiology

Xerophthalmia mainly affects children under the age of 4 years whose diet has been grossly inadequate for a long time (Fig. 13.6). The protective effect of breast feeding (West et al 1986), even into the third year of life (Mahalanabis 1991), has been repeatedly demonstrated. The severity of the eye lesions is in general inversely proportional to age, the blinding corneal

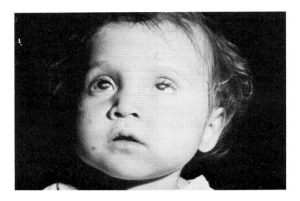

Fig. 13.5 Child blinded in infancy by keratomalacia.

changes targeting young children. Males are almost always more affected than females and this quite consistent characteristic has never been fully explained (McLaren 1986). Seasonal variation is usually present, and although fluctuation in the dietary intake of rich sources of the vitamin probably plays a part, the most important cause is the precipitating role of infections such as measles, gastroenteritis or respiratory infection (Fig. 13.7).

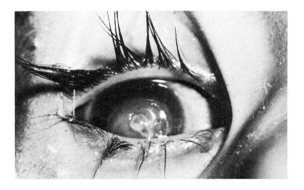

Fig. 13.4 Keratomalacia in a child from Jordan.

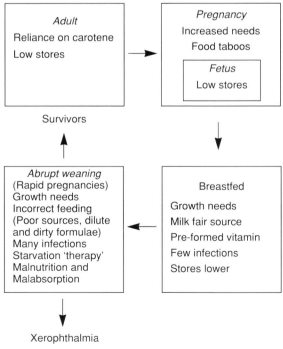

Fig. 13.6 The human xerophthalmia cycle. Reproduced with permission from McLaren (1986).

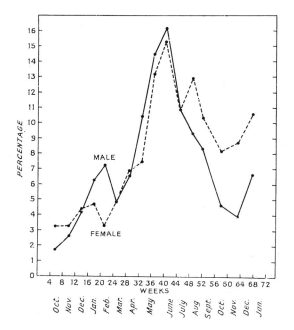

Fig. 13.7 Seasonal prevalence of vitamin A deficiency.

Several national surveys have been conducted over a limited period of the year, and a nutritional blindness problem has been overlooked because the survey happened to coincide with a trough in xerophthalmia prevalence. To assist in reaching a conclusion concerning the presence of a problem of public health magnitude WHO (1982) developed the set of criteria shown in Table 13.5. All of the indicators shown have weaknesses, but taken together they have proved to be reliable on the many occasions on which they have been employed. Conjunctival xerosis (X1A) is not recommended as its inter- and intra-observer reproducibility is very low; night blindness (XN) cannot be tested objectively in young children; Bitot's spots (X1B) may not be caused by vitamin A deficiency, as mentioned above, and are quite superficial lesions which may be easily removed; active corneal changes (X2,X3a+b) occur very infrequently in the field, and in the criteria 10 000 young children have to be examined to produce each case; corneal scars (XS) due to vitamin A deficiency in the past can only be suspected from a suggestive history and some characteristic features. Frequently other causes cannot be ruled out. Inclusion of the serum retinol criterion provides another parameter for assessment, and as an indicator of severe deficiency it is probably reliable, although some have suggested that serum retinol 10–20 µg in 15% of a population at risk (usually

children aged 1–6 years) should also be used (PAHO 1970).

Treatment

Children between 1 and 6 years of age should receive 200 000 IU (66 000 µg) of retinyl palmitate by mouth immediately for any stage of xerophthalmia. Persistent vomiting or profuse diarrhoea necessitate the use of intramuscular injection, which must be of a water-miscible form as the oily form does not leave the muscle. The dose is repeated the next day and again about 4 weeks later to provide liver stores against relapse. Children younger than 1 year or weighing less than 8 kg receive half the dosage. Older children and adults (except women of reproductive age) receive the same regimen as children aged 1–6. Because of the known teratogenic effect of large doses of vitamin A, care has to be exercised in prescribing for women of reproductive age. While active corneal lesions should receive full treatment, XN and X1B are treated with 10 000 IU (3300 µg) daily for 2 weeks (WHO/UNICEF/IVACG 1988).

Morbidity and mortality

In the past few years the whole emphasis of research into vitamin A deficiency has shifted away from xerophthalmia and now centres on child survival. Numerous animal experiments have documented the high mortality in severe vitamin A deficiency (Moore 1957) and this was also found in young children (McLaren et al 1967). A group working in Indonesia, and more recently Nepal, has reported a greatly increased mortality risk and rates of respiratory and gastrointestinal disease in mild xerophthalmia, and at least a 30% reduction in mortality due to the vitamin A supplementation of subclinical deficiency along the

Table 13.5 Prevalence criteria (in percentage of the preschool-age population, 6 months–6 years old, at risk) for determining the public health significance of xerophthalmia and vitamin A deficiency

Night blindness (XN) in >1%

Bitot's spot (X1B) in >0.5%

Corneal xerosis/corneal ulceration/keratomalacia (X2/X3A/X3B) in >0.01%

Corneal scar (XS) in >0.05%

Plasma vitamin A of <0.35 µmol/l (10 µg/dl) in >5%

Reproduced with permission from WHO/UNICEF/IVACG 1988

lines used in prevention programmes (Sommer et al 1986, West et al 1991). One study in India claimed a 60% reduction with a weekly dose (Rahmathulla et al 1990) and another found no significant effect (Vijayaraghavan et al 1990). At the present time there are several more studies that have not yet been completed, and it is not possible to come to a firm conclusion as to the relative importance of subclinical vitamin A deficiency in child morbidity and mortality, in comparison with other forms of nutritional deficiency and infectious disease. Experience with periodic megadose vitamin A supplementation (West & Sommer 1985, see also below) suggests that this is not a feasible solution to the problem over the long term.

Prevention

There is some evidence that xerophthalmia has become less prevalent in recent years in former hyperendemic areas such as Indonesia and south India. Although capsule distribution and other measures may have been responsible to some extent, it is more likely that general development and the improvement of living conditions have played the major part. In the past, nutritional deficiencies have disappeared from some countries without any specific measures having been taken.

Periodic megadose vitamin A supplementation

In the form of capsule, syrup or multiple dispenser 200 000 IU (66 000 µg) has been delivered at 4–6 monthly intervals either to high-risk preschool children or by universal distribution to preschool children and lactating mothers (WHO/UNICEF/IVACG 1988). This approach has been in operation in about 30 developing countries over periods of time that vary by more than 20 years. It is well documented that once the measure becomes a part of routine primary health care, efficiency of delivery sinks so low as to make the operation ineffective (West & Sommer 1985). This intervention is intended to be an emergency measure to save sight and lives on a large scale, while more radical measures are sought. It can never control the problem because fresh subjects continuously enter the system.

Food fortification

In Central America (Arroyave et al 1981) and Indonesia (Muhilal et al 1988) the addition of vitamin A to an item of diet universally consumed – sugar and monosodium glutamate, respectively – has had a favourable impact on the vitamin A status of whole populations. The problems to be overcome are mainly logistical and technical; it does not require the continuing cooperation of the people, but even when successful it improves only a single aspect of a multi-deficiency situation.

Nutrition education

There can be little doubt that this is really what is required. Vitamin A deficiency is nearly always 'poverty in the midst of plenty' – vegetable sources of the vitamin abound but are not being incorporated into the diet of the young child, due to lack of knowledge of infant feeding. Nutrition education, together with practical advice and help with growing cheap, nutritious vegetables and fruits in home and school gardens, could eradicate severe deficiency by the year 2000, in line with the goals set at Alma Ata (WHO 1988). However, at the present time less than a third of most of these populations receive any kind of health care whatsoever, and for those that do its efficacy in improving lifestyle is doubtful.

TOXICITY (HYPERVITAMINOSIS A)

Acute toxicity (Bendich & Langseth 1989) following ingestion of several hundred thousand units of vitamin A has caused a rise in intracranial pressure, especially in young children, with vomiting, headache and papilloedema. With very large doses drowsiness, repeated vomiting and skin exfoliation have occurred. Spontaneous recovery without residual damage usually follows on stopping the vitamin. The death of a 1-month-old baby was attributed to his receiving one million units over 11 days (Bush & Dahms 1984). Arctic explorers and Eskimos have learned not to eat polar bear or seal liver because of the extremely high vitamin A content (see Table 13.1).

Chronic toxicity is more common, and is caused by the regular ingestion over a period of months or years of a dose usually in excess of 10 times the RNI (reference nutrient intake). Signs and symptoms occur insidiously, and the syndrome of headache, loss of hair, dry and itchy skin, hepatosplenomegaly, and bone and joint pains may not suggest the correct diagnosis unless a careful history of drug use is sought and serum sent for retinol determination. Cessation of the vitamin is usually followed gradually by complete recovery, but in some cases liver damage, bone and muscle pain and impaired vision persist.

Congenital malformations in the offspring of mothers receiving large doses of vitamin A during the organogenetic period in utero have been long recognized to occur in animals, but there are only anecdotal reports in man. However, the retinoids accutane (13-*cis*-retinoic acid and etretinate (an aromatic analogue of the ethyl ester of all-*trans*-retinoic acid), used in the treatment of severe acne and some other skin conditions, have produced a set of characteristic birth defects in the offspring of women treated with them (Rosa et al 1986).

Hypercarotenosis results from the prolonged ingestion of large amounts of carotenoids in green and yellow leafy vegetables, or of carrots (often as carrot juice by food faddists), citrus fruits or tomatoes. Total blood carotenoids are also sometimes raised (>250 µg/100 ml) in hypothyroidism, diabetes mellitus, some hyperlipidaemic states and anorexia nervosa, whether from excessive ingestion or defective metabolism is not clear. Yellow or orange discoloration of the skin (xanthosis cutis, carotenodermia) is especially prominent on the nasolabial folds, forehead, axillae and groins, and on the palms and soles. This distribution is related to the secretion of carotenoids in sweat and sebum, and reabsorption by the stratum corneum. The condition appears to be quite harmless and does not lead to hypervitaminosis A.

VITAMIN D (CALCIFEROLS)

N. Loveridge

The first description of a rickets-like bone disease is attributed by Hess (1929) to Soranus of Ephesus, who practised medicine in Rome during the reigns of Trajan and Hadrian. Further description of the disease did not occur until two French (Guillimeau 1609 and Pare 1633) and two British (Whistler 1645 and Glisson 1650) physicians described a disease which by then was endemic in Europe (Hess 1929). However, it was not until the early 1900s that the disease was given a rigorous scientific basis with the work of Mellanby and colleagues (Mellanby 1919a,b). The concept of 'vital amines' was advanced by Funk (1911) and a factor in butterfat and cod liver oil which was essential for growth was described by McCollum & Davis (1913) and termed vitamin A. Mellanby produced a rachitic disorder in dogs and, as he was able to cure it with cod liver oil, assumed that vitamin A prevented or cured rickets.

McCollum then showed that even if the vitamin A activity of cod liver oil was destroyed by oxidation, the oil could still prevent the onset of rickets, suggesting the presence of a different factor, which he called vitamin D (McCollum et al 1922). Clinical studies also showed, however, that the exposure of rachitic children to sunlight or ultraviolet light prevented or cured the disease. Thus the cure of rickets appeared to be related both to sunlight exposure and substances associated with cod liver oil.

Vitamin D is the generic term for two molecules. Ergocalciferol (vitamin D_2) was obtained by irradiating the plant sterol ergosterol, which for many years was the major form of vitamin D used for the prevention and treatment of rickets. Cholecalciferol (vitamin D_3) is the major form of vitamin D in nature, but it can be made by irradiating 7-dehydrocholesterol and is more effective in preventing and curing rickets in chicks than vitamin D_2. DeLuca showed that vitamin D is hydroxylated at the 25 position (Blunt et al 1968) in the liver and Fraser & Kodicek (1970) showed that it was further hydroxylated at the 1 position in the kidney to produce an active hormone (Fig. 13.8).

CHEMISTRY

The first stage of vitamin D_3 synthesis (Fig. 13.8) is the photoconversion of provitamin D_3 (7-dehyrocholesterol) to previtamin D_3 within the stratum basale and stratum spinosum of the skin (DeLuca 1979, Webb & Holick 1988). The amount of photoconversion depends on both the quantity and the quality of the radiation reaching these layers of the epidermis. Wavelengths of the order of 280–320 nm are required, with the maximum conversion occurring at 295 nm. After photoconversion this previtamin D_3 can either undergo further photoconversion to tachysterol and lumisterol, or a heat-induced isomerization to vitamin D_3. At normal body temperatures, 50% of this isomerization takes place within 28 h, with lower rates being achieved at lower temperatures. Thus, production of vitamin D_3 within the skin can take a period of several days. Vitamin D is stored in various fat depots throughout the body. The lipid nature of vitamin D and its metabolites limits their concentration within the circulation, but a specific vitamin D transport protein (an α_2 globulin that corresponds to the G_c system of plasma proteins) binds a number of metabolites with varying degrees of efficacy. There are at least 37 metabolites of vitamin D (Norman 1990) but only three – 25-hydroxyvitamin D_3 ($25(OH)D_3$), 1,25-dihydroxyvitamin D ($1,25(OH)_2D_3$) and 24,25-dihydroxyvitamin D_3 ($24,25(OH)_2D_3$) – are of any major importance for biological activity, the role of the

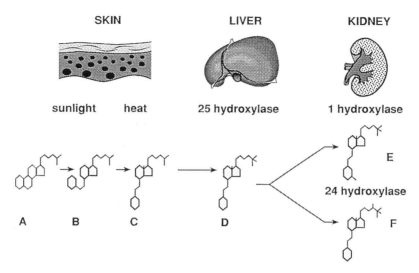

Fig. 13.8 Synthesis of vitamin D and its biologically active metabolites. The action of sunlight on the skin converts 7-dehydrocholesterol (A) to previtamin D (B) which is metabolized to vitamin D (C) by a temperature-dependent isomerization. The vitamin D is then transported via the general circulation to the liver where the enzyme 25-hydroxylase converts it to 25-hydroxyvitamin D (D). Further conversion to the biologically active metabolite $1,25(OH)_2D_3$ (E) or 24,25-dihydroxyvitamin D (F), which may also have a physiological role, occurs in the kidney.

last remaining controversial. The other metabolites seem to represent pathways of inactivation of the various active forms of the molecule.

Conversion of vitamin D_3 to $25(OH)D_3$ occurs in the liver. The enzyme 25-hydroxylase is found primarily in the microsomes and requires NADPH, molecular oxygen, magnesium ions and a cytosolic component (DeLuca 1979). The circulating level of $25(OH)D_3$ is higher than that of vitamin D (Stanbury & Mawer 1990). The circulating $25(OH)D_3$ is further hydroxylated by one of two enzymes: 1α hydroxylase is a classic mixed function oxidase similar to other steroid hormone hydroxylases and is a cytochrome P–450 enzyme which involves NADPH and an adrenodoxin component which incorporates molecular oxygen into the 1α position of $25(OH)D_3$; 24α hydroxylase is a similar enzyme which incorporates the oxygen molecule into the 24α position of $25(OH)D_3$ to yield $24,25(OH)_2D_3$.

CONTROL OF SYNTHESES

Because $1,25(OH)_2D_3$ is the most biologically active form of cholecalciferol, its circulating concentration is tightly controlled. Although the kidney produces both dihydroxylated forms of the vitamin, the dominant

form is determined by both the level of circulating parathyroid hormone (PTH) and the body's vitamin D status. In a vitamin-D-deficient state $1,25(OH)_2D_3$ production is high, while that of $24,25(OH)_2D_3$ is low. This is because $1,25(OH)_2D_3$ controls its own production in a negative feedback loop by suppressing the 1α hydroxylase enzyme. When vitamin D status is adequate more $24,25(OH)_2D_3$ is produced. PTH, the production of which is stimulated by a fall in plasma calcium (see Chapter 11), increases the kidney's hydroxylase activity: when the body's vitamin D status is low the 1α hydroxylase is stimulated, but if vitamin D status is high then $24,25(OH)_2D_3$ production is increased. $1,25(OH)_2D_3$ also directly reduces PTH production within the parathyroid gland. Hypophosphataemia can also induce $1,25(OH)_2D_3$ production. Thus a series of controls regulates the production of the major active form of vitamin D, $1,25(OH)_2D_3$.

This hormone is normally produced solely by the kidney, but during pregnancy the placenta also secretes significant amounts of $1,25(OH)_2D_3$ into the circulation. Patients with sarcoidosis and extensive renal disease can be hypercalcaemic due to high plasma levels of $1,25(OH)_2D_3$ derived from 1α hydroxylase activity in activated macrophages (Reichel et al 1989).

MECHANISM OF ACTION

Being lipid-soluble, vitamin D and its metabolites readily pass through the cell membranes to interact with a specific receptor, which is similar in many respects to other steroid hormone receptors (Haussler et al 1988). This receptor binds $1,25(OH)_2D_3$ avidly and more readily than $24,25(OH)_2D_3$; $25(OH)D_3$ is least actively bound. In the blood, however, the vitamin-D binding protein binds $24,25(OH)_2D_3$ and $25(OH)D_3$ more avidly than $1,25(OH)_2D_3$, so the $1,25(OH)_2D_3$ is readily concentrated within the cell. The receptor, with its bound $1,25(OH)_2D_3$ then translocates to the nucleus (Fig. 13.9), where it binds to the DNA of specific responsive genes. Special loops in the receptor, common to all steroid hormone receptors and known as 'zinc fingers' for their zinc content, enable the receptor to interdigitate with the helical structure of DNA. Once bound to the DNA the receptor induces messenger RNA production for the specific protein or peptide which is controlled by

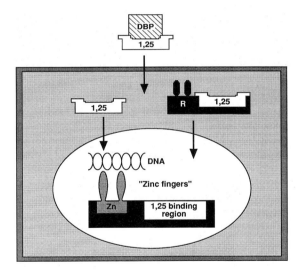

Fig. 13.9 Mechanism of action of $1,25(OH)_2D_3$. The biologically active form of vitamin D, $1,25(OH)_2D_3$ (1,25) is carried in the circulation by a vitamin D binding protein (DBP). At the target cell the $1,25(OH)_2D_3$ is released and enters the cell where it can bind to a specific receptor (R), which then translocates to the nucleus, or passes directly to the nucleus before associating with the receptor. $1,25(OH)_2D_3$ is bound to the carboxyl-terminal portion of the receptor and the amino-terminal portion contains structures which are known as zinc fingers, which interdigitate with the double helix of DNA. This leads to the initiation of the transcription and translation of specific genes and the production of particular proteins involved in the action of $1,25(OH)_2D_3$.

$1,25(OH)_2D_3$. This process of gene transcription and translation takes a number of hours and accounts for the majority of the actions of $1,25(OH)_2D_3$. However, $1,25(OH)_2D_3$-induced calcium uptake by the small intestine can occur within a matter of minutes, so part of vitamin D's effect does not involve the conventional genomic action on the nucleus (see Reichel et al 1989).

ACTIONS OF $1,25(OH)_2D_3$

Vitamin D maintains plasma calcium by stimulating intestinal calcium absorption by the small intestine and by increasing the resorption of calcium from bone (Fig. 13.10).

Intestinal calcium absorption

$1,25(OH)_2D_3$ stimulates calcium transport across the intestinal cells by inducing the production of a calcium-binding protein (CBP) within the villus cells through the normal process of receptor binding, DNA interaction and messenger RNA production. The resulting CBP maintains the usual extremely low concentration of cytosolic calcium within the cell. Calcium probably diffuses into the villus cell passively, but calcium transfer into the blood seems to involve classic ion transport mechanisms such as calcium-activated adenosine triphosphatases. $1,25(OH)_2D_3$ also promotes cell maturation within the intestine (Suda et al 1990). Intestinal mucosa cells have a short half-life and the length of the villus in vitamin-D deficient rats is only some 70–80% of that in normal rates. These effects seem to be related to changes in polyamine metabolism (Suda et al 1990).

Bone resorption

Because appropriate concentrations of calcium are important in vital functions such as nerve and muscle activity, the skeleton is sacrificed when calcium supply is limiting. In a mature adult in normal calcium balance, a demand in excess of the supply of calcium is met by skeletal calcium. As plasma calcium falls, there is a rise in PTH which in turn increases $1,25(OH)_2D_3$ synthesis. This then acts on the bone-forming cells – the osteoblasts – which produce factors that stimulate the activity of the bone-removing cells, the osteoclasts. $1,25(OH)_2D_3$ also promotes bone resorption by increasing the formation of new osteoclasts (Suda et al 1990). $1,25(OH)_2D_3$ therefore leads to an increase in both the number and activity of osteoclasts within the bone, and these remove the bone matrix to release the bound calcium (Fig. 13.11).

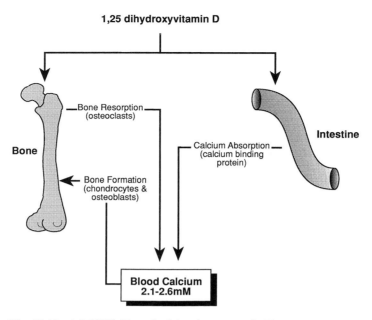

Fig. 13.10   1,25(OH)$_2$D$_3$ and calcium homoeostasis. Plasma calcium is maintained within tight limits. 1,25(OH)$_2$D$_3$ is the principal hormone responsible for calcium absorption from the intestine where it stimulates the production of an intracellular calcium binding protein. 1,25(OH)$_2$D$_3$ also affects bone metabolism, stimulating both resorption and formation.

Growth-plate mineralization and bone formation

1,25(OH)$_2$D$_3$ increases bone formation by providing sufficient calcium within the body to allow calcification to occur. A growing child with vitamin D deficiency fails to absorb enough calcium and will have a poorly mineralized skeleton. 1,25(OH)$_2$D$_3$ also stimulates the production of osteocalcin. This protein is formed by osteoblasts and binds up to four calcium molecules: it is found exclusively in bone (Fig. 13.12). 1,25(OH)$_2$D$_3$ also affects other processes involved in bone formation, including alkaline phosphatase activity and collagen synthesis. Within the growth plate, chondrocytes proliferate, differentiate and finally become calcified to form bone. This process results in longitudinal growth (Fig. 13.12). As they mature the chondrocytes release matrix vesicles, which are considered to be the sites at which the calcification begins. Vitamin D metabolites may affect the mineralization of the skeleton by altering chondrocyte differentiation. The need for 24,25(OH)$_2$D$_3$ as well as 1,25(OH)$_2$D$_3$ in calcification is disputed (DeLuca 1988).

Other actions of 1,25(OH)$_2$D$_3$

It is now clear that 1,25(OH)$_2$D$_3$ has many actions as well as those regulating calcium metabolism.

Numerous tissues respond to 1,25(OH)$_2$D$_3$ and, in common with vitamin A, vitamin D seems to have a role in the processes of cell proliferation and maturation (Reichel et al 1989, Suda et al 1990).

Children with rickets often have abnormalities associated with the immunohaematopoietic system, with increased frequency of infections, impaired neutrophil phagocytosis, anaemia and decreased bone marrow cellularity. These are corrected by vitamin D administration. 1,25(OH)$_2$D$_3$ receptors are found in activated but not quiescent lymphocytes, and 1,25(OH)$_2$D$_3$ stimulates cell proliferation, so this may in part explain a rickety child's susceptibility to infection. Another role for 1,25(OH)$_2$D$_3$ is in the control of cell maturation in the skin. Neonatal skin cells responsible for keratin production produce 1,25(OH)$_2$D$_3$ under experimental conditions, but this does not occur in adulthood. 1,25(OH)$_2$D$_3$ may also have a role in the treatment of leukaemia and lung and colon cancers, where it may inhibit proliferation.

ASSAY OF VITAMIN D METABOLITES

The conversion of vitamin D to the 25-hydroxylated form seems to reflect the supply of cholecalciferol, so

OSTEOCLAST ACTIVATION

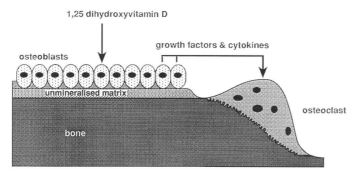

OSTEOCLAST ACTIVATION

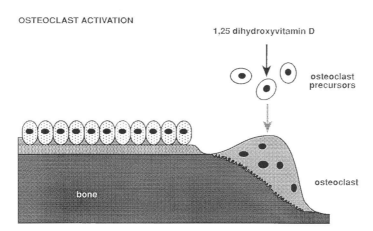

Fig. 13.11 $1,25(OH)_2D_3$ and bone resorption. $1,25(OH)_2D_3$ increases bone resorption by stimulating both the activity and the number of osteoclasts which remove bone matrix. The stimulation of osteoclastic activity is indirect relying on the initial stimulation of the bone forming cells, called osteoblasts, which in turn release cytokines and growth factors which stimulate osteoclastic activity.

assessment of the $25(OH)D_3$ concentration in plasma is a good index of the availability of vitamin D for conversion to its active metabolites. The half-life of $25(OH)D_3$ is about 3 weeks. With so many factors influencing the production of $1,25(OH)_2D_3$, the level of this metabolite does not reflect vitamin D status except in severe vitamin D deficiency.

Vitamin D status is therefore assessed by measuring $25(OH)D_3$ (Holick 1990). A vitamin-D binding protein, which has a very high affinity for $25(OH)D_3$ is often used as the basis of an assay of lipid extracts of serum or plasma. Unfortunately other vitamin D metabolites, although present at less than 10% of the concentration of $25(OH)D_3$, can interfere in this

assay unless a preliminary chromatographic separation of $25(OH)D_3$ is used. The other major method of assessing $25(OH)D_3$ levels combines the initial separation of the lipid extract with HPLC and UV absorbance. The normal range for $25(OH)D_3$ is usually between 20 and 150 nmol (8–60 ng/ml) with concentrations below 25 nmol (10 ng/ml) being indicative of impending or frank vitamin D deficiency (Holick 1990). In hypervitaminosis D, levels are usually above 375 nmol (150 ng/ml) with high plasma calcium and phosphorus levels.

Circulating levels of $1,25(OH)_2D_3$ are measured with lipid extracts of plasma or serum, from which the $1,25(OH)_2D_3$ is separated by HPLC and then

GROWTH PLATE MINERALISATION

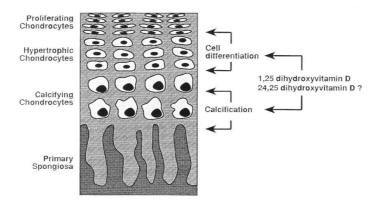

OSTEOBLAST ACTIVITY

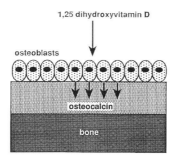

Fig. 13.12   Vitamin D metabolites and growth-plate mineralization and bone formation. Longitudinal growth depends on the proliferation, maturation and calcification of chondrocytes within the ends of the long bones. Both maturation and calcification involve the action of $1,25(OH)_2D_3$. A further vitamin D metabolite, 24,25-dihydroxyvitamin D, may also play an important role in calcification. Bone formation within the skeleton is controlled by osteoblasts and $1,25(OH)_2D_3$ is essential for this process by controlling the formation of certain proteins and enzymes, such as osteocalcin and alkaline phosphatase.

assayed using a receptor purified from bovine thymus, which reacts equally well to the $1,25(OH)_2D_3$ metabolites of both ergocalciferol and cholecalciferol. The half-life of $1,25(OH)_2D_3$ in the circulation is between 4 and 6 hours, and the normal circulating concentrations are 38–144 pmol/l (16–60 pg/ml). The low plasma calcium in vitamin D deficiency leads to a release of PTH, which increases $1,25(OH)_2D_3$ production. Since the plasma concentration of $25(OH)D_3$ is 1000 times greater than $1,25(OH)_2D_3$, even low levels of $25(OH)D_3$ provide enough substrate for conversion. Thus, a patient with vitamin D deficiency can have low or undetectable levels of $25(OH)D_3$ but normal or even elevated levels of $1,25(OH)_2D_3$ (Holick 1990).

SOURCES OF VITAMIN D

Although vitamin D is present in a number of foods such as egg yolk, oily fish, and to some extent milk (Table 13.6), the natural human diet can only be considered as a trivial source of the vitamin (Fraser 1983). Vitamin D, either natural or added, is stable in foods and storage; processing or cooking do not affect its activity. The major source of vitamin D in the normal ambulatory adult is exposure to sunlight, and therefore the use of the word vitamin is not strictly appropriate (Fraser 1983) and $1,25(OH)_2D_3$ should be classified as a hormone (Kodicek 1974, DeLuca 1979).

Vitamin D production by the skin is related to latitude, and the further away from the equator the lower the proportion of the year during which vitamin D can be synthesized. This is because the short UV wavelengths of light necessary for the photoconversion of 7-dehydrocholesterol are absorbed as they pass through the atmosphere. At higher latitudes the angle of the sun's rays is greater, so the path through the atmosphere is longer and less UV-B reaches the earth's surface. In Scandinavia and the UK, plasma $25(OH)D_3$ levels vary from winter to summer (Stamp & Round 1974). Similarly in Boston, USA, at 42.2°N, the photoconversion of 7-dehydrocholesterol occurs only between March and October, with a maximum in June and July (Webb & Holick 1988). Further north in Edmonton, Canada (52°N), conversion only occurs from April to September while in Los Angeles (34°N) there is a low level of conversion even in January. By contrast, in Puerto Rico (18°N) in the Caribbean, 7–dehydrocholesterol conversion in January is similar to that in Boston during the peak summer months.

NUTRITIONAL REQUIREMENTS

With the major source of vitamin D derived from the skin, establishing any requirement or allowance for vitamin D is difficult. Vitamin D toxicity can also occur when levels are only around five times normal, so judging the correct oral dose needs care. The effectiveness of dietary supplementation has also been questioned, as studies on the addition of vitamin D to the diet of either submariners or astronauts (with no exposure to natural sunlight) at 2.5 μg/day (similar to UK requirements) showed that a fall in plasma $25(OH)D_3$ levels was not prevented (Fraser 1983). Different policies regarding dietary allowances exist in different countries, and the following gives some idea of the guidelines issued to particular population groups in three countries with different degrees of sunlight exposure.

Adults

In the USA, where cow's milk (10 μg (400 IU) /quart) and margarine are supplemented, the most recent report on recommended dietary allowances (1989) sets the recommended daily allowance (RDA) for adults (aged 24 years and over) at 5 μg (200 IU)/day even though the estimated dietary intake is of the order of 1.25–1.75 μg/day, and clinical nutritional osteomalacia is rare in the USA. In Australia, with high levels of natural sunlight and consequently an increased risk of toxicity, it is only the housebound who are at any significant risk of vitamin D deficiency (Fraser 1987). The average dietary intake within the UK, where the levels of sunlight are low and margarine is the only food fortified, ranges from 0.5 to 8 μg/day, with a mean of around 3 μg/day. The most recent COMA report (1991) sets no dietary reference value (DRV) for those aged between 4 and 50 years of age, with the exception of those confined indoors where the intake was set at 10 μg/day.

Pregnancy and lactation

In pregnancy and lactation there is a heavy demand for calcium, and in the USA the RDA is doubled to 10 μg (400 IU)/day in women over 24 years of age. No supplementation is considered necessary in Australia, provided there is reasonable exposure to sunlight. In the UK the recommended intake during pregnancy and lactation is 10 μg/day.

Table 13.6   Vitamin D content of food (μg/100 g)

Cereals	
Grain, flours, starches	0
Milk & milk products	
Cow's milk	0.01–0.03
Human milk	0.04
Dried milk	0.21
Cream	0.1–0.28
Cheese	0.03–0.5
Yoghurt	Trace–0.04
Eggs	
Whole	1.75
Yolk	4.94
Fats and oils	
Butter	0.76
Cod liver oil	210
Margarines and spreads*	5.8–8.00
Meat & meat products	
Beef, lamb, pork, veal	Trace
Poultry, game	Trace
Liver	0.2–1.1
Fish & fish products	
White fish	Trace
Fatty fish	Trace–25
Crustacea & molluscs	Trace
Vegetables	0

*Added during production (vitamin D_2). Source: Holland et al 1991

Infants and children

For breast-fed infants under 6 months where exposure to sunlight may be low, and because maternal milk contains only small amounts of vitamin D, the RDA in the USA is set at 5–7.5 μg (200–300 IU)/day. Because of the increased demand of calcium for the growing skeleton, and because peak bone mass is not attained until the third decade, the RDA for the ages 6 months–24 years is 10 μg (400 IU)/day. In the UK, a similar intake level of 10 μg/day was set for babies and young children up to the age of 3 years. Provided there is sufficient exposure to sunlight, no supplementation is recommended in Australia.

The elderly

In Australia this is the only group for whom supplementation, at a level of 10 μg/day, is considered necessary. In the UK adults over the age of 65 are set a recommended intake of 10 μg/day, while in the USA additional supplementation over the 5 μg/day recommended for all adults is not considered necessary (Appendix 2).

PATHOPHYSIOLOGY

The pathophysiology of abnormal vitamin D metabolism is set out in Chapter 11. Asian children living in temperate climates such as the UK can develop vitamin D deficiency, with rickets occurring because of growth failure and poor mineralization of the growth plate. Skeletal deformity, with bone pain or tenderness and muscle weakness, is part of the clinical picture. In florid rickets, tooth eruption may be delayed and the patient may have a low plasma calcium. They are also anaemic and prone to respiratory infections.

In adults, vitamin D deficiency results in osteomalacia which is characterized by a wide seam of unmineralized matrix (osteoid) lining the bone surfaces. Bone pain or tenderness, particularly in the shoulder, hip or spine, is common. $25(OH)D_3$ levels in the plasma are generally below 4 ng/ml, and hypocalcaemia and hypophosphataemia may also occur. Treatment with vitamin D is generally sufficient to cure these disorders.

Vitamin-D resistant rickets (vitamin-D dependent rickets type II) is an inherited disorder which is apparently caused by defective receptors for $1,25(OH)_2D_3$. The symptoms of this disease are similar to those for conventional rickets, with the exception that the levels of $1,25(OH)_2D_3$ are normal or elevated. The molecular defects associated with this disease are related to the inability of the receptor to form the 'zinc fingers' needed for the receptor to bind to the DNA. Vitamin-D dependent rickets type-I is a rare autosomal disease where there is a defect in the 1α hydroxylase system within the kidney. $1,25(OH)_2D_3$ levels are therefore low, but $25(OH)D_3$ levels are elevated. A similar picture occurs in X-linked hypophosphataemic rickets, where the presumed defect is an abnormality of phosphate anion transport in the renal tubule. This hypophosphataemia results in a decrease in 1α hydroxylase activity. Oncogenic osteomalacia is a rare disease, with a tumour of mesenchymal origin presumed to secrete a factor that induces symptoms similar to those in hypophosphataemic rickets; the problem regresses with removal of the tumour. The involvement of reduced levels of $1,25(OH)_2D_3$ in the aetiology of both postmenopausal and senile osteoporosis has been proposed. However, there is still controversy over whether $1,25(OH)_2D_3$ levels are reduced and whether treatment with vitamin D is of any benefit.

VITAMIN E (TOCOPHEROLS)

G. Duthie

In 1922, a fat-soluble dietary constituent was found to be essential for the prevention of fetal death and sterility in rats. This was originally called 'factor X' and 'antisterility factor', but was later named vitamin E. When finally isolated from wheatgerm oil in 1936, vitamin E was called 'tocopherol' from the Greek words *tokos* and *pherein,* meaning to bring forth children (Mason 1977). There are now known to be several forms of tocopherol and the term vitamin E is often used to denote any mixture of biologically active tocopherols. Animals cannot synthesize vitamin E, and to avoid deficiency have to consume diets containing the vitamin. Vitamin E deficiency contributes to many syndromes in animals, but the dietary requirement for the vitamin by humans has yet to be firmly established.

CHEMISTRY

Pure vitamin E is odourless and colourless, although commercial preparations are usually pale yellow/brown at room temperature. It is fully soluble in most organic solvents and is insoluble in water. There are eight naturally occurring vitamin E compounds (Fig.

13.13), which are synthesized by plants from homogenistic acid. All are derivatives of 6-chromanol and differ in the number and position of the methyl groups on the ring structure. The four tocopherol homologues (dα-, dβ-, dγ-, dδ-) have a saturated 16-carbon phytol side chain, whereas the tocotrienols (dα-, dβ-, dγ-, dδ-) have three double bonds on the side chain. These structural differences have important effects on the biological activity of the vitamins. There is also a widely available synthetic form, dlα-tocopherol, prepared by coupling trimethylhydroquinone with isophytol. This consists of a mixture of eight stereoisomers in approximately equal amounts; these isomers are differentiated by rotations of the phytol chain in various directions which do not occur naturally. The synthetic preparation is often used in the fortification of animal feeds and is available in capsules as a nutritional supplement. As tocopherols and tocotrienols are readily oxidized to quinones, dimers and trimers by light, heat, alkali and divalent metal ions such as copper and iron, commercial preparations of vitamin E are often protected by acetylation and succinylation. The resultant esters are hydrolysed by pancreatic enzymes in the gut to yield the biologically active free tocopherol.

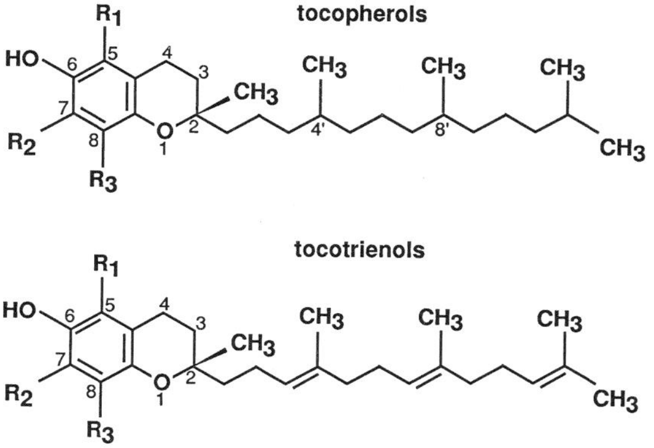

Fig. 13.13 The chemical structure of naturally-occurring tocopherols and tocotrienols. The tocotrienols differ from the tocopherols in that the 16-carbon phytol chain contains three unsaturated double bonds. The number and position of the methyl groups on the chromanol ring denotes the different homologues as follows:

Homologue	Formula	R_1	R_2	R_3
α-	5,7,8-Trimethyl	CH_3	CH_3	CH_3
β-	5,8-Dimethyl	CH_3	H	CH_3
γ-	7,8-Dimethyl	H	CH_3	CH_3
δ-	8-Methyl	H	H	CH_3

BIOCHEMICAL ROLE

Function

The structure of vitamin E (Fig. 13.13) means that it is a highly effective antioxidant, readily donating the hydrogen from the hydroxyl (OH) group on the ring structure to free radicals; these are reactive and potentially damaging molecules with an unpaired electron which, on receiving the hydrogen, become unreactive. On donating the hydrogen, vitamin E itself becomes a relatively unreactive free radical because the unpaired electron on the oxygen atom can be delocalized into the aromatic ring structure, thereby increasing its stability. Vitamin E has a major biological role in protecting polyunsaturated fats and other components of the cell membranes from oxidation by free radicals, and is therefore primarily located within the phosholipid bilayer of the cell membranes (Fig. 13.14).

Free radicals

The production of free radicals which can initiate damage to biological material occurs during normal aerobic metabolism. Activated oxygen species are formed during the stepwise reduction of oxygen to water, and by secondary reactions with protons and transition metals such as copper and iron. For example, the superoxide anion (O_2^-) is produced in many cell redox systems, such as those involving xanthine oxidase, aldehyde oxidase, membrane-associated NADPH oxidases and the cytochrome P-450 system. About 1–4% of the total oxygen taken up by mitochondria may be used for O_2^- production, and about 20% of this may be ejected into the cell. Stimulated macrophages and monocytes also release large amounts of O_2^-. As this radical is not particularly reactive, it can diffuse relatively large distance through the cell, where it is converted in a metal catalysed reaction into the more reactive hydroxyl radical ($OH^\bullet$). Potentially injurious free radicals are also present in pollutants, halogenated anaesthetics and cigarette smoke.

Lipid peroxidation and vitamin E

Polyunsaturated fatty acids (PUFA:H) are major constituents of cell membranes. They are particularly susceptible to free-radical mediated oxidation because of their methylene-interrupted double-bond structure. Thus the process of lipid peroxidation can lead to disturbances in membrane structure and function (Halliwell 1987). Briefly, the process is

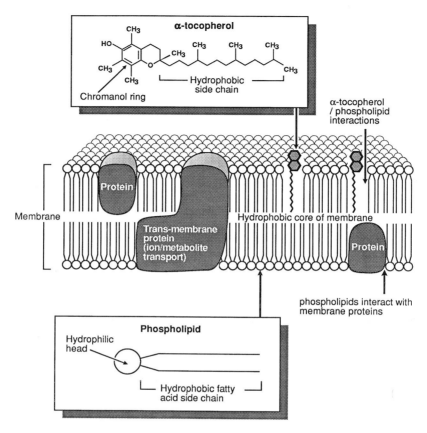

Fig. 13.14   Schematic representation of the lipid bilayer of a cell membrane, showing the possible position of the tocopherol molecule. The phytol side chain intercalates with the membrane phospholipids.

initiated by a free radical such as OH$^{\bullet}$ extracting a hydrogen from PUFA:H, with the formation of a PUFA radical (PUFA$^{\bullet}$). This is followed by the rearrangement of the double bond to form a conjugated diene, which then combines with oxygen to produce a peroxyl radical (PUFAOO$^{\bullet}$), which in turn reacts with more PUFA:H to form a hydroperoxide (PUFA:OOH) and another PUFA$^{\bullet}$. The reaction is now self-propagating:

$$PUFA:H \rightarrow PUFA^{\bullet}$$
$$PUFA^{\bullet} + O_2 \rightarrow PUFA:OO^{\bullet}$$
$$PUFA:OO^{\bullet} + PUFA:H \rightarrow PUFA:OOH + PUFA^{\bullet}$$

Moreover, in the presence of iron or copper PUFA:OOH can undergo a fission of the double bonds and one electron reduction to form more free radicals, including the highly reactive OH$^{\bullet}$.

$$PUFA:OOH \rightarrow PUFA:O^{\bullet} + OH^{\bullet}$$

Such autoxidation will continue unless all the free radicals are scavenged by antioxidants. Therefore, a major biological role for vitamin E is to break the chain of events leading to the formation of PUFA:OOH by donating the hydrogen atom of the hydroxy group on its chromanol ring to the free radical to form a stable species. The resulting vitamin E radical is fairly stable and therefore does not contribute to the propagation of the chain reaction.

Complementary antioxidant defence systems

If vitamin E fails to prevent the formation of PUFA:OOH in the cell membrane, there is a second line of defence (Fig. 13.15): the PUFA:OOH can be released from phospholipids by phospholipase A_2 and then degraded by selenium-containing glutathione peroxidase in the cell cytoplasm. Thus the antioxidant activities of vitamin E and selenium through glutathione peroxidase are closely related. Other important antioxidant enzymes include superoxide dismutase, catalase and glucose-6-phosphate dehydrogenase, and compounds such as carotenoids, ubiquinone, uric acid, glutathione, carnosine and ascorbic acid (vitamin C) also have antioxidant properties.

Although vitamin E is the major lipid-soluble antioxidant in cell membranes, its concentration may only be one molecule per 2000–3000 phospholipid molecules. This suggests that it is regenerated in vivo, otherwise the vitamin would be rapidly used up. Consequently, the well documented regeneration of vitamin E by vitamin C in vitro may also occur in vivo, and/or as yet unidentified reductases may reduce the vitamin E radical back to its native state.

Other roles of vitamin E

Vitamin E may also play important roles in other biological processes which do not necessarily involve its antioxidant function. These include:

1. Structural roles in the maintenance of cell membrane integrity;
2. Anti-inflammatory effects by direct and regulatory interaction with the prostaglandin synthetase complex of enzymes that participates in the metabolism of arachidonic acid;
3. DNA synthesis;
4. Stimulation of the immune response.
   However, further research is required to confirm these functions.

ABSORPTION AND TRANSPORT

Tocopherols are absorbed from the gut in micelles, whose formation depends on bile salts and pancreatic lipase. Since such micelles are also necessary for the absorption of dietary lipids, vitamin E deficiency can occur in patients with fat malabsorption. Animal studies suggest that maximum absorption of tocopherol occurs in the upper and middle thirds of the small intestine. Tocopherol uptake appears to be enhanced by medium-chain triglycerides but inhibited by long-chain polyunsaturated fatty acids. Micelles containing tocopherol may passively diffuse through the brush border, but the mechanism by which vitamin E is then transported across the intestinal epithelial cells is poorly understood. The vitamin is released from the enterocyte into the lymph within chylomicrons which subsequently appear in the circulation, where they are catabolized by lipoprotein lipase (Fig. 13.16) (Bjorneboe et al 1990). The resulting chylomicron remnants are then taken up by the liver, which preferentially secretes the α-form into the plasma in newly formed very low-density lipoproteins (VLDL), but excretes most of the γ-tocopherol into the bile (Traber & Kayden 1989). This explains why the γ-homologue, although absorbed, only accounts for 10% of plasma tocopherol. It is somewhat paradoxical that the organism discriminates against γ-tocopherol, which is abundant in the diet and is also the most effective antioxidant in vitro.

Tocopherols incorporated within plasma lipoproteins are taken up mainly by the low-density lipoprotein receptors on peripheral cells, but little is known of how

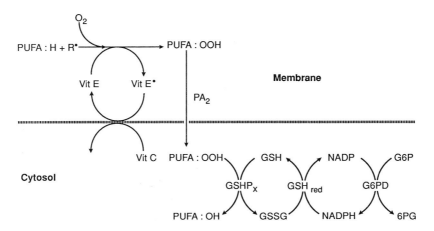

Fig. 13.15   Some of the major antioxidant defence mechanisms within the cell. R•, free radical; PUFA:H, polyunsaturated fatty acid; PUFA:OOH, fatty acid hydroperoxide; GSH, reduced glutathione; GSSG, oxidized glutathione; GSHPx, glutathione peroxidase; PA₂, phospholipase A₂; GSH$_{red}$, glutathione reductase; G6PD, glucose-6-phosphate dehydrogenase; 6PG, 6-phosphogluconate.

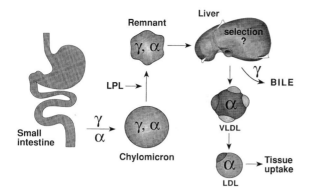

Fig. 13.16 Both α- and γ-homologues are absorbed from the intestine and appear in the circulation in chylomicrons. However, most of the γ-form appears to be rapidly excreted in the bile, whereas α-tocopherol appears in the low density lipoproteins (LDL). Other abbreviations; LPL, lipoprotein lipase; VLDL, very low density lipoprotein.

they are transported within the cell and incorporated into the cell membranes. There is some evidence that cytosolic proteinaceous binders (molecular weight approximately 32 000) and membrane receptors which favour the dα-form are involved (Behrens & Madere 1982, Kitabchi & Wimalasena 1982). The tocopherols then accumulate at those sites in the cell where oxygen radical production is greatest and where they are most needed, viz. in heavy mitochondria, light mitochondria and endoplasmic reticulum.

METABOLISM OF VITAMIN E

Little is known about the metabolic fate of vitamin E. The primary oxidation product of α-tocopherol may be α-tocopherol quinone which can be reduced to a hydroquinone by quinone reductase. The detection of α-tocopherol hydroquinone glucoronate in the faeces suggests that there is some conjugation of the hydroquinone with glucoronic acid. The quinone may also be degraded through a β-oxidation pathway in the kidney to α-tocopheronic acid, followed by conjugation and elimination in the urine as α-tocopheronic acid glucoronate.

NUTRITIONAL ASSESSMENT AND REQUIREMENTS

Deficiency

There are many signs of vitamin E deficiency in animals (Table 13.7), most of which are related to

damage to cell membranes and leakage of cell contents to external fluids. Common disorders are myopathies, neuropathies and liver necrosis. Early diagnostic signs of deficiency include leakage of muscle enzymes such as creatine kinase into plasma, increased levels of lipid peroxidation products in plasma and increased erythrocyte haemolysis.

The assessment of the vitamin E requirement for humans is confounded by the infrequent occurrence of clinical signs of deficiency, since these usually only develop in premature infants or in adults with fat malabsorption. Although this suggests that modern diets contain sufficient vitamin E to satisfy nutritional needs, there is growing epidemiological evidence that intakes of vitamin E and other antioxidants are inversely correlated with the risk of intestinal, breast and lung cancer and coronary heart disease (Diplock 1987, Duthie et al 1989). Thus there may be a distinction between the amount of vitamin E required to avoid overt deficiency and the optimum intake needed to reduce the risk of the development of these diseases.

Problems of estimating requirement

Estimating the dietary requirement of vitamin E is difficult not only because the clinical signs of

Table 13.7 Diseases and syndromes associated with vitamin E deficiency in animals

Syndrome	Affected organ or tissue	Species
Encephalomalacia	Cerebellum	Chick
Exudative diathesis	Vascular	Turkey
Microcytic anaemia	Blood, bone marrow	Chick
Macrocytic anaemia	Blood, bone marrow	Monkey
Liver necrosis	Liver	Pig, rat
Pancreatic fibrosis	Pancreas	Chick, mouse
Muscular degeneration	Skeletal muscle	Pig, rat, mouse
Microangiopathy	Heart muscle	Pig, lamb, calf
Kidney degeneration	Kidney tubules	Monkey, rat
Embryonic degeneration	Vascular system	Pig, rat, mouse
Steatitis	Adipose tissue	Pig, chick
Testicular degeneration	Testes	Pig, calf, chick

deficiency are infrequent, but also because it is affected by the composition of the diet and the different biological activities of the homologues. Thus high dietary intakes of polyunsaturated fatty acids will tend to increase the requirement for vitamin E because of the increased susceptibility of tissues to peroxidation. The biological activity of the homologues of tocopherol can differ by more than thirtyfold, as estimated by tests for fetal resorption in pregnancy studies, the susceptibility of red cells to haemolysis, and the ability to prevent muscular dystrophy. Generally, these tests indicate that d-α-tocopherol has the greatest biopotency of the naturally occurring isomers (Table 13.8). The biological activity of vitamin E can be expressed as International Units (IU), 1 IU of vitamin E being equivalent to 1 mg of synthetic d-α-tocopherol acetate. For example, the biological activities of d-α-tocopherol and d-γ-tocopherol are 1.49 and 0.15 IU/mg, respectively. Alternatively, vitamin E activity is also quoted as tocopherol equivalents (TE), 1 mg TE being the amount of a compound with vitamin E activity nutritionally equivalent to 1 mg d-α-tocopherol. Thus 1 mg of TE is equal to 1.49 IU. The difference in biopotencies of the homologues probably reflects the ease with which they can achieve the orientation within the cell membranes that results in optimum biological function. Intercalation within the phospholipid bilayer (see Fig. 13.14) may be affected by the position of the methyl groups on the chromanol ring and by the configuration of the carbons of the phytol side chain (Kagan et al 1990).

Arguments for increasing vitamin E intake

Cross-cultural epidemiological studies have shown statistically significant inverse associations between plasma vitamin E concentrations and mortality from heart disease and certain cancers. This has led to suggestions that the dietary requirement for health, rather than the avoidance of chronic deficiency, should be increased. Thus it has been suggested that the US figure for the RDA for vitamin E of 10 mg TE/day should be increased fourfold (Diplock 1987).

There is another argument for increasing the RDA. The mean vitamin E intake in the USA is close to the RDA, but a fifth of it comes from fats and oils. As the general population responds to nutritional advice to reduce total fat intake and increase the proportion of unsaturated fat in the diet, total vitamin E intake may fall, while the requirement for vitamin E will increase. Moreover, the high consumption of soya oil in the USA means that over 50% of total tocopherol intake is accounted for by the less biologically active γ-form. It has therefore been proposed that there is a base daily requirement of 5.96 IU plus a factor for the polyunsaturated fatty acid component of the diet (Horwitt 1988):

$$\text{Requirement (IU)} = 5.96 + 0.25 \ (\% \ \text{PUFA kcal} + \text{g PUFAs})$$

The Nutrition Working Group of the International Life Sciences Institute Europe (1990) has similarly suggested that until such time as optimum intakes of vitamin E have been established by long-term intervention trials, the RDA is calculated assuming a daily intake of 14 g of polyunsaturated fatty acid (5% of energy intake), an energy intake of 2400 kcal/day, and with 40% of the energy derived from fat with a P:S (PUFA: saturated fatty acid) ratio from 0.33 to 0.40. This gives a vitamin E requirement of 18 IU/day (12 TE/day).

In the UK, dietary reference values (DRV), which have recently superseded the RDA, also attempt to take into consideration the practical difficulties of setting the vitamin E requirement. A range of acceptable intakes has been derived from a survey of serum tocopherol:cholesterol ratios and dietary records. The dietary requirement is regarded as that needed to maintain a serum tocopherol:cholesterol value above 2.25 μmol/mmol and the DRV are 3.5–19.5 and 2.5–15.2 mg α-tocopherol/day for men and women, respectively (Appendix 2).

Requirements for smokers

Although the benefits to the general population of increasing vitamin E intake are contentious, it is likely that this would aid smokers, a group at high risk of developing heart disease and lung cancer, since

Table 13.8 Approximate biological activity of naturally occurring tocopherols and tocotrienols

Common name	Biological activity	
	(IU/mg)	Compared with d-α (%)
d-α-tocopherol	1.49	100
d-β-tocopherol	0.75	50
d-γ-tocopherol	0.15	10
d-δ-tocopherol	0.05	3
d-α-tocotrienol	0.75	30
d-β-tocotrienol	0.08	5

tobacco smoke contains vast quantities of reactive free radicals in both the tar phase and gas phase. Consequently, alveolar fluid in smokers is deficient in vitamin E and they exhibit signs of increased lipid peroxidation, such as pentane expiration, erythrocyte lipid peroxidation and plasma concentrations of conjugated dienes. Supplementation with vitamin E reduces free radical activity in smokers (Duthie et al 1991), although the significance of these observations in terms of disease prevention requires further study.

Problems of assessing vitamin E status

An individual's vitamin E status is often estimated from the plasma vitamin E concentrations. Current and somewhat contentious European guidelines suggest the following categories: deficient, <6.5 µg/ml; marginally deficient, 6.5–8.6 µg/ml; normal, 8.6–10.8 µg/ml; optimum, > 10.8 µg/ml. Such a system needs to be treated with caution, as plasma vitamin E concentrations may not accurately reflect intakes or tissue reserves. This is demonstrated by data for swine (Fig. 13.17). Plasma vitamin E concentration increases only twofold over a wide range of vitamin E intakes; in contrast, over the same range of intakes there are markedly greater increases of vitamin E in tissue such as heart, skeletal muscle and liver. In humans, where access to tissue samples is often difficult, platelet and red-cell vitamin E contents may be more valid predictors of nutritional status than plasma concentrations (Lehmann et al 1988). In the clinical environment the ratio in serum of tocopherol to total lipid or to (cholesterol + triglyceride) may be useful in identifying vitamin E deficiency (Thurnham et al 1986).

FOOD SOURCES

Fats and oils are major sources of tocopherols in food products. The relative abundance of the tocopherol homologues depends on the species of plant and the extraction procedures. For example, the γ-form accounts for about 60% of total tocopherol in soya oil, whereas the α-homologue is predominant in safflower and olive oil (Tables 13.9 and 13.10). Palm oil, which is used as a base for many foodproducts in the UK, contains significant quantities of tocotrienols (Jacobsberg et al 1978). Little is known about the nutritional significance of tocotrienols. Other major food sources of vitamin E are vegetables, poultry and fish, fortified breakfast cereals and wholegrain bread (Table 13.11 and Murphy et al 1990).

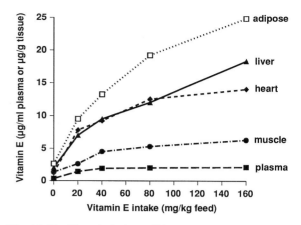

Fig. 13.17   The relatively small increase in vitamin E in the plasma of pigs compared to the increases in the major tissues over an increasing range of dietary vitamin E intakes. Data courtesy of Peter P. Hoppe, BASF Animal Nutrition Research Station, Germany.

TOXICITY

Vitamin E is well tolerated even in pharmacological doses. Acute and chronic toxicities of oral vitamin E are low and animal studies indicate that high doses are not mutagenic, carcinogenic or teratogenic. Relatively few side effects have been observed in humans, even at intakes as high as 3200 IU/day, although some case reports suggest that vitamin E causes breast soreness, emotional disorders, muscular weakness and gastrointestinal disorders in some individuals. One double-blind study among college students indicated that a daily intake of 600 IU for 28 day significantly decreased serum thryoid hormone levels. Moreover, administration of vitamin E to vitamin K-deficient subjects can exacerbate coagulation defects (Bendich & Machlin 1988). At present there are no hard data on

Table 13.9   Total vitamin E content of vegetable oils (mg/100 g)

Oil	Total tocopherol
Soya	56–160
Cotton seed	30–81
Corn	53–162
Coconut	1–4
Peanut	20–32
Palm	33–73
Safflower	25–49
Olive	5–15

Data adapted from Chow (1985)

Table 13.10 Individual isomers as a % of total vitamin E

Oil	Tocopherols				Tocotrienols			
	α	β	γ	δ	α	β	γ	δ
Soya	4–18	-	58–69	24–37	-	-	-	-
Cotton seed	51–67	-	33–49	-	-	-	-	-
Corn	11–24	-	76–89	-	-	-	-	-
Coconut	14–67	-	-	<17	<14	<3	<53	-
Peanut	48–61	-	39–52	-	-	-	-	-
Palm	28–50	-	-	<9	16–19	4	34–39	-
Safflower	80–94	-	6–20	-	-	-	-	-
Olive	65–85	-	15–35	-	-	-	-	-

Data adapted from Chow (1985)

Table 13.11 Concentration of α- and γ-tocopherols in common foods

Food	α-tocopherol (mg/100 g edible portion)	γ-tocopherol (mg/100 g edible portion)
Cereals	0.88	0.77
Pulses	0.27	5.66
Nuts and seeds	9.92	10.97
Vegetables	0.81	0.14
Fruits	0.27	No data
Meat	0.31	0.21*
Eggs	1.07	0.35
Milk	0.34	No data
Lard	1.37	0.70
Butter	1.95	0.14
Hard margarine	9.09	19.38
Soft margarine	18.92	26.02

Data compiled from several sources by Mary Bellizzi
*Value obtained from 3rd revised version of German Food Composition and Nutrition Tables, 1986/87

the beneficial or detrimental effects of long-term consumption of pharmacological levels of vitamin E, but daily intakes of 200–700 mg of TE appear to be free of side effects (Fig. 13.18).

THERAPEUTIC USES

As free radicals have been implicated in many diseases, vitamin E supplements have frequently been used as a therapeutic agent. Early studies involving mega dose supplements of vitamin E were invariably anecdotal, ill-controlled and lacking in scientific consistency. However, more recent studies (Diplock et al 1989) suggest that high doses of vitamin E may slow down the progression of Parkinson's disease, reduce the severity of neurological disorders such as tardive dyskinesia, prevent periventricular haemorrhage in preterm babies, reduce tissue injury arising from ischaemia and reperfusion during surgery, ameliorate malignant hyperthermia syndrome, delay cataract development and improve mobility in arthritis sufferers.

Tappel (1972) remarked that 'The more research is done on the substance (vitamin E), the more intriguing it appears. Thus there is a nagging suspicion that there is a very important use for the vitamin and we are just not smart enough to see it'. Despite the recent explosion in vitamin E research, and its undoubted role in protecting the body from high free-radical concentrations, that comment is still largely true. Many questions still remain unanswered and further research is needed to elucidate the mechanisms whereby tocopherols react with lipid radicals in membrane bilayers, and to establish how tocopherols are regenerated and metabolized in vivo and transported through plasma and cellular fluids to membranes. Furthermore, the role of vitamin E in delaying or preventing the development of major diseases such as coronary heart disease and cancer has yet to be established.

VITAMIN K

C. Bolton-Smith

A dietary-derived coagulation factor was first described by Dam and Schonheyder in Denmark. They observed a bleeding disorder in chickens which was corrected by feeding a variety of foods, but most effectively lucerne (alfalfa) or putrid fish meal. Dam termed the active factor Koagulation-vitamin (Dam 1935), and with the help of Swiss chemists (Karrer and co-workers) he isolated the newest fat-soluble

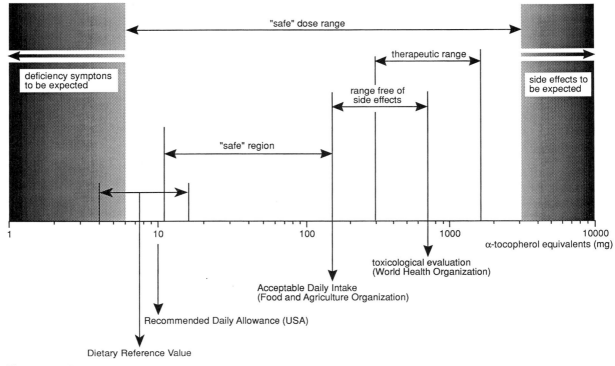

Fig. 13.18 Suggested oral intakes of vitamin E required to avoid deficiency and toxicity. The data have been assembled from several sources and do not constitute an official set of guidelines.

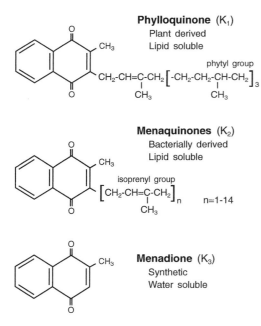

Fig. 13.19 Structures of vitamin K.

vitamin (K) in 1939. It was synthesized shortly after in America by several groups.

CHEMISTRY

Vitamin K exists in two forms; both are 2-methylnaphthoquinone rings with side chains at position three (Fig. 13.19). Vitamin K_1 (phylloquinone) has a phytyl side chain and occurs only in plants; vitamin K_2 is a family of compounds called menaquinones (MK), whose side chain consists of a number of isoprene units, varying from 1–14 (MK1–14). They are synthesized by bacteria, some of which occur naturally in the intestine of animals. Menadione (vitamin K_3) is a synthetic form of vitamin K. It consists of the naphthoquinone ring without a side chain and so is water-soluble. It only becomes biologically active after alkylation in vivo. Vitamin K is progressively destroyed on light (UV) exposure.

BIOCHEMISTRY

The biological activity of vitamin K is due to its ability to change between the oxidized forms (quinone and epoxide) and the reduced form (quinol) in the vitamin K cycle (Fig. 13.20). The conversion of quinol to the epoxide form is catalysed by an enzyme (or enzymes) with epoxidase and carboxylase activity. The carboxylase converts glutamate (glu) residues of proteins to γ-carboxyglutamate (gla) residues. These proteins are termed vitamin K-dependent or gla-proteins. All gla-proteins so far identified have a highly conserved sequence of amino acids near the amino terminal. The enzymes of the vitamin K cycle are found in rough endoplasmic reticular membranes of liver and bone, and to a lesser extent in other tissues. The gla-proteins are able to bind calcium ions very readily, and it is this property which gives them their biological activity (Vermeer 1990).

VITAMIN K-DEPENDENT PROTEINS

Plasma proteins

The first established gla-proteins were the coagulation proteins, Factors II (prothrombin), VII, IX and X (Senflo et al 1974). Their calcium-binding properties enable them to associate specifically with the acidic phospholipids on cell and platelet membranes, a step which is essential to the coagulation cascade. More recently, two further plasma vitamin K-dependent proteins, C and S, have been characterized, which inhibit coagulation by blocking the activation of factors V and VIII. The function of a further gla-protein, Z, is currently unknown. A small amount of the bone gla-protein, osteocalcin (see

below) also circulates in the plasma and may be a useful marker of osteoblast activity and bone function.

Bone proteins

The main gla-protein of mineralized tissue (bone and dentine) is osteocalcin, which is produced by osteoblast and odontoblast cells respectively. A further gla-protein, which is found in both mineralized tissue and cartilaginous tissues, is matrix gla-protein. Osteocalcin and matrix gla-protein bind hydroxyapatite, and while their precise function is still unclear, they are involved with bone mineralization (Price 1988).

Other proteins

Gla-proteins have been identified in many other tissues, such as kidney, placenta, pancreas, spleen, lung, testis and antherosclerotic plaques; their functions are as yet unknown. A gla-protein in brain may be important for the metabolism of sulphatides which are vital for brain development.

SOURCES OF VITAMIN K

Dietary sources

Vitamin K_1 occurs in plants in the quinone form and is particularly abundant in green leafy vegetables such as broccoli (150–200 μg/100 g), spinach (300–400 μg/

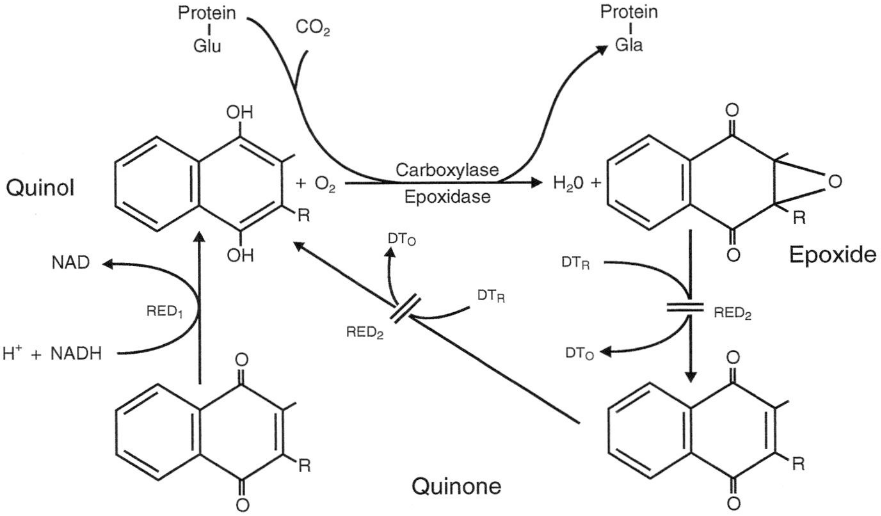

Fig. 13.20   The vitamin K cycle. Glu, glutamate residues; Gla, γ-carboxyglutamate residues; $RED_{1/2}$, reductases; $DT_{O/R}$, oxidized/reduced dithiol; // site of warfarin inhibition.

100 g), parsley (500–600 µg/100 g), cabbage, etc. The greener the leaves the higher the content of vitamin K, thus the outer leaves of cabbage (around 200 µg/100 g) are a richer source than the pale inner ones (50 µg/100 g). Margarines (20–150 µg/100 g) and vegetable oils, particularly those based on soya oil (around 130 µg/100 g) are also good vitamin K_1 sources, but freshness is important for oils, and a long shelf-life is not ideal since exposure to light destroys vitamin K. Other vegetables and fruits contain varying smaller amounts, and a cup of tea contains around 0.4 µg (food composition data: MJ Shearer, personal communication). Cow's milk provides small but significant quantities of vitamin K in the diet. Milk composition shows seasonal variations which probably reflect the summer (grass) and winter (dry fodder) feeding of cattle. Some fermented milk products and cheeses contain bacterially-derived vitamin K_2 which contributes to total vitamin K intake. The liver is the major storage site of vitamin K in animals, and is a dietary source of vitamins K_1 and K_2.

Human colostrum milk contains around 1.8 ng/ml and mature milk 1.2 ng/ml; the concentration in mature milk changes slightly with variations in maternal intake (von Kries et al 1987).

Non-dietary sources

Bacteria in the intestine, and especially in the colon, synthesize menaquinones and may contribute to the physiologically available pool of vitamin K in the body.

REQUIREMENTS

The dietary requirement for adults is thought to be about 1 µg/kg body weight (COMA 1991). The average daily dietary intake of adults in the UK is probably between 50 and 100 µg, which meets the recommended level. For infants a higher value of 2 µg/kg body weight (10 µg/day) is recommended, since their liver stores are lower and their gut flora is poorly developed (Appendix 2).

FROM ABSORPTION TO EXCRETION

About 50–80% of the vitamin K in the small intestine is absorbed and this requires bile salts and pancreatic enzymes, as in the absorption of fat and other fat-soluble vitamins. It is transported to the liver in chylomicrons via the lymphatics and circulates in the plasma predominantly in the triacylglycerol-rich VLDL. Any condition which impairs fat absorption, such as biliary obstruction, pancreatic insufficiency and coeliac disease, will decrease absorption.

The liver provides the major store of vitamin K, of which around 90% are menaquinones. Fasting plasma levels in healthy adults range between 0.2 and 0.7 ng/ml, while those in infants are lower (16 pg/ml) and can be undetectable. Conditions with hypertriglyceridaemia result in correspondingly higher levels of circulating vitamin K (up to 13 ng/ml) (Shearer et al 1988).

After recycling many times over, vitamin K is metabolized to a variety of water-soluble, bile acid-conjugated products which are excreted in the urine and faeces (Barkhan & Shearer 1977).

FACTORS INFLUENCING VITAMIN K STATUS

Effect of diet

The experimental use of vitamin-K deficient diets in humans has demonstrated elevated levels of partially γ-carboxylated prothrombin and depressed plasma vitamin K levels; these effects are reversed on vitamin K supplementation (Suttie et al 1988). The relationship between dietary or gut microbially derived vitamin K and circulating levels of vitamin K is currently unknown. Diets that enhance colonic fermentation (high in soluble non-starch polysaccharides and resistant starch) may increase menaquinone production. However, the absorption of vitamin K_2 from the colon and lower ileum appears to be by passive uptake and, although its precise bioavailability is presently unclear, it is unlikely that gut menaquinones can meet the human requirements for vitamin K in the absence of any dietary intake of vitamin K.

Effect of drugs and surgical interventions

The classic anticoagulant drugs are dicoumarins (e.g. warfarin) which were first isolated from spoilt sweet clover in 1941. They block the recycling of vitamin K (see Fig. 13.20) and result in bleeding. Warfarin poisoning (rat poison) may be overcome by large oral or intramuscular (i.m.) doses of vitamin K, 10–20 mg every 8 hours. Poisoning by the newer 'super' warfarins such as difenacoum and flocoumafen poses a greater problem, as their biological half-life is extremely long and multiple blood transfusions are necessary (Vermeer & Hamulyak 1991).

Broad-spectrum antibiotics destroy the MK-producing intestinal bacteria, and those which contain the N-methylthiotetrazole derivative may also inhibit the functioning of vitamin K itself. Overt deficiency is rare in adults, except in patients with fat malabsorption syndromes or post-intestinal surgery who are taking antibiotics. The combination of inadequate absorption of dietary vitamin K and reduced MK production in the gut is thought to be predisposing.

DISEASES ASSOCIATED WITH VITAMIN K

Haemorrhagic disease of the newborn

Levels of vitamin K in human milk vary and appear inadequate for some babies who are solely breast-fed. This syndrome, termed haemorrhagic disease of the newborn (HDN), or idiopathic late-onset HDN when it occurs between 3 and 8 weeks of life, is characterized by spontaneous bruising/bleeding or intracranial haemorrhage, which can result in death. In the UK it is now uncommon (prevalence of 1.62/100 000 live births between 1988 and 1990) because vitamin K is commonly given as prophylaxis (McNinch & Tripp 1991). However, prophylaxis is neither universal nor standardized, and until recent reports of increased incidence of cancers in children who received i.m. injection of vitamin K (1 mg) at birth (Golding et al 1992), this was the favoured form of prophylaxis in the USA, and is still used in the UK. The recommended forms of prophylaxis are now an oral dose (1mg) to the infant at birth or 20 mg doses to the mother for several days before parturition. It is unclear whether the vitamin K deficiency is due to poor maternal nutrition, inadequate placental transfer or intestinal malabsorption. Detection of HDN is complicated by the normal hypoprothrombinaemic state of newborns.

Thrombosis-associated diseases

These include coronary heart disease (CHD) and veno-occlusive disease (VOD): it is considered that the hypercoagulable state that predisposes to CHD and VOD may be contributed to by relatively high levels of the functional vitamin K-dependent proteins (Factors II, VII, IX and X). Oral anticoagulant therapy appears to reduce the risk of secondary myocardial infarction (but a moderate tendency to bleed is the usual side effect). More evidence is required before it is known whether low-dose oral anticoagulation regimens are definitely beneficial for primary and secondary prevention of thrombosis and CHD (Poller et al 1990). Future possibilities remain for dietary rather than drug administration for regulating coagulation.

Osteoporosis

There is some evidence of lower vitamin K status in patients with osteoporosis (Knapen et al 1989). However, given the uncertainty about the physiological role of osteocalcin and bone matrix gla-protein, it is not yet possible to say whether vitamin K is an important factor in the aetiology of osteoporosis.

DETECTION AND ASSAY

Historically, vitamin K activity in foods was detected using a chick bioassay and this led to high estimates of dietary intakes and of dietary requirements. Vitamin K status has traditionally been assessed by determining the plasma prothrombin time. This is the time taken for fresh plasma to clot in the presence of calcium and a source of thromboplastin. The time to clotting is an inverse measure of the amount of active prothrombin in the blood. This method is still routinely used but it is insensitive and only capable of detecting overt clinical deficiency.

Newer immunological techniques are based on the detection of partially γ-carboxylated prothrombin. This abnormal prothrombin can be detected in advance of a prolongation in bleeding time, and so is a more sensitive, but not more specific, assay of vitamin K status. Direct measurement of vitamin K in foods, plasma and other tissues has only become possible with the advent of HPLC and highly sensitive and specific methods for detection: vitamin K is extracted with hexane, passed through a reversed-phase HPLC column and detected either electrochemically or fluorometrically (Shearer 1991). The interest in the role of sub-clinical vitamin K deficiency in disease processes now depends on these recently developed and more precise methods of measuring vitamin K status.

REFERENCES

Ahmed F, Ellis J, Murphy J et al 1990 Excessive faecal loss of vitamin A(retinol) in cystic fibrosis. Archives of Disease in Childhood 65: 589–593

Arroyave G, Mejia LA, Aguilar JR 1981 The effect of vitamin A fortification of sugar on serum vitamin A levels of preschool Guatemalan children: a longitudinal evaluation. American Journal of Clinical Nutrition 34: 41–49

Barkhan P, Shearer MJ 1977 Metabolism of vitamin K_1 (phylloquinone) in man. Proceedings of the Royal Society of Medicine 70: 93–96

Behrens WA, Madere LT 1982 Transfer of α-tocopherol to microsomes mediated by a partially purified liver α-tocopherol-binding protein. Nutrition Research 2: 611–618

Bendich A, Langseth L 1989 Safety of vitamin A. American Journal of Clinical Nutrition 49: 358–371

Bendich A, Machlin LJ 1988 Safety of oral intake of vitamin E. American Journal of Clinical Nutrition 48: 612–619

Berstein PS, Law WC, Rando RR 1987 Isomerization of all-*trans* retinoids to 11-*cis* retinoids in vitro. Proceedings of the National Academy of Sciences (USA) 84: 1849–1853

Bhat PV, Sundaresan PR 1988 High-performance liquid chromatography of vitamin A compounds. CRC Critical Reviews in Analytical Chemistry 20: 197–218

Bhat PV, Poissant P, Falardeau P, La Croix A 1988 Enzymatic oxidation of all-*trans* retinol to retinoic acid in rat tissues. Biochemistry and Cell Biology 66: 735–740

Bjorneboe A, Bjorneboe GA, Drevon CA 1990 Absorption, transport and distribution of vitamin E. Journal of Nutrition 120: 233–242

Blomhoff R, Green MH, Berg T, Norum KR 1990 Transport and storage of vitamin A. Science 250: 399–404

Blunt JW, DeLuca HF, Schnoes HK 1968 25-hydroxycholecalciferol. A biologically active metabolite of vitamin D_3. Biochemistry 7: 3317

Bush ME, Dahms BB 1984 Fatal hypervitaminosis in a neonate. Archives of Pathology and Laboratory Medicine 108: 838–842

Carlier C, Moulia-Pelat J-P, Ceccon J-F et al 1991 Prevalence of malnutrition and vitamin A deficiency in the Diourbel, Fatick and Kaolack regions of Senegal: feasibility of the method of impression cytology with transfer. American Journal of Clinical Nutrition 53: 66–69

Chow CK 1985 Vitamin E and blood. World Review of Nutrition and Dietetics 45: 133–136

Committee on the Medical Aspects of Food Policy 1991 Dietary reference values for food energy and nutrients for the United Kingdom. HMSO, London

Dam H 1935 The antihaemorrhagic factor of the chick. Biochemistry Journal 29: 1273–1285

DeLuca HF 1979 Vitamin D: metabolism and function. In Gross F, Grumbach MM, Labhart A et al (eds) Monographs on endocrinology Vol 13. Springer-Verlag, Berlin

DeLuca HF 1988 The vitamin D story: a collaborative effort of basic science and clinical medicine. Faseb Journal 2: 224–236

Diplock AT 1987 Dietary supplementation with antioxidants. Is there a case for exceeding the recommended dietary allowance? Free Radical Biology and Medicine 3: 199–201

Diplock AT, Machlin LJ, Packer L, Pryor WA 1989. Vitamin E: biochemistry and health implications. Annals of the New York Academy of Sciences 570: 555

Duthie GG, Wahle KJ 1990 Smoking, essential fatty acids and coronary heart disease. Biochemical Society Transactions 18: 1051–1054

Duthie GG, Wahle KWJ, James WPT 1989 Oxidants, antioxidants and coronary heart disease. Nutrition Research Reviews 2: 51–62

Duthie GG, Arthur JR, James WPT 1991 Effects of smoking and vitamin E on blood antioxidant status. American Journal of Clinical Nutrition 53: 1061S–1063S

Flores H, Campos F, Araujo CRC, Underwood BA 1984 Assessment of marginal vitamin A deficiency in Brazilian children using the relative dose response. American Journal of Clinical Nutrition 40: 1281–1289

Food and Agriculture Organization/World Health Organization 1989 Requirements of Vitamin A, iron, folate, and vitamin B_{12}. Report of a joint FAO/WHO Expert Committee FAO Food and Nutrition Series 23. FAO, Rome

Fraser DR 1983 The physiological economy of vitamin D. Lancet i: 969–971.

Fraser DR 1987 Vitamin D. Journal of Food and Nutrition 44:3–9

Fraser DR, Kodicek E 1970 Unique biosynthesis by kidney of a biologically active vitamin D metabolite. Nature 228: 764–766

Funk C 1911 On the chemical nature of the substance which cures polyneuritis in birds induced by a diet of polished rice. Journal of Physiology 43: 395–400

Giguere V, Ong ES, Segiu P, Evans RM 1987 Identification of a receptor for the morphogen retinoic acid. Nature 330: 624–629

Golding G, Greenwood R, Birmingham K, Mott M 1992 Childhood cancer, intramuscular vitamin K, and pethidine given during labour. British Medical Journal 305: 241–346.

Goodman DS 1984 Plasma retinol-binding protein. In Sporn MB, Roberts AB, Goodman DS (eds) The retinoids, vol 2. Academic Press, Orlando, pp. 41–88

Halliwell B 1987 Oxidants and human disease: some new concepts. FASEB Journal 1: 358–364

Haussler MR, Mangelsdorf DJ, Komm BS et al 1988 Molecular biology of the vitamin D hormone. Recent Progress in Hormone Research 44: 263–305

Hess AF 1929 Rickets including osteomalacia and tetany. Lea and Febinger, Philadelphia

Holick MF 1990 The use and interpretation of assays for vitamin D and its metabolites. Journal of Nutrition 120: 1464–1469

Holland B, Welch AA, Unwin ID, Buss DH, Paul AA, Southgate DAT (eds) The Composition of Foods 5th edn. Royal Society of Chemistry, and Ministry of Agriculture Fisheries and Food, London

Horwitt MK 1988 Supplementation with vitamin E. American Journal of Clinical Nutrition 47: 1088–1089

Hume EM, Krebs HA 1949 Vitamin A requirement of human adults: an experimental study of vitamin A deprivation in man. Special Report Series, Medical Research Council No 264

International Vitamin A Consultative Group 1982 Biochemical methodology for the assessment of Vitamin A status. Nutrition Foundation, Washington DC

Jacobsberg B, Delmide P, Gapor A 1978 Tocopherols and tocotrienols in palm oil. Oleagineax 33: 239–247

Kagan VE, Serbinova EA, Packer L 1990 Recycling and antioxidant activity of tocopherol homologs of differing hydrocarbon chain lengths in liver microsomes. Archives of Biochemistry and Biophysics 282: 221–225

Kitabchi AE, Wimalasena J 1982 Specific binding sites for $d\alpha$-tocopherol on human erythrocytes. Biochimica et Biophysica Acta 684: 200–206

Knapen MHJ, Hamulyak K, Vermeer C 1989 The effect of vitamin K supplementation on circulating osteocalcin (bone gla-protein) and urinary calcium excretion. Annals of Internal Medicine 111: 1001–1005

Kodicek E 1974 The story of vitamin D: from vitamin to hormone. Lancet i: 325–329

Lehmann MS, Rao DD, Canary JJ, Judd JT 1988 Vitamin E and relationships among tocopherols in human plasma, platelets, lymphocytes and red blood cells. American Journal of Clinical Nutrition 47: 470–474

McCollum EV, Davis M 1913 The necessity of certain lipids in the diet during growth. Journal of Biological Chemistry 15: 167–175

McCollum EV, Simmonds N, Becker JE, Shipley PG 1922 Studies on experimental rickets. XXI. An experimental demonstration of the existence of a vitamin which promotes calcium deposition. Journal of Biological Chemistry 53: 293–312

McLaren DS 1980 Nutritional ophthalmology. Academic Press, London

McLaren DS 1986 Pathogenesis of vitamin A deficiency. In: Bavernfeind JC (ed) Vitamin A deficiency and its control. Acadamic Press, Orlando, pp. 153–176

McLaren DS, Zekian B 1971 Failure of enzyme cleavage of β-carotene: the cause of vitamin A deficiency in a child. American Journal of Diseases of Childhood 121: 278–280

McLaren DS, Shirajian E, Tchalian M, Khoury G 1967 Xerophthalmia in Jordon. American Journal of Clinical Nutrition 17: 117–130

McNinch AW, Tripp JH 1991 Haemorrhagic disease of the newborn in the British Isles: two-year prospective study. British Medical Journal 303: 1105–1109

Mahalanabis D 1991 Breast feeding and vitamin A deficiency among children attending a diarrhoea treatment centre in Bangladesh: a case-control study. British Medical Journal 303: 493–496

Mason KE 1977 The first two decades of vitamin E history. Federation Proceedings 36: 235

Matsuo T, Matsuo N, Shirago F et al 1988 Keratomalacia in a child with familial hyporetinol-binding proteinemia. Japanese Journal of Ophthalmology 32: 249–254

Mejia LA, Hodges RE, Rucker RB 1979 Clinical signs of anemia in vitamin A-deficient rats. American Journal of Clinical Nutrition 32: 1439–1444

Mellanby E 1919a A further determination of the part played by accessory food factors in the aetiology of rickets. Journal of Physiology 52: 1iii

Mellanby E 1919b An experimental investigation on rickets. Lancet i: 407–412

Moore T 1957 Vitamin A. Elsevier, Amsterdam

Muhilal, Permeisih D, Idjradinata YR, Muherdiyantiningsih, Karyadi D 1988 Vitamin A-fortified monosodium glutamate and health, growth, and survival of children: a controlled field trial. American Journal of Clinical Nutrition 48: 1271–1276

Murphy SP, Subar AF, Block G 1990 Vitamin E intakes and sources in the United States. American Journal of Clinical Nutrition 52: 361–367

Natadisastra G, Wittpenn JR, West KP Jr, Muhilal, Sommer A 1987 Impression cytology for detection of vitamin A deficiency. Archives of Ophthalmology 105: 1224–1228

Norman AW 1990 The vitamin D endocrine system and bone. In: Pecile A, de Bernard B (eds) Bone regulatory factors: morphology, biochemistry, physiology and pharmacology. Nato ASI series vol 184, Plenum, New York, pp93–109

Nutrition Working Group of International Life Science Institute Europe 1990 Recommended daily amounts of vitamins and minerals in Europe. Nutrition Abstracts and Reviews (Series A) 60: 827–842

Olson JA 1987 Recommended dietary intakes (RDI) of vitamin A in humans. American Journal of Clinical Nutrition 45: 704–716

Olson JA 1989 The provitamin A function of carotenoids. Journal of Nutrition 119: 105–108

Olson JA 1990 Vitamin A. In: Brown ML (ed) Present knowledge in nutrition, 6th edn. Nutrition Foundation, Washington, DC, pp. 96–107

Pan American Health Organization 1970 Hypovitaminosis A in the Americas. PAHO Scientific Publications No. 198, Washington, DC

Panel on Dietary Reference Values of the Committee on Medical Aspects of Food Policy 1991 Dietary reference values for food energy and nutrients for the United Kingdom. HM Stationery Office, London

Petkovich M, Brand NJ, Krust A, Chambon P 1987 A human retinoic acid receptor which belongs to the family of nuclear receptors. Nature 330: 444–450

Pilch SM 1987 Analysis of vitamin A data from the Health and Nutrition Examination Surveys. Journal of Nutrition 117: 636–640

Poller L, MacCallum PK, Thomson JM, Kerns W 1990 Reductions of factor VII coagulant activity (VIIC), a risk factor for ischaemic heart disease by fixed-dose warfarin: a double-blind crossover study. British Heart Journal 63: 231–233

Price PA 1988 Role of vitamin K-dependent proteins in bone metabolism. Annual Reviews of Nutrition 8: 565–583

RDA 1989. Vitamin D. National Academic Press, Washington, pp92–98

Rahmathullah L, Underwood BA, Thulasiraj RD et al 1990 Reduced mortality among children in southern India receiving a small weekly dose of vitamin A. New England Journal of Medicine 323: 929–935

Reichel H, Koffler HP, Norman AW 1989 The role of the vitamin D endocrine system in health and disease. New England Journal of Medicine 320: 980–991

Rosa FW, Wilk AL, Kelsey FO 1986 Teratogen update: vitamin A congeners. Teratology 33: 355–364

Sauberlich HE, Hodges RE, Wallace DL et al 1974 Vitamin A metabolism and requirements in the human studied with the use of labeled retinol. Vitamins and Hormones 32: 251–275

Senflo J, Fernlund P, Egan W, Roepstorff P 1974 Vitamin K-dependent modifications of glutamic acid residues in prothrombin. Proceedings of the National Academy of Science USA 71: 2730–2733

Shearer MJ 1991 Phylloquinone (vitamin K_1) in serum or plasma by HPLC. In: Fidanza F (ed) Nutritional status assessment. Chapman and Hall, London

Shearer MJ, McCarthy PT, Crampton OE, Mattock MB 1988 The assessment of human vitamin K status from tissue measurements, In: Suttie JW (ed) Current advances in vitamin K research. Elsevier, New York, pp 437–452

Sommer A, Hussaini G, Muhilal, Tarwotjo I, Susanto D, Saroso JS 1980 History of nightblindness: a simple tool for xerophthalmia screening. American Journal of Clincal Nutrition 33: 887–891

Sommer A, Tarwatjo I, Djunaedi E et al 1986 Impact of vitamin A supplementation on childhood mortality: a randomized controlled community trial. Lancet i: 1169–1173

Stamp TCB, Round JM 1974 Seasonal changes in human plasma levels of 25-hydroxyvitamin D. Nature 247: 563–565

Stanbury W, Mawer B 1990. Metabolic disturbances in acquired osteomalacia. In: Cohen RD, Lewis B, Alberti KGMM et al (eds) The metabolic and molecular basis of acquired disease, Vol 2. Bailliere Tindall, London, pp 1717–1782

Suda T, Shinki T, Takahashi N 1990 The role of vitamin D in bone and intestinal cell differentiation. Annual Review of Nutrition 10: 195–211

Suttie JW, Mummah-Schendel LL, Shah DV, Lyle BJ, Greger JL 1988. Development of human vitamin K deficiency by dietary vitamin K restriction. American Journal of Clinical Nutrition 47: 475–480

Tanumihardjo SA, Koellner PG, Olson JA 1990 Application of the modified relative dose response (MRDR) assay as an indicator of vitamin A status in a population of well-nourished American children. American Journal of Clinical Nutrition 52: 1068–1072

Tappel AL 1972 Vitamin E and free radical peroxidation of lipids. Annals of the New York Academy of Sciences 203: 12–28

Thurnham DI, Davies JA, Crump BJ, Davis M 1986 The use of different lipids to express serum tocopherol: lipid ratios for the measurement of vitamin E status. Annals of Clinical Biochemistry 23: 514–520

Traber MG, Kayden HJ 1989 Preferential uptake of α-tocopherol vs γ-tocopherol in human lipoproteins. American Journal of Clinical Nutrition 49: 517–526

Underwood BA 1984 Vitamin A in animal and human nutrition. In: Sporn MB, Roberts AB, Goodman DS (eds) The retinoids, Vol. 1 Academic Press, Orlando, pp. 281–392

Vermeer C 1990 γ-Carboxyglutamate-containing proteins and the vitamin K-dependent carboxylase. Biochemistry Journal 266: 625–636

Vermeer C, Hamulyak K 1991 Pathophysiology of vitamin K-deficiency and oral anticoagulants. Thrombosis and Haemostasis 66:153–159

Vijayaraghavan K, Radhaiah G, Prakasam BS, Sarma KVR, Reddy V 1990 Effect of massive dose vitamin A on mortality in Indian children. Lancet 336: 1342–1345

von Kries R, Shearer MJ, McCarthy PT, Haug M, Harzer G, Gobel U 1987 Vitamin K_1 content of maternal milk: influence of the stage of lactation, lipid composition, and vitamin K_1 supplement given to the mother. Pediatric Research 22: 513–517

Wald G 1943 Photoreceptor function of carotenoids and vitamin A. Vitamins and Hormones 1: 195–227

Webb AR, Holick MF 1988 The role of sunlight in the cutaneous production of vitamin D_3. Annual Review of Nutrition 8: 375–399

West KP Jr, Chirambo M, Katz J, Sommer A 1986 Breast-feeding, weaning patterns, and the risk of xerophthalmia in southern Malawi. American Journal of Clinical Nutrition 44: 690–697

West KP Jr, Sommer A 1985 Delivery of oral doses of vitamin A to prevent vitamin A deficiency and nutritional blindness. Food Reviews International 1: 355–418

West KP Jr, Pokhrel RP, Katz J et al 1991 Efficiency of vitamin A in reducing preschool child mortality in Nepal. Lancet 338: 67–71

World Health Organization 1982 Control of Vitamin A deficiency and xerophthalmia. Technical Report Series 672. WHO, Geneva

World Health Organization 1988 From Alma Ata to the year 2000: reflections at the midpoint. WHO, Geneva

World Health Organization 1991 Prevention of childhood blindness. WHO, Geneva

WHO/UNICEF/IVACG Task Force 1988 Vitamin A supplements. WHO, Geneva

14. Water-soluble vitamins

C. H. Halsted

The discovery of vitamins involved new approaches to clinical investigations over a period of 200 years. Probably the first controlled trial of dietary prevention was James Lind's search in 1747 for the cause of scurvy, a disease recognized since the 15th century. Eijkman's animal experiments with chickens and small birds in 1897 tested the hypothesis that beriberi was of dietary origin, and was an early approach to clarifying the cause and cure of a human disease. Then Castle in 1929 discovered an 'intrinsic factor' for the absorption of vitamin B_{12}, having generated a hypothesis from 75-year-old observations that pernicious anaemia affected otherwise well-nourished people who were unable to manufacture gastric acid.

The science of biochemistry was founded in the first half of this century on the identification, extraction and purification of the water-soluble vitamins. The synthesis and production of these essential nutrients resulted in cures for many classic nutritional diseases, including scurvy, beriberi and pellagra. With the decline in the importance of nutrition as a scientific component of clinical medicine in the second half of the century (see Chapter 51), only now are new ideas emerging, with more refined discoveries of the biochemical bases of disease and the roles of vitamin cofactors. New methods for assessing vitamin status have allowed a re-evaluation of vitamin deficiencies and their role in disease.

Water-soluble vitamin deficiency is now recognized as likely in anorexia associated with malignancy or other chronic disease, coeliac sprue and other small intestinal diseases, postsurgical patients receiving inadequate or improper prolonged nutritional support, and chronic alcoholism. Vitamin deficiency is induced by drugs which antagonize vitamin absorption or metabolism, and occurs in those with odd dietary habits. Scurvy, pellagra and beriberi are found worldwide and new syndromes of vitamin abuse, including hyperoxaluria from vitamin C and sensory neuropathy from pyridoxine toxicity, have emerged from vitamin overdosing by enthusiasts.

VITAMIN C

History

From the 15th century, scurvy was dreaded by seamen and explorers forced to subsist for months on diets of dried beef and biscuits. Progressive weakness and pallor, followed by bleeding gums, haemorrhaging into tissue, oedema and ulcerations was followed by death. The Scots physician James Lind in 1772 published a lengthy treatise on scurvy, which included his feeding trials of British seamen given daily supplements of vinegar, seawater or two oranges and one lemon. The citrus group was rapidly cured of scurvy and was able to return to sea duty within 6 days.

On the North American continent, scurvy took the lives of many of the first French settlers in Newfoundland before they recognized the native practice of eating fermented spruce needles and bark. In 1840, the American writer Dana (1937) described a miraculous cure of scurvy in a young sailor after the acquisition of a supply of fresh raw onions. Scurvy was also a common hazard for mid-19th-century emigrants journeying across the continent to California by wagon train and eating dried beef and breadstuffs (Stewart 1962).

Holst & Frölich (1907) then made guinea pigs scorbutic by feeding them cereal diets. The antiscorbutic factor was extracted from lemons (Zilva 1921) and later isolated from diverse sources and characterized by two independent groups (Svirbely & Szent-Györgyi 1932, King & Waugh 1932). Following the synthesis of vitamin C (Haworth & Hirst 1933), it was apparent that the tissue-extracted antiscorbutic factor, vitamin C, ascorbic acid, and hexuronic acid were all the same.

Biochemistry

Ascorbic acid is a crystalline sugar which can be synthesized from D-glucose or D-galactose in most organisms except primates, guinea pigs, an Indian fruit-eating bat and certain birds (Fig. 14.1). Ascorbic

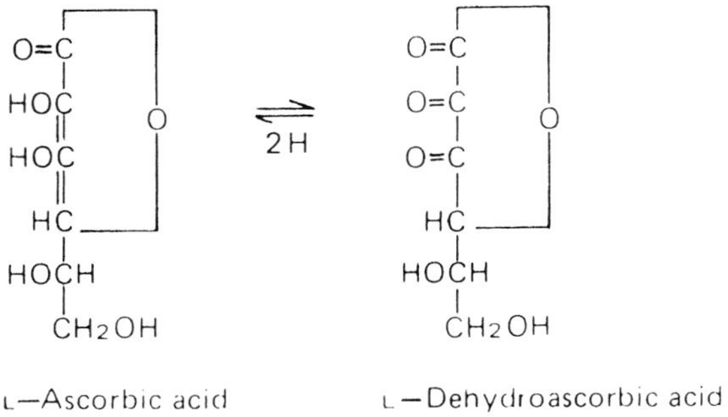

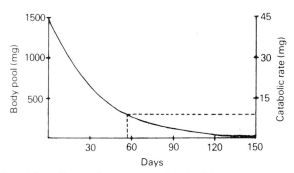

L—Ascorbic acid   L—Dehydroascorbic acid

Fig. 14.1 Structure of L-ascorbic acid and its reversible oxidation to L-dehydroascorbic acid.

acid is reversibly oxidized to L-dehydroascorbic acid on exposure to copper, heat and/or mildly alkaline conditions. Both L-ascorbic acid and L-dehydroascorbic acid are physiologically active forms of vitamin C. Further oxidation of L-dehydroascorbic acid to 2, 3-diketo-L-gulonic acid and oxalate is irreversible.

Ascorbic acid, a strong reducing agent, serves as an antioxidant (see Chapter 13) and as a cofactor in hydroxylation reactions. Many processes are influenced by ascorbic acid but its quantitative role remains poorly understood. Its role in non-haem iron absorption is considered in Chapter 12.

Collagen synthesis

Many aspects of ascorbic acid deficiency are related to impaired collagen synthesis or deposition. Ascorbic acid is essential for the hydroxylation of proline and lysine to the hydroxyproline backbone and the hydroxylysine cross-linkage needed for normal collagen fibre formation. This action may be secondary to the reducing effect of ascorbic acid on the iron cofactor of prolyl hydroxylase (Myllylä et al 1978, Hornig et al 1988). Defective hydroxylation increases the intracellular degradation of collagen fibre precursors and the formation of various cross-linking amino acids in collagen is disturbed.

Carnitine and noradrenaline synthesis

This also involves ascorbic acid. Carnitine plays a central role in transporting long-chain fatty acids into mitochondria for oxidation. Carnitine depletion precedes the development of clinical signs of experimental scurvy in guinea pigs (Nelson et al 1981) and carnitine depletion with weakness and fatigue may be an early symptom of ascorbic acid deficiency (Hornig et al 1988). The ascorbic acid-dependent conversion of dopamine to noradrenaline is impaired in ascorbic

acid-deficient guinea pigs, but human responses are unclear (Deana et al 1975).

Ascorbic acid is absorbed by an active, sodium-dependent process (Stevenson 1974). Following absorption, ascorbic acid circulates freely in plasma, leukocytes and red blood cells, and enters all tissues with maximum concentrations of 1.2–1.5 mg/dl being achieved with oral intakes of 90–150 mg/day (Olson & Hodges 1987). The highest concentrations are found in the adrenal, pituitary and retina. Excess is excreted by the kidney, which conserves the vitamin at plasma levels up to 0.8–1.5 mg/dl (Ralli et al 1938). Its metabolites, principally oxalate, appear in the urine at all levels of intake, but unchanged ascorbic acid excretion increases when intake rises from 80 to 200 mg/day (Kallner et al 1979).

The total body pool size of ascorbate is affected by limited intestinal and renal tubular absorption. Body ascorbate reaches a maximum of 20 mg/kg body weight, i.e. with a total pool size of about 1.5 g, when ascorbate intakes are increased from 30 to 180 mg/day; above this level of intake ascorbic acid excretion in the urine rises rapidly (Kallner et al 1979).

Clinical deficiency

Hodges studied metabolic turnover when healthy adult volunteers ate a diet containing less than 10 mg/day of vitamin C (Fig. 14.2). The plasma and urinary output of ascorbate fell rapidly in the first week, reaching deficient levels by 40 days. The body ascorbate content declined by 3%/day until, at 300 mg on day 55, clinical signs of scurvy appeared, with skin bruises from defective capillary basement membranes, perifollicular haemorrhages, and bleeding gums. More severe changes, including joint pains and effusions, occurred by day 80, when the body pool

Fig. 14.2 Curve of ascorbate pool derived from data on nine men whose body pool of ascorbate was labelled with ^{14}C-L-ascorbic acid. See text for details. (Data from Hodges et al 1971.)

size was below 100 mg. 10 mg a day of vitamin C was the minimal dose to produce clinical improvement (Hodges et al 1971).

Scurvy also impairs the collagen formation needed for wound healing, and the defective extracellular bone matrix impairs osteoblast function and results in pathological bone fractures. Scurvy is confirmed if plasma ascorbate levels are less than 0.10 mg/dl and leukocyte levels below 7 mg/dl (Säuberlich et al 1974) (Chapter 37).

Scurvy is also seen with other nutrient deficiencies, in intestinal malabsorption syndromes such as severe coeliac sprue, and in chronic alcoholics. Alcohol depresses vitamin C absorption (Fazio et al 1981). Low plasma ascorbate levels (0.10–0.19 mg/dl) without signs of scurvy have been described in patients with rheumatoid arthritis, in anorectic patients with cancer (Hornig et al 1988), and in heavy smokers (Smith & Hodges 1987). Cigarette smoking may increase ascorbate turnover by more than 40% because of free-radical scavenging (Kallner et al 1981) (Chapter 13, Vitamin E).

Nutritional status

Ascorbic acid is measured in plasma or leukocytes by a colorimetric assay that uses a dinitrophenylhydrazine reagent. In general, plasma levels reflect the daily intake of vitamin C, whereas leukocyte levels are a better index of tissue stores (Säuberlich et al 1974). Plasma values over 0.2 mg/dl are normal, whereas levels below 0.1 mg/dl indicate deficiency (Hodges et al 1971). Fatigue and depression with a plasma level between 0.1 and 0.2 mg/dl usually reflects a clinical condition other than ascorbate deficiency itself.

Dietary sources of vitamin C

The major sources of vitamin C are vegetables and fruits, especially spinach, tomatoes, potatoes, broccoli, strawberries, oranges and other citrus fruit. Meat and dairy products contain little vitamin C, and none is found in unfortified cereals and grains.

Recommended dietary allowance (see Appendix 2)

The USA National Research Council (Subcommittee on the Tenth Edition of the RDAs 1989) re-established the recommended dietary allowance (RDA) for vitamin C at 60 mg/day for adults of all ages, on the basis of the early turnover studies, an estimated absorption of 85% of dietary intake, and variable losses during food preparation. The US Committee

increased the RDA of smokers to 100 mg/day. Women were also advised to increase their intake of vitamin C by 10 mg/day during pregnancy to meet increased fetal demand, and by 35 mg/day during lactation to maintain ascorbate levels in human milk. Infants should receive 30 mg/day, and children older than 6 months should receive the adult amount.

Therapeutic uses and toxicity

Of all the vitamins, ascorbic acid is probably the most controversial because it is claimed, on the basis of in-vitro or animal experimentation but not clinical studies, to have wide-ranging effects. When the double Nobel Prize winner Pauling published his book *Vitamin C and the common cold* (1970) he transformed the public's attitudes to vitamin C by claiming that large daily doses of vitamin C reduced the likelihood of contracting the common cold. The popularity of this concept prompted at least 14 clinical trials, which failed to show an effect of vitamin C (Chalmers 1975), yet large segments of the population believe that daily vitamin C in amounts far exceeding the RDA is essential to maintain health (Council on Scientific Affairs 1987).

It is accepted that vitamin C may play a role in neutrophil migration as a result of its antioxidant effect on free-radical metabolism. Ascorbic acid improves neutrophil migration in chronic granulomatous disease in vitro, and decreases the frequency of bacterial infection when used clinically in this condition (Anderson 1981), but the effects of vitamin C on immune functions are unproven in other clinical conditions (Hornig et al 1988).

Ascorbic acid is concentrated in the adrenal gland, and adrenocorticotropic hormone (ACTH) stimulates the release of ascorbic acid, perhaps because it serves as a reductant in hydroxylation reactions in the formation of adrenaline and noradrenaline. A role for the vitamin in cortisone metabolism remains to be established (Hornig et al 1988).

In some individuals raised serum triglyceride levels may decrease after large doses of vitamin C (Ginter et al 1977), but this effect has not been proven in clinical trials. A potential role for vitamin C in cancer therapy is also suggested by its effect in vitro in inhibiting nitrosamine formation from naturally occurring nitrates. This effect is quite different from claims that vitamin C may prolong the survival of terminal cancer patients (Cameron et al 1979).

Vitamin C's absorption threshold occurs at intakes of 2–3 g/day (Kübler & Gehler 1970), so massive oral doses are likely to produce unpleasant diarrhoea from the osmotic effects of the unabsorbed vitamin in the intestinal lumen. The physiologically efficient renal tubular reabsorption mechanism also maintains the pool size at about 20 mg/kg body weight (Kallner et al 1979, Olson & Hodges 1987), but as intakes rise the kidney acts as though safeguarding against the tissue accumulation of ascorbic acid by increasing urinary output.

The potential toxicity of excessive doses of vitamin C relates to intraintestinal events and to the effects of metabolites in the urinary system. Within the intestine, iron overload may be accentuated by the permissive effect of ascorbic acid on iron absorption (Cook & Monsen 1977). Excessive daily amounts of vitamin C produce hyperoxaluria and an increased risk of kidney stones, because oxalate is the major metabolite of ascorbic acid and accounts for most of the normal ascorbic acid catabolism. A modest increase in urinary oxalate excretion occurs when the oral intake of vitamin C is increased from 5 to 10 g/day (Schmidt et al 1981). The risk of oxalate stones with excessive vitamin C intake is therefore low, but it may become significant if the subject has a tendency to stone formation (Chalmers et al 1986).

Excessive ascorbate intake also interferes with several common laboratory tests. For instance, megadoses of ascorbate inhibit the faecal test for blood, and ascorbate, through its reducing power, also inhibits the dipstick colour reaction for glucose in the urine. This is commonly used to regulate the insulin dose of diabetics. The reducing property of ascorbate may also provoke haemolysis in individuals with glucose-6-phosphate dehydrogenase deficiency (Woolliscroft 1983).

VITAMIN B$_1$ (THIAMIN)

History

Beriberi occurred in epidemic proportions in Japan, China, and southeast Asia in the 19th century. Osler (1893) characterized 'wet beriberi' as a condition with 'general oedema, shortness of breath and sensory disturbances with paralysis'. Takaki (1906) demonstrated that the disease in Japanese sailors could be reduced by substituting wheat bread for part of a monotonous diet of polished rice, and Eijkman (1897), a Dutch physician working in Java, induced profound weakness in domestic fowls by feeding them the diet of polished rice consumed by his patients. Funk (1911) then isolated the anti-beriberi factor from rice polishings and first used the word 'vitamine' to describe this 'amine', i.e. 'essential for life', and Jansen and Donath (1926) isolated, in Eijkman's laboratory, the crystallized form of thiamin and tested it in deficient small birds. The structure of thiamin was elucidated and its synthesis accomplished by Williams and Cline (1936).

Biochemistry

The thiamin molecule consists of a pyrimidine ring joined to a thiazole ring (Fig. 14.3). Thiamin pyrophosphate (TPP) serves as a coenzyme for many reactions in carbohydrate metabolism, e.g. as a complex in the TPP-dependent pyruvate dehydrogenase reaction in mitochondria. In addition to supplying the Krebs cycle, acetyl-CoA produced by this enzyme is an important precursor for lipids and acetylcholine, providing a biochemical link of TPP to the normal functioning of the nervous system. Within the Krebs cycle, TPP is a cofactor for the oxidative decarboxylation of α-ketoglutarate to succinyl-CoA. TPP is also required for decarboxylation of the ketoacids of the branched-chain amino acids and for several cytosolic transketolase reactions in the hexose monophosphate pathway of glucose oxidation. This pathway supplies the reduced form of nicotinamide-adenine dinucleotide phosphate for lipid biosynthetic reactions.

The essentiality of TPP for carbohydrate metabolism accounted for the development of brain anoxia and lactic acidosis in thiamin-deficient pigeons (Peters 1953) and for the clinical observation that lactic acidosis follows excessive carbohydrate administration

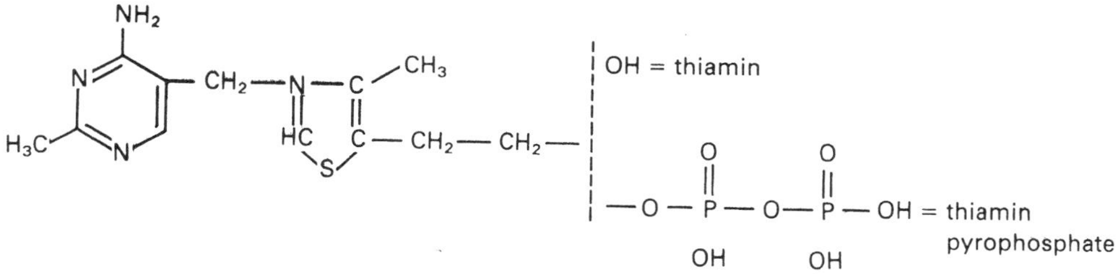

Fig. 14.3 Structure of thiamin.

to severely malnourished patients (Williams et al 1942).

Absorption, metabolism and excretion

Thiamin is absorbed in the proximal small intestine by an active process involving sodium-dependent adenosine triphosphatase (ATPase) on the basolateral membrane of the absorbing enterocyte. A second, passive process of absorption operates at thiamin concentrations >1 µmol or at oral intakes >5 mg/day. This dual mechanism has clinical implications because ethanol inhibits the active but not the passive process of thiamin absorption (Hoyumpa et al 1977). Following absorption, about 30 mg of thiamin is phosphorylated and stored as TPP in different proportions in heart (2.7 µg/g), brain (1.2 µg/g), liver (1.0 µg/g) and skeletal muscle (0.7 µg/g) (Ferrebee et al 1942). Thiamin circulates in the blood in the free form and is excreted in the urine intact with small amounts of its metabolites, primarily thiamin diphosphate and disulphide. Urinary thiamin excretion decreases rapidly in thiamin deficiency, indicating a renal conservation mechanism (McCormick 1988a).

Clinical deficiency

Thiamin deficiency occurs because of inadequate intake, poor absorption or increased metabolic demand. Clinical thiamin deficiency is seen in poor malnourished individuals in many parts of Asia, in patients with chronic disease and anorexia, in chronic alcoholism and intestinal malabsorption, and when there is an increased demand for thiamin during excessive carbohydrate therapy in the malnourished patient with marginal thiamin stores. Acute symptoms with peripheral neuropathy and lactic acidosis may occur.

Beriberi is subclassified into wet and dry forms. Wet beriberi is characterized by the development of progressive dyspnoea and oedema after several years of progressive weakness. Physical signs are indicative of high-output cardiac failure, with a wide pulse pressure, tachycardia, enlarged heart, vasodilation, pulmonary congestion, venous distension and peripheral oedema. Electro- and echocardiograms reveal low voltages and a large dilated heart. Dry beriberi is usually superimposed on wet beriberi and consists of extreme muscle weakness and progressive polyneuropathy. Features of the Wernicke–Korsakoff syndrome (described below) may intervene. The differential diagnosis of beriberi depends upon the clinical setting. In the less developed world, alternate diagnoses would include protein–calorie malnutrition, in which oedema is not associated with cardiac failure, and other vitamin deficiencies associated with peripheral neuropathy. Among alcoholic patients, cardiomyopathy may be caused by the toxicity of chronic exposure to ethanol in the absence of thiamin deficiency. The diagnosis of wet beriberi may be confirmed by appropriate laboratory tests for thiamin deficiency and by the rapid cardiac response to thiamin therapy.

Wernicke–Korsakoff syndrome

Thiamin deficiency is extremely common among chronic binge-drinking alcoholics, especially those who have developed liver disease. About one-third of chronic alcoholics have low circulating levels of erythrocyte TPP. There is a 50% reduction in hepatic thiamin concentration in alcoholic hepatitis, although levels may be normal in patients with stable cirrhosis. Autopsy studies from Australia (Harper 1983) and the USA indicated a prevalence of pathological features of Wernicke disease in more than 2% of the general population, in most cases among chronic alcoholics undiagnosed during life.

Clinical features of Wernicke–Korsakoff syndrome include a horizontal nystagmus of the eyes and paralysis of one or more ocular muscles, a wide-based gait, and a global confusional state (Reuler et al 1985). Neurological changes affect the ocular muscles, cerebellum and brain stem with haemorrhages and necroses of the nerves and myelin, particularly the mammillary bodies of the thalamus. Involvement of the brain stem may result in hypothermia and hypotension. The majority of patients who remain untreated eventually develop Korsakoff psychosis, a condition characterized by amnesia for the recent past and the inability to memorize new information. The symptom of confabulation, or storytelling, represents a defence mechanism to hide the profound memory defect. A genetic predisposition to Wernicke disease is suggested by decreased transketolase reactivity (Blass & Gibson 1977) and by different isoenzymes for this enzyme (Nixon et al 1984).

The reversibility of Wernicke disease depends on its stage. Thus, the ocular changes usually respond dramatically to one or more injections of thiamin, whereas the cerebellar gait may require months of thiamin treatment (with abstinence from alcohol). Tragically, Korsakoff psychosis is usually irreversible.

Chronic alcoholism

The multifactorial cause of thiamin deficiency is now accepted (Halsted & Heise 1987). Ethanol induces malabsorption of thiamin by an acute inhibition of the thiamin-transporting enzyme sodium-dependent ATPase, and a reduced active transport of thiamin across the basolateral membrane of the enterocyte. The inhibition of thiamin absorption in chronic alcoholism may also be mediated by associated folate deficiency. Alcohol does not block the entry of thiamin into the liver, nor impair its hepatic storage or metabolism. Thus, it appears that decreased liver thiamin in alcoholics with liver disease is mainly the result of years of poor intake and absorption, with the added effects of acute hepatic inflammation (Chapter 7).

Other clinical conditions

Beriberi or Wernicke syndrome may occur in patients with coeliac sprue and even in patients undergoing renal dialysis (Raskin & Fishman 1976).

Methods of assessment

The old microbiological assay of serum thiamin has been replaced with a high-performance liquid chromatography method (Kawasaki 1986). Urinary excretion of thiamin and its metabolites before and after oral loading reflects tissue depletion and retention, but is cumbersome and may not detect marginal deficiencies (Säuberlich et al 1974).

The best functional test of thiamin status is the assay of erythrocyte transketolase (ETKA), an enzyme in the hexose monophosphate pathway, which measures the availability of TPP for generating hexoses (Säuberlich et al 1974). ETKA activity is more specific when values are obtained before and after the in-vitro addition of TPP. In this stimulation test, a >20% elevation of ETKA activity after the addition of TPP indicates thiamin deficiency, whereas a rise of 0–15% indicates thiamin sufficiency (Säuberlich et al 1974).

Dietary sources

Although thiamin is present in all natural foods, the most important sources are plant seeds, e.g. unrefined cereal grains, organ meats, pork flesh, nuts and legumes. Because thiamin is soluble only in water, it is not present in animal or vegetable oils. Thiamin is stable in slightly acid water up to the boiling point but may be leached from food by boiling. Thiamin is removed from cereals by refining and from alcohol by grain distillation. Much of the dietary thiamin in western diets appears in fortified cereals and breads.

Recommended dietary allowance (see Appendix 2)

In view of the essential role of thiamin in carbohydrate metabolism, intakes are expressed on the basis of energy intake. Clinical signs of thiamin deficiency occur at intakes of 0.12 mg/1000 kcal, and intakes >0.3 mg/1000 kcal are compatible with good health (Säuberlich et al 1979). The US recommendations are more generous than the British, which rely on both urinary thiamin excretion and transketolase activities in specifying 0.4 rather than the US 0.5 mg/1000 kcal. To accommodate the energy needs of pregnancy and the demands of the growing fetus, an additional 0.4 mg/day is recommended during pregnancy by the US Committee, but no extra allowance is made by the UK in view of the modest effect of pregnancy on energy requirements (Chapter 25). To meet secretory losses, the lactating mother in the USA is advised to consume a total of 0.5 mg/day above the adult requirement, whereas the UK presupposes increased food intake at the RNI of 0.4 mg/1000 kcal. Other small differences in the recommendations are listed in Appendix 2.

Therapeutic uses and toxicity

Patients with wet beriberi respond dramatically to intramuscular doses of 25 mg, followed by thrice-daily oral doses of 10 mg, with a marked increase in urinary output and an improvement in cardiac function. Peripheral neuropathy (dry beriberi) is more resistant to treatment. Patients with the ocular disturbance of Wernicke disease usually respond to 2–3 daily injections of 50 mg thiamin. Oral doses of 50 mg/day should be prescribed for patients with other manifestations of Wernicke–Korsakoff syndrome, although the benefit is variable and is probably considerably influenced by their ability to avoid ethanol consumption.

No known toxicity is associated with the oral administration of thiamin, but parenteral doses >400 times the RDA were reported to cause nausea and mild ataxia (McCormick 1988a).

VITAMIN B$_{12}$ (COBALAMIN)

History

Pernicious anaemia was originally described by Thomas Addison in 1855 as a disease with insidious onset which affected middle-aged or elderly subjects who were always fat. In 1860, the American physician Austin Flint recognized that pernicious anaemia coexisted with 'degenerative diseases of the glandular tubuli of the stomach'. In his textbook of medicine, Osler (1893) described the pathology of fatal pernicious anaemia as including 'a lemon tint of the skin', extensive atrophy of the stomach and occasional 'sclerosis in the posterior columns' of the spinal cord.

These observations set the stage for the Nobel Prize-winning discovery by Minot and Murphy (1926) that pernicious anaemia was a nutritional disorder that could be cured by the oral administration of a diet containing massive daily amounts (100–200 g) of whole calf liver. This was followed by the development of a water-soluble liver extract, which was effective in treating pernicious anaemia when given by injection. Recognizing the key association between pernicious anaemia and the lack of secretion of gastric acid, Castle (1929) cured pernicious anaemia by orally giving beef muscle, which he termed 'extrinsic factor', together with normal human gastric juice, which contained an 'intrinsic factor'. The extrinsic factor vitamin B_{12} was later isolated from the liver by American (Rickes et al 1948) and British (Smith & Parker 1948) groups. Castle's description of the central role of the stomach in the absorption of vitamin B_{12} led to the eventual isolation and purification of intrinsic factor (IF), a glycoprotein secreted by parietal cells of the stomach (Gräsbeck et al 1966). The role of vitamin B_{12} and folate in blood diseases is also discussed in Chapter 39.

Biochemistry

Vitamin B_{12} or cobalamin consists of a porphyrin-like ring, which contains cobalt and is linked to ribose and phosphoric acid (Fig. 14.4). Vitamin B_{12} analogues have the same structure in the absence of cobalt. The anionic R group takes several forms. Cyanocobalamin, the commercial and therapeutic product, is present in minimal amounts in the diet and tissue. The principal natural and dietary forms of vitamin B_{12} are 5-deoxyadenosylcobalamin, methylcobalamin, and hydroxocobalamin.

Vitamin B_{12} is a cofactor for only two known human enzymes, methionine synthetase and methylmalonyl-CoA mutase (Cooper & Rosenblatt 1987).

Methionine synthetase reaction

This cytoplasmic reaction also involves folate (see Fig. 14.6). The methyl group of 5-methyltetrahydrofolate (5-methyl-H_4 folate) is transferred to cobalamin to form methylcobalamin, which then donates the methyl group to homocysteine. The end products of the reaction are methionine, cobalamin, H_4 folate, which is required for the formation of polyglutamyl folates, and 5,10-methylene-H_4 folate, the cofactor for thymidylate synthetase and ultimately for DNA synthesis. The essentiality of vitamin B_{12} in the methionine synthetase reaction accounts for the development of megaloblastic anaemia in deficiencies of both vitamin B_{12} and folate (Shane & Stokstad 1985).

Methylmalonyl coenzyme A mutase reaction

This reaction occurs in the mitochondria, using deoxyadenosylcobalamin as cofactor, and results in the conversion of methylmalonyl-CoA to succinyl-CoA. The reaction is essential for the degradation of propionate and odd-chain fatty acids, especially in the nervous system. The essentiality of vitamin B_{12} for this reaction may account for the accumulation of methylmalonic acid, with acidosis and high serum glycine and glucose concentrations in B_{12} deficiency (Cooper & Rosenblatt 1987). It is generally held that reduction of this enzyme's activity accounts for the neurological changes, but recent studies in animal models of nitrous oxide-induced vitamin B_{12} deficiency challenge this concept (Weir et al 1988).

Absorption, metabolism and excretion

At physiological levels of intake, the overall efficiency of vitamin B_{12} absorption is about 70%, decreasing to less than 10% at intakes greater than five times the RDA (Herbert 1987a). Dietary vitamin B_{12} is liberated from its protein binders by gastric acid and pepsin, then immediately bound avidly to R (rapid electrophoretic mobility) proteins in the stomach. These R proteins are secreted in saliva, gastric juice and bile. In the alkaline environment of the duodenum, pancreatic proteases, particularly trypsin, release the vitamin B_{12} from the R factor, but it is immediately bound to IF. The vitamin B_{12}–IF complex binds to a specific receptor on the brush-border membrane of the terminal ileum, where it is taken up and split within the enterocyte (Kapadia et al 1983). The B_{12} is then transferred to another protein (transcobalamin II or TC-2) at the basolateral border, and transported to the liver (Chanarin et al 1978, Rothenberg et al 1978). The entire absorptive process, from ingestion of the vitamin to its appearance in the portal vein, takes 8–12 hours (Cooper 1968). The TC-2 bound vitamin B_{12} is taken

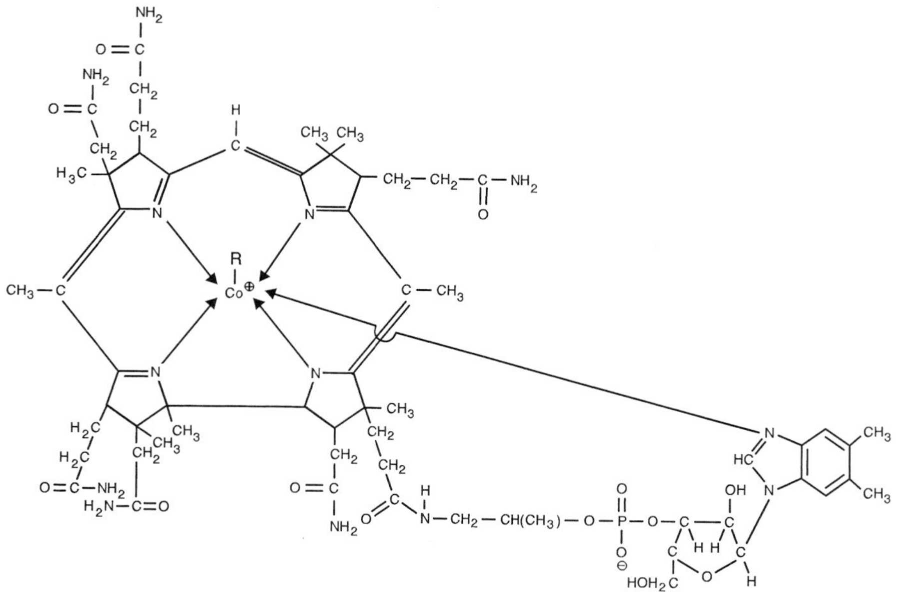

Fig. 14.4   Structure of vitamin B_{12}. Substitutions at R-position include: -CN (cyanocobalamin); -OH (hydroxocobalamin), 5'-deoxyadenosyl (5'-deoxyadenosylcobalamin), and -CH_3 (methylcobalamin). (Modified and reproduced with permission from Herbert 1987.)

up into tissues by specific receptors (Nexo & Hollenberg 1980). R factors, TC-1, TC-3, and haptocorrin are names for glycosylated binding proteins found in plasma and in most secretions. In addition to their role in vitamin B_{12} absorption, R proteins are thought to play a role in the transport of vitamin B_{12} analogues and their disposal in the bile (Kanazawa et al 1983). In pregnancy, the placenta transports vitamin B_{12} released from maternal TC-2 to a separate fetal TC-2 pod (Seligman & Allen 1978).

More than 95% of intracellular vitamin B_{12} is bound to either cytoplasmic methionine synthetase or to mitochondrial methylmalonyl-CoA mutase (Cooper & Rosenblatt 1987).

The body pool of vitamin B_{12} is 2–3 mg, with a daily excretion of 1.2–1.3 µg divided equally between urine and faeces (Hall 1964). Four to ten years are required for the development of vitamin B_{12} deficiency when intestinal absorption is interrupted by lack of IF (Herbert 1987a). Unlike its analogues, endogenous vitamin B_{12} is efficiently absorbed in the ileum (Kanazawa & Herbert 1983). Vitamin B_{12} deficiency therefore develops more rapidly if the enterohepatic circulation is interrupted by ileal disease or surgery. Conversely, efficient conservation of vitamin B_{12} in the enterohepatic circulation may preserve stores for longer than 10 years in individuals whose diet is devoid of the vitamin but whose absorptive capacity is intact (Herbert 1987a).

Clinical deficiency

Vitamin B_{12} deficiency usually occurs as a result of acquired gastrointestinal disease and rarely as a result of inadequate diet or congenital disorders of absorption and transport.

Inadequate diet

Because dietary vitamin B_{12} is exclusively of animal origin, strict vegetarians are at risk for vitamin B_{12} deficiency after many years on their diet. In practice, deficiency is rare because many vegetarians in the developed world ingest multivitamin supplements containing vitamin B_{12} (Council on Scientific Affairs 1987) and because many vegetarians in the less developed world have enough bacterial contamination of the diet to obtain bacterially synthesized vitamin B_{12}.

Gastric abnormality

Pernicious anaemia (PA), with gastric atrophy and deficient IF secretion, usually occurs after age 40. About half the cases are hereditary and mostly of Scandinavian descent; the other cases result from the progressive acquired atrophy of ageing (Herbert & Colman 1988). Circulating antibodies to IF are found only in patients with hereditary pernicious anaemia. The autoimmune nature of the hereditary form of the disease is suggested by the frequent finding of anti-bodies to IF in other tissues. In both types of PA, gastric atrophy is associated with destruction of the gastric parietal cell and an absolute lack of gastric acid, even in response to stimulation. Gastric atrophy predisposes to gastric cancer, which may occur in as many as 10% of patients with PA (Deren 1972).

Juvenile PA refers to a rare congenital condition, occurring before age 5, in which the gastric parietal cells are normal in number and capable of normal acid secretion, but incapable of secreting physiologically active IF (Cooper & Rosenblatt 1987). IF deficiency also occurs in all patients who have had surgical total gastrectomy, and in about 20% of patients who have had partial gastrectomy for peptic ulcer disease (Herbert & Colman 1988). Between 30 and 50% of cases with a gastric bypass for treating obesity become deficient after 5 years (Flickinger et al 1987).

Small intestinal abnormality

Vitamin B_{12} deficiency is one consequence of the bacterial stasis syndrome, which occurs in individuals with small intestinal diverticulosis, strictures or fistulas, and in scleroderma with abnormal intestinal motility (Toskes & Donaldson 1983). In these syndromes, contaminating bacteria are presumed to take up and utilize vitamin B_{12} as it passes through the intestinal lumen. Bacteria that overgrow the small intestine are also capable of the efficient conversion of vitamin B_{12} to metabolically inactive analogues (Brandt et al 1977). The fish tapeworm *Diphyllobothrium latum*, which is endemic in Finland, also utilizes vitamin B_{12}, thus producing deficiency in the human host.

Ileal abnormality

Because of the exclusive presence of the vitamin B_{12}–IF receptor on the ileal surface, vitamin B_{12} malabsorption occurs when the ileum is diseased or surgically resected. Immerslund–Gräsbeck syndrome, an extremely rare congenital disorder, produces vitamin deficiency as a result of an absent or malfunctioning ileal receptor (Cooper & Rosenblatt 1987). Vitamin B_{12} malabsorption is nearly universal in tropical sprue (Klipstein 1983) but rare in coeliac disease, because the former mainly affects the ileum and the latter the jejunum. Patients with Crohn's disease or radiation enteritis, both chronic inflammations of the ileum, are at risk for vitamin B_{12} malabsorption and deficiency. Unless prevented by appropriate therapy, vitamin B_{12} deficiency is predictable in patients who have had more than

50 cm of terminal ileum removed surgically for any cause (Trier 1983b).

Drug interactions

Several drugs, e.g. colchicine, neomycin, ethanol and *p*-aminosalicylic acid, produce vitamin B_{12} deficiency, presumably by interacting with the ileal vitamin B_{12}–IF receptor (Halsted & McIntyre 1972).

Megaloblastic anaemia follows repeated exposure to the anaesthetic nitrous oxide. The anaemia results from the oxidative conversion of vitamin B_{12} to a form incapable of binding to methionine synthetase, the enzyme required for converting circulating 5-methyl-H_4 folate to H_4 folate, the metabolically active form of folate essential for subsequent DNA synthesis (Horne et al 1989). Nitrous oxide exposure has also caused subacute combined degeneration of the spinal cord in humans, and in several experimental animals. A recent report suggests that the neurological defect is caused by inhibition of vitamin B_{12} dependent methionine synthetase, resulting in reduced levels of *S*-adenosylmethionine in pig brain; this effect was prevented by the administration of methionine (Weir et al 1988). Methionine is an important precursor for phospholipid and neurotransmitter metabolism in the brain. Studies with the nitrous oxide model suggest that a deficiency of methionine synthetase may be of equal or greater importance than deficiency of methylmalonyl-CoA mutase in the aetiology of neurological changes that occur in all cases of vitamin B_{12} deficiency.

Congenital disorders

In addition to juvenile PA and the Immerslund–Gräsbeck syndrome, congenital deficiencies of TC-2 or R binder and mutations of both vitamin B_{12}-dependent enzymes are recognized causes of vitamin B_{12} deficiency. These defects are thoroughly reviewed elsewhere (Cooper & Rosenblatt 1987).

Clinical features and treatment

Vitamin B_{12} deficiency can result in abnormalities in bone marrow, small intestine and nervous system. The typical patient with untreated PA develops weakness, glossitis (a sore tongue), and diarrhoea. These symptoms result from the defect in DNA synthesis that causes cell enlargement (megaloblastosis) of the red-cell precursors in the bone marrow and of the absorbing enterocytes in the intestinal lining. Megaloblastosis leads to anaemia, whereas the defect in the small intestine may cause generalized intestinal malabsorption (Lindenbaum et al 1974). Neurological symptoms are less common and consist of paresthesiae of hands and feet, abnormal vibratory and proprioceptive sensation with loss of postural sense, and spastic ataxia. These symptoms result from subacute combined degeneration, with myelin degeneration in the dorsal and lateral tracts of the spinal cord. Tobacco amblyopia, a disorder characterized by myelin degeneration of the optic nerve, may occur in vitamin B_{12}-deficient smokers. The disorder is attributed to the cyanide in tobacco smoke, which converts the limited vitamin B_{12} stores to metabolically inert cyanocobalamin (Beck 1988).

Lindenbaum et al (1988) described a group of patients with neuropsychiatric disorders, including paresthesiae, weakness, ataxia, dementia and psychosis. These patients were not anaemic but had biochemical evidence of vitamin B_{12} deficiency, with subnormal serum vitamin B_{12} levels and elevated serum methylmalonic acid and homocysteine. Therapy with vitamin B_{12} corrected the biochemical abnormalities in every case and improved the neuropsychiatric symptoms in most cases. This study underscores the requirement of the nervous system for vitamin B_{12} and suggests a need for the clinician to investigate vitamin B_{12} status in patients with unexplained neuropsychiatric disorders (see Chapter 42).

Methods of assessment

Functional changes in B_{12}-related metabolism occur as tissue B_{12} levels fall and only later is there a fall in serum B_{12} to below 200 pg/ml (Herbert 1989). Radioassay has supplanted the microbiological method for measuring serum vitamin B_{12}. Pure IF is needed as a vitamin B_{12} binder: other binders detect vitamin B_{12} analogues produced endogenously by intestinal bacteria and yield falsely normal or elevated values (Herbert & Colman 1988).

Functional deficiency of vitamin B_{12} is signalled by the appearance of hypersegmented polymorpho-nuclear neutrophils in the circulating blood, with an increased 'lobe average' (number of lobes per cell nucleus) to >3.5 (Herbert & Colman 1988). At this time, the red-cell folate level falls below 140 ng/ml. The requirement of vitamin B_{12} for the conversion of circulating 5-methyl-H_4 folate to metabolically active H_4 folate results in a normal or elevated serum folate and a decreased red-cell folate level. The deoxyuridine (dU) suppression test becomes abnormal. This test of either vitamin B_{12} or folate deficiency measures the in-vitro suppression of ^3H-thymidine incorporation into DNA when deoxyuridine is converted, with folate

dependent methyl transfer, into additional thymidine after the introduction of the deficient vitamin (Herbert 1989). Anaemia, the final stage of deficiency, is characterized by the appearance of enlarged red blood cells with an increased mean corpuscular volume, low haemoglobin level, and megaloblastic red-cell precursors in the bone marrow.

Other functional tests have recently been developed to detect deficiency earlier and to discriminate between deficiencies of B_{12} and folate. Because both vitamins interact in the synthesis of methionine, a deficiency of either is associated with elevated serum levels of the precursor homocysteine (Stabler et al 1988). Under these conditions, increased urinary excretion of methylmalonic acid distinguishes B_{12} deficiency, which is specific for the conversion of methylmalonyl-CoA to succinyl-CoA (Stabler et al 1986). In these studies, homocysteine and methyl-malonic acid were measured by capillary gas chromatography–mass spectrometry. A simpler and more economical test is needed.

The cause of B_{12} deficiency is best defined by the Schilling (1953) test, which measures the absorption of a physiological labelled amount of the vitamin; 0.1–2.0 μg of isotope-labelled vitamin B_{12} is given by mouth, together with a 1000 μg dose of intramuscular B_{12}, which saturates binding sites in tissues. Normally >9% of the labelled dose is absorbed and excreted in the urine in the first 24 hours. A normal test suggests an inadequate diet as the cause of B_{12} deficiency, whereas a low result from IF deficiency can be corrected in a second step in which IF is given orally with the labelled dose of vitamin B_{12}. A persistently abnormal test suggests ileal disease or a rare receptor defect. In patients with malabsorption due to bacterial stasis syndrome, the abnormal test will be corrected in the third stage after a 2-week course of oral antibiotics.

Dietary sources

All natural B_{12} is synthesized by bacteria, fungi or algae, and reaches the human diet after incorporation into animal protein following intestinal bacterial synthesis. Human intestinal bacteria may also synthesize small amounts of B_{12} of uncertain avail-ability as well as variable amounts of vitamin B_{12} analogues (Herbert et al 1984). The amount of B_{12} consumed in the diet varies with the amount of dietary protein and ranges from 3 to 15 μg/day (Herbert 1987a). The forms of B_{12} in the diet include mainly 5-deoxyadenosyl- and hydroxocobalamin, with lesser amounts of methylcobalamin in dairy products and little or no cyanocobalamin. Dietary B_{12} may be partly destroyed by heating in an alkaline medium.

Recommended dietary allowance (see Appendix 2)

The current recommendations are based on studies of body-pool size and turnover and of the minimal amounts required to maintain normality or to treat pernicious anaemia. Patients with PA may be maintained in remission with parenteral doses of 0.5–1.0 µg/day (Sullivan & Herbert 1965), whereas vegetarians may develop vitamin B_{12} deficiency on diets containing 0.5 µg/day or less (Stewart et al 1970). The RDA is set in the USA at 2 µg/day for adults, but a RNI of 1.25 mg is proposed in the UK (see Appendix 2).

Additional B_{12} is recommended to meet the demands of fetal growth and, based on B_{12} excretion in breast milk (Thomas et al 1980), lactating women are advised to consume more B_{12} in the diet or, if vegetarian, in a vitamin supplement.

Therapeutic uses and toxicity

Vegetarians should be advised to include a multivitamin supplement containing vitamin B_{12} in their daily routine. Patients with IF deficiency can theoretically be treated with large (>300 µg/day) doses of oral B_{12} because about 1% of the vitamin can be absorbed without IF binding (Herbert & Colman 1988). However, this approach is less reliable than the practice of administering 100–1000 µg of vitamin B_{12} by intramuscular injection each month (Herbert & Colman 1988). The improvement in wellbeing within days of receiving B_{12} injection is well recognized but unexplained. There is no known toxicity in administering vitamin B_{12} in single doses up to 1000 µg.

FOLATE (FOLIC ACID)

History

Lucy Wills, a British physician, studied the origins of a macrocytic anaemia prevalent among pregnant textile workers in Bombay. The anaemia was associated with poverty and a diet deficient in animal protein and vegetables. Macrocytic anaemia could be induced by feeding the diet to rats and monkeys, and cured with yeast or liver extract. These remedies also cured anaemic patients in Bombay (Wills 1933). There was no neurological change in the human anaemia of pregnancy and poverty, and deficient monkeys responded to a soluble fraction of liver or yeast that was ineffective in patients with PA (Wills et al 1937). When folic acid was later discovered, both Wills (Roe 1978) and Spies (1945) demonstrated its specific effects on the macrocytic anaemia of poverty.

Biochemistry

The active form of folate consists of a substituted pteridine ring linked to p-aminobenzoic acid (pABA) (together forming pteroic acid) and glutamic acid (Fig. 14.5). The term folic acid refers to pteroyl-

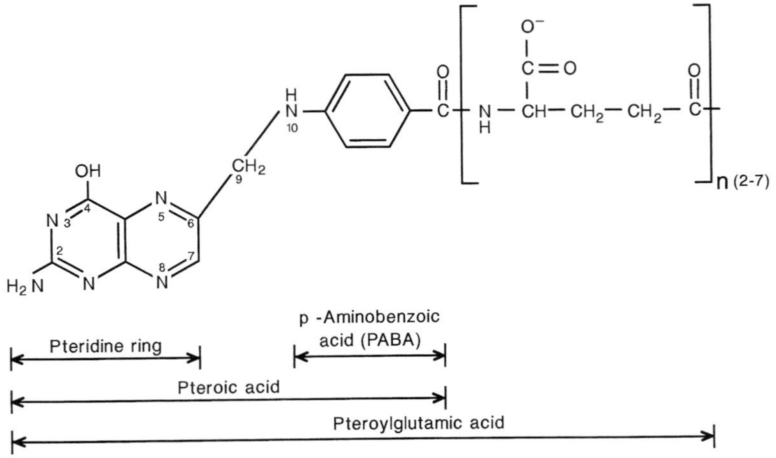

Fig. 14.5 Structure of folate. Monoglutamyl folate (pteroylglutamic acid) is reduced at the 5-, 6-, 7-, and 8-positions of the pteridine ring to form H_4 folate and substituted at the 5-position to form 5-methyl-H_4 folate, the circulating form of the vitamin. Addition of 2–7 glutamates in the gamma linkage results in polyglutamyl folate (pteroylpolyglutamate), the main dietary and intracellular form of the vitamin. (Modified and reproduced with permission from Shane & Stokstad 1985.)

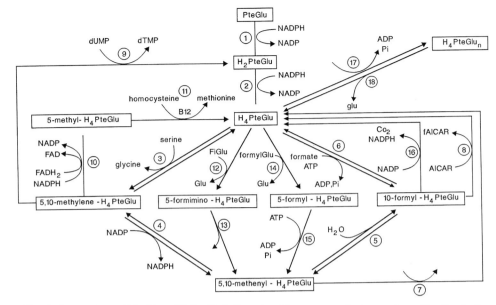

Fig. 14.6 Metabolic reactions of H_4 folate ($H_4PteGlu$). Reaction 11 represents the interaction with vitamin B_{12} which utilizes 5-methyl-$H_4PteGlu$ in the synthesis of methionine from homocysteine. $H_4PteGlu$ produced from this reaction is the substrate for synthesis of polyglutamyl folate ($H_4PteGlu_n$, reaction 17) and for generation of 5,10-methylene-$H_4PteGlu$ (reaction 3), which in turn is essential for production of thymidylate (reaction 9) and synthesis of DNA. Details of the other reactions are described in Shane & Stokstad (1985). (Reproduced with permission from Shane & Stokstad 1985.)

glutamate (PteGlu), which is the monoglutamyl form of the vitamin. Reductions and substitutions in the pteridine ring constitute 5-methyl-H_4 folate, the circulating form of the vitamin. The addition of up to seven glutamates in gamma-carboxyl linkage enhances folate-dependent reactions by producing polyglutamyl folate (PteGlun), the major form in which both dietary and intracellular folates occur. The principal function of the folate coenzymes is the transfer of single-carbon atoms in reactions essential to the metabolism of several amino acids and to nucleic acid synthesis (Shane & Stokstad 1985). The principal interaction with vitamin B_{12} is in the action of methionine synthetase (Fig. 14.6, reaction 11). H_4 folate is essential in turn for polyglutamation (reaction 17) and for the synthesis of 5,10-methylene-H_4 folate (reaction 3), a cofactor of thymidylate synthetase that converts deoxyuridylate into thymidylate in the process of DNA synthesis (reaction 9). Lack of either folate or vitamin B_{12} decreases the supply of H_4 folate, thus limiting the production of both polyglutamyl folate and DNA.

Absorption, metabolism and excretion

Dietary folates exist as polyglutamated, reduced and substituted forms of pteroylglutamate (folic acid) which

have to be hydrolysed to the monoglutamyl form before being actively transported into the absorbing enterocyte. In humans, there are two folate hydrolases in the intestinal mucosa, one in the brush-border membrane and the other in the intracellular lysosomes. Clinical studies and experiments with pigs show that the brush-border hydrolase or 'conjugase' enzyme, localized in the proximal jejunum, is the key to the digestion of dietary folates (Halsted 1990).

Intestinal zinc from endogenous or dietary sources is essential for polyglutamyl folate hydrolysis. Following hydrolysis, the monoglutamyl folate derivative is bound to a specific folate receptor on the brush border of the enterocyte, which probably also transports the vitamin (Mason 1990). Folate is reduced and methylated intracellularly and reaches the liver via the portal circulation as 5-methyl-H_4 folate. The total body folate pool size is estimated at 7.5 ± 2.5 mg for healthy adults (Herbert 1987b).

The liver is the principal site of folate storage and contains about 7 pg folate/g (Hoppner & Lampi 1980). In the liver, 5-methyl-H_4 folate is converted to H_4 folate while donating its methyl group to methionine. H_4 folate then reacts with polyglutamate synthetase to re-establish polyglutamyl folates, which are bound to several enzymes and serve most metabolic functions of the vitamin. Hydrolysed folate leaves the liver to circulate in both plasma and bile as 5-methyl-H_4 folate. Following bone marrow uptake and utilization, folates circulate as polyglutamates in the red-cell pool. 5-methyl-H_4 folate is concentrated in the bile but is conserved by efficient reabsorption from the intestine (Steinberg 1984). Folate as 5-methyl-H_4 folate is excreted in both faeces and urine, the latter by a process of renal glomerular filtration and tubular reabsorption. Approximately equal amounts of the body folate pool are excreted daily in stool and urine, with a biological half-life of labelled stores of about 100 days (Krumdieck et al 1978).

Clinical deficiency

Herbert (1962) measured the progression of folate deficiency in himself when eating a monotonous diet of thrice-boiled and extracted food. Serum folate levels fell by 3 weeks and there was evidence of tissue depletion by 7 weeks. Hypersegmented nuclei in circulating neutrophils and a fall in red-cell folate occurred by 17 weeks, and megaloblastic changes in the bone marrow and anaemia by 20 weeks.

Because folate is required for DNA synthesis, its deficiency is clinically expressed in tissues with high rates of cell turnover. The principal sign of deficiency is megaloblastic anaemia, but jejunal biopsy will show megaloblastosis of the absorbing intestinal enterocytes in folate-deficient alcoholics (Hermos et al 1972) and in tropical sprue (Klipstein et al 1983).

The aetiologies of folate deficiency can be grouped into five categories, as described below:

Decreased dietary intake. Dietary folate deficiency occurs among populations ingesting inadequate or improper diets, such as elderly people who subsist on tea and toast, alcoholics who substitute alcoholic beverages for nutritional energy sources, and impoverished populations who cannot obtain an adequate supply of folate-containing foods.

Decreased intestinal absorption. Intestinal malabsorption causes nearly universal folate deficiency in patients with coeliac disease or tropical sprue. Absorption of both polyglutamyl and monoglutamyl folate is markedly reduced (Corcino et al 1976). Specific therapy of each disease corrects the folate absorption (Halsted et al 1977).

Increased requirements. Increased requirement for folate, and hence an increased risk of dietary deficiency, occurs in multiple pregnancies, in unsupplemented lactation, in haemolytic anaemia, and in leukaemia (Herbert & Colman 1988). Because folate stores are depleted in 20 weeks, unmet increased requirements can result in relatively rapid folate deficiency in these situations.

Effects of drugs. The chronic use of certain drugs is associated with folate deficiency. Patients with inflammatory bowel disease receiving salicylazosulphapyridine are at risk for folate deficiency, because this drug blocks both hydrolysis and intestinal uptake of dietary folate (Halsted et al 1981). Epileptic patients receiving diphenylhydantoin are often folate-deficient, although the mechanism of altered absorption and/or metabolism is less clear (see Chapter 50).

Alcoholism. Chronic alcoholism is the most common cause of folate deficiency in the USA (Halsted & Tamura 1978). The incidence of folate deficiency among chronic alcoholic patients has been described at 30–80%, based on surveys from urban hospitals for predominantly impoverished patients. The presence of alcoholic liver disease increases the likelihood of folate deficiency. Megaloblastic bone marrow changes and anaemia occur in a third of chronic alcoholics.

The aetiology of folate deficiency in chronic alcoholism is multifactorial. Acutely administered ethanol appears to decrease folate availability to the bone marrow and inhibits the normal reticulocyte response to therapy in folate-deficient alcoholics, perhaps as a result of acetaldehyde destruction of the folate molecule (Shaw et al 1989). Chronic alcoholic patients with alcoholic liver disease have lower stores of folate. Alcoholic beverages other than beer are devoid of folate, and heavy drinkers are unlikely to include fresh vegetables or other sources of folate in their diet. As indicated in a recent review (Halsted 1990), clinical and experimental studies indicate that chronic exposure to ethanol decreases the transport of folic acid across the intestine, reduces hepatic uptake, and increases the excretion of folic acid by the kidney.

Methods of assessment

The most common is the measurement of the serum folate level by a microbiological (*Lactobacillus casei*, normal >5 ng/ml) assay or radioassay. Tissue folate deficiency is reflected in the red cell (normal >160 ng/ml). Hypersegmentation of neutrophil nuclei develops and ultimately megaloblastic bone marrow and anaemia occur. These signs are identical to those in B_{12} deficiency and PA patients may also present with low red-cell folate. Thus the accurate diagnosis of folate deficiency requires evidence of morphological signs, low serum and red-cell folate levels, with a normal level of serum vitamin B_{12} (Herbert & Colman 1988).

Dietary sources

Folates are found in a variety of foods, including green leafy vegetables, nuts, grains and liver (its major site of animal storage). Three-quarters of dietary folate occurs in polyglutamyl forms and one-quarter in monoglutamyl form. The folate content of food is measured microbiologically with *L. casei* after treatment with an endogenous source of folate hydrolase, because the growth of this organism is supported only by polyglutamyl folates with three or fewer glutamyl residues. Food preparation, particularly boiling, is known to destroy dietary folates (Herbert 1987b). The availability of folate from different food sources is also limited by the presence of endogenous inhibitors of folate hydrolase and other factors. Thus, in a study of changes in urinary folate excretion (an index of absorption) following intakes of different foods of known folate content, the availability of folate from lettuce, eggs, oranges and wheatgerm was found to be about half that from lima beans, liver, yeast and bananas (Tamura & Stokstad 1973). It is assumed, for the purposes of estimating requirements, that about 50% of polyglutamyl dietary folate is absorbed.

Folate requirements

Metabolic ward studies established that daily intakes of 200–250 μg of dietary folate were sufficient to sustain normal red-cell folate levels and, in Canada, where median folate intakes are 150–200 μg/day, the folate content of liver autopsy samples was greater than 3 μg/g and only 8–10% of the population's red-cell folate fell below 150 μg/ml. On this basis, the UK set its RNI at 200 pg/day and the USA an RDA of 3 pg/kg body weight for adults of all ages (see Appendix 2).

Pregnancy substantially increases folate requirements due to the demands of the growing fetus, and unsupplemented pregnant women carry the risk of premature birth (Baumslag et al 1970) or bearing small-for-dates babies (Iyengar & Rajalakshmi 1975). A recent study of more than 20 000 pregnant women appears to confirm the risk of neural tube defects in the offspring of folate-deficient mothers; the incidence of this anomaly was reduced by three-quarters when 4 mg/day folate supplements were used in early pregnancy (Milunsky et al 1989). This has led to substantial ethical and policy issues (see Chapter 25). Red-cell folate levels can be maintained at normal by supplements of 100μg/day (Chanarin et al 1968). Lactation also represents an increased drain on folate stores, as human milk contains about 50 μg folate/l

and thus provides 40–45 μg folate/day (Matoth et al 1965).

Assuming a minimal 50% absorption of dietary folate, the US RDA for pregnancy and for the first 6 months of lactation is set at 400 μg/day and 280 μg/day respectively, whereas the UK RNI increases to 300 and 260μg/day (Appendix 2). Since oral folate supplementation may reduce zinc absorption (Simmer et al 1987), zinc supplements also have to be considered if folate supplements are to be given routinely before and during pregnancy.

Folate stores in the newborn are small and rapidly used for growth, putting the child at risk of megaloblastic anaemia. Infants fed human milk grow well on about 40 μg/day folate, without anaemia. Formula feeds, despite providing a higher folate intake, induce red-cell folate levels lower than those in breastfed babies, so the UK set the RNI at 50 μg/day. Goat's milk contains substantially less folate than human or cow's milk (Herbert 1987a). Folic acid supplements are recommended for infants fed boiled milk or goat's milk.

Therapeutic uses and toxicity

Folic acid supplements of 1mg/day are indicated in chronic diseases associated with risks of deficiency. The malabsorption, anaemia and intestinal pathology of patients with tropical sprue usually responds to a regimen of 5 mg/day of folic acid, together with the antibiotic tetracycline (Klipstein 1983).

Toxicity is extremely rare. Patients receiving the folate antagonist diphenylhydantoin for epilepsy may have convulsions on excessive doses of folic acid (Hommes et al 1979) which both decrease the drug's concentration in the cerebrospinal fluid and experimentally increase excitatory effects. Conversely, diphenylhydantoin may result in folate-deficiency anaemia (Reynolds 1968). Patients with epilepsy need their folate levels monitored so that a moderate dose of 400 μg/day can be used if biochemical signs of deficiency occur.

VITAMIN B_6 (PYRIDOXINE)

History

György identified and separated the heat-labile vitamin B_6 that cured a scaly dermatitis in rats fed purified diets (György 1934). The structure and synthesis of vitamin B_6 or pyridoxine was established in 1939 and additional forms of pyridoxine and its active form as pyridoxal phosphate were defined during World War II.

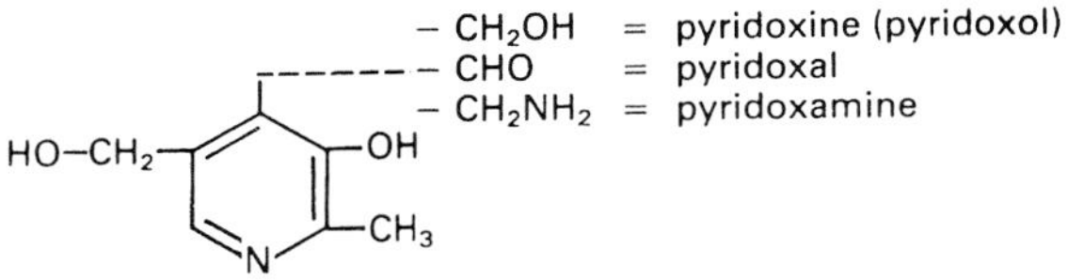

Fig. 14.7   Structure of pyridoxine (vitamin B_6).

Biochemistry

Vitamin B_6 occurs naturally in three forms: pyridoxine, pyridoxal and pyridoxamine (Fig. 14.7). Pyridoxine hydrochloride is the synthetic pharmaceutical form of vitamin B_6. All three natural forms of vitamin B_6 undergo phosphorylation in the 5-position and oxidation to the active coenzyme pyridoxal phosphate PLP. Several drugs (isoniazid and penicillamine) produce vitamin B_6 deficiency by binding to PLP, and a number of natural moulds and fungi are phosphorylation inhibitors (McCormick 1988b).

PLP is a coenzyme for numerous reactions related to protein metabolism, e.g. aminotransferases and decarboxylases. PLP-dependent decarboxylation is central to the formation of several amines, including epinephrine, norepinephrine and serotonin. PLP is required for aminolevulinic acid synthetase activity in the initial synthesis of haem from glycine and succinyl coenzyme A. PLP also plays a role in glycogen metabolism and in sphingolipid synthesis in the nervous system (McCormick 1988b). PLP is also intimately involved in the synthesis of niacin from tryptophan (see Fig.14.9).

Absorption, metabolism and excretion

The predominantly phosphorylated forms of dietary B_6 are hydrolysed by intestinal alkaline phosphatases before being absorbed in proportion to the luminal concentration. Rephosphorylation occurs in the liver, kidney and brain before conversion to the common form of the vitamin PLP by an oxidase. Regulation of hepatic PLP concentration appears to depend on control of the PLP degradative processes; hepatic PLP is bound to its apoenzymes and circulates in the blood tightly bound to serum albumin. Phosphorylation and oxidative conversion of vitamin B_6 may also occur in red blood cells, where PLP is bound to haemoglobin.

An alkaline phosphatase converts B_6 to free pyridoxal, and hepatic and renal aldehyde oxidase converts unbound PLP to pyridoxic acid, the principal metabolite excreted by the kidney (McCormick 1988b).

Clinical deficiency

The causes of pyridoxine deficiency include drug antagonists, congenital disorders, certain chronic diseases, intestinal malabsorption, and alcoholism. The clinical signs of pyridoxine deficiency include inflammation of the tongue, lesions of the lips and corners of the mouth, and peripheral neuropathy. B_6 deficiency usually occurs clinically with other water-soluble vitamin deficiencies. Infants fed formula diets deficient in pyridoxine have seizures, with decreased activity of PLP-dependent glutamate decarboxylase (Henderson 1984). Sideroblastic anaemia may result from deficient PLP-dependent aminolaevulinic acid synthetase and is expressed as unincorporated iron granules in the red-cell precursors of the bone marrow (Lindenbaum 1987).

Biochemical B_6 deficiency is more common than clinical deficiency. Abnormalities occur within 2 weeks on a B_6-free diet, with abnormal excretion of xanthurenic acid following tryptophan loading due to decreased activity of PLP-dependent kynurinase. There is also a decrease in plasma PLP, and decreased urinary excretion of pyridoxic acid (Baker et al 1964).

Drug interactions

Isoniazid, used for treating tuberculosis, forms inactive complexes with PLP. Penicillamine, used in the treatment of Wilson's disease and rheumatoid arthritis, is also a PLP antagonist (Rivlin 1985). Women taking oral contraceptive agents have developed abnormalities of tryptophan metabolism consistent with vitamin B_6 deficiency, but other metabolic measurements were unaffected (Leklem et al 1975). Contraceptive agents do not increase B_6 requirements but pharmacological doses may help suppress some of the symptoms induced by the drugs.

Neurological disorders

Because PLP is involved in the synthesis of neurotransmitters and sphingolipid, its deficiency has been suggested but unproven in neurological disorders, including Down's syndrome (McCoy et al 1969) and epilepsy (Ebadi et al 1981). Pyridoxine deficiency may occur in patients with Parkinson's disease receiving levodopa treatment (Rivlin 1985).

Congenital disorders

Homocystinuria, usually a congenital disorder in the conversion of homocysteine to methionine, may result from pyridoxine deficiency, with implications for the accelerated development of atherosclerosis (McCully 1969).

Other disorders

Pyridoxine deficiency has been reported in patients undergoing dialysis for chronic renal failure because of accelerated destruction of PLP (Kopple et al 1981), in coeliac disease (Reinken & Zieglauer 1978), in patients with biliary obstruction and/or cirrhosis (Mitchell et al 1976), because of the accelerated destruction of PLP by elevated hepatic levels of alkaline phosphatase, and in many chronic alcoholic patients.

Chronic alcoholism

Low serum levels of PLP occur in 50–80% of alcoholics, depending on the presence of liver disease (Halsted & Heise 1987). Multiple deficiencies are, however, common. Pyridoxine deficiency alters the pattern of serum aminotransferases with a 2:1 ratio of aspartate to alanine aminotransferase in patients with alcoholic liver disease. The alanine aminotransferase is more dependent on PLP, so the routine measurement of these enzymes is a useful clue to the diagnosis of pyridoxine deficiency. B_6 deficiency in alcoholism is multifactorial, including poor diet, decreased release of the vitamin from binding proteins in food, and increased degradation and excretion of the vitamin.

Methods of assessment

Direct tests include a microbiological measurement of different forms of vitamin B_6 in serum and urine, a fluorometric assay of 4′-pyridoxic acid in urine, and an assay of serum PLP that measures the metabolism of labelled tyrosine by apodecarboxylase. The plasma PLP measurement using labelled tyrosine is direct and reliable, and normal plasma PLP values are 5–23 ng/ml (McCormick 1988b). Indirect functional tests measure PLP-dependent metabolites in the tryptophan–niacin pathway (see Fig. 14.9). Tryptophan loading and urinary tests are too cumbersome for routine use. Another method measures PLP-dependent aspartate or alanine aminotransferases in red blood cell lysates. Activity coefficients are obtained by measuring enzyme activities before and after adding PLP in vitro, with normal values being <1:5 (McCormick 1988b).

Dietary sources

Poultry, fish, pork, eggs, liver and kidney are all rich sources of vitamin B_6. Soybeans, oats, peanuts, walnuts and unpolished rice are also good sources. The availability of pyridoxine from different foods is variable; absorption of the vitamin from dietary sources is only 60–80% of absorption from the pure vitamin (Tarr et al 1981). Freezing and thawing may cause considerable loss of the vitamin (Schroeder 1971).

Requirements and allowances

Minimal requirements in both men and women are directly proportional to the amount of protein in the diet (see Appendix 2). Increases are estimated for both pregnancy and lactation.

Therapeutic uses and toxicity

Pyridoxine should only be used in cases of suspected or proven deficiency, in doses of 2–10mg/day. Larger doses of up to 100 mg/day may be required to treat peripheral neuropathy in association with chronic alcoholism, coeliac sprue, or when isoniazid or penicillamine are used. Oral vitamin B_6 is usually given routinely with these drugs, but patients receiving levodopa for Parkinson's disease should only receive moderate doses of vitamin B_6, because it may interfere with the effectiveness of this drug (Rivlin 1985).

Severe toxicity has resulted from attempts to treat premenstrual syndrome with B_6; a severe sensory neuropathy of hands and feet may develop with chronic doses of 100–200 mg of pyridoxine (Dalton & Dalton 1987).

NIACIN

History

Pellagra was first recognized to occur in poor people on a corn-based diet (Roe 1973). Corn was introduced to Europe by Spanish explorers returning from the Yucatan, where maize, prepared by soaking corn in lime, was a dietary staple. Two centuries later, in 1739, the Spanish physician Gaspar Casal described pellagra as a disease of malnutrition occurring among corn eaters who developed a particular red rash in sun-exposed areas of the skin ('Casal's collar') and glossitis. The disease of the '3 Ds' – dermatitis, diarrhoea and dementia – was described throughout Europe and the southern USA, and deficiency probably killed many prisoners during the Civil War in 1860–64 (Roe 1973).

Goldberger, in the US Public Health Service, showed in 1914 that pellagra in mental hospital patients could be treated by substituting a diet of mixed grains for corn. Feeding convicts diets devoid of animal protein caused pellagra. Goldberger established black tongue in dogs as an experimental model in which a pellagra-like syndrome could be cured by feeding various sources of animal protein, or a boiled extract of yeast that was almost devoid of protein (Goldberger 1922).

Nicotinamide was isolated from nicotinamide adenine dinucleotide phosphate (NADP) and nicotinamide adenine dinucleotide (NAD). The relationship of dietary tryptophan to niacin was established through human experiments that measured niacin metabolism following different doses of tryptophan. In human experimentation, Goldsmith et al (1961) reported that 60 mg of dietary tryptophan produced the same metabolic effect as 1 mg of niacin (see Fig. 14.9).

Biochemistry

Niacin is the generic description for the specific vitamin nicotinic acid as well as its natural derivative nicotinamide or niacinamide (Fig. 14.8). Nicotinamide is incorporated within NAD or NADP, where it functions as a factor for numerous oxidoreductases involved in glycolysis, fatty acid metabolism, tissue respiration and detoxification.

Present in the diet protein-bound to coenzymes, niacin is hydrolysed and absorbed as nicotinic acid, nicotinamide and nicotinamide mononucleotide (NMN).

Clinical deficiency

Pellagra occurs in parts of India and the African continent. The disease was particularly prevalent in the southeastern USA until its aetiology and dietary cure were discovered. It is occasionally found in malnourished alcoholic patients. Pellagra occurs in Hartnup's disease, an autosomal recessive disorder with impaired absorption of several amino acids, including tryptophan. Similarly, pellagrous symptoms may be seen in carcinoid syndrome, in which endogenous tryptophan is diverted into excessive

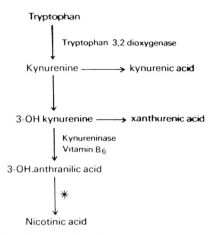

Fig. 14.9 The conversion of tryptophan to nicotinic acid. In vitamin B_6 deficiency, kynurenic acid and xanthurenic acid appear in the urine in increased amounts. * = several intermediary steps.

production of serotonin and away from the niacin pathway.

Methods of assessment

No satisfactory specific direct measurements of blood niacin are available. Urinary excretion of the metabolite 1-methylnicotinamide is decreased in experimental niacin deficiency to <0.5 mg/g creatinine (Säuberlich et al 1974).

Dietary sources

The tryptophan content of dairy products is more than 1% of protein, so that 60 g of milk or egg protein converts to 10 niacin equivalents (NE) or 600 mg niacin. Meat in general is a rich source of both tryptophan and niacin. Cereals such as oatmeal, rice or wheat provide moderate amounts of niacin, with lesser amounts in corn. The bioavailability of niacin from cereals is variable and is increased by treatment with lime. This practice accounts for the absence of pellagra among ancient Mayans and modern-day Mexicans.

Requirements and allowances (see Appendix 2)

The requirement and allowance values for niacin are based on studies in which blood and urinary niacin metabolites are measured as an index of tissue saturation after volunteers have eaten varied amounts of dietary tryptophan and niacin, and a more recent study which measured dietary effects on blood and urinary metabolites of niacin (Jacob et al 1989). An additional 2 NE are recommended during pregnancy

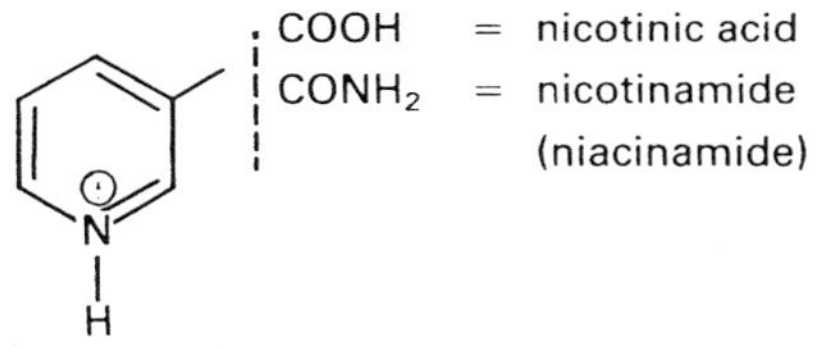

COOH = nicotinic acid
CONH$_2$ = nicotinamide (niacinamide)

Fig. 14.8 Structure of niacin.

in the USA but not the UK, where enhanced tryptophan conversion in pregnancy was deemed sufficient.

Therapeutic use and toxicity

Classic pellagra responds dramatically to nicotinamide or niacin (nicotinic acid) in doses of 100 mg at 4-h intervals or, more slowly, to dietary animal protein (Halsted et al 1969); 40–200 mg niacin/day treats pellagra symptoms in Hartnup's disease or in the carcinoid syndrome. Doses up to 1–2 g/day are used to manage patients with hypertriglyceridaemia and/or hypercholesterolaemia. However, niacin in these large doses carries significant side effects of flushing, and may stimulate gastric acid secretion, with an increased risk of peptic ulceration (Woolliscroft 1983).

VITAMIN B$_2$ (RIBOFLAVIN)

Riboflavin (vitamin B$_2$) was discovered as a yellow growth factor isolated from milk, eggs and liver (György 1971).

Biochemistry

Riboflavin is composed of an isoalloxazine ring linked to a ribityl side chain (Fig. 14.10). Modifications of the ribityl side chain include ester phosphate linkage to form flavin mononucleotide (FMN), which can be linked with adenine monophosphate to form flavin adenine dinucleotide (FAD). Flavoprotein enzymes containing FMN or FAD are bound to many apoenzymes and are involved in oxidation–reduction reactions that enter many metabolic pathways and affect cellular respiration (McCormick 1988c).

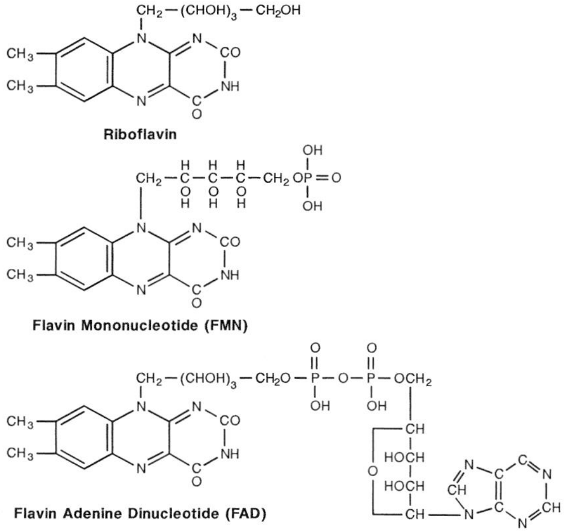

Absorption, metabolism and excretion

Riboflavin is released as FAD and FMN from protein binders in the acid conditions of the stomach and then hydrolysed by a pyrophosphatase and phosphatase to free riboflavin in the intestine. Riboflavin is absorbed in the proximal intestine by a sodium-dependent and saturable process, i.e. phosphorylation to FMN within the enterocyte.

Riboflavin and FMN both circulate bound to albumin and, to a lesser extent, to a subfraction of immunoglobulin G. Riboflavin and its metabolites are stored mainly in the liver and also in the kidney and heart (McCormick 1988c). FAD is the principal storage form; it represents 70–90% of the vitamin, and its concentration is fivefold greater than FMN

Fig. 14.10 Structure of riboflavins. (Reproduced with permission from Rivlin 1970a.)

and 50-fold greater than riboflavin. Riboflavin may be partly conserved by an enterohepatic cycle. About 200 µg of riboflavin and its metabolites are excreted daily in the urine by a process that includes active tubular secretion. Riboflavin constitutes one-half to two-thirds of the vitamin in urine, the rest appearing as its oxidation products (Chastain & McCormick 1987).

Clinical deficiency

The principal signs of riboflavin deficiency in humans include a rash around the nose, angular stomatitis and intense glossitis. The lack of specificity of these signs for riboflavin deficiency may be the result of vitamin interactions, such as the involvement of FMN and FAD in pyridoxine and tryptophan (to niacin) metabolism and coexisting vitamin deficiencies in malnourished people. Anorexia, intestinal malabsorption, chronic alcoholism and biliary atresia all precipitate deficiency (McCormick 1988c). In experimental deficiency induced by a riboflavin antagonist, glossitis was followed by seborrhoeic dermatitis, peripheral neuropathy and hypoplastic anaemia (Lane et al 1964).

Thyroxine deficiency may impair the conversion of riboflavin to FMN, and diabetics are at risk because of high urinary excretion of the vitamin (Cole et al 1976). The drug chlorpromazine may impair FAD synthesis, and barbiturates induce microsomal oxidation and therefore riboflavin catabolism (McCormick 1988c).

Methods of assessment

Assessment involves measuring riboflavin in urine and red blood cells by fluorometric and microbiological techniques (Säuberlich et al 1974) or determining the activity of the riboflavin-dependent enzyme erythrocyte glutathione reductase (EGR). Urinary excretion, the more sensitive measure, reflects daily intake of the vitamin.

The EGR assay, a functional test of FAD availability, measures the oxidation of NADPH to NADP by the FAD-dependent enzyme. The in-vitro addition of FAD provides an activity coefficient, which is inversely proportional to urinary excretion of riboflavin. Riboflavin deficiency is indicated by an activity coefficient >1.2, while tissue saturation of riboflavin with adequate FAD results in no additional stimulation and an activity coefficient of 1.0.

Dietary sources

The principal dietary sources of riboflavin include dairy products, poultry, meat, fish, asparagus, broccoli and spinach. Unless fortified, cereals are a poor source of riboflavin.

Requirements and allowances

Because of the limited storage capacity for FAD, FMN and free riboflavin, the margin between dietary intake resulting in deficiency (0.55 mg/day) and that resulting in tissue saturation (1.1 mg/day) is very small (Horwitt et al 1950).

The US National Research Council (Subcommittee on the Tenth Edition of the RDAs 1989) recommends an intake of 0.6 mg riboflavin/1000 kcal with a minimum of 1.2 mg/day for adults (see Appendix 2). The riboflavin requirement may increase with physical activity and in patients with negative nitrogen balance, because of increased urinary excretion of riboflavin. Higher intakes are recommended in pregnancy and lactation.

Therapeutic use and toxicity

There is no evidence of riboflavin toxicity or therapeutic benefit at doses greater than the RDA.

BIOTIN

History

Biotin was discovered from bacterial and yeast growth factors which prevented a skin condition induced by

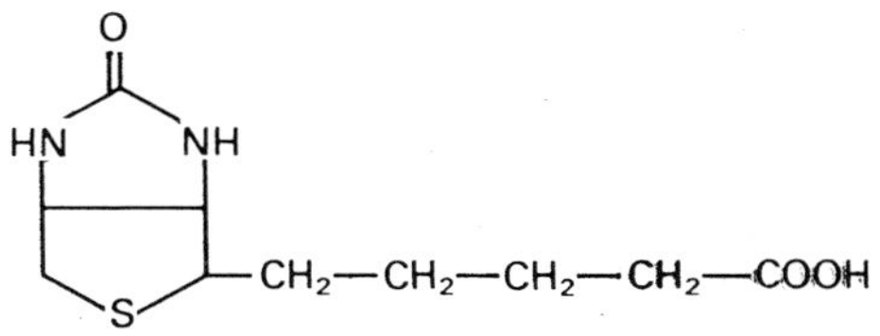

Fig. 14.11   Structure of biotin.

feeding a diet of egg whites to experimental animals. The structure of biotin was determined by du Vigneaud (1942), and the vitamin was synthesized soon after by Harris and coworkers (1943).

Biochemistry

Biotin consists of an imidazole ring fused to a tetrahydrothiophene ring with a valeric acid side chain (Fig. 14.11). The imidazole moiety is important as the binding site to avidin, a major protein in egg white. Biotin is a cofactor for several carboxylases used in fatty acid synthesis and metabolism, gluconeogenesis and branched-chain amino acid metabolism (McCormick 1988d).

Absorption, metabolism and excretion

The protein-bound vitamin is hydrolysed to biocytin, which is absorbed with free biotin in the upper intestine. The biotin–avidin complex, which occurs with a raw egg diet, resists hydrolysis (McCormick 1988d). Biotin is actively absorbed in the duodenum and upper jejunum (Said & Redha 1988), and stored, or utilized after conversion to biotinyl-5'-adenylate in liver, muscle and kidney. Biocytin is hydrolysed to biotin within the plasma. Biotin and its metabolites are excreted in the urine in amounts of 6–50 μg/day (Baker 1985). Biotin is also synthesized by colonic bacteria, so daily faecal biotin excretion is 3–6 times greater than dietary intake (McCormick 1988d). The availability to the human host of biotin from intestinal bacterial synthesis is unknown.

Clinical deficiency

Human biotin deficiency is rare and has been reported to result from bizarre dietary practices or improper use of total parenteral nutrition. Symptoms include fatigue, nausea, anorexia, muscle pains, paraesthesiae, dry scaly skin, alopecia, anaemia and elevated serum cholesterol. The dry scaly dermatitis of biotin deficiency is similar to that of essential fatty acid deficiency, and is characterized by abnormalities in fatty acid composition in the blood (Mock et al 1988).

Methods of assessment

Biotin can be measured in whole blood or urine by microbiological assay (Säuberlich et al 1974). Normal individuals have whole-blood levels of 0.22–0.75 μg/ml, with urinary excretion of 6–50 μg/day (Baker 1985).

Dietary sources

Liver, egg yolk, soy flour, cereals and yeast are excellent sources of biotin, whereas fruit and meat are poor sources. The availability of biotin is governed in part by binders in food. Wheat contains biotin in an unavailable bound form. Although biotin is tightly bound to avidin in raw egg white, it is freed by cooking.

Requirements and allowances

Requirements for biotin are based on incomplete data from studies of patients receiving total parenteral nutrition and from studies of volunteers being measured for urinary excretion as a function of oral intake (see Appendix 2).

Toxicity

There are no reports of toxicity of biotin in amounts up to 10 mg/day.

PANTOTHENIC ACID

History

Pantothenic acid was discovered during investigations of an antidermatitis growth factor from yeast.

Biochemistry

Pantothenic acid is a dimethyl derivative of butyric acid linked to β-alanine (Fig. 14.12). The vitamin is linked through phosphate to form 4'-phosphopantetheine and CoA, the primary active form. As a constituent of CoA and its esters, the vitamin is essential for numerous reactions involved in lipid and carbohydrate metabolism, including fatty acid synthesis and degradation, steroid hormone synthesis and gluconeogenesis. The 4'-phosphopantetheinyl moiety also binds to acyl carrier protein, which functions in acyl-group transfer reactions (McCormick 1988e).

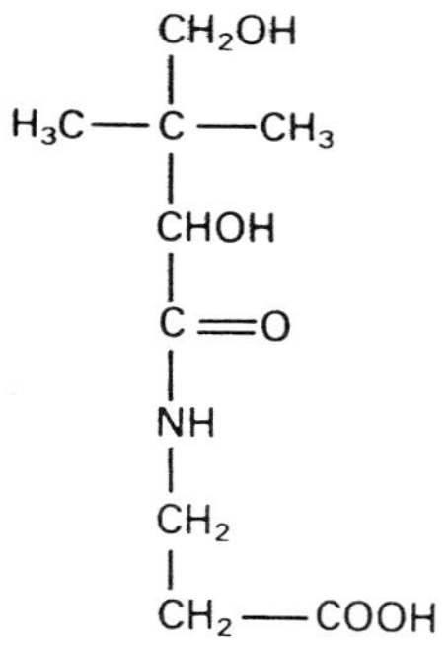

Fig. 14.12   Structure of pantothenic acid.

Absorption, metabolism and excretion

Pantothenic acid is ingested as part of CoA, which is hydrolysed by intestinal phosphatases to yield 4-phosphopantetheine and pantothenic acid, the absorbable form of the vitamin (Rose et al 1984). CoA is resynthesized in liver cells. Pantothenic acid is excreted in the urine, mainly as a metabolic product of CoA.

Clinical deficiency

Human deficiency is very rare, except perhaps in the syndrome of 'burning feet' paraesthesiae, observed in starving prisoners of war (Glusman 1947). Deficient diets produce dermatitis and myelin degeneration in chickens, with more profound deficiencies producing adrenal insufficiency (McCormick 1988e). In two human experiments involving a vitamin antagonist or a deficient diet, deficiency signs included paraesthesiae with 'burning feet', postural hypotension, and impaired eosinophilic response to adrenocorticotropic hormone (ACTH) (Hodges et al 1959, Fry et al 1976). A clinical deficiency syndrome has not been clearly defined.

Methods of assessment

Pantothenic acid in urine and blood is measured by microbiological assay or by radioimmunoassay (Wyse et al 1979). Normal blood values are >100 μg/dl, and urinary excretion is normally 1–15 mg/day (Säuberlich et al 1974). On adequate diets, 2–7 mg/day are excreted in the urine and 1–2 mg/day in the faeces (Fox & Linkswiler 1961). Urinary values are considered a sensitive indicator of dietary intake. CoA in red blood cells is an imprecise measure of status (McCormick 1988e).

Dietary sources

As implied by its name, pantothenic acid is widely distributed in nature, especially in animal products, whole grains and legumes. Additional CoA may be synthesized by intestinal bacteria.

Recommended dietary allowance

With a paucity of data, no RDA or RNI for pantothenic acid has been derived, but intakes between 3 and 7 mg/day seem safe for adults. The US Subcommittee noted that >5 mg/day is adequate for pregnancy and lactation and that 2–3 mg/day is adequate for children up to age 11 (Subcommittee on the Tenth Edition of the RDAs 1989).

Therapeutic uses and toxicity

There are no specific therapeutic uses for pantothenic acid nor reports of serious toxicity with excessive intakes of up to 10 g/day.

REFERENCES

Anderson R 1981 Ascorbate-mediated stimulation of neutrophil motility and lymphocyte transformation by inhibition of the peroxidase/H_2O_2 halide system in vitro and in vivo. American Journal of Clinical Nutrition 34: 1906–1911

Baker EM, Canham JE, Nunes WT, Säuberlich HE, McDowell M E 1964 Vitamin B_6 requirement for adult men. American Journal of Clinical Nutrition 15: 59–66

Baker H 1985 Assessment of biotin status: clinical implications. Annals of the New York Academy of Sciences 447: 129–132

Baumslag N, Edelstein T, Metz J 1970 Reduction of incidence of prematurity by folic acid supplementation in pregnancy. British Medical Journal 1: 16–17

Beck WS 1988 Cobalamin and the nervous system. New England Journal of Medicine 318: 1752–1754

Blass JP, Gibson GE 1977 Abnormality of a thiamine-requiring enzyme in patients with Wernicke–Korsakoff syndrome. New England Journal of Medicine 297: 1367–1370

Brandt LJ, Bernstein LH, Wagle A 1977 Production of vitamin B_{12} analogues in patients with small-bowel bacterial overgrowth. Annals of Internal Medicine 87: 546–551

Cameron E, Pauling L, Leibovitz B 1979 Ascorbic acid and cancer: a review. Cancer Research 39: 663–681

Castle WB 1929 Observations on the etiologic relationship of achylia gastrica to pernicious anemia. I. The effect of the administration to patients with pernicious anemia of the contents of the normal human stomach recovered after the ingestion of beef muscle. American Journal of Medical Science 178: 748–764

Chalmers AH, Cowley DM, Brown JM 1986 A possible etiological role for ascorbate in calculi formation. Clinical Chemistry 32: 333–336

Chalmers TC 1975 Effects of ascorbic acid on the common cold: an evaluation of the evidence. American Journal of Medicine 58: 532–536

Chanarin I, Rothman D, Ward A, Perry J 1968 Folate status and requirement in pregnancy. British Medical Journal 2: 390–394

Chanarin I, Muir M, Hughes A, Hoffbrand AV 1978 Evidence for an intestinal origin of transcobalamin II during vitamin B_{12} absorption. British Medical Journal 1: 1453–1455

Chastain JL, McCormick DB 1987 Flavin catabolites: identification and quantitation in human urine. American Journal of Clinical Nutrition 46: 832–834

Cole HS, Lopez R, Cooperman JM 1976 Riboflavin deficiency in children with diabetes mellitus. Acta Diabetologica Latina 13: 25–29

Cook JD, Monsen ER 1977 Vitamin C, the common cold, and iron absorption. American Journal of Clinical Nutrition 30: 235–241

Cooper BA 1968 Complex of the intrinsic factor and B_{12} in human ileum during vitamin B_{12} absorption. American Journal of Physiology 214: 832–835

Cooper BA, Rosenblatt DS 1987 Inherited defects of vitamin B_{12} metabolism. Annual Review of Nutrition 7: 291–320

Corcino JJ, Reisenauer AM, Halsted CH 1976 Jejunal perfusion of simple and conjugated folates in tropical sprue. Journal of Clinical Investigation 58: 298–305

Council on Scientific Affairs, American Medical Association 1987 Vitamin preparations as dietary supplements and therapeutic agents. Journal of the American Medical Association 257: 1929–1936

Dalton K, Dalton MJT 1987 Characteristics of pyridoxine overdose neuropathy syndrome. Acta Neurologica Scandinavica 76: 8–11

Dana RH Jr 1937 Two years before the mast and twenty-four years after. PF Collier & Son, New York, p 341

Deana R, Bharaj BS, Verjee ZH, Galzigna L 1975 Changes relevant to catecholamine metabolism in liver and brain of ascorbic acid deficient guinea-pigs. International Journal for Vitamin and Nutrition Research 45: 175–182

Deren JJ 1972 Pernicious anemia: a digestive disorder. Viewpoints on Digestive Disease 4: 1–4

du Vigneaud V 1942 The structure of biotin. Science 96: 455–461

Ebadi M, Itoh M, Bifano J, Wendt K, Earle A 1981 The role of Zn^{2+} in pyridoxal phosphate mediated regulation of glutamic acid decarboxylase in brain. International Journal of Biochemistry 13: 1107–1112

Eijkman C 1897 Ein Versuch zur Bekämpfung der Beri-beri. Virchows Archiv für Pathologische Anatomie und Physiologie und fur Klinische Medizin 149: 187–194

Fazio V, Flint DM, Wahlqvist ML 1981 Acute effects of alcohol on plasma ascorbic acid in healthy subjects. American Journal of Clinical Nutrition 34: 2394–2396

Ferrebee JW, Weissman N, Parker D, Owen PS 1942 Tissue thiamin concentrations and urinary thiamin excretion. Journal of Clinical Investigation 21: 401–408

Flickinger EG, Sinar DR, Swanson M 1987 Gastric bypass. Gastroenterology Clinics of North America 16: 283–292

Fox HM, Linkswiler H 1961 Pantothenic acid excretion on three levels of intake. Journal of Nutrition 75: 451–454

Fry PC, Fox HM, Tao HG 1976 Metabolic response to a pantothenic acid deficient diet in humans. Journal of Nutrition Science and Vitaminology 22: 339–346

Funk C 1911 The chemical nature of the substance which cures polyneuritis in birds induced by a diet of polished rice. Journal of Physiology (London) 43: 395–400

Ginter E, Cerna O, Budlovsky J et al 1977 Effect of ascorbic acid on plasma cholesterol in humans in a long-term experiment. International Journal for Vitamin and Nutrition Research 47: 123–134

Glusman M 1947 The syndrome of 'burning feet' (nutritional melalgia) as a manifestation of nutritional deficiency. American Journal of Medicine 3: 211–223

Goldberger J 1922 The relation of diet to pellagra. Journal of the American Medical Association 78: 1676–1680

Goldsmith GA, Miller ON, Unglaub WG 1961 Efficiency of tryptophan as a niacin precursor in man. Journal of Nutrition 73: 172–176

Gräsbeck R, Simons K, Sinkkonen I 1966 Isolation of intrinsic factor and its probable degradation product, as their vitamin B_{12} complexes, from human gastric juice. Biochimica et Biophysica Acta 127: 47–58

György P 1934 Vitamin B_2 and the pellagra-like dermatitis in rats. Nature 133: 498–499

György P 1971 Discoveries leading to the metabolic role of vitamin B_6. American Journal of Clinical Nutrition 24: 1250–1256

Hall CA 1964 Long-term excretion of Co^{57}-vitamin B_{12} and turnover within the plasma. American Journal of Clinical Nutrition 14: 156–162

Halsted CH 1990 Intestinal absorption of dietary folates. In: Picciano MF, Stokstad ELR, Gregory JF (eds) Folic acid metabolism in health and disease. Contemporary issues in clinical nutrition. Alan R Liss, New York

Halsted CH, Heise C 1987 Ethanol and vitamin metabolism. Pharmacology and Therapeutics 34: 453–464

Halsted CH, McIntyre PA 1972 Intesinal malabsorption caused by aminosalicylic acid therapy. Archives of Internal Medicine 130: 935–939

Halsted CH, Tamura T 1978 Folate deficiency in liver disease. In: Davidson CS (ed) Problems in liver disease. Stratton Intercontinental, New York, pp 91–100

Halsted CH, Sheir S, Sourial N, Patwardhan VN 1969 Small intestinal structure and absorption in Egypt: influence of parasitism and pellagra. American Journal of Clinical Nutrition 22: 744–754

Halsted CH, Reisenauer AM, Romero JJ, Cantor DS, Ruebner B 1977 Jejunal perfusion of simple and conjugated folates in coeliac sprue. Journal of Clinical Investigation 59: 933–940

Halsted CH, Gandhi G, Tamura T 1981 Sulfasalazine inhibits the absorption of folates in ulcerative colitis. New England Journal of Medicine 305: 1513–1517

Harper C 1983 The incidence of Wernicke's encephalopathy in Australia – a neuropathological study of 131 cases. Journal of Neurology, Neurosurgery and Psychiatry 46: 593–598

Harris SA, Wolf DE, Mozingo R, Folkers K 1943 Synthetic biotin. Science 97: 447–448

Haworth WN, Hirst EL 1933 Journal of the Society of the Chemical Industry 52: 645–646

Henderson LM 1984 Vitamin B_6. In: Present knowledge in nutrition, 5th edn. Nutrition Foundation, Washington DC, pp 303–317

Herbert V 1962 Experimental nutritional folate deficiency in man. Transactions of the Association of American Physicians 75: 307–320

Herbert V 1987a Recommended dietary intakes (RDI) of vitamin B_{12} in humans. American Journal of Clinical Nutrition 45: 671–678

Herbert V 1987b Recommended dietary intakes (RDI) of folate in humans. American Journal of Clinical Nutrition 45: 661–670

Herbert V 1989 Pathogenesis of megaloblastic anemias. In: Halsted CH, Rucker RB (eds) Nutrition and the origins of disease. Academic Press, San Diego, pp 47–55

Herbert V, Colman N 1988 Folic acid and vitamin B_{12}. In: Shils ME, Young VR (eds) Modern nutrition in health and disease, 7th edn. Lea & Febiger, Philadelphia, pp 388–416

Herbert V, Drivas G, Manusselis C, Mackler M, Eng J, Schwartz E 1984 Are colon bacteria a major source of cobalamin analogues in human tissues? 24-h human stool contains only about 5 μg of cobalamin but about 100 μg of apparent analogue (and 200 μg folate). Transactions of the Association of American Physicians 97: 161–171

Hermos JA, Adams WH, Lin YC, Tries J 1972 Mucosa of the small intestine in folate-deficient alcoholics. Annals of Internal Medicine 76: 957–965

Hodges RE, Bean WB, Ohlson MA, Bleiler R 1959 Human pantothenic acid deficiency produced by omega-methyl pantothenic acid. Journal of Clinical Investigation 38: 1421–1425

Hodges RE, Baker EM, Hood J, Säuberlich HE, March SC 1969 Experimental scurvy in man. American Journal of Clinical Nutrition 22: 535–548

Hodges RE, Hood J, Canham JE, Säuberlich HE, Baker EM 1971 Clinical manifestations of ascorbic acid deficiency in man. American Journal of Clinical Nutrition 24: 432–443

Holst A, Frölich T 1907 Experimental studies relating to ship beri-beri and scurvy. Journal of Hygiene (London) 7: 634–671

Hommes OR, Hollinger JL, Jansen MJT, Schoofs M, vanderWiel Th, Kok JCN 1979 Convulsant properties of folate compounds: some considerations and speculations. In: Botez MI, Reynolds EH (eds) Folic acid in neurology, psychiatry and internal medicine. Raven Press, New York, pp 285–316

Hoppner K, Lampi B 1980 Folate levels in human liver from autopsies in Canada. American Journal of Clinical Nutrition 33: 862–864

Horne DW, Patterson D, Cook RJ 1989 Effect of nitrous oxide inactivation of vitamin B_{12}-dependent methionine synthetase on the subcellular distribution of folate coenzymes in rat liver. Archives of Biochemistry and Biophysics 270: 729–733

Hornig DH, Moser U, Glatthaar BE 1988 Ascorbic acid. In: Shils M E, Young V R (eds) Modern nutrition in health and disease, 7th edn. Lea & Febiger, Philadelphia, pp 417–435

Horwitt MK, Harvey CC, Hills OW, Liebert E 1950 Correlation of urinary excretion of riboflavin with dietary intake and symptoms of ariboflavinosis. Journal of Nutrition 41: 247–264

Hoyumpa AM Jr, Nichols SG, Wilson FA, Schenker S 1977 Effect of ethanol on intestinal (Na, K) ATPase and intestinal thiamine transport in rats. Journal of Laboratory and Clinical Medicine 90: 1086–1095

Iyengar L, Rajalakshmi K 1975 Effect of folic acid supplement on birth weights of infants. American Journal of Obstetrics and Gynecology 122: 332–336

Jacob RA, Swendseid ME, McKee RW, Fu CS, Clemens RA 1989 Biochemical markers for assessment of niacin status in young men: urinary and blood levels of niacin metabolites. Journal of Nutrition 119: 591–598

Jansen BCP, Donath WF 1926. Proceedings of Koninklijke Nederlandse Akademie van Wetenschappen (Amsterdam) 29: 1390

Kallner A, Hartmann D, Hornig D 1979 Steady-state turnover and body pool of ascorbic acid in man. American Journal of Clinical Nutrition 32: 530–539

Kallner AB, Hartmann D, Hornig DH 1981 On the requirements of ascorbic asid in man: steady-state turnover and body pool in smokers. American Journal of Clinical Nutrition 34: 1347–1355

Kanazawa S, Herbert V 1983 Mechanism of enterohepatic circulation of vitamin B_{12}: movement of vitamin B_{12} from bile R-binder to intrinsic factor due to the action of pancreatic trypsin. Transactions of the Association of American Physicians 96: 336–344

Kanazawa S, Herbert V, Herzlich B, Drivas G, Manusselis C 1983 Removal of cobalamin analogue in bile by enterohepatic circulation of vitamin B_{12}. Lancet 1: 707–708

Kapadia CR, Serfilippi D, Voloshin K, Donaldson RM Jr 1983 Intrinsic factor-mediated absorption of cobalamin by guinea-pig ileal cells. Journal of Clinical Investigation 71: 440–448

Kawasaki T 1986 Determination of thiamine and its phosphate esters by high-performance liquid chromatography. Methods in Enzymology 122: 15–24

King CG, Waugh WA 1932 The chemical nature of vitamin C. Science 75: 357–358

Klipstein FA 1983 Tropical sprue. In: Sleisenger MH, Fordtran JS (eds) Gastrointestinal disease: pathophysiology, diagnosis, management, 3rd edn. vol II. WB Saunders, Philadelphia, pp 1040–1049

Kopple JD, Mercurio K, Blumenkrantz MJ et al 1981 Daily requirement for pyridoxine supplements in chronic renal failure. Kidney International 19: 694–704

Krumdieck CL, Fukushima K, Fukushima T, Shiota T, Butterworth CE Jr 1978 A long-term study of the excretion of folate and pterins in a human subject after ingestion of ^{14}C folic acid, with observations on the effect of diphenylhydantoin administration. American Journal of Clinical Nutrition 31: 88–93

Kübler W, Gehler J 1970 On the kinetics of the intestinal absorption of ascorbic acid: a contribution to the calculation of an absorption process that is not proportional to the dose. International Journal for Vitamin and Nutrition Research 40: 442–453

Lane M, Alfrey CP, Mengel CE, et al 1964 The rapid induction of human riboflavin deficiency with galactoflavin. Journal of Clinical Investigation 43: 357–373

Leklem JE, Brown RR, Rose DP, Linkswiler HM 1975 Vitamin B_6 requirements of women using oral contraceptives. American Journal of Clinical Nutrition 28: 535–541

Lind J 1772 A treatise on the scurvy in three parts. Crowder, London, pp 149–153, 177–180

Lindenbaum J 1987 Hematologic complications of alcohol abuse. Seminars in Liver Disease 7: 169–181

Lindenbaum J, Pezzimenti JF, Shea N 1974 Small-intestinal function in vitamin B_{12} deficiency. Annals of Internal Medicine 80: 326–331

Lindenbaum J, Healton EB, Savage DG et al 1988 Neuropsychiatric disorders caused by cobalamin deficiency in the absence of anemia or macrocytosis. New England Journal of Medicine 318: 1720–1728

McCormick DB 1988a Thiamin. In: Shils ME, Young VR (eds) Modern nutrition in health and disease, 7th edn. Lea & Febiger, Philadelphia, pp 355–361

McCormick DH 1988b Vitamin B_6. In: Shils ME, Young VR (eds) Modern nutrition in health and disease, 7th edn. Lea & Febiger, Philadelphia, pp 376–382

McCormick DB 1988c Riboflavin. In: Shils ME & Young VR (eds) Modern nutrition in health and disease, 7th edn. Lea & Febiger, Philadelphia, pp 362–369

McCormick DB 1988d Biotin. In: Shils ME, Young VR (eds) Modern nutrition in health and disease, 7th edn. Lea & Febiger, Philadelphia, pp 436–439

McCormick DB 1988e Pantothenic acid. In: Shils ME, Young VR (eds) Modern nutrition in health and disease, 7th edn. Lea & Febiger, Philadelphia, pp 383–387

McCoy EE, Colombini C, Ebadi M 1969 The metabolism of vitamin B_6 in Down's syndrome. Annals of the New York Academy of Sciences 166: 116–125

McCully KS 1969 Vascular pathology of homocysteinemia: implications for the pathogenesis of atherosclerosis. American Journal of Pathology 56: 111–128

Mason JB 1990 Intestinal transport of monoglutamyl folates in mammalian systems. In: Picciano MF, Stokstad ELR, Gregory JF (eds) Folic acid metabolism in health and disease. Contemporary issues in clinical nutrition. Alan R Liss, New York, pp 47–63

Matoth Y, Pinkas A, Sroka C 1965 Studies on folic acid in infancy. III. Folates in breast fed infants and their mothers. American Journal of Clinical Nutrition 16: 356–359

Milunsky A, Jick H, Jick SS et al 1989 Multivitamin/folic acid supplementation in early pregnancy reduces the prevalence of neural tube defects. Journal of the American Medical Association 262: 2847–2852

Minot GR, Murphy WP 1926 Treatment of pernicious anemia by a special diet. Journal of the American Medical Association 87: 470–476

Mitchell D, Wagner C, Stone WJ, Wilkinson GR, Schenker S 1976 Abnormal regulation of plasma pyridoxal 5'-phosphate in patients with liver disease. Gastroenterology 71: 1043-1049

Mock DM, Mock NI, Johnson SB, Holman RT 1988 Effects of biotin deficiency on plasma and tissue fatty acid composition: evidence for abnormalities in rats. Pediatric Research 24: 396–403

Myllylä R, Kuutti-Savolainen ER, Kivirikko K I 1978 The role of ascorbate in the prolyl hydroxylase reaction. Biochemical and Biophysical Research Communications 83: 441–448

Nelson PJ, Pruitt RE, Henderson LL, Jenness R, Henderson PM 1981 Effect of ascorbic acid deficiency on the in vivo synthesis of carnitine. Biochimica et Biophysica Acta 672: 123–127

Nexo E, Hollenberg MD 1980 Characterization of the particulate and soluble acceptor of transcobalamin II from human placenta and rabbit liver. Biochimica et Biophysica Acta 628: 190–200

Nixon PF, Kaczmarek MJ, Tate J, Kerr RA, Price J 1984 An erythrocyte transketolase isoenzyme pattern associated with the Wernicke–Korsakoff syndrome. European Journal of Clinical Investigation 14: 278–281

Olson JA, Hodges RE 1987 Recommended dietary intakes (RDI) of vitamin C in humans. American Journal of Clinical Nutrition 45: 693–703

Osler W 1893 The principles and practice of medicine. D Appleton, New York, pp 689–696, 780

Pauling L 1970 Vitamin C and the common cold. WH Freeman, San Francisco

Peters RA 1953 Significance of biochemical lesions in the pyruvate oxidase system. British Medical Bulletin 9: 116–122

Ralli EP, Friedman GJ, Rubin SH 1938 The mechanism of excretion of vitamin C by the kidney. Journal of Clinical Investigation 17: 765–770

Raskin NH, Fishman RA 1976 Neurologic disorders in renal failure (second of two parts). New England Journal of Medicine 294: 204–210

Reinkin L, Zieglauer H 1978 Vitamin B_6 absorption in children with acute celiac disease and in control subjects. Journal of Nutrition 108: 1562–1565

Reuler B, Girard DE, Cooney TG 1985 Wernicke's encephalopathy. New England Journal of Medicine 312: 1035–1039

Reynolds EH 1968 Mental effects of anticonvulsants, and folic acid metabolism. Brain 91: 197–214

Rickes EL, Brink NG, Koniuszy FR, Wood TR, Folkers K 1948 Crystalline vitamin B_{12}. Science 107: 396–397

Rivlin RS 1985 Disorders of vitamin metabolism: deficiencies, metabolic abnormalities, and excesses. In: Wyngaarden JB, Smith LH (eds) Cecil textbook of medicine, 17th edn. Saunders, Philadelphia, pp 1197–1208

Roe DA 1973 A plague of corn: the social history of pellagra. Cornell University Press, Ithaca, NY

Roe DA 1978 Lucy Wills (1888–1964): a biographical sketch. Journal of Nutrition 108: 1379–1383

Rose RC, Hoyumpa AM, Allen RH, Middleton HM, Henderson LM, Rosenberg IH 1984 Transport and metabolism of water-soluble vitamins in intestine and kidney. Federation Proceedings 43: 2423–2429

Rothenberg SP, Weiss JP, Cotter R 1978 Formation of transcobalamin II-vitamin B_{12} complex by guinea-pig ileal mucosa in organ culture after in vivo incubation with intrinsic factor-vitamin B_{12}. British Journal of Haematology 40: 401–414

Said HM, Redha R 1988 Biotin transport in rat intestinal brush-border membrane vesicles. Biochimica et Biophysica Acta 945: 195–201

Säuberlich HE, Dowdy RP, Scala JH 1974 Laboratory tests for the assessment of nutritional status. CRC Press, Cleveland

Säuberlich HE, Herman YF, Stevens CO, Herman RH 1979 Thiamin requirement of the adult human. American Journal of Clinical Nutrition 32: 2237–2248

Schilling RF 1953 Intrinsic factor studies: II. Effect of gastric juice on urinary excretion of radioactive vitamin B_{12}. Journal of Laboratory and Clinical Medicine 42: 860–866

Schmidt K-H, Hagmaier V, Hornig DH, Vuilleumier J-P, Rutishauser G 1981 Urinary oxalate excretion after large intakes of ascorbic acid in man. American Journal of Clinical Nutrition 34: 305–311

Schroeder HA 1971 Losses of vitamins and trace minerals resulting from processing and preservation of foods. American Journal of Clinical Nutrition 24: 562–573

Seligman PA, Allen RH 1978 Characterization of the receptor for TC II isolated from human placenta. Journal of Biological Chemistry 253: 1766–1772

Shane B, Stokstad ELR 1985 Vitamin B_{12}-folate interrelationships. Annual Review of Nutrition 5: 115–141

Shaw S, Jayatilleke E, Herbert V, Colman N 1989 Cleavage of folates during ethanol metabolism. Role of acetaldehyde/xanthine oxidase-generated superoxide dismutase. Biochemical Journal 257: 277–280

Simmer K, Iles CA, James C, Thompson RPH 1987 Are iron–folate supplements harmful? American Journal of Clinical Nutrition 45: 122–125

Smith EL, Parker LFJ 1948 Purification of anti pernicious anaemia factor. Proceedings of the Biochemical Society 43: viii-vix

Smith JL, Hodges RE 1987 Serum levels of vitamin C in relation to dietary and supplemental intake of vitamin C in smokers and nonsmokers. In: Burns JJ, Rivers JM, Machlin LJ (eds) Third conference on vitamin C. Annals of the New York Academy of Sciences 498: 144–152

Spies TD, Vilter CF, Koch MB, Caldwell MH 1945 Observations of the anti-anemic properties of synthetic folic acid. Southern Medical Journal 38: 707–709

Stabler SP, Marcell PD, Podell ER, Allen RH, Lindenbaum J 1986 Assay of methylmalonic acid in the serum of patients with cobalamin deficiency using capillary gas chromatography–mass spectrometry. Journal of Clinical Investigation 77: 1606–1612

Stabler SP, Marcell PD, Podell ER, Allen RH, Savage DG, Lindenbaum J 1988 Elevation of total homocysteine in the serum of patients with cobalamin or folate deficiency detected by capillary gas chromatography-mass spectrometry. Journal of Clinical Investigation 81: 466–474

Steinberg S 1984 Mechanisms of folate homeostasis. American Journal of Physiology 246: G319-G324

Stevenson NR 1974 Active transport of L-ascorbic acid in the human ileum. Gastroenterology 67: 952-956

Stewart GR 1962 The California trail. McGraw-Hill, New York, p 283

Stewart JS, Roberts PD, Hoffbrand A V 1970 Response of dietary vitamin-B_{12} deficiency to physiological oral doses of cyanocobalamin. Lancet 2: 542–545

Subcommittee on the Tenth Edition of the RDAs, Food and Nutrition Board, Commission on Life Sciences, National Research Council 1989 Water-soluble vitamins. In: Recommended dietary allowances, 10th edn. National Academy Press, Washington, DC, pp 115–173

Sullivan LW, Herbert V 1965 Studies on the minimum daily requirement for vitamin B_{12}. Hematopoietic responses to 0.1µg of cyanocobalamin or coenzyme B_{12}, and comparison of their relative potency. New England Journal of Medicine 272: 340–346

Svirbely JL, Szent-Györgyi A 1932 CV. The chemical nature of vitamin C. Biochemistry Journal 26: 865-870

Takaki K 1906 The preservation of health among the personnel of the Japanese Navy and Army. Lancet 2: 1369–1374, 1451–1455, 1520–1523

Tamura T, Stokstad ELR 1973 The availability of food folate in man. British Journal of Haematology 25: 513–532

Tarr JB, Tamura T, Stokstad ELR 1981 Availability of vitamin B_6 and pantothenate in an average American diet in man. American Journal of Clinical Nutrition 34: 1328–1337

Thomas MR, Sneed SM, Wei C, Nail PA, Wilson M, Sprinkle EE III 1980 The effects of vitamin C, vitamin B_6, vitamin B_{12}, folic acid, riboflavin and thiamin on the breast milk and maternal status of well-nourished women at 6 months postpartum. American Journal of Clinical Nutrition 33: 2151–2156

Toskes PP, Donaldson RM Jr 1983 The blind loop syndrome. In: Sleisenger MH, Fordtran JS (eds) Gastrointestinal disease: pathophysiology, diagnosis, management, 3rd edn. vol II. WB Saunders, Philadelphia, pp 1023–1030

Trier JS 1983a Celiac sprue. In: Sleisenger MH, Fordtran JS (eds) Gastrointestinal disease: pathophysiology, diagnosis, management, 3rd edn. vol II. WB Saunders, Philadelphia, pp 1050–1069

Weir DG, Keating S, Molly A et al 1988 Methylation deficiency causes vitamin B_{12}-associated neuropathy in the pig. Journal of Neurochemistry 51: 1949–1952

Williams RD, Mason HL, Smith BF, Wilder RM 1942 Induced thiamine (vitamin B_1) deficiency and the thiamine requirement of man. Archives of Internal Medicine 69: 721–738

Williams RR, Cline JK 1936 Synthesis of vitamin B_1. Journal of the American Chemical Society 58: 1504–1505

Wills L 1933 The nature of the haemopoietic factor in Marmite. Lancet 1: 1283–1285

Wills L, Clutterbuck PW, Evans BDF 1937 A new factor in the production and cure of certain macrocytic anaemias. Lancet 1: 311–314

Woolliscroft JO 1983 Megavitamins: fact or fancy. Disease-A-Month 29: 7–56

Wyse BW, Wittwer C, Hansen RG 1979 Radioimmunoassay for pantothenic acid in blood and other tissues. Clinical Chemistry 25: 108–111

Zilva SS 1921 The influence of aeration on the stability of the antiscorbutic factor. Lancet 1: 478

15. Food composition tables

D. A. T. Southgate

A knowledge of the composition of foods is essential in the dietary treatment and management of disease and in most quantitative studies of human nutrition (McCance & Widdowson 1940). Compilations of the nutrient composition of individual food items provide the source of this information for a range of nutritional purposes, although for work demanding a high level of accuracy direct analyses of the foods actually consumed are essential.

The first compilation of this kind was published in Germany by Konig in 1878, and this was followed by tables in the USA compiled by Atwater and Woods (1896). Since then a number of tables have been compiled and published in many countries (Infoods 1986). Table 15.1 summarizes the range of tables presently available. Tables for regional use have also been prepared by the Food and Agriculture Organization of the United Nations (FAO 1968, 1972).

The information in successive compilations has grown in volume, both in the numbers of foods for which compositional information is given, and especially in the range of nutrients covered. This has been due to the development of nutritional science and the recognition of the nutritional importance of a greater number of food constituents, and also to the development of nutritional analysis of food.

The number of food items eaten in a country may be very large, especially if different methods of preparing and cooking foods are taken into account. A food composition table that gave values for all the foods eaten in the UK, for example, would need to list something in excess of 100 000 items, and such complete coverage is rarely seen (Southgate 1985).

Since the 1960s, developments in computer technology have provided an alternative to the printed food composition table; computerized databases are widely available and for many uses are the preferred medium for providing nutritional data on foods. Nutritional databases are especially useful when the data have to be manipulated, for example in calculating nutrient intakes from records of food intake. Computerized systems have many advantages over the printed word: the amount of information that can be stored is virtually infinite, access to large compilations is very rapid, and revising and updating is much easier. Furthermore, very sophisticated calculations and manipulations of the data can be made that are virtually impossible with a printed table.

It is, however, important to remember that the limitations of printed tables are equally applicable to the most perfect database. Food composition tables and databases are valuable tools for the nutritionist, but like all tools, their proper use requires some basic understanding of how they should be used. Many of the following comments apply to both printed tables and computerized databases, and the two terms will be used interchangeably; where the remarks apply to printed compilations, 'tables' will be so qualified.

CONSTRUCTION OF FOOD COMPOSITION TABLES

It is useful for the potential user of food compositional data to have an understanding of the ways in which the tables have been constructed, since this determines the applications to which the data can be put, and the limitations of the particular dataset.

Databases can be assembled in one of two ways; either *direct*, where an analytical program is set up to generate data specifically for use in the database, or *indirect* where the data are compiled from other sources (Southgate 1974). The first series of tables were often prepared by the former method, frequently by an investigator who had a specific need for them. As the scope of the information in the tables has grown, the increasing use of a combination of the two approaches has become necessary, and direct analysis is usually restricted to 'new' foods, that is, items for which no compositional information is available, or existing items where there is reason to believe that the composition of the food has changed significantly. New analyses may also be undertaken in order to include additional nutrients, or when analytical procedures have improved or changed.

Table 15.1   A selection of food composition tables

Food table	Source
AFRICA *Food Composition Table for use in Africa* (1968) Leung, Woot-Tsuen Wu	FAO and US Dept Health, Education and Welfare, Bethesda Maryland, USA
EGYPT *Food Composition Table* Nutrition Institute, Cairo (1985)	Nutrition Institute, Cairo
GAMBIA *Foods of Rural Gambia* McCrae J E, Paul AA (1979)	Dunn Nutrition Unit Cambridge, UK
SOUTH AFRICA *NRIND Food Composition Tables* Gouws E, Langenhoven ML (1981)	National Research Institute for Nutritional Diseases South African Medical Research Council, Tygerburg, South Africa
ASIA CHINA *Food Composition Tables of Peoples' Republic of China* Beijing (1982)	Beijing
EAST ASIA *Food Composition Table for Use in East Asia* Leung, Woot-Tsuen Wu, et al. (1972)	FAO and US Dept Health, Education and Welfare, Bethesda, Maryland, USA
INDIA *Nutritive Value of Indian Foods* Gopalan C, Rama Sastri B V, Balasubramanian S C (1984)	National Institute of Nutrition Indian Council of Medical Research, Hyderabad
JAPAN *Standard Tables of Food Composition in Japan* (1982)	Resources Council, Science and Technology Agency Tokyo
PAKISTAN *Food Composition Table for Pakistan* Hussain H (1985)	Ministry of Planning And Development, Government of Pakistan, Department of Agricultural Chemistry and Human Nutrition, Agricultural University, Peshawar
THAILAND *Thai Food Composition Table* (1981)	Division of Nutrition Department of Health, Ministry of Public Health Bangkok
EUROPE DENMARK *Levnedsmiddeltabeller* (1989) (Food Composition Tables 1989) Moller A (ed)1989	Storkokkencentret, Soborg
FEDERAL REPUBLIC OF GERMANY *Food Composition and Nutrition Tables* (1986/1987) Souci, Fachman and Kraut Scherz H, Kloss G, (eds) (1986/87)	Bundesministerium fur Ernahrung, Landwirtschaft und Forsten, Wissenschaftliche Verlagsgesellschaft mbH, Stuttgart
FINLAND *Ruoka-Ainetaulukko* (Food Composition Table) Turpeinen O (1983)	Helsingissa Keuruu, Otava
FRANCE *Les aliments - Tables des valeurs nutritives* Ostrowski Z L, Josse M C (1978)	Jacques Lanore, Paris
ITALY *Tabelle di composizione degli alimenti* Carnovale E, Miuccio F C (1983)	Ministero dell 'Agricoltura e delle Forete, Istituto Nazionale della Nutrizione, Rome
POLAND *Sklad i Wartosc Odzywcza Produktow Spozwczych* Piekarska J, Los-Kuczera M (1983)	PZWL, Warsaw
SPAIN *Tables de Composicion de Alimentos* Arias D M A, Moreiras-Varela O, Extremera F G (1983)	Instituto de Nutricion, Madrid

Table 15.1 *Cont'd*

Food table	Source
SWEDEN *Livsmedelstabeller* (1986)	Statens Livsmedelverk Uppsala
MIDDLE EAST ARABIAN GULF STATES *Composition of Mixed Dishes Commonly* *Consumed in the Arabian Gulf States* Musaiger A O, Sungpuag P (1985)	Gordon Breach, UK
REGIONAL TABLES NEAR EAST *Food Composition Tables for Use in* *The Near East* (1982)	FAO and US Dept Agriculture, Rome
WESTERN HEMISPHERE CANADA *Canadian Nutrient File* (1985)	Department of National Health and Welfare Ottawa
MEXICO *Valor Nutritivo de Los Alimentos* *Mexicanos. Tablas de Uso Practico* Hernandez M, Chavez A, Bourges H (1980)	La Division de Nutricion, Instituto Nacional de la Nutricion Mexico
UNITED STATES OF AMERICA *Composition of Foods, Agriculture Handbook No 8* Published in Several Parts from 1976 to 1984	Nutrition Monitoring Division, US Department of Agriculture, Washington DC
SOUTH AMERICA BRAZIL *Tabela de composicao de Alimentos* Azoubel L M O, et al. (1982)	Sarvier SA, Sao Paolo
REGIONAL TABLES LATIN AMERICA *INCAP–ICNND Food Composition Table for Use* *in Latin America* Leung, Woot-Tseun Wu (1961)	INCAP and NIH, Guatemala City
OCEANIA AUSTRALIA *Composition of Foods Australia* *Vol I 1989 II* (1990) Cashel K, English R, Lewis J	Australian Government Printing Service, Canberra
NEW ZEALAND *Food Composition Tables and Database* (1989)	Department of Scientific and Industrial Research, Palmerston North, NZ
PACIFIC ISLANDS *Food Composition Tables for Use in* *the Pacific Islands* (1983)	South Pacific Commission, Noumea, New Caledonia

This is a selected list. More complete lists are given by Arab et al (1987) and in the Infoods Directory (1986). Both these publications give details of coverage, especially the former.

OBJECTIVES OF THE COMPILERS OF FOOD COMPOSITION TABLES

The primary objective of the compilers is to produce a database that meets the needs of the users; in practice, the wide range of uses made of the data makes this difficult to achieve, and some compromises are inevitable. Most users, however, expect the tables to provide reliable information; this means that the data must be representative of the foods in question, which must also be properly identified.

In the *direct analytical* method, the compiler has close control over the selection of the food samples, their collection and their analysis. It is thus easier for the compiler to be certain about the identity of the food, and to know whether or not the samples were representative. In addition, closer control of the analytical operations is possible, for example, the choice of analytical methods, the mode of expression of the values, and the quality assurance procedures used during sample preparation and analysis. The direct method of preparation provides the easier route to achieving the main objectives. It is, however, demanding on resources and thus tends to limit the coverage, both of foods and nutrients, that can be achieved. It also could be argued that absolute reliance on this approach neglects the large volume of equally reliable information available from other sources. The indirect method seems at first sight to be much simpler; however, this is far from the truth because the data from other sources must be subjected to close scrutiny before they can be used. The criteria that must be applied are given in Table 15.2.

ORGANIZATION OF FOOD COMPOSITION TABLES

Most compilations have some introductory text that describes how the data have been obtained and gives information on the nutrients covered, the modes of expression used, and often the sources of the data. The user needs to be aware of these sources in order to be sure that the data apply to the foods being consumed. Many tables give indications of the analytical methods used: this, again, is useful because for some nutrients different methods give quite different values, and this can lead to confusion.

The foods are usually arranged in groups. The actual groupings used vary from table to table and are, to a certain extent, arbitrary, because many foods, especially composite dishes, could fall into several groups; in general the basic foods are more easily categorized and the groups adopted in FAO tables follow the major commodities. Table 15.3 gives some examples of the groupings adopted. Most tables are indexed, but finding a particular food can sometimes require a degree of familiarity with the particular tables. In this respect computerized databases have the advantage as they can be searched rapidly. A database may retain the food groupings used in the printed tables, but this is not essential and the groupings usually reflect the origins of the database. In essence, a nutritional database consists of a simple matrix of food items and nutrient values, and the major differences between different databases are the coverage of foods and nutrients and the software available to manipulate the data. Many users of food composition data find it useful to have access to a number of different compilations, and translations of the introductory texts of the more important European tables are available to assist them (Arab et al 1987).

APPLICATIONS OF FOOD COMPOSITION TABLES

Food composition databases have many applications, the major ones of which are the calculation of nutrient intake data from information on food intakes, and the construction of diets, menus or rations that provide specified amounts of nutrients.

Calculation of nutrient intakes

These can be carried out for an individual, for example when a diet history is used to assess the normal intake of a patient, or in a dietary survey where food intakes have been recorded over a period of time. This application is also used for groups of individuals where the food consumption for the group has been measured. Thus the nutrients of a household can be estimated from household purchases of food, as is done in the National Food Survey in the United Kingdom (MAFF 1989). Calculations of this kind are made for countries and regions using food supplies and food disappearance data. Each of these applications measures food intake at a different level and requires a different range of foods and a different database, however, such

Table 15.2 Criteria for scrutiny of data

Parameter	Criteria
Sample identity	Unequivocal identification of sample
Sampling protocol	Collection of representative sample
Preparation of sample	Methods used Precautions taken Material rejected as inedible etc.
Preparation of analytical sample	Nature of material analysed
Analytical procedures used	Choice of method Quality assurance procedures
Mode of expression	Compatible with that used within the data system

Table 15.3   Examples of major food groups used in current tables of food composition

FAO tables	UK tables
Cereals and grain products	Cereals and cereal products
Starchy roots, tubers and fruits	(within vegetables)
Grain legumes and legume products	(within vegetables)
Nuts and seeds	Nuts
Vegetables and vegetable products	Vegetables
Fruits	Fruits
Sugars and syrups	Sugars, preserves and confectionery
Meat, poultry, game	Meat and meat products
Eggs	Eggs
Fish and shellfish	Fish and fish products
Milk and milk products	Milk and milk products
Oils and fats	Oils and fats
Beverages	Beverages
	Alcoholic beverages
Miscellaneous	Sauces, soups and miscellaneous foods

databases are usually subsets of a more comprehensive one.

Construction of diets of specified nutrient composition

The second major group of applications concerns the construction of diets with a defined nutrient composition; examples of this are a diet with a known energy and carbohydrate content for a diabetic; a low-sodium diet for a hypotensive, or a controlled-energy diet for weight reduction.

At the group level the data may be used to design menus in an institution or ration scales for troops in combat, providing a defined supply of nutrients. Internationally this application is used for forecasting food requirements in time of shortage and to aid in agricultural planning.

Nutritional research and teaching

Food tables find application in research and teaching by providing the basic tool for understanding the relation between foods and nutrients, using the tables in one or both of the ways described above.

As a primary source of information on food composition

Nutritional databases have recently begun to be used in another way. The introduction in the USA of nutritional labelling of foods, created a demand for nutrient composition data that had been validated, so that it could be used in labelling with all its attendant regulatory implications. National nutritional databases were pressed into service for this purpose: in many countries the data used on a nutritional label can be taken from an 'authoritative' source, rather than from analysis of the food itself; the nutritional database has thus developed from being a nutritionists' tool to having a place in food regulation.

LIMITATIONS OF FOOD COMPOSITION TABLES

Understanding the limitations of food composition data is one of the keys to making proper use of the data.

Variability in the composition of foods

Foods are biological materials, and as such show the expected natural variations in composition; even processed foods produced under strict quality control show variability in composition, because the ingredients vary and process conditions cannot be controlled absolutely. In preparing food composition tables, the compilers attempt to produce values that are representative of the food item in general, and therefore the tables cannot be expected to predict accurately the composition of a single sample. This leads to the view that food tables are of little value, as McCance and Widdowson have aptly stated: 'there are two schools of thought about food tables. One tends to regard the figures in them as having the accuracy of atomic weight determinations; the other dismisses them as valueless on the grounds that a foodstuff may be so modified by the soil, the season or its rate of growth that no figure can be a reliable guide to its composition. The truth, of course, lies somewhere between these two points of view' (Widdowson & McCance 1943). Ideally a table should present the average value for a nutrient, accompanied by some statistical measure of its variability; this would provide the user with some idea of how the value would apply to the particular sample of food in question. Some compilations are moving in this direction, and this kind of information will become increasingly important as food tables are used in a regulatory way. Many users, however, only require a single value, and the analytical sources needed to generate such a database are very large indeed. Therefore, the user of current compilations must recognize that there are limitations; all calculations made from tables have a limited predictive accuracy and data should be presented and used accordingly. The predictive accuracy should improve with the length of measurement or the number of people studied, since this effectively increases the amount of food being sampled. Some examples of the effects of variations in the composition of foods in calculations of intake are given by Paul & Southgate (1988). The different components of food show different degrees of variability, and a knowledge of these is valuable to the user.

Water

This is one of the most important variables because it produces variations in all the other constituents – variations are often seen in vegetables, due to maturity and the conditions under which they have been stored. Cereal foods in the form of grains and flours have a low water content and thus are less variable in composition; once the cereals have been cooked however, the water content does become more variable. As a general principle, the composition of diets that are rich in cereal foods can be predicted more accurately than those which are rich in other plant foods. Some compilations of food composition, mainly those used in animal feeding, express composition on a dry-matter basis. This reduces variability but the compilations are less useful.

Proximates

The protein content of many foods varies over a fairly narrow range, and food tables predict protein intakes with reasonable accuracy. Fat however, is a different matter and this is primarily due to the variable fat/lean ratio in meats and to wide variations in the fat content of meat products and many other prepared foods. The accurate use of food tables to measure fat intakes therefore requires close attention to the meats consumed, and especially recording fat and lean separately and recording fat not eaten, that is, left as plate waste. Total available carbohydrate values are usually predicted with reasonable accuracy, but sugar values may be underestimated because of the widespread use of sucrose and glucose syrups in processed foods. Few studies of the use of food tables for predicting dietary fibre have been made, but provided cereal foods are correctly identified food tables should be reasonable guides. There are some problems regarding the compatibility of values, which are discussed later.

Energy values

In virtually all tables of food composition the energy values are for *metabolizable energy*, that is, they are estimates of the energy the body can obtain from the food. They are derived values calculated from the proximate composition of the food using energy conversion factors; the factors used vary in different compilations, and thus it is important for the user to be aware of the actual factors being used. Because the values are derived they are estimates, and the energy values are approximate and extreme accuracy should never be ascribed to them.

Inorganic constituents – minerals

The inorganic constituents in foods vary for one of two reasons: first, naturally because the uptake of inorganic constituents into a plant depends on the rate of growth, the soil conditions, the fertilizer treatment the soil has received, climatic conditions during growth and uptake into animal tissues, on the feeding regime of the animal; secondly because of human intervention in processed and cooked foods, on the recipe used. As a general rule the major nutrients – potassium, calcium, magnesium and phosphorus – in unprocessed foods vary within narrow limits, and therefore food composition tables give reasonable indications. Trace constituents (iron, copper, zinc, manganese, iodine and chromium) are much more variable, and tables can only give general guidance. In processed and cooked foods, salt is a common addition and this means that tables only give approximate values for sodium and chloride. Phosphates are also widely used in processed foods and the tables may underestimate phosphorus intake. Many countries have food fortification, and this may produce errors when values from tables prepared for other countries are used. For example, in the UK calcium and iron are added to all wheat flours other than wholemeal. It should also be remembered that the values in food tables are *total values* and do not provide indications of how much of the nutrient is bioavailable.

Vitamins

The vitamins in foods are subject to the same causes of variation that affect minerals; furthermore, many vitamins are labile and prone to destruction during processing, cooking and storage, this means that food tables can only give approximate information on the vitamin content of foods. The water-soluble vitamins are also lost by leaching into the cooking water. Very few studies have been made of the predictive accuracy of tables in respect of vitamins, but it is unreasonable to expect them to be more than a guide for the most labile – vitamin C and the folates – where oxidation and leaching occur. In the case of the fat-soluble vitamins, the storage of these in animal tissues is very dependent on the diet consumed and wide variations in vitamin A have been observed. This emphasizes the desirability of the provision of estimates of variation in tables.

Incomplete coverage

Many users feel that a major limitation of all food tables is the fact that the coverage of foods is never complete, and that values for nutrients are frequently missing. This can limit the accuracy of calculations unless the user adopts an appropriate strategy, because complete compilations – whether of foods or nutrients – will never be practicable.

In the case of foods, the number available for consumption is very large indeed. If one thinks of the range of food items in the typical supermarket and the permutations and combinations of ingredients that take place in the average kitchen, it will be clear that something in excess of 100 000 food items would be needed. In addition, new brands of foods are continually being developed by food manufacturers, formulations are being modified and ingredients are being replaced. Since sampling and analysis take a finite time it is impossible for a compilation to be complete at any one time, even given unlimited analytical resources.

Fortunately, within the context of a day's diet an individual food item rarely makes a major contribution to intake, and therefore, provided the tables contain the foods most frequently consumed and those that are the major sources of particular nutrients, a compilation will usually meet most users' require-

ments. The majority of the intake of most nutrients is provided by relatively few foods, and therefore compilers of food composition tables focus their resources on those foods (Greenfield & Southgate 1989). Where an individual consumes a large amount of a 'missing food' it is important to assign a composition to that food, either by using the values for a similar food or by giving it the average composition of the remainder of the diet. Where it is essential to have accurate compositional data, for example if the food forms more than about 10% of the intake, or where it is likely to be a major source of a particular nutrient, then analysis is essential. However, it is important to make sure the food in question is not recorded in another database, and every nutritionist is advised to have access to a range of tables. Incomplete coverage of nutrients can lead to the underestimation of nutrient intakes or an incorrect dietary prescription. The elimination of 'missing values' for nutrients presents smaller resource problems than missing foods, because the number of nutrients is finite. The gaps usually arise when older data are used which were obtained before the nutrient became of interest, or before adequate methods of analysis were available. A compiler using literature values is limited by the nutrients the original author decided to measure. It is common for many laboratories to have a limited analytical repertoire, and complete coverage is rare unless the analysis is being carried out specifically for the construction of a nutritional database. Analyses do require resources, and a decision not to measure a particular nutrient may be made because of limited resources; this is often the case where a food has been judged not to be an important source of a nutrient. When making calculations from a database it is important to note 'missing values' and to adopt a strategy that minimizes their influence. The use of values from a related food is one approach, as is assigning a value that is the mean for those foods where a value is given. Neither of these approaches is valid if the food forms a major part of the diet, or where it is probably an important source of the nutrient. In most large databases the latter is often unlikely, but must always be considered. Where these strategies are judged inadequate the only recourse is to analysis. This should be carried out on a representative sample using a validated method, and the values added to the database as provisional values.

Identity of foods

In order to use a set of tables with confidence, the user must be certain that the food item whose composition is given corresponds to the food eaten by the person being studied or prescribed for. It can be critically important to identify foods precisely, and this is the reason why tables such as 'McCance & Widdowson' (Paul & Southgate 1978) include information on the sample analysed, and particularly the part of the food that was regarded as edible. The rejection of parts of foods before consumption is highly idiosyncratic, and the accurate use of tables must allow for this. The compilers of tables aim to give representative values, and these may not correspond exactly with a single sample of a food. Therefore, for accurate metabolic studies it is usually necessary to carry out one's own analyses.

Whether this is necessary in any particular application depends on the variation in the composition of foods, discussed earlier. It is important to remember that the measurement of food intake is frequently associated with considerable inaccuracies, and that the errors arising from this are much greater than those arising from errors due to analysis or variations in the food composition. The values in a table for prepared dishes may well have come from dishes prepared to different recipes, and many regular users recalculate the values using their own recipes, thus producing a database specific to their own situation. In nutritional investigations of a special group of subjects, it is frequently more economical of analytical resources to prepare a specific database than to analyse a large number of dietary collections.

Incompatibility of nutrient values

This is not often a problem if only one database is being used; it is, however, a major limitation when using values from different databases. There are two principal types of incompatibility, assuming that the foods are correctly identified. First, the analytical methods used have generated different values; this could be because the methods were attempting to measure different constituents: dietary fibre is one common example, where crude fibre, acid–detergent fibre, unavailable carbohydrate, or non-starch polysaccharide values may all be listed under the heading

'fibre'; carbohydrate values may be direct analytical measurements of the available carbohydrates, or values derived by difference. These problems rarely arise within one database, but they may do and the user must be aware of this. Careful scrutiny of the introductory text or documentation is vital to avoid problems of this kind. The second source of incompatibility lies in the modes of expression. This is usually most common for the vitamins, but can be seen with minerals where SI units, mg/100 g or mg/1000 g are used. Available carbohydrates can be expressed as the monosaccharides or as the disaccharide or polysaccharide. Once again the user must know the conventions being used. This is particularly important for derived values such as protein, where the conversion factors used can differ, and energy where different series of energy conversion factors are used. When Infoods considered the matter of data interchange between databases, it was necessary to define a series of 'tags' that specified precisely the nature of the nutrient, its method of determination (where appropriate) and the mode of expression. These tags were therefore unique, and ensured that incompatible values were not transferred or used together.

THE PROPER USE OF FOOD COMPOSITION DATA

The proper use of any dataset, whether printed or computerized, depends on the user as much as the compilers. It is important first to be familiar with the conventions that have been used; this applies particularly to the way energy values have been derived and the factors used to calculate protein. One feature that can cause error is the way in which traces of nutrients have been transcribed in a computerized system. Missing values in a computerized system are often given a zero value; this practice is wrong and can lead to serious error. Missing values should be tagged to avoid this. The user is most strongly advised to read the introductory text or documentation before using the data, and to recognize the limitations that apply.

REFERENCES

Arab L, Whittler M, Schettler G 1987 European food composition tables in translation. Springer-Verlag, Berlin

Atwater WO, Woods CD 1896 The chemical composition of American food materials. US Department of Agriculture Office Experimental Stations Bulletin 28.

Food and Agriculture Organisation 1968 Food composition tables for use in Africa. FAO, Rome

Food and Agriculture Organisation 1972 Food composition table for use in East Asia. FAO, Rome

Greenfield H, Southgate DAT 1992 Food composition data. Production management and use. Elsevier Applied Science, London

Holland B, Welch AA, Unwin ID, Buss DH, Paul AA, Southgate DAT 1991 McCance and Widdowson's The

Composition of Foods 5th edn. Royal Society of Chemistry, Cambridge

Infoods 1986 International directory of food composition tables. International Network of Food Data Systems, Cambridge, Mass

Konig J 1978 Chemie der menschlichen Nahrungs- und Genussmittel. Springer-Verlag, Berlin

McCance RA, Widdowson EM 1940 The chemical composition of foods. MRC Special Report 235. HMSO, London

Ministry of Agriculture Fisheries and Food 1989 Household food consumption and expenditure: 1987 Annual report of the National Food Survey Committee. HMSO, London

Paul AA, Southgate DAT 1978 McCance and Widdowson's the composition of foods, 4th edn. HMSO, London

Paul AA, Southgate DAT 1988 Conversion into nutrients. In: Cameron ME, Van Staveren WA, (eds) Manual of methodology for food consumption studies. Oxford Medical Publications, Oxford, pp 121–144

Southgate DAT 1974 Guidelines for the preparation of tables of food composition. Karger, Basel

Southgate DAT 1985 Criteria to be used for acceptance of data in nutrient database. In: West CE (ed) Towards compatibility of nutrient data banks in Europe. Annals of Nutrition and Metabolism (suppl) 29, 49–53

Widdowson EM, McCance RA 1943 Food tables, their scope and limitations. Lancet 1: 230–232.

16. Cereals and cereal products

D. A. T. Southgate

The most important plant foods in the human diet are those derived from the seeds of domesticated members of the Gramineae, the grasses – the cereals (Masefield et al. 1969). By convention the cereals group covers a few foods derived from the seeds of other plants, such as buckwheat and quinoa, and this convention will be followed in this chapter. The discovery of the cultivation of cereals, probably in the near east, was a key stage in the development of human society, the ability to cultivate successive crops marking the development of agriculture and permitting settled development. The cereal crop could also be stored between harvests, providing stability in the supply of food.

Cereals remain an important staple food in most countries, and in many parts of rural Africa and Asia provide more than 70% of the energy in the diet. As countries become more affluent the importance of cereals, and plant foods in general, declines; notwithstanding, cereal foods provide approximately 30% of the energy, 25% of the protein and nearly 50% of the available carbohydrate in the UK diet. Wheat is the most important source of cereal foods in the UK, but rice is more important in the far eastern countries, and maize in much of Africa and central America.

The distribution of production, and to a certain extent the importance of the different cereals, is in part due to climatic constraints on the growth of the different species. Wheat production is limited to temperate zones; rye has a wider northern range and can be grown up as far as the Arctic circle, and rice can be grown in standing water in tropical and subtropical climates and, less commonly, on dry uplands. Barley and oats have a similar range to wheat, although oats thrive on poorer soils. Maize and the millets are major crops in the tropics and subtropics, although some varieties can be grown in temperate climates.

On the basis of overall production wheat is the major cereal, making up about a quarter of the total, closely followed by maize and rice. Substantial amounts of maize and barley (the next most produced crops) are used in animal feeds, and therefore wheat and rice are the major cereals in the human diet.

A very large proportion of the world's wheat is grown on the prairies of North America and the steppes of the Soviet Union, and the North American wheat is a major export commodity.

PRODUCTION OF CEREAL GRAINS AND FLOURS

The cereal grains are seeds and contain the embryo of the future plant and food reserve materials to meet the requirements of germination. Although the actual structures of the different cereal grains show some important differences, the anatomy of the wheat grain shows the typical features of a cereal grain (Fig. 16.1). The embryo consists of a thin-walled, slightly differentiated structure which is separated from the endosperm by a structure called the scutellum, an organ that is involved in the mobilization of the food reserves of the grain during germination. The major part of the grain is made up of the endosperm, which consists of thin-walled cells packed with starch grains. The outer layers of the grain comprise the pericarp, derived from the ovary of the flower, surrounding the testa which is the true seed coat. The outer thick-walled structures form the bran, the embryo the germ, and the endosperm provides the starch-rich white flour.

Wheat

The cultivated bread wheats appear to have evolved from their wild ancestors by interspecific breeding and polyploidy, because all the cultivated wheats exhibit polyploidy. One of the wild ancestors is known, but the other hypothetical ancestor is not. The first major bread wheat to be cultivated was *Triticum dicoccum*, which was a tetraploid wheat; the modern species

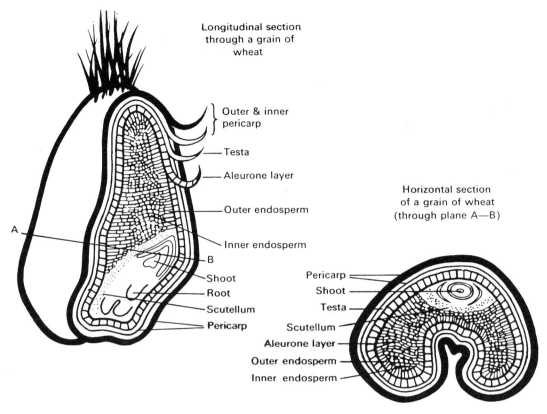

Fig. 16.1   Structure of the wheat grain (from McCance 1946).

T. aestivum is a hexaploid, and many different varieties have been produced by selective plant breeding to produce wheats with special characteristics such as short straw, increased protein content, flour characteristics and improved disease resistance (Von Bothmer 1987).

The varieties can be distinguished by the milling and baking characteristics of the flour produced: hard wheats give a strong flour which is relatively rich in gluten and is preferred for bread making; soft wheat flours contain less gluten and are suitable for use in biscuits and confectionery. Durum wheats are a different species, *T. durum*, very rich in gluten and preferred for the production of pasta.

Wheat is almost invariably milled before use in foods. In prehistoric times the grain was ground by hand using flattened stones called querns. The development of water, wind and steam power led to milling between stones. The stones were dressed to give a ridged surface that breaks the grain, which is fed in at the centre of the stone; the flour is conveyed across the stone to the edge. The flour produced by stone-milling is a wholemeal one and different flours are produced by sieving. The finer, whiter flours are produced by sieving through fine cloth sieves; such flours are termed 'low-extraction' flours, since they represent a small proportion of the original grain; 'high extraction' flours contain more of the outer branny layers of the grain, so that a wholemeal flour is nominally a 100% extraction flour.

At the beginning of the 20th century the stone mills were progressively replaced by roller mills, and the bulk of flour milled in the UK is now produced in this type of mill (Kent 1983). Here the grain is milled by a series of steel rollers, which have progressively smaller clearances between them. The first set of rollers are ridged and break open the grain with a shearing action, which separates most of the branny layer as a flake; the next series of rollers scrape the floury endosperm from the bran. The endosperm is initially broken into fragments called semolina. The output of each set of rollers is sieved and the fine flour removed. The larger fragments pass on to the next series of rollers where the processes of grinding and sieving are continued, finishing with a series of reduction stages which crush and reduce the endosperm into flour of the required particle size. Roller mills produce a series of streams, ranging from the bran fragments through germ to progressively finer flours. These are mixed to produce the various types of flour required by the customer. Wholemeal flours are produced by combing all the different streams in the correct proportions. The characteristics of the flours produced can also be varied according to the variety of wheat grains going into the original grist.

Rice (*Oryza sativa*)

Rice forms the second major cereal in the human diet. The plant originated in Asia and was established as the staple food in the Chinese diet by 2800 BC, and soon after in India. Rice is grown under two different systems. Most of the crop is grown in standing water, the traditional paddy fields, usually maintained by irrigation or by enclosing the water in river deltas with low walls. Most of the rice plants are produced in nurseries and planted out as young seedlings. The water level is maintained for most of the growing period and drained prior to harvesting. Some rice is grown in upland areas where the seed is planted in dry soil similar to the other cereal crops.

The rice grain, although it has many of the structures seen in the wheat grain, has an important difference in that the grain has the inner leaves of the flower fused to the pericarp, which necessitates a different milling process. The first stage involves the removal of these leaves, or husk, traditionally by pounding the grain to break off the husk, producing brown rice where the bran remains attached to the grain. This is now carried out mechanically in hullers. The bran layers are removed in a rice mill which is said to 'pearl' the grain by abrading away the pericarp, testa and some germ, leaving a polished grain. The polishing can be repeated, giving a progressively whiter grain. The grain can be milled to produce flour, but this is not usual.

A number of different varieties of rice are cultivated and in West Africa a different species is grown (*O. glaberrima*), which has a red testa.

Maize (*Zea mays*)

This is the major cereal in many parts of Central and South America and is widely cultivated in Africa. Large amounts of the crop are also grown in the southern USA. The plant originated in the Americas and was brought to Europe by Columbus. The wild ancestor of the cultivated species has not been identified, and the cultivated species is polyploid. The crop is grown for both animal and human food and also as a green crop to produce silage for animal feed. Some of the crop is harvested before the grains have matured, for the production of sweetcorn which is eaten as a vegetable.

The crop is grown from seed and produces a head where modified leaves surround the ear, with the male flowers forming the tassel. The grains form in rows on the central cob. When mature the grains are stripped from the cob mechanically. There is a considerable variety in the appearance of the grains, even from one ear, due to cross-pollination. Maize is milled to produce maize meal, which may be sieved to remove the pericarp and germ.

Rye (*Secale cereale*)

The northern limit for growing rye is considerably higher than for wheat, and rye is still important in Scandinavia and central Europe as an alternative cereal crop to wheat, although production in the UK is mainly for special purposes, such as the production of crispbreads. The cultivated species are diploid.

The grain of rye is similar to that of wheat and the milling processes adopted are generally similar, although the range of extractions produced is lower, with much use of high-extraction flours.

Much of the rye crop is not used directly as food but fermented to produce alcohol.

Barley (*Hordeum spp*)

Barley has been cultivated since neolithic times; the remains of barley and the early wheat species have been found at sites dating from around 6000 BC. There are two major species, the two-rowed (*H. distichon*) and the six-rowed (*H. vulgare*). Most of the modern cultivars grown in the UK are two-rowed, whereas the six-rowed is preferred in more northern countries. The barley grain has a husk which is removed by abrasive processes called blocking or pearling. It is, however, grown mainly for animal feed and only indirectly for human consumption in the production of malt for brewing beer or fermenting whisky. The quality of the barley for malting has to meet strict standards, and unsuitable crops join the major part of the barley crop in animal feeds.

Oats (*Avena sativa*)

Oats are also a cereal that has been cultivated by man for many thousands of years. The cultivated species appears to be closely related to the wild oats which still flourish as a weed. The plant grows well on poor soils and has a slightly higher northern limit than wheat, and was widely cultivated for human and animal consumption in Scotland. Oats are first dehusked to remove a very tough and silicified husk, and then usually rolled to split the grain. The grain can be milled to produce a flour, but this has a restricted use. The cultivation of oats for human use had been quite limited until recently, but the special qualities of the dietary fibre it contains has increased interest in the crop for human consumption.

Sorghum (*Sorghum vulgare*)

Sorghum is a staple crop in many parts of Africa, where it has the advantage of being resistant to drought conditions. It has been cultivated since about 3 000 BC. The grain is round and may have a white or pigmented seed coat. The white-coated varieties are preferred for food as the polyphenolics in the red-coated varieties give a bitter flavour. Traditionally the grains are pounded to produce a flour, the husk being separated by winnowing. Commercial milling uses an initial pearling stage to remove the husk, followed by reduction of the grain by crushing in a roller or hammer mill. A considerable amount of the sorghum crop is used in the production of beers.

Millets

Millets include the grains of several species cultivated in the tropics, especially in Africa. Like sorghum they produce small round grains, often with a coloured coat. They have been cultivated since prehistoric times. The major species are *Eleucine coracana* (finger millet) and *Pennisetum typhoideum* (Bulrush millet), both of which have white-seeded varieties. The 'tef' of Ethiopia, *Eragrostis abyssinia*, produces very fine grains that may be white or red. The millet grains are dehusked before they are ground to flour. This is traditionally done by pounding and winnowing, but commercially a wet-milling process to soften the husk has produced promising results.

COMPOSITION OF CEREAL GRAINS AND FLOURS

Comparison of the range of cereals used as foods shows many similarities, stemming from the fact that they are all seeds of the members of one plant family. The grains show anatomical variations and the different parts of the grain show different relationships to

the total (Kent 1983). In general the pericarp and testa account for about 8–10% of the total; the amount of germ varies considerably: in maize it is about 12% and in sorghum 10%, but in the others it is between 2% and 3%. The endosperm accounts for the remainder, making up between 63% and 80% of the whole grain. The proportions of endosperm are naturally lower in rice, barley and oats, where the grain has a husk attached to it.

The proximate compositions of the grains (Table 16.1) show many similarities. The values in the table are expressed on a dry-matter basis for ease of comparison, although the grains usually have between 11 and 16 g/100 g moisture content when harvested, depending on the conditions at harvest. Cereals will not store satisfactorily above 15% moisture. The grains typically contain 8–16% protein and 2–7% fat, with oats and maize having the highest values. The inorganic matter is around 2% in most grains. The available carbohydrates are principally starch, with small amounts of free sugars, which include glucose, fructose and sucrose, and in grains that have been harvested with a high water content, some maltose may also be present. Many cereals contain low concentrations of glucofructans. The table gives crude fibre values for the whole grain, depending very much on whether or not the husk is present. Oats and rice for example, as harvested, have very high levels but since these cereals are not used as human foods without removal of the husks these high values are not nutritionally relevant.

DISTRIBUTION OF NUTRIENTS WITHIN THE GRAIN AND THE EFFECTS OF MILLING

Cereals are rarely consumed as foods without some form of processing – typically milling – to produce a flour of some kind. During this process the grain is disrupted physically, but the milling process as such does not have any major effects on its nutrients. However, milling is often followed by some kind of fractionation of the grain, to remove less desirable components or to produce specific products for other uses, for example, the production of bread, biscuits or pasta. This fractionation separates the components of the grain and is important nutritionally because the nutrients are not distributed uniformly throughout the grain.

Proteins

The proteins in the grain are present in higher concentrations in the aleurone layer, which is situated immediately below the testa and which usually sepa-

Table 16.1   Composition of some typical cereal grains per 100 g dry basis

Cereal	Protein	Fat	Carbohydrate	Crude fibre	Ash
Wheat					
Manitoba	16.0	2.9	74.1	2.6	1.8
English	10.5	2.6	78.6	2.5	1.8
Rice					
paddy	9.1	2.2	71.2	10.2	7.2
brown	11.1	2.7	83.2	1.8	1.8
Maize					
flint	11.1	4.9	80.2	2.1	1.7
dent	10.0	4.5	80.0	3.5	2.0
sweet	12.1	9.1	74.5	2.2	2.0
Rye	15.0	1.7	80.1	2.6	2.1
Oats					
whole	11.6	5.2	69.8	10.4	2.9
groats	14.9	7.0	74.6	1.3	2.1
Barley	11.8	1.8	78.1	5.3	3.1
Sorghum	12.4	3.6	79.7	2.7	1.7
Millets					
pearl	13.6	5.4	77.9	1.3	1.8
finger	8.4	1.5	82.9	4.1	3.1

From Kent (1983)

rates with the bran layer, which is poor in proteins. The germ has the highest concentration of protein, and the endosperm has the lowest. However, because the endosperm is the largest part of the grain, it contains over 70% of the total protein present. The proteins in the different fractions differ in amino-acid composition, that of the endosperm being richer in glutamic acid and lower in lysine than the protein in the germ.

Lipids

The lipids in the grain are present mainly in the germ and bran fractions, with little in the endosperm. In maize the germ contains 35 g/100 g. The milling process, by crushing the grain, tends to distribute some of the lipids into other fractions.

Carbohydrates

One of the major effects of fractionation of the grain is on the carbohydrates. The starch is primarily located in the endosperm, where the cell walls are thin; the thicker cell walls of the pericarp and testa separate into the bran.

Inorganic constituents

The minerals in the grain are present in higher concentrations in the pericarp, testa and germ.

Vitamins

The grains contain many of the B-vitamins, which are present in the highest concentrations in the germ and the aleurone layer. The endosperm contains significant concentrations of riboflavin and pantothenic acid. Milling and fractionation therefore produce widely different nutritional compositions, but these should not be regarded as processing losses in the strict sense because the nutrients are not destroyed but distributed according to their location in the grain.

COMPOSITION OF CEREALS AND CEREAL PRODUCTS

The range of cereal products consumed in the human diet is very large, and while generalizations are possible it is preferable to discuss them under headings corresponding to the major cereals.

Wheat

The major part of the wheat crop is milled to produce flours which are then used as ingredients in other foods. The flours are produced at a range of extraction rates, including wholemeal. The compositions of flours of different extraction rates are shown in Table 16.2, which illustrates the effects of fractionation.

Table 16.2　Composition of wheat flours per 100 g

Flour	Water	Protein	Fat	Carbohydrate available	Dietary fibre		Energy	
	(g)	(g)	(g)	(g)	(g)	(NSP)	(kcal)	(kJ)
Wholemeal (100%)	14.0	13.7	2.0	63.5	9.6	9.0	318	1351
Brown (85%)	14.5	12.8	2.0	66.9	7.5	6.4	327	1392
White bread-making (72%)	13.0	12.8	2.0	73.3	3.4	3.1	337	1433
Patent (45%)	14.1	10.8	1.3	79.2	—	—	347	1480

From Paul & Southgate (1978)

The flours may be treated to improve or modify their properties. White flours have been highly prized for prestige reasons since Roman times (McCance & Widdowson 1956) and various bleaching agents have been used, including nitrous oxide, nitrogen trichloride (Agene), chlorine dioxide and benzoyl peroxide, the latter two being those permitted in the UK. A range of other improvers is permitted; these agents are believed to modify the cysteine sulphydryl groups in the flour and improve its breadmaking qualities. Chlorine is used to improve the quality of high-volume cake flours.

The protein content of hard wheats is considerably higher than that of most soft wheats, and most flours are milled from a mixture producing flours with the appropriate quantity and quality of proteins. Wheat proteins have particularly important properties: they include the soluble albumins and globulins derived from the cytoplasm of the cells, and the insoluble proteins, prolamins and glutenins. The latter are the storage proteins of the grain, which are deposited in protein bodies compressed together in the aleurone layer of the mature grain. The prolamins contain aqueous-alcohol soluble components called gliadins, and the glutenins are insoluble in aqueous alcohol but soluble in acid and alkali. The insoluble proteins produce gluten when the flour is kneaded with water, and it is the elastic properties of the wheat gluten that makes the production of bread possible.

Bread

Bread can be produced from a wide range of extractions; white bread is most commonly produced from a flour of 72% extraction using the appropriate mixture of wheats to give proteins with the appropriate properties. In the traditional process the flour is mixed with water, yeast and salt and the resultant dough

kneaded to develop the gluten. It is then left to stand in a warm environment for the yeast to start fermenting; the dough is kneaded again to further develop the gluten, and then is left to prove. When the required expansion has occurred the dough is then baked. Baking causes the expansion of the carbon dioxide in the dough and the elasticity of the gluten retains the gas to produce the crumb structure of the bread; the external surface caramelizes to produce a crust of partially gelatinized starch granules. This long fermentation process is very time-consuming and labour-intensive and has now largely been replaced by the Chorleywood process (Kent 1983). In this the dough is mixed mechanically, using a reducing agent L-cysteine, to promote the uncoiling and reorientation of the protein molecules, and oxidizing additives such as ascorbic acid, often with potassium bromate, to reform the disulphide links which are essential to the formation of the gluten network in the dough during mixing. A little fat is also added to improve gas retention. The process produces bread with a slightly higher water content, and also permits the use of a higher proportion of home-produced soft wheats.

Breads can be produced using wheat mixed with other cereals, the most commonly used being rye: wheat/rye breads are very popular in Germany and other European countries. The addition of other cereals tends to reduce the volume of the loaf and the quality of the crumb.

The composition of some typical breads produced in the UK is illustrated in Table 16.3. The importance of bread in the diet is such that its sale and composition have been the subject of legislation since the Middle Ages. Current regulations control the use of additives in the production of bread, and also require that all flours other than wholemeal are fortified with calcium, iron, thiamin and nicotinic acid. The breads in other countries may not contain these additional nutrients

Table 16.3   Composition of some breads per 100 g

Bread	Water	Protein	Fat	Carbohydrate available	Dietary fibre		Energy	
	(g)	(g)	(g)	(g)	(g)	(NSP)	(kcal)	(kJ)
Wholemeal	38.3	9.2	2.5	41.6	7.4	5.8	215	914
Brown	39.5	8.5	2.0	44.3	5.9	3.5	218	927
White	37.3	8.4	1.9	49.3	3.8	1.5	235	1002
Wheatgerm	38.9	9.2	2.5	42.5	5.1	3.3	232	937
Currant	29.4	7.5	7.6	50.7	3.8	—	289	1220
Malt	25.8	8.3	2.4	56.8	6.5	—	268	1139
French	29.2	9.6	2.7	55.4	5.1	1.5	270	1149
Rolls								
white, crusty	26.4	10.9	2.3	57.6	4.3	1.5	280	1192
white, soft	32.7	9.2	4.2	51.6	3.9	1.5	268	1137

From Holland et al (1988)

and some caution is necessary when using UK data for nutritional studies in other countries. In the USA, for example, milk solids are used in many white breads, and the amounts of added fat also differ.

Bread rolls are prepared in a similar way, but their lower volume usually leads to a lower water content on baking. Soft rolls are produced by increasing the fat added.

Breads from high-extraction flours tend to have a lower volume and more dense crumb structure. Wholemeal bread is usually prepared with the minimum of additives – in the UK only vitamin C is permitted. Brown breads of lower extraction are required by legislation to be made from flours with at least 0.6% of crude fibre, although it is anticipated that in the future dietary fibre levels will form the basis of the requirement. A wide range of extractions is used, ranging from almost wholemeal to the minimum allowed by law. Some breads include added softened grains or bran to increase dietary fibre levels. Speciality breads include those with added germ and others with added fruit.

Biscuits

Wheat flours are used in the production of many types of biscuit (cookies). These require a dough mix that retains its shape during cooking and a low-protein flour is preferred. The biscuit mix typically contains fat and sucrose and the baking process leads to a low-moisture product.

Cakes and pastries

These form a group of cooked foods in which wheat flour is the major component, usually in conjunction with fat, egg, dried fruit and often baking powder. Although many of these foods were originally prepared domestically, they are increasingly produced commercially in an industrial setting rather than the domestic kitchen or local bakery. The compositions of a large range of cereal products are given by Holland et al. (1988).

Chappatis

These are prepared from high-extraction wheat flours. The dough is mixed with water and a little salt and in some cultures oil is also added. The mixture is flattened and cooked on a flat heated metal surface.

Pasta

Pasta is prepared from durum wheats, which are hard, high-protein wheats. When mixed with water the flour produces a stiff paste which can be formed into a wide range of shapes which are retained when the product is dried. The mixture can be extruded through a die to produce spaghetti, or tubed structures such as macaroni. In the traditional pastas only flour and water were used, but pastas with added egg and spinach are now very popular. Wholemeal pastas can be prepared, but these may be made using other wheats mixed with the durum wheat.

Wheat-based breakfast cereals

A number of breakfast cereals are prepared from wheat, including some prepared from whole wheat. Puffed products are prepared by subjecting cooked and hydrated grains to a sudden change of pressure, which causes the moisture to expand very rapidly within the grain. Shredded products are made by cooking a starchy variety of wheat with the addition of water; the cooked grains are held for a while and then passed through shredding rollers and the mats of shredded grain are baked. Flaked products are prepared by cooking doughs in an autoclave or extrusion cooker. The dough is flaked on rollers and the flakes are then baked to a low moisture content.

Bran

The development of the dietary fibre hypothesis by Burkitt & Trowell (1975) has led to a substantial increase in the use of wheat bran for human consumption, when previously it was used primarily as animal feed. Bran can be produced by sieving wholemeal flour but most is derived from the bran streams from roller milling. The sieved products often contain more endosperm (and starch) than roller-milled products, where the removal of endosperm is very efficient. Bran contains a relatively high lipid content and this unsaturated lipid rapidly becomes rancid unless the bran is stabilized by heat to inactivate the lipases. Wheat bran is sold in a number of particle sizes and is increasingly used as an additive to increase dietary fibre, particularly in breakfast cereals. Because it forms the outer layer of the grain, bran can become contaminated with agrochemicals and moulds.

Isolated wheat products

Wheat is used as a source of starch and gluten. The starch is separated by fractionating the flour, either by wet or dry air classification methods. Gluten is prepared by washing the soluble components from the flour. The gluten may be used as an additive to low-protein flours to improve their bread-making qualities.

Rice

In contrast to wheat, most rice is not milled into flour but is used as the polished grain. Polishing removes the branny layers and the germ, with consequent substantial loss of the B-vitamins. Other losses occur due to leaching when rice is soaked in water before cooking. The unhusked rice is also subjected to parboiling, where the grains are steamed or boiled after soaking. The process softens the husk but produces other changes, because the water-soluble components, especially the vitamins, migrate into the grain together with some of the oil. The grain structure is modified so that the aleurone layer is retained with the grain when the bran layers are milled off. Parboiling thus changes the nutritional value of the polished grain. The compositions of some rice products are given in Table 16.4.

The bulk of rice is eaten in cooked dishes prepared from the polished or parboiled grains. A number of different varieties of rice are produced, with specific properties or textures. Long-grain rice, which is produced in the USA and Pakistan (Basmati rice), when cooked produces grains that remain separate, whereas the medium and short-grained varieties when cooked produce fluffy grains that clump together. Glutinous, sweet or waxy rice has a chalky endosperm and is widely used as a thickener in processed foods because it does not retrograde. Some use of rice flours is made in infant foods, and rice grains are puffed for breakfast cereal products. Rice bran is a rich source of B-vitamins and dietary fibre and has some use as a supplement.

Maize

Although maize is primarily used for animal feeding in the developed countries, it is a major component of the diet in southern Africa and Latin America. In African diets it is often consumed as a porridge-like

Table 16.4 Composition of some rice products per 100 g

	Water (g)	Protein (g)	Fat (g)	Carbohydrate available (g)	Dietary fibre (g) (NSP)		Energy (kcal) (kJ)	
Brown rice	13.9	6.7	2.8	81.3	3.8	1.9	357	1493
White rice								
polished	11.7	6.5	1.0	86.8	2.2	0.5	361	1510
parboiled	12.4	6.7	1.0	79.3	—	—	364	1523
long-grain	10.5	7.4	0.5	79.8	—	—	359	1502
glutinous	13.9	8.4	1.6	74.9	—	—	359	1502

From Holland et al (1988)

mixture prepared by boiling the meal with water. In central America the maize is widely consumed as unleavened flat breads such as tortillas.

Tortillas

The traditional preparation of tortillas involves steeping the maize meal in water overnight. The water is heated initially to 100°C and contains lime (Ca(OH)$_2$) at a concentration of 0.5–1.5%. The steeped maize meal is then passed through heated rollers to partially gelatinize the starch, ground and dried. This meal is then used with water to prepare a dough which is baked in thin layers on a heated plate.

Cornflakes

These were amongst the first processed breakfast cereals and still the most popular product of this kind in the UK. Flaked grits, preferably from yellow maize, are sieved from the milled maize and cooked with the addition of malt, salt and sugar, and then partially dried to 15–20% moisture content. In the traditional process this is done at elevated temperatures in an autoclave; extrusion cooking is also being used to a limited extent. The mixture is conditioned by holding for a period and is then flaked on rollers, toasted in a continuous oven, cooled, and packed in impervious packs of waxed paper or plastic. The flakes are often fortified with vitamins and minerals which are added towards the end of the processing.

Isolated maize products

The fine meal sieved from the milled grain, cornflour, is the major ingredient in custard powder. Maize starch is prepared from the milled grain by steeping the meal in water with added sulphur dioxide. The suspension is treated to adjust the density and the starch is separated from the protein by continuous high-speed centrifu-gation. The starch is recentrifuged to remove residual protein and then dried, initially in ovens or kilns and finally by vacuum techniques. The starch is widely used as a food ingredient and for the production of glucose and high-fructose syrups by a combination of acidic and enzymatic treatments. The compositions of some maize products are given in Table 16.5.

Oats

Oatmeal was a staple food in Scotland during the 17th and 18th centuries, being consumed in mixtures with hot water as porridge, and in oatcakes. While porridge survives as a breakfast cereal, the traditional overnight heating has largely been superseded by the use of processed precooked ready-to-eat products (Table 16.6). In these the starch is partially dextrinized by steaming the meal.

Some fine oat flours are used in infant cereal mixes. A variety of oat-bran products is being used for dietary fibre ingredients.

Rye

The proteins in rye contain relatively little gluten and only produce satisfactory loaf volumes and crumb structures when mixed with wheat; often as little as 25% wheat results in a substantial improvement. Rye breads are often prepared using a sour-dough process, in which the dough is left to stand to allow a natural lactic acid fermentation to take place. Bread baked in this way has a rather dense crumb structure. Pumpernickel is a dense-textured product produced from a coarse rye meal.

Rye flour is also used to produce crispbreads. In these the flour is mixed vigorously with salt and water to produce a stiff dough. In some products yeast is added and the dough is fermented briefly before baking. The dough is baked as a thin sheet in a continuous oven. The sheets are dusted with ground

Table 16.5 Composition of some maize products per 100 g

	Water (g)	Protein (g)	Fat (g)	Carbohydrate available (g)	Dietary fibre (g)
Wholemeal	12.0	9.2	3.9	73.7	4.4
Hominy grits	12.0	8.7	0.8	77.7	—
Cornflour	12.5	0.6	0.7	92.0	traces
Cornflakes	3.0	10.2	1.9	69.0	3.4

From Paul & Southgate (1978); Kent (1983)

Table 16.6 Composition of some oat, rye and barley products (g/100 g)

	Water	Protein	Fat	Carbohydrate available	Dietary fibre DF	NSP
Oats						
oatmeal	8.8	11.8	6.8	68.4	6.3	6.8
rolled	10.1	12.0	6.8	67.2	—	—
quick-cook	8.2	11.2	9.2	66.0	6.8	7.1
Rye						
wholemeal flour	15.0	8.2	2.0	66.0	—	11.7
bread	37.4	8.3	1.7	45.8	5.8	4.4
crispbread	6.4	9.4	2.1	70.6	11.7	—
Barley						
whole-grain	11.7	10.6	2.1	64.0	—	14.8
pearled	10.6	7.9	1.7	83.6	5.9	—

From Paul & Southgate (1978); Holland et al (1988)

trimmings from earlier bakings, and cut into sheets and packed. Table 16.6 includes some typical rye products.

Barley

Barley, like rye, does not produce breads of high volume and open crumb structure, and little barley is used in this way. The major human use for barley is in the production of beer and whisky.

Pearl barley

The barley grain has a fused husk and pearling involves two stages – dehusking and the abrasion of the bran. The pearl barley is used in soups and other products. Some fine flours are used in infant foods.

Sorghums and millets

The foods prepared from these grains are most commonly porridge-like mixtures prepared by heating the meal with water. The mixtures range in consistency from thin gruels to thick pastes. In many African cultures the cereal foods are consumed with a range of sauces, and the name of the dish varies with the sauce rather than the cereal used.

CEREALS AS SOURCES OF NUTRIENTS

Cereals form the staple foods in virtually all populations, and the dietary patterns and types of meals eaten – and indeed diet in its true sense as a way of life – are greatly determined by the type of cereals used. It is therefore useful when considering the nutritional properties of cereals to examine them as a group, and to compare the different cereals as sources of nutrients. At the same time it is important to remember that the type of staple cereal also plays a major role in determining the other foods that are consumed.

Protein

In many popular texts cereals are labelled as carbohydrate foods, and although this is compositionally correct such a classification tends to discount the importance of the proteins in cereals. Table 16.1 showed that in many cereals protein provides around 10% of the energy value. Many cereals show considerable variations in protein content, and a twofold range is quite common. In the preparation of processed foods, the protein content is one factor in the selection of the variety used, but in many rural diets the differences in protein content can produce uncertainties when making assessments of the diet. Milling and fractionation of the grain separates the protein-rich germ and aleurone layers, so that low-extraction flours have reduced protein concentrations.

The proportions of soluble cytoplasmic proteins and insoluble storage proteins differ between cereals. In most cereals the soluble proteins account for about 25–30% of the total; rice and sorghum have lower levels and in oats the soluble proteins account for around 60%. Wheat and rye contain significant quantities of gluten, but the levels in oats and rice are very low. The variations in amino acid composition of the cereal proteins is partly a consequence of the varying distribution of the cytoplasmic and storage proteins, and species differences, the insoluble storage proteins being richer in glutamic acid and proline and lower in lysine and cystine. Comparison of the amino acid compositions (Table 16.7) shows that in most cereals the limiting amino acid is lysine, with rice being relatively low in threonine as well. Maize is the exception in having tryptophan as the first limiting amino acid and lysine the second. Maize, sorghum and the millets are also richer in leucine. All the cereals contain substantial amounts of glutamic acid, usually present as glutamine in the intact protein.

The total nitrogen content of cereal proteins is significantly higher than 16%, and for this reason the conversion factors used to calculate protein values for cereals in many food composition tables are lower than 6.25 (FAO 1973).

The processes used in the production of many cereal products are quite severe, and can damage the biological value of the protein. The major reaction involves the lysine residues when the cereal is heated in the presence of carbohydrate, and the formation of unavailable lysine. As this is the limiting amino acid the reductions can be nutritionally significant. The dry heating involved in toasting and the puffing process seems to have the most effect.

Gluten

The special properties of this mixture of proteins make it particularly important in bread-making; isolated gluten is also used as an additive in high-protein breads. The gliadin components of the mixture appear to be the precipitating agent in gluten intolerance.

Lipids

The total lipid content of the various cereals varies between the low (1–3%) levels in wheat, rice, rye and barley, and higher levels in oats (5–10%) and maize (5–9%). The lipids include triglycerides and phospholipids, the latter making up to 4% of the isolated cereal oils. The fatty acid composition of the lipids in the different cereals shows some species differences, but all are rich in oleic and linoleic acids with linolenic acid making up between 1–8% of the total fatty acids (Paul & Southgate 1978). The major saturated fatty acid is palmitic acid.

In themselves, cereals are low-fat foods, their endogenous fats making only a very minor contribution to total intake and being overshadowed by the amounts and compositions of the fats used in cooking and preparation processes.

Carbohydrates

These form the major part of the cereal grain, and especially the endosperm. Cereals contain free sugars, starches, and a range of non-starch polysaccharides, and the different characteristics of these three groups make it inappropriate to consider them together. In discussing the carbohydrates, the available and

Table 16.7 Amino acid composition of cereal protein (mg amino acid/g nitrogen)

	Wheat	Rice	Maize	Rye	Oats	Barley	Sorghum	Millet (pearl)
		hulled			hulled			
Isoleucine	210	240	230	220	240	220	238	269
Leucine	420	510	780	390	450	420	850	819
Lysine	150	230	170	210	230	160	125	106
Methionine	100	130	120	90	110	100	94	150
Cystine	160	100	100	120	170	140	69	113
Phenylalanine	280	300	310	280	310	320	306	350
Tyrosine	190	250	240	120	210	190	95	231
Threonine	170	210	230	210	210	210	194	194
Tryptophan	70	80	40	70	80	100	63	88
Valine	280	360	300	300	320	310	312	338
Arginine	290	470	260	290	390	300	163	206
Histidine	130	150	170	140	130	130	131	144
Alanine	230	360	470	270	280	260	593	706
Aspartic acid	310	600	390	450	480	350	394	400
Glutamic acid	1710	1200	1180	1510	1310	1470	1356	1388
Glycine	250	270	230	270	290	240	194	143
Proline	660	290	560	590	320	680	494	431
Serine	330	290	310	240	290	250	269	431

From Paul & Southgate (1978); Kent (1983)

unavailable categories of McCance & Lawrence (1929) form a convenient starting point.

Available carbohydrates

Free sugars. The free sugars are present in low concentrations in most cereal flours, concentrations of between 0.8 and 2.7 g/100 g being typical. The concentrations of glucose and fructose are usually very low, with sucrose usually being the major sugar. Raffinose and other oligosaccharides of the series are common, together with higher glucofructans (Kent 1983). Maltose levels are low, rising on germination due to the activation of amylases.

Starches. These are the major components of the grains themselves and the endosperm, where they may account for over 70% of the total dry matter. They are contained in granules in the endosperm cells. These granules contain linear amylose and branched amylopectin, the latter playing an essential role in the organization of the granule. The ratio of amylose to amylopectin differs for the different cereals and between varieties. In the common varieties, between 25 and 27% of the starch is amylose, whereas in the waxy varieties (barley, maize, rice and sorghum) the starch is virtually entirely amylopectin, and high-amylose varieties of maize and barley have been bred. The type of starch determines the behaviour of the cereal food when cooked, for the starch granule when heated in an aqueous mixture absorbs water and swells, rupturing the granule. The amylose leaches out as a sol, which gels on cooling; further heating 'melts' the granule and the amylopectin forms a sol. This process is known as gelatinization. Amylose molecules aggregate on cooling to form insoluble, partially crystalline aggregates, a process known as retrogradation. During the preparation and baking of bread the granules are not fully gelatinized and the crust usually contains a mixture of granules in various states of disruption. The starch granules are slightly damaged mechanically during milling, and these damaged granules play an important role during the initial stages of baking. Ungelatinized starch is partially resistant to enzymatic hydrolysis in vitro, but the cereal starches appear to be well digested in vivo, apart from any retrograded amylose which is very resistant to enzymatic hydrolysis both in vitro and in vivo (see also Chapter 5). Enzymatically resistant starch is formed in most processed cereal products (Bailey 1986), and this starch is measured as unavailable carbohydrate in methods such as Southgate (1969), and when these methods are used in the analysis of dietary fibre the values are higher than those for non-starch polysaccharides (Southgate & Englyst 1985).

Unavailable carbohydrates

Dietary fibre. The cereal grain contains a range of cell-wall structures that are a source of non-starch polysaccharides (NSP), which are the major components of dietary fibre as originally defined (Trowell et al 1976). The highest concentrations are found in the outer bran layers of the grain, where the walls often have thickened, lignified walls (Selvendran 1984). The aleurone layers also have thickened walls. The cells of the embryo and the scutellum are thin walled and relatively undifferentiated. The endosperm cell walls are also thin, but often have rather specialized compositions. The amounts of non-starch polysaccharides in the different cereals show considerable variation, and milling and fractionation result in great differences in the quantities in flours of different extraction rates. When the concentrations are plotted against extraction rate, it can be seen that the amount of dietary fibre falls very rapidly when the extraction rate falls below 85% (Nyman et al 1984).

The composition of the NSP in the different cereals shows considerable variation (Table 16.8). In wheat, rye and barley the major matrix polysaccharides are arabinoxylans; in oats there are significant amounts of beta-glucans located in the thickened layers below the aleurone layer. The arabinoxylans and beta-glucans form the major water-soluble NSP in the cereals, which are higher in oats, barley and rye than in wheat (Southgate & Englyst 1985). The insoluble NSP in most of the major cereals show considerable similarities.

Lignin. The outer tissues of the grain contain lignified walls and the dietary fibre in the whole grain, and high-extraction flours are the major sources of lignin in the diet. The cereals contain other phenolic materials (Selvendran 1984) and these appear to be covalently linked to the polysaccharides and modify their susceptibility to enzymatic hydrolysis and bacterial degradation (see also Chapter 5).

Energy

Although in many popular views of nutrition the provision of energy by a food is seen as a negative attribute, in a staple food this is essential. Cereal flours are relatively low in fat and the metabolizable energy is provided by the carbohydrates and protein. Cereals are, however, used as ingredients in composite foods that are rich in fat, so that these foods act as vehicles for bringing fat into the diet. The fats used in cereal-based foods are usually strong determinants of the texture of those foods, and these textures are difficult to achieve without the use of fats. The type of fat can be selected to increase the level of unsaturation, although the physical attributes of the fat used are

Table 16.8   Composition of non-starch polysaccharides (NSP) in cereals

	Total NSP (g/100 g dm)	Non-cellulosic polysaccharides (percentage of total NSP) soluble	insoluble	Cellulose (% total NSP)
Wheat bran	41.6	8	73	19
Wholemeal	10.5	26	57	17
White flour	2.69	71	22	8
Brown rice	2.02	7	58	35
White rice	0.67	24	52	24
Oatmeal	7.22	55	41	4
Rye	13.7	34	56	10

From Southgate & Englyst (1985) (See also Table 4.3)

critical for the textures of some products. Cereal-based foods such as biscuits, cakes and confectionery frequently include sucrose as an ingredient: again this has a textural and bulking function and is not primarily used to create sweetness. The replacement of sucrose in these foods can therefore not be achieved by the use of artificial sweeteners alone, but also requires the use of a bulking agent.

Inorganic constituents

The cereals, in common with most plant foods, are low in sodium, with potassium, magnesium and phosphorus being the major inorganic constituents. Table 16.9 gives some representative values, showing

that calcium concentrations are relatively low but that the whole-grain cereals contain appreciable amounts of iron and zinc, together with low levels of many trace elements. The inorganic constituents are located in the outer layers and germ of the grain, and milling and fractionation produce substantially lower values in the low-extraction flours. The pearling process used in the production of cereals with fused husks produces the flours with the greatest reductions. The husks of rice and oats are particularly rich in silica, and their removal is essential for the production of acceptable foods, so that one cannot regard the reductions as losses of edible matter. Nevertheless the production of low-extraction flours does reduce the contribution of these flours to the consumption of total inorganic nutrients.

Table 16.9   Inorganic constituents in cereals of different extractions (mg/100 g)

	Na	K	Ca	Mg	P	Fe	Zn
Wheat							
wholemeal	3	360	35	140	340	4.0	3.0
brown	4	280	150*	110	270	3.6*	2.4
white	3	130	140*	36	130	2.2*	0.9
patent	3	100	110*	19	89	1.7	—
Rice							
paddy	30	216	15	118	260	2.8	1.8
brown	8	257	22	187	315	1.9	1.8
polished	6	110	4	13	100	0.5	1.3
Maize	40	342	20	143	294	3.1	—
Rye	1	410	32	92	360	2.7	—
Oats							
whole	28	450	94	138	385	6.2	2.0
rolled	33	370	55	110	380	4.1	—
Barley							
whole	49	534	52	145	356	4.6	3.1
pearl	2	120	10	20	210	0.7	—
Sorghum	11	277	30	148	305	7.0	3.0
Millet (pearl)	11	454	36	149	379	11.0	2.5

From Paul & Southgate (1978); Kent (1983)
Unless stated the values apply to the whole-grain cereal
* Signifies that the constituent includes the statutory additions in the United Kingdom

A substantial proportion of the phosphorus in the cereal grain is present as the inorganic salts of phytic acid (*m*-inositol hexaphosphate) which provides the germinating embryo with a source of phosphate ions. Phytic acid reacts with many divalent cations to form insoluble salts, and in the presence of phytates the bioavailability of iron, calcium and zinc is substantially reduced. The phytates in the grain are associated with the outer layers, and so the higher levels of these inorganic nutrients in the high-extraction flours are not always indicative of higher nutritional value.

Fortification

In the UK the fortification of cereal flours was introduced in the early years of the 1939–45 war, when it was anticipated that the supply of dairy products, and therefore calcium, might be reduced and the extraction rate of cereals would be increased, and that these two factors would lead to a reduction in the availability of calcium in the diet. Accordingly all flours other than wholemeal were fortified with calcium as the carbonate to remedy this anticipated reduction (DHSS 1981). During the war, the extraction rate of bread flour was increased to 85%, and after the war to 90% when the calcium addition was increased. Discussions were held at the end of the war about the return to lower-extraction bread flours and it was decided to restore the levels of iron (and some vitamins) in these low-extraction flours to the level found in 85% extraction. The fortification regulations have been reviewed on several occasions but continue to this day. Fortification with iron is permitted in the USA, but this is not a general practice and care is needed when making comparisons between the contributions of cereals to the dietary intake in other countries.

Vitamins

The whole-grain cereals are the source of most of the B-vitamins; they contain virtually no vitamin C and of the fat-soluble vitamins only the tocopherols (vitamin E) are present in appreciable quantities in the lipid fraction. Yellow maize varieties are a source of carotenoids: Table 16.10 illustrates some typical values. The vitamins are present in the highest concentrations in the aleurone layers and the germ, and therefore milling and fractionation lead to low concentrations of most vitamins in the low-extraction flours. The pearling process used, for example, in the production of polished rice produces a reduction of over 80% in the thiamin content of rice. The reductions in wheat flours are of a similar order, with very low extraction

(40%) patent flours containing only a quarter of the concentrations seen in the wholemeal flours.

Fortification

The importance of bread in providing thiamin led to fortification at the start of the 1939–45 war in the UK, and this was continued during the post-war years on the return to lower-extraction bread flours, when thiamin and nicotinic acid were added to all flours except wholemeal. In 1981 a review of these additions concluded that the nutritional reasons for the addition of vitamins had disappeared (DHSS 1981), but their perceived contribution to the nutritional image of white bread among the general public was such that the additions continue.

The nicotinic acid in wheat and some other cereals is not present in a form that can be readily absorbed unless the flour is treated with alkali (as in the production of tortillas). Several complexes containing nicotinic acid have been isolated from the flours but the structures of the complexes have not been established. It is probable that much of the endogenous nicotinic acid is biologically unavailable.

Effects of processing and cooking

Many cereal-based foods are subjected to heat-processing in baking, frying and extrusion cooking, and these affect the more labile vitamins. In processes involving boiling, the losses are of the order of 40% for most of the B-group vitamins, losses of folates are slightly higher at around 50%. In baking the losses are

Table 16.10   The major vitamins of the B-group in cereals of different extraction rates (mg/100 g)

	Thiamin	Riboflavin	Niacin
Wheat flours			
wholemeal	0.46	0.08	5.6
brown	0.30	0.06	1.7
white bread-making	0.10	0.03	0.7
patent	0.10	0.02	0.7
Rice			
paddy	0.40	0.05	5.5
brown	0.34	0.05	4.7
polished	0.07	0.03	1.6
parboiled	0.44	0.03	3.5
Maize			
whole, sieved	0.30	0.08	1.9
degermed	0.14	0.05	1.0

From Paul & Southgate (1978); Kent (1983)

generally lower, except for the folates. The losses during the more vigorous conditions of extrusion cooking are of the same order, primarily because the cooking times are generally shorter than the more conventional cooking procedures.

NUTRITIONAL ROLE OF CEREALS AND CEREAL-BASED FOODS

In the United Kingdom, in common with most industrialized countries, the consumption of bread in particular and cereal products in general, has declined in the present century as the standard of living has increased and animal products have become a greater part of the diet. Between 1880 and 1973 the consumption of wheat very nearly halved (Wardle 1977) and the decline continues. Part of this reflects a general reduction in total food consumption, which itself reflects decreased energy needs. In the past 3 years there has been some evidence that the consumption of cereal foods in general has stabilized (MAFF 1989), although the consumption of white bread continues to decline. Bread accounts for just over half the total cereal consumption at the present time, with white bread accounting for half of the total breads. Cakes and biscuits make up about 7% and 10% of the cereals respectively, and breakfast cereals about 8% (MAFF 1989).

The proportions of the nutrients supplied by cereals have varied a little over the past few years, providing about 30% of the energy, 25% of the protein and about 50% of the available carbohydrates. Cereals provide about 10% of the total fat intake, with most of this coming from biscuits. Contributions to the intake of inorganic constituents are somewhat distorted by the constituents added to flour, so that white breads provide around 38% of the calcium and 26% of the iron. The position with the vitamins is similarly affected by the added vitamins: cereals provide about half of the total thiamin intake and about 20% of the intakes of riboflavin and nicotinic acid. If thiamin was not added to wheat flours, it has been estimated that thiamin intake would fall by about 0.2 mg/person/day (DHSS 1981) and nicotinic acid by about 1 mg.

The cereals make a major contribution to the intake of dietary fibre: in 1987 the contribution was 31% of the total intake of about 13 g/person/day of non-starch polysaccharides, with white bread providing half of the cereal contribution.

Despite the importance of other foods in the diet, cereal foods retain their importance as a staple food. Current nutritional advice (Health Education Council 1983, DHSS 1984) reinforces the importance of cereal foods as a source of complex carbohydrates and foods that should replace the energy currently provided by the fat in the diet.

REFERENCES

Bailey CS 1986 Resistant starch: formation and measurement of starch that survives digestion with amylolytic enzymes during the determination of dietary fibre. Journal of Cereal Science 4: 301–314

Burkitt DP, Trowell HC 1975 Refined carbohydrate foods and disease: some implications of dietary fibre. Academic Press, New York

Department of Health and Social Security 1981 Nutritional aspects of bread and flour. Reports on Health and Social Subjects 23. HMSO, London

Department of Health and Social Security 1984 Diet and cardiovascular disease. Reports on Health and Social Subjects 28. HMSO, London

Food and Agriculture Organisation 1973 Energy and protein requirements. FAO Nutrition Report Series No. 41. WHO Technical Report Series No. 522. FAO Rome, WHO Geneva

Health Education Council 1983 Proposals for nutritional guidelines for health education in Britain. National Advisory Committee on Nutrition Education, London

Holland B, Unwin ID, Buss DH 1988 Cereals and cereal products. Third supplement to The composition of foods. Royal Society of Chemistry, London

Kent NL 1983 Technology of cereals, 3rd ed. Pergamon, Oxford

McCane RA 1946 Bread. Lancet I: 77–81

McCance RA, Lawrence RD 1929 The carbohydrate content of foods. MRC Special Report No. 135, HMSO, London

McCance RA, Widdowson EM 1956 Breads white and brown. Pitman, London

Masefield GB, Wallis M, Harrison SG, Nicholson BE 1969 The Oxford book of food plants. Oxford University Press, Oxford

Ministry of Agriculture, Fisheries and Food 1989 Household food consumption and expenditure 1987. Annual Report of the National Food Survey Committee. HMSO, London

Nyman M, Siljestrom M, Pedersen B et al 1984 Dietary fiber content and composition in six cereals at different extraction rates. Cereal Chemistry 61: 14–19.

Paul AA, Southgate DAT 1978 McCance and Widdowson's The composition of food, 4th ed. HMSO, London

Selvendran RR 1984 The plant cell wall as a source of dietary fiber: chemistry and structure. American Journal of Clinical Nutrition 39: 320–327

Southgate DAT 1969 Determination of carbohydrates in foods. II, Unavailable carbohydrates. Journal of Science of Food and Agriculture 20: 331–335

Southgate DAT, Englyst HN 1985 Dietary fibre: chemistry, physical properties and analysis. In: Trowell H, Burkitt D,

Heaton K (eds) Dietary fibre, fibre-depleted foods and disease. Academic Press, London

Trowell H, Southgate DAT, Wolever TMS, Leeds AR, Gassull MA, Jenkins DJA 1976 Dietary fibre redefined. Lancet I: 967

Von Bothmer R 1987 The evolutionary history of the cereals. In: Munck L (ed) Cereal science and technology. Danish Cereal Society, Copenhagen, pp. 47–60

Wardle C 1977 Changing food habits in the UK. Earth Resources Research, London

17. Vegetables, fruits, fungi and their products

D. A. T. Southgate

Plants provide a major part of the diet of most of the world's population, and are the major sources of energy in most of the developing countries. The range of plants consumed is very large and the *Oxford Book of Food Plants* (Masefield et al 1969) is a useful reference for identifying the different plants that are eaten. All parts of plants are consumed and the mature seeds of one plant family, the Gramineae, are so important in the diet that they justify a separate chapter (Chapter 16) to discuss them.

A formal classification of vegetables and fruits for nutritional or food compositional purposes is difficult to devise without resorting to arbitrary groupings, and in this chapter the various plant foods are discussed in groups that broadly relate to the structure of the plant. Even this creates some difficulties, however, because many foods considered as vegetables in the UK are botanically fruits.

VEGETABLES

Tubers

The underground organs of many plants are widely consumed; in addition to true roots, the storage tubers are extremely important in many diets because they are rich in starch. These vegetables were especially important before the development of refrigerated storage, because they can be stored under simple conditions for quite long periods, and together with cereals, provided a staple supply of food energy throughout the winter.

Potato (Solanum tuberosum)

In the UK diet potato is a stem tuber of major importance; the plant is native to the high Andes, where a number of species are cultivated as food (Wolfe 1987). The tubers were imported into Europe by the early explorers of the Americas, and became estab-lished as a food crop in the late 17th and early 18th centuries. The potato gives a high yield of biomass, and it rapidly became established as a staple that supplemented the cereal crops as a source of energy. The cultivation of the potato as a cheap food led to its becoming the major component of the diet in many peasant communities, and the destruction of the crop by the fungus *Phytophthora infestans*, in 1845–87 in Ireland, caused one of the most disastrous famines in history and was a major factor in mass emigration to the USA.

The potato is grown as a crop throughout northern Europe and also in Cyprus and Egypt. Two main types of crops are grown: the first 'early' or 'new' potatoes are sown in the spring and are lifted in the early summer and usually eaten without being stored; in the UK the local crops are supplemented with imports from the Channel Islands and Cyprus. The maincrop potato varieties are harvested in the autumn, and the bulk of this crop goes into store.

Selective breeding of the potato has produced a range of varieties with higher yields and improved disease resistance. Selection is becoming increasingly focused on the eating and processing quality of the varieties grown, because approximately one-third of the crop goes into some form of processing. This has led to the selection of potatoes with a high proportion of dry matter (and therefore starch content), and to varieties where the content of free sugars does not increase on storage, because this leads to darkening of cooked products such as crisps and chips. Since the main crop is for the most part stored, attention has been given to varieties that are late in sprouting, which is associated with the mobilization of starch and increased sugar content. These selection criteria, which have not included nutritional attributes, have fortunately led to only minor changes in the nutritional composition of the potato (Finglas & Faulks 1984).

The potato is a storage organ and its composition is affected by cultural conditions, especially the latitude at which it is grown, which affects the solar radiation the plant receives and thus the accumulation of dry matter. Table 17.1 gives the typical values for the composition of a number of starchy tubers, including some potatoes. In the potato starch is the major component, with relatively small amounts of protein. The nitrogenous material is made up from true protein and free amino acids. The biological value of potato protein is quite high, and in experimental studies subjects have subsisted on potato protein as the sole source of protein.

The potato contains significant amounts of vitamin C and the amounts consumed in the UK make it a major source of this vitamin. The potato is also an important source of thiamin and iron in the diet.

Like all plants, the potato contains cell-wall material and therefore is a source of dietary fibre. The walls of the potato are very thin and unlignified; the suberinized periderm changes on cooking to produce a thickening of the skin and a minor increase in the dietary fibre content of potatoes eaten with their skins. The potato contains alkaloids of the solanidine group, the levels of which vary between varieties, but which are higher in the skin and sprouts. Greening of the potato on exposure to sunlight leads to increased concentrations, as does physical damage. These glycoalkaloids make the potato bitter and at high intakes are toxic, so that the consumption of green and damaged potatoes should be avoided.

Cooking and processing of potato The tubers of the potato are not eaten raw and a variety of cooking methods are used. The simplest is boiling in water: early potatoes are usually cooked without peeling as they have a very thin skin; maincrop potatoes are usually peeled, a process that results in wastage of the order of up to 15% depending principally on the care of the peeler, but also on the presence of physical damage and the number of buds (eyes) that are also customarily removed. The cooking water leaches out the water-soluble vitamins and this loss adds to the thermal losses of vitamin C (Table 17.2). The boiled potato may be eaten whole or mashed, a process that disrupts the cell walls and increases the absorption of water by the starch. Milk or a fat such as butter or margarine is often added to improve the physical texture. The whole potato may be baked; this produces a floury starch interior and a toughened skin; baked potatoes that are eaten with their skins contribute a little more dietary fibre than those eaten without, but also contribute increased amounts of glycoalkaloids, and unless thoroughly washed may be contaminated with agrochemicals. The levels of glycoalkaloids in the skins of most varieties consumed in the UK are not likely to provide intakes above the safe limits (Davies & Blincow 1984), but some varieties commonly grown in the USA have very much higher levels.

The most frequently used method of cooking is frying, usually in deep fat or oil to produce chips (french fries). The frying process causes two major changes in the composition of the potato: first, the frying temperature drives off water as steam, and secondly, the potato absorbs fat from the frying medium. The

Table 17.1 Composition of starchy tubers (per 100 g raw edible matter)

Constituent	Potato		Sweet potato	Taro	Yam
	Early	Main			
Water (g)	82.6	75.8	70.0	75.4	73.0
Energy					
(kcal)	66	87	91	94	131
(kJ)	276	372	387	393	560
Protein (g)	1.6	2.1	1.2	2.3	2.0
Fat (g)	trace	0.1	0.6	0.2	0.4
Sugars (g)	1.3	0.5	9.5	—	1.0
Starch (g)	14.6	20.3	11.8	—	31.4
Carbohydrate (g)	15.9	20.8	21.5	21.0	32.4
Dietary fibre (g)	1.1	1.7	—	—	—
Calcium (mg)	6	8	22	34	10
Iron (mg)	0.3	0.5	0.7	1.2	0.3
Carotene (µg)	trace	trace	4000	trace	12
Vitamin C (mg)	16	8–20	25	8	10
Thiamin (mg)	0.2	0.2	0.10	0.12	0.10
Riboflavin (mg)	0.02	0.04	0.06	0.04	0.03
Niacin (mg)	0.6	1.2	0.8	1.0	0.4

Table 17.2 Losses of vitamins in potato on storage and cooking

	Thiamin	Riboflavin	Vitamin C	Folates
Storage				
freshly harvested			18.7 mg	
stored 3 months			8.85 mg	
stored 5–6 months			7.75 mg	
stored 7–8 months			7.60 mg	
Cooking		% of raw		
boiled	20	20	40	20
baked	10	30	30	0
roast	10	15	30	0
chipped, fried	10	15	20	0

From Finglas & Faulks (1984)

kinetics of these two processes are not properly understood, but the uptake of fat to replace the water is determined by the variety of potato, the temperature of frying, and the fat or oil used. The fat content of the final chip can vary over a wide range, higher frying temperatures usually leading to less uptake, but in commercially prepared chips a range of 7–15 g/100 g can be found. The fatty acid composition of the fat present depends entirely on the fat used, so that it can be highly saturated or unsaturated, although in commercial frying the very unsaturated oils have a shorter life than the more saturated fats. Frying 'seals' the chip and the high temperature and oxygen-poor environment of the hot oil lead to good retention of vitamin C in these foods.

Processed potato products Approximately one-third of the potato crop is processed in some way. This may be a relatively simple process involving the commercial peeling of potatoes for the catering industry, or more sophisticated processes where the potato is used as a source of starch which is isolated and then 'reformed' to produce extruded snacks. Commercial peeling usually involves mechanical abrasion of the skin, although alkali is sometimes used. The peeled products are very prone to discoloration, and the peeled materials are treated with sulphite to control this.

A wide range of fried snack products is based on potato, the potato crisp (chips in the USA) being the most familiar. In the production of crisps the potato variety must have a high dry-matter content and a low free-sugar content. The latter is essential for the desired final colour – too-high sugars lead to unacceptably dark crisps. The oil most frequently used is a plant oil rich in tocopherols which virtually completely replaces the water, leading to a fat content of about 35 g/100 g; the process leads to very high retention of

vitamin C. Other snack products may often rely on isolated potato starch which is formed into the desired shape, commonly by extrusion through a specially designed die, followed by frying in deep fat.

Nutritional role of potato In the UK diet the potato has a unique place among vegetables, primarily because it is very widely consumed and is commonly served at main meals, accompanying meat or fish. It remains a cheap, abundant food consumed by large, low-income families that have generally lower intakes of fresh fruits and vegetables, so that although on average it contributes about a quarter of total vitamin C intake, for some sections of the population it is a much more important source (MAFF 1989). The popularity of high-fat fried products is viewed by many nutritionists with concern, but it is possible to see the potato as a vehicle for increasing the intake of unsaturated oils, and its value of a source of complex carbohydrates is a positive attribute. The starch of the potato contains phosphate groups and raw potato starch is poorly digested by many animals; cooked potato starch is readily digested, and the rise in blood glucose following the consumption of freshly cooked potato is as rapid as that following the equivalent amount of glucose. On cooling however, the amylase in starch retrogrades and the starch then becomes highly resistant to enzymatic digestion, and can contribute to fermentable carbohydrate in the large intestine, thus having analogies with the non-starch polysaccharides (see Chapter 4).

Sweet potato (Ipomoea batatas)

This plant produces tubers that are widely eaten in the tropics; the tubers are similar to the potato in composition but have higher dry-matter, and therefore higher starch, content. The tubers contain a little protein and the vitamin C content is a little higher. The flesh of the sweet potato may be white or yellow, and the latter varieties provide a source of carotenes. Sweet potatoes are usually eaten boiled or in mashed dishes.

Yam (Dioscorea spp)

The yam is also an important tuber-producing crop that is widely cultivated across the tropical world. The plant may produce one large brown wrinkled tuber, or a number of smaller ones. The yam contains mainly starch, with little protein, and yellow-fleshed varieties provide carotenes. The tubers are commonly eaten boiled or mashed.

Taro (Colocasia antiquorum)

Taro forms a minor root crop in many parts of the wet tropics, and uncultivated taro forms a component of the diet eaten in Papua New Guinea and of residual populations of hunter-gatherers. The tubers are strictly corms formed by the thickening of underground stems. These corms are sources of starch and a little protein.

Jerusalem artichoke (Helianthus tuberosus)

This plant produces stem tubers that are consumed as food. The tubers are unusual in having the fructosan inulin as their storage polysaccharide. The tubers are eaten boiled, baked and as components of stews, and have a sweet taste from the fructose produced by hydrolysis.

Arrowroot (Maranta arundinacea)

This plant produces starchy rhizomes that contain very fine starch grains. The rhizomes are not used as food as such, but as a source of starch.

Root crops

In addition to the tubers there is a large number of important foods that are botanically roots, albeit specialized and selected structures. In addition to their role as foods, they are also important sources of food products, particularly cassava from manioca and sugar from the sugar beet. The major root crops are members of two plant families: the Cruciferea, which includes turnips and swedes, and the Umbelliferea, including carrots and parsnips. The composition of some typical roots is given in Table 17.3. Typically they are rather high in water, with low protein contents. The carbohydrates include free sugars and some starch in the more mature roots. They contain relatively low amounts of dietary fibre and most other nutrients, carrots being the exception, being very rich in carotenoids. Beetroots are very rich in anthocyanin pigments, but contain virtually no carotenoids.

Cassava (Manihot utilissima)

The roots of the manioca tree are a very important food. The tree was native to South America but is now widely cultivated in tropical Africa and Asia. The trees are propagated from stem cuttings and harvested

Table 17.3 Composition of some root vegetables (per 100 g edible portion)

Constituent	Beetroot	Carrot		Parsnip	Swede	Turnip
		young	old			
Water (g)	87.1	88.8	89.8	77.4	95.8	91.2
Energy						
(kcal)	45	30	35	73	11	23
(kJ)	188	125	146	305	46	98
Protein (g)	1.7	0.7	0.6	1.7	0.3	0.9
Fat (g)	trace	0.5	0.3	1.1	0.1	0.3
Sugars (g)	7.0	5.8	7.6	6.7	2.2	4.5
Starch (g)	0.6	0.2	0.3	8.4	0.1	0.2
Dietary fibre (g)	1.9	2.4	2.2	3.8	0.7	1.6
Calcium (mg)	20	34	25	41	26	48
Iron (mg)	1.0	0.4	0.3	0.6	0.1	0.2
Carotenes (µg)	140	6310	9330	150	350	20
Vitamin C (mg)	5	4	6	17	31	17
Thiamin (mg)	0.01	0.04	0.10	0.23	0.15	0.05
Riboflavin (mg)	0.01	0.02	0.01	0.01	trace	0.01
Niacin (mg)	—	0.2	0.2	—	1.2	0.4
Folates (µg)	148	28	—	87	31	14

when they are 6–12 feet high. The fresh roots contain mainly water (50–75 g/100 g) with about 1 g/100 g protein, the remainder being starch. However they also contain the cyanogenic glyceride linamarin, which is highly toxic, and the roots are ground, washed and dried to hydrolyse the major part of this toxin. Cassava is the staple food of many people in the tropics, despite the need to prepare it very carefully to prevent toxicity. It is, however, a low-protein food and communities relying on cassava as a staple often have a high incidence of protein-energy malnutrition. Tapioca is a starch product prepared from cassava. Sago is an analogous starchy product produced from the washed pith of the sago palm.

Sugar beet (Beta vulgaris subsp. cicla)

Although not consumed as a vegetable the sugar beet is one of the most important root crops cultivated in northern Europe. Its cultivation became common in France during the Napoleonic wars, and throughout Europe during the two world wars when imports from the West Indies and other cane sugar-producing regions were restricted. The sugar beet is a subspecies of the common beetroot, which has been selectively bred to increase the content of sucrose. The roots are harvested in the late autumn and processed until February. The processing campaign continues until all the beet have been processed or frost damage to the roots makes processing inefficient. The washed roots are sliced into slivers, which are washed in a countercurrent process with hot water; the extracts are treated with lime and carbon dioxide, which removes unwanted constituents as an insoluble mass which is separated by filtration. The extract is then heated to concentrate it sufficiently to induce crystallization. The sucrose crystals form on these nuclei to produce the familiar granulated table sugar. The syrup contains residual sucrose and partially inverted sugar; the syrups are further clarified and sold as invert sugar syrups, which are important food ingredients in many products. The residual molasses is usually added back to the dried sugar beet pulp to produce animal feed. A small fraction of the pulp produced is processed to produce a dietary fibre fraction for use in human foodstuffs.

Sugar cane (Saccharum officinarum)

The stem of this plant provides more than half the world's supply of sugar. The crop is cultivated principally in the tropics, where it gives its best yields, but it can be grown in the subtropics. Sugar cane is propagated using stem cuttings, and the first cut is made after about a year, with successive crops at yearly intervals. The leaves are removed before harvesting the stems or canes. The canes are crushed to extract the sugar-rich juice. The woody residual matter, bagasse, is used mainly as fuel. The raw juice is clarified by the addition of lime, followed in some cases by carbon dioxide to remove the excess lime. The mixture is then filtered and the extract evaporated to sugar strengths that will induce crystallization; this is usually carried out in vacuum vessels to reduce caramelization. The sugar crystals are separated by centrifugation and the residual extract is further concentrated to give a second and further crops of crystals. The final residual molasses is used in animal feeding. The later crops of sugar crystals contain more residual colour from the molasses and form the speciality brown sugars. These contain minor quantities of iron and other trace elements and other sugars. Sucrose produced in this way is a very pure substance, and is chemically identical to beet sucrose except in one respect: the sugar-cane plant (and maize) belongs to the group of plants which have a distinctive carbon metabolism in photosynthesis known as C_4, where the first product of carbon dioxide fixation contains four carbon atoms; this results in an increased proportion of the natural C^{13} isotope in the sucrose.

Leafy vegetables

This category includes the wide range of foods consisting of the leaves and stems of the food plant. It also includes modified buds and flowers, and is very heterogeneous. The plants are drawn from several families, but even so the number of plant species used for food is restricted when one looks at the plant kingdom as a whole. The reason for this is that many plants contain natural toxicants and these are often bitter to taste. The plants that are consumed are those that experience has shown to be safe to eat, although they still contain some natural biologically active components.

Cruciferae

These include the brassicas and many other important vegetables.

Brassicas A large number of vegetables are varieties of *Brassica oleracea*; these include the cabbages, which are enlarged terminal buds; Brussels sprouts, which are enlarged axial buds; the kales, which are leafy crops that can withstand freezing; cauliflowers and sprouting broccoli and calabrese, where the flowering head and leaves are consumed; and kohlrabi, which resembles a root crop but is in fact a swollen stem. Other cruciferous vegetables include watercress, mustard, and the young leaves of turnips, often included in spring greens.

Compositeae

Lettuce, endive and chicory fall within this family.

Umbelliferous vegetables

These include plants grown for their leaves, such as parsley, dill, chervil and samphire, and others that are grown for their leaf stems such as celery, angelica and fennel. The plants of this family have strong flavours and many are consumed as herbs.

Other leafy vegetables include spinach and the leaves of a range of beets.

Nutritional role of leafy vegetables

Some typical values are given in Table 17.4, which shows that as a group the leafy vegetables are relatively low in dry matter and therefore energy; the leaves contain protein, sugars and cell-wall material, although on a weight basis the levels are relatively low. The vegetables are usually consumed in large portions

and do make significant contributions as a whole to intake. Their major importance lies in the contribution of vitamins, as they contain carotenoids, vitamin C and folates in particular, together with minor amounts of B-vitamins. Potassium and magnesium are present at significant levels and the vegetables contain a range of trace elements absorbed from the soil. Many of the leafy vegetables are cooked before consumption, and cooking in water can lead to leaching and thermal losses of vitamin C, especially if the vegetables are left standing when cooked, prior to consumption. Conservative cooking using pressure cookers or the minimum of water reduces vitamin losses, as does microwave cooking.

The freezing of vegetables involves minor losses of the labile vitamins which are of the same order as those occurring domestically. Canning produces slightly greater losses and drying may result in the complete loss of vitamin C and folates.

Onions (Allium spp)

This is a group of vegetables that are widely consumed, often because of the flavours they contribute. They are formed from the fleshy bases of the leaves (bulbs). A number of species are used as foods: *A. cepa* is the main one, the bulb being covered with a dry brown or purple skin when mature. Some varieties

Table 17.4 Composition of some leafy vegetables (per 100 g edible portion)

Constituent	Broccoli (sprouting)	Brussel sprouts	Cabbage (summer	white)	Cauliflower	Lettuce	Spinach
Water (g)	85.7	84.3	92.0	90.7	88.4	94.7	89.7
Energy							
(kcal)	35	43	24	27	34	16	25
(kJ)	148	177	100	113	142	65	103
Protein (g)	3.9	3.5	1.6	1.4	3.6	1.0	2.8
Fat (g)	1.1	1.4	0.4	0.3	0.9	0.6	0.8
Sugars (g)	2.4	3.4	3.6	4.9	2.6	1.7	1.5
Starch (g)	0.2	0.8	0.1	0.4	trace	0.1	trace
Dietary fibre (g)	3.5	4.0	1.2	2.1	2.2	1.2	2.1
Calcium (mg)	204	26	38	49	21	21	171
Iron (mg)	1.9	0.8	0.4	0.5	0.7	0.6	2.1
Carotenes (µg)	2060	215	200	40	50	290	3550
Vitamin C (mg)	—	115	48	35	43	6	26
Thiamin (mg)	0.04	0.15	0.11	0.12	0.17	0.12	0.0
Riboflavin (mg)	0.12	0.06	0.03	0.01	0.05	0.02	0.09
Niacin (mg)	0.1	0.2	0.7	0.3	—	0.6	1.2
Folates (µg)	—	137	40	34	15	—	150

are consumed immature in salads as spring onions. Chives, *A. schoenprasum*, and garlic, *A. sativum*, are principally used to provide strong characteristic flavours to cooked dishes. Leeks, *A. ampeloprasium* var. *porrum*, are unusual in that the bulb and leaves are customarily eaten together.

The nutritional composition of the onion group is similar to the leafy vegetables.

Legumes

A major group of vegetables is provided by the plants of what used to be the Leguminosae, but now according to the systematologists, the Fabaceae, although for nutritional purposes they remain 'the legumes'. These vegetables are derived from the fruits and seeds of a number species.

Peas (Pisum sativum)

These are the seeds of the pea plant, an important crop in the UK and Europe which probably originated in the near east. The species *P. arvense* is grown as animal feed. The crop may be harvested when the seeds are mature, when they go for processing, but it is increasingly common for the crop to be harvested for deep-freezing when the seeds are relatively immature; a substantial volume of this production still goes for canning. Canned peas are also prepared from dried mature seeds, which are then called 'processed peas'. The immature pods are cooked and consumed as 'mange-tout'.

Lentils (Lens culinaris)

This is a food which has been consumed for several thousand years. The mature seeds are usually dehusked prior to retail sale.

Beans (Phaseolus spp and Vicia spp)

The beans may be consumed as the fruit and seeds, the immature seeds, or the mature seed. The runner bean (*P. coccineus*) is usually consumed as the immature fruit or pod, whereas the French bean (*P. vulgaris*) may be consumed in this form or allowed to mature to give the kidney bean. In practice, different varieties are grown for the two types of consumption. The *P. vulgaris* varieties are very diverse both in size and coloration of the seed coat, so that both white-coated haricot and smaller 'navy beans' have the same systematic name. Many tropical species are commonly consumed. *P. lunatus* may be known as butter or lima beans; *P. mungo* is the black gram, and *P. aureus* is the mung bean or green gram. The chickpea, *Cicer arietinum*, is also widely cultivated in India. The sprouted seeds of the beans are also used as foods, having compositions similar to the leafy vegetable but with very high water contents.

Nutritional role of the peas, beans and lentils

The legumes, particularly the seed legumes, are of major nutritional importance, especially in the developing world. They have a low water content when mature, and store well, and in many diets are a staple food alongside cereals. The seed legumes are important because they have high protein contents and the protein is of good biological value, with the sulphur-amino acids being limiting. The seeds are rich in complex carbohydrates, both starch and dietary fibre. Some typical values for the composition of legumes are given in Table 17.5, which shows that they provide significant quantities of vitamins and inorganic nutrients. Most legumes are cooked before consumption and where it is customary to consume the dish without discarding the cooking water, leaching losses are avoided.

The legumes as a group contain a range of toxic constituents which act as haemagglutinins and trypsin inhibitors. Many of the mature seeds contain toxic levels of these constituents, and thorough soaking and cooking is essential to avoid toxic effects.

Soya bean (Glycine max)

Although the soya bean has been an important element in Chinese cooking for many thousands of years, the major importance of soya as a food crop lies in its use in the production of oil and protein concentrates. Soya-bean oil is widely used in blended plant oils for cooking, and as an ingredient in processed products. The defatted meal is rich in protein and is used in animal feeds as a cheap source of good biological value protein; the limiting amino acids can be added to the feed, thus resulting in very good protein quality, provided that the meal has been properly heat-treated to inactivate the trypsin inhibitors. The meal can also yield protein isolates, which can be used as ingredients in human foods and spun to produce texturized protein analogues of meat.

Groundnuts (Arachis hypogea)

The groundnut or peanut is also a legume, which is widely grown as a food crop. After flowering the flower stalks bend down to the soil and the pods are pushed underground as they develop. Groundnuts are rich in oil (typically 40%) and although they are consumed in

Table 17.5   Composition of some legumes (per 100 g edible portion)

Constituent	Beans			Pea	Dry seed legumes[*]		
	broad	French	runner		haricot	lentil	mung
Water (g)	80.3	90.9	91.2	74.6	11.3	12.2	12.0
Energy							
(kcal)	59	24	22	83	271	304	231
(kJ)	247	99	93	348	1151	1293	981
Protein (g)	5.7	1.9	1.6	6.9	21.4	23.8	22.0
Fat (g)	1.0	0.5	0.4	1.5	1.6	1.0	1.0
Sugars (g)	1.8	2.3	2.8	3.2	2.8	2.4	1.2
Starch (g)	5.4	0.9	0.4	8.1	42.7	50.8	34.4
Dietary fibre (g)	4.5	2.2	2.0	4.7	25.4	11.7	—
Calcium (mg)	36	33	33	21	180	39	100
Iron (mg)	1.2	1.2	1.2	2.8	6.7	7.6	8.0
Carotene (µg)	190	150	150	310	trace	60	24
Vitamin C (mg)	32	12	18	24	—	trace	trace
Thiamin (mg)	0.04	0.05	0.06	0.74	0.45	0.50	0.45
Riboflavin (mg)	0.04	0.07	0.03	0.02	0.13	0.20	0.20
Niacin (mg)	3.2	0.9	—	2.5	2.5	2.0	2.0
Folates (µg)	146	44	35	62	—	35	140

[*]The cooked values for these dried seeds are approximately 0.31 times these raw values

significant quantities as snack foods, the major use of the crop lies in the production of groundnut or arachis oil, which is used for cooking and as an ingredient for margarines. The defatted meal is used as a protein concentrate for compounded animal feeds. It is said that the strong flavour precludes its use for making protein isolates for human use. Groundnuts are also ground with a little extra oil to produce peanut butter, which is widely used as a spread.

Groundnuts are grown in tropical humid environments, conditions that favour the growth of moulds; contamination with moulds that produce mycotoxins such as aflatoxin has been the cause of mortality in poultry fed with contaminated meal, and the potency of aflatoxin as a carcinogen is such that contaminated groundnuts are rejected for use in human foods.

Vegetables consumed as their fruits

Some foods commonly considered as vegetables are botanically fruits, and this section considers these particular foods.

Cucurbitaceae

This family includes the cucumbers, courgettes (zuccini), marrows, pumpkins and squashes (and

incidentally the melons!). Cucumbers (*Cucumis sativus*) probably originated in southern Asia; they are usually eaten raw in salads or pickled in vinegar. The marrows, on the other hand, are usually cooked before consumption. These foods are characterized by being very high in water content and provide minor amounts of sugars and dietary fibre. The vitamin C contents are low, but the pumpkin and the squashes with coloured flesh provide some carotenoids. The nutritional value of these vegetables lies principally in their provision of variety of taste and texture to meals.

Capsicums

Capsicums are another group of fruits considered to be vegetables. They include sweet peppers (*Capsicum annuum*), chilli (*C. frutescens*) and black pepper (*Piper nigrum*). The sweet peppers are used as a salad vegetable and have a high vitamin C content; chilli and black pepper are primarily used as flavouring ingredients and spices.

FRUITS

This section of the chapter deals with those plant foods that are conventionally described as fruits.

These are drawn from a number of plant families and a formal systematic classification is not especially necessary for the nutritionist. A classic text on the chemistry and biochemistry of fruits, which includes descriptions of their production, is that of Hulme (1970).

Fruits are specialized plant structures that surround the seeds; the structures are often derived from the ovary or the base of the flower itself. The tissues are usually parenchymatous with thin cell walls, although the tissues adjacent to the seeds may be lignified and there are usually lignified vascular elements. The epidermal structures are often specialized to protect the fruit from desiccation, and the outer surfaces are often cutinized or secrete waxy substances. Table 17.6 gives some typical values for the composition of fruits.

Tomatoes (Lycopersicon esculentum)

Although sometimes considered a vegetable, the tomato is clearly a fruit. It was imported into Europe from South America and was originally known as the love-apple. Selective breeding has produced a range of fruit colours and sizes, and high-yielding crops are usually grown under glass in the UK. The tomato has a highly cutinized skin and both skin and seeds are virtually indigestible. The sugars present are a mixture of glucose and fructose, with small amounts of sucrose. The tomato contains a little carotene and is a significant source of vitamin C.

Apples and pears

These are important crops in the UK and many temperate and subtropical countries. The cultivated varieties are derived from the wild crab-apple, *Malus pumilla*, and the common pear, *Pyrus communis*, although centuries of selective breeding makes formal classification of the cultivated varieties very difficult. Apples and pears are pome fruits formed from the receptacle which surrounds the ovary and expands as the fruit matures. The cells of the ovary develop as lignified parchment tissues, and thin strands of vascular tissue run through the flesh from the stalk. The skins are relatively thin and waxy; in the pear and some apples there is a suberinized periderm, and the flesh of the pear contains lignified sclerides. A large number of different varieties are grown commercially. Cooking apples tend to be larger and have a lower sugar concentration than eating varieties. Apples contain traces of starch, especially during development, and the major sugar is characteristically fructose with some sucrose and glucose. Pears have a similar mix-

Table 17.6 Composition of some fruits (per 100 g edible portion)

Constituent	Apple (eating)	Banana	Black-currant	Grape (black)	Melon (honeydew)	Orange	Plum	Strawberry
Water (g)	84.3	70.7	77.4	80.7	94.2	86.1	84.1	88.9
Energy								
(kcal)	46	79	28	61	21	35	38	26
(kJ)	196	337	121	258	90	150	164	109
Protein (g)	0.3	1.1	0.9	0.6	0.6	0.8	0.6	0.6
Fat (g)	trace	0.3	trace	trace	trace	trace	trace	trace
Sugars (g)	11.8	16.2	6.6	15.5	5.0	8.5	9.6	6.2
Starch (g)	0.1	3.0*	0	0	0	0	0	0
Dietary fibre (g)	2.0	—	8.7	0.4	0.9	2.0	2.1	2.2
Calcium (mg)	4	7	60	4	14	41	11	22
Iron (mg)	0.3	0.4	1.3	0.3	0.2	0.3	0.4	0.7
Carotenes (µg)	30	200	200	trace	100	50	220	30
Vitamin C (mg)	3–20	10	200	4	25	50	3	60
Thiamin (mg)	0.04	0.04	0.03	0.04	0.05	0.10	0.05	0.02
Riboflavin (mg)	0.02	0.07	0.06	0.02	0.03	0.03	0.03	0.03
Niacin (mg)	0.1	0.6	0.3	0.3	0.5	0.2	0.5	0.4
Folates (µg)	5	22	—	6	30	37	3	20

*As the banana ripens the starch content declines, and in the very ripe fruit all the carbohydrates are present as sugars. From Paul & Southgate (1978)

ture of sugars. The non-starch polysaccharides of apples are rich in pectin and some varieties, particularly those used for cider production, are an important source of pectin as a food ingredient. Apples are a source of vitamin C but are not as rich as the citrus fruits: the levels show variation by variety but within one variety there is also considerable variation. Pears have lower levels of vitamin C.

Stone fruits

These include a number of different species of the genus *Prunus* which are characteristically one-seeded drupes with a thick fleshy layer surrounding a hard lignified stone. They include cherries, plums, peaches and apricots. Cherries and plums have cutinized waxy skins, whereas the peaches and apricots have a downy appearance. The flesh of the fruit is rich in juice and sucrose is the most abundant sugar in most species – cherries are the exception, having a mixture of glucose and fructose with a low sucrose concentration. The stone fruits contain modest levels of vitamin C, but the coloured flesh of peaches and apricots contains appreciable concentrations of carotenoids.

Berries

Those fruits commonly called berries are botanically two different types of fruit. The strawberry is strictly not a berry, because it has single-celled ovaries resembling seeds embedded in a swollen receptacle which forms the flesh of the fruit. The strawberry contains glucose and fructose as its major sugars, with sucrose forming about 20% of the total sugars. The non-starch polysaccharides contain pectin with a low methoxyl content, which is the reason why strawberry jam is often difficult to set. The 'seeds', like all highly lignified seeds, are virtually indigestible. Nutritionally strawberries are most remarkable for their high vitamin C content; the fact that they are a highly perishable crop ensures that losses of the vitamin due to storage are minimal. It is worthy of note that irradiation of strawberries to prolong their shelf life produces a considerable loss of vitamin C.

True berries are many-seeded drupes, and raspberries, blackberries and related fruits of the genus *Rubus* are widely consumed, both fresh and conserved in jams and jellies. The fruits contain a range of sugars, with blackberries tending to have less sucrose. The pectic substances of the true berries are highly methoxylated and form strong gels in sugar solutions. Berries are good sources of vitamin C, with levels sometimes approaching those seen in citrus fruits.

Currants

These are the fruits of the *Ribes* genus, which includes red, white and blackcurrants and gooseberries. The fruits typically have a thin translucent skin and contain many seeds. The mixture of sugars usually have glucose and fructose as the major components, although sucrose is always present. The pectic substances of the currants form strong gels in sugar solutions. Blackcurrants contain very high concentrations of vitamin C; the levels in red and white species are lower, but these fruits are still very good sources.

Citrus fruits

On a worldwide basis the citrus fruits as a whole are probably the most important fruit crop. The various species of the *Citrus* genus probably originated in China, and they are cultivated mainly in subtropical regions throughout the world. They can be grown in heated glasshouses in temperate climates such as the UK, but modern transportation has removed these fruits from the luxury category and production in temperate climates is no longer anything other than a test of ingenuity. The citrus fruits typically have a waxy skin that is rich in oil sacs, and the lime and the bergamot are cultivated as sources of essential oils. The interior of the skin has an albedo layer of parenchymatous tissue surrounding the segmented flesh, which contains the specialized juice sacs. Selective breeding has reduced or eliminated the seeds in many varieties. The flesh may contain anthocyanin pigments, as in 'blood' oranges. The levels of sugar are dependent on variety and species: the sweet orange contains sucrose as the major sugar, with substantial concentrations of glucose and fructose; the lemon, on the other hand, has only half the sugar concentration and high levels of acidity. The amounts of non-starch polysaccharides in the flesh are low. The skin is the major source of citrus pectin, which is usually highly methoxylated and forms strong gels in sugar solutions. The citrus fruits are rich sources of vitamin C. In addition to their use as fruits, a large proportion of citrus crops is used in the production of juice.

Grapes

Although most grapes are cultivated for use in wine production, the so-called dessert grapes are widely consumed as fruit. They are also processed on a very large scale to give raisins, sultanas and currants, which are produced by sun-drying. The grape is rich in sugars, the concentrations being about 12–16 g/100 g.

The concentrations of non-starch polysaccharides are low and the levels of vitamin C are also low.

Bananas

The banana is a popular and unusual fruit which is cultivated throughout the tropics. The plants are propagated vegetatively and the banana tree grows very rapidly: the flower is produced after a year and the fruit grows from the female flowers without fertilization, in characteristic bunches. The fruit is picked green and transported under closely controlled temperatures. Ripening is carried out in the importing country. The banana is unusual in that it contains starch in the immature fruit; during the process of maturation the starch is converted into sugars and in the fully ripened fruit a mixture of glucose, fructose and sucrose is present, with sucrose the principal sugar. The unripe banana contains a starch that is highly crystalline and therefore resistant to enzymatic hydrolysis in vitro, and partially in vivo. The fruit contains relatively low levels of carotene and vitamin C.

Pineapple

The pineapple is an important tropical fruit that originated in South America. It is formed by the coalescing of the fruits of several hundred flowers on a spike surmounted by spiny leaves. The fuit has a high sugar content, of which sucrose is the major component. It is a modest source of vitamin C.

Dates

The fruit of the date palm is an important crop in the Middle East, where it is a valued source of sweetness, and in many countries fresh dates are eaten as snacks with drinks. The dates are compressed and partly dried before export, as fresh dates need to be stored under refrigeration. Dates in this form are very rich in sugars, but contain only low concentrations of vitamins.

Melons

These fruits are produced by plants of the same family that gives marrows and related 'vegetables', and differ principally in the fact that they are grown in subtropical climates and so produce higher levels of sugars, otherwise they are notable for their very high water content. The coloured-fleshed varieties provide a significant source of carotenoids, and all varieties contain some vitamin C.

Other imported fruits

The development of improved post-harvest storage and the application of these conditions during transport has resulted in many tropical and other fruits being imported into the UK at prices which make them generally available, rather than exotic luxuries. Thus mangoes, guavas, persimmons, akees and lychees are now quite common. The avocado has also become more common; this fruit is unusual because it contains fat and heptulose and higher monosaccharide sugars.

NUTS

Nuts are botanically seeds with a specialized toughened, often lignified, seed coat. Like most seeds they contain a food reserve to meet the needs of the germinating embryo. In many nuts this is fat, although some have starch or other polysaccharides. Most nuts are consumed in relatively small quantities as snacks, or on special occasions.

The coconut is not truly a nut but is the endosperm of a stone fruit. The material is unusual in that the fat is rich in medium-chain saturated fatty acids, and the storage polysaccharide is a substituted mannan.

The lipids in nuts are frequently highly unsaturated and the oils are considered of special value in the preparation of salad dressings.

FUNGI

Although many fungi are edible (Ramsbottom 1953) the population of the UK is unadventurous when it comes to eating any species other than the field mushroom (*Agaricus campestris*). Most of the mushrooms eaten are cultivated. The major constraint on the consumption of other species is the justifiable fear of consuming toxic species, especially *Amanita phalloides*, the death-cap mushroom, which is superficially similar to the field mushroom. Compositionally the field mushroom is uninteresting, being low in available carbohydrate and fat. The nitrogenous components include urea, and less than half is true protein. The cell-wall material is primarily chitin, and although analysing as dietary fibre its physiological effects are unknown. Potassium and phosphorus are the major inorganics and the concentration of B-vitamins is low, with the exception of folates. The role of fungi in the diet is quite clearly limited to their sensory contribution to the diet. This is especially true of one of the most prized foods, the truffle (*Tuber aestivum*), which is a subterranean tuberous fungus located by its aroma by trained pigs or truffle-hounds.

Yeast has been used as a dietary supplement for a considerable time; the dried product is a concentrated source of several of the B-vitamins, notably thiamin, nicotinic acid and vitamin B_6, but the concentrations are comparable with many other foods (Bender 1986) and therefore yeast is not a unique food. It is, however, the source of a popular product, an extract prepared by autolysis, and is usually very rich in salt but which provides an attractive vitamin-rich product that can be used as a spread or mixed with water as a beverage.

NUTRITIONAL COMPOSITION AND ROLE IN THE DIET OF VEGETABLES, FRUITS, NUTS AND FUNGI

Considered individually, the plant foods described in this chapter, with the exception of the potato, have a very minor role in the diet and it is important to consider them as a group, because they share many common features.

Nutritional composition

The fruits and vegetables are characterized by being high in water content; this together with their low fat content makes the foods high in bulk and of low energy density. The seed legumes are not consumed in the dry state and also fall into the low energy density category. The lipids naturally present in these foods are often unsaturated. The protein concentrations are low, with the exception of the seed legumes, but the biological values are generally quite good.

The available carbohydrates provide the major sources of energy in these foods; fruit contains a mixture of glucose, fructose and sucrose, with the proportions varying according to the fruit; vegetables contain a mixture of sugars and starch, the tubers being major sources of the latter.

The non-starch polysaccharides are present to the extent of 2–4 g/100 g in all except the seed legumes. The cell walls are typically undifferentiated parenchymatous cells, and the non-starch polysaccharides are rich in water-soluble pectic subtances (galacturonans and arabinogalactans). Most of the seed legumes eaten as food are not rich in the viscous galactomannans found in the locust and cluster beans.

These foods are low in sodium and high in potassium; magnesium and phosphorus are the other major inorganic constituents. The plants take up trace elements from the soil, so that there is considerable variation in composition.

The fruits and vegetables are primarily seen as a source of vitamins; however, the concentrations of most of the B-vitamins are low, with the exception of folates where the leafy vegetables are important sources. The fruits and vegetables are the most important sources of vitamin C, although the concentrations in the different foods show wide variations. The variation within the fruits on a single plant can vary depending on the position on the plant, which affects the amount of solar radiation the fruit can receive. In the metabolism of the plant, vitamin C is essentially a carbohydrate and the concentrations vary in a similar way. Green and yellow-coloured fruits and vegetables are also important sources of carotenoids and therefore have a very important nutritional role in diets that are poor in sources of retinol. The carotenoids are believed to have protective roles other than acting as pro-vitamin A.

The plant foods contain a very wide range of other substances which contribute to their flavour; many of these are biologically active and fall into the category of 'natural toxicants', which are discussed in another chapter. It is, however, probable that the biological activity may contribute to the protective effects of these foods.

STORAGE AND PROCESSING OF PLANT FOODS

The production of plant foods is usually seasonal, and the high moisture content of most of them means that they are very prone to microbial attack and spoilage. The availability of these foods between harvests is therefore dependent on the development of storage conditions that prevent or minimize spoilage and maximize the retention of eating and nutritional quality.

Until the development of refrigerated storage and, more recently, modified-atmosphere storage, the only crops that could be stored were those with a naturally low water content and those that could tolerate being covered with soil in clamps - the roots and tubers. All other crops had to be processed in some way and it is important to recognize that the essential and most important effect of processing is to extend the availability of food crops.

Refrigerated storage has only a limited applicability to plant foods, because temperatures around freezing damage many crops: potatoes, for example, become sweet and many plants lose turgor and their textural properties. Controlled-temperature storage, on the other hand, has been successfully used to maintain the eating quality of many fruits. These foods are still alive and undergoing metabolism, and to be effective the storage conditions must control metabolism but prevent senescence or ripening until it is required. Regulating the levels of carbon dioxide and oxygen surrounding the food has been remarkably successful in increasing the high quality of storage life, and usually the nutritional value, of many fruits and vegetables. This approach was aided by the discovery that the concentration of ethylene rose in the atmospheres above fruits that were ripening, and it is now known that ethylene can be used to initiate the ripening stage. While these storage conditions maintain the plant food in good condition, they do not control fungal growth to any extent, and there is widespread use of fungicides to control fungal contamination at all stages of production and storage.

Processing

Drying

Drying in air was probably the earliest form of preservation of plant foods, and it is still used in the production of prunes and other dried fruits. The process results in substantial changes in the product and different foods result.

Drying with heat is still used in the production of some vegetable products, principally those to be used as ingredients in soup mixes and similar products. The drying is usually carried out using a continuous process such as a fluidized bed in a forced draught to minimize localized heat damage and facilitate the drying process. Drying causes the loss of the more labile vitamins, such as folates and vitamin C, and thiamin losses can also be substantial, particularly when sulphite is used to preserve the fresh produce during storage prior to drying.

Freeze-drying leads to minimal losses of nutrients but is too expensive on a large scale to be used for plant crops which are not high-value foods.

Bottling

The preservation of fruit by heating in water to destroy spoilage organisms is still used domestically, but the process does not kill sporing organisms and is only safe if the fruit is sufficiently acid.

Pickling

This form of preservation has a long history. The simplest process uses vinegar and depends on acidity to control bacterial and mould growth; some pickling solutions use vinegar-and-sugar mixtures. The acidic conditions lead to good retention of vitamin C, and Captain Cook found that pickled cabbage as sauerkraut was highly protective against scurvy (Carpenter 1986).

Conservation with sugar – jams and marmalades

This is another preservation method with a long history. Many fruits, when heated with large amounts of sugar, produce a mixture that sets on cooling because of the acidity and pectin content of the fruit and the high sugar concentration (68 g/100 g). The high sugar content reduces the water activity and inhibits microbial spoilage. Jams can be prepared from fruits with low concentrations of, or unsuitable, pectins by the addition of pectin, either of apple or citrus origin. It is customary to add citric or tartaric acid to improve setting. Marmalades are prepared from citrus fruits. Low-sugar jams rely on the use of preservatives for product stability.

Salting

Vegetables can be stored in salt, which reduces the water activity to a level that inhibits bacterial growth.

Canning

Canning provides a safe process for the long-term preservation of many plant foods. It usually involves a preliminary washing and blanching of the food before the can is filled, heat-treated and sealed. Some products are cooked during the canning process, for example baked beans. Until relatively recently, vegetables were canned in salt solutions that raised the sodium content of the finished product to around 300 mg/100 g, but many now use lower concentrations of salt, in response to consumer demand. Fruits were usually canned in syrup, the strength of which varied depending on the type of fruit. The current tendency is to use lower-strength syrups, and some canned fruits are available in fruit juice – often apple. During the canning process and subsequent storage the syrup and fruit come into equilibrium, so that the sugar content of the strained fruit is very similar to the syrup.

Canning causes losses in the heat-labile vitamins, thiamin, vitamin C and the folates in particular; in addition there are leaching losses into the canning media. Table 17.7 summarizes the typical losses seen in the different processes.

Table 17.7 Losses of vitamins in cooked and processed vegetables (percentage of raw values)

Vitamin	Root	Leafy	Legumes	
Carotene	0	0	0	Some isomerization may occur on frying
Thiamin	25	40	30	Addition of bicarbonate results in total loss
Riboflavin	30	40	30	
Niacin	30	40	40	
Vitamin C	40	70	50	Losses are lower at low pH
Vitamin E	0	0	0	
Vitamin B_6	40	40	40	
Folates	50	20–40	90	
Pantothenate	30	30	30	

These values show considerable variation due to the fact that they include leaching losses as well as thermal ones. Leaching losses are dependent on the ratio of vegetable to water and to the state of division of the vegetable. Warm-holding will greatly magnify the losses of vitamin C and folates. From Paul & Southgate (1978)

Freezing

The development of rapid cooling of foods to temperatures around −20°C has resulted in the widespread use of deep-freezing as a method for processing vegetables and fruits. The produce is washed and blanched to inactivate enzymes, and then rapidly frozen using a device such as a blast freezer. The frozen product must be stored in an airtight container to prevent water loss by sublimation during frozen storage. The loss of labile nutrients during storage is low, most losses occurring during blanching and thawing. The retention of eating quality is good, provided that the produce is rapidly processed after harvest and the commercial production of frozen vegetables is highly geared to harvesting at the optimum time. This means that the original plant material often has a higher vitamin C content than fresh produce that has been harvested and passed through the normal marketing chain.

Role in the diet

The consumption patterns of these foods in the diet in the UK have been relatively constant over the past 5 years, although there have been substantial changes over the past 20 years.

The consumption of fresh vegetables has declined substantially since 1965 but has been virtually constant since 1975 (MAFF 1989). Potatoes are the single most important vegetable, accounting for nearly half of the total consumption. Table 17.8 gives the information from the latest published report of the National Food Survey. Of the leafy vegetables, cabbages are the most important, with carrots the most important root crop. Processed vegetables account for about 20% of the total, with frozen products accounting for a third of this. The consumption of frozen vegetables has increased by a factor of six since 1965, and frozen peas, which were the first to become popular, now account for about 25% of the consumption of frozen foods.

The consumption of fruits has increased a little since 1965 but this increase is due entirely to the rise in the popularity of fruit juices. Apples are the major fruit consumed, representing some 35% of the total, with bananas and oranges being the next most popular. Fruit juices account for nearly 75% of fruit pro-

Table 17.8 Consumption of vegetables and fruits in the UK (g per person per week)

	1965	1975	1985	1987	1991
Vegetables					
Potato	1510	1244	1163	1070	958
Fresh green	407	329	278	283	259
cabbage	138	131	102	98	77
Brussel sprout	76	44	33	34	25
cauliflower	78	67	55	57	76
Other fresh	407	391	446	473	461
carrot	89	65	108	115	114
onion	88	83	95	96	85
tomato	111	110	103	102	96
Frozen	25	93	170	191	200
Processed	279	326	355	362	345
Fruits					
Fresh	534	497	526	575	610
apple	209	192	197	200	190
banana	101	82	80	91	129
orange	90	98	70	77	76
Processed	192	183	242	306	341
fruit juice	19	38	148	203	249

Recalculated from MAFF (1989)

Table 17.9 Contributions of vegetables and fruits to nutrient intakes in the UK (percentage of total)

	Vegetables			Fruits		
	Potato	Green	Total	Fresh	Processed	Total
Energy	5.0	0.2	8.9	1.1	1.8	2.9
Protein	3.6	1.0	9.3	0.5	0.7	1.2
Carbohydrate	10.6	0.2	15.1	2.4	2.9	5.3
Dietary fibre	10.7		16.6			10.4
Iron	5.9	1.5	17.5	1.8	2.4	4.2
Carotene	—	6.3	82.9	2.5	1.1	3.6
Thiamin	8.4	1.1	16.7			3.6
Riboflavin	2.7	1.1	8.1			1.6
Vitamin C	21.7	6.5	49.5	29.0	11.2	40.2

From MAFF (1986, 1989)

ducts (other than jams), with canned peaches, pears and pineapple accounting for about 10%. Consumption of fruit and vegetables is much lower in the UK than in Southern Europe.

Nutritional contributions

The contribution of fruit and vegetables to the overall supply of nutrients is given in Table 17.9, which shows that collectively they make only minor contributions to the proximate constituents and energy intake.

Fruits and vegetables are important contributors to the intake of dietary fibre and provide about a third of the total. The dietary fibre from these foods is rich in the water-soluble components which have been shown to be most effective in lowering serum cholesterol levels and slowing glucose absorption. Potatoes are also a rich source of starch.

The contribution to iron intakes approaches 16%, with the potato being the major contributor. Although vegetables contribute vitamins of the B-group, only that of folate – which was estimated by Tan et al (1984) to be approximately 30%, but which is probably higher because of the underestimation of folates in the compositional data used (Paul & Southgate 1978, Phillips & Wright 1982) – may be judged to be nutritionally important.

Fruits and vegetables provide the major part of the vitamin C intake, with the proportion provided by potatoes becoming less important as the consumption of fruit juices increases.

Plant foods provide nearly 90% of the intake of carotenoids, and this is equivalent to about 25% of the retinol activity of the diet as a whole. There are good arguments for the proposition that there is a specific requirement for carotenoids in their own right (Hautvast 1987), and if this is accepted then fruits and vegetables have an even more important part in the diet than they are credited with at present.

The long-standing advice in Northern Europe to increase the consumption of fruits and vegetables as part of a proper balanced and healthy diet clearly warrants continued support (see also Chapters 13, 14, 41, 45 and 51).

REFERENCES

Bender AE 1986 Health or hoax. Sphere Books, London
Carpenter KJ 1986 The history of scurvy and vitamin C. Cambridge University Press, Cambridge
Davies AMC, Blincow WPJ 1984 Glycoalkaloid content of potatoes and potato products sold in the UK. Journal of Science of Food and Agriculture 35:553–557
Finglas PM, Faulks 1984 Nutritional composition of UK retail potatoes, both raw and cooked. Journal of Science of Food and Agriculture 35:1347–1356
Hautvast JGAJ 1987 Proteins and selected vitamins. In: Siminopoulos AP (ed) Diet and health: scientific concepts

and principles. American Journal of Clinical Nutrition 45 (suppl):1044–1045
Hulme AC 1970 (ed) The biochemistry of fruits and their products, Vols 1 & 2. Academic Press, London
Masefield GB, Wallis M, Harrison SG, Nicholson BE 1969 The Oxford book of food plants. Oxford University Press, Oxford
Ministry of Agriculture, Fisheries and Food 1989 Household food consumption and expenditure 1987. Annual Report of the National Food Survey Committee. HMSO, London

Paul AA, Southgate DAT 1978 McCance and Widdowson's The composition of food, 4th edn. HMSO, London

Phillips DR, Wright AJA. 1982 Studies on the response of *L.casei* to different folate monoglutamates. British Journal of Nutrition 47:183–189

Ramsbottom J 1983 Mushrooms and toadstools. Proceedings of the Nutrition Society 12:32–44

Tan S, Wenlock R, Buss DH 1984 Folic acid content of the diet in various types of British household. Human Nutrition: Applied Nutrition 389:17–22

Wolfe J 1987 The potato in the human diet. Cambridge University Press, Cambridge.

18. Meat, fish, eggs and novel proteins

D. A. T. Southgate

MEAT AND MEAT PRODUCTS

Meat has formed an important part of the human diet throughout history. There is, moreover, considerable evidence that non-human primates also eat meat in an opportunistic fashion, and may even exhibit hunting types of behaviour. In the early stages of human development – the 'hunter-gatherer' – meat consumption was somewhat erratic, depending on the frequency of success in killing an animal, and the remainder of the diet consisted of roots, tubers and fruits – foods that are characteristically low in energy. Meat and its associated fats may have provided about a third of the total energy intake (Eaton & Konner 1985).

Hunter-gatherers eventually began to follow the herds of game, and some, such as the Lapps, developed techniques for controlling herds and became pastoralists to what were, and still are, essentially wild animals. In other cultures the animals were domesticated and came closely under the influence of man, who controlled their breeding and patterns of movement. In these cultures the animals provide food and clothing, and their bones are used to make ornaments and tools; the animals also become the units of exchange in trade, and measures of wealth – factors that are of critical importance nutritionally in times of drought, when the death of the herds deprives the community of food and the means to purchase other foods.

The production of animals in the next, 'agricultural', phase of development changed because of the cultivation of cereals, which allowed communities to give up the nomadic existence, settle and cultivate the land. Animals became slightly less important in the diet as cereal and root crops increased in importance. In northern climates forage was not available throughout the winter months, and animals were therefore culled in the autumn and the techniques of drying and salting meats for preservation were developed. The production of root crops that could be stored over the winter for animal fodder produced radical changes in animal husbandry, in that the stock could be maintained in good condition, thus increasing the variety of foods available.

In all these cultures animals had an importance greater than that of food providers, so that the slaughter of an animal became associated with ritual and the consumption of meat was often an integral part of festive occasions. Many of these cultural factors associated with meat and its consumption persist to the present day (Fieldhouse 1986); meat is still regarded by many people in the UK as being an essential part of a 'proper' meal (British Nutrition Foundation 1982).

Major carcase meats

In Europe and the USA these are produced from cattle, sheep and pigs, whereas in the Middle East, Africa and the Indian subcontinent goats, camels and water buffalo are more important.

Beef

The systems for beef production range from extensive ranging of cattle to very intensive production on 'feed-lots' in the USA. The economic pressures on farming communities have led to the introduction of sophisticated selective breeding programmes, to produce animals that grow rapidly and produce the desired carcase composition, such as the Charolais and Limousin breeds. Substantial numbers of beef animals are produced from dairy herds by artificial insemination using the semen from beef bulls.

The animals are usually raised initially on grass, which may be grazed or fed as conserved hay or silage, with cereal-based concentrates fed during the finishing stages. In the 'feed-lot' system the animals are fed concentrates under very closely controlled conditions.

Veal is produced from calves under semi-intensive systems using milk-based concentrated rations to produce very light-coloured meats.

In addition to the use of breeding and controlled feeding to improve growth rates and carcase composition, implants of anabolic steroids – either the natural substances or synthetic analogues – are used in some countries to produce the desired muscle growth.

Sheep and lambs

These are usually farmed extensively, often on land that would not support any other kind of agriculture. The production of sheepmeat is closely integrated with the production of wool, and lambs are the major meat product. The lambs grow rapidly on grass and it is common in the UK to move lambs produced by hill sheep to fatten on lowland pastures, and as future breeding stock. During the autumn and early winter the later lambs are fed on conserved grass and forage crops such as kale. Once again current selective breeding aims at producing rapid growth of lean carcases.

Pigmeat

Most pig production in the UK is intensive, with the pigs kept in environmentally controlled housing and fed compound rations with the objective of producing rapid growth and controlled carcase composition. Selective breeding and feeding are used to optimize performance and carcase conformation, especially in bacon pigs. Very fat animals are economically undesirable, as the carcases are only suitable for manufacturing operations.

Other domesticated species

Horsemeat, although mainly used for animal food in the UK, is widely consumed in continental Europe. Goats and camels are major meat animals in many Arab countries; the animals are usually managed traditionally, as free foraging herds. Mature camels produce rather tough meat and young animals are preferred for meat. Water buffalo are important in the Middle East and Asia, and are usually farmed extensively in traditional ways.

Perception of which animals or parts of animals are acceptable as foods varies considerably with national preferences and religious beliefs. Thus the consumption of horsemeat, dogmeat and guineapigs is not regarded as normal in the UK, although these are foods prized by others. The Jewish food laws proscribe a number of animals whose flesh was regarded as unclean, for example those animals that chewed the cud but did not have cloven feet, such as the coney (the rock hyrax), the hare and the camel, and those with cloven feet that did not chew the cud, i.e. pigs. The rules also forbade the consumption of many other animals, including birds of prey or carrion eaters, waterfowl, snakes and marine mammals (Leviticus 11).

In the Islamic religion the proscriptions include the pig, again because it is regarded as unclean (Qur'an, Al-Baqara (The Cow)). Both Judaism and Islam prescribe a ritual protocol for the slaughter of animals for human consumption, thus contributing to the cultural significance of meat as a food.

In discussing topics of nutritional importance it is convenient to consider how the range of meats consumed is produced, their composition and the overall nutritional role of meats and meat products in the diet.

Wild animals and game

Worldwide a large number of species are taken as food from the wild by hunting, and in countries such as the USA careful management of the wildlife produces a regular crop of animals that can be culled in this way to provide meat. In Sweden the picture is similar, with deer and reindeer providing a good source of meat. Wild animals can frequently flourish on poor forages and the composition of their meat is attractive to many consumers. This has led to several attempts at farming wild animals; the reindeer are handled in this way by the Lapps, and experiments in Scotland with red deer and in Zimbabwe with eland (Talbot 1964) show that this approach is viable and may be very useful where it has proved difficult to introduce dairy cattle, because of endemic cattle diseases

Rabbit

Rabbits were introduced to England by the Normans and were farmed in warrens as a source of meat; the wild rabbit population was greatly reduced by myxomatosis in the 1960s, and is slowly re-establishing itself. Domestic rabbit production is relatively small and not intensive.

Venison

Much of the venison produced in Scotland is exported, and venison makes only a small contribution to total meat consumption in the UK, the culling of deer from forestry plantations being one source.

Poultry

One of the major changes in diet in the UK, and indeed in many countries, is the growth in importance of poultry meat, initially from chickens but increasingly from turkeys and ducks. Poultry were domesticated many centuries ago, probably in China, and were commonly kept under free-range foraging conditions as a source of eggs and meat. In the UK before the 1939–1945 war their consumption was often associated with festive occasions. The development of intensive systems to produce 'broiler chickens' has transformed the position of poultry meat in the market. Under these systems growth is rapid and feed-conversion efficiency is high, so that large-scale production at low prices is possible.

Turkeys and ducks cannot be produced under such intensive regimes, but many of the selective breeding principles and feed formulations evolved for chickens can be used to give rapid and economical production.

Offal

In addition to the muscles which form the bulk of the carcase meat, animal production and slaughter produces a wide range of by-products, some of which are edible and considered delicacies in many cultures. Many religious traditions place restrictions on the consumption of offals which are regarded as unclean, for example blood and blood products. Liver, kidneys, brain and pancreas (sweetbreads) are often consumed, but other organs may be associated with taboos or cultural limits. Thus intestine (tripe), pigs trotters, and cow heel are delicacies with restricted consumption.

The organs can form the foci of infection in an animal, and most developed countries have veterinary inspections at slaughterhouses to eliminate this possibility.

Meat production

In developed countries the slaughter of animals for meat takes place under closely regulated conditions in slaughterhouses. Cattle and sheep may be humanely killed with a captive bolt, but pigs and some lambs are stunned electrically; the animal is then strung up and bled. The abdominal cavity is opened and the viscera are removed; pigs are usually scalded in hot-water to remove the bristles before being cleaned. The carcases are then usually split longitudinally and chilled. However, there is a substantial amount of hot boning, where the meat is separated from the bone before chilling. Rapid chilling tends to make the meat tougher, but is often used to improve throughput; electrical stimulation is widely used in New Zealand to reduce the cold-shortening that accompanies very rapid chilling.

The carcase may be divided into primal cuts, which are distibuted to the retail meat trade. Some trimming of the carcase to remove fat may take place at this level, but trimming usually takes place when the carcase or primal cuts are further butchered.

The pattern of butchering and the naming of the cuts produced varies in different countries; in the UK and the USA the cuts divide the carcase into anatomical regions, but in Europe, butchering follows the muscle boundaries, a process known as muscle seaming. One consequence of these differences is that it is difficult to compare the composition of meat cuts in different countries or regions on the basis of their names alone.

However expert the butcher, the division of the carcase invariably leaves relatively large amounts of fat, both subcutaneous and deep-body, and muscle on and off the bone, which cannot be sold in its unprocessed state. This includes parts of the animal that are unattractive to the consumer, such as heads, intestines and feet. These by-products of the butchering process are the source materials for a wide range of products such as sausages, where the meat is finely ground into an emulsion; in the UK cereal or soya rusk are added, but continental sausages are made without these additions. The emulsion is then extruded into a case of gelatin or cellulose to produce the conventional sausage. In the UK it is customary to cook sausages before consumption, but continental sausages are cooked before retail sale and eaten cold. Meat pies, where the chopped or minced meat is encased in pastry and baked, are another use of these by-products. Much other meat, including the tougher meats from older animals, is manufactured into canned meats.

Conventional knife trimming of the bony residual carcase leaves a considerable quantity of muscle and connective tissue on the bone, and new techniques have been developed to recover this material. Mechanical recovery involves massive maceration of the residual carcase, followed by extrusion through an apparatus that identifies and rejects bone fragments; the mechanically recovered meat emerges as an emulsion which can be used in meat products.

Other techniques for using small pieces of meat have been developed, although they have been used fraudulently and have received less publicity recently. The process involves 'tumbling' the pieces of meat in a hot phosphate buffer which solubilizes the actomysin, which subsequently acts as an adhesive when the meat is cooled and compressed. This reformed meat is very difficult to distinguish visually from steak or ham.

Composition of meats and meat products

The composition of all meats is dependent on the ratio of fat to lean, which determines the energy value and the concentrations of virtually all nutrients, because the nutrients are present in different concentrations in the fat and the lean. It is consequently difficult to give a mean or typical values for meats as a whole without specifying the fat:lean ratio. At the present time the nutritional advice to reduce saturated fat intake has intensified consumer demand for leaner retail cuts of meats, and this demand is reflected back to the producer in a demand for leaner carcases, because the fat has increasingly less commercial value. Most countries operate grading schemes for carcases which determine the payments to producer: these have usually been based on carcase composition and fat content, and have discriminated against very fat and very lean carcases. There is pressure from nutritional and public health bodies to make these grading schemes more responsive to nutritional and medical opinion, which means that in future, as a result of breeding and selection to reduce the fat in carcases, one should expect the fat:lean ratio to fall. There is considerable evidence that this change is taking place quite rapidly (Greenfield 1987, Wood et al 1986).

This has important nutritional implications for those involved in dietary surveys because it makes it more difficult to estimate the fat intake from meats unless the lean and fat are measured separately, or the fat:lean ratio is estimated. This is possible, but not easy, with meats served as such, but the same caveats apply to meat products, where unless the product carries a nutritional label, the fat content can vary widely.

Table 18.1 gives the compositions of the separable lean and fat of the more important meats in the UK. The separation was made by domestic-type procedures, not by careful dissection. The table shows that the lean of the three major carcase meats is similar in gross composition, which should not be unexpected because they are in effect mammalian muscle; the poultry muscles have less intramuscular fat and most of the fat is associated with the skin, although it is not subcutaneous as seen in mammals.

The ratio of lean to fat varies between the different retail cuts of meat, depending on the anatomical position of the cut and also on the extent to which the joint has been trimmed. Paul & Southgate (1977)

Table 18.1 Typical composition of some meats (raw) (per 100 g edible material)

Meat	Separable components*	Water (g)	Protein† (g)	Fat (g)	Energy (kcal)
Beef	Lean	74.0	20.3	4.6	123
	Fat	24.0	8.8	66.9	637
Lamb	Lean	70.1	20.8	8.8	162
	Fat	21.2	6.2	71.8	671
Pork	Lean	71.5	20.7	7.1	147
	Fat	21.1	6.8	71.4	670
Veal fillet		74.9	21.1	2.7	109
Chicken meat		74.4	20.5	4.3	121
meat and skin		64.4	17.6	17.7	230
Turkey meat		75.5	21.9	2.2	107
meat and skin		72.0	20.6	6.9	145

From Paul & Southgate (1978). Data refer to uncooked meat
* By usual 'domestic' procedures, not rigorous dissection
† N × 6.25

obtained values on typical retail cuts purchased in the 1960s, and these may not be representative of typical cuts available now or in the future, but the values serve to illustrate the relative ranking of cuts. In the case of beef the leanest cuts were silverside and rump steak, and the fattest forerib; for lamb they were leg and chops respectively, and for pork, leg and belly respectively.

Information on the composition of the less common meats and those eaten in the developing countries is very much less extensive, but some examples for the proximate composition of a selection are given in Table 18.2, with the caveat that the fat:lean ratios will also vary in these species.

Table 18.2 shows that it is possible to make some generalizations about meats. First, as one would expect, the water content declines as the fat increases; second, the protein contents are around 20% in most fresh meats; and third, the fat content of wild animals is usually lower than comparable domesticated species. Domesticated species have been selected for growth rate, and until recently the ideal animal was a fat one; the use of the terms 'fatstock prices' in the marketing of animals, and 'fattening livestock' during finishing reflect this preference. In mediaeval times fat breeding stock had advantages in maintaining condition over the winter, and even now, the survival of hill cattle and sheep under extreme conditions may depend on an adequate covering of subcutaneous fat. The fat content of a retail joint is an important factor in the development of flavour during cooking, and there is a widely held view in the meat trade that adequate fat levels are required to produce acceptable eating quality.

Table 18.2 Composition of some other meats (per 100 g edible matter)

Species	Energy (kcal)	(kJ)	Water (g)	Protein (g)	Fat (g)
Dog	274	1146	60.8	14.5	23.5
Camel	267	1117	59.1	19.6	20.3
Frog	68	285	83.6	15.3	0.3
Goat					
lean	179	749	69.2	18.0	11.3
medium	357	1494	51.6	15.2	32.4
Hare	115	480	75.0	21.5	3.1
Horse	170	713	70.0	19.0	10.0
Moose, lean	111	420	76.0	22.0	1.2
Rabbit	126	529	74.6	22.2	4.0
Reindeer	117	490	74.0	21.0	3.6
Roe deer	120	500	74.0	21.0	4.0
Snake	94	393	75.0	14.4	3.3
Squirrel	110	460	72.2	26.3	0.4
Venison	120	500	74.0	21.0	4.0
Water buffalo	120	502	76.5	17.7	4.9

The composition of the organs which are collectively described as offal shows much smaller variations; kidney and hearts often have adhering fat, but the organs themselves have characteristic compositions and more constant lean:fat ratios. Table 18.3 gives the ranges of compositions for heart, kidney and liver in the major meat species. These values are for trimmed organs taken from young animals; the fat content of the hearts of very mature animals may be over 17 g/100 g. Brain is exceptional in having a fat content of the same order as protein; in brain, however, a large proportion of the fat is made up of complex phospholipids and glycolipids.

The very wide range of meat products available (Paul & Southgate 1978) is a testimony to human ingenuity in using as much as possible of the whole animal. It is therefore impossible to make generalizations about their proximate composition. Many contain substantial concentrations of fat but this is very variable, and there is a tendency for the cheaper products to contain more fat and connective tissue because these are cheaper

Table 18.3 Ranges of composition in organs (per 100 g edible matter)

	Heart	Kidney	Liver
Energy			
(kcal)	86–150	86–90	153–179
(kJ)	363–629	363–380	567–683
Water	73.6–79.2	78.8–79.8	67.3–72.9
Protein	15.2–17.1	15.7–16.5	19.1–21.3
Fat	2.6–9.3	2.6–2.7	6.3–10.3

ingredients than steak. Meat products often contain cereal, and statistics on meat comsumption are very slightly distorted if the amounts of meat products eaten are taken as being entirely meat.

Nutrients in meat and meat products

Meats are conventionally seen as protein foods, and this is true for the lean, which contains substantial amounts of high biological value protein. The amino acid composition shows that when compared with the amino acid requirements of man, and the ideal reference protein, the balance of amino acids is very close to the reference. The concept of first-class proteins has, however, been superseded as information on amino acid composition has become available. The major proteins of connective tissue, collagen and elastin, have imbalanced and inadequate amino acid compositions and will not support growth. There is some evidence that meat products prepared from joints where the connective tissue content is high, do have a slightly inferior biological value in the standard NPU (net protein utilization) assay, but this is of little real nutritional significance in the context of the whole diet.

Meats as a whole are important sources of fat in the diet. A range of different classes of lipid is present in animal tissues: triglycerides, which form the fat stores in adipose tissues in subcutaneous fat; the abdominal fats surrounding kidney and the intestines, and marbling fats between the muscle blocks; phospholipids within cell membranes and nervous tissues; glycolipids in brain and other neural tissues; and lipoproteins in many tissues. In lean tissues that have been carefully dissected the major lipids are phospholipids (Sinclair & O'Dea 1987), but in adipose tissue the triglycerides are the most abundant and the fat in meat is principally triglyceride.

The fatty acid composition of the fat in meats depends on whether or not the species is a ruminant. The fat in non-ruminants is dependent on the composition of the fats in the animal's diet, whereas that of the ruminant is affected by the activities of the microflora in the rumen, which hydrogenate much of the ingested fat, so that the fats of ruminant animals are usually highly saturated. This is illustrated in Table 18.4 (British Nutrition Foundation 1988), which also shows that liver lipids are less saturated than the fat in the animal as a whole because they contain phospholipids in their cell membranes. The fats in wild ruminants also appears to be less saturated, because the fat contents are lower and the phospholipids consequently form a greater proportion of the total.

Table 18.4 Fatty acid composition of some meats (lean plus fat portion of the meat) (fatty acid per 100 g total fatty acids and percentages of total as saturated, monounsaturated and polyunsaturated)

| | Saturated | | | | | | Monounsaturated | | | | | Polyunsaturated | | | | | | |
	14:0	15:0	16:0	17:0	18:0	(%)	16:1	17:1	18:1	20:1	(%)	18:2	18:3	20:3	20:4	20:5	22:5	(%)
Beef	3.2	0.6	26.9	1.2	13.0	(44.9)	6.3	1.0	42.0	tr	(49.3)	2.0	1.3	tr	1.0	tr	tr	(4.3)
Lamb	5.4	0.6	24.2	1.0	20.9	(52.1)	1.3	1.0	38.2	tr	(40.5)	2.5	2.5	0	0	tr	tr	(5.0)
Pork*	1.6	tr	27.1	tr	13.8	(42.5)	3.4	tr	43.8	0.7	(47.9)	7.4	0.9	0	tr	tr	tr	(8.3)
Chicken*	1.3	tr	26.7	tr	7.1	(35.1)	7.2	tr	39.8	0.6	(47.6)	13.5	0.7	tr	0.7	tr	tr	(14.9)
Turkey	1.0	tr	25.0	0.5	10.0	(36.5)	5.0	tr	21.5	0.4	(26.9)	20.0	1.0	tr	5.0	1.5	2.0	(29.5)
Calf liver	0.8	tr	16.5	0.6	23.3	(41.2)	1.9	0.7	20.8	tr	(23.4)	15.0	1.4	2.1	9.0	0.3	4.0	(16.8)
Lamb liver	1.3	0.5	20.4	1.0	18.3	(41.5)	3.5	1.6	29.7	0	(34.8)	5.0	3.8	0.6	5.1	0	3.0	(17.5)

From Paul & Southgate (1978)
* Composition depends on diet being fed
tr = trace

Meats also contain a range of inorganic constituents; they are relatively low in sodium and calcium, and high in potassium, phosphorus and magnesium. However it is the amount of essential micronutrients they provide that is of nutritional importance; iron levels are high in meats that have not been bled out at slaughter, and in blood products; zinc, copper and several trace elements are present in meat. The inorganic constituents are mostly found in the lean portion, so concentrations are lower in high-fat meats. One very important nutritional characteristic of meats is the high bioavailability of the inorganic nutrients they contain.

Meats contain most of the B-vitamins and they are especially important as a source of vitamin B_{12}. The fat-soluble vitamins are present in the fat, the concentrations being highly dependent on the diet eaten by the animal. Retinol is stored in the liver, and very high concentrations can be seen in animals given supplemented rations and among wild animals that eat fatty fish.

Nutritional role of meats and meat products

In the developed countries meat consumption is substantially higher than in the less developed countries, where plant products and the carbohydrates they supply provide up to 80% of the total energy intake, and the major protein sources are plants. Meat is not an essential component of the diet and societies that have adopted vegetarian diets for religious or other reasons do not show evidence of malnutrition when the supply of total food is adequate.

In the UK, total meat consumption as estimated from the National Food Survey (MAFF 1986) shows that meat provides 16% of the energy, 30% of the protein and 26% of the fat. In food purchased for the home, poultry is the most important single type of meat, but the total usage of carcase meats greatly exceeds poultry. Meat products account for nearly half of total meat consumption, with bacon and ham making up about a quarter of this. Meat fat provides about 23% of saturated fat intake, and is less important than separated fats and dairy products in this respect; it also provides 16% of the polyunsaturated fat intake. It is important to recognize that the amount of fat in meat that is actually consumed is highly idiosyncratic and much fat served ends up as plate waste; it is also difficult to estimate the losses of fat at the preparation level, both from trimming and during cooking.

Meat is an important source of highly bioavailable inorganic nutrients, and provides 26% of the zinc, 29% of the copper, 28% of the selenium and 24% of the iron intakes in the UK. In the case of the vitamins, meat provides 55% of B_{12}, 36% of vitamin A, 26% of niacin, 23% of B_6, 18% of riboflavin and 14% of thiamin intakes.

FISH AND FISH PRODUCTS

Fish and a wide variety of other seafoods have always been important in the diets of communities living close to the sea, rivers and lakes. The development first of refrigerated transport and then of on-board refrigeration on fishing vessels, has both improved the quality and shelf-life of fish and made it more available to populations distant from water. The development of attractive processed products has also been instrumental in widening fish consumption. Although fish catches worldwide are increasing (FAO 1985, British Nutrition Foundation 1986), fish stocks in some waters are declining due to overfishing, and much of the fish caught is manufactured into animal feeds. In the UK fish is a relatively minor component of the diet, although it is widely consumed (MAFF 1988).

Fish are unusual for a major a commodity because, with the exception of farmed trout and salmon, they are wild creatures that have to be located and taken from their natural environment – they are in fact one of the few animal foods that are hunted.

A very large number of species of fish are taken for food by the world's population as a whole, the numbers of species being more limited in the colder waters surrounding the UK, which may account for the limited range of fish in the UK diet.

Although there are still some fish caught in coastal waters, most fishing is done from deep-sea trawlers which either have on-board processing and refrigeration or are accompanied by factory ships that process the catch at sea. In all vessels the fish are cooled as quickly as possible after catching, in order to minimize postmortem deterioration. Fish are an unstable commodity, and among the early products of spoilage are trimethylamine and ammonia, which reduce consumer acceptability. Furthermore the fish may struggle when netted, and usually die from asphyxiation, which produces metabolic changes that are disadvantageous to the shelf-life of the fish as food.

The custom of linking the other seafoods with fish has been continued in this chapter, but it is more logical to discuss their composition and nutritional role in the diet seperately.

Composition of fish

There are three main categories of fish used as foods; the bony fishes, the Teleosts, fall into two composi-tional groups, white fish such as cod, haddock, halibut, lemon sole, plaice (and most other flat fish), saithe and whiting; and fatty fish such as eels, herring, pilchards, salmon, sardines, sprats, trout, tuna and whitebait. The third category contains the cartilaginous Elasmobranch fish, such as dogfish, shark and skate.

White fish

The flesh of these fish is very low in fat and consists primarily of muscle blocks surrounded by thin sheets of connective tissue. The concentrations of most of the B-vitamins are lower than in mammalian muscle, with the possible exception of vitamin B_6. The mineral levels are similar, although the very fine bones in fish are often eaten with the flesh, raising the calcium content slightly but significantly. Fish, in common with most marine organisms, accumulate trace elements from seawater and are a rich source of iodine and, less fortunately, of toxic metal contamination if taken from heavily polluted waters (MAFF 1980). These fish accumulate fats, or more correctly oils, in their livers, which are a rich source of vitamin A, retinol and vitamin D, and long-chain polyunsaturated fatty acids in their triglycerides.

Fatty fish

These fish have fat in their flesh, which is usually much darker with similar blocks of muscle interspersed with connective tissue. The amount of fat is related to the breeding cycle of the fish, and after breeding the fat content falls considerably. Thus herring may have only 5% of fat from February to April, rising to 20% from July to October. Herring are normally fished in the seasons when they are fat, so that the typical value for fat in herrings as purchased is around 19%. The flesh of the fatty fish is usually richer in the B-vitamins than white fish, and there are significant amounts of vitamins A and D present. The mineral concentrations are not markedly different. The fat of these fish is particularly rich in very long-chain polyunsaturated fatty acids and thus very prone to develop rancidity, which may be one reason why many of these fish are traditionally smoked or pickled to preserve them.

Cartilaginous fish

These fish are almost exclusively marine and include the sharks and rays, which are among the most successful of all fish in their mastery of the seas. The flesh of these fish is relatively low in fat, although they do accumulate oils in their livers; compositionally the concentrations of the vitamins and minerals are very similar to those in white fish. These fish are remarkable in that they maintain the osmolality of their extracellular fluids by increasing the urea content, so that protein values based on total nitrogen values are substantially overestimated.

Table 18.5 gives some representative values for the composition of a range of fish, showing that within the major groups there is considerable similarity.

Invertebrate seafoods

The species popularly known as shellfish include species from two major and distinctive phyla, the Mollusca, the true shellfish and the Arthropoda, order Crustacea, which includes crabs, shrimps, prawns and lobsters.

Molluscs

A wide range of molluscs is eaten by man, including bivalves such as mussels, oysters and scallops, gastropods such as winkles and whelks, and molluscs that have lost their external shells but retain an inner pen – the squids and octopuses. The true shelled molluscs are often eaten whole after boiling, and sometimes raw. The flesh is very muscular, with low levels of fat, the mineral levels are usually higher than in true fish, and the vitamin levels are low. Molluscs are generally filter feeders and accumulate trace elements, both essential and contaminant, from the seawater. They are also very prone to contamination from pathogenic organisms in the water, and most countries have regulations about the sites where molluscs can be taken, and some require the animals to be 'rested' in unpolluted water for a period before sale. Usually only the muscular mantles of squids and octopuses are eaten, after cooking.

Crustacea

These include a range of species, both freshwater – crayfish – and marine – crabs, shrimps, prawns and lobsters. These animals are characterized by tough exoskeletons composed of chitin and protein; the parts eaten are the muscular parts of the thorax and the muscles of the specialized appendages: the claws of crabs and lobsters. The animals may be trapped from the wild but techniques for farming them are under development, because in some communities they are gastronomically very highly valued.

The flesh is characteristically low in fat and high in minerals, especially sodium from marine species. The

Table 18.5 Composition of some fish, molluscs and crustaceans (per 100 g edible matter)

	Energy (kcal)	Energy (kJ)	Water (g)	Protein (g)	Fat (g)
White fish					
cod	76	322	82.0	17.4	0.7
haddock	73	308	81.3	16.8	0.6
halibut	92	390	78.1	17.7	2.4
lemon sole	81	343	81.2	17.1	1.4
plaice	91	386	79.5	17.9	2.2
catfish	90	376	78.1	16.1	2.7
carp	115	481	77.8	18.0	4.2
bream	103	430	78.0	16.7	4.0
perch	84	355	81.0	18.1	1.3
pike	81	343	80.0	18.4	0.7
Fatty fish					
eel	168	700	71.3	16.6	11.3
herring	234	970	63.9	16.8	18.5
mackerel	223	926	64.0	19.0	16.3
salmon	182	761	65.4	18.8	12.0
trout, rainbow	160	670	71.0	18.6	9.6
tuna	185	770	65.0	24.2	9.9
Cartilaginous fish					
dogfish	156	653	72.3	17.6	9.9
shark	100	418	77.0	20.6	1.3
skate	98	410	77.8	21.5	0.7
Molluscs					
abalone	98	410	75.8	18.7	0.5
clam	82	343	80.8	14.0	1.9
cockle	81	339	79.9	16.8	1.0
mussel	95	397	78.6	14.4	2.2
oyster	73	276	84.6	8.4	1.8
scallop	81	339	79.8	15.3	0.2
whelk	69	289	83.6	11.6	0.6
cuttlefish	81	339	81.0	16.1	0.9
octopus	73	305	82.2	15.3	0.8
squid	75	314	82.0	15.3	0.8
Crustaceans					
crab	100	418	76.8	17.9	2.0
crayfish	69	285	82.0	14.6	0.5
lobster	87	365	79.0	16.9	1.9
shrimp	87	365	79.0	18.1	0.8

animals also accumulate trace elements from the water, and the vitamin levels are similar to those in white fish.

Nutrients in fish

The major part of fish eaten as food, both the true fish and the molluscs and crustacea, is a muscle, and fish are quite properly seen as important sources of good-quality protein, weight-for-weight providing similar amounts to lean meats. The amino acid composition of the proteins in most fishes is very similar, and although the molluscan and crustacean proteins are distinctive they are all rich sources of essential amino acids (Paul & Southgate 1978) (Table 18.6). The protein is accompanied by very low amounts of fat in white fish, crustacea and molluscs, and the fat from fish as a whole is characterized by the high proportion of long-chain polyunsaturated fatty acids. Table 18.7 provides a selection of values that illustrate the fatty acid composition of a number of fats from fish compared with typical values for carcase meat. The concentrations of the inorganic nutrients in fish are not particularly unusual when compared with meats, with the exception of calcium in fish with fine bones, such as herring, where the bones are eaten with the flesh. The levels of sodium are higher in marine species, and the levels of the intercellular elements potassium and phosphorus are higher than in meats. The iron and zinc levels tend to be lower, except for the shellfish, which tend to accumulate trace elements, so that oysters have the distinction of being one of the richest sources of zinc eaten, with levels of up to 100 mg/100 g being recorded (it is possible that these rich sources contain high levels of other trace elements, some of which are less desirable). Fish are a major source of iodine, again being accumulated from their environment.

Nutritional role of fish

Despite being a country surrounded by sea, the consumption of fish by the UK population as a whole is relatively small compared with countries such as Spain, Portugal and Italy. It is true that these countries have access to a wider range of species, and the dietary culture in these countries is probably more dependent on fresh foods. In 1991 the average consumption of fish in the UK amounted to about 20 g/person/day, and of this 18% was frozen convenience products (MAFF 1992); shellfish accounted for about 2.5% of total fish consumption. Consumption appears to have increased very slightly over recent years, but over the longer term has remained relatively low. It is interesting to note that fish consumption was higher in unemployed households, with an income over £95 per week, where purchases of fresh, frozen and prepared fish were greater than in the higher income groups. At these levels of consumption it is not unexpected that the contribution to nutrient intakes from fish is relatively minor, providing about 1% of energy, 4.7% of protein and 1.3% of fat (3.2% of polyunsaturated fatty acid intakes). The only vitamin provided in significant quantity was vitamin D, where fish provides 14% of the total.

EGGS

The eggs of a range of species are eaten in many human cultures, and although in some cultures eggs are proscribed for women, in most they form a common, if not important, part of the diet. In the UK hens' eggs are the most important, with minor usage of duck, goose, and quail eggs.

Most hens' eggs are produced intensively under battery conditions, although there is a growing

Table 18.6 Amino acid composition of some fish compared with other protein foods (mg/g total N)

Amino acid	Fish	Crustacea	Molluscs	Beef	Milk	Egg	Wheat
Essential							
histidine	180	120	150	230	190	150	130
isoleucine	330	290	300	320	350	350	210
leucine	530	540	480	500	640	520	420
lysine	610	490	500	570	510	390	150
methionine	180	180	170	170	180	200	100
phenylalanine	260	250	260	280	340	320	280
threonine	300	290	290	290	310	320	170
tryptophan	70	70	80	80	90	110	70
valine	360	300	390	330	460	470	280
Nonessential							
arginine	400	520	470	420	250	380	290
alanine	430	420	350	440	240	340	230
aspartic acid	650	680	700	600	530	670	310
cystine	70	80	100	80	60	110	160
glutamic acid	950	980	880	1080	1440	750	1710
glycine	290	410	320	350	140	190	250
proline	260	270	260	320	590	240	660
serine	310	320	320	280	370	490	330
tyrosine	220	230	260	240	280	250	190

Table 18.7 Fatty acid composition of the lipids of some fish compared with other foods*

	Fatty acid[†]	Cod	Herring	Beef	Milk	Corn (maize)
Saturated	C16:0	21.5	13.7	26.9	26.0	14.0
	C18:0	3.5	1.2	13.0	11.2	2.3
	Others	1.1	7.4	5.0	26.0	0.9
Monounsaturated	C16:1	2.3	10.0	6.3	2.7	0.3
	C18:1	11.0	15.2	42.0	27.8	30.0
	C20:1	1.8	13.2	—	—	0.2
	C22:1	0.8	17.4	—	—	0.2
	Others	—	—	2.5	3.2	—
Polyunsaturated	C18:2	0.5	1.4	2.0	1.4	50.0
	C18:3	0.1	1.2	1.3	1.5	1.6
	C18:4	0.2	1.8	—	—	—
	C20:4	3.9	0.6	1.0	—	—
	C20:5	17.2	7.0	—	—	—
	C22:5	1.5	1.1	—	—	—
	C22:6	33.4	6.5	—	—	—

* Values expressed as % total fatty acid content (approx)
† The nomenclature used for the fatty acids in this table may need explanation: a C16:0 acid contains 16 carbon atoms, no double bonds between carbon atoms and is described as saturated; a C18:1 acid contains 18 carbon atoms with one double bond and is monounsaturated; a C20:5 acid contains 20 carbon atoms with five double bonds and is polyunsaturated (i.e. containing more than one double bond)

demand for eggs produced under less intensive systems, such as deep-litter where the hens are enclosed in a controlled environment, sometimes known as 'barn' eggs; or range eggs, where the hens are allowed access to open space to forage, although they are fed specially formulated rations. True free-range production, where the hens are not confined and range freely in search of food, is seen as the ideal by many animal welfare organizations, but such systems are not common. Detailed comparisons of the composition of eggs produced by the different systems show no nutritionally significant differences (Tolan et al 1974, Holland et al 1989). Differences in yolk colour can be seen when free-range hens have access to greenstuff, where the carotenoids pass into the yolk; natural and synthetic pigments are commonly incorporated into the rations fed to battery hens to produce acceptable yolk colours. The white of freshly laid eggs has better functional properties, for example when whipped to produce a foam. This property deteriorates when the egg is stored, as is common in the production and distribution of battery eggs; it is not, however, a direct effect of the system.

Composition of eggs

Some typical values for the composition of different eggs are given in Table 18.8, which shows a remarkable similarity between the eggs of different species.

The proteins of eggs contain the amino acids essential for the complete development of the embryo, and for this reason egg protein was seen as having the perfect amino acid composition; the reference protein for biological evaluation and assessing amino acid patterns was, for a considerable period, egg protein. It is now recognized that it is perfect for the chicken, but not necessarily for other species, and other amino acid compositions are now seen as ideal for humans.

The lipids in eggs are rich in phospholipids and the fatty acid composition shows quite a high P/S ratio. Cholesterol is present in the egg lipid, where it forms a key percursor for membrane synthesis in the chick. It is possible to manipulate the cholesterol content of the egg by dietary means, but it is not yet clear whether this is a useful or stable change. The eggs contain the range of minerals and vitamins necessary for the development of the chick, and thus eggs are a valuable food. The iron in eggs has been shown to have a low bioavailability, possibly because it is bound to the egg proteins. Egg white contains the protein avidin, which binds to biotin and makes it unavailable to man; cooking the egg denatures the avidin and abolishes the effect.

Nutritional role of eggs

Eggs provide a versatile food of high biological value. They can be produced efficiently and relatively

Table 18.8   Composition of eggs of different species (per 100 g)

	Hen	Duck	Pigeon	Quail	Goose	Turkey	Turtle
Water (g)	74.8	70.6	79.8	73.7	70.4	72.2	75.6
Energy							
(kcal)	147	188	116	161	185	171	148
(kJ)	615	787	485	674	774	715	619
Protein (g)	11.8	13.2	10.7	13.1	13.9	13.1	12.0
Fat (g)	9.6	14.2	7.0	12.1	13.9	12.1	10.0
Calcium (mg)	52	64	62	49	56	49	84
Iron (mg)	2.0	3.6	3.5	4.1	2.8	4.1	1.3
Retinol (µg)	140	370	95	—	—	—	445
Vitamin D (µg)	1.75	—	—	—	—	—	—
Thiamin (mg)	0.09	0.16	0.13	—	0.18	0.11	0.11
Riboflavin (mg)	0.47	0.40	0.65	—	0.36	0.47	0.46

From various food composition table references

cheaply and many developing countries have established egg production as a means of improving the supply of animal protein. In the developed world the focus on cholesterol in the diet as a potential risk factor for coronary heart disease has led to a fall in egg consumption and, although the climate of opinion regarding the effects of dietary cholesterol on blood levels has changed, a negative view is still taken by many consumers of the cholesterol levels in eggs. Changes in dietary patterns in the UK have also led to reduced consumption and among these decline in the consumption of the traditional English cooked breakfast is possibly the most important (British Nutrition Foundation 1982). Household purchases of eggs average around 3 per head per week; as the usual size of an egg is between 50 and 60 g this represents 20–24 g per day. However, there is considerable usage of eggs in processed foods and the actual consumption of eggs will be higher.

NOVEL PROTEIN FOODS

The widespread prevalence of protein-energy malnutrition in the developing world has created a considerable interest in the development of protein supplements for use in weaning foods. This interest coupled with demographic and protein supply predictions in the 1960s have combined to provide the stimulus for research on the development of alternative sources of protein. Increasing the production of animal protein was seen as an inefficient use of plant protein, and two lines of research developed, the first to produce isolates of plant proteins and the second to explore the production of protein microbiologically using bacteria, yeast and other fungal organisms.

Plant protein isolates

Two avenues have been tried; the use of seed legumes which are rich sources of both protein and oils, and the use of leaves. In both the principles of production are similar: the plant source is extracted with alkali to solubilize the protein, filter off the structural plant material and adjust the pH of the filtrate to the isoelectric point of the protein and precipitate a protein curd, which is then washed and dried. The leaf protein concentrates retain the plant pigments and are therefore green in colour – this has been seen as a disadvantage precluding their use in many foods. The concentrates can, however, be produced with simple equipment and some consider that a low-technology approach is better for developing countries. The protein isolates from legumes are amorphous, lightly coloured powders, and soya isolates in particular have wide use as food ingredients in this form. There has been considerable interest in using these isolates to produce meat analogues, but the main technological problems have been the introduction of the essential sensory characteristics, texture and flavour. Textures have been developed by spinning fibres, initially using textile machinery: alterations in the alignment of the fibres can produce a range of textures simulating different types of meat. The addition of flavours was in principle easy, the major problem being to make the flavours stay with the simulated meat when it is chewed, and this is possibly why simulated stewing-steak type products have been acceptable. Nutritionally the protein isolates from legumes have lower biological values than meat proteins, with the sulphur amino acids being limiting; in a mixed diet this is not really of great importance, but the levels of B-vitamins, especially B_{12}, are very dissimilar and fortification was considered desirable in the UK (DHSS 1980); the levels of iron and zinc are low in these isolates and the presence of phytates reduces the availability of these nutrients.

Microbiological proteins

The rapid microbiological production of biomass makes this approach attractive, particularly if the substrate is of low value. The chance discovery of a yeast growing in oil pipelines led to the development of a protein concentrate from hydrocarbon wastes. The material was developed as an animal protein supplement because it was considered that the possibility of hydrocarbon residues in the product would create toxicological problems. Methane was also used as a substrate to produce protein for animal feeding, but changes in the value of oil-based products in the 1970s made these approaches uneconomical. The use of a filamentous mould to produce protein from carbohydrate sources was developed by Rank Hovis Macdougal in the UK: the

advantage of such a mould is that it produces its own texture. The major problems in the production of microbial protein are the selection of a species that does not produce any toxic metabolites or unusual amino or fatty acids, and secondly the high concentrations of nucleic acids associated with the protein. It was necessary to develop processes to reduce the nucleic acids before the material could gain approval for food use. The protein quality is similar to that of other plant proteins and the product is naturally low in fat and contains the fungal cell-wall material chitin, which has some of the properties of dietary fibre.

These novel protein foods require sophisticated technology for their production and do not provide the ideal solution to the need for protein-rich weaning foods in the third world; nevertheless, they have their role to play in the diet of the developed countries, where they are attractive alternatives to meat for those who do not wish to eat meat. Their nutritional composition does, however, need to be regulated to protect the consumer, who may come to rely heavily on these novel foods.

REFERENCES

British Nutrition Foundation 1982 Eating behaviour and attitudes to food, nutrition and health. BNF, London

British Nutrition Foundation 1986 Nutritional aspects of fish. BNF Briefing paper No.10. BNF, London

British Nutrition Foundation 1988 Nutritional aspects of meat. BNF Briefing paper No.18. BNF, London

Department of Health and Social Security 1980 Foods which simulate meat. Reports on Health and Social Subjects No.17. HMSO, London

Eaton SB, Konner M 1985 Paleolithic nutrition. New England Journal of Medicine 312: 283–289

Fieldhouse P 1986 Food and nutrition:customs and culture. Croom Helm, London

Food and Agriculture Organisation 1985 Fishery commodity situation and outlook report 84–85. FAO, Rome

Greenfield H (ed) 1987 Composition of meat in Australia. Food Technology in Australia 39

Holland B, Unwin ID, Buss DH 1989 Milk products and eggs, 4th suppl to McCance and Widdowson's The Composition of Foods. Royal Society of Chemistry, London

Ministry of Agriculture, Fisheries and Food, Annually, Household food consumption and expenditure. Annual Report of the National Food Survey Committee. HMSO, London (Reports used to take 2 years but now only 1 – 1992 reports on 1991, etc.)

Ministry of Agriculture, Fisheries and Food, Steering Group on Food Surveillance, Series of Reports published at irregular intervals. HMSO, London

Paul AA, Southgate DAT 1977 A study on the composition of retail meats: dissection into lean, separable fat and inedible portions. Journal of Human Nutrition 31: 259–272

Paul AA, Southgate DAT 1978 McCance and Widdowson's The composition of food, 4th edn. HMSO, London

Sinclair AJ, O'Dea K 1987 The lipid levels and fatty acid compositions of the lean portions of Australian beef and lamb. Food Technology in Australia 39: 229–231

Talbot LM 1964 Wild animals as sources of food. In: Cuthbertson DP, Mills CF, Passmore R (eds) Proceedings of the Sixth International Congress on Nutrition. E & S Livingstone, Edinburgh, pp. 243–251

Tolan A, Robertson J, Orton CR et al 1974 The chemical composition of eggs produced under battery, deep litter and free-range conditions. British Journal of Nutrition 31: 185–200

Wood JD, Buxton PJ, Whittington FM, Enser M 1986 The chemical composition of fat tissues in the pig: the effects of castration and feeding treatment. Livestock Production Science 15: 73–82

19. Milk and milk products; fats and oils

D. A. T. Southgate

Milk and milk products became part of the diet of adult humans when the hunter-gatherer developed into the pastoralist, and the exploitation of animals for products other than meat and skins began. Since that time the milk of many species has been used as a food and as a source of a range of products. Liquid milk is an unstable commodity and many products that evolved were fermented foods that could be stored and transported, thus extending their value. A land 'flowing with milk and honey' was clearly very attractive to the tribes of Israel, and is clear evidence of the value that has been placed on milk in the diet for many thousands of years.

The development of the dairy industry to its present place in the agricultural economy of countries such as the USA, New Zealand and northern Europe was dependent on a combination of factors, including the selection of high-yielding breeds of cattle and their progressive improvement by selective breeding, particularly over the last 40 or so years by the use of artificial insemination from bulls of proven productivity. This was accompanied by close attention to hygiene during the production and distribution of milk. In particular, the introduction of pasteurization was instrumental in reducing the propensity of milk as a cause of bacterial infection. Animal health programmes were also introduced to eliminate milk as a vector for the transmission of disease, especially bovine tuberculosis, to humans.

Milk and other dairy products became important components in programmes to improve the nutritional status of the poor following the depression of the 1930s, and in the UK during the 1939–45 war, and were firmly established in the consumer's perception as 'good' foods.

MILK

Milk is the secretion of the mammary gland and is the staple food for all young mammals, including human infants. The milk of all species has undergone evolutionary pressure during the development of the species, and it is reasonable to argue that the composition of the milk secreted by each species is adapted in some way to the specific needs of the species in question. The milks used as human foods are therefore adapted to the needs of the young animal for which they evolved, and not man, and there are distinct differences between, for example, cows' milk and human milk that can be related to the differences in rates of growth and the ways in which maternal immunity is transferred to the young animal. However, this chapter is concerned with milk as a food and not infant nutrition, which is discussed elsewhere.

Milk in the UK context implies milk from the cow (*Bos domesticus*), with a minor but expanding contribution from goats and sheep. In the Middle East, goats and camels are the milk animals and in the Far East water buffalo are important; the Lapps consume reindeer milk. In some communities other species of cattle are used, for example in Africa *Bos indicus* is important, because it is resistant to many diseases that affect European breeds. The milk from the mare and the ass was important to the herdsman of the Eurasian plains.

The compositions of some milks are given in Table 19.1, illustrating the range of compositions that are seen. Milk production in the UK relies heavily on the Friesian (Holstein) breed. The production of milk is regulated by the Milk Marketing Board, which purchases the bulk of liquid milk production, which is controlled by quotas from the European Community.

Cows are milked by machine – usually twice a day, although improved yields can be obtained by more frequent milking, paralleling the feeding pattern of calves – and the milk is pooled and pasteurized. There is a small amount of raw milk produced without pasteurization. Pasteurization is usually carried out using continuous-flow equipment giving a heat treatment of at least 72°C for 15 s, which is sufficient to kill all

Table 19.1 Composition of milks of different species (per 100 g)

Constituent	Cow	Goat	Sheep	Camel	Buffalo	Human mature
Water (g)	87.8	88.9	83.0	88.8	83.3	88.2
Energy						
(kcal)	66	60	95	63	92	69
(kJ)	276	253	396	264	385	289
Protein (g)	3.2	3.1	5.4	2.0	4.1	1.3
Fat (g)	3.9	3.5	6.0	4.1	5.9	4.1
Lactose (g)	4.6	4.4	5.1	4.7	5.9	7.2
Calcium (mg)	115	100	170	94	175	34

From FAO (1972); Paul & Southgate (1978); Holland et al (1989)

non-sporing pathogens and non-thermoduric organisms; the resistance of spores is one reason why milk needs to be stored at refrigeration temperatures, to prevent the growth of sporing organisms. The hygienic quality of milk is still very dependent on the maintenance of hygienic production standards (Mabbit et al 1987).

Milk products

Whole milk has long had a special status in UK food laws, dating back to the need to control food adulteration, where the addition of water was an early example of fraud. The removal of the separated cream produced skimmed milk, which until recently was of little interest as a human food, and in some countries was used as an animal food. The evolution of dietary guidelines recommending the reduced consumption of saturated fat (Health Education Council 1983, Department of Health and Social Security 1984) radically changed this and there has been a substantial demand for both completely and semi-skimmed milks. The difference in composition of these products is illustrated in Table 19.2.

Dried, condensed and ultra-heat treated milks

Milk has a high water content and is unstable, and a number of processes have been developed to reduce the water content and make the product more stable. Dried milks were originally produced by roller-drying, where the milk passed in a thin film over heated rollers; this was a rather vigorous treatment and produced flavour changes and substantial losses of vitamins. It also caused changes in colour due to the formation of Maillard reaction products between the protein and the lactose, which were associated with a reduction in the biological value of the proteins. Roller-drying has been largely replaced by spray-drying, where a thin spray of milk is passed into a heated chamber. This is a milder treatment that can be more closely controlled, and therefore leads to less nutritional and sensory damage. Evaporated milks have had about a third of their water removed, and are usually canned to ensure stability. Condensed milks have sucrose added. These milks can be prepared from whole or skimmed starting materials. Sterilized milk was widely used before domestic refrigeration became common, and the specific flavour produced by sterilization is still preferred by some consumers. Sterilized milk is now often prepared from ultra-heat treated milk (UHT), where the milk has been treated at 130°C for 1 s. This milk has a very long storage life when packed aseptically in packs that exclude oxygen.

Cream

The separated fat layer of milk is used to produce a range of different types of cream, varying principally in the fat content but also in the methods used in their production, which modify their physical properties. Single cream contains about 18% fat and is usually pasteurized. Double cream contains about 48% fat, whereas whipping cream contains about 39%; both of these products may be pasteurized without it affecting their capacity to form foams. Clotted creams are produced by scalding the milk in heated pans, producing a very efficient separation of fat, and the clotted creams contain 60% fat. Some creams are ultra-heat treated to produce a long-life product. The creams also contain some of the residual aqueous phase of the milk and this contains the water-soluble nutrients in milk in the same proportions.

Cheese

Cheese-making from milk was one of the earliest ways of converting an unstable liquid product into a con-

Table 19.2   Composition of some milk products (per 100 g)

	Milks					Creams	
	Semi-skimmed	Skimmed	Dried skimmed	Evaporated whole	Condensed sweetened whole	Single	Double
Water (g)	89.8	91.1	3.0	69.1	25.9	74.0	48.0
Energy							
(kcal)	46	33	350	159	329	188	449
(kJ)	194	140	1491	664	1390	776	1849
Protein (g)	3.3	3.3	36.0	8.2	8.5	2.6	1.7
Fat (g)	1.6	0.1	1.0	9.0	9.0	18.0	48.0
Lactose (g)	4.7	4.8	50.1	12.0	12.3	3.9	2.6
Sucrose (g)					43.2		

From Holland et al (1989)

Table 19.3   Composition of some cheeses (per 100 g)

	Camembert	Cheddar	Danish blue	Edam	Parmesan	Cottage	Processed
Water (g)	50.7	36.0	45.3	43.8	18.4	79.1	45.7
Energy							
(kcal)	297	412	347	333	462	98	330
(kJ)	1232	1708	1437	1382	1880	413	1367
Protein (g)	20.9	25.5	20.1	26.0	39.4	13.8	20.8
Fat (g)	23.7	34.4	29.6	25.4	32.7	4.0	27.0

From Holland et al (1989)

centrated food that could be stored. It is possible that milk's capacity to undergo fermentation, and the subsequent coagulation of the protein, led to the development of cheese-making. There are a very large number of different types of cheese, which vary because of differences in the treatment of the starting material and the way in which the curd is subsequently treated and matured, and it is not possible to discuss them here. In the traditional Cheddar process the milk is treated with a starter, originally rennet prepared from calf stomach, which coagulates the protein to produce a curd; this is heated to around 30°C and the resultant mass is cut, stirred and reheated at a higher temperature (38.5°C). The cheese curd is then stacked to develop cohesion, milled, salted and pressed into moulds. The finished cheese is traditionally stored to mature and develop its characteristic flavour. The consistency of cheese can be modified by varying the starting milk, the temperature at which the curd is heated, and the efficiency with which the residual whey is expelled. Blue-veined cheeses are produced by inoculating the cheese with bacterial cultures. Because of the many variations in cheese production it is difficult to generalize about its composition. Paul and Southgate (1978) grouped the

cheeses into the major types (Table 19.3), and this classification is adequate for most nutritional purposes because cheese-making is in many cases a relatively small-scale operation. The composition of two samples of the same-named cheese may differ as much as two differently named cheeses. Holland et al (1989) give values for the composition of a number of different cheeses, based on the analysis of a range of samples purchased in the UK.

Fermented milks

The fermentation of milks with lactobacilli leads to the production of lactic acid from the lactose, and the fall in pH inhibits the growth of many pathogenic organisms, so that fermentation provides an early type of milk stabilization. Acidified milks have been prized foods in many cultures, and at one time it was argued that they had a value in infant feeding for encouraging the establishment of a desirable intestinal flora in young infants.

One of the most important fermented foods is yogurt, a food originating in south-east Europe and Turkey, where the milk is fermented with *Lactobacillus bulgaricus*. The acid conditions cause the milk to form a soft curd. Yogurts contain all the constituents present in the original milk, with the exception of the lactose which is substantially reduced; the organism uses the glucose moiety of the lactose preferentially, so that some residual galactose is present, making the carbohydrates of yogurt quite distinctive. Yogurt can be produced from skimmed or whole milk, and there is a large range of flavours used commercially.

Products based on the constituents of milk

Whole milk can be processed to produce products based on its major components, and these are also important in the diet both as foods and as ingredients. Butter is prepared by churning milk or cream to break down the fat emulsion in milk, so that the fat separates and forms a mass that can be worked up into the finished butter. The nutritional aspects of butter are discussed later, with the other fats and oils. The major protein in milk, casein, can be precipitated easily and the isolated protein finds considerable use as a food ingredient, either as the protein or as caseinates. The other major component of the aqueous whey, lactose, is difficult to isolate by chemical means but physical separation by membrane filtration or reversed osmosis is now used on a commercial scale. Lactose is not very sweet compared with sucrose, and has limited value as a food ingredient in its own right; it has been used as a fermentation stock for the production of ethanol, but this is not really economical. Hydrogenation of lactose produces the disaccharide sugar alcohol lactitol, and this is used as a bulk sweetener because it has a lower metabolizable energy value than lactose itself. Its use for this purpose has been approved in several countries.

Nutrients in milk and milk products

Milk is the sole food of virtually all young mammals and contains all the nutrients essential for mammalian growth.

Proteins

The major protein in milk is casein, which in cows' milk is around 80% of the total. The other major proteins are lactalbumin and a range of immunoglobulins. Casein is a phosphoprotein, and the organization of the casein into micelles is responsible for the physical properties of milk. It appears to be a major factor in retaining the calcium and phosphate present in solution above concentrations that would lead to their precipitation in aqueous solution. The casein micelles are stabilized by calcium phosphates. The casein is present in milk as caseinogen, which is converted into casein by gastric enzymes that remove a glycoprotein peptide, leading to the formation of casein clots (Regenstein & Regenstein 1984).

In human milk the proportion of lactalbumin is higher and the proteins are believed to be better digested because of reduced clotting in the stomach. The immunoglobulins are responsible for the transfer of maternal immunity to the young animal in the early stages after birth, when the gastrointestinal mucosa is permeable to large molecules. In the cow some transference of immunity across the placenta also occurs, but in man the immunoglobulins of milk are believed to be very important to neonatal immunity.

Fats

The amount of fat in milk varies between different species. In ruminant milks the fat contains a significant proportion of short-chain volatile fatty acids, derived from the fermentation of carbohydrate in the rumen; this anaerobic fermentation also leads to the saturation of fatty acids in the diet, so that the fat in the milk contains only low levels of unsaturated fatty acids (Table 19.4). In non-ruminants the saturation of the fat can be altered by dietary means. It is possible to feed protected fats to ruminants to increase the levels of unsaturation, but this has not proved to be economically viable because it leads to loss of condition in the cow and reduced yields.

Carbohydrate

Milk contains the disaccharide lactose and is the only known source of this sugar in the diet. The amounts vary in the milks of different species, the level in human milk being among the highest. Human milks also contain small amounts of the higher oligosaccharides, derived from lactose by the addition of fucosyl residues. The role of these oligosaccharides is not known, but they are found in the milks of some other species and may have immunological properties.

Inorganic nutrients

Some typical values for the inorganic nutrients in the milks of different species are given in Table 19.5, and for milk products in Table 19.6. The sodium levels in milks vary over a narrow range, with that of mature (after 10 days' lactation) human milk being substantially lower than that of cow's milk. Human milk also contains lower levels of potassium, calcium, magnesium, and especially phosphorus, where the value is

Table 19.4   Fatty acid composition of cow's and human milk (fatty acids % of total fatty acids)

	4:0	6:0	8:0	10:0	12:0	14:0	16:0	18:0	14:1	16:1	18:1	18:2	18:3
Cow's milk	3.2	2.0	1.2	2.8	3.5	11.2	26.0	11.2	1.4	2.7	27.8	1.4	1.5
Human milk	0	0	tr	1.4	5.4	7.3	26.5	9.5	tr	4.0	35.4	7.2*	0.88

tr = trace
* Value varies over wide range depending on maternal diet
From Paul & Southgate (1978)

only 16% of that in cow's milk. The concentrations in the products are proportional to the protein concentrations (in the terminology used in the dairy industry this corresponds approximately to the 'solids-not-fat levels') because the inorganic nutrients are principally in the aqueous phase. Hence skimmed products contain higher levels of inorganic nutrients. In cheese, the addition of sodium chloride as common salt produces very substantial increases in the sodium level, and the level of addition can vary in the same-named cheese from batch to batch.

Vitamins

Milks contain both fat-soluble and water-soluble vitamins (Table 19.7). The concentrations of fat-soluble vitamins are dependent on the type of feeding the animals are receiving, and are usually higher in the summer months when the animals are grazing and lower in the winter when they are fed concentrates. The levels are broadly proportional to the fat content in both milks and milk products, because these vitamins are essentially stable during the processing of milk. Skimmed milks are consequently low in the fat-soluble vitamins, and many proprietary products using skimmed milks are fortified with a vitamin mix. Milks are a good source of the B-vitamins, but riboflavin levels decline on storage if the milk is exposed to sunlight or fluorescent lighting. Some losses of thiamin occur on pasteurization, and these losses are higher in sterilized and UHT milks, which also show losses of B_6, B_{12} and folates. Raw milk contains significant amounts of vitamin C but substantial losses occur on storage and following heat processing (Holland et al 1989).

Table 19.5   Inorganic constituents in milks of different species (mg/100 g)

	Cow	Goat	Sheep	Human
Sodium	55	42	44	15
Potassium	140	170	120	58
Calcium	115	100	170	34
Magnesium	11	13	18	3
Phosphorus	92	90	150	15
Iron	0.06	0.12	0.03	0.07
Zinc	0.4	0.5	0.7	0.3

Nutritional role of milk and milk products

The nutritional composition of milk and its products clearly demonstrates the fact that these are excellent sources of many nutrients. The milk proteins are of high biological value, and their high lysine content means that when consumed with cereals there is a substantial supplementation between the two sources of protein. The heat processing of milk leads to some loss of biological value, and this often correlates well

Table 19.6   Inorganic constituents of some milk products (mg/100 g)

	Milk			Yogurt whole	Cottage cheese	Cheddar cheese	Parmesan cheese
	whole	skimmed	dried skimmed				
Protein (g)	3.2	3.3	36.1	5.7	13.8	25.5	39.4
Sodium	55	54	550	80	380	670	1090
Potassium	140	150	1590	280	89	77	110
Calcium	115	120	1280	200	73	720	1200
Magnesium	11	12	130	19	9	25	45
Phosphorus	92	94	970	170	160	490	810
Iron	0.06	0.06	0.27	0.1	0.1	0.3	1.1
Zinc	0.4	0.4	4.0	0.7	0.6	2.3	5.3

Table 19.7   Vitamins in some milks and milk products (per 100 g)

	Milks			Creams		Cheeses	
	Whole	Skimmed	Channel Island	Single	Double	Edam	Cheddar
Fat (g)	3.9	0.1	5.1	18.0	48.0	26.0	34.4
Retinol (µg)	52	1	65s 27w	315	600	175	325
Carotene (µg)	21	tr	115s 27w	125	325	150	225
Vitamin D (µg)	0.03	tr	0.03	0.14	0.27	—	0.26
Vitamin E (mg)	0.09	tr	0.09	0.40	1.10	0.48	0.53
Thiamin (mg)	0.03	0.04	0.04	0.04	0.02	0.03	0.03
Riboflavin (mg)	0.17	0.17	0.19	0.17	0.18	0.35	0.40
Vitamin B_6 (mg)	0.06	0.06	0.06	0.05	0.03	0.09	0.10
Vitamin B_{12} (µg)	0.4	0.4	0.4	0.3	0.2	2.1	1.1
Folates (µg)	6	5	7	7	7	40	33

s = summer
w = winter
From Holland et al (1989)

with the proportion of lysine that has become unavailable because of interaction with carbohydrate. Milk and its products are important as sources of inorganic nutrients, especially calcium, and of vitamins. The contribution of dairy products in the UK diet is very important, as illustrated by the data given in the National Food Survey (MAFF 1983–1992).

The current nutritional advice to reduce the consumption of total fat, and especially saturated fats, has focused considerable attention on the fat in dairy products which, as mentioned earlier, is low in unsaturated fatty acids. This has led to a decline in the consumption of dairy products in some sectors of the population, and to an increase in the consumption of skimmed or semi-skimmed products. It is important that the major role of milk in the provision of nutrients such as calcium and riboflavin is not prejudiced by the improper interpretation of nutritional guidance, which recommends a modest reduction in fat intake, not total abstinence (Health Education Council 1983). This caveat is particularly important where the diet of children is concerned, where milk and its products are valuable components (DHSS 1984).

Milk and its products are not without adverse effects in some individuals. Allergic reactions to milk proteins are one of the most common forms of food intolerance in infants, with antibodies to milk proteins frequently being demonstrable (Royal College of Physicians, British Nutrition Foundation 1984); in these infants the use of a soya milk preparation is necessary, although goats' milk appears to be less allergenic.

Infants with the inherited disorder galactosaemia cannot metabolize galactose effectively, and since

the consumption of galactose will lead to cataract formation all lactose-containing foods must be excluded.

The production of cheese leads to the release of free amino acids into the product and the conversion of some of these to amines; the presence of tyramine can stimulate the sympathetic nervous system and is believed to be associated with migraine in susceptible people; patients receiving monoamine oxidase inhibitory drugs must also avoid the consumption of this amine, and therefore cheeses.

FATS AND OILS

A range of separated oils and fats is consumed as food, especially in developed countries such as the UK. In the developing countries the use of separated fats is lower and the major part of the fat intake comes from fats present intrinsically in foods.

Fats and oils are distinguished by their physical characteristics, oils being fluid at ambient temperatures and fats being solid. Chemically they are predominantly triglyceride, with minor amounts of nonsaponifiable matter and very small quantities of mono- and diglycerides. During use some hydrolysis takes place, with the formation of free fatty acids, but the levels in fresh products are very low because even at low concentrations the free fatty acids produce unacceptable flavours and lead to rancidity. The lipids isolated from animal products tend to be solid fats, whereas those from plants are usually oils, but the distinction lies in their fatty acid and triglyceride composition, not their origin.

Animal fats

Butter

The most important fat from animal sources is butter obtained by churning cream or milk vigorously enough to break the emulsion and to separate the fat as a mass; the buttermilk is drained off and the mass washed and then salted. The butter is then worked to distribute the salt and moulded prior to division into packs for retail sale. The amount of salt added varies greatly, depending primarily on the market for which it is intended. Current nutritional concerns about the levels of salt in the diet have made unsalted butter more popular.

Lard

Lard is fat that has been rendered (heated, liquefied and strained) from adipose tissues trimmed from pork carcases.

Ghee

Ghee is used in many Asian cultures; it is prepared by heating and clarifying butter.

Suet

This is obtained from the shredded adipose tissue of cattle or other ruminants, and usually contains a little protein.

Plant oils

The seeds of many plants contain storage lipids and those that are rich in oil are used in the commercial production of oils. The flesh of the fruits of some plants also provides a source of oils.

Olive oil

The flesh of the olive is rich in oil, which is extracted by pressing the pulped flesh. A significant amount of oil can be obtained by mild pressure in the cold; this is known as cold-pressed or virgin oil and is regarded as having the highest culinary quality. The bulk of commercial olive oil is obtained by increased pressure. The expressed oil is usually dark in colour and is clarified by allowing it to settle and then racking-off the supernatant oil; the oil can also be clarified by filtration.

Seed oils

The processes used for the production of seed oils differ for the different oils, but in general the seeds are brought to a suitable moisture content and then crushed. The oil is then expressed using hydraulic pressure or a continuous expeller. The presses require a heated meal and the oil is said to be hot-pressed. The expeller can press unheated meal but precooking the meal can give higher yields. The expressed oil usually contains solid particles; these are separated and the oil is treated with alkali to neutralize any free fatty acids formed during the extraction. The oil may also need decolorizing or some treatment to deodorize it. Treatment with charcoal will adsorb unwanted flavours or colours, and steam treatment is sometimes used to remove volatile components.

Products derived from processed plant oils

The fluidity of oils is due primarily to their fatty acid composition, which is more unsaturated than the solid animal fats. In a programme to develop substitutes for butter, the French chemist Mege-Mourie discovered that by blending a mixture of fats and oils he was able to produce a fat that was similar in texture to butter, and thus invented margarine (Van Stuyvenberg 1969). The process originally used oils of animal origin and involved taking a mixture of fats and oils, rendering them and then allowing the mixture to crystallize under controlled conditions. Salt, colouring and flavouring materials are added to simulate as closely as possible the characteristics of butter. Catalytic hydrogenation enables the controlled hardening of plant oils for use in the production of margarine which have largely replaced the animal fats and marine oils formerly used. The commercial production of margarine demands that the product has closely controlled physical properties, for example, its spreadability at refrigeration temperatures, and the choice of ingredient fats is also closely related to the market, so that sophisticated least-cost programmes are used to control ingredient formulations. In recent years the evidence that polyunsaturated fats have beneficial effects on serum cholesterol levels has led to the production of margarines using highly unsaturated oils such as maize and sunflower oils, although as yet specific claims about these products and health benefits are not permitted in the UK. Despite this there has been a substantial increase in the consumption of margarines in general, and polyunsaturated ones in particular, since the 1984 COMA report on diet and cardiovascular disease (DHSS 1984). The earlier advice to reduce fat intake also acted as a stimulus to the development of low-fat products; in these the fat content is reduced to 40 g/100 g and they contain a range of emulsifiers. These low-fat products are suitable for use as spreads, but heating breaks the emulsion and they are therefore unsuitable for use in frying.

Composition of fats and oils

Butter and normal margarines contain water, small amounts of protein, and added salt. Margarines are required by UK legislation to be fortified with vitamins A and D, so that they are nutritionally equivalent to butter. Plant oils are usually virtually entirely triglyceride, although they often contain significant concentrations of tocopherols which act as natural antioxidants. The main aspect of composition of nutritional importance is the fatty acid composition of the different fats. The chapter on lipids contains an extended account of the fatty acid composition of fats and oils and their metabolism. It must be remembered that all the fats listed are natural products, or derived from natural products, and therefore show variations in composition. This is further complicated by the fact that much blending of oils occurs, and it is often difficult to be absolutely sure that a named oil is authentic; this is not a matter of deception but that different oils are frequently processed in the same industrial plant and carryover occurs.

Nutritional role of fats and oils

Fats provide a source of energy and are the most energy-rich of the proximate nutrients, with a gross energy value of 9.4 kcal/g. The concentration of fat in a food or the diet is the major determinant of its energy density, and in circumstances where the weight of food to be carried is critical, for example in rations for an expedition, or in combat rations, a high fat content is often desirable, since the immediate risks are greater than the longer-term risks associated with high fat intakes. Fats also provide the essential fatty acids and contribute to the absorption of the fat-soluble vitamins. Fats are also important in connection with the palatability of foods. Many of the characteristic aromas associated with cooked foods are due to interactions between the lipids and the amino acids in foods. The fat in foods is also associated with satiety, by mechanisms that are not clearly understood, but which may be related to the effects of fats on gastric emptying (Hunt & Stubbs 1975) and interactions with gastrointestinal hormones.

The links between fat and the palatability of foods have profound nutritional implications because they act as a constraint on the adoption of nutritional advice to reduce total fat intakes. The introduction of low-fat and polyunsaturated margarines is one avenue of attack on this problem, but does not address the use of fats and oils as cooking media in frying, and as ingredients in cakes, pastries and similar foods. Here the approach may lie in the development of oils with physical characteristics that minimize their penetration into foods, or that drain rapidly from the cooked food. Other more sophisticated approaches lie in the development of fat substitutes, and one of these based on fatty acid esters of sucrose has the required organoleptic properties; it now has to meet the food safety and nutritional requirements for a fat substitute.

REFERENCES

Department of Health and Social Security 1984 Diet and cardiovascular disease. Reports on Health and Social Subjects 28, HMSO, London
Health Education Council 1983 Proposals for nutritional guidelines for health education in Britain. National Advisory Committee on Nutrition Education, London Holland B, Unwin ID, Buss DH 1989 Milk products and eggs, 4th Suppl. to McCance and Widdowson's The Composition of Foods. Royal Society of Chemistry, London
Hunt JN, Stubbs DF 1975 The volume and energy content of meals as determinants of gastric emptying. Journal of Physiology 245: 209–225
Mabbitt LA, Davies FL, Law BA, Marshall VM 1987 Microbiology of milk and milk products. In : Norris JR,

Pettipher GL (eds) Essays in agriculture and food microbiology. John Wiley, Chichester, pp.135–166
Ministry of Agriculture, Fisheries and Food 1984–1992 Household food consumption and expenditure 1983–91. Annual Reports of the National Food Survey Committee. HMSO, London
Paul AA, Southgate DAT 1978 McCance and Widdowson's The composition of food, 4th edn. HMSO, London
Regenstein JM, Regenstein CE 1984 Food protein chemistry. Academic Press, Orlando
Royal College of Physicians, British Nutrition Foundation 1984 Food intolerance and food aversion. Journal of the Royal College of Physicians London 18:3–41
Van Stuyvenberg JH 1969 (ed) Margarine. Liverpool University Press, Liverpool

20. Beverages, herbs and spices

D. A. T. Southgate

BEVERAGES

Although not formally a nutrient, water is an essential component of the human diet, required to maintain the hydration of tissues and the composition of the extracellular fluid compartments of the body. While many foods contain substantial amounts of water, additional sources of water are essential, even for infants consuming milk.

The consumption of water alone is not particularly attractive to many people, and indeed the water supply of much of the world's population is unattractive aesthetically, and frequently a source of pathogenic organisms and a major cause of morbidity. Whether these are the reasons for the development of a wide range of alternative beverages is debatable, but certainly humans prefer to drink water flavoured with other substances. The discovery of fermentation and the effects of consuming dilute solutions of ethanol undoubtedly contributed to this popularity, and a range of beverages containing other pharmacologically active components is also widely consumed. In many societies the offering of a beverage is an integral part of welcoming a guest, and beverages often have a central role in their food cultures, so that the consumption of a beverage also has a symbolic role (Fieldhouse 1986).

In the production of virtually all beverages great importance is attached to the organoleptic quality of the finished product, because this is a major factor in the acceptability of the beverage. The human sensory apparatus is extraordinarily discriminating (Barlow & Mollon 1982) and can detect very subtle differences in the flavour of beverages, and in many cases beverage production and consumption has evolved a highly developed language to describe the most critical differences in flavour. This is reflected in the literature, where much attention has been given to the flavour constituents and relatively little to the nutrients the beverages supply. Fortunately for the nutritionist the variation in the nutritional composition of most beverages is not nearly as diverse as the variation in flavour.

Non-alcoholic beverages

Soft drinks

These range from products consisting of water with added sugar and flavouring, to those containing some fruit juice or fruit homogenates. The simplest products, soda waters, contain carbonated water, that is water that has been treated with carbon dioxide under pressure; tonic waters contain a little quinine to give a bitterness and sharpness to the flavour.

The most widely consumed products contain a flavoured mixture in carbonated water – the colas are the major beverages of this kind. The base syrup has a closely guarded composition consisting of a mixture of flavours. Originally the mixture contained an extract of the kola nut which contains alkaloids of the cocaine family, but the present mixtures are more benign, containing caffeine and other flavouring together with caramel as colour. Some of the colas contain appreciable levels of phosphoric acid and are therefore strongly acidic. The original formulations of these products contained sucrose as the carbohydrate; however, some formulations contain high-fructose syrups and consumer demands for low-calorie products led to the development of formulations without carbohydrate, and with the sweetness provided originally by saccharin but now more commonly by aspartame. The syrups are distributed worldwide and bottled locally. Strict quality control is maintained and this may require the use of de-ionized water in the bottling plant. In countries where drinking water is of doubtful quality these products are very attractive because the brand image offers a guarantee of safety.

Lemonade, orangeade and a large variety of proprietary products are similarly carbonated, flavoured, sugary drinks, often with citric and other fruit acids added to enhance the fruit flavour, although in the UK these drinks contain no fruit material. Low-calorie formulations contain saccharin or aspartame, and quite commonly a mixture of the two.

Fruit squashes contain a defined proportion of the named fruit added to a solution of carbohydrate, and comminuted products contain a defined proportion of comminuted, i.e. macerated, fruit. Lower-calorie products utilize sweeteners rather than the sugar solution. These drinks are usually marketed in a concentrated form intended for dilution (one part to four of water is common) before consumption.

The nutritional role of these beverages is essentially limited to making the consumption of water attractive, while the carbohydrate they contain contributes energy. Typically they contain about 10 g/100 ml of carbohydrate (Table 20.1) and therefore provide around 40 kcal/100 ml, so the consumption of a typical can does provide a significant contribution to energy intake. The high acidity of these beverages has caused concern in relation to the possible association with dental caries.

Although sucrose is probably the most commonly used carbohydrate, the acidity of most of these drinks is sufficient to produce inversion to glucose and fructose. In the USA there is a substantial use of high-fructose syrups produced enzymatically from glucose syrups derived from the hydrolysis of starch. These syrups are sweeter than the equivalent sucrose syrup, and are also reported to enhance fruit flavours; tariff barriers currently limit their use in Europe. Glucose syrups are used in some preparations, where they produce 'body' and enhance mouth-feel without sweetness.

Fruit juices

These are produced by expression from the fruits, and the name is reserved in food labelling for products that are derived from fruit, although some additions are permitted and some products are derived by dilution from imported concentrates. The major sources of fruit juice are citrus fruits, with orange, grapefruit, lemon and lime being important. Pineapple, apple and grape juices are all widely consumed. In continental Europe fruit nectars are also popular; these are prepared by mixing fruit juices with a syrup. Apricot, pear and peach varieties are among the more common varieties. In juice production the fruit is washed and then pressed; the equipment to express citrus fruits prevents the expression of the skin, which could impart undesirable bitter flavours. The processes are

Table 20.1   Composition of soft drinks (per 100 ml)

	Cola	Lemonade	Lime juice cordial undiluted	Orange drink undiluted
Water (g)	89.8	94.6	70.5	71.2
Energy				
(kcal)	39	21	112	107
(kJ)	168	90	479	457
Sugars (g)	10.5	5.6	29.8	28.5
Sodium (mg)	8	7	8	21
Potassium (mg)	1	1	49	17
Calcium (mg)	4	5	9	8

These drinks contain only traces of other nutrients
From Paul & Southgate (1978)

designed to maximize the yield of juice; however, the pectic substances in the fruit can act to restrict yield and it is common to use pectolytic enzymes to increase the volume expressed. The concentration processes are designed to minimize the loss of flavour components, and the conditions favourable to flavour retention also favour retention of vitamin C. In the production of apple juice, discoloration due to the activity of polyphenol oxidases is limited by the addition of vitamin C as a processing aid. The developments in processing and packaging of fruit juices over the last decade have played a major role in increasing consumption. Canning was the major form of packaging up to the 1960s, but since that time pasteurization and aseptic packaging in laminated cardboard packs have led to greatly improved quality and lower transport costs.

The fruit juices are very similar in composition to the fruits from which they are derived, because the plant cell-wall material which is separated in the process represents only a small proportion of the fruit. Fruit juices show similar variations in composition to those seen in fruits, where cultural conditions, solar radiation and post-harvest handling can produce significant variations in sugars, organic acids, inorganic constituents and vitamins. Some typical values for the composition of a range of juices are given in Table 20.2 (Southgate et al 1990).

Nutritionally, fruit juices contain all the nutrients present in fruits, with the exception of the dietary fibre; their major role therefore lies in the provision of vitamin C, although they do provide minor amounts of other vitamins and minerals. The consumption of fruit juice as part of a meal such as breakfast results in a substantial improvement in the availability of iron in the meal as a whole. The increased consumption of fruit juices in the UK has been one of the more

Table 20.2   Typical values for the composition of fruit juices (per 100 ml)

Fruit and type of juice	Water	Protein	Sugars	Energy (kcal)	(kJ)	
Citrus						
Orange						
freshly squeezed	87.7	0.6	9.4	39	163	UK
	88.3	0.7	10.4*	42	176	USA
range of US values	87.2–89.6	0.6–1.0	9.3–11.3*			
frozen concentrate	58.2	2.3	38.0*	152	636	USA
diluted ready to consume	88.1	0.7	10.7*	43	180	USA
canned unsweetened	88.7	0.4	8.5	33	138	UK
	87.4	0.8	11.2*	45	188	USA
canned sweetened	85.8	0.7	12.8	51	213	UK
	86.5	0.7	12.2*	49	205	USA
Grapefruit						
freshly squeezed	90.0	0.5	9.2*	37	154	USA
range of values	89.0–90.4	0.4–0.5	8.8–10.2*			
frozen concentrate						
unsweetened	59.1	2.1	34.6*	139	582	USA
sweetened	57.0	1.6	40.2*	157	657	USA
canned unsweetened	89.8	0.7	7.9	32	133	UK
	89.2	0.5	9.8*	39	163	USA
sweetened	87.3	0.5	9.7	38	159	UK
	88.7	0.6	10.1	40	167	USA
Lemon						
freshly squeezed	91.3	0.2	1.6	7	29	UK
	91.0	0.5	8.0*	32	133	USA
frozen concentrate	58.0	2.3	37.4*	150	628	USA
diluted ready to consume	92.0	0.4	7.2*	29	121	USA
canned unsweetened	90.3	0.3	9.0*	35	146	USA
Lime						
freshly squeezed	90.3	0.3	9.0*	35	140	USA
canned unsweetened	90.3	0.3	9.0	35	140	UK
	93.0	0.2	6.7	26	109	USA
Tangerine and other small citrus fruits	89.9	0.5	10.1	40.0	163	
Other						
Grapejuice, canned	82.9	0.2	16.6	63	264	SWE
Apple, canned	88.0	0.2	10.2	39	163	SWE
Apricot, nectar canned	84.6	0.3	14.6	56	234	SWE
Pear, nectar canned	86.2	0.3	13.2	51	213	SWE
Peach, nectar canned	87.2	0.2	12.4	47	197	SWE
Pineapple						
frozen concentrate	53.0	1.3	44.5	172	720	USA
diluted ready to consume	86.0	0.4	12.8	50	210	
canned unsweetened	86.1	0.3	13.4	51	213	UK
	85.6	0.4	13.5	52	278	USA

* These values are measured 'by difference' and include organic acids

striking changes in the UK diet recorded by the National Food Survey (MAFF, 1984–92). The data show that fruit juices now make a major contribution to vitamin C intakes. Fruit juice consumption also tends to remain relatively stable throughout the year, so that it provides vitamin C when fresh fruits are less available (Southgate et al 1989).

Tea, coffee and cocoa

Although these beverages are derived from different plants and their methods of production are very different, they are often considered together because they contain alkaloids of the methyl xanthine group – caffeine, theobromine and theophylline – of which caffeine is the most active and acts as a stimulant, and which can prevent fatigue. In some individuals caffeine produces an increased heart rate and restlessness. Habituation to caffeine is quite common but the substance is not strictly addictive (Nutrition Reviews 1979).

Tea

Tea is produced from the leaves and buds of the tea plant *Thea sinensis*; as the name implies, the plant and the beverage originated in China, where it has been consumed for a very long time. It was introduced into Europe in the 17th century as a luxury commodity. The plant was introduced to Sri Lanka and then into India, Assam and the hilly districts of south India, and large plantations were planted to meet the demands of the then British Empire.

The plant grows as a shrub, requiring a fertile soil, a warm climate and a good rainfall. The tea plants are allowed to grow to a height of about four feet and are then pruned to maintain this size. The leaves are picked by hand, primarily because of the delicacy required to prevent damage to the leaves. After picking the leaves are allowed to wither, then rolled and allowed to ferment, which produces changes in the polyphenolic components and leads to darkening of the leaves, rendering the tannin components more soluble. This process produces black tea; green teas such as those originally used in China are produced by withering the leaves at a higher temperature and omitting the fermentation stage.

The teas produced by the various plantations differ in quality, as judged by the size of the leaf and especially by the flavour of the infusion. Teas are blended to produce the flavours required by different consumers.

Nutritionally these differences are of little significance because the amounts of nutrients extracted into the infusions are very small. The tannins are responsible for much of the astringency of tea, which is desired by some consumers but rejected by others. The polyphenolic materials react with proteins and also with divalent ions, such as iron, and tea produces a reduction in the bioavailability of iron consumed with tea. Small quantities of trace elements present in tea are extracted into the infusions, but these have not been associated with any increased morbidity.

Herbal teas

The leaves of many plants are dried and used to produce flavoured infusions which are drunk in many countries, for example camomile, peppermint, rosemary and jasmine. Many of these are attractive alternatives to conventional teas: they are usually lower in tannins and less astringent; they do not, however, have any proven special nutritional benefits (Bender 1986) and the injudicious selection of a plant leaf for making a tea can lead to infusions that contain pharmacologically active levels of natural toxicants.

Coffee

Coffee is produced from the seeds of cultivated varieties of three species, *Coffea arabica*, *C. liberica* and *C. robusta*, trees that are widely cultivated in the tropics. The major plantations are in Brazil, Kenya, India and Indonesia. The plants grow as evergreen trees, usually in plantations which contain other larger trees to provide shade. The trees produce berries when 6–14 years old. The green berries undergo a natural fermentation after harvesting, which is essential for the development of flavour and aroma. These, however, only become really apparent after roasting, which produces the characteristic flavour volatiles. These aromas are unstable and the flavour of coffee infusions prepared from freshly roasted beans is regarded by many as the ultimate standard of quality. As with tea, considerable skill is exercised in the blending of coffees for retail sale.

Instant coffees These are produced by drying infusions of selected blends of coffee under very carefully controlled conditions, to minimize the loss of flavour volatiles and the development of undesirable flavours. The early production involved the use of spray-drying, but more sophisticated vacuum procedures are now employed and some use is also made of freeze-drying. The processes inevitably lead to some changes in the balance of aromas, but increasingly sophisticated sensory analysis coupled with knowledge of the chemical nature of many of the flavour volatiles has produced a range of products, which because of their convenience have overtaken in popularity the consumption of coffee from infused beans.

Decaffeinated coffee This is prepared by extracting the ground coffee or an infusion with a solvent that selectively removes caffeine. The process is very difficult to carry out without altering the balance of the flavour, and most decaffeinated coffees can be distinguished from traditional infusions; nevertheless, they are useful for those who must, or who wish to, avoid the consumption of caffeine. The choice of solvent has come under scrutiny recently because of the possibility of residues in the final product.

Nutritionally, coffee infusions from ground beans extract only minor quantities of many nutrients, but instant coffees contain significant concentrations of potassium and many other inorganic constituents, which are present in a readily soluble form in the powder. Roasting coffee leads to the production of nicotinic acid, and instant coffees provide an appreciable level when diluted for consumption. Table 20.3 gives some typical values for the nutritional composition of these beverages.

Cocoa (chocolate)

Cocoa is derived from the seeds of a tree native to central America, *Theobroma cacao*, a tree that grows only in tropical regions. The trees are often not cultivated in plantations and the harvesting of the fruit in many areas is still done on a relatively small scale. The exception to this are plantations in Malaysia, where larger-scale production is being developed.

The ripe fruits are split and the pulp and seeds are formed into large mounds, sometimes on the forest floor, and covered with leaves. The pulp attracts insects and the mound undergoes a natural fermentation. The isolated seeds are then dried and packed for the wholesale trade. The beans are roasted and crushed and sieved to produce cocoa nibs, these are then finely ground to produce cocoa mass. This mass sets on cooling and is the basic material from which chocolate is manufactured. Cocoa butter can be expressed from this mass, leaving a residual chocolate powder or cocoa, which was traditionally used as a beverage although in the UK the more important beverages are prepared from a mixture of cocoa and sucrose.

Nutritionally cocoa as a beverage is a significant source of several nutrients (Table 20.3) and its value is often enhanced because it is prepared with milk, which contributes other nutrients. The major alkaloid in cocoa is theobromine, a name ('food of the gods') which is a reflection of the status of cocoa as a food in the ancient cultures of Central America.

Proprietary beverages

A range of products have been produced that are used as beverages in a way somewhat analogous to cocoa. The formulations are designed to produce a nutritious beverage mixture, that when mixed with hot water or milk is suitable for adults and children. The composition of drinking chocolate is included in Table 20.3. The base can be cereal, with the addition of milk solids, soya or egg to provide additional protein; some products are fortified with vitamins to enhance their nutritional value and image.

Mineral waters

Waters from natural springs, particularly those with a pronounced flavour, have been ascribed health-giving properties by many cultures during human development, and in more credulous times were assigned miraculous healing powers. These claims led to the development of spa towns and cities, where the fashionable members of society gathered to 'take the cure'. This custom is still popular on the continent and the health farm is an analogous modern development, where a rigorous regimen of diet and other therapies is believed to repair the damage induced by over indulgence.

Many of these natural waters are rich in mineral salts, and others contain sulphurous compounds;

Table 20.3 Composition of cocoa, coffee and tea (per 100 g)

	Cocoa		Coffee		Tea	
	Powder	Drinking chocolate	Infusion	Instant	Leaves	Infusion
Water (g)	3.4	2.1	—	3.4	9.3	—
Energy						
(kcal)	312	336	2	100	108	< 1
(kJ)	1301	1554	8	424	455	2
Protein (g)	18.5	5.5	0.2	14.6	19.6	0.1
Fat (g)	21.7	6.0	trace	0	2.0	trace
Sugars (g)	trace	73.8	trace	6.5	3.0	trace
Starch (g)	11.5	3.6	0.3	4.5	trace	trace
Sodium (mg)	950	250	trace	41	45	trace
Potassium (mg)	1500	410	66	4000	2160	17
Calcium (mg)	130	33	2	160	430	trace
Phosphorus (mg)	350	190	2	350	630	1
Iron (mg)	1.9	2.4	trace	4.4	15.2	trace

From Paul & Southgate (1978)

many in fact claim slight radioactivity as one of their desirable attributes! The benefits of consuming the spa waters were most probably due to the fact that they replaced excessive alcohol consumption, but the high mineral content that characterizes some of them would have had some purgative properties. Others claim benefits as a diuretic when consumed at 4 litres per day! These waters maintained an image of being fashionable, beneficial and safe, when the public water supply was of doubtful quality.

In recent years bottled water consumption has markedly increased in the UK, and although it is difficult to determine the reasons for this increase, it probably parallels concerns about the quality, particularly the organoleptic quality, of the public water supply. The fashionable image created by advertising must also be a contributory factor.

Some of the longer-established European waters are Appollinarius, Evian, Vichy and Perrier. Malvern and Ashburton are popular English ones. Many retailers produce their own-label brands of bottled water and Scottish Highland water is marketed as the only water that is proper to add to Scotch whisky.

Nutritionally these waters have virtually no special properties, apart from contributing minor quantities of sodium, calcium and magnesium to the diet. Their composition is known, however, and they may have some merits where the water supply is contaminated, for example, with high levels of nitrate.

Tap water

It would be incorrect to leave the discussion of non-alcoholic beverages without some mention of water itself. In the UK this can be quite reasonably be called tap water, because relatively few people rely on wells for their supply. The development of a public supply of clean water was one of the major contributions to public health in the UK in the 19th century. The public water supply is drawn from three major sources in the UK: subterranean aquifers, reservoirs, and to a lesser extent, rivers. The aquifers are often in chalk and the water from these sources tends to be rich in calcium and magnesium and therefore 'hard', but the water having percolated through the subsoil to reach the aquifer is low in bacterial contamination, and usually needs less purification. The major reservoirs collect water from precipitation over hilly catchment areas, and where the water runs over granite rocks it can be very low in mineral content and is characteristically 'soft'. River sources are constrained by the difficulties in controlling pollution from domestic sewage, industrial and farm wastes, and rivers used for

water supply have very closely regulated catchments. Both reservoir and river waters require extensive purification; this may involve the treatment of the water with salts to flocculate particulate matter suspended in the water, which would otherwise slow filtration. The filtration beds are composed of layers of increasingly finer particles of sand, with charcoal to act as a final decolorizer and deodorizer. While these treatments remove most organisms, the water is not sterile and treatment with chlorine is common as a final protective measure.

In many Middle Eastern countries with low rainfall, alternative supplies of drinking water have been developed. These have involved the construction of desalination plants where seawater is distilled and the distilled water is blended with seawater to give water of potable osmolality. The development of solar stills has also made considerable progress; in these the sunlight falls on black-coated panels supported on frames placed on the ground, and the absorbed heat evaporates the water from the soil, which condenses and runs off and is collected. Water, particularly hard water, can provide an appreciable intake of calcium, and water intake cannot be discounted in calcium balance studies. Soft water can solubilize the lead from water pipes, and these older pipes are being replaced in soft-water areas. Some water authorities used to partially soften very hard water using ion-exchange processes, but these have largely been discontinued because the process adds sodium to the water. The epidemiological links between soft water and cardiovascular disease that have been seen in many countries were regarded as sufficiently convincing to lead to official advice to discontinue softening, and current regulations in the UK require an unsoftened supply for drinking in houses fitted with softeners. The widespread use of nitrogenous fertilizers in agriculture has led to some concerns about nitrate levels in drinking water, particularly those derived from rivers and reservoirs whose catchments include agricultural land. The direct links between nitrate levels and morbidity are not strong, but revised standards have been adopted by the European Community as a precautionary measure.

Alcoholic beverages

Fermented beverages containing alcohol appear to have been part of the human diet from very early times and the consumption of these beverages in many cultures is associated with special or festive occasions. Ethyl alcohol is a drug that depresses higher nervous function, and at low doses produces a feeling of well-being and freedom from worry. It lowers inhibitory control, and for this reason acts as a social drug that promotes fellowship. At higher levels of consumption it produces intoxication and unconsciousness, and eventually inhibits the respiratory centre, leading to death. It is interesting to note that whereas in the Judaic-Christian religion wine-drinking is permitted, the Islamic tradition forbids the consumption of alcohol (see Chapter 7).

A very wide range of fermented beverages is consumed by man, most of which involve the use of yeasts. The products of fermentation are principally ethanol and carbon dioxide, but many other substances are also produced, including other alcohols, methanol and higher alcohols, and organic acids. These components interact in the beverage to produce the characteristic flavours and aromas valued by the discerning consumer. The minor components, the congeners, are responsible for some of the unpleasant hangover effects of the over-consumption of these beverages.

Beers, ales and stout

This type of beverage is produced by the fermentation of cereal, usually barley, with yeast. The barley is first malted by allowing the grains to germinate in a warm atmosphere; this activates the amylolytic diastases in the grain, and hydrolysis of the starch begins. At a suitable point the sprouted grains are heated in a kiln to inactivate the enzymes and produce malted barley. The dried malt is then ground and mixed with water to produce a mash. The fluid from this process, the wort, is then heated to stop enzyme activity and kill any adventitious microorganisms. Hops or hop extract are added at this stage to give the characteristic bitter flavour, and the cooled wort is inoculated with a selected yeast culture. *Saccharomyces cerevisiae* is used to make the traditional British beers which have a top

fermentation. Lager-type beers use a bottom-fermenting strain, *S. carlsbergensis (uvarum)*. The character of the finished product is determined by the fermentation conditions and the precise strain of yeast used. The fermented wort is then allowed to stand to flocculate the yeast, and flocculating substances are often employed. Some beers are filtered to produce a clear bright drink, but in traditional beers the clarity is achieved by racking. The beers may be pasteurized before bottling or canning. More traditional producers prefer to maintain the stability of their product by skilled cellar management.

The composition of some typical beers is given in Table 20.4 which shows that the alcohol content usually ranges between 3 and 7 g/100 ml. The alcohol strength is determined primarily by the concentration of carbohydrates in the wort, and in the UK beers are taxed on the basis of the specific gravity of the wort; the higher-gravity worts also contain higher concentrations of the other constituents derived from the original barley. Higher alcohol concentrations can be produced using higher-gravity worts and selected yeasts; these special beers are sometimes called barley wines. Beers contain low concentrations of riboflavin and nicotinic acid, and may provide a good source of available iron whose absorption is enhanced by alcohol. The complete fermentation of the carbohydrates can produce beers with very low concentrations of carbohydrate, which are sometimes promoted for diabetics. Current opinion is that these confer no advantages for the diabetic and that the higher alcohol levels are disadvantageous because of their effects on glucogenesis in the liver.

Other beers

Worldwide, a range of other substrates is fermented to produce products that resemble beer, at least in

Table 20.4 Composition of some beers (per 100 ml)

	Brown ale	Bitter			Lager	Pale ale	Stout	Strong ale
		Canned	Draught	Keg				
Alcohol (g)	2.2	3.1	3.1	3.0	3.2	3.3	4.3	6.6
Energy								
(kcal)	28	32	32	31	29	32	39	72
(kJ)	117	132	132	129	120	133	163	301
Sugars (g)	3.0	2.3	2.3	2.3	1.5	2.0	2.1	6.1
Sodium (mg)	16	9	12	8	4	10	4	15
Potassium (mg)	33	37	38	35	34	49	86	110

Beers contain traces of thiamin and about 0.02 mg riboflavin and 4 µg folates
From Paul & Southgate, 1978

their alcohol content. Cereals such as sorghum, maize and rice are fermented in similar ways: a preliminary germination to initiate starch hydrolysis, followed by drying, mashing and fermentation with yeasts. In many cases wild yeasts are the fermenting agent, and the products of fermentation can be very variable in composition and flavour. These beers are usually richer in other nutrients, and in some parts of Africa the beers are very rich in iron from the vessels used in the process, and have been associated with iron overload. Plant saps that are rich in sugars can be fermented, and toddy is produced in this way from palm-tree sap.

Cider, perry and mead

These beverages have possibly been known for much longer than most alcoholic beverages, especially mead, made from fermenting honey, which is mentioned by Homer and in the Norse sagas. Cider and perry are produced by fermenting the juices from crushed and pressed apples and pears respectively. The alcohol concentrations achieved are usually comparable to beers (Table 20.4) but concentrations comparable to those seen in wines – around 10 g/100 ml – can be achieved.

Wines

The concentrations of sugars in grapes are such that the juice can be fermented by the wild yeasts naturally present on the fruit without the addition of sugar. The name 'wine' is considered to apply only to the liquid produced by the fermentation of grape juice, although it is often applied to the fermented products of other fruits. Wine is another alcoholic beverage with a long history: the *Iliad* contains many references to wine, and the residues in amphoras from ancient shipwrecks in the Mediterranean provide evidence of a flourishing international trade in wine and olive oil.

The vine flourishes on quite shallow soils and can be cultivated in temperate climates. The grapes are harvested in the autumn, and the fruit is crushed to expel the juice. The grape juice or must is fermented traditionally with the yeasts on the surface of the fruit, but in modern wineries with selected strains of yeast. Red wines are produced by fermenting the juice together with the skins and stalks; white wines use the juice alone. The temperature in the fermentation vats must not be allowed to rise too high, or the desired fermentations that control the acidity of the wine will not take their proper course. Once the fermentation is complete the wine is run off into large casks or containers, to allow the yeasts and other particulate matter to settle; fining, the addition of substances such as isinglas to flocculate the sediment, may take place at this stage. The clear supernatant wine is removed, and this process of racking is repeated until the wine is clear. Red wines are usually stored in casks for some time before bottling, during which time a range of interactions occurs between the alcohols and acids in the wine, leading to the development of its aroma and flavour. The composition of the grapes is profoundly influenced by the soil type, cultural conditions and the climate during growth, so that a very large number of subtle variations is possible in the finished wine, producing the daunting number of types of wine available.

As far as the nutritionist is concerned these variations only produce a limited number of nutritionally significant effects. The most important are the variations in alcohol and sugar contents. In a wet season the sugar levels will be lower, producing less alcohol, and the sugar may be fermented out to leave a dry wine with very low carbohydrate concentrations. Minor variations in mineral levels also occur, depending on the soil where the grapes were grown. The major positive nutritional feature of wines lies in its enhancement of appetite. Clearly the over-consumption of wine carries with it the risks of alcoholism and cirrhosis. Table 20.5 gives some typical values for the composition of some wines.

Sparkling wines are produced in a number of ways, the most prestigious being the 'methode champenoise', where additional sugar is added to the fermented wine in the bottle, creating a secondary fermentation which produces the gas under pressure. Other less skilful and cheaper processes produce cheaper sparkling wines.

Fortified wines such as sherry and port contain appreciably higher concentrations of alcohol. The production of sherry in Spain depends on a secondary fermentation of the must after the first racking, when the flor yeast *S. ellipsoideus* develops on the surface. This yeast can tolerate higher concentrations of alcohol. The fermented wine is then blended in the solera system, where the wine passes through a series of casks over a prolonged period, the wine moving down the series to replace evaporative losses. The fermentation continues in the cask until the alcohol levels inhibit further growth of the yeast. The wine from the final series of casks is fined to flocculate particulate matter, and may be filtered and the alcohol content adjusted with highly rectified brandy.

Port is produced by the addition of brandy to a wine must that has only been fermented for a few days

Table 20.5 Composition of some wines (per 100 ml)

	Red	Rosé	Dry	Sweet	Sparkling	Port	Dry	Medium	Sweet
			White			Port	Sherry		
Alcohol (g)	9.5	8.7	9.1	10.2	9.9	15.9	15.7	14.8	15.6
Energy									
(kcal)	68	71	66	94	76	157	116	118	136
(kJ)	284	294	275	394	315	655	481	489	568
Sugars (g)	0.3	2.5	0.6	5.9	1.4	12.0	1.4	3.6	6.9
Sodium (mg)	10	4	4	13	4	4	10	6	13
Potassium (mg)	130	75	61	110	57	97	57	89	110
Iron (mg)	0.9	0.95	0.5	0.58	0.5	0.4	0.39	0.53	0.3

Spirits at 70° proof contain 31.7 g alcohol/100 ml
From Paul & Southgate (1978)

and which therefore still contains sugars. A concentrated syrup is added at the same time, and the wine is first stored in vats and then in casks to mature.

A number of other fortified wines are produced, for example Madeira, Masala and Malaga, which are produced by adding brandy to the wine, together with some sugary, flavoured extracts.

Vermouths are a class of fortified wine where complex mixtures of flavours and herbs, and usually sugars and alcohol, are added to a muscatel wine base.

Spirits

The process of distillation was developed by the early Arab chemists before 900 AD to produce perfumes, and was applied to wine early in the Middle Ages when the distilled beverages came to be popular. Water and alcohol form an azeotropic mixture and the production of pure alcohol is neither achieved nor desired in the production of spirits. The spirits are produced from virtually all carbohydrates that can be fermented, and the carbohydrate source largely determines the flavour and aroma of the different spirits, although there is a substantial production of neutral highly rectified spirits flavoured by the addition of other materials.

Brandy This is traditionally produced from the distillation of wine, the finest brandies being produced from wines produced in the Champagne district of France. The wine is distilled from pot-stills made of copper. Typically a series of distillations is used to increase the alcohol strength and to avoid the presence of unwanted methanol and other higher alcohols. The final distillation produces an alcohol concentration of around 70% by volume. The brandy is stored in cask for up to 20 years, during which time

considerable losses occur and the brandy extracts materials from the wood. A number of subtle reactions occur that produce the prized aromas, and the higher alcohols are oxidized and esterified. The cheaper brandies are distilled from lesser wines and are not aged for such a long time.

Whisky The traditional production of whisky is based on the fermentation of malted barley using relatively simple pot-stills. The malting of the barley, the kilning with peat fuel and the use of water running over peaty soils are responsible for the unique and distinctive flavours of malt whiskies. Much whisky is now distilled in patent or Coffey stills, which produce a higher final alcoholic distillate and one that has lost many of its flavour volatiles. This spirit is blended with malt whiskies to produce the bulk of whisky consumed. The freshly distilled spirit is matured in casks – ideally old sherry casks – during which time colour is extracted from the cask, the concentrations of the higher alcohols are reduced and the flavour and aromas develop. The minimum period in cask is 7 years, although the more expensive malt spirits may spend considerably longer.

Many other spirits are distilled from other carbohydrate sources, usually in patent stills which are run to produce a virtually neutral spirit which is subsequently flavoured with an extract of some kind: gin is flavoured with juniper berries, for example. The essentially neutral spirit is sold as vodka, and is generally mixed with fruit juice or other additions.

Liqueurs are a range of drinks where a strongly flavoured mixture and, usually, sugar, are blended with spirit, most commonly a neutral one but whisky and brandy are also used.

Nutritionally spirits must solely be regarded as a source of energy from the alcohol, as they contain virtually no other nutrients. The liqueurs also provide sugars and minor amounts of inorganic constituents. There are some exceptions, where eggs or cream are used.

The expression of alcohol contents on labels can be made in two ways. The older 'proof' system was based on the percentage of proof spirit present (proof spirit was originally the strength that would ignite when mixed with gunpowder, but is now less prosaically defined as 57.07% by volume at 51°F). This system is being replaced within the European Community by the simpler percentage by volume designation, the former Degrees Gay Lussac. Ethanol has a specific gravity of 0.790 and percentage by volume can be converted into g/100 ml by simple multiplication using this value.

HERBS AND SPICES

These are two groups of commodities used as ingredients to enhance the flavour and aroma of foods. They are produced from plants and this distinguishes them from flavourings in the food-labelling sense, although many food additives used as flavours are chemically identical to substances present naturally in herbs and spices.

Herbs

These are various parts of plants that are added to foods either in their fresh state or, more usually, after drying. Their use in the human diet has a very long history and the records of the ancient world contain many references to herbs, both as articles of commerce and in the preparation of foods. In many cases the development of herb gardens ran parallel with the development of the pharmaceutical use of plants. Herbal remedies are part of many cultures and their use persists today, often on an insecure basis of evidence, although there is no doubt that herbs skilfully used enhance many dishes. Dowell & Bailey (1983) provide a summary of the types of herbs in culinary use. The essential oils are the major source of the flavouring provided by herbs, and the level of use in most dishes is such that their contribution to nutritional value in the conventional sense is negligible, although making foods attractive to the consumer is important nutritionally, for a food that is not eaten has no nutritional value. The plants used as herbs can be a source of physiologically active compounds, as can be deduced from their origins in herbal medicine, and some of these substances are potentially toxic in large quantities; caution is desirable in the use of the leaves of plants other than those whose long history of use in the human diet suggests that they are safe.

Spices

These are dried parts or extracts of aromatic plants usually originating in the tropics. Like herbs, they provided the flavours of dishes in the ancient world and were highly prized, and the spice trade between Europe and the east led to many of the great voyages of exploration, including the discovery of America. As with herbs, a range of spices has been and is used, particularly in the Middle and Far East where the plants are indigenous. The spices owe their properties to essential oils and a range of astringent substances. These include many biologically active substances which at higher levels of consumption can exhibit toxicity (Liener 1969). Although the spices themselves contain significant concentrations of some vitamins (US Department of Agriculture 1977) the normal levels of use in foods makes their nutritional contribution negligible.

REFERENCES

Barlow HB, Mollon JD 1982 (eds) The senses. Cambridge University Press, Cambridge

Bender AE 1986 Health or hoax. Sphere Books, London

Dowell P, Bailey A 1983 The book of ingredients. Mermaid Books, London

Fieldhouse P 1986 Food and nutrition: customs and culture. Croom Helm, London

Liener IE 1969 (ed) Toxic constituents in plant foodstuffs. Academic Press, New York

Ministry of Agriculture, Fisheries and Food 1984–92. Household food consumption and expenditure 1983–91. Annual Reports of the National Food Survey Committee. HMSO, London

Nutrition Reviews 1979 Workshop on caffeine. Nutrition Reviews 37: 124–126

Paul AA, Southgate DAT 1978 McCance and Widdowson's The composition of food, 4th ed. HMSO, London

Southgate DAT, Johnson IT, Fenwick GR 1990 Nutrition, safety and contamination. In: Hicks D (ed) The production and packaging of non-carbonated fruit juices and fruit beverages. Blackie and Son, Glasgow, pp. 309–329

US Department of Agriculture 1977 Composition of foods. Handbook No. 8 revision, 8–2 Spices and herbs. US Government Printing Office, Washington

21. Food processing

D. A. T. Southgate and I. Johnson

Much of the food consumed in a developed country such as the United Kingdom has undergone some kind of food processing. The chapters on the major food groups include brief accounts of the ways in which the foods within those groups are processed and the effects of the processes on the nutrient contents of those foods; in this chapter some of the main features of food processing as a whole are discussed although in a text on nutrition it is clearly impossible to cover the details of the technology of food processing. Detailed accounts of these are available in several excellent specialized texts.

Many of the traditional methods of food processing, such as the milling of cereal grains to produce flours, the fermentation of cereals in the production of breads, the enzyme and heat treatments used in the production of cheeses, for example, are so well established that they are regarded as 'natural' by many critics of food processing. Analogously the traditional techniques for preserving foods, such as drying, smoking or preservation with chemicals such as salt, acetic acid (vinegar) or alcohol, have such an ancient history of use that they are regarded as unexceptional. These traditional forms of food processing came into use gradually, and improved the acceptability and nutritional value of the unprocessed foodstuffs, and also provided a way of extending the availability of the food supply beyond the periods of abundance that occurred at harvest time. This extension of the food supply into periods when plant foods could not be produced or animals maintained because of seasonal changes represents the most important contribution of food processing to human social evolution and the development of civilization, because it freed humans from the virtually continuous search for food which characterizes the life of the hunter–gatherer.

DEVELOPMENT OF URBAN SOCIETIES

While human societies remained close to the sites of food production, the traditional methods of process-

ing foods on a small scale in the village bakery or dairy, and in the home, were adequate to provide the community with a reasonably secure food supply. The distances over which foods had to travel to market were short, and the time between production and consumption were therefore also short, so that the fact that many foods were perishable was not a great cause of health problems. It should, however, be recognized that the failure of a harvest due to adverse weather conditions or plant and animal disease had very severe consequences, just as it does in much of the developing world today. Furthermore, until the introduction of heat processing and canning, and later refrigeration, many animal products were difficult to store safely without recourse to salting or drying. Thus in medieval times, at the end of the winter in northern Europe, many basic foodstuffs were in short supply and the nutritional quality of much of the food that was available would have been rather low.

When the industrial revolution began to draw workers and their families from the countryside into the town, they became isolated from the areas where food was produced. Furthermore, the demand for labour was such that women and children were frequently also employed. These two factors created a need for the safe transport of foods from the farms to the towns, and also made reliance on the traditional ways of preparing foods in the home less secure. The modern food industry arose under these twin pressures, first to process foods so that they could safely be transported without deterioration, and second, to move many of the traditional ways of preserving and cooking foods out of the domestic kitchen into the factories of the food processor.

The processing industry, once established, was responsible for a large number of major technological advances; for example, the development of heat processes for the drying, pasteurization and canning of foods, which proved important in controlling the bacterial deterioration of foods and food poisoning. Refrigeration was developed as a method for controlling the spoilage of meats and other foods during prolonged storage and transport, and later deep-freezing developed as a technique for retaining the quality of the most perishable foods, vegetables and fish.

At the present time, in a country such as the United Kingdom, the majority of the food consumed has been processed in some way. Without the use of many of these processing methods it would be difficult to maintain the population at its present size and nutritional status.

NUTRITIONAL VALUE OF 'PROCESSED', 'NATURAL' AND 'HEALTH' FOODS

As will be evident from the above discussion, many of the foods that are perceived as 'natural' have been processed in some way, even if that processing was, for example, the storage of an apple in controlled atmospheres to prolong its shelf-life. It is extremely difficult to argue that 'natural' has any real scientific meaning, because the techniques of animal and plant production have developed alongside those of the food producer (Southgate 1984). Regulatory bodies such as the UK Ministry of Agriculture, Fisheries and Food's (MAFF) Food Advisory Committee would prefer that the term 'natural' as applied to food was no longer used. The techniques used in food processing do affect the concentrations of some nutrients in food, particularly heat treatment, which causes the loss of the labile vitamins which are discussed later in this chapter.

This does not contradict the argument that there are genuine concerns about the techniques used in the processing of foods. Some of these relate to the nature of the processes themselves, and others to the use of additives of various kinds. These issues relate primarily to the safety of processed foods rather than to their nutritional value. There are other concerns about the nutritional composition of processed foods which relate primarily to their formulation in respect of the major components.

A food producer is in business to make a profit for the shareholders of the company, and to maintain his workforce and the plant in which the company has invested. In order for him to remain in business, therefore, the customers must continue to purchase and consume the foods produced. The producer has a legal obligation regarding the safety and quality of the products, and none would wish to disadvantage the consumers on which the business depends. However, the foods must be attractive to the consumer and appeal to the senses. Obviously the manufacturer has no interest in producing foods whose qualities would limit the amounts consumed. It is in this connection that most nutritional concerns arise. There are great pressures to produce foods that have high hedonic ratings, preferably higher than those of a competitor's product, so there has been a tendency in the past to focus attention on those properties that contribute to the acceptability of foods; for example, to incorporate sweetness from sucrose in products, and to add salt or monosodium glutamate to enhance the flavour of savoury foods. In addition, as all admirers of traditional French cuisine will know, the incorporation of fat has important benefits in terms of postprandial satisfaction.

In nutritional terms, therefore, the pressures on the food producer in the past have not been compatible with the current health messages from the nutritionists. Fortunately, the evidence for a relation between diet and health and disease have been accepted by the consumer and the food industry, so that the nutritional composition of a product is beginning to become a factor in determining consumer choice, thus creating demands for lower levels of fat, salt and sugar in processed foods.

Many of the specific claims about so-called 'health' foods are difficult to substantiate, and current legislation in the European Community (EC) and the United States positively discourages health claims for foods, especially when related to protection from, or treatment of, a specific disease. This is seen as making a medicinal or drug claim for a food and thereby blurs the boundary between foods and medicines. Many plant foods do contain biologically active substances, in fact much of the pharmaceutical industry has developed from the herbal remedies of the past; some of these substances are, however, also toxic and their use carries some risk. The claims for other 'health' foods rest on less substantial evidence, some of which could almost be regarded as magical and sometimes even fraudulent (Bender 1986).

NEW FOODS

The financial pressures on the food processor are such that there is a continual search for new improved products, and innovation is a major feature of a successful food processor. In most cases the changes involve minor alterations in formulation or presentation, but the financial pressures are also to improve the added value given to the basic ingredients by processing; this can lead to the use of lower-quality ingredients or a search for cheaper ingredients to replace expensive ones. The existing food legislation requires the product purchased to 'be of the nature, substance and quality demanded by the consumer', a phraseology originally worded to prevent fraud in the formulation of foods by adulteration.

The food producers, in their search for innovation, may also develop radically new processes or foods; for example, the use of irradiation to extend shelf-life or the development of non-digestible and therefore low-calorie fat substitutes. In the UK these are controlled on an informal basis (at the time of writing, 1992) by the Advisory Committee on Novel Foods and Processes (ACNFP), a joint committee of the Departments of Agriculture and Health which considers whether these novel foods pose safety, nutritional or toxicological hazards, and how their introduction to the food supply should be regulated. In the EC, the Scientific Committee for Food fulfils the analogous function.

One area of current activity concerns the use of genetic modification using techniques such as recombinant DNA technology in the production of novel foods; many of these techniques have close analogies with conventional plant and animal breeding techniques, and are therefore associated with similar risks, but new issues have to be considered such as the possibility of transfer of genetic material into the environment. This is a field that is expanding in importance (World Health Organization 1991).

FOOD LABELLING

So that the consumer is protected against fraudulent formulations and can be aware of the actual nature of a processed product, a series of food labelling regulations is in force in all developed countries. In the UK these are regulated by MAFF, although the national regulations are being progressively replaced by those of the EC. The precise nature of the regulations regarding labelling is in a state of development, but in general the labels are required to include a list of ingredients, including additives, listed in decreasing order of concentration. Nutritional labelling includes the energy values, the protein, fat, carbohydrate and fibre values as a minimum; however, if a nutritional claim is made about a product, then more extensive labelling for vitamins and mineral nutrients would become compulsory. At one time the EC was in favour of developing defined compositional standards for foods with specific names, but this is being replaced by more informative labels of what a product contains.

PROCESSES FOR THE PRESERVATION OF FOODS

The objective of these processes is to arrest the biological deterioration of foodstuffs due either to microrganisms contaminating the foods or to the intrinsic enzymes in the food which would bring about undesirable changes in appearance, odour, taste, texture or nutritional quality.

Heat treatments

In these the foods are either dried, a process which reduces the water activity in the product and so limits bacterial activity and enzymatic changes, or subjected to moist heat sufficient to make a product that is stable under ambient temperature storage. Drying produces changes in the sensory attributes of foods, and modern processes are designed to minimize these changes. Thus a series of high-temperature, short-time processes have been developed for processing liquid foods such as fruit juices and milk. Drying technologies have also been developed to minimize undesirable changes in flavour, the ultimate development in this field being the use of freeze-drying. This process is, however, very expensive and only viable for high-value products. The flavour components these processes are designed to protect are destroyed by factors that also lead to vitamin losses, so these new treatments have also improved nutritional quality.

Canning

This is the most vigorous heat treatment, given to inactive both vegetative and spore-forming bacteria. The canned product is sealed in a container and thus protected from oxidative changes. The can is conventionally made out of tin-plate, which protects the steel from rusting due to the water and residual oxygen in the food. In the sealed can there is a slow loss of tin into the food, which is accentuated when the can is opened – hence the advice not to store foods in cans once opened. The interior surface of the can may be protected with a lacquer. Canning is a rigorous heat treatment as it is essential for the entire contents to reach, and be maintained at, the required temperature. This can be difficult with large cans because of the low thermal conductivity of many foods. Heat treatment in plastic pouches has been developed, which overcomes some of the difficulties, but the materials for the pouches require special formulation and are thus expensive. Canning leads to a safe and stable product but the sensory changes are quite considerable, and there are losses of the more labile vitamins. It would be wrong to dismiss canned foods nutritionally, however, since many nutrients are retained completely in canning and others suffer losses only marginally greater than in some domestic procedures.

Refrigeration

This is another type of thermal processing in which heat is removed from the product. At temperatures of around 3–5°C the growth of most bacteria is slowed considerably, so that refrigeration is a very useful process for prolonging the storage or shelf-life of a product. Nutritionally it is satisfactory because enzyme activity is also lowered, so that the metabolism of nutrients is also reduced. Deep-freezing, where the food is brought to −18–20°C and then stored at these temperatures, extends storage for some food products almost indefinitely if the food is protected from losing water by sublimation. However, oxidative changes in fats still take place at this temperature, so that fatty foods can only be stored for a limited time. Deep-freezing depends on the very rapid removal of heat to reduce the size of ice crystals which form in the food; slow freezing produces larger crystals, which disrupt the texture of the food and can lead to increased enzyme activity on thawing with loss of quality. Many vegetables are blanched with steam or hot water to inactive enzymes before freezing.

Chemical preservatives

Chemicals such as salt, ethyl alcohol and acetic acid have been used for the preservation of foods for many generations, in the domestic salting of meats and vegetables and the preparation of pickles, for example, and their use has continued in the food industry. These methods rely on reducing the water activity or increasing the acidity so that pathogenic organisms cannot grow. A number of other substances have also come into use which directly inhibit bacterial or mould growth in foods; Table 21.1 lists those that are permitted in foods. Their use is closely controlled and the levels at which they are permitted

Table 21.1 Permitted preservatives (UK Preservatives in Food Regulations 1975)

Benzoic acid	Sodium nitrite
Methyl 4-hydroxybenzoate	2-hydroxybiphenyl
Ethyl 4-hydroxybenzoate	Propionic acid
Propyl 4-hydroxybenzoate	Sorbic acid
Biphenyl	Sulphur dioxide
Nisin	2-(thiazol-4-yl) benzimidazole
Sodium nitrate	Hexamine

in different foodstuffs are regulated on the basis of extensive safety evaluation. Some, such as sulphur dioxide and benzoates, have been linked with food intolerance in sensitive individuals. Sodium nitrite and nitrate, together with common salt, are permitted in cured meats where they have a synergistic effect in controlling *Clostridium botulinum*. Although there are concerns that the nitrate and nitrite may increase the levels of nitrosamines in food, the risks of botulism are so great without their use that they are still permitted.

Irradiation

If a food is treated with ionizing radiation from a radioactive source such as ^{60}Co, or an electron beam such as used in X-rays, the bacteria and many enzymes in foods are inactivated. The dose of radiation given to the food can be sufficiently high to sterilize the food, or at lower doses will pasteurize the surface organisms and kill insect pests in grain. It will also delay the ripening of a fruit such as a mango or strawberry, or sprouting in a potato. Table 21.2 gives some of the typical potential applications and the typical dose levels required. The irradiation of food has been considered in great depths by several expert committees. In the UK, the Advisory Committee on Irradiation and Novel Foods recommended that the process should be allowed under licence in the UK with an upper dose level of 10 kGy. This recommendation was reconsidered and endorsed by the Advisory Committee on Novel Foods and Processes (MAFF 1989a).

Cooking

The cooking procedures used in the processing of food are in most cases scaled-up versions of those used in the domestic kitchen. The major differences, apart from the size of the vessel, lie in the close control of the heating and other processes; first to achieve the desired quality of the product both in respect of sensory quality and microbiological safety. Second, because the economic implications of producing a large batch of an unacceptable product are powerful reasons for the levels of control used both in production and packaging. Close control is also exercised on the raw ingredients being used; however, these natural materials do exhibit variations in composition that may affect the final quality of the product. In many circumstances the processor has to either modify the process or use chemical processing aids to ensure that the product conforms to the

Table 21.2 Examples of applications of irradiation in food preservation

General application	Specific examples	Dose (Mrad)
Decontamination of food ingredients	Various spices Onion or cocoa powder Dyes Mineral supplements	1.0 (10 kGy)
Inactivation of salmonella	Meat and poultry Egg products Shrimps and frog legs Meat and fish meal	0.30–1.0 (3–10 kGy)
To extend refrigerated storage (0–4°C)	Prepackaged meat and fish	0.25–0.50 (2.5–5 kGy)
Prolonged storage of fruit, etc.	Strawberries Mangos Papayas	0.20–0.50 (2.5–5 kGy)
Control of insects	Wheat and rice Dates Cocoa beans	0.02–0.30 (0.20–3 kGy)
Inhibition of sprouting or growth	Potatoes Onions Garlic Mushrooms	0.01–0.30 (0.1–3 kGy)

required standards. For example, in making jam the acidity and pectin content of the mixture are critical, so acidity-regulating additives and additional pectin are used to ensure that the jam sets. The household practice of reboiling is uneconomic, and the customer will reject jam that has not set.

Extrusion cooking is a process unlikely to be found in the home. It involves subjecting a mixture to high pressure, and usually high temperature, in the barrel of the extruder using a helical screw that runs through the centre of the barrel. At the exit there is a die that shapes the extruded product, and the fall in pressure as the food leaves the die results in the water 'flashing-off' to give a dry product suitable for packing directly or for further processing, such as deep-frying. Extrusion cooking is widely used for producing snack foods.

FOOD ADDITIVES

Food additives are defined as substances other than nutrients added to foods for technological purposes, which includes organoleptic objectives. Additives are classified according to the purposes for which they are used. Their use in foods is controlled by MAFF on the advice of the Food Advisory Committee, although this control will eventually pass to the EC and the Scientific Committee for Food. Before a new additive is permitted it must satisfy these committees that there is a technological need for it which cannot be met by existing additives, or that the new additive has advantages over those already approved; it must then satisfy the criteria for safety in use. A submission for a new additive therefore requires considerable documentation on its technological uses and advantages or novelty, together with the results of safety evaluation studies. The major categories of additives are listed in Table 21.3.

Preservatives

The major preservatives are listed in Table 21.1 and the objectives for their use discussed above.

Colours

The visual appearance of a food is a major factor in determining its acceptance by the consumer, who has a number of inbuilt expectations regarding the 'proper' colour for a particular type of food; for example, we expect peas to be green and strawberry jam to be red. When conducting the sensory evaluation of foods it is often necessary to carry out the tests under special neutral lighting so as not to bias the results with the consumers' colour expectations. It therefore follows that the food producers are especially concerned with the colour of their products, and colouring agents are a widely used group of additives.

The colours used include organic dyes and natural colouring pigments extracted from foods such as

Table 21.3 Major categories of food additives

Preservatives
Colours
Flavours
Sweeteners
Emulsifiers and stabilizers
Antioxidants
Flour improvers

Processing aids
Acid
Acidity regulators
Humectant
Gelling agents
Antifoaming agents

beetroot. One of the most important types of colouring materials, by volume of usage, is, however, the range of substances classified as caramels, being second only in importance to the yellow dye tartrazine, which in the 1987 review of the usage of colours conducted by the Steering Group on Food Surveillance was reported to be used in over 2000 products (MAFF 1987). The frequency of usage is not a good indicator of the overall dietary intake of these colouring agents, because some of the more intense synthetic dyes are used at a low concentrations whereas some colours derived from natural sources have to be used at higher concentrations to achieve the desired colour.

In all about 30 colours are permitted under current regulations. The synthetic colours have all undergone extensive safety evaluation, but nevertheless there is growing pressure on the food producers to limit the numbers used and to use natural colours if at all possible. Most of the pressure to remove these synthetic colours comes from reports of intolerance reactions to these substances. As with all suspected cases of food intolerance it is extremely difficult to evaluate these claims in formal scientific studies. There are, however, a small number of individuals who exhibit allergic types of symptom (urticaria) to tartrazine and clearly they need to be able to identify foods using this colour. Thus they must be aware of the relevant E-number (E 102). There are a number of published lists available from MAFF, or in more popular format (e.g. Hanssen & Marsden 1987).

Some nutrients are used as colours and it is important for the nutritionist to be aware of their use, as it can cause unexpected sources of nutrient intake; for example, E 101 is riboflavin, which is used in some sauces and mustard pickles, and E 160 (a) is ß-carotene. The red dye erythrosine E 127 contains a high concentration of iodine, but most of this is not absorbable from the intestine.

Flavouring agents

The flavours of most fruits and vegetables are formed by very complex mixtures of aldehydes and esters of organic alcohols and acids, and to a large variety of essential oils which contain complex terpenoid substances. Many of these naturally occurring substances are used by the flavourists who formulate the flavourings used in processed foods. Other savoury flavours are developed from hydrolysates of cereals or proteins. A 1976 review of flavourings used in foods listed more than 2000 substances in use, including natural extracts and synthetic materials (MAFF 1976). The very size of the list is one of the major reasons why a definitive series of regulations on flavours has been so difficult to establish. Many of the synthetic substances are 'nature identical', that is, they are found naturally in foods or are formed during conventional cooking procedures. In addition, many flavours are present in minute quantities in foods, making the enforcement of regulations to control their use difficult.

A closely related group of additives are called flavour improvers, of which the best known is monosodium glutamate (MSG); other salts of glutamic acid are used and some nucleotides also exhibit flavour-enhancing properties by as yet unknown mechanisms. Although there are some individuals who are sensitive to MSG, there is no evidence at the levels used in foods that it causes any lasting effects. The use of all additives is, however, under regular review and (at the time of writing, 1992) a review of evidence relating to reactions to MSG is planned by the FDA in the United States.

Sweetening agents

Sucrose from cane or beet is the most widely used sweetening ingredient in foods, although glucose syrups and high-fructose syrups produced from hydrolysates of starch are being used increasingly. These sugars are, however, also sources of food energy and there is a great demand for products that taste sweet but have a lower energy content from those who wish to regulate or reduce their body weight; patients with diabetes mellitus who need to control their intake of sugars also have a perceived need for sweetness without sugars. To meet these demands a number of artificial sweeteners have been developed. Saccharin was the first to be widely used; it is about 400 times as sweet as sucrose on a weight basis and yields no metabolizable energy. However, saccharin is unstable when heated and this limits its usefulness as an additive.

Cyclamates, which are stable to heat and about 30 times as sweet as sucrose, came into use but concerns about the possible carcinogenicity of their metabolites led to their ban in 1969 in the USA, the UK and some other countries. They are still permitted in some countries provided that the pack carries a warning statement and advice to limit consumption.

When the Food Advisory Committee of MAFF reviewed the use of sweeteners in foods (MAFF 1982), it distinguished between 'intense sweeteners', such as saccharin, and a new category of 'bulk sweeteners', which were coming into use. These included the sugar alcohols, either mono- or disaccharide alcohols such as sorbitol and maltitol. These substances are relatively poorly absorbed from the small intestine and therefore contribute less metabolizable energy than the sugars they replace.

The review also led to the approval of three new intense sweeteners, 'aspartame', which is a dipeptide of aspartic acid and phenylalanine; 'acesulfame K', which is the potassium salt of acetyl sulphame; and a natural extract, thaumatin, from a tropical fruit.

Recently concern has been raised about the possible adverse effects of high intakes of saccharin, and diabetics in particular have been advised to mix their usage of table-top sweeteners as a precaution against excessive intakes.

Emulsifiers and stabilizers

The texture of many processed foods is due to the fact that they are emulsions or foams, and if they are to retain these textural properties they must be stabilized in some way. This group of additives are surfactant, amphipatheic molecules that act at the interfaces of the two phases in the food. The commonly used emulsifiers are mono- and diglycerides and phospholipids such as lecithin, which occurs naturally in many foods.

Stabilizers are usually macromolecules that form a dispersed matrix or gel in which other smaller molecules can be incorporated. Commonly used stabilizers include modified starches, pectins and polysaccharide gums.

Antioxidants

One of the more important types of deterioration that can occur in a foodstuff involves the oxidation of the fats present to produce unpleasant odours which can be detected at very low concentrations by the human senses. The process is known as rancidity, and can take place at low temperatures. It is most commonly a problem with high-fat foods and especially those where the fat is rich in polyunsaturated fats. Most unsaturated plant oils contain natural antioxidants that prevent the development of rancidity, such as the tocopherols, and these are also widely used as antioxidants in processed products. In addition, synthetic antioxidants are permitted, such as butylated hydroxyansole (BHA) and butylated hydroxytoluene (BHT). The levels of usage are closely controlled.

Ascorbic acid and its non-vitamin isomer erythorbic acid and their salts are used as antioxidants in aqueous systems, for example to prevent the darkening of apple juice during processing, and in the retention of colour in processed meats.

Flour improvers

This is a group of additives which are added to flours used in breadmaking, either because they improve the elasticity of the dough and lead to a greater volume of the loaf, or because they improve the stability of the crumb and slow the rate of redistribution of water in the bread, which is associated with staling.

Wholemeal bread is given special attention by the advocates of natural foods, and although it was recommended that the use of flour improvers be permitted, the regulations allow only the use of ascorbic acid, which maintains a reducing environment during dough development in the Chorleywood bread process.

Miscellaneous food additives

A large number of smaller categories of additives are used in foods, which are for the most part essentially processing aids. They include acids such as citric, tartaric and malic acid, which are used to increase the acidity of foods, and a group of acidity regulators, usually the salts of these acids, which buffer the acidity in a food.

Other substances are used as humectants, such as glycerol and sorbitol, to prevent a product drying out. Many polysaccharide additives are used as thickening agents to alter or control the textural physical properties of a food during heating and cooling, and in the stored product.

Polyphosphates may be used in the processing of milk to prevent gelation in the can, and they are also used in some meat products to stablize the water content and prevent water loss. Properly used this can lead to more succulent products, although it can also be used to retain processing water and increase the product weight in a fraudulent manner.

LOSSES OF FOOD AND NUTRIENTS IN FOOD PROCESSING

Measurements of food consumption

Food consumption can be measured at several different levels; while the nutritionist is most often concerned with the amounts of food actually ingested, others are concerned with measurements, or more strictly, estimates, of food consumption at other points in the food chain from production to consumption. Much of the international data on food consumption, although expressed per head of the population and therefore giving the impression that it is a measure of consumption at the individual level, are derived from estimates made higher up the food chain. It is important for nutritionists to understand how these estimates are derived, because it is possible to develop false arguments from them; in particular, deductions about the nutritional adequacy of the diet, or relationships between diet and the incidence of disease.

In many countries there are administrative reasons for obtaining estimates of food consumption; these may be fiscal in origin where there is a need for estimates of food production for taxation or for subsidizing the primary producers of food. The import and export of foodstuffs is also frequently a matter of considerable importance to the economic health of a country. Most industrialized countries, therefore, collect statistics on food production, the import and export of food, and the non-food use of food commodities. The latter includes foods used for animal feeds, crops retained for seed in subsequent years, and the use of food materials for the production of other non-food products; for example, starch is used to prepare adhesives, and fermentable carbohydrates may be used to produce industrial alcohol and many other substances. Statistics of this kind are also used for planning and estimating food needs in the less fortunate regions of the world, and provide the basis for planning agricultural programmes.

These statistics are measured at the wholesale commodity level, for example in tonnes of cereal grains and carcases of animals, and other units in which production, import and export are recorded. The quality of such data is variable but can be very good because of the fiscal and economic implications of the information.

In the UK these data provide an estimate of food moving into consumption, and are called the consumption levels estimates (CLE). When combined with estimates of changes in the stocks of food held in the country, they give an estimate of food disappearance. This approach forms the basis of the Food Balance Sheets prepared by the FAO. The FAO uses data supplied by the different countries and in Europe by the OECD and the EC. The actual method used in the collection of the data differs in different countries, but the FAO has no other sources of information. The development of common custom tariffs in the EC will in future lead to the collection of more consistent information. However, it must be recognized that these measurements, for all their inherent inaccuracies, provide a gross overall picture of food disappearance, and because of the scale on which they are calculated are reasonable indicators of the consumption of foods at the level at which they were recorded.

In the UK and in many countries food consumption is measured at other levels. One widely used approach is the 'household purchases or budget' type of study, where foods purchased by a household unit are recorded over a period of time, most usually 7 days. The National Food Survey conducted by MAFF is a good example (MAFF 1989b). In this, a randomly selected number of households (7000) are surveyed for a week. The study is carried out for the whole year, with only the 2 weeks at Christmas being excluded. The study was originally intended as an economic one but has included a nutritional element from its outset in the early 1950s.

The estimates from the NFS and nutritional studies indicate that measurements of the amounts of food actually eaten are substantially lower than estimates derived from food supplies estimates (CLE). This is not unexpected because of the differences in the levels at which the foods were measured. The supplies estimates cannot take into account the inevitable losses that occur during the movement of foods along the food chain. Nevertheless, between 1972 and 1976, the difference in the energy intakes estimated from supplies and actual consumption was about 25% of the total food moving into consumption. At this time there was a great deal of talk about 'waste' of food, and considerable work was set in hand to identify and measure the reasons for the difference. The loss of food and the associated nutrients along the food chain has considerable significance for the nutritional interpretation of food balance sheets, and for the many international comparisons that are made using these calculations. Alongside this is the related problem of quantifying the nutrient supply from measurements of foods consumed, which raises the issues of nutrient losses during processing of foods in both the factory and the kitchen.

Losses of food along the food chain

Losses of food occur throughout the food chain, some of which are an inevitable consequence of the conversion of the primary produce into edible food. It is incorrect to consider these losses as 'wastage'. There are losses that occur as a consequence of storage, some of which are avoidable. These include losses due to spoilage by rodents or insect pests, or to fungal or bacterial damage of the stored crop, often due to physical damage and contamination during harvesting. These losses are preventable, but at the cost of improved storage facilities, and the use of pesticides and antimicrobial agents. Mechanical damage during harvesting is a common focus for the start of microbial damage, and this represents another means of reducing storage losses. Losses of stored foodstuffs are a major influence on the availability of food in the third world, where temperature and humidity magnify the potential for biological damage.

The processing of foods results in other types of losses: carcases have to be trimmed during butchering, cereal grains have to be cleaned and milled before they can be used as food, and vegetables are trimmed to remove external leaves to prepare them for the retail market. Processes such as cheesemaking and the blanching of vegetables prior to freezing all produce waste products that are not usually recoverable as food. Some of these by-products of processing are suitable for use as animal feeds, and the sale of these can be of major importance to the economy of processing as a whole. For example, the branny layers of the wheat grain went for animal feed before bran became popular for humans as a source of dietary fibre.

The preparation of foods for retail sale produces yet more losses; appearance is a major factor in food choice and blemished fruit and vegetables are frequently discarded or sold on downmarket, where their sale may not produce sufficient return for the producers. This produces an economic 'feedback' that can reduce waste at the earlier stages of the chain. Further trimming of meats and fish is common, as is that of vegetables for the 'prepacked market'.

Further trimming and preparation losses occur in the kitchen, and there are additional losses where all the edible material prepared is not consumed at the meal. These losses are more important in the developed affluent communities, but in many cultures it is considered improper to consume all the food served, or to serve only as much as can be eaten. In large-scale institutional catering, wastage of edible material often substantially reduces the planned nutritional value of the meals served. The study of hospital meals by Platt et al (1963) focused attention on the size of the wastage, which was between 25% and 35% of the food served; the introduction of menu selection has gone some way to improve this situation, but the problem of matching demand remains. In restaurants a similar situation occurs because the proprietor cannot afford to acquire a reputation for appearing mean, and thus must prepare more than the customers can consume. Clearly the price paid allows for the economic consequences of the waste, but not for the discrepancy in the food supply statistics.

The measurement of waste is extremely difficult in most situations, but especially in the home, where 'waste' has a pejorative connotation, and it is one aspect of behaviour that is most likely to be altered by the very act of measurement. In a study in the UK in 1980 several hundred families collected all household food waste. This was analysed for energy and proximate constituents; weekly waste amounted to 6.5% of the energy in summer and 5.4% in winter. As might be expected, wastage was lower in large families. The group studied was highly motivated and aware of the purpose of the study, and may have modified its behaviour, and other investigators have attempted to obtain estimates of waste by the analysis of garbage. A similar approach was used in a study of food consumption in a submarine, which showed substantial losses of edible or potentially edible material (Southgate & Shirling 1970).

In communities living at or near the hunger level there is virtually no waste, and under the extreme conditions seen in prisoner-of-war camps in the 1939–1945 war and in concentration camps, the inmates went to great lengths to husband their meagre food supplies.

Foods fed to pets

In the USA it has been estimated that 22 million dogs and 30 million cats eat food equivalent to 5% of the total human energy intake and 14% of the protein requirement. In Britain there are about 5 million dogs and nearly 5 million cats, and these may eat 3% of the energy and 2% of the protein required by the human population. The expenditure on foods for pets is of major economic importance to the retail food trade, and also, incidentally, to the manufacturers of cans. This food cannot be regarded as waste, and indeed much of the food used is not fit for human consumption – for example, offal such as lungs and trachea and carcase trimmings are used. There is, however, a substantial amount of food prepared, or suitable for human consumption, that is fed to pets, for example scraps from plates and surplus food prepared for the family meal. The measurement of this is difficult because behaviour may change when it is observed, but the major study on domestic waste cited above did take account of food fed to pets.

In addition to the losses of food during the various stages of the food chain there are also losses of specific nutrients.

Proximate constituents, protein, fat and carbohydrates

Many changes in the chemical structure of the molecules of the proximate constituents are brought about by heat, where heat energy is applied to the foodstuff. Similar changes also arise from the application of other forms of energy such as gamma or electron beam irradiation, or the application of microwaves. Some of these changes may reduce the nutritional value of the food and others may produce potentially toxic constituents. These processes are particularly important for the generation of flavour components, in addition to their essential role in destroying harmful microorganisms discussed in Chapter 22. In principle, the only difference between the heating processes used in food processing and in the domestic kitchen is one of scale, and it is possible to consider the effects of these extremes of scale together. In practice there are differences in the levels of control that are used: in the factory there is a need for very close control of the processes themselves, and of the raw ingredients and finished products, to ensure that they will meet the quality standards demanded by the customer.

Proteins

Heating of proteins leads to changes in their tertiary structure and eventually to denaturation. The protein may become insoluble and form precipitate or curd, and the behaviour of the protein is very important in relation to the texture of the cooked food. The denaturation process does not affect the nutritional value of the protein because the initial stages of proteolytic digestion involve similar types of changes. When proteins are heated in the presence of carbohydrate, particularly if reducing sugars are present, a series of reactions known as Maillard reactions takes place (Fig. 21.1). The reducing sugar condenses with free

amino groups on the protein; these are limited in number and the reaction with the epsilon amino group of lysine is the most important nutritionally, since it reduces the biological value of the protein by making lysine unavailable. The effects are directly related to the severity of heating, and excessive heat treatment can drastically reduce the nutritional value of a food. Mild heating produces browning and only slight losses. When milk is roller-dried there is often considerable damage (up to 40% of the lysine) but the milder spray-drying that is more widely used produces only slight losses (10%). The baking and toasting of cereal products is associated with the formation of Maillard products on the surface of the food, and some loss of lysine (10–15%) can be seen. The same effects occur in extrusion cooking if the barrel temperature is high. The reactions between amino acids and other components of foods are important for the generation of flavour compounds.

Fats

The changes that take place in fats during heat processing are greatly dependent on the fatty acid composition of the fat and the other components present. The major changes involve the unsaturated fatty acid constituents of the fats. In the presence of oxygen the double bonds react to form peroxides; these substances are highly reactive and decompose to give a wide range of compounds, some of which are responsible for the flavour of fried foods, but many of which are potentially toxic or cause darkening of the oil. Some free fatty acids are also produced. The reaction occurs slowly at normal frying temperatures

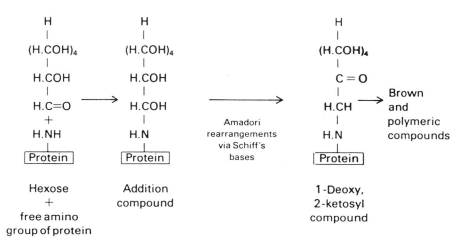

Fig. 21.1 Simplified outline of the Maillard reaction.

in pure fats, but it is catalysed by traces of metals such as iron and copper, which are common constituents of foods. Fats that are abused – that is, overheated or used for a long period – progressively darken and the products of the oxidation accumulate. The fat in this state may well be toxic. Fortunately, foods cooked in these fats have a bitter, unpleasant and often 'rancid' flavour and are rejected, so that poisoning from this cause is very rare. Many processed fats and oils contain antioxidants to minimize these changes, which also take place very slowly at ambient temperatures. Highly unsaturated vegetable oils often contain high levels of the natural antioxidant tocopherol.

Carbohydrates

The effects of heat processing on carbohydrates differ for the three major classes. The sugars take part in Maillard reactions and therefore contribute to browning. Concentrated solutions of sugars also react in the absence of amino acids to form caramel, which is a mixture of a range of condensation products formed between hexose molecules that have lost water to form furfural compounds. The starches in unprocessed foods are present in the form of granules; when heated in an aqueous medium the granules absorb water and smell, and when the swollen granules rupture the linear amylose component leaches out as a colloidal sol. On further heating the remaining amylopectin also 'melts' to give a colloidal sol. These starch sols gel on cooling; the linear amylose molecules retrograde and form an insoluble precipitate, which is only very slowly hydrolysed by alpha amylase. The heating and cooling of starchy foods therefore renders part of the starch resistant to digestion in the small intestine, and this resistant starch is only slowly degraded by the microflora of the large intestine. The heat processing of foods therefore has the effect of making starch as a whole more digestible, but subsequent cooling makes a small proportion resistant. The nutritional significance of this latter effect has yet to be established, but the resistant starch shares some properties with the non-starch polysaccharides of dietary fibre (Chapter 4). The effects of heat treatment on the cell wall polysaccharides have not been fully documented, but the heating of a plant tissue brings about cell death, and a food such as fresh fruit or vegetable loses cell turgor and the tissues collapse. The pectic substances dissolve on heating in water, and this causes the intercellular matrix to break down and cells to separate. Cooking therefore changes the texture of plant tissues very markedly, and extensive cooking produces a soup-like homogenate. The carbohydrates are rather unreactive when compared with fats or proteins, and cooking has only minor effects on their nutritional properties.

Minerals

Heat treatments in themselves have little effect on the minerals in foods. Losses can occur by leaching into the cooking medium, but the major effects are on the organic components, which may restrict the bioavailability of minerals such as iron, calcium and zinc. Heat treatment may, for example, allow the phytase enzymes to hydrolyse phytates in cereal foods and so improve availability. The reverse of this can also occur when the heat treatment inactivates the natural phytases present in the raw food, allowing higher levels of phytate to be present in the processed product.

Vitamins

The effects of heat treatment on vitamins are often quoted as the most deleterious effects of processing on nutritional values. It is, however, not possible to generalize regarding the magnitude of the losses, which depend on the specific vitamin and the conditions employed. Losses can occur by two major routes: first, the vitamin may be soluble in the cooking medium and therefore leach out. If the medium is discarded, as, for example, the water used for cooking vegetables, substantial amounts of the water-soluble vitamins can be lost. Second, many vitamins are unstable and prone to destruction under certain conditions; for example, vitamin C is easily oxidized and destroyed by heating in the presence of air, and thiamin decomposes if heated in alkaline conditions. Table 21.4 summarizes the stability of the major vitamins under different conditions. The most sensitive vitamins are ascorbic acid (vitamin C), folates and thiamin, but losses of the other vitamins can occur under specific conditions.

Ascorbic acid. Losses in processing and cooking can be very large and nutritionally significant. The vitamin is a powerful reducing agent and is readily oxidized. If this proceeds beyond the dehydroascorbic acid stage all vitamin activity is irreversibly lost. Oxidation is accelerated by enzymes present in most plant tissues, heat, alkaline conditions, traces of copper and atmospheric oxygen. These factors therefore need to be taken into account in the operation of cooking and processing to maximize vitamin retention.

The enzyme ascorbic acid oxidase is released from plant tissues when they are cut or macerated. It is rapidly inactivated at temperatures of about 60°C,

Table 21.4 Stability of vitamins under different conditions

Vitamin	pH 7	Acid	Alkaline	Air	Light	Heat	Cooking losses (%)
Retinol	S	U	S	U	U	U	0–40
Carotenes	S	U	S	U	U	U	0–30
Vitamin D	S	U	U	U	U	U	0–40
Vitamin E	S	S	S	U	U	U	0–55
Thiamin	U	S	U	U	S	U	0–80
Riboflavin	S	S	U	S	U	U	0–75
Niacin	S	S	S	S	S	S	0–75
Vitamin B_6	S	S	S	S	U	U	0–40
Vitamin B_{12}	S	S	S	U	U	S	0–10
Vitamin C	U	S	U	U	U	U	0–100

Losses depend on the duration of exposure to the conditions listed (modified from Harris & Loesecke 1960). U = unstable; S = stable

and therefore placing fruits and vegetables into boiling water minimizes enzymatic losses, as does cooking them for the shortest possible time. Warm-holding of cooked dishes is a major cause of loss, and the cooked foods should not be prepared too far in advance of consumption.

In the processing of fruits and vegetables the fresh produce is often blanched to minimize enzymatic activity, and this process and packaging are designed to exclude oxygen. The acidity of fruits is a major factor in the retention of ascorbic acid during the production of fruit juices, and special care is taken to reduce copper levels in the process water and production plant.

Alkaline conditions promote destruction, and the use of bicarbonate to retain the colour of vegetables during cooking is highly undesirable.

Frying in shallow fat can lead to high losses, but deep-fat frying often gives very good retention, as in the preparation of potato crisps (chips).

Thiamin. Thiamin is water-soluble and significant losses can occur when foods such as rice are washed prior to cooking. Alkaline conditions lead to losses, but these are lower than with vitamin C, usually being of the order of 10–20%; thiamin is destroyed by sulphur dioxide and sulphites.

Riboflavin. Although reasonably stable during cooking, riboflavin is sensitive to light as it absorbs UV light and decomposes. Significant losses can occur in milk left in sunlight or under fluorescent lighting.

Folates. These are very susceptible to oxidation when heated in neutral or alkaline conditions, and leaching losses are also important. Dissolved oxygen in a product or a pack that is permeable to oxygen can cause substantial losses in stored foods.

Vitamin B_6. The pyridoxal and pyridoxamine are sensitive to oxidation during heat treatments, particularly those that use very high temperatures, such as canning.

Vitamin B_{12}. Vitamin B_{12} is stable at normal cooking temperatures, but high-temperature, short-time (HTST) processes such as pasteurization and ultraheating (UHT) can result in losses.

Vitamin A and carotenes. These are stable at normal cooking temperatures, but the high temperatures used in frying can produce oxidative losses and isomerization of the carotenoids, with loss of biological activity.

Vitamin E. This is slowly destroyed during frying and is decomposed by light.

OTHER TYPES OF PROCESSING

The previous discussion focused on heat treatment processes that are common to both the factory and the kitchen. However, there are a number of types of process that are rarely if ever feasible in a domestic environment, because of the capital investment required. This was once true for the freezing of foods at temperatures in the region of −20°C, but in many developed countries the domestic deep-freeze is very common. Deep-freezing is now probably the preferred method for the domestic preservation of fruit and vegetables, and to a possibly smaller extent, meat and fish. The effects of this process on nutrients are generally small; some losses occur on blanching, but deep-frozen foods are virtually equivalent to the fresh product nutritionally, if not texturally. There are, however, other processes that are restricted to the factory.

Extrusion cooking

This is an HTST process, and losses of vitamins are comparable to those in conventional baking. The starch and other polysaccharides may undergo some depolymerization due to the shear forces, and proteins are extensively modified physically, but the nutritional changes are slight.

Irradiation

Irradiation is another way of passing energy into a foodstuff and the nutritional effects are very similar to other more conventional thermal treatments. The effects on proteins and their biological values are very small at the dosages currently under discussion (up to 10 kGy). Unsaturated fats undergo oxidation and bond scission, leading to unacceptable flavours, so that applications to fatty foods are limited, but only small depolymerization effects are seen with carbohydrates. The labile vitamins are destroyed to a similar extent to that in normal thermal heating.

CONCLUSIONS

Some food losses are inevitable during the transition from primary produce to food for human consumption. These losses include the parts of foods not usually regarded as edible, although this is greatly conditioned by the prevailing food culture, and losses of notionally edible parts that are damaged or spoiled during storage or processing. In most cases the losses of nutrients due to food processing are of the same order as those that occur during domestic preparation of the same food.

The nutritional significance of these losses depends on the importance of the food in the diet, either as a major item quantitatively, or as a major source of a specific nutrient. Thus losses of vitamin C from strawberries when they are irradiated to increase shelf-life would be of much less significance than losses of vitamin C in potatoes, because the latter are an important source of the vitamin in the UK diet.

Where a food forms a very major part of the diet, either of the population as a whole or a specific group, the losses in processing may be extremely important; for example, losses during the processing of infant formulae are of great nutritional importance, and processing needs to be controlled to minimize them.

It is, however, important to recognize that food processing in some form is essential to the maintenance of urban populations, and also has a major nutritional benefit in increasing the range of foods available for consumption throughout the year.

REFERENCES AND FURTHER READING

Bender AE 1986 Health or hoax. Sphere Books, London

Benterud A 1977 Vitamin losses during thermal processing. In: Hoyem T, Kvale O (eds) Physical, chemical and biological changes in foods caused by thermal processing. Applied Science, London, pp. 185–201

Cameron ME, van Staveren WJ (eds) 1988 Manual on methodology for food consumption studies. Oxford Medical Publications, Oxford

Department of Health and Social Security 1986 Advisory Committee on Irradiated and Novel Foods, Report on the safety and wholesomeness of irradiated foods. HMSO, London

Drummond JC, Wibraham A 1957 The Englishman's food. Jonathan Cape, London

Food and Agriculture Organisation 1980 Carbohydrates in human nutrition. FAO Food and Nutrition Paper No.15 FAO, Rome

Food and Agricultural Organisation 1984 Food balance sheets 1979–1981. FAO, Rome

Gurr MI, James AT 1975 Lipid biochemistry, 2nd edn. Chapman and Hall, Science Paperbacks, London

Hanssen M, Marsden J 1987 The new E for additives. Thorsons, Wellingborough

Hurrel RF, Carpenter KJ 1977 Maillard reactions in foods. In: Hoyem T, Kvale O (eds) Physical, chemical and biological changes in foods caused by thermal processing. Applied Science, London

Karmas E, Harris RS (eds) 1988 Nutritional evaluation of food processing, 3rd edn. Van Nostrand Reinhold, New York

Kelly A 1986 (ed) Nutritional surveillance in Europe: a critical appraisal. CIP-gegevens Koninklijke Bibliotheek, Den Haag

Ministry of Agriculture, Fisheries and Food 1976 Food Additives and Contaminants Committee review of the flavourings in food. HMSO, London

Ministry of Agriculture, Fisheries and Food 1982 Review of Food Advisory Committee on use of Sweetners in Foods. HMSO, London

Ministry of Agriculture, Fisheries and Food 1987 Survey of colour usage in food. Report of Steering Group on Food Surveillance. HMSO, London

Ministry of Agriculture, Fisheries and Food 1989a Annual Report of the Advisory Committee on Novel Foods and Processes. HMSO, London

Ministry of Agriculture, Fisheries and Food 1989b Household food consumption and expenditure. Annual Report of the National Food Survey Committee 1987. HMSO, London

Morton ID 1977 Physical, chemical and biological changes related to different time–temperature combinations. In: Hoyem T, Kvale O (eds) Physical, chemical and biological changes in foods caused by thermal processing. Applied Science, London, pp. 135–151

Paul AA, Southgate DAT 1978 McCance and Widdowson's The composition of food, 4th edn. HMSO, London

Platt BS, Eddy TP, Pellett PL 1963 Food in hospitals. Oxford University Press, Oxford

Regenstein JM, Regenstein CE 1984 Food protein chemistry. Academic Press, Orlando

Roy R 1976 Wastage in the UK food system. Earth Resources, London

Southgate DAT 1984 Natural or unnatural foods? British Medical Journal 288: 881–882

Southgate DAT, Shirling D 1970 The energy expenditure and food intake of the ship's company of a submarine. Ergonomics 13: 777– 782

Statutory Instruments 1984 Food labelling descriptions etc. Food labelling regulations 1984 SI 1305

Wenlock RW, Buss DH, Derry BJ, Dixon EJ 1980 Household wastage in Britain. British Journal of Nutrition 43: 53–70

World Health Organization 1981 Wholesomeness of irradiated food. Report FAO/IAEA/WHO Expert Committee, WHO Technical Report Series No 659

World Health Organization 1991 Strategies for assessing the safety of foods produced by biotechnology. WHO, Geneva

22. Pathogenic agents in food

D.A.T. Southgate

The dangers from pathogenic agents in food far exceed those of toxic agents, either naturally occurring or man-made chemicals added to foods or present as contaminants. There are a large number of organisms, helminth worms, bacteria, protozoa and viruses that may gain access to foods and so enter the body and cause a well-defined disease. Meat, eggs and milk from infected animals may contain pathogens and, when eaten, can cause disease – for example, tapeworms, brucellosis, tuberculosis and salmonella infections are familiar examples of disease in both animals and man (International Commission on Microbiological Specifications for Food 1978).

There are more than 1600 types of salmonella which have been identified and distinguished by serological typing. These organisms are among the commonest causes of food poisoning (Moss 1987). They infect most species of vertebrates and are especially widespread in poultry and many other intensively reared animals. *Salmonella typhimurium* was until recently the type most commonly associated with human infections, but *S. enteriditis* has now become the most common in the UK. The organisms are usually confined to the intestines, where they cause an acute gastroenteritis with diarrhoea and vomiting, but they may enter the bloodstream and invade tissues, causing an enteric fever similar to typhoid. Mice and rats infected with *S. typhimurium* commonly excrete the organism in their faeces and urine, and so infect foods to which they have access. *S. enteriditis* may be spread from the intestines of infected poultry during processing of the carcases, and there is some evidence of vertical transmission to the eggs from the oviducts of infected birds.

Many pathogenic bacteria and viruses are excreted in human faeces and urine. Infection may be spread by transfer of the pathogen by flies or the human hand to foods or food utensils. Infections spread in this way are known as faecal–oral infections. They include the dysenteries and acute gastroenteritis, which are often caused by infection with various viruses and some serotypes of *Escherichia coli*.

All pathogens are destroyed by heat, and food which has been properly cooked and handled is safe. However, in cooking the heat may not penetrate the food sufficiently: for example, a large joint of meat is potentially dangerous because the internal temperature of the food may not have been high enough for the length of time required to kill the organism. Foods may also be contaminated after cooking. Meat, milk and eggs are excellent growth media for bacteria; foods that have been cooked and incorrectly stored and then inadequately reheated are especially liable to be associated with food poisoning.

The prevention of spread of infections in foods depends on scrupulous attention to cleanliness along the whole food chain – primary produce, abattoirs, food manufacturers, warehouses, retail shops, catering establishments, restaurants and domestic kitchens and larders (Hobbs & Gilbert 1978). In all these places care is required to prevent food from being contaminated by rodents, flies, and, most importantly of all, the people who handle and prepare it. Scrupulous attention to personal hygiene is essential, as is the proper provision of facilities for maintaining cleanliness. There is a need to be aware of symptomless carriers among food handlers, who may excrete the pathogens in their urine or carry the organisms in the mucous membranes of the mouth or nose, and thus unknowingly act as a source of infection. Food-borne infections and faecal–oral diseases are especially prevalent in poor urban communities with poor facilities for storing foods, inadequate water supplies and sanitation. In such circumstances infections are common and contribute to the high mortality rates, especially among infants and young children. The prevention and control of outbreaks of bacterial food poisoning is aided by knowledge of the organism responsible, and the route by which the associated foods become infected. The Public Health

Laboratory Service has the expertise for bacterial diagnosis.

Public and Environmental Health Authorities are also responsible for inspecting abattoirs, the premises of food manufacturers, wholesale and retail shops that sell food, and catering establishments and restaurants as part of consumer protection. The safety of the staff within these establishments is the responsibility of the Health and Safety Executive who exert control on microbiological hazards that may affect the staff. In many cases they have the legal right to issue orders closing premises that do not reach the required standards, or notices identifying inadequacies that need correction by a certain date if closure is to be avoided.

BACTERIAL FOOD POISONING

This usually produces an acute gastroenteritis, which is often short and self-limiting. The incidence of reported cases has increased substantially since 1980 and these undoubtedly represent only a proportion of the true incidence. The number of fatal cases is small, deaths usually occuring among the very young or those whose immunological defences are weakened because of some other condition. Nevertheless, food poisoning represents a major cause of morbidity and economic losses, quite apart from the distress and discomfort it causes. The gastroenteritis causes severe dehydration and loss of electrolytes, and these are a major cause of infant mortality in the developing world.

Ecology of food-poisoning bacteria

Many foods provide ideal culture media for the growth of bacteria; the nutrient supply from the food is, however, only one of the factors that control bacterial growth. The physicochemical environment in the food has a major influence and it is by manipulating this environment that the growth of pathogenic organisms can be controlled.

Temperature

As mentioned earlier, the temperatures achieved in cooking will usually kill most pathogens, certainly the vegetative cells. Some organisms produce spores, which are more resistant, and higher temperatures are required such as are reached in canning. Low temperatures slow the rate of growth, and the maintenance of such temperatures in refrigerated storage in a major factor in controlling food poisoning.

pH

The pH of a food is another factor that controls growth; many pathogens will not grow in acid media and synergistic effects that inhibit growth are seen, involving pH and the use of other preservatives such as sodium chloride and nitrates in preserved meats (Egan & Roberts 1987).

Controlled atmospheres

Some pathogens are obligate anaerobes and their growth is encouraged in atmospheres where oxygen concentration is very low. The growth of other species is inhibited by high concentrations of carbon dioxide.

Water activity

Low water activity has an inhibitory effect on growth, and the use of salt and sugar in many foods as preservatives takes advantage of this effect.

Organisms most commonly causing food poisoning

It is customary to divide the bacteria causing poisoning into two categories: those that multiply in the foodstuff and produce toxins (exotoxins) that are subsequently consumed and cause the effects in the body, and those that are consumed with the food and infect the gastrointestinal tract, where they grow and produce the toxins (endotoxins). To produce an exotoxin the bacteria must have multiplied sufficiently within the food without causing spoilage that would lead to food being rejected. The type of bacterial toxin involved in food poisoning determines the interval between ingestion and the appearance of symptoms, and this interval is often of value in investigating the cause of an outbreak. Table 22.1 lists the species and the characteristic symptoms they produce.

Staphylococcus

S. aureus is a widely distributed organism that is frequently a commensal on the skin. It is responsible for many skin infections and can frequently be cultured from nasal swabs. Most outbreaks are the result of contamination of the foods by carriers of the organism, which will multiply within the food if the temperature is not below 7°C, producing a toxin that is partially resistant to normal cooking temperatures that would kill the organism. The ingestion of contaminated food is followed by a reaction within

Table 22.1 Characteristics of bacterial food poisoning

Organism	Sources of infection	Incubation period (hours)	Site of toxin production	Control measures
Staphylococcus aureus	Skin and mucous membranes of carriers	2–6	Food	Store food at below 5°C
Bacillus cereus	Airborne spores	1–16	Food (rapid) Intestine (slow onset)	Refrigerate to control growth
Clostridium perfringens	Soil, raw meat	18–20	Food	Heat to 80°C to inactivate spores which are heat-labile
Clostridium botulinum	Soil, fish	12–96	Food, heat-labile	Store at low temperatures, pH < 4.6, low water activity, curing salts
Salmonella spp.	Excreta, contents of intestine	3–36	Intestine	Thaw and cook food thoroughly
Listeria monocytogenes	Soil, widely distributed	Days to weeks	Intestine	Keep low-acid foods frozen

2–6 hours. Foods that are cooked and eaten cold, such as meats and poultry, or cold desserts such as custards, trifles and creams, are most often associated with this type of poisoning.

Bacillus cereus

This organism results in two types of symptom: a short delayed response suggestive of an exotoxin, followed by a response more typical of an infection and the production of an endotoxin. The organism is widely distributed in the environment. The rapid onset of symptoms is due to growth in the food and the production of heat-stable toxins. The diarrhoeal symptoms appear to be due to the ingestion of very large numbers of organisms; the endotoxin is destroyed by heat. The foods that are most commonly associated with this type of poisoning are meats and rice.

Clostridium botulinum

This organism produces an extremely potent exotoxin, the ingestion of which is often fatal due to its effects on the nervous system. The organism is an anaerobe and produces spores that are heat-resistant. This form of poisoning is rare in the UK but is more common in the USA, where inadequate heat treatment during domestic canning or preservation of meat and fish is often involved. The toxin is destroyed by relatively mild heat treatment.

Clostridium perfringens

This is a widely distributed anaerobic organism that produces heat-resistant spores. Infection typically occurs when cooked meats are allowed to cool under conditions where the spores can form vegetative cells, and the intestinal tract is infected when the food is ingested. Cooked meats should therefore be cooled rapidly under conditions that restrict germination of the spores and growth of the organism.

Salmonella

Salmonella was the major cause of food poisoning outbreaks in the UK; it has now been superseded by *Campylobacter*, but still remains an important problem. The importance of the species has also changed, with *S. enteriditis* rather than *S. typhimurium* now being the most important. The organism is often found in the intestines of animals and contamination with excreta or gut contents is the major route of transfer to foods. The processing of poultry under intensive conditions is a frequent cause of cross-infection. The organism causes poisoning by infecting the intestine and producing an endotoxin, but it can be killed by heat. Proper cooking of all poultry would eradicate this type of poisoning. One major instance of incorrect cooking is that of cooking unthawed frozen poultry, where the frozen meat is a poor conductor of heat so that the inner parts of the meat only reach incubation temperatures. Another example is the transfer of contaminating organisms from raw to cooked meat that is to be eaten without further heating. Catering establishments are forbidden to store raw and cooked meat in the same refrigerator, to prevent this type of transfer.

Campylobacter jejuni

This organism has recently become associated with outbreaks of food poisoning that have overtaken those due to salmonella. The foods involved were initially milks, but other foods have also been implicated. Like salmonella the organism infects the intestinal tract, producing an endotoxin.

Other organisms

A number of other species have been associated with sporadic outbreaks. These include *E. coli* and *Yersinia enterocolitica*, which are infective organisms producing endotoxins. *Vibrio parahaemolyticus* infections are associated with the consumption of raw or undercooked seafoods. There is growing recognition of the potential importance of *Listeria monocytogenes* as an infective organism in foods. The organism is widely distributed in the environment and the contamination of dairy products low in lactic acid-producing organisms has produced outbreaks of listeriosis. The organism is also capable of growth at relatively low temperatures, so incorrect storage can cause outbreaks.

VIRAL INFECTIONS

A large number of different viruses are known to infect man through the intestinal tract, and can be isolated from faeces. Rotaviruses and norwalk virus are established as major causes of gastroenteritis, and others may also be responsible (Blacklow & Cukor 1981). Viruses, unlike bacteria, cannot multiply in foods, but food handlers and dirty utensils are means whereby small doses may be transferred to foods and subsequently ingested. The viruses infect the intestinal tract. The identification of viruses as the cause of gastroenteritis is technically exacting and it remains possible that viruses may be more important than is currently thought to be the case.

DISEASE TRANSMITTED BY FOOD

Bacterial diseases can be transmitted by infected foods, although most countries have some kind of restrictions on the consumption of food from diseased animals. These may be secular, imposed by public health agencies, or they may be religious in origin. Where the animal or its products are not readily identified as being diseased they can still form a disease vector. Tuberculosis is an obvious example of this, where infected milk was the cause of transmission of bovine tuberculosis to man. The introduction of heat treatment in the form of pasteurization was effective as a control measure, and the testing and certification of dairy herds produced a fall in the incidence of the disease in the UK over the past 50 years (Mabbitt et al 1987). Eradication of the disease in cattle should effectively eliminate this type of food-borne disease.

Brucellosis caused by *Brucella melitensis* and *B. abortus* has been traced to infected milks that had not been pasteurized. It is unfortunate that the benefits of some types of food processing are discounted by some who insist on consuming raw milk.

Helminth infections (Passmore & Robson 1974)

Many helminths have complex life-cycles involving more than one host. The major route for transmission of these parasites to man is the consumption of undercooked infected pork and beef, or the consumption of raw salads that have been washed or irrigated with contaminated water.

Undercooked pork and beef

The pig and beef tapeworms, *Taenia solium* and *T. saginata*, form cysts, which are present in muscle. If these are eaten by man, the adult worms develop in the gut. Segments of the worm and ova are shed with faeces. The ova may also develop into larval forms which invade muscle and other tissues, where they form cysts. This condition is known as cysticercosis and may lead to neurological disorders. Undercooked pork may also contain larvae of *Trichinella spiralis*, which can also invade tissues and cause a febrile illness.

Undercooked and raw fish

The fish tapeworm *Diphyllobothrium latum* has a wide distribution in freshwater fish and thus may infect man if the fish are undercooked or eaten raw. The adult worm can reach 15 m in length, and as it competes with the host for dietary vitamin B_{12} has been known to cause a megaloblastic anaemia.

Raw fish and crabs are sometimes eaten in the Far East and these may be infected with two species of liver fluke.

Raw salads

If the ingredients of the salad have been washed in contaminated water or the crops were grown and irrigated with water from a source colonized by the molluscan hosts of the helminthic worms, then it is possible for infection to occur by this route. The infection is unlikely in countries with well established water and sewerage systems, but these are rare in many parts of the world. Here the consumption of raw salads is a finite risk, unless the salads are washed in permanganate first. Raw salads will also carry on their surfaces many saprophytic bacteria; these are normal commensals in the gastrointestinal tract, but could present a hazard to those whose immunological defences have been weakened.

OTHER DISEASE AGENTS

Since its detection in 1985, bovine spongiform encephalopathy (BSE) has excited much speculation as to its cause and its implications for human health. The disease is transmissible between several animal species and is caused by a strain of a scrapie-like agent. Epidemiological studies indicate that the feeding of cattle with protein supplements prepared from the rendered offal derived from scrapie-infected sheep carcasses may have played a role in the establishment of this disease. So far, there is no evidence of its transmission to humans, but a lot more research needs to be done before the public can be reassured.

CONCLUSIONS

The prevention of food-borne disease is a matter of applying a series of well established principles throughout the food chain. Many of these diseases are completely avoidable if the principles are understood and applied by all those who come into contact with foods that are going to be consumed by man.

The most important principle involves the personal hygiene of the food handler – cleanliness, and the avoidance of touching unwashed surfaces or the nose or mouth. The second concerns the thorough cooking of food so that the temperatures achieved throughout the food are adequate to kill the organisms. Hot food that is not going to be used at once should be covered and cooled rapidly. The third concerns proper storage. The temperature of refrigerators should be below 5°C; raw foods should be stored separately from cooked, and cooked foods should not be placed on surfaces that have held raw foods or manipulated with tools that have been used with raw foods, without thorough washing between the operations. 'Cleanliness is indeed next to Godliness', especially in the control of food poisoning.

REFERENCES

Blacklow NR, Cukor G 1981 Viral gastroenteritis. New England Journal of Medicine 304: 397–406

Egan AF, Roberts TA 1987 Microbiology of meat and meat products. In: Norris JR, Pettipher GL (eds) Essays in agriculture and food microbiology. John Wiley, Chichester, pp. 167–197

Hobbs BC, Gilbert RJ 1978 Food poisoning and food hygiene, 4th edn. Edward Arnold, London

International Commission on Microbiological Specifications for Food 1978 Micro organisms in foods. University of Toronto Press, Toronto

Mabbitt LA, Davies FL, Law BA, Marshall VM 1987 Microbiology of milk and milk products. In: Norris JR, Pettipher GL (eds). Essays in agriculture and food microbiology. John Wiley, Chichester, pp. 135–166

Moss MA 1987 Micobial food poisoning. In: Norris JR, Pettipher GL (eds) Essays in agriculture and food microbiology. John Wiley, Chichester

Passmore R, Robson JS (eds) 1974 A companion to medical studies. Blackwell Scientific Publications, Oxford, Vol 3, 12.36–12.64

23. Food toxicity

R. Walker

At a very early age a child learns from his parents that he cannot eat everything and that certain substances are poisonous. An older child hears and reads stories of romance in which kings and courtiers, afraid that their enemies may poison them, employ food tasters at banquets. It is not surprising that many adults have an ingrained fear of poisons in food nor that the widespread dissemination of chemicals in an industrial society and their deliberate addition to food, though proper causes of concern, raise irrational fears and emotions.

A poison is difficult to define and many substances present in food would have adverse or toxic effects if taken in large doses, but the amounts normally present in foods are harmless.

Table 23.1 gives a classification of the ways by which toxic substances may be present in foods.

Toxins naturally present in plant foods, and infection of food by pathogenic bacteria have caused more human disease and mortality than the other categories. Accidental chemical contamination and environmental pollution have been responsible for local disasters from time to time. The intentional additives used in food processing today in well-organised countries are those considered safe by authoritative bodies.

Table 23.1 Toxic substances in foods

NATURAL	
Inherent	Usually present in the food and affects everyone if they eat enough, e.g. solanine in potatoes, and lathyrus toxin
Toxin resulting from abnormal conditions of animal or plant used for food	For example, neurotoxic mussel poisoning, honey from bees feeding on Rhododendron or Azalea nectar
Consumer abnormally sensitive	Constitutional, e.g. coeliac disease from wheat gluten, favism from broad beans, allergy to particular food, or drug-induced, e.g. cheese reaction
Contamination by pathogenic bacteria	Acute illness, usually gastrointestinal, e.g. toxins produced by *Staphylococcus aureus* or *Clostridium botulinum*; food may not appear spoiled
Mycotoxins	Food mouldy or spoiled, e.g. aflatoxin B_1 from *Aspergillus flavus* is a liver carcinogen
Mutagens and carcinogens	Produced by grilling, roasting or frying meat and fish
ACCIDENTAL CHEMICAL CONTAMINATION OR POLLUTION	
Unintentional additives — man made	
Chemicals used in agriculture and animal husbandry	For example, fungicides on grain, insecticides on fruit, antibiotics or hormones given to animals
Environmental pollution	For example, organic mercury, cadmium, lead, aluminium, PCB and PBB and radioactive fall-out can affect any stage of food chain
Intentional food additives	
Preservatives, emulsifiers, flavours, colours, etc	Some have been in use for centuries; many are naturally based and used in small amounts; the most thoroughly tested and monitored of all chemicals in food

Standards of safety are strict and may be getting stricter. The public and their food safety administrations tend to set higher standards of safety for pure synthetic chemicals than for the complex of substances present in natural foods.

As Magnus Pyke (1971) put it, the tests for new foods and additives are now so stringent that if Sir Walter Raleigh turned up now with the potato, as a new and unknown food, he would never stand a chance of having it accepted because of the solanine which it contains.

Disposal of ingested foreign substances

As foreign substances differ greatly in their chemical nature, their fate in the body varies. In general a substance may follow one of five possible sequences, each of which has variants.

1. It may pass through the gastrointestinal tract and not be absorbed. Pectin and other food thickeners are examples. It may, however, be digested by enzymes in the upper gastrointestinal tract or broken down by bacteria in the colon. Even if a substance is not absorbed it can affect the motility of the gastrointestinal tract and cause vomiting, diarrhoea or constipation. It can also irritate the mucous membrane and produce ulceration. Chronic irritation, if caused by a substance ingested over a long period, could lead to cancer formation. Cancer of the gastrointestinal tract occurs at sites where movement is slowed down and gut contents are in prolonged contact with the mucous membrane, e.g. the lower end of the oesophagus, the pyloric end of the stomach and the colon.

2. A substance may be absorbed and pass into the portal vein to the liver. Here it may be metabolised and then excreted back into the gastrointestinal tract in the bile. This sequence may be repeated, in an enterohepatic cycle. The substance or its metabolites can be recovered in the faeces but it has been inside the body and could damage the liver.

3. Water-soluble substances may be absorbed and pass through the liver into the general circulation. In the blood the substance may be partly bound to one of the plasma proteins, but it is excreted by the kidneys and passes into the urine. An example of a substance which follows this sequence is saccharin, which is excreted unchanged. If such a substance should be oncogenic, the organ most likely to be affected is the urinary bladder.

4. Fat-soluble substances after absorption reach the liver. There they are often metabolised in two stages and usually the metabolites are more water-soluble and so more easily excreted and less toxic. The first stage is oxidation by the non-specific microsomal enzyme oxidising system (MEOS) in the hepatocytes. Cytochromes P-450 are an integral part of this system. Some, e.g. cytochrome P-450 1A, are involved in activation of some pro-carcinogens. The second stage is conjugation of the oxidation product, usually with glucuronic acid or sulphate. Some substances wholly or partly bypass the first stage and are conjugated directly. The metabolites are then excreted in the urine or the bile. An example is the antioxidant BHT (butylated hydroxytoluene); its two tertiary butyl groups are partly oxidised and it is excreted in the urine as glucuronic acid conjugates.

5. A substance may be absorbed but neither metabolised nor excreted; it stays in the body and accumulates. Even if harmless in small amounts in acute or subacute tests, it may lead to long-term harmful effects. Toxicologists are naturally concerned about substances that behave in this way. Examples are fat-soluble compounds like DDT and PBB. These are not only stored in the adipose tissue but pass into the milk fat in lactating women. Substances handled like calcium can stay in bone for a long time, e.g. fluoride, lead and radioactive strontium.

Cadmium is a good example of a substance with a long biological half-life (17–33 years in man), where small daily exposure over a long period leads to accumulation of toxic levels in the kidney.

Toxicity testing

Safety is always relative. Despite numerous statutory safety regulations, travellers on land, sea and air are still killed by accidents, and no food can be guaranteed safe. The most an authority can do is to define an acceptable risk. In general, authorities permit substances to be present in foods when the maximum amount likely to be consumed daily is 100 times less than the maximum amount shown not to have an adverse effect on experimental animals with due allowance for the body weight of the animals. Experimental animals are used for toxicity testing of pharmaceuticals, including cosmetics, and foods; such tests form the large majority of over 4 million vivisections carried out annually in the UK. Antivivisectionists protest strongly against this use of animals. The tests are also expensive and add to the price of many products. Hence attempts are being made to find alternative tests which use tissue cultures or isolated cells. These tests may be the main method of testing for toxicity in the future, but cannot wholly replace animal testing until much more is known about their reliability.

Species differ in their tolerance of many poisons, and an equivalent dose of a chemical shown to be harmless in one species of experimental animal may not be safe for man. Most substances are first tested on rats, but none is considered safe for man until the tests have been repeated on a species which is not rodent: rabbits, cats and dogs are most commonly used. Preferably, tests should also be carried out on a primate.

The signs of acute poisoning are usually obvious and it is not difficult to determine the maximum amount of a single dose of a substance that can be taken with safety. Since a potential food toxin is likely to be consumed throughout the life span of consumers, it has to be tested for long periods in animals and over at least two generations. The fetus is especially sensitive to some toxins, as is the ability of mature animals to reproduce. Malignant disease frequently does not arise until an animal has been exposed to an oncogenic agent for a major portion of its life span. A WHO report (1987a) outlines procedures for investigating intentional and unintentional food additives.

Examples are now given of poisoning in man due to natural and artificial toxins in foods. The accounts are of necessity anecdotal and many, it is hoped, are only of historical interest. Characteristically the illnesses present with an unusual combination of symptoms and signs in a community over a considerable time, and the possibility of their being due to a food toxin has been overlooked at first. In any outbreak of an unusual disease, it is wise to consider this possibility.

NATURAL FOOD TOXINS

There are people who are so alarmed at the possible chemical hazards from eating foods grown and prepared with the aid of the modern chemical industry that they wish to return to a simple life and eat only natural foods. Unfortunately the chemical hazards in the fields and woods are also numerous. Table 23.2 gives a list of foods containing pharmacological agents known to have adverse effects on man. The list is far

Table 23.2 Some possible toxic effects of foods

Source	Active agent	Effects
Bananas and some other fruits	5-Hydroxytryptamine; adrenaline; noradrenaline	Effects on central and peripheral nervous system
Some cheeses	Tyramine	Raises blood pressure; enhanced by monoamine oxidase inhibitors
Almonds, cassava and other plants	Cyanide	Interferes with tissue respiration
Quail	Due to consumption of hemlock	Hemlock poisoning
Mussels	Due to consumption of dino-flaggellate, *Gonyaulax*	Tingling, numbness, muscle weakness, respiratory paralysis
Cycad nuts	Methylazoxymethanol (cycasin)	Liver damage; cancer
Some fish, meat or cheese	Nitrosamines	Cancer
Mustard oil	Sanguinarine	Oedema (epidemic dropsy)
Legumes	Haemagglutinins	Red cell and intestinal cell damage
Some beans	Vicine β-Aminopropionitrile β-N-Oxalyl-amino-L-alanine	Haemolytic anaemia (favism) Interferes with collagen formation. Toxic effects on nervous system, lathyrism
Ackee fruit	α-Amino-β-methylene Cyclopropane propionic acid	Hypoglycaemia, vomiting sickness
Brassica seeds and some other Cruciferae	Glucosinolates, thiocyanate	Enlargement of thyroid gland (goitre)
Rhubarb	Oxalate	Oxaluria
Green potatoes	Solanine; possibly other sapotoxins	Gastrointestinal upset
Many fish	Various, often confined to certain organs or seasonal	Mainly toxic effects on nervous system
Many fungi	Various mycotoxins	Mainly toxic effects on nervous system and liver

from complete and monographs are available prepared by the Committee on Food Protection of the US Food and Nutrition Board (1973) and by Liener (1969, 1974). These contain much curious information and are very readable. Here it is only possible to give a brief account of a few somewhat arbitrarily selected toxins which appear of special interest in medicine.

Table 23.2 indicates that there are natural poisons which have a great variety of acute and chronic pharmacological effects. Presumably many of these evolved in plants as protective mechanisms against animals feeding on them. Animals in turn have evolved elaborate biochemical reactions and cellular responses for disposing of the toxins or of at least partially neutralising their effects. Man and many other animals have also learnt by experience to avoid eating some of the foods containing potent toxins. Some of the most potent toxins are found in fungi which may contaminate otherwise healthy foods.

LATHYRUS POISONS

Tares is the traditional English name for the vetches and an old word used loosely for various pulses and legumes. In Biblical times they were poorly regarded. The tendrils by which these plants climb up the wheat stalks certainly hamper reaping. But they may also have been known to be nutritionally unsatisfactory.

For a long time one species of tare (*Lathyrus sativus: Khesari dhal* in Hindustani) has been deliberately sown with the wheat by farmers in dry districts of many countries in Asia and North Africa where the rainfall is uncertain. If the rains are good, the wheat overgrows the lathyrus, of which little is harvested. If the rains fail and there is a poor crop of wheat, a useful harvest of lathyrus may be reaped. Eaten in small quantities, lathyrus seeds are a valuable food. But if they are the main source of energy (providing more than 50 per cent), a severe disease of the spinal cord (lathyrism, Chapter 42) may result, causing crippling and permanent paralysis. An excellent account of the disease and the circumstances under which it arises has been given by a soldier, General Sleeman (1844).

After many failures to find a neurotoxin, two were isolated in succeeding years. In 1962 in the USA β-N-oxalyl-amino-L-alanine (BOAA) was isolated and identified in the common vetch (*Vicia sativa*), which frequently grows as a weed in lathyrus crops (Ressler 1962). The next year in India β-N-oxalyl-L-α,β diaminopropionic acid was isolated from seeds of *Lathyrus sativus* (Adiga et al 1963). Both of these can cause neurological lesions in primates, but over 30

years later the relation between intakes of the two toxins and the incidence and nature of the neurological lesions in man has not been worked out.

Allied vetches, notably the sweet pea, *Lathyrus odoratus*, when fed to rats, readily give rise to a severe disturbance of collagenous structures throughout the body, notably in skin and bones, known as osteolathyrism (Weaver 1967). This is not a natural disease of either man or animals but can be readily produced in laboratory animals. The neurotoxin responsible, β-aminoproprionitrile, is a much used tool in the experimental study of collagen formation.

SEAWATER FISH

Ciguatera

This is an old Portuguese word introduced in 1787 to describe poisoning that arose after eating fish from the Pacific Ocean and the Caribbean Sea. The clinical features are those of an acute neuromuscular disorder with weakness and sensory changes. Most attacks are of moderate severity and the symptoms clear up in a few days, but itching may persist for several weeks and occasionally widespread paralysis is followed by coma and death.

A large number of species of fish may be poisonous. Some of these are always poisonous and others may usually be eaten with safety, but are poisonous at certain times of the year. Poisonous fish have usually been feeding on a coral reef; deep-sea fish are generally safe. The toxin or toxins responsible have not been identified. Fish become poisonous because of factors in their environment which get into their food supply. Jardin (1972) has suggested that the toxins may be organo-minerals. It is possible that natural disturbances in ocean beds may affect the amounts of trace elements in rocks and sediment, which become incorporated into organic material and so into the algae and other basic components of the food of fishes.

Scombrotoxic poisoning

Scombrotoxicosis can occur from eating tuna, mackerel and related fish. It was formerly thought to be due to histamine intoxication from eating spoiled fish but this historical misapprehension should not be perpetuated (Clifford & Walker 1992). Recent results from fish involved in an outbreak of scombrotoxicosis suggest that algal toxins may be relayed to the mackerel, possibly via shellfish and sand eels (Clifford et al 1993). A review of marine toxins is given in Hall & Strichartz (1990).

Mussel poisoning

A toxin, saxitoxin, may be present in plankton, particularly the dinoflagellate *Gonyaulax tamarensis* which is ingested by bivalves such as mussels. The toxin is stable and remains in the tissues of the shellfish which appear to be resistant. It is not destroyed by cooking. Dinoflagellates at times multiply to such an extent that they may colour the sea and such 'red tides' cause a heavy mortality among seabirds, especially shags. Mussels, usually safe to eat, may then become toxic. These conditions occur sporadically along the east coast of Britain between Aberdeen and Yorkshire in the summer. During 1990 and 1991 blooms were particularly dense and extensive and led to the temporary closure of some of the shellfish fisheries. An EC directive now requires regular monitoring of paralytic shellfish poisoning (PSP). A level of 80 µg/100 g in shellfish meat is the action level for increased sampling in an area, and results are made available daily. Diarrhoetic shellfish toxins (DSP) such as okadaic acid produced by *Procentrum* and *Dinophysis* species of phytoplankton. In addition to causing acute gastrointestinal symptoms, okadaic acid is a potent promoter of carcinogenesis.

FRESHWATER FISH

Fishermen and their families around the Koenigsberg Haff in East Germany during the period between World Wars I and II suffered outbreaks of acute paroxysmal myoglobinuria, preceded by severe pain in all muscles. Always on the day before an attack fish, usually eel or burbot, had been eaten. The condition became known as Haff disease, and German investigators concluded that the fish eaten contained a toxin which had entered the Haff with the effluent from nearby industrial works. However, a small outbreak in Sweden affected persons who had eaten burbot from a lake uncontaminated by industrial waste. Berlin (1948) suggested that thiaminase present in the fish might be the cause, but this seems unlikely. Haff disease is rarely reported nowadays and the toxin responsible remains unidentified.

MISCELLANEOUS TOXINS IN FOODS

Herbal teas

The promotion of herbal teas, including comfrey tea, in some women's magazines is cause for concern. Comfrey root and leaf contain hepatotoxic and carcinogenic pyrollizidine alkaloids, and cases of fatal

human intoxication from these and related sources are known. Other herbal teas may contain other toxins and have not been analysed and tested, so caution is essential (WHO 1989a).

Argemone contamination of edible oils

In Bengal and Bihar mustard oil is the chief cooking fat. In the same part of the world epidemic dropsy has been endemic for a long time. In a series of investigations in which the clues were analysed in the best detective manner, Lal and his colleagues (Lal & Roy 1937, Lal et al 1940) showed that mustard oil was responsible for this disease. The toxin was not present in the oil from the mustard seeds themselves, but in oil from the seeds of a poppy weed (*Argemone mexicana*). This weed commonly grows in the mustard crops. Its seeds contain a toxic alkaloid, sanguinarine (Sarkar 1948). Sanguinarine inhibits the oxidation of pyruvic acid and, as in wet beriberi, cardiomyopathy may follow (Chapter 14). Other edible oils, such as groundnut oil, can be contaminated with argemone oil.

Ackee fruit (*Blighia sapida*)

The fruit grows profusely in Jamaica and is eaten by large numbers of people, especially children. Yet it is widely credited with being responsible for a form of food poisoning, 'vomiting sickness' (Jelliffe & Stuart 1954). Dr Cicely Williams undertook an investigation of the disease for the Jamaican Government (Williams 1954). She was able to study numerous patients and a few outbreaks in detail. In some, the symptoms could be attributed to other diseases. Yet there were several patients in whom no definite cause could be found, despite thorough investigation. A specific poison from the ackee fruit could not be excluded. She concluded that if such poison were indeed responsible, large amounts would have to be consumed, and the patients must be peculiarly susceptible to the poison, probably because of their undernourished state. Ackee fruit contains a water-soluble substance, α-amino-β-methylene cyclopropyl-proprionic acid, that causes accumulation of branched short-chain fatty acids and acute hypoglycaemia and is known as hypoglycin (Holt et al 1964). This substance is now believed to be responsible for the clinical features of vomiting sickness.

Brassica species

Brassica is a large genus which includes cabbages, mustards and rapes. Rabbits and other laboratory animals fed large amounts of raw leaves develop goitre, which may also occur after feeding the seeds. This is due to the presence of glucosinolates and thiocyanates. Glucosinolates act on the thyroid gland like thiouracil by preventing the synthesis of thyroxine. Thiocyanates reduce the concentration of iodine in the thyroid gland. Some of the brassicas, notably cabbage, are common human foods, but there is no evidence that when eaten in normal amounts, as part of a balanced diet, they are anything but beneficial. Goitrogens in foods are further considered in Chapter 36.

Potatoes

It has been known for a long time that potatoes contain an alkaloid, solanine, that is potentially toxic. In normal potatoes there is about 7 mg/100 g, mostly in the skin, but also in eyes and sprouts. Potato poisoning is very rare, but an outbreak occurred in a London school affecting 78 boys (McMillan & Thompson 1979). The main symptoms were headache, vomiting and diarrhoea. Fever and circulatory collapse led to 17 of the boys being admitted to hospital, of whom three were dangerously ill with neurological disturbances, stupor and hallucinations. A sample of the potatoes that had been served at the school, when peeled and boiled, contained 33 mg of solanine per 100 g. There is little doubt that solanine poisoning was responsible for the outbreak, but how these particular potatoes came to have such a high solanine content is a mystery.

A suggestion that solanine in potatoes eaten by mothers in early pregnancy might be responsible for spina bifida and other abnormalities of the central nervous system received much publicity in the lay press. There is no epidemiological or other evidence to support it. Folate deficiency is now thought to be involved (Chapter 14).

Cycads

There has been a high incidence of a form of motor neurone disease and of a disease known as Parkinsonism dementia among the Chamorro people on the island of Guam and the neighbouring Mariana islands. It has been suspected that the traditional high consumption of the seeds of the cycad, *Cycas circinalis*, might be responsible. Certainly cycad seeds contain a toxin, cycasin, which in experimental animals is a potent hepatotoxin and is also carcinogenic. Yet hepatic disease, including carcinoma, is only slightly more common in Guam than in the USA; feeding adult animals with cycasin has not produced neurological damage, and it has not been shown that the victims of the motor neurone disease have eaten more cycad seeds or prepared them in a different way from unaffected islanders (Kurland 1972).

Spices

Spices and flavouring agents contain volatile and essential oils and hydrocarbons which stimulate glandular secretion and may have a weak action on the nervous system. Many of them if taken in large doses have toxic actions.

There are literally thousands of components of the essential oils of herbs and spices. This poses something of a problem, since essential oils and their individual components derived from herbs and spices may also be used as food additives (flavours) and most components have not been tested toxicologically – which raises difficulties in framing a Flavours Directive in the EC, particularly in establishing a permitted list on a rational scientific basis.

Oestrogens

Some plant foods, including soya bean, contain traces of oestrogens, but the amounts are so small that no adverse effects follow the consumption of such foods. Larger amounts may be present in meat from animals previously dosed with oestrogens to promote growth. This practice is now not permitted in most countries.

Carcinogens

Many natural foods have been shown to contain substances which produce tumours in experimental animals. Potent mutagens and carcinogens like the aminoimidazo-aza-arenes are produced by high temperature cooking (grilling, roasting, frying) of meat and fish (Sugimura 1982). The extent to which they may be responsible for malignant disease in man is discussed in Chapter 45.

Antivitamins

Attention was first drawn to the antivitamins in veterinary practice. Cattle fed on spoiled sweet clover develop a haemorrhagic disease. This is due to the presence in the clover of dicoumarol, a substance chemically related to vitamin K (Link 1945). It produces haemorrhages by causing vitamin K deficiency in the tissues. Synthetic analogues of dicoumarol are used in clinical practice to reduce the liability to coagulation.

Natural substances can act as antivitamins by preventing their absorption or by destroying them in the gut. For example in 1936 an outbreak of paralysis, 'Chastek paralysis', developed in silver foxes on a farm in the USA belonging to Mr Chastek. The foxes had been fed on carp. The presence of a thiaminase was demonstrated in the flesh and viscera of these fish (Green et al 1942). Additional thiamin both prevented and cured the disease. Thiaminase has been found in several species of fish. A different substance (3, 4-dihydroxy cinnamic acid) with thiaminase activity occurs in bracken and other plants. Thiamin deficiency due to consumption of thiaminase has not been reported in man. Fish is used as a food in zoos and nature reserves, as well as in commercial animal production, and those who use it should be aware of the hazard from thiaminase.

Hallucinogenic substances

In 1676 British soldiers engaged in putting down a rebellion in Virginia ate a salad containing the Jimson weed *Datura stramonium*. Some of them were reported to have been turned into natural fools performing many simple tricks, but they remembered nothing of this when they recovered. The weed contains alkaloids, such as scopolamine, which produce hallucinations. Cases of poisoning have been reported in 'beatniks' who have eaten the weed for its psychic effects and in children who have tasted its fruits out of curiosity.

The Mexican plant peyote, which contains mescaline, and the hemp plant, *Cannabis indica*, widespread in Asia and Africa, are two examples of plants which have been consumed deliberately for their psychic effects.

The fly toadstool, *Amanita muscaria*, contains muscarin, but only in small amounts and the characteristic symptom of poisoning is cerebral excitement, which is due to mycetoatropine. An example of its action was a young man admitted to a Glasgow hospital in a confused and drowsy state (Horne & McCluskie 1963). By occupation he was a salmon poacher, and he and his brother used to eat deliberately *A. muscaria* because they enjoyed the feeling of unreality and detachment which it gave. Others have become addicted, including apparently the Russian Empress Catherine the Great.

TOXINS OF FUNGAL ORIGIN

Mushrooms

Some mushrooms and many other species of fungi are excellent eating but others are poisonous. The mushroom commonly responsible for poisoning in Britain is *Amanita phalloides* and in America *Amanita serna*. Each contains two types of toxin. Phallotoxins are heptapeptides that act quickly, causing vomiting, diarrhoea and abdominal pain. Amatoxins are octopeptides and act after they have been taken up by hepatocytes and renal tubular cells. Oliguria and other evidence of renal failure may appear only after the gastrointestinal symptoms have subsided. Damage to the kidney may be fatal unless haemodialysis is available. Treatment is by washing out the stomach repeatedly and replacing losses of fluid and electrolytes. Haemodialysis should be started early in severe cases. Antidotes that may be useful are penicillin in large doses, silymarin and thioctic acid.

The dangers of eating any unfamiliar mushroom are illustrated by the story of three young people on holiday in the north of Scotland (Short et al 1980). They had gathered and eaten mushrooms with orange gills (*Cortinarius speciosissimus*). Gastrointestinal symptoms of varying severity followed and 10 days later all three were admitted to the Edinburgh Royal Infirmary. One of the party showed evidence of only slight renal damage and recovered fully. The other two are now also alive and well, thanks to haemodialysis and subsequent renal transplantation.

Ergot

Epidemics of the disease known as St Anthony's fire was described in France in the eleventh century. The disease was called 'fire' because of the intolerable burning pain in the limbs, which became black, shrivelled and dropped off. Convulsions, palsies and disordered movements affected some patients, indicating that the central nervous system as well as the peripheral vascular system were affected. Epidemics were frequent in many countries in Europe, but it was not until the beginning of the eighteenth century that it was associated with eating rye infected by a fungus, *Claviceps purpura*. The disease, especially the convulsive form, was severe in Germany in the eighteenth century and persisted in Poland and Russia until well into the twentieth century. A classic book by Barger (1931) describes the features of the disease and his work with Dale on the ergot alkaloids present in the fungus and responsible for its toxicity.

Occasional outbreaks are reported still. Thus in Ethiopia five cases of gangrenous ergotism occurred, associated with eating wild oats infected with *Claviceps* species (King 1979). In India outbreaks have occurred associated with the millet (*Pennisetum typoides*), known as bajra, infected with *Claviceps fusiformis* (Krishnamachari & Bhat 1976). This fungus produces alkaloids of the clavine group, which are different from the ergot alkaloids. The clinical features of poisoning are severe nausea and vomiting, accompanied by giddiness and drowsiness, but recovery is rapid and complete. Hence it is a much less serious disease than classical European ergotism.

Aflatoxins

In 1960 a widespread outbreak of a fatal disease characterised by acute enteritis and hepatitis occurred in England among young turkeys which had been fed a ration containing imported groundnut meal (Allcroft et al 1961). The groundnuts concerned had been harvested, stored and processed under conditions of high humidity. The toxic factors were produced by *Aspergillus flavus*, a mould contaminating the nuts. They are brightly fluorescing furanocoumarin compounds known as 'aflatoxins'. Aflatoxins are now known to contaminate human foods. Nuts and grains produced and stored in warm moist climates are most likely to be affected. Aflatoxins damage the liver and lead to carcinoma in many animals. Aflatoxin B1 is the most potent known natural hepato-carcinogen, at least in susceptible species such as the rat and duckling. The toxic dose in primates is about 0.05 mg/kg daily. There has been much conjecture about the possible role of aflatoxin in primary carcinoma of the liver in man in Africa and Asia (Chapter 45).

Maize contaminated with aflatoxin appeared to be responsible for an epidemic of an acute illness which occurred in 1974 and affected 200 villages in Gjarat and Rajasthan, India. The clinical features were jaundice, ascites, portal hypertension and a high mortality. It was estimated that patients had consumed from 2 to 6 mg of aflatoxin daily for one month (Krishnamachari et al 1975). Aflatoxins have also been detected in autopsy liver samples from some cases of the Reye-Johnson syndrome, acute encephalopathy with fatty liver (Chaves-Carballo et al 1976). Aflatoxins are of great importance in animal husbandry, and a review is available (Ueno 1985).

Other mycotoxins

The discovery of aflatoxins means that mouldy food and fodder is not merely unattractive; it may be dangerous. Other potentially dangerous mycotoxins may be produced by moulds that can grow on foods. Sterigmatocystin from *Aspergillus versicolor* on maize is carcinogenic in animals but much less potent than the aflatoxins. Patulin from *Penicillium expansum*, found in rotten apples, may occur in apple juice and is also carcinogenic.

The trichothecenes, produced by species of *Fusarium* on mouldy cereals, appear to be responsible for a human disease, alimentary toxic aleukia, in Russia. Ochratoxin from *Aspergillus ochraceus* on mouldy barley has been responsible for kidney disease in swine in Denmark. Evidence is accumulating that Balkan nephropathy, a slowly progressive nephropathy without hypertension which is endemic in parts of the Danube valley, may be due to toxins from *Penicillium cyclopium* on stored maize (Barnes et al 1977). The list of mycotoxins is long and recent additions are the fumonosins. It will take a long time to work out which are of importance in human disease. Meanwhile all mouldy food should be regarded with caution. It would be salutary for the enthusiasts for natural foods to ponder that mycotoxins are more likely to contaminate foods grown and processed without fungicides, preservatives and chemical additives.

AGRICULTURAL CHEMICALS

A farmer has to worry about his crops. Weeds, insects, fungi, bacteria and viruses can all seriously reduce the yield in the fields. After harvest, rodents, moulds and putrefying bacteria may cause further loss. His animals may suffer from external parasites, ticks, lice and maggots in the skin and many species of worms and other organisms in the alimentary canal and internal organs. These dangers can be prevented or at least reduced by chemical agents which, if improperly used, can reach a final food product in amounts which may be toxic to consumers. Modern farming is a highly technical business which depends on the chemical industry. The very high yields now obtainable would be impossible without the use of chemicals.

PESTICIDES AND WEED KILLERS

The danger from these is mainly to manufacturers, distributors and farm workers; acute poisoning is well known to occur amongst them and has been responsible for several deaths. Only very rarely has the residue left on a crop been responsible for acute poisoning. Two such outbreaks are now described.

One evening in 1959, 13 children and one adult were admitted to a hospital in Singapore (Karagaratnam et al 1960). They had been taken ill suddenly and most of them had collapsed. Examination showed signs of overactivity of the parasympathetic system – sweating, dilated pupils, excessive salivation and increased secretions in the lungs. Many had fits and those severely affected became unconscious; four children died. Acting with commendable speed, the medical staff of the hospital suspected organo-phosphate poisoning and warned the public health authority. Early on the next morning, after it had been discovered that all the patients had eaten barley recently imported from Europe, instructions were issued making 'barley poisoning' notifiable. Subsequently the barley was found to be contaminated with the insecticide Parathion, which is a powerful anticholinesterase agent. Prompt action contained the outbreak to 38 cases with nine deaths.

Another dramatic story comes from Sri Lanka 22 years later (Senanayake & Jeyaranam 1981). Young Tamil girls from tea estates complained of pain in the calves and weakness of the feet and hands; they had absent ankle jerks, wrist drop and other signs suggesting a toxic polyneuropathy. In all cases the symptoms had first appeared two to four weeks after the menarche. At this time it was the custom to prohibit meat and fish and to give the girls raw eggs and gingili oil. This cooking oil was used sparingly in the community but the girls after eating a raw egg were served the oil in the shell, filled to the brim. This ritual continued for two weeks and ended with a ceremonial bath. Enquiries at the oil merchants revealed that oil had been stored in metal drums originally used for mineral oils. The insecticide tri-cresyl phosphate was detected in the samples of oil. It was calculated that during the two weeks the girls had each received 2.8 to 5.6 g of the poison, a dose probably sufficient to cause neuropathy.

There are many pesticides in use. The organochlorine insecticides such as DDT were formerly used widely, but because of their toxicity their use is banned in most developed countries. Because of their persistence they are still detected in the food chain. The widespread use of DDT has had adverse effects on hawks, eagles and other birds that live on the flesh of small animals. In some areas many of their eggs did not hatch and this led to a reduction in numbers. The eggs may be defective due to a deficiency of oestrogens which may be metabolized at an increased rate by microsomal enzymes of the liver induced by DDT.

More modern pesticides such as carbamates and organophosphorus pesticides are much more toxic than the organochlorines but, because of their low persistence, present less of problem to the consumer (although perhaps more to the agricultural worker). Current issues are considered by MAFF (1992), and regulatory safety assurance systems are leading to the establishment of ADIs and Maximum Residue Levels (WHO 1990).

ANTIBIOTICS

Antibiotics are used to treat infectious diseases in farm animals. They have also been incorporated into animal foodstuffs because in some way, not yet fully explained, they promote growth; thus they are of economic value in the rearing of pigs and poultry. They have also been used in food preservation. In these ways foods may become contaminated, but there is no evidence that this has had any direct adverse effect on man.

A serious indirect effect of the indiscriminate use of antibiotics in animal husbandry is the development of bacterial resistance to their action. Strains of *Salmonella typhimurium* and *Escherichia coli* which may infect both man and livestock are liable to acquire such resistance. This is carried in the genetic material of the bacteria and may be transferred to different bacteria, which then become resistant, although not previously exposed to the antibiotic.

The problems of regulating the veterinary drug residues in food are discussed by the Joint European Committee on Food Additives (JECFA) and published by WHO (1991). The situation in the UK is monitored by MAFF (1992). Illegal use of the β-agonist clenbuterol in beef production does occur (Martinez-Navarro 1990). It is now illegal to add antibiotics to animal foodstuffs but unfortunately strains of *Salmonella* resistant to antibiotics continue to be found.

HORMONES

Steroid sex hormones act as anabolic agents in beef cattle. Their use has been banned in the EEC but not in the USA. Bovine somatotropin (BST) is used in the US to improve milk production in dairy cattle. Although there is little scientific evidence that it is harmful, public opinion finds it unacceptable so there is currently a moratorium against its use in Europe. The ban on oestrogens in beef production is not really logical. Comparable amounts of oestrogens are naturally present in soya beans and in eggs; endogenous production in women and the amounts used in oral contraceptives are much larger. The ban is being challenged but meanwhile hormonal feed additives are not permitted in the EEC.

FUNGICIDES ON SEED GRAIN

Several tragic accidents have affected peasant farmers who were supplied with new types of seed grain that had been treated with chemicals to prevent fungus disease of the young wheat plant. If the previous harvest was small and instructions poor, people have eaten some of the seed grain. Alkyl mercury poisoning occurred in Iraq in 1972 for this reason. In Turkey hexachlorobenzene was used as the fungicide. Ingestion of treated grain led to 3000 cases of porphyria with skin lesions precipitated by sunlight in the late 1950s (Peters 1976).

INDUSTRY

Foods may be contaminated by industrial poisons in various ways – improper disposal of industrial waste and accidents and crime at a plant. Fortunately all of these are rare but, as the scale of industrial processing gets bigger, the wider the effect when something goes wrong.

Industrial waste

Outbreaks of poisoning by food contaminated by failure to dispose of industrial waste containing mercury and cadmium in a safe manner sometimes occur. Lead from car exhausts has been recognized as a serious problem and the apparent fall in food lead levels may be associated with the introduction of unleaded petrol and non-soldered can seams (MAFF 1989). However, there is increasing concern about lead since the most recent data suggest that a threshold cannot be determined for impairment of mental performance in infants and young children, with deleterious effects noted at very low exposure levels (WHO 1989b). A recent scandal of lead in animal feed resulted in milk from several affected herds having to be withdrawn from the market in the Netherlands and the UK (Baars et al 1992, Crews et al 1992).

Polychlorinated biphenyls from electrical insulation and plasticizers can cause contamination of fish and the problem was recognized by Skene et al (1989) and WHO (1992a). Dioxins (TODD) and tetrachlorodibenzofurans produced in incinerators and paperworks cause dangerous contamination of agricultural areas. A tragic example of this was the Seveso disaster (WHO 1989c).

Accident

Widespread poisoning of farm animals with lesser effects on man occurred in the USA in 1973. An illiterate truck driver in Michigan delivered 2000 lb of Firemaster, a fire retardant made of polybrominated biphenyls (PBB), instead of Neutromaster, a magnesium oxide supplement, from a chemical firm to an animal feed depot. Here the employees assumed it was an improved version of the feed supplement. In consequence, poisoned grain was delivered to hundreds of farms and fed to many thousands of animals. Animals became ill but it took a year before the poison was identified. By that time much farm and dairy produce had become contaminated with PBB, which is metabolised extremely slowly and tends to accumulate in the body. Some people in the area lost weight and became disorientated. Three years later PBB could be detected in most samples of mother's milk in Michigan State (Brilliant et al 1978). A similar recent example was the incident of aluminium sulphate in drinking water at Camelford (Cornwall and Isles of Scilly District Health Authority 1989).

CRIMINAL ADULTERATION

A mysterious new disease broke out in Spain in May 1981. There were 13 000 cases admitted to hospital and over 100 deaths. People in the poorer quarters of Madrid were most affected but some cases occurred in the provinces. The agent responsible was soon identified as a cooking oil, sold fraudulently by doorstep traders in unlabelled bottles as pure olive oil. In fact it was mostly rapeseed oil with some other oils as ingredients. It contained aniline, which is used to denature rapeseed oil for industrial purposes (WHO 1992b). However, the nature of the chemical poison remains unknown.

The clinical features were diverse and not explicable by any known pathology (Toxic Epidemic Syndrome Group 1982). In May acute cases presented with fever, rashes, myalgia and respiratory distress; most of the deaths were due to a pneumonopathy. Although the oil was quickly identified as the responsible agent and ceased to be used, cases continued to present in June and July but with new features. Intense muscular pain and numbness of the arms and legs were common. Thromboembolism was a serious but uncommon complication. The disease changed again in August and September when patients presented with scleroderma-like skin lesions, Raynaud's phenomenon, dysphagia, severe motor weakness with muscular atrophy and weight loss. Some died of respiratory failure. In each of these stages there was no consistent change in laboratory findings. At autopsy vascular changes with endothelial swelling and cellular infiltration of the vessel wall was seen in all organs.

Crime will always be with us but this strange and tragic consequence of it could have been averted by rapid enforcement of the law. The lesson is that local authorities should have the staff to detect promptly all breaches of food safety laws and regulations, together with the power to enforce them strictly.

RADIOACTIVE FALL-OUT

For 18 years from 1945 when an atomic bomb was dropped on Hiroshima until 1963 when the Nuclear Test Ban was signed by the governments of the United States, the Soviet Union and the United Kingdom, atomic explosions periodically liberated radioactive dust into the atmosphere. This dust rose into the stratosphere, where it might drift for many thousands of miles before sinking into the lower atmosphere and finally to the earth's surface. After each nuclear explosion, fall-out contaminated a large area determined mainly by local meteorological conditions. In an affected area, cereal crops, vegetables and fruits which may be eaten by man were contaminated, and also grasses and herbage eaten by cattle. Their milk and meat then contains radioactive material. In general, foods of animal origin become more dangerous to man than those of plant origin because the radioactive material is concentrated in milk and meat.

The main potentially dangerous radioisotopes in fall-out are iodine-131 (^{131}I), strontium-90 (^{90}Sr) and caesium-137 (^{137}Cs). ^{131}I has a half life of only 8 days and so most of that liberated by an explosion becomes inactive in the upper atmosphere. Nevertheless, unacceptable amounts were found in some samples of milk. ^{90}Sr and ^{137}Cs have half lives of 28 and 30 years respectively and so are potentially greater dangers. The absorption, storage and excretion of strontium is similar to that of calcium and so ^{90}Sr is concentrated in milk. The body deals with caesium as it deals with potassium and so caesium is concentrated in muscle and all meats may be contaminated. ^{90}Sr is especially dangerous because it is stored in bone, and the adjacent bone marrow is very susceptible to damage by radiation. The concentration of ^{90}Sr in milk makes it especially dangerous to infants and children.

Before 1963 radioactive fall-out caused significant contamination of food in many countries and was a real cause of concern. An account of the situation in the United Kingdom at that time is given by Hawthorn (1959). The Nuclear Test Ban Treaty in 1963 was an event of major importance to the world but the protection provided by the ban is as secure, and no more, as any other international treaty.

An accident in a nuclear power station can also be followed by contamination of foods produced in its vicinity. The Chernobyl disaster is a recent incident in which food was contaminated with radionuclides over a wide area (Fry & Britcher 1987, Mondon & Walters 1990).

In 1969 WHO and the International Atomic Energy Agency (IAEA) established an International Reference Centre for Environmental Radioactivity at Le Vesignet, France. This assists national governments in collecting information about all forms of radiation in the environment which are a potential danger to health and gives advice on control measures. It publishes periodically reports on the concentrations of ^{90}Sr and ^{137}Cs in samples of milk from various countries.

In an emergency, it is safe to eat foods which have been stored or packed in airtight tins or jars or otherwise protected from atmospheric dust. Tinned foods which have been exposed to intense radiation do not become radioactive. Other remedial measures are uncertain. Since calcium and strontium use the same transport mechanism, increasing the dietary calcium might be expected to reduce intestinal absorption of ^{90}Sr.

FOOD ADDITIVES

No chemical can be deliberately added to foods until it has been through extensive tests for toxicity. Yet, experience may lead to reassessment.

Some current examples of problems with food additives are sulphiting agents and nitrates. Some groups of people are particularly sensitive to sulphiting agents, and deaths occurred among a group of severe, steroid-dependent asthmatics following the use of sulphite to treat salads in salad bars to prevent enzymic browning, never a practice in the UK (Federation of American Societies of Experimental Biology 1985, Walker 1988). The concern about nitrates in food arises because nitrates can be converted to nitrites in the body and these can combine with amines to form nitrosamines, which have been linked with stomach cancer. A recent review and safety evaluation is given by Walker (1990).

Cyclamate

The Soft Drinks Regulations (1964) permitted the use of cyclamate as an artificial sweetener. The maximum amount that could be added to soft drinks was 1.35 g/litre. The regulation was based on the advice of the Food Additives and Contaminants Committee, who were aware that cyclamates were already permitted in the USA and in a report published in 1966 they give extensive evidence based on tests on rats, mice, cats, dogs, rabbits and man that cyclamate is not toxic. A 1969 study on rats in the USA reported that high levels of cyclamate produced bladder cancer in eight out of 240 rats. As a result, cyclamate was banned immediately in the USA and soon after in the UK. In fact the study was carried out on a mixture of cyclamate and saccharine; cyclamate alone has never been shown to produce bladder tumours, whereas saccharine has. Cyclamate has since been reinstated. European committees (SCF and JECFA) have allocated an ADI of 11 mg/kg body weight based on its metabolism to cyclohexylamine and the No Observed Adverse Effect Level for cyclohexylamine (WHO 1982). However, the Committee on Toxicity in the UK have used a rather more conservative interpretation of the metabolic data and have set an ADI of 1.5 mg/kg body weight.

Monosodium glutamate

In 1968 Dr Kwok (1968) reported that for several years he had suffered 'from numbness of the back of the neck, gradually radiating to both arms and back, general weakness and palpitation'. The symptoms came on while eating in a Chinese restaurant, lasted two hours and left no hangover. The syndrome is now well known and presumed to be due to monosodium L-glutamate (MSG). The Chinese have used seaweeds and soya beans, both of which contain sodium glutamate, as natural condiments for generations. MSG is a permitted flavouring enhancer widely used for savoury foods in the food industry. There is no certainty that it is responsible for the symptoms as double-blind trials have generally been negative or inconclusive (Kenney 1986, WHO 1987b). As the symptoms are transient, only affect a minority of consumers, lead to no permanent damage, are early associated by the sufferer with excess consumption of highly flavoured foods and so can be avoided, there seems no case for banning the use of glutamate as a flavouring agent – at least for adults. Glutamate has been added to many infants foods, but most manufacturers of these foods have now ceased to use it. This seems a wise decision until more is known about its possible actions.

The stories of cyclamate and of monosodium glutamate are worth pondering on for they have several messages for nutritionists. First, they show the uncertainty of contemporary knowledge; reports of new observations may at any time challenge accepted opinions of the day. They illustrate the value of a careful study of unusual and unexplained symptoms when these appear either in man or in any other animal species. The difficulty in making a decision as to what is an acceptable risk, and the need to proceed slowly before making a judgement on any chemical, is well demonstrated. Consumers may take comfort from the fact that we are unable to provide evidence that any human being has suffered in health in any serious way as a consequence of taking a permitted food additive, although occasionally an individual is found to be allergic to one of them (Chapter 44). This, of course, must not be used as an excuse for relaxing present standards of toxicity testing. The need to make present tests more precise and to devise better tests continues.

REFERENCES

Adiga PR, Rao SLN, Sarma PS 1963 Some structural features and neurotoxic action of a compound for *L. sativus* seeds. Current Science 32: 153–155

Allcroft A, Carnaghan RBA, Sargeant K, O'Kelly J 1961 A toxic factor in Brazilian groundnuts. Veterinary Record 73: 428–429

Baars AJ, Van Beek H, Visser IJR et al 1992 Lead intoxication in cattle: a case report. Food Additives and Contaminants 9: 357–364

Barger G 1931 Ergot and ergotism. Gurney & Jackson, London

Barnes JM, Austwick PKC, Carter RL, Flynn FV, Peristianis GC, Aldridge WN 1977 Balkan (endemic) nephropathy and a toxin-producing strain of *Penicillium verucosum* var *cyclopium*: an experimental model in rats. Lancet 1: 671–675

Berlin R 1948 Haff disease in Sweden. Acta Medica Scandinavica 129: 560–572

Brilliant LB, Wilcox K, Amburg GV, Eyster E, Isbister J, Bloomer A W et al 1978 Breast-milk monitoring to measure Michigan's contamination with polybrominated biphenyls. Lancet 2: 643–646

Chaves-Carballo E, Ellefson RD, Gomez MR 1976 An aflatoxin in the liver of a patient with Reye-Johnson syndrome. Mayo Clinic Proceedings 51: 48–50

Clifford MN, Walker R 1992 The aetiology of Scombrotoxicosis. International Journal of Food Science and Technology 27: 721–724

Clifford MN, Walker R, Ijomah P et al 1993 Do saxitoxin-like substances have a role in scombrotoxicosis? Food Additives and Contaminants 10 (in press)

Committee on Food Protection, Food and Nutrition Board, National Research Council 1973 Toxicants occurring naturally in foods, 2nd edn. National Academy of Sciences, Washington DC

Cornwall and Isles of Scilly District Health Authority 1989 Water pollution at Lowermoor North Cornwall; report of the Lowermoor Incident Health Advisory Group, July 1989, Truro

Crews HM, Baxter MJ, Bigwood T et al 1992 Lead in feed incident – multi-element analysis of cattle feed and tissues by inductively coupled plama-mass spectometry and co-operative quality assurance scheme for lead analysis of milk. Food Additives and Contaminants 9: 365–378

Federation of American Societies of Experimental Biology 1985 The re-examination of the GRAS status of sulfiting agents. Report by Life Sciences Research Office, FASEB, prepared for the Center for Food Safety and Applied Nutrition, US Food and Drug Administration, Washington, DC

Fry FA, Britcher A 1987 Doses from Chernobyl radiocaesium. Lancet 2: 160–161

Green RG, Carlson WE, Evans CA 1942 The inactivation of Vitamin B_1 in diets containing whole fish. Journal of Nutrition 23: 165–174

Hall S, Strichartz G (eds) 1990 Marine toxins: origin, structure and molecular pharmacology. American Chemical Society Symposium Series No. 418. American Chemical Society, Washington

Hawthorn J 1959 The occurrence of radiostrontium in foodstuffs. Proceedings of the Nutrition Society 18: 44–49

Holt C von, Chang J, Holt M von, Bohm H 1964 Metabolism and metabolic effects of hypoglycin. Biochimica et Biophysica Acta 90: 611–613

Horne CHW, McCluskie JAW 1963 The food of the gods. Scottish Medical Journal 8: 489–491

Jardin C 1972 Organo-minerals and ciguatera. FAO Nutrition Newsletter 10(3): 14–25

Jelliffe DB, Stuart KL 1954 Acute toxic hypoglycaemia in the vomiting sickness of Jamaica. British Medical Journal 1: 75–77

Karagaratnam K, Bron WK, Hoh TK 1960 Parathion poisoning from contaminated barley. Lancet 1: 538–542

Kenney RA, 1986 The Chinese restaurant syndrome: an anecdote revisited. Food and Chemical Toxicology 24: 351–354

King B 1979 Outbreak of ergotism in Wollo, Ethiopia. Lancet 1: 1411

Krishnamachari KAVR, Bhat RV 1976 Poisoning by ergoty bajra (pearl millet) in man. Indian Journal of Medical Research 64: 1624–1628

Krishnamachari KAVR, Bhat RV, Nagaragan V, Tilak TBG 1975 Hepatitis due to aflatoxicosis: an outbreak in western India. Lancet 1: 1061

Kurland LT 1972 An appraisal of the neurotoxicity of cycad and the etiology of amyotrophic lateral sclerosis in Guam. Federal Proceedings 31: 1540–1542

Kwok RHM 1968 Chinese-restaurant syndrome. New England Journal of Medicine 278: 796

Lal RB, Roy SC 1937 Investigations into the epidemiology of epidemic dropsy. Indian Journal of Medical Research 25: 163–259

Lal RB, Makherji SP, Das Gupta AC, Chatterji SR 1940 Quantitative aspects of the problem of toxicity of mustard oil. Indian Journal of Medical Research 28: 163

Liener IE (ed) 1969 Toxic constituents in plant foodstuffs. Academic Press, New York

Liener IE (ed) 1974 Toxic constituents of animal foodstuffs. Academic Press, New York

Link KP 1945 the anticoagulant 3,3'-methylene bis(4-bis (4-hydroxycourmanin)). Federal Proceedings 4: 176–182

McMillan M, Thompson JC 1979 An outbreak of suspected solanine poisoning in schoolboys. Quarterly Journal of Medicine 227–243

Martinez-Navarro JF 1990 Food poisoning related to the consumption of illicit β-agonist in the liver. Lancet 336: 1311

Ministry of Agriculture, Fisheries and Food 1989 Lead in food: progress report. The twenty-seventh report of the Steering Group on Food Surveillance; the Working Party on Inorganic Contaminants in Food, third supplementary report on lead. HMSO, London

Ministry of Agriculture, Fisheries and Food/Health and Safety Executive 1992 Annual Report of the Working Party on Pesticide Residues: 1991. Supplement to the Pesticides Register. HMSO, London

Ministry of Agriculture, Fisheries and Food 1992 Veterinary residues in animal products 1986–1990. Thirty-third report of the Steering Group on Chemical Aspects of Food Surveillance. Food Surveillance Paper No. 33. HMSO, London

Mondon KJ, Walters B 1990 Measurement of radiocaesium, radiostrontium and plutonium in whole diets following deposition of radioactivity in the UK originating from the Chernobyl power plant accident. Food Additives and Contaminants 7: 837–848

Peters HA 1976 Hexachlorbenzene poisoning in Turkey. Federal Proceedings 35: 2400–2403

Pyke M 1971 Food and society. Murray, London, p. 102

Ressler C 1962 Isolation and identification from common vetch of the neurotoxin β-cyano-1-alanine, a possible factor in neurolathyrism. Journal of Biological Chemistry 237: 733–735

Sarkar SN 1948 Isolation from argemone oil of disanguinarine and sanguinarine: toxicity of sanguinarine. Nature 162: 265–266

Senanayake N, Jeyaranam J 1981 Toxic polyneuropathy due to gingili oil contaminated with tri-cresyl phosphate affecting adolescent girls in Sri Lanka. Lancet 1: 88–89

Short AIK, Watling R, Macdonald MK, Robson J S 1980 Poisoning by *Cortinarius speciosissimus*. Lancet 2: 942–944

Skene SA, Dewhurst IC, Greenberg M 1989 Polychlorinated dibenzo-*p*-dioxins and polychlorinated dibenzofurans: the risks to human health. A review. Human Toxicology 8: 173–203

Sleeman WH 1844 Rambles and reflexions of an Indian official. (New edition 1893 Smith V A (ed).) Westminster Press, London

Sugimura T 1982 Mutagens, carcinogens and tumour promoters in our daily food. Cancer 49:1970–1984

Toxic Epidemic Syndrome Study Group 1982 Toxic epidemic syndrome, Spain, 1981. Lancet 2: 697–702

Ueno Y 1985 The toxicology of mycotoxins. CRC Critical Reviews in Toxicology 14: 99–132

Walker R 1988 Toxicological aspects of food preservatives. In: Walker R, Quattrucci E (eds) Nutritional and toxicological aspects of food processing. Taylor and Francis, London, pp. 25–49

Walker R 1990 Nitrates, nitrites and *N*-nitroso compounds: a review of the occurrence in food and diet and the toxicological implications. Food Additives and Contaminants 7: 717–768

Weaver AL 1967 Lathyrism: A review. Arthritis and Rheumatism 10: 470–478

Williams CD 1954 Report on vomiting sickness in Jamaica. Government Printer, Jamaica

World Health Organization 1982 Evaluation of certain food additives and contaminants. Twenty-sixth report of the Joint FAO/WHO Expert Committee on Food Additives. Technical Report Series No. 683. WHO, Geneva, pp. 27–28

World Health Organisation 1987a IPCS Environmental Health Criteria No. 70. Principles for the safety assessment of food additives and contaminants in food. WHO, Geneva

World Health Organization 1987b Toxicological evaluation of certain food additives. Food Additive Series No. 22. WHO, Geneva, pp. 97–161

World Health Organization 1989a Environmental Health Criteria No. 80. Pyrollizidine alkaloids. WHO, Geneva

World Health Organization 1989b IPCS Environmental Health Criteria No. 85. Lead – environmental aspects. WHO, Geneva

World Health Organization 1989c IPCS Environmental Health Criteria No. 88. Polychlorinated dibenzo-para-dioxins and dibenzofurans. WHO, Geneva

World Health Organizations 1990 IPCS Environmental Health Criteria No. 104. Principles for the Toxicological Assessment of Pesticide Residues in Food. WHO, Geneva

World Health Organization 1991 Evaluation of certain veterinary drug residues in food. Thirty-eighth report of the Joint FAO/WHO Expert Committee on Food Additives. Technical Report Series No. 815. WHO, Geneva

World Health Organization 1992a IPCS Environmental Health Criteria No. 140. Polychlorinated biphenyls and terphenyls. WHO, Geneva

World Health Organization 1992b Toxic oil syndrome: current knowledge and future perspectives. Regional Publication Series No. 42. WHO, Copenhagen

24. Consumer protection

D. A. T. Southgate

Consumer protection has its origins in the need to protect the purchaser of foodstuffs from fraud due to the adulteration of food. The record of history shows that there have always been those who are ready to make a 'fast buck' by trick or fraud. Short weight and the dilution of milk with water are ancient practices, and almost everywhere there have been laws against them; these practices still continue in countries which lack adequate means of enforcement. In Europe in the middle ages, pepper and other costly spices imported from the east were frequently adulterated by mixing them with local seeds, leaves, flour or even sand. Sugar, coffee and tea were similarly diluted. There were also old laws against the sale of unsound meat and other foods.

In the period 1750–1850 the industrial revolution caused large numbers of people to leave the countryside to work in the new towns. Separated from the fields where their food was grown, and from local markets and shops where they could purchase fresh foods, industrial workers became increasingly dependent on food manufacturers, some of whom were fraudulent. Foods were often adulterated and some adulterants were new chemicals which were poisonous. The medical profession then knew little about toxicology, and analytical methods for detecting and identifying adulterants did not exist. In Britain the problem came to a head in 1851, when Dr Wakeley, the owner and first editor of the *Lancet*, published the names of over 3000 tradesmen whose wares had been found by private investigators to be adulterated. Many people thought that libel actions would kill the *Lancet*, but it was never sued, probably because it had the support of the medical profession. Instead, his crusade led to the passage by parliament of the 1860 *Adulteration of Food and Drink Act*, and when this proved ineffective, of the 1875 *Sale of Food and Drugs Act*, the basis from which modern laws have developed. By 1875 new chemical knowledge had enabled the science of food analysis to develop, and the appointment of public analysts to local government authorities enabled the law to be enforced. Similar laws were passed in other countries and fraudulent adulteration of food on a large scale ceased. Analogous situations arose in the 1950s with the rapid growth of towns in Africa and Asia, where there was a lack of suitable trained personnel to enforce the regulations. It appears that the problem seems to be characteristic of rapid urbanization, where large numbers of people become separated from the site of food production and there is a growth in the demand to transport and supply food to the urban areas before an adequate infrastructure has been developed.

In 1875 knowledge of bacteriology was rudimentary, but the next 25 years was a golden age and by 1900 most of the bacteria commonly involved in food poisoning had been identified, together with some understanding of how they were spread and the nature of the diseases they caused. Food hygiene then became a science, and this made possible the control of the spread of food poisoning by inspection of slaughterhouses, food warehouses, retail shops and kitchens in restaurants, hotels and other public institutions. Although the principles of control are well understood, their application still shows many lapses and new processes and methods of animal husbandry have been responsible for other organisms becoming sources of food poisoning (Hobbs & Gilbert 1978). Pathogenic agents constitute the greatest immediate danger to health from foods, against which the consumer needs protection. The 20th century has seen the rise of new chemical hazards from foods. A large number of substances are used during the production, storage and processing of foods, ranging from the pesticides and weedkillers used on crops to improve yields by reducing losses due to disease and competition, and the antibiotics used in animal feeds to control disease and improve growth, some of which may carry over into foods. Other substances are used during storage: pesticides to control losses due to infestation, and a range of other compounds to control losses due to senescence, ripening or sprouting. Many of these 'agrochemicals' are highly active substances and their use is closely controlled, first because they can be hazardous to the person applying them, and second to control the levels of residues in the food for consumption. These controls usually take the form of prescribed intervals between application to crops and entry into food distribution. Many countries also have a surveillance programme that samples imported foods and foods in the market place for residue analysis. In the UK and many other countries, 'market basket' studies are undertaken where samples of a typical day's intake of food are collected for residue analysis to determine the typical daily intake (MAFF 1988).

In an agricultural community food is bought and sold in local markets and shops. The consumer can see what he or she is purchasing and judge its quality. Formerly, retail shops purchased most of their food in bulk from wholesalers and a purchase was weighed and wrapped before the consumer's eyes. Nowadays foods are supplied, for the most part, to the retailer and thence to the purchaser in prepacked form, and the consumer has to rely on the label for information on what the purchase provides. It is therefore essential that this information is accurate and not misleading. This applies particularly when the package contains a food prepared from many ingredients, or consists of a whole meal. Customers are also influenced in their choice of food by a number of external factors, including advertising. A main concern of contemporary food legislation to protect the consumer is therefore concerned with the control of food labelling and advertising.

Although the introduction and growth of food legislation was due to the fraudulent practices of tradesmen and manufacturers, their modern counterparts should not be regarded in this light. The greater majority of food manufacturers and retailers are greatly concerned with the quality of their products; in a competitive market any disclosure of an unsatisfactory or unsafe product usually has disastrous effects on sales, not only of the product in question but frequently of other products from the same source or type of food. Modern legislation arises from a continuing dialogue between trade associations, consumer bodies and enforcement authorities. These dialogues are in general harmonious, because there is a common interest that foods should be safe and of good quality. In a country the size of Britain there are a great many people whose work in some way or other ensures the quality of food. Most of these have spe-

cialist knowledge and some have experience in judging complex issues. The rest of this chapter provides a resumé of how this work is organized. Each country has its own institutions for dealing with food legislation and a complete account of the position internationally would require several large volumes and would probably be of interest only to food legislators. The control of food quality is very highly developed in the USA, and a brief account of the situation there is also given; in Europe the formation of the Economic Community has had a profound effect on food legislation, and some of the main features of the way that legislation is developing are described.

UK LEGISLATION

The *Sale of Food and Drugs Act* 1875 was replaced by the *Food and Drugs (Adulteration) Act* 1928, and later by the *Food and Drugs Acts* of 1938 and 1955. The drugs aspects of the 1955 act were superseded by the *Medicines Act* in 1968. Each act is amplified by regulations which cover specific commodities or foods, e.g. the Bread and Flour Regulations, the Condensed Milk Regulations and the Soft Drink Regulations, which set out the compositional standards that apply to these foods and specify the permitted additives that can be used. Food hygiene is dealt with under separate regulations. These regulations are reviewed at intervals, or whenever current scientific developments in processing or nutrition indicate that revision is desirable. Proposals for new legislation are prepared by the Ministry of Agriculture, Fisheries and Food and laid before parliament. Before the legislation is drawn up there is a period of discussion, where interested parties can express their views.

Between 1948 and 1983 the revisions were channelled through the Food Standards Committee (FSC); this consisted of a number of independent scientists from a range of disciplines, including food scientists from the food industry. These were chosen on the basis of their expertise as individuals and they did not represent the industry as such. The committee was served by a secretariat and received advice on health and nutritional matters from the Department of Health (and Social Security) usually via two committees, the Committee on Medical Aspects of Food Policy (COMA) and the Committee on Toxicity (COT). The FSC produced reports on specific topics, such as bread and flour, novel protein foods, labelling, and claims and misleading descriptions. These reports were then open for a period of consultation and often formed the basis for new legislation. An independent committee was set up in

1964, the Committee on Food Additives and Contaminants (FACC), acting in a similar way to the FSC, preparing reports on specific topics such as preservatives, antioxidants and flavourings, which were open for consultation before forming the basis for legislation. In receiving submissions regarding new additives the cardinal criteria which had to be satisfied were evidence of technical need (to provide evidence that the new substance was required for a new process, or that it was markedly superior to the substance in current use), and that it was safe to use (this would require evidence from toxicological studies in animals and estimates of the likely human exposure that would follow its use). The reports of the FACC usually contain detailed discussions of the evidence and its recommendations often specify the foods in which the additive may be used and the levels that are permitted.

Regarding contaminants, the FACC was concerned with establishing sound agricultural, manufacturing and handling techniques, so that contamination at all levels of the food chain should be minimized.

Since 1983 the functions of these two committees have been merged in the Food Advisory Committee (FAC), constituted in a similar way to the two committees it replaced and carrying out its responsibilities in the same way.

Enforcement

The best-intentioned and soundest legislation will not achieve its purposes unless it is enforced, and indeed, one factor in drawing up food legislation is the consideration of how it *can* be enforced. Enforcement is in the hands of the local government authorities. They inspect, analyse and initiate legal action where necessary. Environmental health officers are responsible for inspection, and consumer protection officers are responsible for ensuring that food labelling is not misleading and that prescribed standards are being met; the duties of these officers are thus approximately equivalent to the former sanitary inspectors and weights and measures inspectors respectively. The officers inspect premises and take samples for analysis; they also respond to complaints about composition, labelling and advertising made to the local authorities. The cases are heard at magistrates' courts.

EUROPEAN COMMUNITY

Although the individual member states of the community still retain their own legislative framework for food legislation, the community is playing an increasingly important role. The Treaty of Rome called for the establishment of a common market with free movement of all commodities, including foods. This ideal carries with it the implicit obligation to remove any restrictions to the free movement of foods by regulations relating to the composition or labelling of foods. One major activity of the European Commission (the administrative apparatus of the Community, responsible for preparing proposals for legislation for the Council of Ministers, which is the decision-making body), has been the 'harmonization' of regulations relating to food. The Commission prepares draft directives to this effect; these relate to specific commodities or classes of foodstuffs. The directives are then considered by the different members and after discussion in committee, and usually after considerable argument, the directives are approved by the Council of Ministers. Each member state is then expected to incorporate the substance of the directive into its own legislation. The year set for achieving the free market was 1992, and now in principle, all legislation relating to food should be common across the European Community. National legislation reflects the preferences for specific foods and often the national attitudes to foods. It is unrealistic and probably unnecessary to expect these differences to disappear at a stroke, and the principle being followed is that foods that may legally be sold in one country must not be prevented from being sold in another.

Initially the Commission focused its attention on harmonizing compositional standards, which created considerable resentment in some quarters because it appeared that national preferences – for example sausages, chocolate and ice cream in the UK – were being disregarded, and that national standards were being radically changed for the sake of uniformity. In other instances direct translation from one language to another produced problems; for example, the word 'cream' was considered to imply the presence of butter fat in a product, whereas the word was also being used to imply a texture. In recent years the thrust of the harmonization process has moved away from compositional standards towards informative labelling, based on the concept that if labelling is explicit the consumer can impose the compositional standards that he or she wishes at the point of sale. This approach has much to recommend it, because it will enable more informed choice and also it will not pose a restraint on innovation by the food industry. This may prove to be of considerable nutritional importance, because the production of low-fat cheeses, for example, has been constrained by rigid compositional standards.

One field where the harmonization of labelling has reached an advanced stage is that of food additives, where the Commission has developed a unified system for designating food additives which have been subjected to safety evaluation. The system has caused some unfavourable consumer reaction due to misapprehension of the reasons behind the scheme, which was intended to reassure consumers that the additives had been evaluated.

UNITED STATES

As in many other countries, food legislation in the USA has its origins in the prevention of fraud. The federal structure of the USA, where the individual states have considerable legal autonomy, led to a very diverse approach to food legislation. In 1906 the first federal *Food and Drugs Act* was introduced, with a considerable emphasis on preventing the use in foods of undesirable toxic substances. The act was revised in 1938 to strengthen its powers and establish the Food and Drugs Administration (FDA), which is still responsible to the Department of Health, Education and Welfare for protecting public health.

Originally the onus of proof that a drug or additive was harmful lay with the FDA, but in 1958 the act was amended to place the onus on the manufacturer to prove that a proposed additive is safe before it can be cleared for use. Obtaining the evidence for this can be very onerous, since the FDA has developed a very strict code which often provides a model adopted, in whole or in part, by other regulatory bodies. Additives that have been used for many years, including natural and traditional ingredients, are placed on the GRAS list (generally recognized as safe). One feature that has dominated food legislation in the USA is the Delaney Clause, which was inserted into the 1958 act; this states that 'No (food) additive shall be deemed safe if it is found to induce cancer when ingested by man or animal'. This absolute proscription, irrespective of the level of feeding required to induce cancer, prevented the FDA from using its own judgement over cyclamates when very large doses were found to produce bladder cancers in rats. The situation is made more difficult by advances in modern analytical techniques, which can often detect substances at the parts per billion level (micrograms per kilogram). An additional anomaly arises because many naturally occurring substances are also capable of producing cancers. In recent years considerable attention has been given to the matter of developing more rational approaches based on risk assessment, where the question of whether an additive or ingredient can be used in foods is based on the probability that an unacceptable level of risk of cancer or some other condition will arise. The risk would need to be judged against some level of risk that is perceived as acceptable.

The major public health risk from foods in the USA, as in the UK, is that from food-borne infections. There is, for example, a higher level of botulinum poisoning, possibly because of the home canning or curing of meat.

Another aspect of food labelling in the interest of the consumer that was introduced in the USA was nutritional labelling. When first introduced it was not regarded with much enthusiasm in the UK, where it was argued that the consumer was not capable of making proper use of the information. However, the situation is now radically different, as will be discussed later.

INTERNATIONAL ACTIVITY

Many of the developing countries now face the same problems of food adulteration and contamination that affected Europe and the USA in the 19th century. It is much easier to transfer legislation to these countries than it is to train and develop the personnel to enforce it.

These countries frequently depend on exporting foods for their development, and these exports have to meet the quality and hygienic standards imposed by the importing country. To facilitate international trade and to assist in economic and technical development, the FAO and WHO agencies of the United Nations Organization established in 1963 a *Codex Alimentarius*. This is concerned with standards for the composition of all major foods and, with provisions affecting food hygiene, additives, pesticide and other residues, methods of analysis and labelling. Codes of Principles in these various areas are developed and submitted for adoption by each country. Quite clearly the extension of these considerations to all foods is a monumental task, but the organization does provide a valuable forum where issues that relate to food quality in all its aspects can be discussed.

It is important to recognize that there is considerable interchange of information between governments, both formally and informally, on issues of food safety; the evaluation of an additive by, say, the FDA, while not necessarily being regarded as definitive by the European Community, does provide guidance and can expedite the work of approval in Europe. This is becoming a matter of great importance in the light of the considerable international trade in foods.

LABELLING OF FOODS

The provision of accurate and informative labels on foods is a major part of consumer protection; this is particularly true where a food contains several ingredients. In the UK most foods must have a list of ingredients on the label, in order of the relative amounts present. In some foods this requirement is waived, if, for example, there are precise compositional standards for the food. In many foods water is the major ingredient, but it is rarely listed. Additives are usually minor ingredients and therefore appear toward the end of the list. Either the approved name for an additive or its E number may be used.

Many food labels are required by law to give an indication of the acceptable period of storage, either in the shop as a 'sell by' designation, or before consumption – a 'best before' statement; these labelling statements usually include the appropriate conditions for storage.

In the UK and many other countries there are restrictions on the claims, particularly nutritional ones, that may be made about a product. This is designed to protect the consumer from misleading claims about the benefits that may follow the consumption of the food. It must be said that this type of claim frequently escapes prosecution unless a major food producer is involved, which is fortunately very rare. The reason for this is that a misleading claim must be brought to the attention of the authorities, and frequently the time taken to bring a case enables the offending food to be withdrawn.

Nutritional labelling

Nutritional labelling was introduced in the USA over the period 1973–1975. It was intended to provide compositional information that would permit the consumer to judge the nutritional value of foods and choose a dietary mixture that would meet nutrient requirements. Nutritional labelling was optional for many foods unless a nutritional claim regarding the food was being made. The regulations effectively prescribed the format and mode of expression, and hence values for proximate constituents, energy (kcal), protein, fat and carbohydrate were given in grams, and protein, vitamins and calcium as percentages of the recommended daily allowances. The values chosen for these recommendations were the highest amounts for

an adult in the National Research Council's Recommended Dietary Allowances. The values were expressed per unit serving, which had to be given on the label.

The growth of knowledge about the relationship between diet and the incidence of chronic diseases has introduced a new dimension into nutritional labelling, which enables the consumer to choose foods to minimize the risks of chronic diet-related diseases. Nutritional labelling thus becomes part of public health strategy, where the target is not the short-term issue of preventing bacterial food poisoning or the slightly longer-term effects of contaminants, but the reduction in the long-term incidence of disease, for example, coronary heart disease and some cancers.

In the UK, nutritional labelling was seen as an essential part of implementing nutritional guidelines, such as those proposed in the NACNE discussion document (Health Education Council 1983). The report of the COMA panel on cardiovascular disease (DHSS 1984) formally recommended the introduction of fat labelling of foods, so that the consumer could adopt the recommendation to reduce fat intake and modify the degree of unsaturation of the fats eaten. The recommendation was accepted by the Government and discussions followed involving the food industry to examine how the recommendations could be implemented. This led to the present position, where MAFF, the department responsible for food labelling, has produced guidelines for nutritional labelling. At present these are voluntary and prescribe the format and mode of expression. The values must be expressed per 100 g of food and per portion if the package contain less than 100 g. Three levels of information are envisaged; the first gives energy, protein, fat and carbohydrate; the second includes dietary fibre and sodium; and the third permits sugars, vitamins and minerals, the latter only when the amounts present are greater than one-sixth of the recommended dietary intake (as is the position under current legislation regarding nutritional claims). Under current proposals from the FAC, the nutritional labelling would become obligatory when a nutritional claim is made. The regulations will include obligatory fat labelling that lists the percentages of saturated fatty acids at the first level of labelling; the other levels can include a more detailed breakdown of the fat.

At the same time the European Community Scientific Committee for Food is also developing proposals for nutritional labelling. Again these would be voluntary, unless a claim was being made. These proposals include energy, protein, fat, carbohydrates, total sugars, sodium and dietary fibre in the minimum statement, but as yet no breakdown of the fat present.

It is clear from pilot studies of nutritional labelling in the UK that consumers can find such labelling difficult to use in the way the advocates of nutritional labelling would like; to be effective, a parallel-running scheme of nutritional education will almost certainly be essential. Retailers who have introduced nutritional labelling have supplemented it with booklets containing nutritional information, to assist the consumer in choosing an appropriate diet.

FOOD ADVERTISING

Advertising can be seen as an extension of food labelling, where claims about the product are made in ways that have direct analogies with the label. In the UK all advertising is supervised by a Code of Advertising Practice Committee, which is a self-regulating body formed from the advertising profession and the media. There is a higher, independent Advertising Standards Authority that acts on complaints that particular advertisements are not honest and truthful. The advertisements about foods may offend under the misleading claims regulations developed from the reports of the Food Advisory Committee.

DIETARY SUPPLEMENTS AND 'HEALTH FOODS'

These constitute a heterogeneous group of products which, as far as the consumer is concerned, fall on the boundary between foods and medicines. In many cases their advertising usually includes the implication, which may be explicit, that the consumption of the product will confer health benefits on the consumer. These claims may be generalized or specifically related to a disease state. As mentioned earlier, most food legislation in Europe and the USA does not permit specific health claims because they blur the distinction between foods and medicines, for which there are very strict requirements to demonstrate effectiveness.

Nutrient supplements

In the case of nutrient supplements it is clear that the nutrients have a specific function related to health, and consumer protection is concerned with the levels of usage, that is, the dosage recommended, and with the implicit assumption that a consumer's diet is inadequate without the addition of the supplement. In some cases a nutritional supplement would clearly be of potential benefit; for example, the supplementation of pregnant women with folate and iron, or where there is good dietary evidence that the diet is inadequate with respect to a specific nutrient, and for some reason the nutrient cannot be supplied by normal foods. Examples are iodine as iodized salt where the soil is a poor source of iodine, or vitamin A where the supply of fats and dairy foods is not adequate. In a developed country such as the UK, specific nutrient deficiencies are rare, and the case for supplements often rests on concepts of optimal intakes rather than intakes to prevent deficiencies. Consumer protection therefore has to ensure that unwarranted claims for the benefits of supplementation are not made, and to control the amounts available in products to prevent hazardous overdosing. In a review of supplements, a Working Party of the Ministry of Agriculture Fisheries and Food (1991) recommended that the amounts of nutrients in supplements should be limited to one-tenth of the undesirable dose levels for nutrients where adverse effects of high doses were known (Table 24.1).

Health foods

The same report (MAFF 1991) considered health foods; here it was recognized that many of the claims made for 'health' foods were extremely difficult to substantiate. Many of these 'natural' foods contain biologically active substances, some of which are toxicants and many of which have undesirable effects at high doses. The Working Party considered that these 'health foods' should be regulated within the existing food legislation, and there are no good arguments for creating a special category for them. There was considerable concern at the continued sale of products that contained toxic constituents and that there was a need to increase awareness of the potential hazards of some products.

European community activities

At the time of writing (1993), the EC Scientific Committee for Food is undertaking a consultation concerning the possible regulation of supplements, 'health' foods and the fortification of foods. The views on nutrient supplements differ between members of the community, and considerable discussion will be necessary before a common view emerges. One can have no doubt, however, that the legislation will

Table 24.1   Recommended levels of nutrients in foods

Nutrient	UK RNI	US RDA	Undesirable dose	
			chronic (per day)	acute
Vitamins:				
retinol	700 μg	800–1000 μg	6000 μg (3300 μg)**	
vitamin D	10 μg	10 μg	50 μg	
vitamin B$_6$	1.4 mg	1.4–2 mg	100 mg	
vitamin C	40 mg	50–60 mg	6 g	
niacin	17 mg	13–20 mg	500 mg†	
Minerals:				
iron	14.8 mg	10–15 mg	40 mg	20 mg/kg
copper	1.2 mg	1.5–3 mg*	30 mg	
zinc	7–9.5 mg	12–15 mg	20 mg	
selenium	60–75 μg	40–70 μg	1 mg	
sodium	1.6 g	x	8 g	
cobalt	x	x	300 mg	
chromium	>2.5 μg	50–200 μg	1 g	
iodine	140 μg	150 μg	1 mg	
fluorine	x	1.5–4 mg*	10 mg	
molybdenum	50–400 μg	75–250 μg*	10 mg	

x   no recommended daily amount (RDA) set. Historically, previous UK committees felt either that not enough evidence was available to set RDAs for a number of nutrients, or that there was no public health need to do so. However, more evidence is now available about human needs and in COMA's current review of RDAs, it is expected that the range of nutrients covered will be more extensive.

*   no RDA set, but an estimated safe and adequate daily dietary intake.

**   during pregnancy.

†   high doses of nicotinic acid have been associated with liver damage, sometimes severe. Most, but not all of the formulations responsible for this association have been sustained-release products. It is not yet known whether the critical factor is the dose or the formulation or both.

include regulations to prevent the consumer being given false claims for a product and that the levels of nutrients will be controlled in some way by reference to nutrient requirements for health, and that the sale of potentially toxic materials will be closely regulated.

SUMMARY

Consumers in the industrialized countries are protected by an intricate system involving central and local government, food manufacturers, advertisers and the media, and operating through statutory regulations and voluntary codes of practice. In common with all human systems it involves some compromises, particularly when the information needed for a rational judgement is not available and a decision has to be made on the basis of the evidence available at the time. This is the reason why all food legislation is subject to regular review, so that new evidence and developments in scientific understanding can be incorporated. At the present time few scientists actually involved in the evaluation of the safety of food ingredients believe that current methods of assessment are ideal, and considerable research is in progress and much thought is being given as to how safety can be better judged. However, the protection of the consumer is a primary concern of all involved, not least the food industry, whose economic livelihood depends on the continued purchasing of their products. The major hazard to health from foods in the short term is that from microbial contamination, and the limitation of the effects of this depends on the activity of all those concerned with food throughout the food chain, not least those concerned with food preparation in the kitchen, at home, in restaurants and in all catering institutions.

REFERENCES

Department of Health and Social Security 1984 Diet and cardiovascular disease. Report on Health and Social Subjects 28. HMSO, London

Health Education Council 1983 Proposals for nutritional guidelines for health education in Britain. National Advisory Committee on Nutrition Education (NACNE)

Hobbs BC, Gilbert RJ 1978 Food poisoning and food hygiene. Edward Arnold, London

Ministry of Agriculture, Fisheries and Food 1988 The British diet: finding the facts. Food Surveillance Paper No. 23. HMSO, London.

Ministry of Agriculture, Fisheries and Food and Department of Health 1991 Dietary supplements and health foods. Report of the Working Group. HMSO, London

25. Pregnancy and lactation

C. Garza

Successful pregnancy and lactation require a continuum of adjustments in maternal body composition, metabolism and the functions of various physiological systems (e.g. cardiovascular and renal). A diet that meets maternal nutritional needs is required for these adjustments so that maternal wellbeing is safeguarded with the birth of a healthy, thriving infant. Other factors (see Table 25.1) also influence maternal and infant outcomes, and the role of nutrition in promoting maternal and infant wellbeing must always be considered within a broader context.

Nutrient needs during pregnancy and lactation are presented for distinct phases of each physiological state. Pregnancy usually is divided into quarters of 10 weeks, or trimesters of approximately 13-weeks' duration. The duration of lactation is highly variable. Generally, infants are expected to be predominantly breastfed for the first 4–6 months and may be partially breastfed for periods up to 2 or 3 years. Nutrient needs during lactation, therefore, usually are presented for the first 4–6 months and for the subsequent duration.

PRINCIPLES FOR ESTIMATING NUTRIENT NEEDS DURING PREGNANCY AND LACTATION

The current approach to estimating nutrient needs emphasizes the principle that nutrient intakes should be consistent with long-term health and in energy terms allow for the maintenance of 'economically necessary and socially desirable physical activity' (FAO/WHO/UNU 1985). The goal of promoting the wellbeing of not one individual but two (i.e. mother and fetus, or infant), complicates the estimate. The nutritional wellbeing of the fetus and the exclusively breastfed infant is totally dependent on the mother. The biological mechanisms which allow healthy outcomes for both, or that explain unequal outcomes, are not always well understood. It is clear that for some nutrients, the infant's status is maintained at the expense of the mother; for other nutrients mother and offspring compete more evenly, and for others the infant suffers more severe consequences of deficiency than the mother.

Nutrient needs are usually estimated by factorial approaches, balance methods and dietary surveys of presumably well-nourished populations. Factorial approaches are commonly used to estimate nutrient needs during pregnancy and lactation, i.e. the extra nutrient needs imposed by pregnancy or lactation are added to the baseline estimates for non-pregnant, non-lactating women. Thus, to estimate energy needs during lactation, the sum of energy secreted into milk and the energy required to synthesize all the milk components are calculated. The difference between the energy cost of milk production and secretion and

Table 25.1 Factors that influence maternal and infant outcomes

Demographic/ socioeconomic/ lifestyle characteristics	Medical history	Previous reproductive history	Complications	
			Intrapartum	Postpartum
Maternal age Unwanted pregnancy Education Income Illicit drug addiction Alcohol consumption Smoking	Chronic diseases such as diabetes, hypertension, anatomical abnormalities of the mammary gland	Spontaneous abortion Premature delivery Uterine anomalies Successful attempt to breastfeed	Premature rupture of amniotic sac membranes Amnionitis Vaginal bleeding	Mastitis Nipple erosion Breast engorgement

the energy represented by the weight lost during lactation is added to the baseline energy needs of non-pregnant, non-lactating women.

BODY COMPOSITION: CHANGES DURING PREGNANCY AND LACTATION

The amount and composition of the weight gained during pregnancy are major determinants of the extra energy and nutrient needs, and the amount of weight gained significantly influences pregnancy outcomes. Gestational weight gain associated with a desirable pregnancy outcome, i.e. a full-term infant weighing 3–4 kg, is also influenced by the mother's pre-pregnancy weight. A greater gain is needed in women with a low prepregnancy body mass index (BMI) to achieve a desirable birth weight (SNSWGDP & SDINSDP 1990) (Fig. 25.1). There are also various sociodemographic characteristics that significantly affect gestational weight gain. Examples are summarized in Table 25.2.

The rate of weight gain is not uniform throughout pregnancy. Approximately 5% of the total is usually gained in the first quarter and the remainder is gained fairly evenly throughout the rest of pregnancy. The distribution of weight gain among maternal and fetal tissues is illustrated in Figure 25.2. Of the total weight increase, about 62% is water, with increased blood volume accounting for about 10% and extracellular

Table 25.2   Factors that influence weight gain during pregnancy

Individual characteristics	Socioeconomic
Maternal age	Diet
Genetic differences	Smoking
Ethnicity	Physical activity
	Prepregnancy weight-for-height

fluid for 13%; fat contributes 30% and protein 8% (Hytten & Chamberlain 1980). The gain in body water is larger than that occurring during normal weight gain, so measurements of body composition which rely on assuming a constant proportion of water in lean tissue, e.g. underwater weighing or derivations of body composition from measurements of total body water, are difficult to evaluate. Applying the usual factors leads to underestimations of the fat component.

Gains in maternal body fat are not constant during pregnancy, nor are such gains distributed uniformly (Taggart et al 1967). Adipose tissue accumulates most rapidly in midpregnancy. The most marked increases in body fat occur in abdominal, subscapular and upper thigh areas.

The fetus accounts for about 25% of the total weight gained, but for only 10% of the fat stored during pregnancy. However, 60% of the protein gained is in fetal and placental tissues (Hytten & Chamberlain 1980).

Changes in body composition during lactation are less well described. The expansion of extracellular

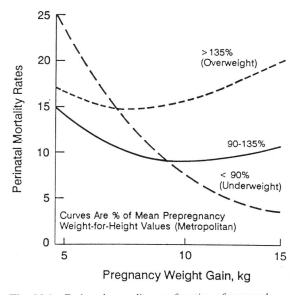

Fig. 25.1   Perinatal mortality as a function of maternal weight gain. (Reproduced with permission from Naeye (1979).)

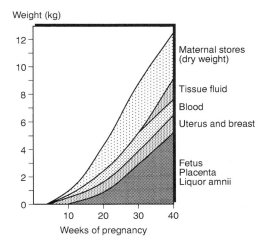

Fig. 25.2   The components of weight gain in normal pregnancy (Hytten & Chamberlain 1980).

and blood volumes during pregnancy are not reversed immediately after delivery. In both animals and humans, plasma volume appears to be increased during lactation, but the increase seems to be modest.

The adipose tissue stored during early pregnancy is available to meet the needs for fetal growth in the last quarter of gestation and the increased energy demands of lactation. Breastfeeding, therefore, may be viewed as potentially beneficial in preventing the progressive weight gain and obesity associated with multiple pregnancies. However, food intake also increases during lactation, and the gap between total expenditure and energy intake is often not great enough to ensure the loss of all the fat gained during pregnancy. Women in western societies who breastfeed their infants exclusively during the first 4–6 months lose 0.6–0.8 kg/month, with a slower weight loss later (Heinig et al 1990). In western societies, each pregnancy *on average* leads to 1 kg weight gain in excess of that expected for a woman's age. The expected modulation of lactation on that average estimate is not well defined.

The energy content of the weight lost during lactation varies between individuals (Butte et al 1984, Brewer et al 1989), but over 90% is usually fat, and the subscapular and suprailiac fat depots are the most labile.

ENERGY COST OF PREGNANCY

The UK COMA Report (1991) estimates the average cost of pregnancy at about 293 MJ for women with a prepregnancy weight of approximately 60 kg. About 60% of this energy cost is accounted for by the energy content of the fetus and increments in maternal tissues. The remaining 40% is due to a higher basal metabolic rate (BMR) and the extra cost of moving a heavier body. Variations in maternal weight gain and increases in BMR, however, account for wide differences in the estimated costs of pregnancy. Table 25.3 illustrates an approximate fourfold difference in the energy content of maternal adipose tissue gained during pregnancy, and an eightfold difference in added basal metabolic costs in women living in very diverse environments. The range in the energy content of maternal fat stores is a reflection of weight gained during pregnancy. The energy content of fetal and maternal tissues approached the expected 167 MJ only for the group studied in Scotland. With the exception of the Gambian women, the energy content of fetal and maternal tissues in the other groups was about 105 MJ.

An increase in basal metabolism is expected through most of pregnancy because of the increased metabolic activity of maternal and fetal tissues and because of the extra work done by the maternal cardiovascular, renal, respiratory, and other systems. Nevertheless, metabolic efficiency during pregnancy may change at low planes of nutritional status, as seen in the Gambia (Table 25.3), so that the BMR is reduced in early pregnancy and other metabolic processes may slow down. The reduction in BMR is, however, partially reversed when food supplements are provided (Lawrence et al 1984). Any functional costs of this adaptation have not been described.

Increases in the energy cost of moving during pregnancy may be compensated for by decreased levels of activity, but this generalization may not hold in all societies, especially where women are responsible for farming and other energetic tasks.

Detailed studies of postprandial thermogenesis show that this is reduced in well-fed pregnant and lactating women, so this is another metabolic adaptation which seems to occur in response to the different physiological states of the mother. The energy

Table 25.3   Energy requirements of pregnancy as estimated by the five-country study

Factor	Energy cost and additional intake during pregnancy by country (MJ)				
	Scotland	The Netherlands	The Gambia	Thailand	Philippines
Energy cost					
Fetus	34	34.5	30	30	29
Placenta	3	3.1	2	2.5	2.5
subtotals:	37	37.6	32	32.5	31.5
Maternal tissues	12	12.3	10	10.5	10
Maternal fat	106	59.9	28	64.5	60
subtotals:	118	72.2	38	75	70
Basal metabolism	126	144.2	8	100.5	79.5
Total energy cost:	281	254	78	208	181

Adapted from Durnin (1986)

saving may, however, only amount to 2–5% of the total food eaten (Illingworth et al 1986).

With the potential for metabolic adaptation and physical activity changes, the known costs of accumulating the extra tissues during pregnancy may not be matched by a need to increase food intake by an equivalent amount. It is, therefore, perhaps not surprising that direct measurements of food intake in pregnancy usually show only a small increase, and that in late pregnancy. Underreporting of intake may, however, be common (Mertz et al 1991), so it is unwise to assume that pregnancy does not require an increase in intake. Food supplements are known to benefit maternal weight gain and infant birthweight in the most undernourished women. Committees therefore differ in their assessment of the extra energy needs of pregnancy (see Appendix 2). The FAO/WHO/UNU report (1985) recommended the highest increment (1.3 MJ, 300 kcal) daily throughout pregnancy, whereas the UK panel recommended only 0.84 MJ (200 kcal) daily for the last trimester.

Fasting should be minimized during pregnancy because there is a more rapid fall in circulating glucose, insulin and gluconeogenic amino acids than in non-pregnant women (Tyson et al 1976). Ketone production is also accelerated, with the ketones being transferred easily to the fetus. Worries about possible fetal metabolic derangements and even brain damage in fasting women has led to the recommendation that pregnant women should not fast for more than 6–8 hours.

ENERGY COST OF LACTATION

Lactation requires much more energy than pregnancy, with 1 month's lactation being equivalent to the full cost of pregnancy if maternal fat storage is neglected. The major determinant of the extra energy needed during lactation is the energy content of the milk produced. Milk production in well nourished women is approximately 750 ml/day for the first 4–6 months of full lactation. Following the introduction of solid foods, milk production tends to fall to approximately 600 ml/day. Since the gross energy content of milk is approximately 2.8 kJ/ml, approximately 2.1 MJ/day are secreted in milk. Estimates of the efficiency of milk production range from 80% to 95% (NRC 1989, Frigerio et al 1991a); the energy cost to synthesize 750 ml of milk with the indicated energy content may vary from 0.1 to 0.5 MJ/day, depending on the efficiency factor chosen.

The BMR falls to normal levels after delivery in well nourished lactating women, but the low BMRs in pregnant Gambian women persisted into lactation if the usual diet was maintained (Whitehead et al 1986). Estimates of the cost of milk synthesis and secretion differ (Illingworth et al 1986, Motil et al 1990, Frigerio et al 1991b), so estimates of the full energy costs of lactation do not allow for possible changes in BMR or postprandial thermogenesis. In the first 6 months of full lactation, energy costs range from 2.2 MJ (525 kcal/day) to 2.6 MJ (625 kcal/day). If 146 MJ (35 000 kcal) are stored in adipose tissues during pregnancy and are mobilized during lactation at a steady rate for 6 months, energy costs would be offset by about 0.84 MJ (200 kcal/day). Additional dietary energy needs during lactation, therefore, are approximately 1.4–1.8 MJ (325–425 kcal/day) above pre-pregnant levels, as long as full lactation persists and the extra energy stores are available.

Successful lactation is possible with gradual weight reduction. A weight loss of up to 2 kg/month is unlikely to affect milk volume or composition, but more rapid weight loss is not advisable (SNDL 1991). The total intake of dietary protein, carbohydrate or fat has no detectable impact on milk quantity or quality under normal dietary conditions. The fatty acid composition of the diet does, however, affect the composition of milk fat. It is difficult to establish a link between total energy intake and milk production because of differences between women in their size, BMR, physical activity patterns, and the demands of their infant. However, poorly nourished women produce less milk (Brown et al 1986) and in these women indices of body fatness seem to link with better lactation performance.

Food supplementation trials yield variable results, but in general undernourished women produce more milk when supplemented during either pregnancy or lactation. Animal studies show that adequate diets given during pregnancy buffer the effects of inadequate postpartum energy intakes on milk production. The most severe effects on milk production are observed when poor intakes during pregnancy are followed by poor intakes during lactation.

PROTEIN REQUIREMENTS

Extra protein is gained during pregnancy at a variable rate; there is a marked increase during the second trimester and a slower increase in the last, a total of 925 g of protein being accumulated in all. From these assessments of protein storage it is possible to estimate the protein requirements and allowances of pregnancy (see Appendix 2 and Table 25.4). The average rate of nitrogen accumulation is first estimated and then this value is increased by 30% to cover the +2 SD limits of the variability in protein accumulation expected in healthy women. Their variable needs are estimated from the ±15% coefficient of variation in birthweight. This allowance is adjusted further because there is about a 70% conversion efficiency of dietary protein to body protein.

Generally, populations with a ready access to food consume more protein than the RNI, and protein supplements given to mothers in developing countries do not increase the amounts stored (Lechtig et al 1975, Delgado et al 1982). In poorer communities, however, dietary adequacy may be more of a problem.

The protein costs of lactation are also calculated by the factorial method based on milk volumes of 750 ml/day for the first 6 months and 600 ml/day thereafter. It is assumed that the mean protein concentration of milk is 1.1 g/dl, with a 30% interindividual variability in milk production, and again an efficiency of 0.70 in the conversion of dietary protein to milk protein. The allowance or RDI is thereby estimated as 15 g of protein/day for the first 6 months of full lactation, and 12 g/day thereafter (NRC 1989).

Animal data indicate that improvements in total protein intake or protein quality may increase lactation performance, and there are some limited data on the beneficial effects of protein supplementation in women (SNDL 1991).

FAT REQUIREMENTS

There is increasing interest in the role of essential fatty acids in pregnancy and how these fatty acids are transferred by the placenta to sustain fetal cell division and brain growth. The role of n-3 fatty acids in

Table 25.4 Safe levels of additional protein during pregnancy (From FAO/WHO/UNU (1985)).

Trimester	N gain (g/d)[1]		Efficiency[2]	Additional protein required[3] (g/day)
	(Average)	(+30%)	(0.70)	
1	0.104	0.14	0.20	1.2
2	0.525	0.68	0.98	6.1
3	0.922	1.20	1.71	10.7

[1] Estimated tissue N gained in a pregnancy producing a 3.3 kg infant; CV of birthweight 15%
[2] Assuming 70% efficiency of conversion of dietary to tissue protein
[3] In terms of absorbed protein

altering the time of delivery and in promoting fetal growth is being assessed (Olsen et al 1992). The long chain n-3 fatty acids are particularly needed for neuronal structures and the fetal requirements are high in the latter stage of pregnancy (Nettleton 1993). Thus the premature infant is vulnerable (see Chapter 46).

ASSESSING VITAMIN AND MINERAL NEEDS DURING PREGNANCY AND LACTATION

The nutrient concentrations of vitamins and minerals in blood or plasma are often used to assess nutrient status, but this is difficult in pregnancy and lactation. The normal expansion of blood volume during pregnancy dilutes circulating nutrient concentrations, and there is also a highly efficient placental transport of some nutrients to the fetus. The concentrations of some nutrients are therefore higher in the fetal than in the maternal circulation. The activation coefficients of vitamin-dependent enzymes are frequently higher in pregnant than in non-pregnant women, but the effects of pregnancy on the enzyme–coenzyme relationships are unknown, so again interpretation is difficult.

Comparing nutrient intakes and/or blood or plasma levels with specific outcomes, e.g. infantile congenital malformations or maternal bone density, is inconclusive without a controlled, double-blind supplementation trial to evaluate rigorously epidemiological associations of this type.

Fat-soluble vitamins

The American recommended allowances for the fat-soluble vitamins during pregnancy include substantial increases above non-pregnant levels for vitamins D (100%) and E (25%), but no increase for vitamins A and K (NRC 1989). The allowances during lactation are the same or higher than in pregnancy (see Appendix 2).

Vitamin D

Maternal vitamin D deficiency during pregnancy has been linked to maternal osteomalacia, reduced birthweight, and neonatal hypocalcaemia and tetany. The maternal effects of vitamin D deficiency during lactation have not been well described. Low sun exposure, dark skin and living in a northern climate are risk factors for vitamin D deficiency. Vitamin D toxicity can cause hypercalcaemia in women. Aortic malformations have been observed in the offspring of animals fed high levels of vitamin D, but its occurrence in human infants is not documented clearly (SNSWGDP & SDINSDP 1990).

Most studies indicate that the placental transfer of vitamin D to the infant is particularly important because of low vitamin D levels in human milk. Concentrations of vitamin D vary substantially (0.3–0.9 µg/l), in part because of differences in maternal vitamin D status, which is related to vitamin D intake and sun exposure.

Exclusively breastfed infants are at risk of vitamin D deficiency if maternal vitamin D intake is limited and maternal and infant sun exposure is low. A fully clothed infant without a hat requires approximately 2 hours of sun exposure per week to maintain normal serum 25-OH vitamin D levels (Specker et al 1985).

Vitamin E

The general expectation that higher vitamin E levels are needed to promote fetal growth is the basis for the increased American RDA for vitamin E during pregnancy (NRC 1989). Maternal consequences of vitamin E deficiency during pregnancy or lactation are not described in humans.

Vitamin E status is of importance in the management of premature infants. As with other nutrients, most vitamin E transfer from mother to fetus probably occurs in the last quarter of pregnancy, so premature infants are likely to be born with inadequate stores. Haemolytic anaemia in the premature infant is often responsive to vitamin E administration. Inadequate vitamin E status in premature infants has also been linked to bronchopulmonary dysplasia, retinopathy and intraventricular haemorrhage. A causative role for vitamin E deficiency, however, has not been demonstrated conclusively.

Maternal requirements for vitamin E during lactation are based on the expected amount of milk produced and its mean tocopherol content (NRC 1989).

Vitamin K

Vitamin K intake during pregnancy is of particular concern because a vitamin K-deficient neonate may develop a haemorrhagic disease with intracranial haemorrhage, which can be fatal. Babies are born with inadequate stores of vitamin K (see Chapter 13) and a vitamin K injection for the infant at birth is recommended by both USA and UK expert committees (Committee on Nutrition 1985, COMA 1991). Giving vitamin K to pregnant women at term

does not appear to affect the activities of the clotting factors II, IX, and X in their infants. However, giving vitamin K to women who deliver prematurely may offer some short-term protection to the infant (Pomerance at al 1987).

Vitamin K output in milk is approximately 1.5 µg/day, mostly in the phylloquinone form, but its concentration does not appear to be tightly regulated. Maternal supplementation with vitamin K can increase its milk concentrations markedly, but a seemingly adequate vitamin K status in the mother (see Chapter 13) does not appear to ensure adequate vitamin K intakes for the exclusively breastfed neonate. A failure to provide supplemental vitamin K to the neonate significantly increases its risk of vitamin K-responsive bleeding in the first month of life. The relative importance of placental transfer of vitamin K, the vitamin K intake from milk, the limited ability of the neonate's intestinal microbes to synthesize vitamin K, and the neonate's ability to absorb vitamin K are unknown. Similarly, the role of a single injection of vitamin K at birth in the prevention of late-onset vitamin K deficiency is uncertain (SNDL 1991).

Vitamin A

In western countries, the usual intakes of retinol and its precursors meet baseline needs and the additional requirements imposed by pregnancy (NRC 1989). Intakes may be inadequate in less developed countries or among other populations where there is restricted access to vitamin A-containing foods. Vitamin A deficiency during pregnancy has been linked with increased rates of intrauterine growth retardation and premature birth (Shah & Rajalakshmi 1984). The recent associations between subclinical vitamin A deficiency in children and increased childhood mortality (see Chapter 13) have heightened interest in the preventive role of vitamin A supplementation during pregnancy. Supplementation may, however, induce teratogenicity and this is of special concern among malnourished women who may be at increased risk of vitamin A toxicity (Malheiros et al 1988).

Maternal vitamin A needs during lactation are determined from estimates of milk output of vitamin A. The expected vitamin A output in milk is approximately 500 µg/day. Under conditions of marginal vitamin A adequacy, vitamin A levels in milk respond to maternal supplementation. Vitamin A deficiency in breastfed infants is not reported commonly even among populations with low vitamin A intakes, and breastfeeding appears to protect infants against vitamin A

Table 25.5   Recommended dietary allowances of vitamins (From National Research Council, Recommended Dietary Allowances (1989))

	Fat-soluble vitamins				Water-soluble vitamins						
	A (μg RE)[1]	D (μg)[2]	E (mg α-TE)[3]	K (μg)	C (mg)	Thiamin (mg)	Riboflavin (mg)	Niacin (mg NE)[4]	B$_6$ (mg)	Folate (μg)	B$_{12}$ (μg)
Pregnant	800 (0%)[5]	10 (100%)	10 (25%)	65 (0%)	70 (17%)	1.5 (36%)	1.6 (23%)	17 (13%)	2.2 (38%)	400 (122%)	2.2 (10%)
Lactating											
1st 6 mos	1300 (62%)	10 (100%)	12 (50%)	65 (0%)	95 (58%)	1.6 (45%)	1.8 (38%)	20 (33%)	2.1 (31%)	280 (45%)	2.6 (30%)
2nd 6 mos	1200 (50%)	10 (100%)	11 (38%)	65 (0%)	90 (50%)	1.6 (45%)	1.7 (31%)	20 (33%)	2.1 (31%)	260 (44%)	2.6 (30%)

[1]   Retinol equivalents. 1 retinol equivalent = 1 μg retinol or 6 μg β-carotene
[2]   As cholecalciferol. 10 μg cholecalciferol = 400 IU of vitamin D
[3]   α-Tocopherol equivalents. 1 mg α-α tocopherol = 1 α-TE
[4]   1 NE (niacin equivalent) = 1 mg niacin or 60 mg of dietary tryptophan
[5]   Percentage increase above levels for non-pregnant, non-lactating women

deficiency following weaning (Sommer 1982), perhaps because of the infant's ability to store the vitamin.

Water-soluble vitamins

Special allowances for pregnancy and lactation are proposed for water-soluble vitamins by both USA and UK committees. Allowances during pregnancy are increased by 10–100% or more above those for non-pregnant women, and sometimes further increased to meet the needs during lactation (see Appendix 2 and Table 25.5).

Folate

Folate is the only vitamin whose allowance is set substantially higher in pregnancy than in lactation, reflecting the key role of folate in cell division and development. Folate deficiency during pregnancy causes megaloblastic anaemia and is linked with high rates of spontaneous abortion, toxaemia, intrauterine growth retardation, premature delivery, fetal malformation and antepartum haemorrhage. The inference of a causal relationship between folate supplementation and reductions in the occurrence of neural tube defects has remained particularly controversial. A recent panel in the USA concluded that 'scientific evidence does not provide a sufficient basis for making recommendations concerning the periconceptual use of vitamins and minerals for the prevention of neural tube defects' (SNSWGP & SDINSDP 1990). This group recognized the need for additional studies and endorsed

recommendations for increased consumption of foods rich in folates. The RDA of 400 μg/day is in excess of the average amount consumed in North America (NRC 1989), where intake ranges are more compatible with the British RDI of 200–300 μg/day. If an adequate folic acid intake is needed to avoid neural tube defects, then it is important to ensure an adequate folate status before pregnancy, because by the time a women realizes she is pregnant the critical stage when the fetal neural tube closes by further cell division has passed. This explains the new medical and public interest in prepregnancy nutritional counselling and the widespread use and abuse of periconceptual vitamin supplementation.

A recent European double-blind controlled trial of 4 mg of folate daily in women who had already had a child with a neural tube defect showed a highly significant reduction in the chances of the mother having a second abnormal child (MRC 1991). Unfortunately, the dose used was large so a pharmacological effect in women with unmet metabolic needs for folic acid may have been responsible.

Extrapolating the results of this trial to all women is difficult, although Smithells, in his original studies, claimed that women on poor diets were particularly liable to have a child with neural tube defects (Smithells et al 1976). His uncontrolled trial with supplements containing 0.36 mg of folate seemed to be protective (Smithells et al 1981). New controlled trials (Czeizel & Dudas, 1992) help to resolve the issue. The US Department of Health now recommends consumption of at least 0.4 mg (but less than 1 mg) of folic acid per day to reduce the risk of neural tube defects (Rosenberg 1992). A UK report (Department of Health 1992) recommends that all young women should consume 0.4 mg folic acid daily to ensure adequate folate stores should they have either a planned or unplanned pregnancy. To prevent a recurrence of neural tube defects 4 mg should be taken (see also Chapter 39).

Folic acid needs in lactation Recommended folate intakes during lactation are calculated on the basis of the expected output of folate in milk, i.e. about 40 µg/day, an estimated efficiency of absorption of food folate of 50%, and a coefficient of variation of 12.5% in the interindividual variability in milk production, milk content and absorption efficiency (NRC 1989).

Folate concentrations in milk appear to be regulated, because concentrations are not correlated with the mother's plasma folate concentrations, nor does milk folate increase with maternal folate supplementation. Correlations between maternal and infant serum folate levels suggest that folate stores accumulated during fetal life are affected by maternal folate status, and that stores transferred to the infant in utero play a significant role in maintaining folate status in infancy (SNDL 1991).

Vitamin B_{12}

Neither pregnancy nor lactation appears to deplete the substantial hepatic vitamin B_{12} stores of omnivorous women. However, pregnancy or lactation in vegetarians can impair B_{12} status. The vitamin B_{12} output in milk from well nourished women is approximately 0.4 µg/day but it may drop to one-tenth of that level in depleted women. Concentrations of urinary methylmalonic acid (an index of deficiency, see Chapter 14) are higher in ovo-lacto vegetarian mothers and their breastfed infants compared to those in omnivorous subjects and their infants (Specker et al 1988). Infants are more vulnerable than are mothers to B_{12} deficiency. Infantile clinical B_{12} deficiency occurs before any clinical manifestation of maternal B_{12} deficiency; the infant will use up fetal stores by about 6 months of age.

Vitamin B_6

The increased protein needs during pregnancy and the role of pyridoxal phosphate (PLP) and pyridoxamine phosphate as coenzymes of transamination and other products of protein metabolism probably increase the requirements for this vitamin (NRC 1989). However, direct evidence for this is lacking. Inadequate maternal vitamin B_6 status has been linked to toxaemia, low birthweight, and to a poor general condition of the infants of deficient mothers at birth (SNSWGDP & SDINS 1990).

Concentrations of vitamin B_6 in mature milk vary substantially and depend on maternal dietary intake. Output in milk is approximately 70 mg/day. Reductions in milk B_6 levels may be sufficiently severe to cause abnormalities in central nervous system functions (Kirksey & Roepke 1981).

Thiamin

Studies of the thiamin status of pregnant women, assessed by erythrocyte transketolase activation (see Chapter 14), indicate that thiamin requirements are increased throughout pregnancy. Severe cardiac decompensation occurs in pregnant women with marked thiamin deficiency, and congestive heart failure may occur in their newborn babies. Reductions in stillbirths, maternal and perinatal mortality and toxaemia have been linked to thiamin supplementation programmes in populations at risk of thiamin deficiency, but no conclusive evidence for a causative role has been published.

Recommended thiamin intakes during lactation are derived from the estimated milk thiamin outputs at 160 µg/day. Since thiamin requirements are related to energy needs, there is an additional increment needed for the extra energy requirement of lactation (see Appendix 2). Milk thiamin concentrations are influenced by maternal intakes and may fall so low in women who consume high carbohydrate diets with low thiamin levels that their breastfed infants develop beriberi.

Riboflavin

Longitudinal studies of pregnant women indicate that urinary excretion of riboflavin falls and erythrocyte glutathione reductase activation coefficients rise as pregnancy progresses, suggesting developing deficiency. These findings have not, however, been related to adverse outcomes (SNSWGDP & SDINSDP 1990), but the activation coefficients do respond to riboflavin supplementation.

Recommended riboflavin intakes during lactation are derived from estimates of riboflavin output in milk (about 260 µg/day) and adjustments for an efficiency factor of 70% in the utilization of riboflavin for milk products (NRC 1989). Milk riboflavin concentrations are influenced by the mother's riboflavin intake. Transient periods of subclinical riboflavin deficiency have been described in otherwise healthy, full-term newborn babies, but the condition appears to resolve spontaneously with or without riboflavin supplementation (SNDL 1991).

Niacin

Requirements for niacin during pregnancy may not be increased significantly because oestrogens induce a higher rate of conversion of tryptophan to the derivatives of niacin (NRC 1989). The increased efficiency is expected to partially compensate for the additional needs of fetal growth and maternal metabolism, so the niacin allowance for pregnancy is increased by approximately 13%. Niacin deficiency during pregnancy has been linked inconclusively to toxaemia.

The output of niacin in human milk is approximately 2.3 mg/day but the US allowance is increased to 4 mg/day because niacin requirements are expressed in terms of dietary energy needs. The higher niacin output in milk and the assumption of a normal tryptophan-to-niacin conversion rate in lactation explain the increased allowance.

Vitamin C

Plasma ascorbic acid concentrations fall during pregnancy, probably because of the normal expansion of blood volume and the concentration of vitamin C in the fetus by special placental transfer mechanisms (NRC 1989). To account for this transfer and for the presumably higher metabolic demands of pregnancy for vitamin C, the USA recommends an increase of 10 mg/day. The UK chose a similar figure for the last trimester of pregnancy. The increased needs of lactation led the USA to recommend an increase of 30 mg/day to allow for maternal loses of about 2 mg/day in milk and the range in milk output where 2 SD is

taken as about 25%. This increment, plus an allowance for an ascorbate absorption efficiency of 85%, brings the final figure to 35 mg/day. The COMA DRV report chooses a value of 30 mg/day. Ascorbic acid output in milk is highly variable and responsive to levels of maternal intake.

Mineral needs during pregnancy and lactation

Minerals have three general roles in metabolism: as structural components (e.g. calcium and phosphorous), as cofactors to metalloenzymes (e.g. zinc and selenium), and as constituents complexed or covalently bound to hormones (e.g. iodine) and various other functional molecules (iron and cobalt). These roles are unaltered by pregnancy and lactation, but mineral needs in pregnancy and lactation must take account of fetal transfer and milk losses. Table 25.6 summarizes recommended intakes for minerals during pregnancy and lactation. The functional impacts of changes in maternal mineral content have not been identified, but it is recognized that there are adaptive mechanisms which alter the rates of mineral absorption and utilization during pregnancy and lactation.

Calcium

The calcium content of adults is approximately 23 g/kg fat-free mass, thus the total body calcium content of a 55 kg woman with 25% body fat is approximately 0.9–1.0 kg. The neonate's calcium content is approximately 30 g, most of which is deposited in the last trimester. This high demand for fetal calcium in the last few weeks of pregnancy means that the maternal skeleton has to provide the mineral. Maternal calcium stores therefore decline, despite the increased efficiency of calcium absorption (Purdie 1989).

Table 25.6 Recommended dietary allowances of minerals (From National Research Council Recommended Dietary Allowances (1989))

	Calcium (mg)	Phosphorus (mg)	Magnesium (mg)	Iron (mg)	Zinc (mg)	Iodine (µg)	Selenium (µg)
Pregnant	1200 (50%)[1]	1200 (50%)	320 (14%)	30 (100%)	15 (25%)	175 (17%)	65 (18%)
Lactating							
1st 6 mos	1200 (50%)	1200 (50%)	355 (27%)	15 (0%)	19 (58%)	200 (33%)	75 (36%)
2nd 6 mos	1200 (50%)	1200 (50%)	340 (21%)	15 (0%)	16 (33%)	200 (33%)	75 (36%)

[1] Percentage increase above levels for non-pregnant, non-lactating women

Enhanced calcium absorption in early pregnancy may boost maternal stores for transfer to the fetus in late pregnancy. The loss of maternal calcium explains why calcium balance in late pregnancy is not sufficiently positive to account for the calcium transferred to the fetus during that period. Since the fetal accumulation of calcium amounts to only 2.5% of maternal stores, detecting calcium loss from the skeleton in pregnancy is difficult.

Calcium losses during 6 months of lactation are approximately 40 g (about 210 mg/day). Taken together, potential calcium losses from repeated pregnancies and lactations can be significant. At present, however there are no conclusive data showing that pregnancy and lactation contribute significantly to bone loss under most dietary conditions in developed countries. Various investigators have speculated about the possibility of compensatory mechanisms between successive pregnancies and lactations which result in the repletion of maternal calcium status (SNDL 1991). Allowances during pregnancy and lactation are increased by 400 mg/day.

Iron

Iron needs during pregnancy total approximately 800–900 mg. Changes in maternal erythrocyte volume and haematopoietic tissues account for approximately 500 mg of iron, and the placenta and fetus for the additional 300–400 mg. Blood loss at delivery results in iron losses of approximately 250 mg. The net loss of iron to the mother after parturition, therefore, is approximately 550–650 mg.

The normal newborn baby's body iron concentration is approximately 50% greater than that of the normal adult. Infants at term, therefore,

have significant iron reserves. These reserves and the high bioavailability — approximately 50% — of iron in human milk are sufficient to maintain iron status within normal limits in exclusively breastfed infants for approximately 6 months. The iron content in human milk does not appear to be influenced by maternal iron status, and the daily output of iron in milk is approximately 0.2 mg/ day, which is substantially below the normal average menstrual losses of 0.7 mg/day. Unlike most other nutrients, iron demands are greater in pregnancy than lactation.

Iron deficiency remains the most common nutrient deficiency in both economically developing and developed countries. Iron deficiency in pregnant women usually results from the combination of low iron stores induced by menstrual losses, inadequate iron intakes, and the high demands of the fetus. Fetal iron needs are met at the expense of maternal stores, so that iron stores are similar in the infants of both iron-sufficient and iron-deficient mothers. Women in lower socio-economic groups, teenagers and multiparous women are at the highest risk of iron deficiency. Symptoms of iron deficiency during pregnancy are similar to those seen in non-pregnant women. Iron-deficient women, however, risk greater complications from the blood loss that accompanies parturition. Maternal iron deficiency (haemoglobin <10 mg/dl) has been associated with increased rates of prematurity, low birthweight and perinatal mortality (NRC 1989, SNDL 1991, SNSWGDP & SDINSDP 1990).

Acknowledgement

This project has been supported in part by Hatch funds and NIH grant no. HD 21049.

REFERENCES

Brewer MM, Bates MR, Vannoy LP 1989 Postpartum changes in maternal weight and body fat depots in lactating vs. nonlactating women. American Journal of Clinical Nutrition 49: 259–265

Brown RH, Akhtor NA, Robertson AD, Ahmed MG 1986 Lactational capacity of marginally malnourished mothers: relationships between maternal nutritional status and quantity and proximate composition of milk. Pediatrics 78: 909–919

Butte NF, Garza C, Stuff JE et al 1984 Effect of maternal diet and body composition on lactational performance. American Journal of Clinical Nutrition 39: 296–306

Committee on Medical Aspects of Food Policy (COMA) 1991 Reference values for food energy and nutrients for the United Kingdom. HMSO, London

Committee on Nutrition 1985 Pediatric Nutrition Handbook, 2nd edn. American Academy of Pediatrics, Elk Grove Village, IL

Czeizel AE, Dudas I 1992 Prevention of the first occurrence of neural tube defects by periconceptual vitamin supplementation. New England Journal of Medicine 327: 1832–1835

Delgado HL, Valverde VE, Martorell R, Klein RE 1982 Relationship of maternal and infant nutrition to infant growth. Early Human Development 6: 273–286

Department of Health, Scottish Office Home and Health Department, Welsh Office, Department of Health and Sosial Services Northern Ireland 1992 Folic acid and the prevention of neural tube defects. Report from an expert advisory group. Department of Health, London

Durnin JVGA 1986 Energy requirements of pregnancy. An integrated study in 5 countries: background and methodology. Nestlé Foundation Annual Report 1986. Nestlé Foundation, Lausanne

FAO/WHO/UNU Expert Consultation 1985 Energy and protein requirements. Technical Report Series 724. World Health Organization, Geneva

Frigerio C, Schutz Y, Prentice A et al 1991a Is human lactation a particularly efficient process? European Journal of Clinical Nutrition 45: 459–462

Frigerio C, Schutz Y, Whitehead R, Jéquier E 1991b Lactation and infant feeding. American Journal of Clinical Nutrition 54: 526–533

Heinig MJ, Nommsen LA, Dewey KG 1990 Lactation and postpartum weight loss. FASEB Journal 4: 362A

Hytten FE, Chamberlain G 1980 Clinical physiology in obstetrics. Blackwell Scientific, Oxford, pp. 193–228

Illingworth PJ, Jung RT, Howie PW et al 1986 Diminution in energy expenditure during lactation. British Medical Journal 292: 437–441

Kirksey A, Roepke JLB 1981 Vitamin B_6 nutrition of mothers of three breastfed neonates with central nervous system disorders. Federation Proceedings, FASEB 40: 864

Lawrence M, Lawrence F, Lamb WH, Whitehead RG 1984 Maintenance energy cost of pregnancy in rural Gambian women and influence of dietary status. Lancet ii: 363–365

Lechtig A, Habicht JP, Delgado H et al 1975 Effect of food supplementation during pregnancy on birthweight. Pediatrics 56: 508–520

Malheiros LR, Paumgartten FJ, Riul TR, da Silva VA 1988 Protein-energy malnutrition increases teratogenicity of hypervitaminosis A in rats. Brazilian Journal of Medical Biology Research 21: 659–662

MRC Vitamin Study Research Group 1991 Prevention of neural tube defects: results of the Medical Research Council Vitamin Study. Lancet 338: 131–137

Mertz W, Tsui JC, Judd JT et al 1991 What are people really eating? The relationship between energy intake derived from estimated diet records and intake determined to maintain body weight. American Journal of Clinical Nutrition 54: 291–295

Motil KJ, Montandon CM, Garza C 1990 Basal and postprandial metabolic rates in lactating and nonlactating women. American Journal of Clinical Nutrition 52: 610–615

Naeye RL 1979 Weight gain and outcome of pregnancy. American Journal of Obstetrics and Gynecology 135: 3–9

National Research Council 1989 Recommended Dietary Allowances, 10th edn. National Academy Press, Washington, DC

Nettleton JA 1993 Are n-3 fatty acids essential nutrients for fetal and infant development? Journal of the American Dietetic Association 93: 58–64

Olsen SF, Sorenson JD, Secher N J et al 1992 Randomised controlled trial of effect of fish-oil supplementation on pregnancy duration. Lancet 339: 1003–1007

Pomerance JJ, Teal TG, Gogolok JF et al 1987 Maternally administered antenatal vitamin K: effect on neonatal prothrombin activity, partial thromboplastin time, and intraventricular hemorrhage. Obstetrics and Gynecology 70: 295–299

Purdie DW 1989 Bone mineral metabolism and reproduction. Contemporary Reviews in Obstetrics and Gynaecology 1: 214–221

Rosenberg IH 1992 Folic acid and neural tube defects – time for action. New England Journal of Medicine 327: 1875–1877

Shah RS, Rajalakshmi R 1984 Vitamin A status of the newborn in relation to gestational care, body weight and maternal nutritional status. American Journal of Clinical Nutrition 40: 794–800

Smithells RW, Sheppard S, Schorah CJ 1976 Vitamin deficiencies and neural tube defects. Archives of Diseases of Childhood 51: 944–950

Smithells RW, Sheppard S, Schorah CJ 1981 Apparent prevention of neural-tube defects by periconceptual vitamin supplementation. Archives of Diseases of Childhood 56: 911–918

SNDL (Subcommittee on Nutrition During Lactation) 1991 Nutrition during lactation, Institute of Medicine. National Academy Press, Washington, DC

SNSWGDP (Subcommittee on Nutritional Status and Weight Gain During Pregnancy) and SDINSDP (Subcommittee on Dietary Intake and Nutrient Supplements During Pregnancy) 1990 Nutrition during pregnancy. Institute of Medicine, National Academy Press, Washington, DC

Sommer A 1982 Nutritional blindness: xerophthalmia and keratomalacia. Oxford University Press, New York

Specker BL, Miller D, Normal EJ et al 1988 Increased urinary methylmalonic acid excretion in breastfed infants of vegetarian mothers and identification of an acceptable dietary source of vitamin B_{12}. American Journal of Clinical Nutrition 47: 89–92

Specker BL, Valanis B, Hertzberg V et al 1985 Sunshine exposure and serum 25-hydroxy vitamin D concentrations in exclusively breastfed infants. Journal of Pediatrics 107: 372–376

Taggart NR, Holiday RM, Billewicz WZ et al 1967 Changes in skinfolds during pregnancy. British Journal of Nutrition 21: 439–451

Tyson JE, Austin K, Fairnholt J et al 1976 Endocrine-metabolic response to acute starvation in human gestation. American Journal of Obstetrics and Gynecology 125: 1073–1084

Whitehead RG, Lawrence M, Prentice AM 1986 Maternal nutrition and breast feeding. Human Nutrition: Applied Nutrition 40A, (Suppl 1): 1–10

26. Infant nutrition

B. E. Golden

At no time in life is nutrition more important than in infancy. During the first few months after birth, tissue and organ synthesis rates are high, while the processes of maturation continue rapidly. These changes require a balanced and relatively large intake of specific nutrients and energy, but the infant's tolerance to 'food' is limited by the immaturity of the gastrointestinal tract, liver and kidneys. Unlike adults, young infants cannot consume solids and do not tolerate foods containing large amounts of fibre, toxins or foods which provide a high renal solute load: they rely, for at least the first few months, on just one liquid food – milk – for all their nutritional needs. It is vital that the composition and supply of this milk is as near optimal as possible. Table 26.1 shows the average requirements of energy and selected nutrients for infants growing normally.

BREASTFEEDING

Within the first hour of life, a normal human neonate, put on its mother's chest, spontaneously roots, finds a nipple and starts to suckle (Widstrom et al 1987). This behaviour is common to all mammalian species and, in many, both the action of suckling and the initial milk, called colostrum, are necessary for the neonate to survive. This is not the case in humans, but both early suckling and the intake of early maternal milk play important roles in infants' development, both psychological and physical.

The suckling of breastfeeding allows mutual somatosensory stimulation and responsiveness between mother and child (Uvnas-Moberg & Winberg 1989). Immediately postpartum, the sensitivity of the mother's nipples and surrounding skin increases dramatically. The infant's buccal mucosa is also particularly sensitive. When stimulated by mutual contact, hormonal responses occur, e.g. the infant's somatostatin levels fall while gastrin and cholecystokinin levels rise: in the mother, prolactin

Table 26.1 Estimated requirements of energy and selected nutrients in normal infants

	Age (months)	
	0–6	6–12
Based on normal infants' intake[1]		
Energy (MJ/kg)	0.42	0.38
Protein (g/kg)	1.46	1.16
RDA[2] Fat-soluble vitamins		
Vit A (μg RE[3])	375	375
Vit E (μg α-TE[3])	3	4
Vit K (μg)	5	10
Vit D (μg)	7.5	10
RDA[2] Water-soluble vitamins		
Vit C (mg)	30	35
Thiamin (mg)	0.3	0.4
Riboflavin (mg)	0.4	0.5
Niacin (mg NE[3])	5	6
Pyridoxine (mg)	0.3	0.6
Folic acid (μg)	25	35
Vit B_{12} (μg)	0.3	0.5
RDA[2] Major and trace elements		
Calcium (mg)	400	600
Phosphorus (mg)	300	500
Magnesium (mg)	40	60
Iron (mg)	6	10
Zinc (mg)	5	5
Iodine (μg)	40	50
Selenium (μg)	10	15

[1] Fomon 1991
[2] Food and Nutrition Board 1989
[3] 1 RE = 1 μg retinol or 6 μg β-carotene
1 α-TE = 10 g d-α tocopherol
1 NE = 1 mg niacin or 60 mg dietary tryptophan

and oxytocin levels also rise. The effects of these changes are many and include, in the mother, stimulation of milk production, a let-down reflex which brings milk to the point of delivery, milk ejection, local skin vasodilatation which provides warmth for the infant in contact and, usually, a pleasurable, sleepy sensation. In the infant, these endocrine changes help to stimulate the growth and development of the gastrointestinal tract, increase nutrient absorption and then induce satiety and sleepiness. These effects in the infant are independent of the provision of maternal milk. When breastfeeding is the only source of food, the infant lies in close contact with his mother for at least 2 hours a day. This ensures rapid 'bonding' between mother and infant: the infant learns to trust early and such a relationship fosters normal psychological development. Breastfeeding also depresses the mother's reproductive system, thereby delaying further conception. This is associated with increased basal circulating prolactin levels postpartum; these fall with time, as fertility improves. This phenomenon appears to be exaggerated in poorly nourished mothers (Uvnas-Moberg & Winberg 1989).

MATERNAL MILK

Human milk provides sufficient energy and essential macro- and micronutrients for rapid growth and development for at least the critical first 4 months. It also contains a repertoire of antimicrobial substances and cells, hormones, enzymes, growth factors and binding proteins, as well as many substances of indeterminate function. However, human milk appears not to provide sufficient vitamin K or fluoride for optimum health (Williams 1991), nor does it supply enough iron after about 4 months, and it may not supply sufficient vitamin D. The approximate concentrations of the constituents are shown in Table 26.2, but the ranges are wide as the composition varies from mother to mother, with the time of day and with the time into a feed, as well as with the length of time postpartum.

Colostrum, or the milk produced during the first 5 days, contains relatively large amounts of protein, particularly secretory immunoglobulin A (secr IgA), but also albumin, serum immunoglobulins and lysozyme (Williams 1991). It also contains higher concentrations than does mature milk of cholesterol and several trace elements including zinc and selenium (Hambraeus 1991). It contains relatively little fat. Carnitine concentration is maximal at 2 weeks of age: newborns have a limited capacity for its synthesis. Jaundice during the first few days of life in breastfed babies is a well recognized occurrence of no pathological consequence. The cause of this prolonged unconjugated hyperbilirubinaemia is not clear. Several factors in breast milk have been implicated, including raised levels of pregnane-3(α),20(β)-diol, free fatty acids and β-glucuronidase (Freed et al 1987). The jaundice is familial in that, if it occurs in

Table 26.2 Approximate composition of mature human milk, unmodified cow's milk and a cow's milk whey-based infant formula (selected constituents)[1]

Constituent	Human milk	Cow's milk	Typical formula[3]
Energy[2] (MJ/l)	3.1	2.9	2.8
Total protein (g/l)	8.9	31.4	15.0
Total whey (g/l)	6.4	5.8	9.0
α-lactalbumin (g/l)	2–3	1.1	9.0
β-lactoglobulin (g/l)	0	3.6	0
Lactoferrin (g/l)	1–3	Trace	0
secr IgA (g/l)	0.5–1.0	0.03	0
Lysozyme (g/l)	0.05–0.25	Trace	0
Total caseins (g/l)	2–3	27.3	6.0
Non-protein nitrogen % total N	18–30	5	–
Total fat (g/l)	42	38	36
Cholesterol (mg/l)	160	110	–
Essential fatty acids (g/100 g fatty acids)			
18:2 linoleic	7.2	1.6	–
18:3 linolenic	0.8	0.4	–
20:4 arachidonic	0.3	0.1	–
Carbohydrate			
Lactose (g/l)	60–70	47	72
Oligosaccharides (g/l)	12–13	1	0
Fat-soluble vitamins			
Vit A (μg/l)	600	350	605
Vit E (μg/l)	3500	1400	7400
Vit D (μg/l)	0.1	0.8	10
Vit K (μg/l)	2.1	35	40
Water-soluble vitamins			
Vit C (mg/l)	38	18	60
Thiamin (μg/l)	160	430	400
Riboflavin (μg/l)	300	1700	500
Niacin (μg/l)	2300	950	4000
Pantothenic acid (μg/l)	2600	3600	4000
Biotin (μg/l)	7.6	40	11.3
Folic acid (μg/l)	52	55	100
Vit B$_{12}$ (μg/l)	0.1	4.5	1.5
Major and trace elements			
Sodium (mg/l)	150	450	180
Calcium (mg/l)	350	1200	590
Phosphorus (mg/l)	150	940	350
Magnesium (mg/l)	28	120	60
Iron (mg/l)	0.8	0.6	8
Zinc (mg/l)	3	3	4
Iodine (μg/l)	70	80	40
Selenium (μg/l)	14	30	–

[1] Williams 1991
[2] George & DeFrancesca 1989
[3] Cow's milk whey-based formula (Aptamil, Milupa)

one infant, it is also likely to occur in the breastfed siblings.

Human milk fat is 98% triacylglycerols and contributes 50–60% of total milk energy. It contains substantial amounts of unsaturated fatty acids, particularly oleic and linoleic acids. The fat occurs as globules enclosed in membranes, which help protect it from lipolysis and oxidation (Chan 1992). Within the membranes are also phospholipids, cholesterol, proteins and trace elements: the membranes play several important physical roles. Human milk fat is hydrolysed mainly to β-monoglycerides, which are more easily absorbed than α-monoglycerides, the main products of fat hydrolysis in cow's milk.

The fat content and composition of 'mature' milk, i.e. that produced after the first 10–15 days, are particularly variable (Jensen 1989). For example, the fat concentration increases during a feed and usually during the morning. The fat content and fatty acid composition vary among different populations on different diets. However, when a mother is semi-starving, her milk composition reflects that of her own adipose tissue which is being catabolized. Maternal diet also affects the milk content of fat-soluble vitamins.

Mature milk protein comprises whey proteins and caseins in a 60:40 ratio. Of the whey proteins, over a third is α-lactalbumin which, with the caseins, is the main source of essential amino acids. Other important whey proteins are lactoferrin and secr IgA. Their main functions are non-nutritional. Maternal milk contains secr IgA antibodies to the microorganisms to which both mother and infant are exposed, in their gastrointestinal tracts and probably also their respiratory tracts (Hanson et al 1988). These antibodies bind bacterial antigens, preventing them from attaching to the intestinal mucosal cell membrane. They also neutralize toxins and viruses, including poliovirus. This latter effect may interfere with oral immunization by live poliovirus vaccine (Plotkin et al 1966). It has also been postulated that secr IgA plays a role in the prevention of allergic food sensitization in infants, particularly relevant in those with a family history of atopy. The manifestations of food sensitivity, particularly diarrhoea and vomiting but also eczema and asthma, are markedly reduced in breastfed infants, especially when their mothers exclude potent allergens, such as cow's milk and eggs, from their diets. This subject is dealt with in Chapter 44. Lactoferrin is also bacteriostatic: it binds iron, thus withholding it from bacteria so that their intestinal growth is inhibited. Its other postulated roles include effects on iron absorption and mitogenic or trophic activities on the intestinal mucosa. Both lactoferrin and secr IgA resist acid and peptic digestion and therefore appear, to a significant extent, in the stools of breastfed infants (Samson et al 1980). Whey proteins, present in minor quantities, also bind corticosteroids, thyroxine and vitamins, e.g. folate,

vitamin D and vitamin B_{12}. Many proteins act as enzymes, e.g. lysozyme, which is also bacteriostatic, and lipases, α-amylase, antiproteases and lactoperoxidase. The caseins comprise mainly β-casein with minor amounts of κ-casein, linked together with inorganic ions, largely calcium and phosphate, to form small micelles. These result in a soft, flocculant coagulum in the infant's gastrointestinal tract which aids casein digestion. Around a quarter of total N in human milk is not in the form of protein (Carlsson 1985). It is largely present as N-acetyl glucosamine and urea, neither of whose functions are yet clear. Other non-protein nitrogen compounds include amino acids, of which taurine is important for bile salt formation, peptides, which include epidermal growth factor, somatomedins, insulin, thyroxine, thyroid-stimulating hormone and thyrotrophin-releasing hormone, carnitine, creatinine and creatine.

Carbohydrate in human milk is mainly lactose which, unlike the other constituents, varies little in concentration. Lactose accounts for about 38% of the total energy in human milk. Unabsorbed lactose is converted to lactic acid by the intestinal microflora: this reduces the pH, increasing the solubility and therefore the absorption of calcium. The functions of other oligosaccharides and other glycoproteins are ill understood.

The major and trace elements in human milk are shown in Table 26.2: calcium and phosphorus are associated with the casein fraction whereas the others are associated mainly with the whey fraction. The essential trace elements are also associated with the fat globules. 28% of zinc and 40% of copper are bound in part to serum albumin in the milk, and 30–40% of iron is bound to lactoferrin: this protein also binds manganese and, perhaps, zinc as well (Hambraeus 1991). Selenium is found largely in selenomethionine and selenocysteine. The concentrations of these elements are low but their availability (percentage absorption) appears to be extremely high: the reasons are still not clear. Fluoride is present in low concentration: the American Academy of Pediatrics (1979) recommends that fluoride supplements are given to infants who are solely breastfed after 6 months of age.

The vitamin content of human milk is related closely to the vitamin status of the mother (Hambraeus 1991). In general, the levels of water-soluble vitamins are adequate, but thiamin deficiency (beriberi) has been described in a SE Asian breastfed infant (Rascoff 1942). Vitamin E levels tend to be high, vitamin A levels are moderate but particularly variable, and vitamins D and especially K tend to be low. Vitamin D deficiency – rickets – classically occurs in Middle

Eastern breastfed infants, even when they are resident in the UK. The main reason is lack of exposure to sunlight (for skin production of cholecalciferol) of both the mother and the child, and not dietary deficiency (Bachrach et al 1979). Rickets is now very uncommon in Caucasian infants. However, several authorities recommend vitamin D supplements for breastfed infants (American Academy of Pediatrics 1985). Haemorrhagic disease of the newborn continues to occur in breastfed rather than in bottle-fed infants (Motohara et al 1984). This is entirely preventable by vitamin K administration just after birth, which implies that human milk is, indeed, an inadequate source of vitamin K. It is usually given by intramuscular injection, but the oral route is safer and also seems to be effective.

Other important components of human milk include water, cells and 'contaminants'. The water intake of an entirely breastfed infant is adequate, even in very hot climates: water supplementation is unnecessary. There are several cell types whose main function appears to be antimicrobial in the infant's gastrointestinal tract. The majority are macrophages and polymorphonuclear leucocytes, with smaller numbers of lymphocytes, of which over half are T-lymphocytes. Their numbers fall dramatically during the first month of lactation; however, there are a few epithelial cells in colostrum and these increase to appreciable numbers in mature milk. As yet, the precise roles of the different cells are poorly defined. The major function of macrophages is probably phagocytosis and the killing of microorganisms. Unlike the polymorphs, they are more motile than those in blood and may be active in the mucosa as well as in the intestinal lumen (Goldman & Goldblum 1989). One of the functions of the lymphocytes is the production of interferons, a group of glycoproteins that render cells less susceptible to viral infection. There are numerous other antimicrobial substances produced by the different cell types (Ogra & Ogra 1988).

Possible contaminants are many and varied. Some residues are actively secreted, others are passively diffused into the milk. They include hormones, drugs, pesticides and other pollutants and viruses. Oral contraceptives appear to suppress milk volume (Hambraeus 1991), probably due to the effect of their oestrogens on prolactin; whether they affect milk composition is unclear. Drugs, alcohol and smoking have clear effects. Acidic drugs pass readily into milk. The concentration of lipid-soluble drugs depends on the milk fat content. Breastfeeding is generally contraindicated when the mother is receiving phenobarbitone, thiouracil or cytotoxic drugs, but alcohol and many other drugs also appear in significant amounts in human milk. Smoking reduces milk volume. Most chemical pollutants are lipid-soluble and therefore pose a real risk if they have accumulated in the mother's adipose tissue and are released during lactation. This can be avoided to some extent if the mother continues to eat adequately, so that her own fat is not being catabolized (Hambraeus 1991). In fact, there is little clinical evidence of the toxic effects of pollutants in breastfed infants. Unfortunately, there is evidence of transmission of a variety of viruses, including the human immunodeficiency virus (Oxtoby 1988). As a result, infected mothers in the UK are advised not to breastfeed their offspring (DHSS 1988). However, for poor communities in most parts of Africa, the risk of HIV infection from breastfeeding is still less than the risks of other infections and undernutrition associated with bottle-feeding (Lederman 1992).

COW'S MILK

Cow's milk is made for calves and is different from human milk in many respects (Table 26.2). Unmodified, it is inappropriate for young infants, as its associated renal solute load is too large – nearly three times that of human milk, due to its high concentrations of protein and inorganic ions. Nowadays, skimmed milk is popular in adults' diets, but this is even more inappropriate for infant feeding. However, by manipulating the casein/whey ratio and adding specific essential nutrients, e.g. linoleic acid, iron, zinc, copper and vitamins, and subsequently diluting, formula manufacturers have now produced good substitutes for human milk. As our knowledge of infants' requirements improves, so the composition of these formula milks is changing. At present, there remain several problems: the biggest is the fact that they must be fed by bottle. This loses the advantages of suckling to both infant and mother. Bottled feeds are much more likely to become contaminated by local organisms, especially where hygiene is poor and the ambient temperature is high, as in many underdeveloped regions. Bottled feeds are also much more expensive than the extra cost of feeding the mother sufficiently to permit normal lactation and maintain her health. The composition of milk formulae remains suboptimal in several circumstances. Some infants quickly become milk-intolerant. The basic aetiology is not yet clear because, by the time the infant is investigated, there are secondary effects of the intolerance. Nevertheless, sensitivity of the infant's gastrointestinal tract to bovine protein, probably β-lactoglobulin, seems to play a part. Other infants develop secondary, or, rarely, are born with primary, disaccharidase deficiencies. 'Specialized' formulae are therefore being made, e.g. with the protein hydrolysed to reduce its antigenicity, with different carbohydrates and fat or with extra trace elements and/or vitamin supplements. Formula milks are extremely convenient because they allow the mother freedom to work outside the home and increase the number of possible carers for her child. However, formulae will probably never match the remarkable properties of maternal milk. Every mother (except those with particular infections, severe illnesses, or those on certain drugs, as described above) should be recommended to breastfeed initially and, if possible, for the first 4 months. By 4 months, the non-nutritional advantages of human milk are becoming less important and after this, many, but not all, infants gain weight faster if supplemented with or changed to formula milk. Whether this is an advantage or not is unclear.

OTHER MILKS

Although recommended in the folklore of some cultures, goat's and sheep's milk should not be fed to young infants as, like cow's milk, the resultant renal solute loads are too high and the mineral and vitamin, especially folate, contents are inappropriate (Taitz & Armitage 1984).

Soy-based formulae have been promoted for infants being reared as vegetarians and for those intolerant of cow's milk-based formula. Soy 'milk' is very different from both cow's and human milk. For example, it is short of methionine and carnitine. Thus, soy-based formulae are now supplemented with both (Fomon et al 1979). Soy 'milk' also contains phytates which bind cations, especially calcium and zinc, also iron, and thus reduce their availability (Lonnerdal 1985). This occurs even at low phytate concentrations. As phytates are difficult to remove completely from soy milk, most formulae still contain some. Soy protein is also antigenic, like cow's milk protein (Eastham et al 1978). Thus, if an infant is cow's milk-intolerant due to protein sensitivity, he or she is likely also to become soy milk-intolerant. Recently, it has been noted that soy formulae contain high concentrations of aluminium (Bishop et al 1989). The newer cow's milk formulae containing hydrolysed protein are usually better tolerated and should be recommended rather than soy formula in cases of protein sensitivity. Much intolerance, however, is due to secondary lactase deficiency following gastrointestinal infection. In this case, soy formulae can be recommended as they generally contain sucrose, glucose or polysaccharides, rather than lactose. Transient intolerance to a range of carbohydrates developing as a result of infection is quite common in young children.

WEANING

Weaning is the name given to the infant's gradual transition from a single-food milk diet to a mixed diet containing a variety of foods. In very traditional societies, this occurs late: in the UK, it is occurring earlier and earlier; in poor urbanized communities in the tropics, it is also occurring early. It is in these latter communities that the weaning period is a particular time of risk for the infant's nutrition (Rowland 1986).

The range of time over which weaning may occur successfully is wide but, clearly, there are limits. Weaning too early is not tolerated by the young infant's immature gastrointestinal tract, liver and kidneys. Weaning is too late if the milk is insufficient to permit normal growth, development and metabolism. For example, human milk provides little iron and copper, but young breastfed infants normally use their haemoglobin and hepatic stores of these elements; eventually, these are depleted and a low serum ferritin develops as iron stores are used up by 6 months. Serum ferritin in infants fed unmodified cow's milk is low by 4 months (Wharton 1991). However, infant formulae are now supplemented with iron and copper, as well as vitamins A, D and K. Thus, from present knowledge of nutritional requirements, breastfed infants should probably start weaning at an earlier age than formula-fed infants. Present knowledge, however, is limited: we still do not know what governs nutrient availability from human milk. The general consensus is that infants should commence weaning between 4 and 6 months of age. Since milks of all types are excellent sources of energy and essential nutrients and are still available, almost worldwide, at reasonable cost, their intake should not fall significantly during weaning, if possible. Also, maternal milk is likely to continue to confer some protection against infection; although secr IgA and lactoferrin levels fall during the first 6 months of lactation, lysozyme levels rise and remain high 2 years postpartum! Prolonged breastfeeding – for at least up to a year – should therefore be encouraged in poor households where nutrition and hygiene are compromised, usually in developing regions.

Weaning foods are chosen on the basis of their flexible consistency and their taste and acceptability by the infant. They should aim to be more energy-dense than milk, to be well balanced with respect to essential nutrients, but to improve the status of those nutrients in short supply from milk. Usually, the staple food of the region, being a bland cereal or rootcrop, is offered early during weaning. Guidelines are available for the manufacture of commercial early weaning foods (ESPGAN Committee on Nutrition 1981): these are also usually based on cereals (except wheat), pre-cooked, with milk or soya to improve nutrient quality and supplemented with specific micronutrients. Initially, weaning foods can be prepared as a fluid gruel given once a day; later, a thicker gruel is given more often. To reduce cereal viscosity without altering its energy density, germination of the cereals can be used (Rowland 1986). 'New' foods should be introduced in small quantities at intervals of several days. Feeding should be slow and care is needed to avoid choking. Other common early weaning foods include milk-based custards, other cooked cereals and rootcrops, egg and banana, but not high-fibre foods, highly acidic fruits or vegetables, or highly seasoned food. Until the eruption of the infant's deciduous teeth is complete (30–36 months), solid foods should be crushed or, later, cut into small pieces. By this stage, weaning is almost complete.

The result of successful infant nutrition is a healthy child who has gained weight and height normally and has a normal body composition. If breastfeeding fails, or bottle-feeding is inappropriate or infection occurs, then undernutrition can develop rapidly. This occurs particularly in underdeveloped regions in association with poverty and frequent infection (see Chapter 30).

In the developed world, however, the obvious immediate adverse effects are feed intolerance, as described above, and obesity.

LONG-TERM EFFECTS OF INFANT NUTRITION

Recently evidence of possible long-term adverse effects has emerged: if verified, these may be extremely important. Thus, Barker's group (Barker et al 1989, Hales et al 1991) has shown statistically significant associations between birthweight and weight at 1 year on the one hand, and cardiovascular disease and impaired glucose tolerance on the other; these data imply that growth and, therefore, nutrition pre- and postnatally may be affecting morbidity and mortality many decades later. From another point of view, it is clear that the composition of the infant's diet affects his or her lipid metabolism: breastfed infants have higher circulating total, low-density lipoprotein (LDL) and very low-density lipoprotein (VLDL), cholesterol than those fed commercial formulae. Some researchers have suggested that this pattern in breastfed infants may reduce their serum cholesterol in adulthood, and therefore their risk of ischaemic heart disease, by chronically suppressing hepatic HMG CoA reductase activity, which is required for cholesterol synthesis (Barclay et al 1991). Again, this suggests the possibility of long-term adverse effects of infant nutrition.

REFERENCES

American Academy of Pediatrics 1979 Fluoride supplementation: revised dosage schedule. Pediatrics 63: 150–152

American Academy of Pediatrics, Committee on Nutrition 1985 Pediatric Nutrition Handbook. American Academy of Pediatrics, Illinois

Bachrach S, Fisher J, Parks JS 1979 An outbreak of vitamin D deficiency rickets in a susceptible population. Pediatrics 64: 871–877

Barclay S, Ralph A, James WPT 1991 Childhood diet and adult disease. In: McLaren DS, Burman D, Belton NR, Williams AF (eds) Textbook of paediatric nutrition, 3rd edn. Churchill Livingstone, Edinburgh, pp 531–556

Barker DJP, Winter PD, Osmond C et al 1989 Weight in infancy and death from ischaemic heart disease. Lancet 2: 577–580

Bishop N, McGraw M, Ward N 1989 Aluminium in infant formulas. Lancet 1: 490

Carlsson SE 1985 Human milk non-protein nitrogen: occurrence and possible functions. In: Barness LA (ed) Advances in pediatrics, Vol. 32. Year Book Medical, Chicago, pp 43–70

Chan GM 1992 Human milk membranes: an important barrier and substance. Journal of Pediatric Gastroenterology and Nutrition 5: 521–522

DHSS 1988 Present-day practice in infant feeding: third report. Report on Health and Social Subjects 32. HMSO, London

Eastham EJ, Lichauco T, Grade MI, Walker WA 1978 Antigenicity of infant formulas: role of immature intestine on protein permeability. Journal of Pediatrics 93: 561–564

ESPGAN Committee on Nutrition 1981 Guidelines on infant nutrition. II: Recommendations for the composition of follow-up formula and Beikost. Acta Paediatrica Scandinavica 287 (suppl): 1–36

Fomon SJ 1991 Requirements and recommended dietary intakes of protein during infancy. Pediatric Research 30: 391–395

Fomon SJ, Ziegler EE, Filer L J et al 1979 Methionine fortification of a soy formula fed to infants. American Journal of Clinical Nutrition 32: 2460–2469

Food and Nutrition Board, National Academy of Sciences – NRC 1989 Recommended dietary allowances, Revised 1989. National Academic Press, Washington

Freed LM, Moscioni D, Hamosh M et al 1987 Breast milk jaundice revisited: No role for β-glucuronidase or 'unstimulated lipase'. Pediatric Research 21: 167A

George DE, DeFrancesca BA 1989 Human milk in comparison to cow milk. In: Lebenthal E (ed) Textbook of gastroenterology and nutrition in infancy, 2nd edn. Raven Press, New York, pp. 239–261

Goldman AS, Goldblum RM 1989 Immunologic system in human milk: characteristics and effects. In: Leventhal E (ed) Textbook of gastroenterology and nutrition in infancy, 2nd edn. Raven Press, New York, pp. 135–142

Hales CN, Barker DJP, Clark PMS et al 1991 Fetal and infant growth and impaired glucose tolerance at age 64 years. British Medical Journal 303: 1019–1022

Hambraeus L 1991 Human milk: Nutritional aspects. In: Brunser O, Carrazza FR, Gracey M et al (eds) Clinical nutrition of the young child. Raven Press, New York, pp. 289–301

Hanson LA, Carlsson B, Jalil F et al 1988 Antiviral and antibacterial factors in human milk. In: Hanson LA (ed) Biology of human milk. Nestlé Nutrition Workshop Series Vol. 15, pp. 141–156

Jensen RG 1989 Lipids in human milk composition and fat-soluble vitamins. In: Lebenthal E (ed) Textbook of gastroenterology and nutrition in infancy, 2nd edn. Raven Press, New York, pp. 157–208

Lederman SA 1992 Estimating infant mortality from human immunodeficiency virus and other causes in breast-feeding and bottle-feeding populations. Pediatrics 89: 290–296

Lonnerdal B 1985 Dietary factors affecting trace element bioavailability from human milk, cow's milk and infant formulas. Progress in Nutrition and Food Science 9: 35–62

Motohara M, Matsukura M, Matsuda I et al 1984 Severe vitamin K deficiency in breast-fed infants. Journal of Pediatrics 105: 943–945

Ogra PL, Ogra SS 1988 Cellular aspects of immunologic reactivity. In: Hanson LA (ed) Biology of human milk. Nestlé Nutrition Workshop Series Vol 15, pp. 171–184

Oxtoby MJ 1988 Human immunodeficiency virus and other viruses in human milk: placing the issues in broader perspective. Pediatric Infectious Diseases Journal 7: 825–835

Plotkin SA, Katz M, Brown RE, Pagano JS 1966 Oral poliovirus vaccination in newborn African infants. The inhibitory effect of breastfeeding. American Journal of Diseases in Childhood 111: 27–30

Rascoff H 1942 Beriberi heart in a 4-month-old infant. Journal of the American Medical Association 120: 1292–1293

Rowland MGM 1986 The weanling's dilemma: are we making progress? Acta Paediatrica Scandinavica 322 (Suppl): 33–42

Samson RR, Mirtle C, McLelland DBL 1980 The effect of digestive enzymes on the binding and bacteriostatic properties of lactoferrin and vitamin B_{12} binder in human milk. Acta Paediatrica Scandinavica 69: 517–523

Taitz LS, Armitage BL 1984 Goats' milk for infants and children. British Medical Journal 288: 428–429

Uvnas-Moberg K, Winberg J 1989 Role for sensory stimulation in energy economy of mother and infant with particular regard to the gastrointestinal endocrine system. In: Lebenthal E (ed) Textbook of gastroenterology and nutrition in infancy, 2nd edn. Raven Press, New York, pp. 53–62

Wharton BA 1991 Weaning and early childhood. In: McLaren DS, Burman D, Belton NR, Williams AF (eds) Textbook of paediatric nutrition, 3rd edn. Churchill Livingstone, Edinburgh, pp. 47–58

Widstrom A-M, Ransjo-Arvidson AB, Christensson K, Matthiesen A-S, Winberg J, Uvnas-Moberg K 1987 Gastric suction in healthy newborn infants. Effects on circulation and developing feeding behaviour. Acta Paediatrica Scandinavica 76: 566–572

Williams AF 1991 Lactation and infant feeding. In: McLaren DS, Burman D, Belton NR, Williams AF (eds) Textbook of paediatric nutrition, 3rd edn. Churchill Livingstone, Edinburgh, pp. 21–45

27. Childhood, youth and old age

J. T. Dwyer

CHILDHOOD

Late infancy

By 4–6 months of age the infant's needs and developmental readiness are such that supplements to breast milk are necessary (American Academy of Pediatrics 1980a). The transition to family diets begin with the gradual weaning of the infant from the breast or bottle to drinking from a cup. Slow, stepwise introduction of solid foods which have the appropriate texture, consistency and non-allergic characteristics helps the infant learn to chew, eat solid foods, and to use fingers, spoons and other eating utensils.

Supplementary feeding of puréed or semi-solid baby foods in addition to breast or bottle adds needed energy and other nutrients, and permits the mastery of these new eating skills while minimizing the risks of aspiration. As the infant gains experience in eating, foods which must be chewed, chopped foods and small pieces of food can be safely introduced. As long as growth continues to be appropriate this is no reason for concern. Parents need guidance in monitoring child growth and health so that they can identify when growth problems are sufficiently severe to warrant seeking medical advice. Since children differ in their genetic potential for growth, a group of normal children of the same age will vary in weight and height, as shown in Figs 27.1 and 27.2. However, a normal child should be in a similar centile band for weight as for height, and should show the rate of weight and height gain which will maintain that centile ranking.

Parents need to become sensitive to their child's ways of expressing hunger, so that both over- and underfeeding are avoided. Poor appetites may be associated with growth, teething, growing independence, attempting to change too many aspects of the child's diet at once, or illness. The infant and young child should not be forced to finish every bit of food on their plate, or drop of milk in their cup, nor should the child constantly be fed when he expresses discontent for any reason.

Poverty groups in the USA are eligible for continued food assistance, nutrition education and health surveillance of their infants from the Women's Infant's and Children's supplementary feeding program (WIC). This has positive effects on infant nutritional status and growth (Rush 1985). The WIC food package includes items appropriate for the older infant. The parents of infants with handicaps or other health problems may also require special medical advice to ensure that such special developmental needs are met. By 18 months of age, most normal infants have successfully completed the transition to family fare. After about the age of 2, moderation is in order with respect to several dietary components, such as fat, cholesterol, sugar and sodium, but they should not be severely restricted. Before 2 years of age, modified diets should not be attempted without medical supervision.

Preschool children continue to be nutritionally vulnerable even though their growth rates are slower than they were in infancy, and their nutrient needs are reduced correspondingly. Surveys in the USA find that, as a whole, most preschool children are in relatively good nutritional health, although those in poor families sometimes show poor growth and less desirable nutrient intakes (Surgeon General's Report 1988a,b). Toddlers and preschool children require a physical and social environment that supports their physical growth as well as their emotional, intellectual and motor skill development.

Parental role

Family structures and lifestyles today present new challenges in ensuring that the nutritional needs of young children are met. These include alterations in sex roles relating to child care, increases in the care of young children outside the home, with more working

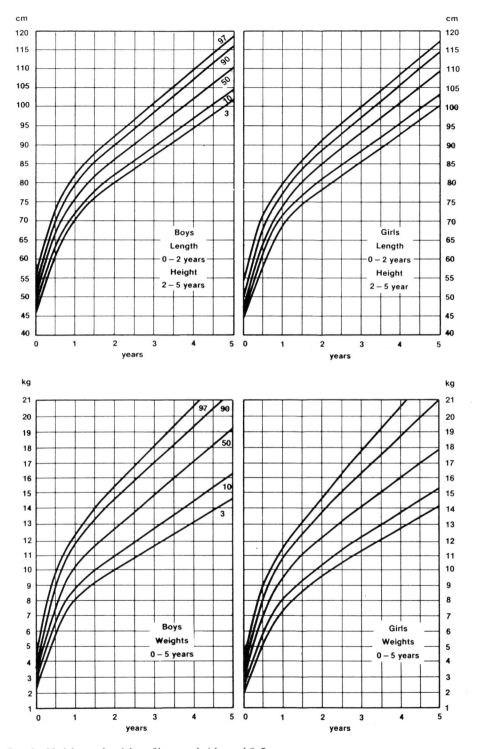

Fig. 27.1   Standard heights and weights of boys and girls aged 0–5 years.

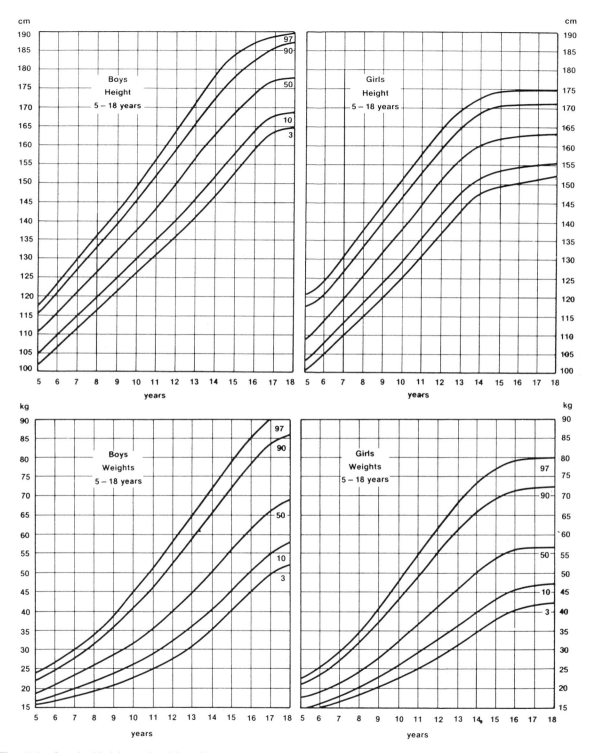

Fig. 27.2   Standard heights and weights of boys and girls aged 5–18 years old.

mothers, more single parent families, and more strains on working parents in both single and dual wage-earning households. Child feeding is less likely to be solely a maternal affair than it was formerly. More and more children eat one or more meals a day outside the home. The appropriate role of government in preschool child care and feeding continues to be debated, but many families need some sort of care outside the home by individuals other than the parents. Parents and other caretakers play a powerful role in ensuring that nutrition enhances development during the preschool years. There are a number of positive steps they can take to do this. Parents must ensure that the child's levels of physical activity and rest each day are sufficient to foster and maintain a good appetite and normal growth. Parents should provide nutritious food in the home, and demand that it is provided in the other settings in which the child eats, such as infant care centres, nursery schools and preschools. Parents must teach the child to choose and eat nutritious food by emphasizing nutrition in family meal and snack planning, and by stocking food supplies to match. Parents should teach the toddler to distinguish between food and non-food objects, and to avoid the mouthing and eating of non-food objects so as to minimize the risk of poisoning.

Families with severe economic constraints should avail themselves of the food stamp programme (in the USA), surplus commodity foods when they are available, preschool and other child nutrition programmes such as Head Start (USA), school breakfast and lunch, and free or low-cost health services.

Preschool programmes outside the home are increasing in popularity. Good ones share some common characteristics, including a strong nutritional component. Such programmes should screen and identify children at nutritional or health risk because of poor growth, disorganized or disrupted families, poverty, or other easily identifiable characteristics, and refer them for assistance. Such assistance should include early intervention and social welfare services.

Preschool child feeding outside the home should be an adjunct to and not a substitute for home efforts. Home food intakes should be supplemented with healthy food which is provided in a timely, safe, sanitary manner in the child care setting outside the home. Meals in preschool programmes should provide proportions of protein, vitamins and minerals which are in line with energy supplied, nutrient needs and meals eaten at home. Preschool programmes should include nutrition education components that expose the child to new eating experiences in a supervised and safe environment, and also include involvement in preparation and clean-up.

Preschool children who have special developmental and health needs involving nutrition are increasingly 'mainstreamed' into regular preschool programmes. There should be referrals to experts when special problems arise.

Food refusal

Parents and others who feed children need to avoid counterproductive behaviour as well as acting to promote good nutrition by more active means. Parents must distinguish between expressions of real physiological need on the child's part, and other emotional and physical needs that are sometimes expressed in food terms. The child's normal strivings for greater independence mean that temporary refusals to eat, dawdling, and the use of food and eating to attempt to exert control over the parent are inevitable. Parents should handle such food-related struggles calmly and without becoming emotionally involved in the issues themselves, to avoid the development of long-term feeding problems in their children. Appropriate parental behaviours include recognizing that child appetites wax and wane from day to day; that some food waste is inevitable; taking a child dawdling and toying with food in their stride; and developing a 'take it or leave it' attitude toward feeding the child. Parents should not become unduly concerned about the ill effects of short-term (e.g. meal to meal or a few days) fluctuations in their child's food intakes. It is best to avoid counterproductive measures such as forcing, coaxing, nagging and above all physical punishment or emotional isolation to remedy food refusal, which is unlikely to be a serious problem to begin with. Parental feelings and emotions directed toward the child should not be expressed through the use of food alone. When food is used excessively for rewarding, pacifying or punishing the young child, the stage is set for emotional battles which often result in both immediate and more long-term feeding problems. Parents should recognize and deal with feeding problems before they become well established. Refusals of specific foods during temporary periods of negativism on the child's part are best coped with by ignoring them and waiting for a better time to introduce the food again. More generalized poor appetite may be due to many causes, and steps should be taken to eliminate those which are remediable. These causes include small size for age, or small appetite compared to other children in the family; poor appetite at a particular time of day, such as supper (especially after exhausting play and numerous snacks in the late afternoon); poor appetite due to falling ill or recovering from an illness; and wide variations in physical activity from day to day.

Persistent negativism and multiple food dislikes on the child's part indicate that parents need to re-evaluate the strategies they are using in dealing with their child's eating. Excessive coaxing, cajoling or forcing the child to eat virtually never succeed. In the long run the parent or caretaker who attempts to force a child to eat will end up with a worse problem that he began with. The emotional costs to the parent as well as to the child in such battles are enormous. In addition, they set the stage for later feeding problems. Thus if the parent has fallen into the trap of food forcing, advice should be sought from a nutritionist, psychologist or paediatrician who is skilled in dealing with and resolving feeding problems.

Bizarre food habits such as pica, rumination, hyper-phagia, or polydipsia that continue for longer than a few days may signal undetected health problems or increased health risks. These require immediate advice from a physician.

Ingestion-related poisoning accidents are common among infants and toddlers. Special care needs to be taken by the parents of children of this age to teach them to avoid harmful substances, including the 'pretty poisons' such as lemon-coloured floor wax, blue window-cleaning fluid, and the like. These are best kept out of the child's reach and sight, and hope-fully also out of his mind.

SCHOOLCHILDREN

The health of school-aged children today, as revealed in national surveys, is generally excellent. Children in poverty groups tend to be at higher risk of inadequate nutrient intakes and poor growth, but even in these groups their general status is good. Dietary deficiency diseases are rare. Vitamin or mineral supplements do not produce biochemical or functional improvements (Surgeon General's Report 1988a,b), therefore vita-min and mineral supplementation is not recommend-ed, except for high-risk children such as those from very poor families, those with poor appetites and eat-ing habits, and those who are ill (American Academy of Pediatrics 1980b). Nevertheless, many children are given such supplements by their parents, especially those from affluent families whose diets are already the most likely to be adequate (Denner 1991).

Dietary excess is more common than insufficient dietary intakes in children. Obesity is relatively common, and intakes of total fat, saturated fat, sodi-um and cholesterol are often excessive. Action to prevent obesity and to intervene by non-pharmacolog-ical means to decrease the diet-related risk of hyper-lipidaemia and hypertension in high-risk children is recommended by virtually all health authorities. However, there is still controversy about how much stress should be placed on fat- and sodium-modified diets for schoolchildren in general (American Academy of Pediatrics 1983, 1985, 1986, National Cholesterol Education Program 1991).

Causes of poor nutrition

Recent surveys of schoolchildren 8 years of age and older in the USA reveal that their cognitive knowledge of nutrition, both with respect to avoiding deficiency diseases and diet-related chronic degenerative diseases and obesity, is good. However, their food choices are not in line with this knowledge, nor with expert recommendations. Poor choices are due in part to not knowing the nutritional value of some foods, or which food choices are the most appropriate. However the relative unavailability of more appropriate choices at home, in fast-food restaurants, in schools and other institutions also is a strong determinant (Harris Scholastic Research 1989). Social pressures, adver-tising and personal preferences no doubt also play a part. These findings point to the need for more attention to be paid to promoting good nutrition by example, and by altering food availability in the physi-cal and social environments in which children live.

Parents continue to play a pivotal role in the nutrition of their children during the school years. In addition to their own efforts they should arrange for periodic monitoring of growth in weight, height and fatness, and ongoing paediatric surveillance to help ensure that the child's nutritional status and health are satisfactory (Baumgartner et al 1986). By precept and example, parents must provide guidance and instill healthy habits and attitudes to food and eating in their children. Guidelines should be set down that govern eating away from home. Parents should be open-minded and accommodating in coping with child preferences for favourite foods in planning home diets, but this does not mean that the parent must capitulate to the child's food whims, or become a short-order cook because the child refuses to eat all that is served at family meals.

Diet provided at home

Home diets should be planned to provide variety, balance and moderation in nutrient intakes. They should provide moderate amounts of energy, total fat, saturated fat, sodium and cholesterol, so that excesses and imbalances do not result. Good choices include low-fat or skimmed milk products, lean meats and skinned poultry.

In addition to menus which are reasonable from the nutritional standpoint, meal scheduling is important, so as to encourage regular eating patterns. Children with irregular meal patterns, or who skip meals, are less likely to have diets that meet recommended nutrient intakes than children with more regular patterns. Insistence on attendance at most meals, even if the child does not wish to eat, helps to establish regular patterns. Parents control the home eating environment and have some influence about what is eaten in other environments outside the home. Thus they can exert considerable influences on children's diets by stocking pantries and refrigerators with foods they want children to eat, and never buying foods they do not approve of.

Special attention needs to be paid to providing plenty of choices that fulfil the 'basic four' food groups. A basic four food guide for young children is four servings of breads and cereals, four servings of fruits and vegetables, three servings of milk and milk products, and two servings of meat, poultry, fish, eggs and beans a day. Remaining choices can come from these groups or from sweets, fats and oils, which contribute primarily calories to the diet. The use of such a food guide helps to ensure that intakes of protective nutrients, especially iron and foods rich in vitamin A and ascorbic acid, are encouraged. Family meals can be planned around such a food guide. It is more difficult to ensure that it is used to plan snacks and meals outside the home, and to control their nutritional quality. Several steps in the right direction may be helpful. Parents can pack nutritious snacks, brown-bag breakfasts, lunches and even dinners for the child to eat away from home. An alternative is to make sure that the child participates in organized school lunch or breakfast programmes. In addition, parents should let those in institutions outside the home who feed children know their views on what they regard as appropriate foods and eating times for children.

Schoolchildren themselves must take an active role on their own behalf, and learn to pay attention to nutrition throughout the day. By school ages children are old enough to keep track of what they eat at meals and snacks, and to compare their intakes to simple food guides. This sort of exercise forms the basis for helping the child plan meals and between-meal eating to emphasize fulfilling the basic four while using moderation in the fats and sweets group.

Snacking

Child snacking is inevitable, and therefore it does parents little good to worry about it, to condemn the fact that children snack, or to forbid them from eating snacks. There is no evidence that snacking is unhealthy so long as snack choices are appropriate and carry their share of vitamins and minerals as well as calories, and are without excessive amounts of saturated fat, sodium and cholesterol. Children need help in making wise snack choices. The notion that foods at meals should be healthy and nutritious but that snack foods need not be so violates the principles of moderation and balance in total intake, since for many children snacking is extremely common and meals are frequently missed. Healthy snacks include fruit, vegetables, bread and low-fat milk products, and should be readily available in the home for after-school eating, so that the child's appetite for dinner will not be blunted by overindulgence in the late afternoon. Snack foods high in energy and sticky, sugary and starchy ingredients should be de-emphasized in home pantries and left for children to buy on their own if they must have them. Family policies on sweets that limit them to once or twice a week at family meals, or to special occasions, might be considered. If sweet foods are packed as desserts in bag lunches, and provided even when the child has not specifically requested them, this is another area for cutting back. In addition to their high calories content and low contributions of other nutrients, such items also increase the risk of dental caries. When sticky, sugary snacks are eaten, children should be urged to rinse out their mouths with water and to brush their teeth afterwards to minimize this risk.

Food as a reward

Moderation on the part of parents and other adults in the use of food rewards, especially sweets, is important. Parents and other adults in the family need to review the uses to which they put foods in dealing with their children, and they themselves should moderate their own use of foods for these purposes. Expressing affection and rewarding good behaviour on the part of the child by verbal praise and non-food treats are preferable to constant rewards with candy or sweets. Others, such as grandparents, should be encouraged to use non-food rewards as well.

Meal planning

It is important for children to eat breakfast because this provides a good portion of total intakes of ascorbic acid and other nutrients, which are often lower than recommended levels in children's diets. Without breakfast children may find it difficult to pay attention to morning tasks in school. Mornings are hurried and often hectic in families with young children. Waking the child early enough so that there is time for him to eat something, putting out quick-to-prepare breakfast foods the night before so that family members can make their own breakfasts, packing breakfasts to eat as they travel, and the use of non-traditional foods, may encourage breakfast eating.

A decade ago, over 50% of commercials on programmes directed toward children were for food products and the situation has not improved much since then. Half or more of these are for sugary foods, snacks and fast foods, whereas advertisements for fruit, vegetables and the like were few in number (Council on Children, Media and Merchandising 1977). Many different advertising strategies are employed to encourage children to buy and eat these branded products. They include the use of superheroes who eat the food in commercials; clever commercials in which adventures, fantasies and humour dramatize the importance of the product; the use of cartoons, music, singing and jingles incorporating the product name; endorsements by celebrities; magical promises about the good effects of eating food; appeals to the child's self esteem; and tie-in promotions for popular toys (Langbourne Rust Research 1986). Parents can help children be good consumers by resisting the pressures of advertising themselves and not buying foods they do not wish their children to eat.

Parents especially need to alter their family food-buying practices if a review of their diet reveals that family consumption is excessive in costly high-calorie, sweet-starchy-sugary items, which are low in protective nutrients. Parents should make sure their children understand what is undesirable in these foods, and why it is that consumption needs to be altered. They should use judgment in acceding to children's requests for specific brands of food, especially if they are expensive or undesirable from the parent's standpoint.

Obesity in schoolchildren

Obesity is all too common in schoolchildren, and reflects the interaction of genetic predisposition and permissive environments (Rosenbaum & Leibel 1989). In spite of continuing emphasis on prevention and treatment, the prevalence of child and adolescent obesity may be increasing (Gortmaker et al 1987,

Shear et al 1988), but this is still disputed. However, increases do seem to be apparent among the massively obese and among some minority groups, such as blacks (Harlan et al 1988). In part this is because of increasingly sedentary lifestyles, which for many children include excessive amounts of television viewing and other sedentary activities (Dietz & Gortmaker 1985, Tucker 1986). The root causes of childhood obesity are rarely endocrine. Low energy outputs relative to needs are more frequently involved than high energy intakes.

Obesity has adverse effects on child development, even in the school years. Obesity stimulates and reinforces patterns of physical inactivity, intensifies family tensions, and contributes to the development of a negative and distorted body image and sense of individual worth in the obese child. Children who are consistently obese throughout primary school are at higher risk of obesity in later life, although correlations are not high (Johnston 1985). Obesity continued into adult life has very negative effects upon social mobility and physical and mental health. Therefore, even if obesity cannot be eliminated, efforts to reduce its severity and progression are desirable. The focus should not be solely medical. It is also necessary to address psychosocial factors, to foster more tolerance of diversity in bodily appearance, emphasize prevention by manipulation of the food environment, to educate parents and children about food and physical activity, and to prevent the development of unhealthy relationships between parents and children which revolve around food. It is important to address such issues as the use of food for emotional purposes such as rewards, punishments, pacification and affection, and the use of food for conveying other emotional messages to the exclusion of other channels of communication. Non-food-oriented forms of emotional release must be found, and distorted communications between children and parents re-established (Peck & Ulrich 1988).

In preventing and treating obesity in children the goal is fat loss, not necessarily weight loss. By very modest alterations in energy inputs and increased emphasis on physical activity the child is permitted to grow up into his fatness. Weight-reduction diets, particularly when they are rigid and below 1000 calories, are unwarranted except in medical emergencies, as linear growth and lean body mass growth may be retarded (see Chapter 32). All schoolchildren need social and physical environments that promote moderation in eating, and vigorous physical activity. These are conducive to maintaining normal body fatness and cardiovascular fitness. Recent surveys of

American children show that at present many are unfit. Healthy family attitudes and practices, including regular and vigorous physical activity several times a week, can do much. Parents and others in the family should act as positive role models for schoolchildren by practising moderation in their own food intakes, adopting physically active lives themselves, and maintaining their own body weights at normal levels. They can also plan their children's lives to ensure that the child engages in vigorous physical activity on a year-round basis.

ADOLESCENCE

The pubertal growth spurt that heralds adolescence is the period of most rapid growth after infancy that the human being experiences. Growth charts for height and height velocity for following an individual child's growth through adolescence are now available (Tanner & Davies 1985). These are helpful in problem cases to judge whether or not a child's growth is abnormal.

Nutritional needs during adolescence

Adolescents have unique nutritional needs from the biological, psychological and social points of view. Biologically speaking, adolescents' nutrient needs are similar in the types of nutrients they need, but they need larger amounts of protective nutrients such as protein, vitamins and minerals per unit of energy consumed, than prepubertal children and adults. Energy needs are only slightly increased, whereas the needs for other nutrients imposed by growth and sexual maturation are much increased over younger individuals (see Appendix 2). By late adolescence, nutrient needs approach those of adults. Adolescents need diets that are high in nutritional quality. The growth spurt itself requires energy and nutrients as structural materials. Once laid down, the large size and altered body composition resulting from pubertal and later growth must be maintained. Changes in physiological function after sexual maturity also alter nutrient needs, such as the requirement for iron after the menarche, which increases due to menstrual losses (see Chapter 12). Changes in lifestyle, especially in physical activity, affect energy needs. Finally, in some adolescents, diseases are present that alter nutrient needs because of the changes they induce in absorption, nutrient metabolism or excretion.

Physical growth during adolescence consists of pubescence, during which linear growth is rapid, and a later and slower period of growth after the menarche or adrenarche is reached (Tanner 1962). Nutrient needs correlate rather poorly with chronological or calendar age during adolescence, and are more closely linked to biological or maturational age as determined from bone age or sexual maturity ratings. However, because of the difficulty in determining biological age, recommendations for nutrient needs are currently given by sex on a chronological age basis in the Recommended Dietary Allowances (see Appendix 2). The margins of safety in these recommendations are sufficiently large to be satisfactory for most purposes. For very early or very late maturers special attention to their individual problems is necessary in the application of the recommended dietary allowances. Sexual maturity ratings or other clinical indices of sexual maturation are helpful in assessing biological age, and in making appropriate recommendations on a clinical basis. From the quantitative standpoint, adolescent nutrient needs differ by sex, and change with growth during adolescence. These differences also depend on individual variability in the timing of adolescent growth (Slap 1987). Females reach their full height about 2 years before males. Although adult men are an average of 6 in (15 cm) taller, and over 30 lbs (15 kg) heavier than women, for a brief period during puberty girls are often larger than boys (Tanner 1962).

From their own particular psychological and sociological perspectives, adolescents believe that they have unique nutritional needs. Most adolescents are not primarily concerned with health in making their eating decisions. As with adults, hedonistic, social, environmental and other factors are stronger influences. Nevertheless, they are both concerned and aware of the importance of eating a balanced diet, avoiding cholesterol and salt, avoiding excess snacks, having a regular meal pattern, and more general issues such as getting enough exercise, maintaining the right weight for health, and dental health (Yankelovich et al 1979).

State of health and nutrition among adolescents

Since the turn of the century, the decline in poverty and disease-related forms of malnutrition among adolescents in western countries has been profound. Adolescents who live in poverty, or have other social or health disadvantages, are more likely to be malnourished than their affluent counterparts, but the prevalence and severity of such problems is less. Those at high risk include ethnic or racial minorities, especially if they are also poor and have chronic illnesses or other special developmental and health needs. Much progress has been made in improving adolescent nutrition and health. The dietary deficiency diseases, which were rampant in the entire population in the early 1900s, are now rare. Undernutrition due to lack of money or environmental access to food is also rare. Inadequate intakes, when they do occur, are more likely to be due to intentional dieting of various types, or to occur secondarily to other pathophysiological and social problems. However, inappropriate food choices due to lack of access, lack of knowledge, habit, or cultural and other influences, is common. In contrast to the progress made in dealing with dietary deficiency disorders and undernutrition, adolescent food habits leading to overnutrition and imbalances are more common, and are increasing in all social classes and ages (Surgeon General's Report 1988, Committee on Diet and Health 1989). Excessive intake of total and saturated fat, cholesterol, sodium and energy is common by mid to late childhood and early adolescence, and can occur as early as the preschool and school years. Excessive energy intakes coupled with low energy outputs give rise to adolescent obesity. Also, toxicity due to alcohol abuse or acute intoxication affects teenagers at younger ages. It is reaching epidemic proportions in some subgroups of the population, such as among native Americans and other poor minority group adolescents. Outcomes are particularly poor when alcohol abuse is coupled with drug abuse.

Body weight issues

Years ago it was popular to distinguish between the poor, who were expected to be those who suffered solely from problems of dietary inadequacy, and more affluent groups, whose problems were assumed to consist primarily of disorders associated with dietary excess. Such distinctions are no longer valid. In certain subgroups of adolescents, such as teenage girls, emaciation due to anorexia nervosa is more common among the more affluent, and obesity is more common among the poor. Poor adolescents are at greater risk for both poverty-related malnutrition and the forms of overnutrition common in an affluent society. Co-morbidities which combine both under - and overnutrition, such as iron-deficiency anaemia and obesity, may exist in a single person. Adolescents themselves, parents, and others who deal with adolescents, all need anticipatory guidance to enhance the nutrition and fitness status of teenagers. Adolescents need assistance in monitoring their own growth on charts which plot height and weight. They also need

to understand why nutrient needs change with growth, and how body composition and nutrient needs change during adolescence.

In order to adopt and maintain healthy dietary habits during adolescence, needs for energy and protective nutrients such as protein, vitamins and minerals, must be met. An environmental context that permits adolescents to find ways to eat which fulfil their own individual needs, philosophies and wants without doing violence to their nutritional status, should be established. Eating habits which are not conducive to good nutrition should be identified and altered. These include excessive intakes of high-calorie low nutrient-density foods, high-fat foods, highly irregular food habits with totally unplanned intakes, and alcohol abuse. Many adolescents need help in maintaining their weight at appropriate levels for their growth status, and in altering weight either upwards or downwards to achieve a healthier nutritional status. If weight problems are complained about, their presence must be objectively determined before treatment begins. Adolescents themselves, especially girls, often have extremely unrealistic views of what they look like and how they can change their body shapes by gaining or losing weight. Often there is no health reason for doing so.

Obese adolescents need help to reduce their fatness. Physical activity is to be encouraged in all adolescents. It helps to prevent obesity, helps the already obese to lose weight, and also has its own intrinsic health benefits. Vigorous aerobic physical activity for at least 20 min at 60% or more of maximal aerobic capacity is especially important among obese adolescents, since their problems with fatness are usually associated with low energy outputs rather than with dramatically elevated intakes. Moderation in dietary habits should be encouraged, rather than periods of strict dieting alternating with binges and dietary excess. In practice this means that reductions in caloric intakes by perhaps 50, or not more than 100, calories are in order, with very much increased energy outputs until linear growth has ceased. Decreasing fatness by dietary means during puberty must not stunt growth. Unless obesity is very pronounced, dietary treatment is often best delayed until physical maturity is reached. The goal of dietary treatment is not weight loss, but fat loss and the growth of lean tissue. In most cases a programme that includes social and psychological support of the obese adolescent, modest caloric reductions, and a vigorous physical activity programme that expends energy, favours the development of muscles and bones, and includes a social component is most likely to be successful. Obese adolescents also need help in recognizing and avoiding ineffective reducing diets, and the perils of fasting and self-induced vomiting to achieve weight control.

Very lean adolescents need help in assessing their weight status and reaching more healthy weights. Scrawny late maturers, especially boys, have only transient problems which are easily remedied by time. Adolescents on therapeutic diets for chronic disease which have not been adjusted to cope with the increased needs of puberty may be excessively lean. Other adolescents suffering from chronic diseases may fail to adhere to therapeutic diets because of the psychological or social constraints they impose. Chronic drug and alcohol abuse, untreated mental illness and intentional dieting for quasi philosophical or religious reasons may also be associated with emaciation on some occasions. Other excessively lean teenagers who may need special help include teenagers suffering from anorexia nervosa – a form of self-induced starvation due to psychiatric causes (see Chapter 49) – teenagers who have become fanatical about a vigorous sport such as swimming or running, and who have lost large amounts of weight, and some pregnant and lactating teenagers.

Adolescent pregnancy

Adolescent pregnancy and lactation further increase the need for many nutrients over the already considerable increases that occur in the second decade of life in all human beings. Thus pregnant adolescents may need special help in meeting their nutrient needs while increasing both the quality of their diets and satisfying their food preferences. Some adolescents, such as the chronically ill, may need help in planning their intakes to include therapeutic considerations. Others who are at high risk although they are not yet ill, such as adolescents who are hyperlipidaemic or who are overweight and hypertensive, also need special assistance in formulating realistic and healthy food plans for themselves.

Fitness

The development of a healthy body includes, but is not limited to, nutritional wellbeing. Aerobic fitness, muscle strength, flexibility and adequate fatness are also important. Adolescents need help in assessing their own lifestyles and fitness levels in all these respects. They need to become aware of the immediate benefits of physical fitness. These include fun, new ways to combat boredom, social networking through a group, exercise, stress or tension relief, and a positive mental attitude. Over the longer terms the benefits include better physical appearance, increased self confidence, better tolerance of physical exertion, and possibly better control of weight.

In order to become more fit, the first step teenagers can take themselves is to recognize and overcome problems and fears which often pose as barriers to physical activity. These include lack of time, fear of soreness or overheating and, among girls, concerns that exercise will make them unfeminine and cause ravenous appetites, which in turn will lead to excessive weight gain. At the same time overemphasis on achieving the cosmetic aspects of fitness using 'short cuts' such as fasting, self-induced vomiting, anabolic steroids and the like, must be discouraged. Differences between fitness and leanness may also need to be clarified.

The easiest way to improve fitness is for adolescents to increase their daily physical activities, as well as exercise training. Any activity involved in moving the body qualifies, especially every day activities such as walking, lifting objects, climbing stairs and the like, since the total time spent in these is considerably more than that spent in vigorous exercise. Thus they too can lead to considerable energy outputs, even though outputs per minute are lower than they are for the most vigorous exercise. It is also important that adolescents develop lifelong aerobic exercise patterns that foster cardiovascular fitness, and which can continue throughout life, such as bicycling, walking, jogging, soccer and tennis. The key is to make sure that adolescents themselves are involved in choosing the types of physical activity and exercise which best meet their needs, and that they consider and optimize the costs, opportunity, time and locations available for performing those activities.

Teenage athletes

Good nutrition for optimal fitness also needs attention. The energy needs of teenage athletes are increased, often greatly, if very heavy training and competitive sports are involved (see Chapter 28).

Teenage athletes are often the targets for those marketing questionable nutritive substances which are often suggested for use as ergogenic aids to increase performance. Some of the many unproven substances include galatic, carnitine, wheatgerm oil, bee pollen, honey, vitamin 'B_{15}' (calcium pangamate, which is not a vitamin for human beings), phosphorus, lecithin, aspartate, amino acid supplements, branched-chain amino acids, ginseng, inosine, lipotropic factors and succinate. None of these products boosts performance. Adolescent athletes and their coaches need to be aware of the fact that the use of these substances is a form of economic exploitation. More dangerous are drugs used as ergogenic aids. The growing use of anabolic steroids among adolescents to increase lean body mass and to improve muscular strength is alarming. The practice is banned by both the US and International Olympic Committees. It is extremely dangerous from the health standpoint. Among other ill effects it may impair normal sexual function, and may stunt growth if it is used before maturity is attained.

In summary, the importance of good nutrition in childhood and adolescence in determining later health is becoming increasingly apparent. Examples include alterations in risk factors for coronary artery disease associated with dietary fat and cholesterol intakes in early life and, more recently, the importance of achieving high peak bone mass on later risk for osteoporosis. Therefore adolescent nutrition deserves attention.

AGEING

As the human organism ages qualitative needs for all the essential nutrients remain, but quantitative changes do occur in some instances – most notably energy. The energy intakes of the elderly are usually less than earlier in life, thus the nutrient density of needs rises. Foods with high nutrient density and low in fat, such as lean meat, fish, eggs, low-fat milk, and vegetables or fruits are helpful in that they provide the protein, vitamins and minerals the ageing need with relatively few calories.

Diet-related diseases and other conditions afflict many of the aged. Many of the elderly require therapeutic diets (US Senate 1987–88, Gaffney & Singer 1985). Approximately three million elderly Americans have difficulties in undertaking the purchase, preparation and cooking of food (Posner & Krachenfels 1987). In addition, the elderly's eating difficulties mean that alterations in food constituents, the physical form of food or manner of feeding may also be called for.

The overriding goals for nutrition among individuals over 65 years of age are improved quality of life and the promotion of continued autonomy, not simply cost containment. Good nutritional status is essential for a high quality of life, since food contributes to the quality of life through psychological, social and physical mechanisms (Surgeon General's Workshop on Aging 1988a,b). To implement these goals among the aged, several assumptions must be kept in mind.

First, in terms of functional capacity, physical conditions, social, economic and lifestyle situations, the elderly population is more heterogeneous than any other age group. Secondly, the research base for making nutritional recommendations for older adults is evolving. Therefore, specific recommendations must be periodically updated. Finally, there is the issue of finding ways not only to lessen the ageing process but to lessen the consequences of disease. Diseases that are identical from the medical standpoint have very different consequences with respect to day-to-day function, and on such components of it as work performance, feelings of wellbeing and quality of life. That is, the impairments, disabilities and handicaps arising from even the same disease with respect to their impacts on the activities of daily living, including but not limited to, eating, are quite disparate. In the next few years increasing attention needs to be paid to examining nutritional problems of the elderly in this context.

Nutritional requirements

In the latest (1989) Recommended Dietary Allowances, recommended intakes for most nutrients other than energy for individuals 55 years and older are not broken down separately by decade, since data upon which to permit such discriminations are lacking (see Appendix 2). As more experimental evidence becomes available more specific recommendations may be possible. Current knowledge on how requirements for vitamins and mineral change with age are available (Suter & Russell 1987). In general energy needs decrease with age, owing to decreases in physical activity and in resting energy expenditure. The major reason for this is that, after retirement, physical activity related to work usually declines, as do optional household tasks. Also, lean body mass, which is the metabolically active tissue of the body, decreases by about 3 kg per decade after age 50. It is likely that these declines in lean body mass are not totally inevitable, but rather that they reflect the more sedentary lifestyle of older people. To a lesser extent, they may also signal the presence of disease (Parizkova 1989, Powell et al 1989, Ravussin & Bogardus 1989). Cellular metabolic rates also decrease with ageing, but these declines are much smaller than physical activity decrements. Currently it is assumed that energy allowances should decrease by about 6% between 51 and 75 years of age, and by another 6% after age 76, about two-thirds of the decrease being due to decreased physical activity, and one-third to decreases in resting metabolism (McGandy et al 1966).

Little direct information on the protein needs of ageing adults is available. The current Recommended Dietary Allowance of 0.8 kg/day of high-quality protein is reasonable. However, some researchers think that older adults may require more protein than do younger adults (Young 1990).

There are only a few other quantifiable changes in nutritional requirements in old age. For the nutrients involved in energy metabolism (thiamin, riboflavin and niacin), requirements are lower than those of young adults, whereas calcium needs may be higher in oestrogen-deprived postmenopausal women (Recker & Heaney 1989). Iron requirements are reduced, due to a gradual accumulation of iron stores throughout life and cessation of blood loss in postmenopausal women. Dietary inadequacy of iron is therefore rare in the elderly, and other factors such as blood loss, drug therapy or disease are the principal causes of iron deficiency in this age group. Vitamin D nutrition may be impaired in old age due to a combination of factors: low intakes, inadequate sunlight exposure, reduced vitamin D synthesis in ageing skin, and impaired hydroxylation of 26-OH vitamin D by the kidney (Suter & Russell 1989). For institutionalized or housebound elderly, vitamin D status can best be improved through low-level vitamin D supplementation (10 mg/day), especially during the winter months, and increased sunlight whenever possible.

With respect to meeting their nutrient needs, food guides stressing the basic four are helpful to ensure that needs for protective nutrients are met. The recent recommendations of the Committee on Diet and Health (1989) are designed for adults of all ages, including the elderly, and stress the avoidance of excess and imbalances, as well as achieving sufficiency.

There is increasing evidence that the marked declines in physical activity which are observed among the elderly today are undesirable. Reasonable, individually tailored physical activity and exercise programmes are in order, but these should only be attempted after consultation with a physician.

Healthy weights for the elderly

Desirable weights for the elderly are currently a matter of considerable debate. Overweight tends to peak in men at ages 35–64, but rates for women continue to rise throughout the ages in which they are measured, at least to age 65 years. There is also a slight lifetime loss in stature, probably about 3 cm in men and 5 cm in women (McDowell et al 1981,

National Center for Health Statistics 1987). Weight for height reference standards based on desirable weights for lowest mortality are derived from insured people aged 25–59 years. Their younger age, and the fact that weight for height relationships may be different, call into question the use of these standards among the elderly (Russell & McGandy 1984). Normative standards, such as the HANES surveys, do include data on people up to age 75. However, normative standards also have disadvantages, since such data simply report the weights and heights of those who are elderly, and they are based on what is rather than on an actuarial standard of lowest mortality, or some other index showing that at these weights function is improved. As part of the work of the National Institutes on Agings's longitudinal study, Andres summarized data from several studies which argued that minimal mortality did not occur in the leanest segments of the population, as was commonly averred, but in individuals who are somewhat plumper (Andres 1980a, 1981, Andres et al 1985). Also, data from the longitudinal ageing study indicated that mild or moderate overweight among the elderly was not a potent risk factor, even after correcting for smoking (Andres 1980b). However, the longitudinal data in the series Andres studied were small and were not drawn from a population-based sample, the number of subjects in the study was small, and other confounding variables may have accounted for the effects observed. Also, other studies suggest that in fact the very old have mean weights which are close to or even lower than desirable (Russell & Sahyoun 1988). Therefore, until better data are available the NCHS data should be used (National Center for Health Statistics 1987), as suggested by Frisancho (1984). Actual measurements are divided by the NCHS reference standard and the quotient multiplied by 100 to get the percentage of the standard. The recommended reference standards for body mass index are the HANES II 50th centile for age groups 55–64 and 65–74 years (National Center for Health Statistics 1987).

Weight should be maintained at desirable levels. The optimal weights from the standpoint of morbidity and improved functional status appear to be in the range of the adjusted values presented by Frisancho (1984) using HANES data. It is well known that height decreases with age, and when it is impossible to obtain weights for height since height cannot be measured, segmental measurements, such as lengths from ankle to knee, can be made, and these related to overall height. Tables are available for making these conversions.

Goals for macronutrient intake

There is no recommended allowance for carbohydrate, apart from ensuring that intakes are at least 100 g/day to avoid ketosis. The dietary guidelines for Americans suggest that among most Americans intakes of complex carbohydrates and fibre should increase, and those of simple sugars should decrease. Fibre intakes in the range of 25–30 g/day from naturally occurring sources should permit normal laxation with recourse to medication. Increases in fibre intake should be gradual, to avoid discomfort and to ensure that tolerance is satisfactory, particularly among the ageing, who sometimes have used laxatives for many years.

Sugary starchy mixtures provide the food for cariogenic bacteria, to produce acid and caries of the tooth root as well as the crown. Root caries is the type of caries likely to afflict the elderly, as gums recede from remaining teeth and the roots of the tooth are exposed. Crown caries may also occur on the remaining teeth. Therefore, avoidance of a diet – especially between meals – which is high in fermentable carbohydrates, and the importance of good oral hygiene, should be stressed. Maintenance of ideal weight and modest reductions in sugar in the diet are suggested for individuals suffering from diabetes mellitus, especially of the type II (non-insulin-dependent) variety. Also among most diabetics, increased calories from carbohydrates are called for, and decreased proportions of calories from fat, since diabetics of all types are at high risk for artherosclerosis. For recommendations for fat intake to reduce the risk of heart disease, see Chapter 41 and Appendix 2.

The rationale for the recommendation is that the type and amount of dietary fat and cholesterol are risk factors for elevated serum cholesterol, at least among middle-aged persons. There is reason to suspect that they may also be so among older individuals, especially since most of the age-related rise in serum cholesterol is in low-density lipoprotein (LDL) cholesterol, levels of which can be modified by such dietary alterations. Although it is important to emphasize moderation with respect to fat and cholesterol consumption, it is vital to set these and other dietary recommendations in the context of overall risk reduction. For example, it makes little sense for the elderly to strictly control their diets while they continue to smoke cigarettes and fail to take their antihypertensive medications, two health behaviours which are likely to have very great and well documented impacts on arteriosclerotic as well as cardiovascular disease, even among the elderly.

Attention to some simple precepts can help the elderly person maintain or enhance nutritional status with advancing age. More societal attention to the nutritional and health needs of our elderly citizens can make further improvements (Surgeon General's Workshop on Aging 1988a,b).

First, it is important that the economic wherewithal be present for the elderly person to buy a nutritious diet. Most of the elderly are on fixed incomes. When they are faced with meagre resources, housing and other fixed expenses are often coped with first, and food budgets must shrink to absorb increases in these other items. Food stamps, community meals for the poor, and other government-sponsored programmes in food, nutrition and health can ease the burden for those with incomes below the poverty line.

Fluids and alcohol

The water content of the body decreases with age and urine-concentrating capacity often decreases, so that more water is needed to excrete smaller quantities of wastes. It is thus important that fluid needs are liberally met by the elderly.

Special caution is warranted in the use of alcohol among the aged. Some of the medications they take, such as the barbiturates (see Chapter 50), interact adversely with alcohol. Also, because of the lower body water of the ageing individual, the same amount of alcohol leads to far greater blood alcohol levels in older than younger individuals from the same amount of alcohol. Therefore, moderation is warranted for all, and for some, such as those on medications, those who are severely depressed, or those who have a history of alcohol abuse, alcohol should be eschewed entirely.

Factors influencing nutrition

Drug–drug and drug–nutrient interactions need to be discovered and measures taken to avoid or minimize them. Since the elderly are often on several medications, this is a frequent problem (see Chapter 50).

Ensuring that the home, or other environments in which the elderly live, are safe is another priority. Kitchens, pantries and dining rooms should be checked to make sure that high cupboards, narrow stairs, unlit food storage areas or the like do not increase the likelihood of accidents. For the absent-minded, automatic shutoffs on water taps and stoves may be considered, or the addition of microwave ovens and cookers which have built-in timers and are suitable for cooking for one or two people.

Swallowing is sometimes made more difficult by stroke, other illnesses, or the effects of medication, and choking accidents also need to be guarded against. Both the elderly person and those who care for them or live with them should learn the Heimlich manoeuvre to dislodge food or other particles which may stick in the throat.

It is easier to prevent infectious diseases such as pneumonia or influenza than it is to attempt to revitalize an elderly person who has lost large amounts of weight and strength from its ravages. Therefore all elderly people should be vaccinated against these diseases.

Supplement use

The elderly should be advised to use vitamins and mineral supplements in moderation. A multivitamin–multimineral supplement in levels which do not exceed the recommended dietary allowances (Committee on Dietary Allowance 1980) will do little harm. However, amounts 10–100 times these levels may have undesirable pharmacological effects on health. Also, self-treatment may cause the older person to wait too long before seeking health care for problems which have no nutritional cause or remedy, but which need immediate attention.

CONCLUSION

Childhood, youth and old age are all periods during the lifecycle when physiological needs for nutrients, the psychological aspects of food, and health need special attention.

REFERENCES

American Academy of Pediatrics, Committee on Nutrition 1980a The feeding of supplemental foods to infants. Pediatrics 65:1178–1181

American Academy of Pediatrics, Committee on Nutrition 1980b Vitamin and mineral supplement needs in normal children in the United States. Pediatrics 66:1015–1021

American Academy of Pediatrics, Committee on Nutrition 1983 Toward a prudent diet for children. Pedriatics 71:78–80

American Academy of Pediatrics, Committee on Nutrition 1985 Pediatric nutrition handbook, 2nd edn. American Academy of Pediatrics, Elk Grove Village, IL

American Academy of Pediatrics, Committee on Nutrition 1986 Prudent life style for children: dietary fat and cholesterol. Pediatrics 78:521–525

Andres R 1980a Effect of obesity on total mortality. International Journal of Obesity 4:381–386

Andres R 1980b Influence of obesity on longevity in the aged. In: Borek C, Frengolio CM, King DW (eds) Aging, cancer and cell membranes. Thieme-Stratton, New York

Andres R 1981 Aging, diabetes, and obesity: standards of normality. Mount Sinai Journal of Medicine 48:489–495

Andres R, Elahi D, Tobin JD, Muller DC, Brant L 1985 Impact of age on weight goals. Annals of Internal Medicine 103:1030–1033

Baumgartner RN, Roche AF, Himes JH 1986 Incremental growth tables: supplementary to previously published charts. American Journal of Clinical Nutrition 43:711–722

Committee on Dietary Allowances 1980 Food and Nutrition Board recommended dietary allowances, 9th edn. National Academy of Sciences, Washington, DC

Committee on Diet and Health 1989 Diet and health – implications for reducing chronic disease risk. National Research Council. National Academy Press, Berkeley, CA

Committee on Medical Aspects of Food Policy 1991 Dietary reference values for food energy and nutrients in the United Kingdom. Department of Health Report 41. HMSO, London

Council on Children, Media and Merchandising 1977 Edible TV: your child and food commercials. Prepared for the Select Committee on Human Needs. US Senate, Washington DC

Denner WHB 1991 Dietary supplements and health foods: report of the working group. Ministry of Agriculture, Fisheries and Food, London

Dietz WH, Gortmaker SL 1985 Do we fatten our children at the TV set? Obesity and television viewing in children and adolescents. Pediatrics 75:807–812

Frisancho AB 1984 New standards of weight and body composition by frame size and height for assessment of nutritional status of adults and the elderly. American Journal of Clinical Nutrition 40:808–819

Gaffney JT, Singer GR 1985 Diet needs of patients referred to home health. Journal of the American Dietetic Association 85:198–202

Gortmaker SL, Dietz WH, Sobol AM, Wehler CA 1987 Increasing pediatric obesity in the US. American Journal for Diseases of Children 141:535–540

Harris Scholastic Research 1989 The Kellogg Children's Nutrition Survey. Louis Harris and Associates Inc., New York

Harlan WR, Landes JR, Flegal KM, Davis CS, Miller ME 1988 Secular trends in body mass in the US 1960–180. American Journal of Epidemiology 128:1065–1074

Johnston FE 1985 Health implications of childhood obesity. Annals of Internal Medicine 103:1068–1072

Langbourne Rust Research 1986 Children's advertising: how it works, how to do it, how to know if it works. Journal of Advertising Research 26:15

McDowell A, Engel A, Massey JT, Mauer K 1981 Plan and operation of the second national health and nutrition examination survey 1976–1980. Vital and health statistics series 1, no 15, DHHS Publication no (PHS) 81–1317. US Department of Health and Human Services, Washington, DC

McGandy RB, Barrows CH, Spanias A, Meredith A, Stone JL, Norris AH 1966 Nutrient intakes and energy expenditure in men of different ages. Journal of Gerontology 21:581–587

National Centre for Health Statistics 1987 Anthropometric reference data and prevalence of overweight, United States 1976–1980. National Health Survey Series 11, no. 128 DHSS Publication No (PHS) 87-1688. National Center for Health Statistics, Hyattsville, MD

National Cholesterol Education Program 1991 Report of the Expert Panel on Blood Cholesterol Levels in Children and Adolescents. US Department of Health and Human Services, Public Health Services, National Institutes of Health

Parizkova J 1989 Age-dependent changes in dietary intakes related to work output, physical fitness and body composition. American Journal of Clinical Nutrition 49:962–967

Peck EB, Ulrich HD (eds) Ad Hoc Interdisciplinary Committee on Children and Weight 1988 Children and weight: a changing perspective. Nutrition Communications Associates, Berkeley, CA

Posner BM, Krachenfels MM 1987 Nutrition services in the continuum of health care. Clinics in Geriatric Medicine 3:261–275

Powell KE, Caspersen CJ, Koplan JP, Ford ES 1989 Physical activity and chronic disease. American Journal of Clinical Nutrition 49:999–1006

Ravussin E, Bogardus C 1989 Relationship of genetics, age and physical fitness to daily energy expenditure and fuel utilization. American Journal of Clinical Nutrition 49:968–975

Recker RR, Heaney RP 1989 Calcium nutrition and its relationship to bone health. In: Munro HN, Danford DE (eds) Human nutrition: a comprehensive treatise, Volume 6: Nutrition, aging and the elderly. Plenum Press, New York, pp. 245–291

Rosenbaum M, Liebel RL 1989 Obesity in childhood. Pediatrics in Review 11:43–55

Rush D 1985 The National WIC Evaluation Office of Analysis and Evaluation, Food and Nutrition Service. US Department of Agriculture, Washington DC

Russell RM 1983 Evaluating the nutritional status of the elderly. Clinical Nutrition 2:4–8

Russell RM, McGandy RB 1984 Reference weights: practical considerations. American Journal of Medicine 76:767–769

Russell RM, Sahyoun NR 1988 The elderly. In: Paige D (ed) Clinical nutrition, 2nd edn. C.V. Mosby, St. Louis, pp. 110–119

Shear CL, Freedman DS, Burke GL, Harsha DW, Webber LS, Berenson GS 1988 Secular trends of obesity in early life: the Bogalusa Heart Study. American Journal of Public Health 78:75–77

Slap GB 1987 Normal psychological and psychosocial growth in the adolescent. Journal of Adolescent Health Care 7 (Suppl):135–235

Surgeon General of the United States, US Department of Health and Human Services 1988a The Surgeon General's Report on Nutrition and Health. US Government Printing Office, Washington, DC, pp. 595–628

Surgeon General of the United States, US Department of Health and Human Services 1988b The Surgeon General's Report on Nutrition and Health. US Government Printing Office, Washington, DC, pp. 539–594

Surgeon General's Workshop on Aging 1988, Surgeon General's Workshop: Health promotion and Aging. US Department of Health and Human Services, Public Health Service, Washington, DC

Suter P, Russell RM 1987 Vitamin requirements of the elderly. American Journal of Clinical Nutrition 45:501–512

Suter PM, Rusell RM 1989 Vitamin nutriture and requirements in the elderly. In Munro HN, Danford DE (eds) Human nutrition. A comprehensive treatise, Volume 6: Nutrition, aging and the elderly. Plenum Press, New York, pp. 245–292

Tanner JM 1962 Growth at adolescence, 2nd edn. Blackwell Scientific Publications, Oxford

Tanner JM, Davies PSW 1985 Clinical longitudinal standards for height and weight velocity for North American children. Journal of Pediatrics 107:317–329

Tucker LA 1986 The relationship of television viewing to physical fitness and obesity. Adolescence 21:797–806

US Senate 1987–1988 US Senate Special Committee on Aging: 1988 Aging America: trends and projections LR 3377 (188) D 12198. US Department of Health and Human Services, Washington, DC

Yankelovich, Skelly and White Inc. 1979 Family health in an era of stress: General Mills American family report 1978–1979. General Mills, Minneapolis, MN

Young VR 1990 Protein and amino acid metabolism with reference to aging and the elderly. In: Prinsley DM, Sandstead HH (eds) Progress in clinical and biological research, Volume 326: Nutrition and aging. Alan R Liss, New York, pp. 279–300

28. Exercise, sport and athletics

D. S. Tunstall Pedoe

Sporting competition has attracted nutritional rituals for centuries. The primitive and understandable belief that 'You are what you eat' and that certain constituents of the diet can confer exceptional virtues or abilities is illustrated by the Zulus who reputedly increased their valour by cutting out and eating the hearts of their prisoners. Ancient gladiators and classic Olympic competitors ate bulls' testicles for strength (the first use of anabolic steroids).

Success and failure in modern sport can be separated by millimetres or 100ths of a second. Performance differences of fractions of 1% may separate fame and fortune from anonymity. These small differences are often attributed to a champion's diet, especially if this contains anything exotic. Lasse Viren, Finnish Olympic champion at 5000 and 10 000 m in both 1972 and 1976, claimed his achievement was based on a diet which included reindeer milk. Sceptics suggested it was due to blood doping – the infusion of extra blood a few days before competition.

Modern athletes may have their dining tables covered with nutritional supplements. A quick browse through any sport and body-building magazines reveals a plethora of advertisements for a multitude of vitamin, protein, carbohydrate, amino acid and mineral formulations, all designed to cater for what appears to be the special needs of athletes who want to have the 'edge' over the competition. Also advertised are total dietary packages catering specifically for the 'special needs' of the athlete and including all the daily requirements of certain nutrients.

Computerized assessment of energy expenditure during football has been used to produce precisely calculated diets for individual players. Dr Roy Shephard (Toronto) has suggested (in public discussion) that as this method has an accuracy of perhaps 20% in calculating energy expenditure, and as there is only 20% accuracy in following a feeding formula, the average athlete would be some 10 or 20

times more accurate in the long term by relying on their body mechanisms and appetite than with such a 'high tech' system.

Does exercise create special nutritional requirements? Has millions of years' evolution of the human body developed metabolic pathways that make it uniquely sensitive to performance-enhancing aids such as Ginseng, trace elements or amino acid supplementation?

Before dismissing such supplements as being expensive forms of placebo for gullible athletes and their advisors, it is necessary to examine the background against which such claims have to be judged, and to appreciate that many athletes suffer from failures of performance and 'overtraining states', which may have a variety of causes, of which dietary factors may be the easiest to remedy.

NUTRITIONAL EFFECTS OF MODERN TRAINING SCHEDULES

The modern athlete is very much a victim of the hard work approach to training, which developed in the 1960s and 1970s. It appeared then that he who trained hardest and longest triumphed, resulting in training schedules for many athletes consisting of several hours per day of severe exertion. These training loads can only be achieved if they are split into two or more sessions per day, each lasting as long as 2 h. Since exercise should only be taken more than 1–2 h after meals, just fitting in the meals between the training sessions can be a major problem, so meals are often skipped. If the athlete is an 'amateur' and has to support himself financially by other means, or is a student with inflexible meal times, arranging the training and adequate meals can be very difficult and expensive.

Training itself may produce several other problems. Severe exertion burns up a large amount of carbohydrate, depleting muscle glycogen stores. Running or jogging a mile is estimated to expend 100 kcal. Some runners run 20 miles per day and triathletes and other sportsmen may even exceed this 2000 kcal additional metabolic demand. Cyclists in the Tour de France may require more than 6000 kcal/day (Saris et al 1989), a caloric intake which is very difficult to achieve by conventional means.

Exertion raises body temperature for long periods. Does this shorten the life of heat-sensitive vitamins?

Severe exertion has a catabolic effect on muscle. It also subjects muscles, joints and ligaments to repeated microtrauma. Does repair of these tissues raise the protein and vitamin requirements of the body?

Athletes sweat to maintain body temperature. Prolonged severe exertion may generate several litres of sweat per day. Sweat contains not only salt and water but a number of other plasma constituents such as iron and water-soluble vitamins. Do large volumes of sweat act as an avenue for depletion of body stores of vital nutrients?

TYPES OF EXERCISE AND THEIR METABOLIC REQUIREMENTS

(For a fuller treatment of these topics the reader is referred to Astrand & Rodahl (1986).)

Exercise can be classified as aerobic or anaerobic.

Aerobic exercise

Aerobic exercise is a sustained level of exertion, usually of large muscle groups, such as walking, jogging, swimming or cycling, which can be maintained for several minutes without excessive breathlessness. The exertion is performed with aerobic metabolism of glycogen and fat and without the accumulation of lactic acid from anaerobic glycolysis.

If an incremental exercise load is performed, such as on a treadmill with stepwise increases in speed and gradient, or on a bicycle ergometer with increments in resistance every 1.5–3 min, as shown in Fig. 28.1,

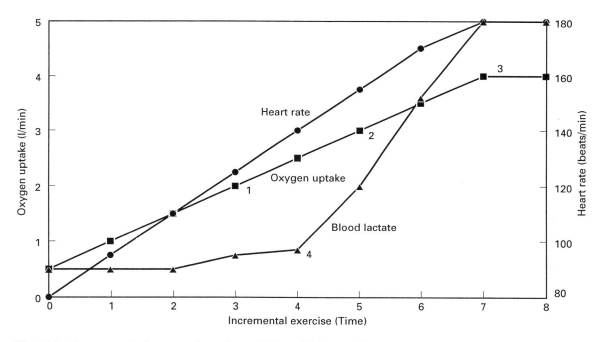

Fig. 28.1   Oxygen uptake, incremental exercise and $VO_{2\,max}$ With a steadily increasing exercise load on an ergometer, e.g. bicycle or treadmill with increasing speed/gradient, the oxygen uptake gradually increases to a maximum (3), in this case of 4 litre/min. The oxygen uptake then plateaus as does the heart rate. 50% (1) and 75% (2) of maximum oxygen uptake are marked. The blood lactate remains steady during the early totally aerobic phase of the exercise but begins to increase at point (4) and then increases rapidly. This is the anaerobic threshold, or in this case lactate threshold. (No units are given for this idealized representation.) The lactate threshold in this case is at about 65% of $VO_{2\,max}$ and can be increased with aerobic training. Close to $VO_{2\,max}$ glycogen is the sole muscle fuel but at lower levels fat contributes up to 50% of the energy (see text).

aerobic exertion can be performed only until a certain point. Then there is a sudden increase in the ventilation which becomes more laboured and is associated with a large increase in the level of perceived exertion. At this point glycogen is metabolized anaerobically as well as aerobically and lactic acid accumulates in the muscles and in the blood. This is called the *anaerobic threshold*. Incremental exercise after this point is usually of limited duration and the rate of oxygen consumption plateaus at a high level of perceived exertion, with the heart rate close to its maximum. Any further exertion renders the subject severely short of breath. The acidity of the blood becomes more marked with the normal pH of about 7.35 dropping down towards 7.0 or even lower on extreme exertion. The low pH causes breakdown of carbonic acid, with the release of carbon dioxide and an increasingly high respiratory quotient with more carbon dioxide being expired than oxygen being taken up. Exertion above the level at which the oxygen consumption plateaus becomes increasingly anaerobic and is eventually limited by fatigue in the muscles from an excess of protons generated by anaerobic glycolysis. Further severe exertion is not usually possible until the lactic acid in the muscles and the blood has been cleared and metabolized by aerobic processes in the liver.

Anaerobic exercise

Anaerobic exercise is exercise at a level above the anaerobic threshold in which the predominant source of energy is anaerobic glycolysis of glycogen. It is usually short lasting as it is limited by accummulation of lactic acid. Typical examples are a 'sprint' or a series of press ups.

This picture of aerobic and anaerobic exercise is based on whole body measurements. Below the anaerobic threshold some individual muscle fibres will be functioning anaerobically and the lactic acid will be metabolized by other fibres or by the liver without the blood lacatate level rising. Above the anaerobic threshold there will still be many muscle fibres working aerobically. Which fibres do what will depend on their fibre type, the intensity of the exercise, the degree of 'training' of the muscle and the muscle perfusion.

Maximum oxygen uptake

The level of exertion at which the oxygen uptake plateaus is called the *maximum oxygen uptake*, the

$VO_{2\,max}$ which is expressed in litre/min, e.g. 4 litre/min, or very often in order for comparisons to be made between people of different build, as ml of oxygen/kg body wt/min. Thus an 80 kg man with this $VO_{2\,max}$ would have a value of 50 ml/kg body wt/min. Values vary between 20 and 95 ml/kg/min, with the highest values being found in exceptional athletes with very little body fat. The maximum oxygen uptake is related to lean body mass and the lowest values for $VO_{2\,max}$ expressed per kg body weight are not suprisingly found in the obese. Thus, although a value of 4 litre/min gives a respectable value of 50 in an 80 kg subject, the same value in a 160 kg man would give the very low value of only 25 ml/kg body wt/min. $VO_{2\,max}$ indicates the potential for aerobic exercise and can be increased with training by up to 20% in the previously unathletic subject.

Exercise at 100% of maximum levels of oxygen uptake cannot be sustained for long. The stimulus to maximum oxygen uptake appears to be partly anaerobic and this level of exertion can be maintained for about 7 min in the well-trained athlete. The anaerobic threshold is a better measure of what can be sustained for long periods and is usually expressed as a percentage of the $VO_{2\,max}$. The value varies greatly with the degree of training. The elite marathon runner can run for >2 h at 80–90% of $VO_{2\,max}$. The untrained have difficulty maintaining 60%.

The importance of the $VO_{2\,max}$ is that comparisons between different subjects exercising are best made on the basis of the exercise load they are performing, not in terms of the load in units of work but between the loads expressed in terms of the percentage of the individual's $VO_{2\,max}$. This is particularly important in terms of metabolic demands of exercise and the physiological response. High levels of exertion redistribute blood away from the gastrointestinal tract and kidneys and have a profound influence on both utilization and absorption of food. Anaerobic exercise and exercise close to the $VO_{2\,max}$ is almost entirely catered for by glycogen metabolism, whereas the fuel for aerobic exercise at levels below 60% of $VO_{2\,max}$ is about 50% fat, although the percentage used varies with training, the state of the glycogen stores and recent feeding. Aerobic training increases the percentage of fat used.

Levels of exertion can be expressed in various ways apart from relating them to the $VO_{2\,max}$. A common method is to use the oxygen demand in ml/kg body wt, which can then be expressed in terms of multiples of the resting oxygen uptake, which is 200–250 ml/min for the average man or 3.5 ml/kg/min for a 70 kg man. Severe exertion in an elite endurance athlete would be 20 times this (20 metabolic equivalents (METS)) and give totals of 70 ml/kg/min or 5 litre/min. This is about the level of oxygen uptake needed to run 11–12 mile/hour (17.5 km/h) on a flat surface. This level of exertion generates about a kilowatt of heat.

Moderate exercise is 10 METS or 2.5 litre/min and is the level that can be sustained by the moderately fit.

IMMEDIATE REQUIREMENTS OF EXERCISING MUSCLE

Energy stores in muscle supply requirements for both immediate and prolonged exertion. These energy stores can be replaced or supplemented over the course of time by stores outside the muscle. The energy sources, ATP, creatine phosphate, muscle glycogen used anaerobically and aerobically and finally fat are described in detail in Chapter 8. What this variety of sources achieves is a graded response from immediate extreme exertion, such as a sudden jump, to the other extreme of prolonged low level endurance, lasting several days. Sudden exertion is catered for by ATP, a very short burst of exercise by creatine phosphate, and longer periods of exercise by anaerobic and then aerobic utilization of glycogen and an increasing utilization of fat as the exercise becomes less intense and more prolonged (Krogh & Lindhard 1920).

The relatively very much smaller stores of energy in the form of ATP and creatine phosphate, and the inhibition of further anaerobic metabolism of glycogen by the development of acidosis, all have a protective effect on the muscle which could otherwise overheat and suffer enzyme denaturation.

The divide between aerobic and anaerobic energy sources is found in events involving maximum exertion lasting about 2 min (800 m on the running track), where about 50% of the energy comes from aerobic and 50% from anaerobic metabolism of muscle glycogen.

Fat metabolism on its own can only maintain exercise at about 50% of $VO_{2\,max}$ (Holloszy & Coyle 1984) and exercise of this type with depleted muscle glycogen stores (after a marathon runner has reached the 'wall') is extremely arduous. Fat cannot be metabolized at rates comparable to glycogen. Fat is the most efficient energy store in that it releases more than twice the energy of glycogen for each gram oxidized, and unlike glycogen is stored in the cell as a pure fat, whereas glycogen is stored with about three times its weight of water. Table 28.1 shows the running time and distance that can be supported by the energy stores of an average man.

Table 28.1 Energy stores as fat and glycogen in the average man (adapted from Newsholme & Leech 1983)

	kJ	Running time (min)	Miles
Adipose triglycerides	337 500	4018	550–630
Liver glycogen	1660	20	3–4
Muscle glycogen	5880	71	10–14
Blood glucose	48	<1	0

The much larger energy stores as fat are of limited value in most sports as they do not allow a sufficiently high energy output and have an adverse effect on the power/weight ratio, which is of great importance where mobility is at a premium. Fat is of value as insulation against cold in swimming and is used as a fuel source in all endurance events. However, it is never used as the sole fuel supply and the current belief in health clubs that slow exercise burns fat and vigorous exercise burns carbohydrate and is thus less effective as an aid to slimming, lacks experimental support.

Glycogen used anaerobically would last a comparatively short time as it produces one-thirteenth of the ATP of complete oxidation. Lactic acid accumulation prevents excessive anaerobic utilization of glycogen in one sustained effort. However, team games involving multiple short sprints, such as top-class rugby, football or hockey, and individual games, such as squash and tennis, may burn glycogen rapidly, with the potential for glycogen depletion, particularly if matches are closely spaced.

FLUIDS AND ELECTROLYTES

Adequate fluid replacement is probably the most important dietary essential in maintaining exercise performance. The best general advice for the athlete is to drink sufficient fluid to maintain a pale straw-coloured urine, and plenty of it, and if the volume of urine does reduce and become darker, to drink copiously even if thirst seems to be already quenched.

This priority may be subjugated to meeting weight categories in particular sports, such as boxing, wrestling and light-weight rowing. Jockeys may use fluid deprivation, deliberately induced sweating or even diuretics, 'wasting', to lose several unwanted kilograms in weight before the 'weigh in'. Depending on the sport, and the time of the weigh in with respect to the competition, they may have time to rehydrate themselves before the competition. This practice is potentially dangerous and some authorities are looking at alternative controls which would prevent sportsmen seeking success in lower weight categories than they can easily and safely achieve. Diuretics are now banned substances for Olympic sports.

A 70 kg man has a total body water of 50 litre of which 36 litre is intracellular, 10.5 litre interstitial and only some 3.5 litre is in the blood plasma from which sweat is generated. Water moves between these compartments, so severe dehydration from sweat loss will in time not only deplete plasma and interstitial compartments, but also intracellular water. Total rehydration after severe dehydration is therefore gradual and often takes more than 24 h.

Thirst, which reflects plasma volume, stomach contents and recent mouth breathing, is a poor, usually insufficient guide to fluid requirements and is even worse when there is intracellular water and salt loss and contraction of the plasma volume. Should this occur, water may not be the best fluid replacement for *rapid* correction of the dehydration (Nose et al 1988). In large volumes it renders the blood plasma hypotonic and so promotes a brisk diuresis before the intracellular water depletion is rectified. An electrolyte glucose solution does not promote such a brisk diuresis and so allows greater fluid retention and replacement of intracellular water loss. However most people will be eating and drinking at the same time, so this is of practical importance only where fluids alone are being taken and further competition is imminent. The common athlete's beverage, beer, can potentiate dehydration, since it gives the illusion of satisfying thirst, but may produce a bigger volume of diuresis than the volume consumed.

Sweat and temperature control

Water loss as sweat can be considerable during prolonged exertion with sweat rates between 1 and 2 litre/h. Loss of 8% body water (4 litre) or even more is not uncommon during marathons lasting 2–4 h. Fluid replacement is difficult while running and dehydration can have profound physiological effects, not least in limiting sweat production, which is the main method of temperature control during exertion.

Exercise is thermodynamically very inefficient and generates twice as much heat energy as mechanical energy. Sustained production of as much as 1 kW of heat energy is possible by a well-trained athlete (Nadel et al 1977). A small amount of the heat is stored to produce a temporary rise in body temperature, but most has to be dissipated to the environment by conduction, convection, and radiation, but principally by evaporating sweat. If this heat is not dissipated it could raise body temperature

by 1°C every 5 min, which in theory would be lethal after 30–40 min. In practice it produces heat collapse, and even heat stroke, in athletes who stop sweating or exercise too hard in hot moist conditions, or wear clothing that does not allow heat dissipation.

Sweating is the main mechanism of heat loss for runners unless the environment is cold or wet or extremely windy.

Sweat evaporative heat loss

A 70 kg man running 10 miles (16 km in 1 h) produces a heat output of 1000 kcal (4000 kJ), which has to be dissipated or body temperature would rise. Heat loss from evaporation of 1 litre of sweat if all of it were evaporated from the skin, would be about 600 kcal (2500 kJ), but sweating efficiency is drastically reduced if the sweat drops to the ground or runs into clothing and is not evaporated freely from the skin. To retain thermal equilibrium by sweating alone, the runner would therefore need to sweat at least 1.7 litre and in practice considerably more.

Other cooling mechanisms are involved but sweating is unlikely to be 100% efficient and larger men or a faster pace would generate more heat and thus require a faster sweat rate.

During severe exertion, particularly distance running, practical experience shows that on average runners can only consume about 500 ml of fluid/h without it 'sloshing about in the stomach' and producing nausea and discomfort (Shephard & Kavanagh 1978, Maughan 1985). Drinking on the run may cause much air swallowing, and both gastric emptying and intestinal absorption are rate limited and influenced by the salt content, osmolality and carbohydrate content of the drinks consumed and the intensity of the exercise (Rehrer 1991).

With forced air movements past the runner or cyclist, sweat evaporation may be largely insensible. Further loss occurs as evaporation from the respiratory tract, which may account for 5% of heat loss during exercise (Nadel et al 1977). Cold conditions increase the respiratory tract evaporative losses because cold air has a low water vapour content but is warmed to 37°C and humidified to 100% saturation by the respiratory tract. Dehydration is a common consequence of exercise under cold conditions, and is a major problem at altitude, where the combination of extreme cold and hypoxic ventilation increases respiratory tract water losses even further. Respiratory losses while climbing Everest have been estimated at 200 ml/h.

Where exertion is over 70% $VO_{2\ max}$, sweating becomes profuse and with severe exertion it is even possible to sweat quite markedly when swimming in water cooler than body temperature.

The highest recorded sweat rates (5 litre/h) are not found during exertion, but on exposure to hot environments at rest, where the skin blood flow is at a maximum and not competing with circulation to active muscle. However, athletes may train for as much as 20 h/week with sweat rates of 1–2 litre/h during exertion. Chronic dehydration is therefore common, especially since thirst seems to be a poor guide to fluid requirements.

Daily fluid intake during the Tour de France cycle race in a study of five cyclists averaged over 6 litre, with the extreme individual intake being 11.8 litre (Saris et al 1989). Even allowing for urine production, these values suggest copious volumes of sweat, far exceeding the plasma volume and made possible by repeated drinking during the race as well as afterwards.

Fluid losses are best made good as soon as they occur, and whilst many sports do not officially allow drinks throughout the event, a blind eye may be turned to drinks being consumed by players during injury breaks as well as during official breaks such as half time.

Water and electrolyte 'sports drinks'

Traditional fluid replacement by athletes has consisted of water or fruit cordials of various kinds, supplemented perhaps too frequently by beer after competition, which promotes a diuresis by inhibiting anti-diuretic hormone and so prevents complete rehydration. In the last few years a variety of sports drinks have been heavily promoted and claim to put back fluid faster than water, and replace electrolytes lost in sweat. More recently they have taken on the additional role of supplementing carbohydrate intake and thus delaying fatigue – 'put back lost energy fast!'. This latter role is discussed below. Do they have a role during and after exercise for replacement of water and electrolytes?

Drinking during exercise

In endurance events such as marathon runs, where dehydration can be both a threat to health and a limiting factor in performance, a drink taken frequently during the course of the race containing small quantities of sodium and other electrolytes, and glucose to make it 'isotonic', is absorbed slightly faster than plain water (which is not absorbed from the gut until it has become isotonic), and may have benefits over water in preventing, correcting or delaying dehydration and some of the gastrointestinal symptoms from which some runners suffer, which are apparently more common in more severely dehydrated runners (Rehrer et al 1989). Differences between the rates of absorption of water and electrolyte solutions are not very large. On the negative side, particularly in mass participation events, there are problems in distributing these drinks, correctly diluted, in adequate amounts along the course. There are problems too of palatability, which is a very difficult problem during vigorous exercise, particularly where athletes are already dehydrated.

Different runners like different 'sports drinks' and blame the race organizers for their gastrointestinal symptoms and poor performance if 'the wrong drink' is supplied. The drinks contain carbohydrate and are sticky and 'messy' if spilt or poured over a runner as runners traditionally do with 'spare water' in hot weather. They also make excellent bacterial and fungal culture media if kept at room temperature and therefore need careful handling. Sealed, sterile containers of prediluted drinks are expensive. Water is much more readily available and easier to handle. The International Marathon Medical Directors Association (IMMDA) recommends that water should be available at every feeding station along the route and leave the availability of glucose electrolyte drinks, which are considered more of a luxury, to the generosity of the race organizers and their sponsors, who usually place them less frequently.

Post-competition drinks

There would seem to be little justification for routine use of glucose electrolyte 'sports drinks' post competition or training when there is adequate time for both eating and drinking, and any electrolytes lost are more than compensated for by normal dietary intake. Dressendorfer et al (1982) measured nine minerals in the blood of a group of 12 runners racing 17 miles/day (average) for 20 days and eating and drinking ad libitum, with no special drinks or mineral supplements. No significant changes were found. The runners all maintained normal serum electrolytes. Obviously, if athletes suffer from diarrhoea or vomiting, or if they have several rounds of a competition in close succession, such drinks may serve a very useful role.

Sodium loss in sweat: salt supplements

Sweat sodium content falls with training, acclimatization and the volume produced. An unfit person's sweat contains approx. 80 mmol/l, whereas a fully acclimatized endurance runner's may be as low as 40

(Verde et al 1982) The serum level is 140 mmol/l. Plasma is in equilibrium with the interstitial fluid, which has the same sodium concentration. There is an extracellular sodium pool of approx. 2000 mmol.

Hyponatraemia

Does drinking water to replace sweat loss during marathons and other endurance events cause hyponatraemia? In order to achieve sodium depletion of 10%, causing hyponatraemia of 126 mmol/l, sweat loss (replaced with water alone) would need to be 200 mmol, the content of 5 litre of sweat for the acclimatized runner and 2.5 litre for the unacclimatized. However, during an event such as a marathon, there is usually only partial correction of dehydration (say 50%). In practical terms the inadequate fluid replacement at about 500 ml/h usually causes a rise rather than a fall in serum sodium as secretion of hypotonic sweat causes haemoconcentration.

However, hyponatraemia has been recorded in endurance events lasting >5 h, such as the South African Comrades marathon, a double marathon of 52 miles (Noakes et al 1985), and occasionally in shorter events, usually in athletes who have admitted drinking many litres of fluid over the course of several hours, to replace sweat losses. Mechanisms in addition to an excessive water load appear to be operating, as the kidneys would normally excrete excess water, if not during exercise when renal function may be inhibited, then rapidly afterwards. Exercise perhaps promotes prolonged excretion of antidiuretic hormone in these individuals.

As most runners cannot tolerate > 500 ml/h fluid intake, an event lasting 2–5 h cannot induce significant hyponatraemia, unless the runners stop and force feed themselves with water. In double marathons, the benefits of electrolyte drinks become more obvious. Their use for these should be encouraged and excessive water drinking alone discouraged. Fortunately, in even longer endurance events, food has to be taken as well as drinks, making hyponatraemia most unlikely.

Is salt supplementation required?

The normal diet contains more salt than is likely to be lost in sweat, except under very extreme circumstances. Excess salt, like excess water, is excreted by the kidneys and salt supplementation, especially with salt tablets, may lead to fluid loss from increased urine production and can cause nausea. The much quoted stokers' heat cramps (Talbot 1935), due to hyponatraemia from enormous sweat loss, are *not* the same as cramps in athletes, who usually have normal serum electrolytes, even with severe cramps, and whose cramps are usually uninfluenced by additional salt. Old fashioned stokers were exposed to temperatures of over 100°C and lost as much as 5 litre/h of sweat, which they replaced with water. They really did become salt depleted but their experience does not justify widespread adoption of salt supplementation for very different conditions.

Chronic salt depletion in athletes is very unlikely, but *may* occur, particularly in non-endurance athletes (who unlike endurance athletes are not already heat acclimatized) on sudden exposure to hot conditions. They can be advised to put extra salt on their food and add a little salt to their drinks, but this should not become a life-time habit. The use of slow-release salt tablets, 'slow sodium' has been fashionable in sport but seems extravagant and unnecessary and encourages athletes to take 'pills or medication' contrary to the philosophy of sport. Excess salt intake also encourages diuresis and thus dehydration.

Potassium loss

Excess potassium loss with exercise has been proposed, but again dietary intake is usually adequate and fruit juices and bananas, much favoured by athletes, are a better source than potassium salt or tablets.

CARBOHYDRATE

Sustained exercise at between 60 and 80% of $VO_{2\,max}$ is limited by muscle glycogen stores, which become depleted after 1–3 h of continuous exercise at this level (Bergstrom & Hultman 1966). When muscle glycogen levels are low, exercise is a much greater effort and running or cycling becomes much slower as fat becomes the main fuel source. Exercise can then continue at only about 50% of $VO_{2\,max}$. Indeed, the oxygen cost of running at the same pace is higher with fat as the fuel than with carbohydrate, as more oxygen is used per unit of ATP produced. When muscle carbohydrate is severely depleted, there is a risk of hypoglycaemia (Coyle et al 1983). Liver stores of glycogen are broken down to maintain blood sugar, some of which is taken up by muscle with a fall in blood glucose, but usually not to severely hypoglycaemic levels.

Blood glucose can be used to maintain exercise but only at a slow pace, as it appears to be transferred to muscle at an inadequate rate to maintain exercise at more than about 25% $VO_{2\,max}$ (Coyle 1991).

An instructive example of carbohydrate depletion was seen by the author in the late 1960s in a 24-h running race. The fashion then appeared to be to set off at a pace of about 10 mile/h, which could only be maintained for 50–60 miles. At about this point, each of the runners slowed to almost half the pace or less as they (presumably) ran out of muscle glycogen, so that they eventually covered 120–130 miles in the 24 h. Runners in ultra-endurance races now aim for a much more even pace and set off at a slower pace, burning a lower initial percentage of carbohydrate and thus eking it out much further.

Exercise at 60–80% $VO_{2\,max}$ in trained athletes can be maintained for a greater period of time if the muscle glycogen is at a high level before exercise begins. Higher than normal muscle glycogen levels are found in endurance athletes on a high carbohydrate diet who have rested for a few days.

'Carbo loading'

A regimen for endurance athletes to increase muscle glycogen became popular with marathon runners in particular and was known as 'carbo loading'. Classically, a week before the event, they severely depleted their muscle stores by going on a long run followed by repeated fast strides. For the next 3 days they would train moderately hard while eating a low carbohydrate diet, predominantly composed of protein and fat, to deplete the muscle glycogen even more. For the last 4 days they would train only lightly but eat a very high carbohydrate diet. The muscles deprived of glycogen would be avid for it and super-compensate with much higher than normal muscle glycogen stores (Bergstrom et al 1967, Astrand 1967). This regimen did not suit all runners. Many found that training on a low carbohydrate diet was very uncomfortable and they started the race stiff and heavy.

More recent views are that endurance runners tend to have high muscle glycogen as a result of training and all that is required is for them to taper off their training for the few days before the race and eat a very high carbohydrate diet and equally high levels will be achieved (Brewer et al 1988).

A well-trained endurance athlete can load his muscles with about 2 kg of glycogen, which is bound in the muscle with water which is released as the glycogen is metabolized and acts as an additional source of water. Weight loss in endurance events is partly from loss of muscle glycogen and cannot all be explained by fluid depletion from sweat.

Carbohydrate drinks

A high carbohydrate meal or snack taken in the hour before exercise was shown to carry the risk of producing a dramatic insulin response, increased glycogen utilization and premature fatigue (Foster et al 1979), and even rebound hypoglycaemia. More recent studies have shown that this does not occur with a carbohydrate drink taken just as exercise commences. The circulating catecholamines during vigorous exercise suppress the insulin response and prevent these negative effects of carbohydrate feeding (Galbo 1983). Further studies have shown that these drinks, or indeed solid carbohydrate, may prolong exercise endurance or improve performance if they are taken repeatedly during an endurance event and thus may delay or prevent 'the wall' in the marathon, which is thought to be largely due to muscle glycogen depletion at about 20 miles. Paradoxically, studies by Coyle et al (1986) show no muscle glycogen sparing from glucose ingestion, although the exogenous glucose is used by the exercising muscle.

Another strategy based on experiments by Ivy et al (1979), which is now less favoured, was to drink strong coffee just before the event, on the basis that caffeine would raise serum fatty acids and encourage fatty acid metabolism in the muscle and thus conserve glycogen. This strategy, like much experimental work, was based on cycle ergometry under laboratory conditions quite different from a marathon foot race, but became widely advocated for marathon runners. In the author's experience as a competitor and medical officer observing other marathon runners, it certainly had a powerful diuretic effect and so did not help fluid conservation. It could also aggravate another runner's problem – 'runner's trots'. Studies in runners have not shown the benefit found in laboratory cyclists (Casal & Leon 1985) and a large dose of caffeine is not now pressed on marathon runners by willing sponsors.

Tour de France cyclists drink a high carbohydrate drink during race stages. Studies by Saris et al (1989) have shown that their average requirements of almost 6000 kcal/day could only be met by almost continuous feeding with a high carbohydrate drink, which accounted for 50% of their caloric intake on race days. Simulation of the race in a calorimeter (Brouns et al 1989) showed that without the maltodextrin drink, cyclists could not maintain their energy balance, and catabolized muscle protein. Cyclists who could not maintain the required energy intake in the Tour de France were forced to drop out from fatigue and those who did well matched their caloric intake to the energy expended day by day, presumably conserving and replacing muscle glycogen.

Muscle glycogen repletion

Training at high intensity, both aerobic and anaerobic, can deplete muscle glycogen, and repeated days of heavy training can cause progressive depletion and fatigue. It can take up to 48 h to replace the glycogen and rest days may be essential to do this. Glycogen is taken into muscle most avidly within 2 h of exercise (Ivy et al 1988) and repeated carbohydrate meals are probably better than one or two large ones. A high carbohydrate diet (preferably 60–70%) is essential for rapid replenishment and maintenance of high glycogen levels in muscle.

Protein requirements

The role of protein in the sportsman's diet remains controversial. Whilst some nutritionists have questioned the need for any greater protein intake per kilogram body weight than non-athletes, body builders and strength athletes have traditionally believed that they need to eat vast quantities of protein to maintain their extraordinary bulk and powerful muscles. This belief may well be based on 19th (von Liebig 1842) rather than 20th century theories, but is not easily dispelled. Famous athletes, such as Geoff Capes who competed in gladiatorial television strength contests, were photographed beside their daily dietary intake of several pounds of steak, two dozen eggs, several pints of milk and enormous quantities of other foods. Their successors believe that this is the only way to emulate their gargantuan success.

Where physical bulk is more important than power/weight ratio, some of this excess may be needed. Larger men on average are stronger and sheer bulk wins some competitions.

No one has attempted a controlled trial in such world beaters but many have suggested that these excessive protein loads confer no advantage and that a high carbohydrate intake would benefit them as much as the endurance athlete. This debate has been complicated by the wide use of anabolic steroids by participants in strength events, who may have found an abnormally high protein intake was essential to obtain the maximum very dramatic anabolic effects associated with non-pharmacological, high dosage steroids, plus very heavy training.

It has also become apparent that where there is inadequate carbohydrate intake for a very heavy training load, negative nitrogen balance may occur. This is as easily remedied by increased carbohydrate in the diet as by the apparently more logical increase in protein. Lemon (1991) reviewed this complex area and concluded that endurance athletes require a higher than normal protein intake, probably about twice the usual recommended daily amount (RDA) and this is probably true also of strength athletes, provided both groups have adequate caloric intake from carbohydrate. Where strength athletes are on a muscle building/weight reduction regimen, they may require more than 200% of the RDA to maintain nitrogen balance.

What reasons could there be for extra protein being required? The rate of formation of new muscle tissue accelerated by training would hardly justify these amounts. Studies appear to show an accelerated rate of protein turnover in athletes in training who demonstrate increased protein catabolism.

IRON

The frequency of iron deficiency in athletes appears to vary widely in different studies, depending on the techniques used and the population studied. In the USA, where iron deficiency in students is apparently widespread, as many as 30% of women cross-country runners have been labelled iron deficient (Risser et al 1988), a value that seems very high and may be related to food fads or 'junk food'.

Although there may be some iron loss in sweat, slightly increased gastrointestinal blood loss in runners, particularly if they regularly take aspirin or other non-steroidal anti-inflammatory drugs for an injury or stiffness, occasional frank haematuria from bladder trauma and haemoglobinuria (from red cells being crushed in the plantar fascia in heavy footed runners), this is usually well compensated by the increased total dietary intake associated with their high calorie diet. Iron supplements are therefore not usually considered necessary and can cause gastrointestinal disturbances or even haemosiderosis.

Brotherhood et al (1975) measured haematological parameters in a group of 40 male distance runners and 12 controls and found no significant differences between those on iron, or iron and folic acid supplements, and those on a normal diet.

Iron deficiency may be suspected in athletes who have a slightly lower than average haemoglobin from athletes' anaemia (a haemoglobin of <14 g% in men or <12 in women endurance athletes). This is usually a training-induced physiological condition caused by an increase in plasma volume (from 10 to 30%), which is greater than the training-induced increase in red cell mass. Despite a slightly reduced haemoglobin, the total red cell mass is normal or greater than normal. Although athletes' anaemia may be associated with a low serum ferritin, this physiological condition has not been found to correlate with poor performance and does not respond to iron supplementation. Iron stores are present in the bone marrow (Magnusson et al 1984). This complex subject has been reviewed by Watts (1989). Haemoglobin and ferritin levels can be misleading in athletes, so he suggests that if the mean cell volume (MCV) is <75 fl and the mean cell haemoglobin <25 µg or the ferritin is >5 µg lower than the laboratory lower limit, then a trial of iron therapy for 1 month is justified. If iron deficiency is really present the haemoglobin should rise by 1 g.

Women athletes may have genuine iron deficiency from menstrual losses, dietary fads or a combination of the two. Women endurance athletes who have exercise-induced amennorhoea may appear to be less likely to develop iron deficiency, but they may be on marginal diets that may inhibit iron absorption and may be at risk from this cause.

AMINO ACIDS, VITAMINS AND TRACE ELEMENTS

Amino acids are used as a fuel source by active muscle (Brooks 1987) and are promoted in advertisements as a more accessible method of body building than whole protein. Newsholme et al (1991) have suggested that the overtraining syndrome of endurance athletes with its attendant immune deficiency may be prevented by glutamine supplements.

Extensive work on trace elements and antioxidants, including vitamins C and E, has failed to show any advantages in super supplementation with these substances where the diet is adequate.

Despite the lack of positive findings for a wide variety of nutritional supplements, many athletes dose themselves every day with cocktails of amino acids, vitamins, trace elements, royal jelly, Ginseng, etc. whose promoters can all produce 'scientific evidence' of the benefits. Many of the herbal extracts have traces of drugs that may be banned by the International Olympic Committee and their users face suspension after random drug testing. Unfortunately, some sports doctors have aggravated the situation by giving, for example, B_{12} (cyanocobalomin) injections

as placebos to athletes to boost performance, thereby giving credibility to the idea that something is missing in the normal diet.

The third most common nutritional problem in athletes after dehydration and inadequate carbohydrate intake is overindulgence in dietary supplements.

An International Congress on Sports Nutrition in 1990 produced the following Consensus Statement, which best summarizes current knowledge and addresses these issues.

CONSENSUS STATEMENT

'Diet significantly influences athletic performance. An adequate diet, in terms of quantity and quality, before, during and after training and competition will maximize performance. In the optimum diet for most sports, carbohydrate is likely to contribute about 60–70% of total energy intake and protein about 12%, with the remainder coming from fat.

Total energy intake must be raised to meet the increased energy expended during training and maintenance of energy balance can be assessed by monitoring body weight, body composition and food intake. Where there is a need to reduce body weight, this should be done gradually, and not immediately before competition.

In athletic events of high intensity and long duration (such as multiple sprint and endurance sports), performance is generally limited by carbohydrate availability. High carbohydrate diets (even in excess of two-thirds of total energy) maximize carbohydrate (glycogen) stores and improve performance in such activity. A high carbohydrate diet is also necessary to sustain high intensity training on a daily basis. After each bout of exercise the diet should contain sufficient carbohydrate to replenish the glycogen stores and to maximize subsequent performance. The requirement for sugars and starches, in both solid and liquid forms, will vary depending on the timing and nature of the physical activity.

Increased fluid intake is necessary to avoid dehydration, and may improve performance during prolonged exercise, especially when sweat loss is high. These fluids may contain some carbohydrate, the concentration of which will be dictated by both the duration of exercise and climatic conditions. If exercise is of short duration and sweat losses are small, the replacement of salts can be achieved from a normal food intake after exercise.

Protein requirements are higher in individuals involved in physical training programmes than in inactive people. Most athletes already consume sufficient protein, however, as a consequence of their increased energy intakes.

Fat consumption should be no greater than 30% of total energy intake. Supplementary fat beyond this intake is not recommended for training or competition because the body is able to mobilize its large reserve of this energy store. Except where there is a need to reduce body fat content, it is important to maintain these stores by ingesting sufficient energy between periods of exercise.

Vitamin supplements are not necessary for athletes eating a diet adequate in respect of quality and quantity. Of the minerals and trace elements essential for health, particular attention should be paid to iron and calcium status in those individuals who may be at risk.

There is no good evidence to support the use of other nutritional supplements, including those commonly assumed by athletes to have ergogenic effects.'

REFERENCES

Astrand PO 1967 Diet and athletic performance. Federation Proceedings 26: 1772–1777

Astrand PO, Rodahl K 1986 Textbook of work physiology; physiological bases of exercise, 3rd edn. McGraw Hill, New York

Bergstrom J, Hultman E 1966 The effect of exercise on muscle glycogen and electrolytes in normals. Scandinavian Journal of Clinical Investigation 18: 16–22

Bergstrom J, Hermansen L, Hultman E, Saltin B 1967 Diet muscle glycogen and physical performance. Acta Physiologica Scandinavica 71: 140–150

Brewer J, Williams C, Patton A 1988 The influence of high carbohydrate diets on endurance running performance. European Journal of Applied Physiology 57: 698–706

Brooks GA 1987 Amino acid and protein metabolism during exercise and recovery. Medicine and Science in Sports and Exercise 19: 5150–5156

Brotherhood J, Brozovic B, Pugh LGC 1975 Haematological status of middle and long distance runners. Clinical Science and Molecular Medicine 48: 139–145

Brouns F, Saris WHM, Stroecken J et al 1989 Eating, drinking and cycling: A controlled Tour de France simulation study. 11 Effects of diet manipulation. International Journal of Sports Medicine 10: S41–S48

Casal DC, Leon AS 1985 Failure of caffeine to affect substrate utilization during prolonged running. Medical Science of Sport Exercise 17: 174–179

Coyle EF, Magberg JM, Hurley BF et al 1983 Carbohydrate feeding during prolonged strenuous exercise can delay fatigue. Journal of Applied Physiology 55: 230–235

Coyle EF 1991 Carbohydrate feeding: effects on metabolism, performance and recovery. In: Brouns F (ed) Advances in nutrition and top sport. Medical Sport Sciences, vol 32. Karger, Basal, pp. 1–14

Coyle EF, Coggan AR, Hemnert MK, Ivy JL 1986 Muscle glycogen utilisation during prolonged strenuous exercise when fed carbohydrate. Journal of Applied Physiology 61: 165–172

Dressendorfer RH, Wade CE, Keen CL, Scaff JH 1982 Plasma mineral levels in marathon runners during a 20 day road race. Physician Sportsmed 10: 113–18

Foster C, Costill DL, Fink WJ 1979 Effects of pre-exercise feeding on endurance performance. Medical Science of Sports and Exercise 11: 1–5

Galbo H 1983 Hormonal and metabolic adaptations to exercise. George Thieme Verlag, New York

Holloszy JO, Coyle EF 1984 Adaptations of skeletal muscle to endurance exercise and their metabolic consequences. Journal of Applied Physiology 56: 831–838

Ivy JL, Costill DL, Fink WJ, Lower RW 1979 Influence of caffeine and carbohydrate feeding on endurance performance. Medical Science of Sports 11: 6–11

Ivy JL, Katz AL, Cutler CL et al 1988 Muscle glycogen synthesis after exercise: effect of time of carbohydrate ingestion. Journal of Applied Physiology 65: 1480–1485

Krogh A, Lindhard J 1920 Relative value of fat and cabohydrate as a source of muscular energy. Biochemical Journal 14: 290–298

Lemon PWR 1991 Does exercise alter dietary protein requirements? In: Brouns F (ed) Advances in nutrition and top sport, Medical Sport Sciences vol 32. Karger, Basal pp. 15–37

Magnusson B, Hallberg L, Roossando L 1984 Iron metabolism and "sports anaemia" – a haematological comparison of elite humans and control subjects. Acad Medica Scandinavica 216: 157–164

Maughan RJ 1985 Thermoregulation in marathon competition at low ambient temperature. International Journal of Sports Medicine 6: 15–19

Nadel ER, Wenger B, Roberts MF et al 1977 Physiological defences against hyperthermia of exercise. Annals of the NY Academy of Science 31: 98–109

Newsholme E, Leech T 1983 The runner: energy and endurance fitness. Walter L Meagher, New Jersey and Oxford

Newsholme EA, Parry-Billings M, McAndrew N, Budgett R 1991 A biochemical mechanism to explain characteristics of overtraining. In: Brouns F (ed) Advances in nutrition and top sport. Medical Sport Sciences, vol 32. Basel, Karger, pp. 79–93

Noakes TD, Goodwin N, Rayner BL, Branken T, Taylor RKN 1985 Water intoxication: a possible complication during endurance exercise. Medical Science in Sports and Exercise 17: 370–375

Nose H, Mack GW, Xiangong S, Nadel ER 1988 Role of osmolality and plasma volume during rehydration in humans. Journal of Applied Physiology 65: 325–331

Rehrer NJ, Janssen GME, Brouns F, Saris G 1989 Fluid intake and gastrointestinal problems in runners competing in a 25 km race and a marathon. International Journal of Sports Medicine 10 (Suppl 1): 22–25

Rehrer NJ 1991 Aspects of dehydration and rehydration during exercise. In: Brouns F (ed) Advances in nutrition and top sport. Medical Sport Sciences vol 32. Basel, Karger pp. 128–146

Risser WL, Lee EJ, Poindexter HB W et al 1988 Iron deficiency in female athletes: its prevalence and impact on performance. Medical Science in Sports and Exercise 20: 116–121

Saris VHM, van Erp-Baart MA, Brouns F et al 1989 Study on food intake and energy expenditure during extreme sustained exercise: The Tour de France. International Journal of Sports Medicine 10: S26–S31

Shephard RJ, Kavanagh T 1978 Fluid and mineral needs of middle aged and post coronary distance runners. Physician and Sportsmedicine 6: 90–102

Talbot JH 1935 Heat cramps. Medicine 14: 323–376

Verde TR, Shephard RJ, Corey P, Moore R 1982 Sweat composition in exercise and in heat. Journal of Applied Physiology 53: 1540–1545

von Liebig J 1842 Animal chemistry and its application to physiology and pathology. Taylor and Walton, London

Watts E 1989 Athlete's anaemia. British Journal of Sports Medicine 23: 81–83

RECOMMENDED READING

Brouns F (ed) 1991 Advances in nutrition and top sport. Medicine and Sports Sciences vol 32. Karger, Basel

29. Nutritional management of clinical undernutrition

C. Pichard and K. N. Jeejeebhoy

The malnutrition syndrome is a generic term which encompasses the different clinical manifestations resulting from a lack of nutrients in general. The incidence of malnutrition in hospitalized patients is about 50%, even in countries with a high standard of living (Weinsier et al 1979, Willard et al 1980, Perrot et al 1982). Clinical malnutrition results from a variety of factors, including an inability to eat, malabsorption, loss of endogenous nutrients, prolonged administration of hypocaloric solutions or inadequate use of a defined nutritional mixture. The imbalance between intake and requirements results in wasting of muscle, a negative nitrogen balance (Waterlow & Jackson 1981) and multisystem dysfunction, ultimately promoting clinical complications such as infection, poor wound healing and increased mortality (Mullen et al 1980, Rombeau et al 1982). Nutritional support of patients has become of particular importance because improvements in the treatment of sepsis, cardiorespiratory failure, and electrolyte abnormalities have allowed patients to survive to a point where malnutrition becomes a limiting factor in their progress. Nutritional deficiency is especially likely to occur in patients with prolonged inability to eat, such as those who have undergone surgery and radio-chemotherapy or in those with gastrointestinal diseases compromising absorption of an oral diet (Willicuts 1977, Champault & Patel 1979, Brennan 1979).

During the last decade, malnutrition-related complications are believed to have increased hospital costs and thus nutritional support is believed be a cost-saving strategy (Lennard-Jones 1992).

In this chapter, the general principles of adequate nutritional support will be outlined with reference to the pathophysiology of the malnutrition syndrome.

STARVATION AS A MODEL OF MALNUTRITION

The metabolic changes related to starvation are all designed to decrease energy requirements and loss of lean body mass. Starvation results in reduced insulin levels which promote the mobilization of adipose tissue fat as free fatty acids (FFA). The enhanced output of FFA provides fuel to meet the energy requirements of the individual. Part of the increased FFA output is oxidized by the carnitine-dependent β-oxidation pathway in the liver to ketones. There is a continued hepatic glucose output because of glycogenolysis and gluconeogenesis. Despite the increased output of FFA in early fasting, there is continued catabolism of muscle protein, which is released mainly as alanine and glutamine, but includes other amino acids. Alanine and glutamine are deaminated in the liver and kidneys, and the carbon skeletons of the deaminated ketoacids are converted to glucose, while the nitrogen moiety is excreted as urea and ammonia. Glutamine is also an energy substrate for the intestine. Hence, muscle breakdown provides substrate for gluconeogenesis and other metabolic activities of the liver, kidneys and intestine at the cost of a negative nitrogen balance. The negative nitrogen balance averages 10 g/day during the first 4 days of complete fasting, but subsequently the nitrogen loss tapers off and falls to about 3 g/day when starvation extends beyond 1 week. In addition to a reduction in nitrogen loss, there is a fall in metabolic rate of about 30%, which reduces energy needs. Complete starvation, such as in hunger strikers, leads to death in 40–60 days (Lowe 1982). Survival during starvation depends on conserving body protein as well as supplying fuel to vital organs. These opposing needs are met during starvation by reducing the energy expenditure (up to one-third) and by a reduction in gluconeogenesis. Glucose requirements fall because ketoacids are increasingly used instead of glucose as a brain fuel (normal need ≈ 100 g/day).

The metabolic effect of energy and protein deficits may be aggravated in patients with gastrointestinal disease by an insufficient intake and an increased loss of micronutrients from the gastrointestinal tract (fistula, drainage and diarrhoea). Zinc losses can cause catabolic effects (Wolman et al 1979) and the retention of nitrogen in tissues depends on the availability of several micronutrients (potassium, phosphorus, magnesium and zinc (Rudman et al 1975, Wolman et al 1979)). Insufficiency of these elements can adversely affect nitrogen balance.

CLINICAL MALNUTRITION

Clinical malnutrition tends to be polymorphic because it results from a variety of situations in which there may be combined macro- and micronutrient deficiencies. The effects of such a combined picture on the metabolism of individual nutrients is considered below.

Effects on protein metabolism

When an individual reduces protein intake, the loss of nitrogen initially continues at the previous rate and exceeds the current intake. The discrepancy between intake and output is greatest in those who have previously taken a high protein diet and is least in those already depleted or living on a low protein diet. After a few days the nitrogen excretion progressively falls and, ultimately, the nitrogen excretion plateaus at about 2 mg/cal of metabolic rate (Munro 1964).

The reduction in nitrogen excretion with progressive starvation appears to be mediated in part by the increasing availability of fat energy to meet requirements and in part by a change in the so-called 'labile nitrogen stores', which amounts to between 30 and 50 g of nitrogen (Munro 1964). This finding is of considerable significance in interpreting short-term nitrogen balance studies (up to 5 days) (Jeejeebhoy et al 1976a). During the first week of starvation, individuals taking large amounts of nitrogen prior to the onset of starvation would clearly require a higher nitrogen intake to maintain balance than would those who have previously taken less protein. Correspondingly, the negative nitrogen balance in the former may appear to be grossly exaggerated, during this initial period, in contrast to those who have not been on such a high protein intake prior to starvation. This change in body nitrogen over a short period of time can be easily regained by refeeding the individual, and hence fluctuations of between 30 and 50 g of nitrogen can occur in response to acute dietary changes and need not reflect a major change in the protein content of muscles and somatic tissues. Here again, temporarily positive balances of nitrogen observed with nutritional support should be interpreted with caution

in regard to their significance to the long-term repletion of body protein stores. Studies of body composition in healthy humans have demonstrated that total body potassium (TBK) and total body nitrogen (TBN) exist in a constant proportion (Moore et al 1968, Lukaski et al 1981, McNeill et al 1982, Russell et al 1983). However in malnourished patients, the ratio TBK/TBN is significantly lower in males, but not changed in females, as compared with controls. This highlights the fact that the loss of different body components may vary with malnutrition and may be disproportionate in males but not in females (Lukaski et al 1981, McNeill et al 1982).

Changes in energy metabolism

The fall in metabolic rate due to malnutrition is proportional to the loss of the lean body mass (Kinney 1980), although Rosa & Shizgal (1984) have shown that the lean body tissues in malnourished subjects are relatively hypermetabolic. There is reduced spontaneous physical activity and an altered profile of several hormones, such as catecholamines, thyroid metabolites, insulin, glucagon, glucocorticoids and growth hormone. In addition to changes in the metabolic rate, there is a change in the respiratory quotient, which is the ratio of carbon dioxide excreted to oxygen consumed. Normally, with a mixed carbohydrate-fat diet this ratio varies between 0.85 and 0.90. If carbohydrate is the sole source of energy, then this ratio approaches 1.0, and in contrast, if fat is the main source of energy this ratio drops to 0.70. Malnourished patients have a respiratory quotient of about 0.70. This finding suggests that in such patients fat is the major source of calories.

To provide energy fatty acids undergo β-oxidation in the mitochondria. The entry of fatty acid into mitochondria is under the control of the carrier carnitine. Carnitine is present in most natural foods (meat, vegetables) but is absent in the artificial diets used for nutritional support. Thus it has been suspected that patients receiving total parenteral nutrition (TPN) could develop carnitine deficiency. Studies based on carnitine balance and indirect calorimetry (Pichard et al 1988, 1989) in acutely ill patients receiving TPN for 2 weeks, have shown significant carnitine depletion. Despite carnitine depletion the fat oxidation was unaltered. However, after more prolonged artificial nutrition for up to 9 months in patients undergoing repeated surgery (Roulet et al 1989) or those with renal insufficiency (Bellinghieri et al 1983), carnitine deficiency and slightly altered fat and protein oxidation have been found. These findings suggest that L-carnitine supplementation (20 mg/kg/day) may be beneficial to some patients on TPN.

Interaction of malnutrition with stress and sepsis

In 1932, Cuthbertson showed that trauma caused a rise in the losses of phosphorus, potassium, urea and nitrogen indicative of muscle cell catabolism. These catabolic changes are maximal 4–8 days after an injury (Cuthbertson 1979) and their magnitude is proportional to the level of protein intake before injury (poor nutritional intake is known to reduce the protein catabolic response to injury) (Munro 1964). Studies by Long et al (1977) using isotopic tracers in septic surgical patients have suggested that the observed negative nitrogen balance may be due to increased protein synthesis, with an even greater increase in protein breakdown. It has also been shown that in trauma, hormones (glucagon, glucocorticoids and catecholamines) that oppose the action of insulin are elevated and accelerate nitrogen loss. In addition, Clowes et al (1983) showed that there was a circulating factor in the plasma of septic patients that increased muscle proteolysis in vitro. More recently, it has been shown that infusion of cachectin, a cytokine released by the effect of endotoxin on macrophages, will increase the metabolic rate and flow of amino acids from muscles, decrease fatty acid release, elevate the levels of catabolic hormones and the body temperature (Starnes et al 1988). Thus it is believed that the negative nitrogen balance and muscle wasting seen in sepsis may result from the action of cytokines (see Chapter 31).

A stressed patient often shows a mild-to-moderate hyperglycaemia, which is related to an inability to oxidize glucose. In fact Long et al (1971) showed that stressed patients oxidize glucose at a normal or even an increased rate in the absence of shock. Such patients have an increase in hepatic glucose production despite the presence of hyperglycaemia. The increased glucose output is partly derived from increased recycling of lactate and partly from alanine release from muscle catabolism.

Despite a greater availability of glucose, in a study on unfed surgical patients, indirect calorimetry indicated that up to 90% of the caloric expenditure was from body fat, while protein provided the remainder (Duke et al 1970).

Starvation coupled with stress and sepsis has the effect of mobilizing the energy stored in adipose tissue, but in addition, increased breakdown of muscle protein results in an accelerated loss of muscle mass. While muscle loss is minimized in pure starvation, this is not the case when starvation is combined with trauma or sepsis. Thus malnourished patients who are also stressed represent a group with a high degree of risk for profound muscle wasting.

Electrolytes and micronutrients

In an elegant study of patients receiving parenteral nutrition, Rudman et al (1975) showed that nitrogen retention can occur only when patients were also supplemented with potassium and phosphorus. When these two elements were withdrawn from a parenteral nutrient solution (otherwise adequate in calories and nitrogen), nitrogen retention did not occur. It is therefore clear that positive nitrogen balance is dependent on not only providing calories but also on providing the principal intracellular electrolytes. This concept has been extended by Freeman (1977) to the need for magnesium, who has shown that in the absence of adequate amounts of magnesium, nitrogen retention is reduced.

Trace elements, vitamins and essential fatty acids constitute the three major groups of micronutrients. Trace elements and vitamins frequently act as cofactors of enzymes and are vital for normal cellular activity. Essential fatty acids are required for prostaglandin synthesis.

Seven elements (iron, zinc, copper, chromium, selenium, iodine, and cobalt) are known to be essential in humans. Among the trace elements, zinc is an essential constituent of a number of tissues, including muscle. During the catabolic phase of injury, zinc is lost in proportion to the nitrogen in urine (Cuthbertson 1932). Golden & Golden (1981) have shown that there is a rapid fall in the concentration of plasma zinc when malnourished patients are refed with a zinc-free diet. In contrast, starved individuals have normal zinc levels prior to refeeding. Thus, during the catabolic phase of starvation, zinc appears to be released from tissues and labile zinc stores appear to be adequate. When refeeding produces anabolism, these stores are rapidly depleted, and the patient becomes zinc deficient. Golden & Golden (1981) showed that in the absence of zinc supplementation, even when high energy formulae are fed to children with protein–calorie malnutrition, there is very little change in body weight. Zinc supplementation, keeping all other parameters of energy and protein constant, is associated with an increase in body weight and resumption of growth. Thus, it appears that for nitrogen retention, zinc is very important during refeeding.

These findings have been confirmed by Wolman et al (1979) in patients fed parenterally, who showed that a positive zinc balance resulted in a better nitrogen balance. Thus, the trace element zinc appears to be vital in promoting nitrogen retention and deposition of lean body tissue during refeeding of depleted patients. Another effect of zinc is on energy utilization. Wolman et al (1979) showed that during TPN the attainment of a positive zinc balance was associated with a higher insulin concentration in the plasma and reduced glucose levels. Thus, zinc improves carbohydrate utilization, which is one of the two major substrates given during artificial nutritional support. Prasad et al (1988) showed that T-cell function was altered by zinc deficiency. This alteration was mediated by the effect of zinc thymulin activity.

NUTRIENT REQUIREMENTS

In animals refeeding is associated with rapid weight gain and restoration of lean and fat masses. Human adults who are not growing respond in a different manner. Several studies have shown that both oral and enteral feeding is followed by a rapid improvement in function and rise in intracellular potassium, but only a later modest gain in body nitrogen. In anorexic patients refed over an 8-week period, the mean increase in body nitrogen was only 10% while body potassium and fat increased by 30–40%. At the same time these individuals regained muscle function despite incomplete recovery of body nitrogen. The same observations have been made in patients with a variety of other diseases, including cancer. Chan (1986) showed that a 2-day infusion of glucose, potassium and insulin restored muscle function in malnourished patients who were to undergo surgery. On the other hand, over a longer period of time, patients receiving home parenteral nutrition do gain body nitrogen and weight, and restore both lean and fat masses. Hence, nutrient requirements have to be defined in terms of the goals of feeding and its duration. In addition, excessive feeding of severely malnourished or injured patients may be associated with complications. Hence, a modest balanced nutrient intake is advised for hospital patients receiving short-term feeding. Over the longer term progressive feeding with increased calories and proteins may be used to rehabilitate the patient who has recovered from illness and in whom the aim is to restore the premorbid physical status.

Protein

It was shown by Calloway & Spector (1954) that protein and energy interact to maintain nitrogen balance. They showed that when protein is limiting, an excess of energy does not improve retention of nitrogen. On the other hand, giving protein without significant energy was also ineffective in maintaining nitrogen balance. However, these studies were performed in normal subjects who were replete in body protein, and thus the results showed that both nitrogen and energy are required to maintain normal body nitrogen. In the human, the body cell mass is fixed in relation to the person's stature (Cahill et al 1972), so that in a normal subject there is little potential for long-term nitrogen gain through diet alone. The two ways in which long-term nitrogen retention can occur in normal subjects is the increase in muscle mass with exercise and/or the nitrogenous supporting structure occuring with deposition of adipose tissue. Is this true in malnourished patients?

In the malnourished subject the results are somewhat different. Let us consider the effects of an amino acid (AA) supplementation in depleted postoperative subjects given infusions of AA but insufficient calories. Greenberg et al (1976) randomized preoperative patients into four categories. One group received 5% dextrose alone providing 550 kcal/24 h; the other three groups received 1 g protein/kg/day. Among the protein-fed groups, one group received no additional calories, the second group received an additional 550 kcal as fat, and the third group received an additional 550 kcal as glucose. When nitrogen balances were compared, patients in all groups were in net negative nitrogen balance, but patients in the groups receiving 1 g protein/kg/day had half the negative nitrogen balance of those receiving only 5% dextrose without protein. When the substrate–hormone profiles were examined, the patients who were receiving 5% dextrose had high levels of lactate, pyruvate, and insulin, whereas the groups receiving fat or no additional non-protein energy substrate had high levels of FFA and ketones with lower levels of insulin. Despite these different hormone profiles, the nitrogen balance was determined not by the substrate–hormone profile but by the giving or the absence of nitrogen. Thus it became clear that the main effect of nitrogen was nitrogen-sparing irrespective of the substrate–hormone profile. To confirm this further, patients were studied in a crossover design in which they received either 1 or 2 g protein/kg/day. In this study, Greenberg & Jeejeebhoy (1979) showed that giving the higher amount of AA resulted in a net positive balance of nitrogen in contrast to the negative nitrogen balance with the lower intake. Hence, in postoperative malnourished patients, it was possible to maintain nitrogen balance or even induce a slight positive balance without the provision of added non-protein calories. This finding is in complete contrast to that obtained in subjects who were replete, but has been confirmed by other workers. Bozzetti (1976) and Elwyn (1979) showed in comparable patients a positive nitrogen balance in a situation that was energy deficient in relation to the requirements of the patient. Hill et al (1979) also showed that giving AA without calories maintained total body nitrogen in contrast to unfed controls who lost body nitrogen during the same period. Anderson et al (1974) have shown that the nitrogen requirement for balance in stable adults is only 0.8 g/kg/day. However, there was increased nitrogen retention with increasing intake and the gain was linear over a range of 0.25–2 g/kg/day. The administration of substantial amounts must be tempered by the fact that altered renal and/or hepatic function will reduce tolerance to AA loads. Considering these factors, it seems desirable generally to prescribe 1.0–1.5 g/kg ideal body weight/day of a balanced AA mixture.

Amino acid mixture

The next question concerns the AA profile of the mixture used for refeeding. Protein in human tissue is made up of 20 different AA, of which eight cannot be synthesized by the body and thus are termed essential. Two non-essential AA, arginine and histidine, may become essential under certain circumstances, such as in childhood or in patients with renal failure. Three of the essential AA, the branched-chain AA (BCAA) (leucine, isoleucine, valine), have biochemical properties that distinguish them from others. It was shown by Rose (1949) that for optimum nitrogen balance, AA have to be given in certain proportions and in specified minimal amounts. Mixtures with correct proportions have since been referred to as 'balanced'. Thus the quantity of protein needed to maintain nitrogen balance is dependent on the nutritional quality of the protein given and thus on the AA composition. If an AA mixture is deficient in an essential AA or if there is an imbalance in the essential AA, nitrogen balance is not achieved in experimental animals and in patients receiving parenteral nutrition (Patel et al 1973). It should be noted that AA solutions that contain only the essential AA are probably not as well utilized as more balanced solutions containing essential and non-essential AA (Anderson et al

1974). Leucine and its transaminated analogue, α-keto-isocaproic acid, appear to enhance protein synthesis and inhibit proteolysis (Buse & Reid 1975, Sherwin 1978, Li & Jefferson 1978). There are conflicting data on whether these actions of leucine can be used to improve nitrogen balance in patients with trauma and sepsis (Walser 1984, Hammarqvist et al 1988). At the present time, there is no demonstrated role for the BCAA-enriched solutions in patients with sepsis or injury (Freund et al 1978, Daly et al 1983, Bonau 1984). The efficiency of the branched-chain keto analogues in these patients remains to be demonstrated (Walser 1983).

Patients with renal failure

Predominance of essential AA has reduced azotemia in patients with renal failure. On the basis of this observation, considerable attention has been given to formulating an optimal AA solution for patients in acute renal failure in order to minimize the azotemia and avoid dialysis. A mixture containing only essential AA was shown to improve survival as compared with controls receiving glucose without reduction of the need for dialysis in patients in acute renal failure (Giordano 1963, Abel et al 1973, Saba et al 1983, Walser 1984). However, others have shown no difference between a balanced AA mixture and that containing only essential AA (Feinstein et al 1981).

Our current practice is first to place the patient on alternate day dialysis or ultrafiltration and then to give a balanced AA solution at 1 g/kg body weight/day in a regimen of full TPN. Only Na, K, Mg and P intakes are restricted, in order to maintain normal electrolyte levels. (See Chapter 40.)

Patients in hepatic failure

These patients have a perturbed plasma AA profile and disturbances of water and electrolytes balance. In chronic hepatic encephalopathy, low levels of BCAA are associated with elevated aromatic AA and tryptophan levels. This has led to the use of BCAA-enriched mixtures in such patients. Unfortunately, controlled trials have produced conflicting results. Briefly, BCAA have not consistently resulted in clinical and electroencephalographic improvement (Wahren et al 1983). In addition, when the use of BCAA-enriched solutions has been compared with the use of standard AA solutions, there has been no difference in mortality (Aubin et al 1983). As yet, BCAA-enriched mixtures cannot be considered to be of proven efficiency in patients with liver failure. (See Chapter 48.)

Energy

Basal energy expenditure (BEE) of a fasting subject is dependent on the weight, height, age and sex and can reasonably be predicted by the Harris–Benedict (1919) equation:

Men: kcal/24 h $= 66 + (13.7 \times W) + (5 \times H) - (6.8 \times A)$

Women: kcal/24 h $= 655 + (9.6 \times W) + (1.9 \times H) - (4.7 \times A)$

where W = weight in kg, H = height in cm and A = age in years. More recent WHO equations are given in Chapter 3.

The resting energy expenditure (REE) of the bed-ridden patient can be approximated by adding the specific dynamic activity of food (diet-induced thermogenesis) to the BEE. Alternatively, as suggested by Jéquier (1987), Kinney (1987) and Van Lanschot et al (1986), the REE can be approximated by increasing the BEE by 10%. Malnutrition reduces the BEE to an extent which may be as much as 35%. Physical activity, injury and sepsis, and especially burns, were believed to increase EE by about 30, 60 and 100%, respectively. However, this concept of marked hypermetabolism has been disproved (Askanazi et al 1980a, Roulet et al 1983, Baker et al 1984). In any case, an increase of even 60% in the BEE (about 20–25 kcal/kg/day) works out to be a requirement of only 40 kcal/kg/day or 2800 kcal/day in a 70 kg individual. Hence, there is no evidence for feeding 4000–6000 kcal to critically sick patients as had been previously recommended.

During the last decade, indirect calorimeters have become available for clinical use and have made it possible, at least in theory, to customize nutritional support to the patient's needs. Nevertheless, it has been found that using the Harris–Benedict equation and increasing it at most by 30% will meet the needs of most patients. Precise measurements at this time should be reserved for research studies.

Energy requirements may be calculated also on the basis of body weight. Clearly, these will be less accurate, but adequate in most clinical situations, except in cases of obesity or cachexia. Basal energy requirements can be taken to be about 20 kcal/kg body weight/day, ambulatory or stressed patients require about 25–30 kcal/kg body weight/day, up to a maximum of 35 kcal/kg body weight/day.

Sources of energy: glucose versus fat

The energy intake for restoration of body tissues is provided by carbohydrate and fat. In several refeeding studies, Munro (1964) has shown that surfeit feeding with carbohydrates and fat was equally effective in promoting nitrogen retention. However, Silwer (1937) showed that when dietary carbohydrate was isocalorically replaced by fat there was an initial phase of increased nitrogen excretion, which returned to that before the diet after a few days. This observation suggests that studies comparing the two substrates, carbohydrate and fat, in relation to their nitrogen-retaining properties, should be carried out for a sufficient time to re-establish equilibrium.

In a study using a crossover design for a period of time that exceeded the temporary effects of changing to one substrate from another, Jeejeebhoy et al (1976a,b) showed that the two substrates are comparable in their nitrogen-retaining properties. In this study, depleted patients with a variety of gastrointestinal diseases were given a constant intake of nitrogen in the form of casein hydrolysate together with approximately 60 g of carbohydrate. The patients received a total of 40 kcal/kg ideal body weight. The remaining calories were given either as glucose crossed over with fat or as fat crossed over with glucose. Each energy substrate was given for a period of a week at a time. When glucose was the sole source of energy there were increased plasma levels of lactate and pyruvate, with almost complete suppression of FFA and ketones. Correspondingly, the insulin levels were very high. When fat was the major substrate, the insulin levels were within the normal postprandial range, and the patients had high levels of FFA and ketones. Thus, there were two very different substrate–hormone profiles, each of which was unique to the energy source given. Despite these differences, it was noted that on days 5, 6 and 7 the nitrogen balances were comparable with either substrate.

There were some very interesting correlations (Jeejeebhoy et al 1976a,b) between insulin levels and nitrogen retention. In the subjects given fat as the major source of calories, the nitrogen retention was improved as the concentration of insulin in blood increased from 1.25 to 12.5 µU/ml. Above a concentration of 12.5 µU/ml, further increase in insulin levels did not improve nitrogen retention. Thus, it appears that while minimal amounts of insulin are essential for nitrogen retention, once postprandial levels are attained there is no further benefit from additional insulin. This conclusion has been supported by the findings of MacFie et al (1981), who showed that adding 30 U/l of insulin to parenteral nutrients did not increase the total body nitrogen.

Wolfe et al (1979) showed that when increasing amounts of glucose were infused into normal subjects, there was an increase in carbohydrate oxidation until the rates of infusion reached 4 mg/kg/min. Above this level a further increase in the rate of glucose infusion did not increase the proportion of total energy derived from glucose oxidation. In contrast, the glucose utilization rose linearly as more glucose was given to the subjects. Thus, it appears that glucose retention or glucose utilization may increase without an increase in glucose oxidation rate: at no state was it possible to increase the proportion of calories derived from glucose oxidation to a state exceeding 60%. There appears to be an upper limit to glucose oxidation even when all the calories are given as glucose (Wolfe et al 1979). The need of obligatory fat oxidation was further supported by the studies of Carpentier et al (1979), who showed that fat oxidation and fatty acid turnover continued even when the patients were receiving parenteral nutrition in which all the calorie requirements were met by infused glucose. This finding is supported by the observations of MacFie et al (1981) that the provision of fat calories results in a significant gain of total body nitrogen during TPN, not observed when glucose was the only source of calories. Furthermore, the excess glucose calories are converted to fat in the liver, resulting in hepatic steatosis which disappeared after glucose-only non-protein calories were replaced by a glucose–lipid mixture (Jeejeebhoy et al 1973). Moreover, provision of fat to patients receiving glucose-based TPN reduced the need for insulin (Baker et al 1984) and decreased the production of CO_2 (Askanazi et al 1980b).

In conclusion, malnourished patients receiving glucose-based or lipid-based TPN have shown equivalent nitrogen retention (Nordenström et al 1983, Baker et al 1984). By using a balanced glucose–lipid TPN, the complications associated with the administration of substantial amounts of glucose can be prevented. These include hepatic steatosis, CO_2 retention and essential fatty acid deficiency, hypo- or hyperglycaemia and the need to add insulin to the TPN regimen.

Electrolytes and micronutrients

Electrolytes

The importance of fluid and electrolytes for promoting tissue perfusion and ionic equilibrium is self-evident. Malnutrition is associated with major changes in electrolyte balance. With malnutrition there is a loss of the intracellular ions potassium, magnesium and phosphorus, together with a gain in sodium and water. A positive nitrogen balance during refeeding is achieved when these ions are supplied in sufficient

Table 29.1 Standard electrolyte recommendations (mmol/day) in parenteral and enteral nutrition

Sodium	100–120
Potassium	80–120
Calcium	8–10
Phosphorus	14–16
Magnesium	12–15

amount to be in balance (Rudman et al 1975, Freeman 1977). A positive balance of sodium and water may be seen during refeeding with carbohydrate (MacFie et al 1981). This process is referred to as 'refeeding oedema' and disappears concomitantly with improvement in the nutritional status. In malnourished patients, particularly elderly subjects and those with cardiopulmonary disease or renal insufficiency, refeeding has to be undertaken very carefully because of the risk of pulmonary oedema.

Recommendations for electrolyte supplementations are given in Table 29.1. They have to be altered to meet special needs such as in cardiac, renal and hepatic dysfunction.

Micronutrients

Micronutrients are essential for the proper utilization of protein, carbohydrate, fat and electrolytes. Vitamins, trace elements and essential fatty acids constitute the three major groups of micronutrients. Vitamins and trace elements are essential because they regulate metabolic processes in many different ways, either as co-enzymes or as elemental constituents of enzymes complexes, and so are vital for normal cellular activity. Essential fatty acids are required for prostaglandin synthesis.

Vitamins Vitamins are active in minute quantities. Actions and deficiencies are described in Table 29.2. Vitamins must be given with enteral and parenteral nutrition. Precise vitamin requirements during nutritional support are unknown. Water-soluble vitamins can be given liberally without apparent toxicity, but excesses of fat-soluble vitamins (notably A and D) are toxic. Thus, prolonged parenteral administration of vitamin D has been shown to enhance metabolic bone disease (Shike et al 1981) and has been associated with hypercalaemic pancreatitis, so we do not give this vitamin to our home TPN patients but rather recommend exposure to sunlight. Patients receiving prolonged enteral nutrition, as in the case of permanent coma, tetraplegia or major upper gastrointestinal dysfunction, have similar

Table 29.2 Vitamins: roles and clinical signs of deficiencies

Vitamin	Roles	Symptoms
B₁ (thiamin)	Coenzyme involved in the removal of carbon dioxide (α-ketoacids and glucose metabolism)	Beriberi, hypoglycaemia Blood acidosis
B₂ (riboflavin)	Constituent of flavin nucleotide coenzymes related to energy metabolism	Photophobia, glossitis, cheilosis, skin pruritus
B₆ (piridoxine)	Coenzyme related to amino acid metabolism	Dermatitis, intertrigo, seborrhea, irritability, somnolence, neuropathy
B₁₂ and folic acid	Nucleic acid and amino acid metabolisms	Megaloblastic anaemia, glossitis, diarrhoea, neuromyelopathy
C (ascorbic acid)	Maintenance of intercellular matrix of cartilage, bone and dentine Collagen synthesis Antioxidant	Scurvy
Biotin	Coenzyme related to fat synthesis, amino acid metabolism and glycogen formation	Fatigue, depression, dermatitis, myalgia
Choline	Constituent of phospholipids Precursor of neurotransmitter acetylcholine	Not reported
Niacin	Constituent of NAD and NADP related to reduction-oxidation reactions	Pellagra
Pantothenatic acid	Component of coenzyme A related to energy metabolism	Asthenia, paresthesia, mental problems, epigastric discomfort
A	Constituent of retinal pigment Maintenance of epithelium Infection defence	Xerophthalmia, night blindness, infection
D	Calcium absorption and deposition in bone	Osteomalacia
E (and selenium*)	Antioxidant preventing cell membrane lesions	Myalgia, cardiomyopathy
K	Blood clotting	Blood dyscrasia

*Trace element having a cross-action with vitamin E
See also Chapters 13 and 14

vitamin requirements to those receiving prolonged TPN. Patients with gastrointestinal diseases resulting in specific malabsorption or a loss of vitamins for a prolonged period of time should be given special prescriptions of vitamins after a clinical examination made to detect vitamin deficiencies.

General recommendations for parenteral and enteral intakes of vitamins are listed in Table 29.3.

Trace elements Iron, zinc, copper, chromium, selenium, iodine and cobalt as vitamin B₁₂ are considered to be the essential elements for humans. Iron and zinc deficiencies are especially common and

may develop more rapidly than for other elements. Clinical situations with increased requirements are frequent (iron in chronic bleeding; zinc in diarrhoea, gastrointestinal fistula, surgical drainage, hypermetabolism) and the normal requirements are clearly higher than for other trace elements.

General recommendations for parenteral intakes of trace elements are listed in Table 29.4.

Essential fatty acids The main essential fatty acid is linoleic acid. Linoleic acid is a precursor of arachidonic acid which is needed for prostaglandin synthesis. It has been shown that patients given fat-

Table 29.3 Standard vitamin recommendations in parenteral and enteral nutrition

Vitamin	Recommended dose
Water-soluble	
B$_1$ (thiamin)	5 mg/day
B$_2$ (riboflavin)	5 mg/day
Pantothenic acid	15 mg/day
Niacin	50 mg/day
B$_6$ (pyridoxine)	5 mg/day
Folic acid	0.6 mg/day
C (ascorbic acid)	300 mg/day
Biotin	None (?)
B$_{12}$	12 µg/day
Fat-soluble	
A	Home TPN: 2500 IU/day
D	Home TPN: none added
	Hospital TPN: 400 IU/day
E	50 IU/day*
K	10 mg/week

*Fat emulsions contain vitamin E in different amount (i.e. 35 IU in 1 litre of "Nutralipid ®")

Table 29.4 Standard trace element recommendations in parenteral and enteral nutrition

Element	Recommended dose
Iron	
Men	1 mg/day
Women	Pre-menopausal: 2 mg/day
	Post-menopausal: 1 mg/day
Zinc	2.2 mg/day + 12.2 mg/1 small bowel fluid loss + 17.1 mg/1 stool loss
Copper	300 µg/day
	None with severe liver disease
Chromium	20 µg/day
Selenium	120 µg/day
Iodine	120 µg/day
Molybdenum	20 µg/day
Manganese	700 µg/day
	None with severe liver disease

free TPN develop biochemical evidence of essential fatty acid deficiency within 2 weeks (Goodgame et al 1978) without any change in linoleic acid stores (12% of total fatty acids). Deficiency develops rapidly because of suppressed lipolysis resulting from the high insulin level secondary to the glucose infusion (Wene et al 1975). Clinical deficiency can be avoided by giving 2–4% of total calories as linoleic acid.

NUTRITIONAL SUPPORT

The rational use of nutritional support depends on the identification of malnutrition or the potential for malnutrition, definition of the risks of malnutrition and demonstration of the reversal of such risks by nutritional support. Nutritional support in hospital should be based on the history of the patient's food intake, his present nutritional state and his ability to metabolize nutrients. Clinical nutrition consists of a spectrum of approaches which should be integrated, proceeding from a normal oral diet to parenteral nutrition and vice versa until the patient is discharged. The programme should be initiated on admission of the patient and modified according to the clinical course. Normal or modified oral diet should be used whenever possible and the nutrient intake and tolerance should be monitored. However, if oral intake is consistently poor, enteral feeding should be started. If there is intolerance to enteral feeding or if the gut is not functional, TPN should be given. The critical role of a dietitian on site needs to be emphasized in this context.

Nutritional assessment

Advanced malnutrition is easy to recognize but early malnutrition is difficult to define clinically, especially with a view to initiating nutritional support before the occurrence of complications. The nutritional status can be assessed by a variety of methods. The widely applied traditional methods rely heavily on objective anthropometric measurements and laboratory tests (Table 29.5). Their lack of specificity, in relation to their ability to predict a clinically significant adverse effect, may lead to an erroneous conclusion. These measurements provide more information about body composition than outcome, which is the clinically significant event. A practical way of assessing the risks of malnutrition is to evaluate the patient at the bedside – subjective global assessment (SGA) (Table 29.6). This technique was found to be reproducible,

Table 29.5 Objective parameters for nutritional assessment

Anthropometry (age, sex, weight, height, skin-fold thickness, arm muscle circumference)
Body composition (creatinine–height index, 3-methylhistidine excretion, total body nitrogen and potassium, total body water)
Hepatic secretory proteins levels (albumin, pre-albumin, transferrin, retinol-binding protein, thyroxine-binding protein)
Immunological tests (delayed cutaneous hypersensitivity)
Combination of above (as in the prognostic nutritional index)
Physiological methods (muscle function, dynamometry)

Table 29.6 Methodology for subjective global assessment (SGA)

History	Physical examination
Weight change	Loss of subcutaneous fat
overall loss in past 6 months	Muscle wasting
in kg and in % loss	Ankle oedema
change in past 2 weeks in kg	Sacral oedema
Dietary intake change	Ascites
duration in weeks, gradation	
from none to starvation	
Gastrointestinal symptoms that	*SGA rating*
have persisted for > 2 weeks	Well nourished
none, nausea, vomiting,	Mildly malnourished
diarrhoea, anorexia	Severely malnourished
Functional capacity	
optimal, duration and	
dysfunction, type (working,	
ambulatory, bedridden)	
Disease and its relation to	
nutritional requirements,	
primary diagnosis, metabolic	
demand (none to high stress)	

and predictive of adverse clinical events (Baker et al 1982). The assessment is a composite evaluation of the ability to eat, disease stress, functional impairment and clinical wasting. The benefits of SGA are that it can be performed anywhere, clinical judgement being the only tool required, and the expense involved is that of the examiner's time. We believe that in the usual hospital setting, good clinical judgment is the best available method for assessing nutritional status.

Selection of patients and routes of nutrition

Enteral nutrition

All patients unable to meet nutritional requirements by eating a normal diet are candidates for enteral nutrition (EN). The clinician and the nutritionist should together set a target for the patient's nutrient requirements. After a limited trial period, if nutrient intake is insufficient, nutritional support should be given. In the following situations oral intake is often insufficient even in the presence of a usable gastrointestinal tract, and nasogastric or nasointestinal tube feeding is required:

— severe systemic illness
— anorexia
— neurologic impairment preventing oral feeding
— increased requirements with relative anorexia (e.g. burned patients)
— chronic obstructive lung disease with severe dyspnea or pharyngeal surgery.

Enteral feeding is useful in diseases of the oesophagus, stomach or pancreas, short bowel with more than 60 cm of small intestine available, inflammatory bowel disease, chronic partial bowel obstruction and postoperative reduced bowel motility; tolerance can be promoted and success of enteral feeding assured by delivering diets carefully with the aid of a pump to avoid a surge of nutrient, consequent bowel distension and interruption of feeding (Pichard & Roulet 1984). For inflammatory bowel disease, a greater efficiency has been claimed for an elemental diet (O'Morain et al 1984, Saverymuttu et al 1985), but another trial suggests that remission with a polymeric diet is as good as with TPN (Greenberg et al 1985). A proportion of patients fed by EN will show intolerance and complications. When EN fails or cannot be used for the reasons given below, then TPN must be used.

Parenteral nutrition

The use of this expensive nutritional support became controversial because of conflicting conclusions as to whether or not it alters the patient's outcome (Koretz 1984). However, it has been shown that TPN has positively influenced rehabilitation and morbidity after surgery (Young et al 1979, Bastow et al 1983).

It is clear that TPN is essential in the presence of prolonged bowel obstruction and in patients with extended intestinal resection. In patients with acute pancreatitis and those with high output fistula, TPN is often necessary. In these situations, enteral feeding will not be tolerated and may even aggravate the clinical problem. On the other hand, TPN is a pragmatic approach for the clinical conditions listed below, where TPN should be started to save time and EN instituted if possible. A 'die hard' approach only aggravates patient malnutrition and causes an increase in discomfort.

Starving patients intolerant to enteral nutrition In patients in the intensive care unit (ICU) who are intolerant to enteral feeding, especially those who have starved for a week or more as well those who at the outset are malnourished, TPN is indicated.

Gastrointestinal symptoms compromising oral feeding Critical illness is often associated with gastrointestinal motility disorders, making it impossible to give sufficient enteral feeds because of nausea, vomiting, diarrhoea or bloating. Within this group are patients who, because of chemo- or radiotherapy, are constantly nauseated and unable to eat.

In several GI disorders, symptoms worsen with oral feeding. For example, pain related to acute pancreatitis will be increased by oral feeding. In patients with high small bowel fistula, the output will increase and the fistula will open if oral feeding is undertaken. It is believed, but not demonstrated, that TPN may promote fistula closure. It is also thought that bowel rest, by precluding oral intake, may aid the resolution of Crohn's disease, although controlled trials have not shown this to be the case (Greenberg & Jeejeebhoy 1979, Dickenson et al 1980). It is difficult to believe that bowel 'rest' occurs in the fasting patients because of the existence of migratory myoelectric complexes.

Cancer   Malnutrition in cancer has been considered as an indication for TPN but controlled trials have failed to demonstrate its utility (Shike et al 1984). In cases of cancer producing malnutrition by obstructing the bowel, nutrition appears to be beneficial and the indications for TPN are the same as those for starving patients who cannot be fed enterally and for those with gastrointestinal symptoms that preclude oral feeding.

Renal and hepatic diseases   The parenteral route should be used if the gastrointestinal tract is non-functional and nutrient intake modified because of the metabolic abnormalities of liver and renal diseases. Patients on chronic haemodialysis have high infection potential and if they require TPN (as after major surgery), special attention should be given to avoid infection related to the catheter.

Patients with immunodeficiency or immunosuppression   Severely ill patients and patients receiving chemo- or radiotherapy are mostly anergic. When enteral feeding is not possible, TPN should be routinely used. Nevertheless, in immunosuppressed patients undergoing major surgery for organ transplantation, if TPN is only needed for less than a week, the associated risk of infection should be considered against the beneficial effect of nutrition.

Techniques of administration

Enteral nutrition

The principle of administering nutrients through a nasogastric or nasoenteral tube is to infuse the nutrient at a rate that corresponds to the absorptive capacity of the gastrointestinal tract. The stomach normally releases a constant number of calories into the intestine – about 150 kcal/h. The osmolarity is not of as much concern as the rate at which calories are infused. This is particularly true in patients with a short bowel. To ensure a steady flow of nutrients, nasoenteral rather than nasogastric feeding should be used in patients with a short bowel, gastric stasis or severe systemic illness where gastric stasis is likely,

and in those receiving opiate analgesics. If gastric emptying is erratic, releasing gushes of highly osmolar fluid into the intestine, diarrhoea will occur.

Insertion of nasogastric or nasoenteral tubes

Introduction of nasogastric and nasoenteral tubes   The nasogastric and nasoenteral tubes vary in size from 5 to 8 Fr. They are made of silicone or polyurethane, are 80–110 cm long, are weighted at the end with mercury or tungsten ball, and have a lubricated stylet for introduction.

Before the tube's introduction, the patient should lie on his left side or be seated if possible. The tube is inserted through a nostril, advanced through the pharynx and oesophagus for about 50 cm and positioned close to the pylorus.

In patients with gastric stasis, the tube is passed into the duodenum under fluoroscopy or with the aid of a gastroscope. The tube is advanced with the stylet, then the gastroscope and finally the stylet are withdrawn.

Operative insertion of feeding tube   Cervical pharyngostomy has limited usefulness, but the tube can be inserted during neck dissection. The tube is comfortable and can be kept in place for long periods. Percutaneous gastrostomy has now been shown to be useful for long-term enteral feeding. In brief, a gastroscope is passed and, after transilluminating the stomach, a catheter is inserted transabdominally through an anaesthetized area. This route of feeding avoids nasal irritation and oesophageal ulcer. Needle catheter jejunostomy has also been used but requires surgery. The details of the technique have been described by Delany (1980). In essence, an intramural anti-reflux tunnel is created in the jejunal wall with a 14G needle through which a 16G polyurethane catheter is inserted and the other end pulled through the abdominal wall. The jejunum wall is anchored to the abdominal wall. This technique is useful after surgical procedures where it is anticipated that the patient may not be able to eat for a prolonged period.

Selection of feeding mixture   The feeding mixtures used for enteral feeding can be classified with regard to their composition into the following categories:

1. *Polymeric diets* are composed of whole proteins, oils and corn syrup or sucrose to provide proteins, fats and carbohydrates. They are subdivided into the following categories: 'Blenderized formulae' are composed of whole foods blended into a liquid consistency; 'Lactose-containing milk-based diets',

which cannot be given to lactose-intolerant patients, but are the most palatable and can be taken orally as a supplement; 'lactose-free formulae', some of which are also palatable and which can be given to lactose-intolerant patients. Polymeric diets are suitable for most clinical situations.

2. *Defined formula or elemental diets* are composed of amino acids or short-chain peptides and oligosaccharides or monosaccharides. Fat is present as long- or medium-chain triglyceride oils. Because of their unpleasant taste, these diets must be administered by tube feeding. Their advantage is their good absorbability, which may be useful in cases of a very short bowel or in patients with pancreatic insufficiency.

3. *Modular diets* are composed of separate modules of protein, fat, carbohydrate, electrolytes and trace elements. Because they can be combined in different ratios, they are valuable for feeding patients with specific needs.

Infusion of nutrients   Use of a so-called starter regimen, where the patients is started on diluted diets has been shown to be unnecessary (Keoane et al 1984). While in patients without gastrointestinal disease, full feeding can be undertaken from the first day, this may not be applicable in patients with certain gastrointestinal diseases. In such patients, we start with full-strength feeding, given slowly (25 ml/h) with careful monitoring of the gastric emptying over the first 8 h. Then, the rate is increased rapidly to 125 ml/h over 3 days. Pumps will ensure trouble-free enteral feeding in general, but are mandatory for ventilated patients in the CU and in cases of bowel disease. Pumps are not essential in other situations. Contamination of the diets may be avoided by using prepacked sterile diets and by restricting the bag infusion to a maximum of 8 h.

Parenteral nutrition

Parenteral nutrition requires continuous infusion of hypertonic fluids, which are only tolerated when infused into large veins such as the superior vena cava (SVC) where the rapid blood flow dilutes the incoming hypertonic fluid. It is crucial to position the catheter down into the SVC to avoid venous thrombosis. We usually use a 16 G catheter, made of urethane treated with an hydromer, inserted through a 14 G cannula. For long-term infusions we prefer a Hickman type silicone rubber catheter.

Catheter insertion   Catheters placed in the SVC are less likely to cause infection than when inserted in

other sites. Our preferred route is via an infraclavicular percutaneous puncture because of the reduced sepsis and thrombosis rates, ease of fixation and care. Complications, such as pneumothorax, may occur with this type of insertion but can be limited by employing experienced operators. It is critical that catheter insertion be done with full aseptic precautions. We recommend the following procedure:

1. The operator puts on mask, cap and gloves after hand washing.

2. The patient is placed in a slight Trendelenburg position (10°) with a rolled towel between the shoulder blades to position the shoulders backwards.

3. The skin over the neck, clavicle and chest up to the costal margins is disinfected according to accepted surgical practice.

4. A 26 G needle containing 1% Xylocaine is used to raise a 2 cm diameter skin weal, 1 cm below and 1 cm medial to the middle of the clavicle. A long 22 G needle is used to anaesthetize the subcutaneous tissue, muscle and fascia, as well as the periosteum of the clavicle, with the needle passing towards a finger placed in the suprasternal notch as a landmark. To avoid injuring the pleura, subclavian artery and the brachial plexus, the needle should scrape just under the clavicle and should not be inclined more than 10° posteriorly. If inserted correctly, the needle will often enter the vein and a gush of blood will flow.

5. The 14 G needle with the cannula is inserted in the same direction until the subclavian vein is entered. The needle is withdrawn and the 16 G catheter inserted. It should go smoothly. Then a 500 ml bag of normal saline connected to an i.v. infusion set is connected. By lowering the bag, free backward flow of blood should occur and by raising the bag saline should drip rapidly. If there is pain on advancing the catheter, difficulty in advancing or lack of blood flow, then it should be withdrawn and reinserted.

6. The catheter is properly secured and normal saline is allowed to flow slowly. We place a small gauze coated with povidone–iodine ointment over the site of exit and cover the exit site with an Op-Site film. This is a plastic film which is hypoallergenic and waterproof.

7. The patient is transported to Radiology and a posterior angiogram and lateral chest X-ray taken to demonstrate that the catheter tip is in the SVC, lying just above the atrium. If the tip is high, thrombosis of the central veins may occur. If it is too low then arrhythmias may occur due to atrial irritation.

Nutrition prescription   The requirements should be calculated on the basis of the requirements given above and the prescription sent to the pharmacy. The solutions are sent to the ward ready mixed in plastic bags and the lipid in bottles. There is an increasing tendency to provide all nutrients including the lipid in a 3-in-1 mixture in a 3 litre plastic bag. The mixture is stable for 24 h. Instability may be due to excessive quantities of divalent cations, Ca, Mg and Zn.

Technique of administration   We administer the amino acid–dextrose–electrolyte–trace element mixture with the lipid running in concurrently through a Y connector. This allows the simultaneous infusion of glucose and fat calories, making hyperglycaemia less likely. We do not use pumps but if desired a pump can be used to control the delivery of these solutions. If only one pump is to be used, it should be attached to the tube carrying the amino acid–dextrose mixture as the control of flow for the lipid is not as critical. Alternatively, a 3-in-1 mixture can be used.

Catheter care and tubing change   The dressing around the catheter exit site should be changed at least once a week and more often if the dressing becomes non-occlusive, or there is sweating or skin infection. Women with dry hairless skin need the least frequent changes and hairy men with oily skin require frequent changes. The nurse puts on a mask and gloves after hand washing. Then the old dressing is removed and the exit site inspected for infection. If there is exudation, then a culture is taken and a Gram smear done. If pus cells and bacteria are seen, we prefer to give systemic antibiotics. The skin and exit site are cleaned when the dressing is changed and the connecting tubing is changed every 48 h.

Monitoring

Dedicated nurses are essential to the operation of any successful nutrition programme. They not only provide a liaison between the nutritional service and the ward nurses, but also improve the patient's outcome (Keoane 1984). The nutritional team provides explanations to the ward nurses as well to the patient about the technical aspects of nutrition.

General monitoring includes daily weight, vital signs, daily input and output, and urine testing every 6–8 h for glucose. Blood tests should be done at least twice per week and include haemoglobin, white blood cell count, electrolytes, glucose, urea and creatinine. Weekly blood tests are albumin, iron, iron-binding capacity, calcium, magnesium, phosphorus, triglycerides, cholesterol, alanine aminotransferase, serum glutamic-pyruvic transferase or aspartate aminotrans-

ferase, glutamic-oxaloacetate transaminase, alkaline phosphatase and bilirubin. The above tests should be repeated if the patient is unstable and requires modification of the feeding mixture or needs drug therapy.

Clinical monitoring includes looking for evidence of catheter or systemic sepsis by examining, and if necessary, culturing the catheter sites and performing blood and urine cultures whenever sepsis is suspected. Mouth care is important to prevent inflammation of the mucosal surfaces secondary to dryness.

Complications

Enteral nutrition

Misplaced tube   This problem is avoided by taking an X-ray prior to infusion in all cases. If misplaced, then serious problems can arise by infusing nutrients into a bronchus or peritoneum. With jejunostomy and gastrostomy tubes it is necessary to check displacement from the bowel into the peritoneum.

Gastric retention and aspiration   This problem is avoided by nasoenteral feeding instead of nasogastric feeding of critically sick patients. If gastric feeding is used, then residuals should be checked and if above 150 ml, then infusion is resumed at half the rate and the residue determined every 4 h. Intravenous metoclopramide may help gastric motility. To decrease risk of aspiration the patient can be fed with the head raised to 30° and a check made for gastric residuals.

Diarrhoea, nausea, vomiting and cramps   Factors that can cause diarrhoea and gastrointestinal discomfort during EN, and measures to correct them, are as noted below:

— Lack of sodium in the feed. Add sodium.
— Uncontrolled flow into the intestine. Use pump to regulate flow.
— Bacterial contamination. Change bags and sets every 24 h. Reduce interval to 8 h. Use aseptic preparation of feeds.
— Infusing ice-cold feeds. Warm to room temperature before feeding.
— Broad-spectrum antibiotic administration. Review use of antibiotics and culture stools for *Clostridium difficile* and test for its toxin.
— Intercurrent gastrointestinal problem. Examine patient for gastrointestinal disease.

Electrolyte disturbance   Hypernatraemia, hyperchloraemia and dehydration are caused by osmotic diarrhoea secondary to malabsorption. This should be evaluated and the rate of infusion adjusted. Also, water requirements should be assessed and deficits replaced.

Metabolic complications. These are the same as with TPN (see below).

Parenteral nutrition

The number of complications related to parenteral nutrition may be divided into technical, septic and metabolic. Proper patient monitoring, good observation and good aseptic technique may prevent most complications.

Technical complications related to catheter insertion Pneumothorax is the most common complication of catheter insertion. Usually a pneumothorax will be diagnosed by the chest X-ray taken following catheter insertion. The size of the pneumothorax can be documented by chest X-rays repeated at 24 or 48 h and treated if necessary. If the catheter is in the correct position within the SVC and if the pneumothorax is treated, there is no necessity for catheter removal.

Injury to the subclavian artery with resultant external bleeding can be treated by removing the needle and/or catheter and applying direct pressure. The radial and ulnar pulses on the injured side should be checked frequently. Laceration of a major vein should be controlled by direct pressure. If the tip of the catheter lacerates the vein and terminates in the pleural space, infusion of fluid will quickly produce chest pain, dyspnea and possibly shock. A chest X-ray and aspiration of the chest will confirm this diagnosis. This complication can be avoided if the intravenous infusion bottle or bag is lowered following catheter insertion, to observe reflux of blood. Treatment should include discontinuing the infusion immediately, removing the catheter and monitoring the pleural space by a thoracostomy tube if necessary. Nerve damage reflected by radial, ulnar or median nerve signs can be treated simply by removing the catheter.

Injury to the thoracic duct from a left subclavian catheter is rare and manifests itself by lymph drainage from the insertion site. Treatment involves removal of the catheter. Chylothorax has been reported and should be treated by evacuation and aspiration of the pleural space until lymphatic drainage ceases. Insertion of a catheter into the mediastinum is rare and may result in the production of a mediastinal haematoma. This could cause compression of the SVC and requires emergency surgery to evacuate the haematoma and relieve the obstruction.

Air embolism can occur at the time of catheter insertion when the syringe is removed prior to threading of the catheter. It can be avoided by getting the patient to perform a Valsalva manoeuver during this step in the technique. Catheter embolism is rare and due to pulling back on the catheter and adjusting its position while the needle is still in the vein. The catheter is sheared off against the bevelled tip of the needle and lodges in the vein. The treatment of choice for a catheter embolus is transvenous removal with a guidewire snare technique performed under image intensification in the cardiac catheterization unit.

Malposition of the catheter is observed when the tip is not low down in the SVC. Cardiac arrhythmias may occur if the catheter is positioned within the right atrium or ventricle. In any other location infusion of hypertonic solutions can cause thrombophlebitis. If malposition occurs it should be corrected by repositioning under fluoroscopic control. If this is not possible, the catheter should be removed, the absence of pneumothorax checked by an X-ray and only then a new catheter inserted on the contralateral side.

Complications related to the catheter maintenance If the catheter becomes clotted, an attempt should be made to unplug it. A 1 ml syringe containing sterile normal saline is attached to the hub of the catheter and an attempt made to loosen the clot by irrigation. If this fails, the clotted catheter should be unplugged by instilling urokinase which will dissolve the fibrin. The technique consists of dissolving 7500 IU of urokinase in 3 ml of normal saline and injecting as much of it as will go into the catheter. Then the catheter is capped for 3 h and flushed with a mixture of 10 ml saline containing 1000 U of heparin.

Thrombosis of the SVC and its main tributaries can occur anytime during parenteral nutrition. The usual cause is malposition of the catheter and resultant phlebothrombosis and thrombophlebitis. This complication usually requires the infusion of urokinase and the use of anticoagulants.

Thrombi can also occur at the tip of the catheter. Catheter thrombosis and sepsis are closely related complications of indwelling Silastic catheters. Glynn et al (1980) described a procedure by which thrombi are dispersed with urokinase while the permanent Silastic catheter remains in situ. Urokinase was successful in clearing the catheter in all 20 patients. The concomitant use of antibiotics cleared the sepsis. The procedure resulted in no detectable firbinolysis or other complications.

Air embolism can occur as a late complication if the intravenous line inadvertently becomes detached from the catheter or if the catheter itself is inadvertently removed. The patient is usually found collapsed with the intravenous line detached from the catheter. The catheter must be immediately clamped and the patient place in the Trendelenburg position with the right side up. This positioning is crucial to prevent air obstructing the pulmonary artery.

Septic complications Catheter sepsis can be defined as an episode of clinical sepsis in a patient receiving short- or long-term TPN that resolves after removal of the catheter. Confirmatory evidence includes a positive culture of blood or of removed catheter tip. Its incidence varies from 2% to 7%, depending on the care given to the catheter.

Sepsis is a serious complication of TPN and patients receiving this therapy are susceptible to infection for various reasons. If a fever develops during the administration of TPN, a close examination for focal sources must be carried out. In particular, injection abscesses, phlebitis, chest infection, urinary tract infection and abdominal sepsis should be considered. The fever may also be associated with allergic reactions to the nutrients, an infected central venous line, contaminated fluid, or tubing.

The most common organism involved in catheter sepsis is *Staphylococcus epidermidis*. Less frequently, coliform and enteric organisms and fungi are found. Factors that may contribute to catheter sepsis include poor technique in catheter insertion, lack of adherence to post-insertion protocol, duration of catheterization and patient population. Certain patients are at greater risk for catheter sepsis than others, including anergic patients, those receiving steroids, those with acute pancreatitis and those with severe inflammatory bowel disease. The most common portals of infection are those around the entrance site or the hub connection of the catheter.

A low-grade fever in the absence of any other fever source should alert the physician to the possibility of catheter sepsis. A fever spike to 39°C or above might also occur. If catheter sepsis is suspected and other sources of fever have been ruled out, the TPN should be discontinued and the infusate and tubing sent for culture. Maintenance intravenous fluids should be substituted. Peripheral blood cultures and retrograde cultures through the catheter are obtained. The exit site of the catheter is swabbed and cultured. Routine cultures of urine, sputum, mouth and drainage sites are also obtained. If the blood cultures are positive or if the fever continues, the temporary subclavian catheter should be changed over a guide wire. If despite this the fever continues, then the catheter is removed and reinserted after the fever has subsided for 48 h. If the blood cultures are negative and the temperature returns to normal, The Toronto General Hospital policy is to resume TPN through the same line after 48 h. Sepsis related to a permanent Silastic line has been successfully treated without removal of the catheter in 66% of cases. In this situation, urokinase is used as described above for clotted catheters, and antibiotics are given daily for 4 weeks. If the sepsis is not controlled or fever returns, the catheter must be removed.

However, in certain circumstances fever and positive blood cultures will persist. In this situation, antibiotics are used, and the catheter should *not* be reinserted for at least 48 h after the temperature has returned to normal levels. Patients with established and persistent fungemia should be treated appropriately with intravenous amphotericin B over a 4- to 6-week period depending on the total dose given.

Metabolic complications Hyperglycaemia will occur when the rate of infusion exceeds the rate at which the body can metabolize glucose. It may be caused by too rapid infusion of dextrose or by metabolic complications. The ability to utilize glucose may be decreased by trauma and sepsis. It should be noted that the sudden appearance of hyperglycaemia in a patient who was previously euglycaemic usually heralds an infection. Hyperglycaemia may also appear under the following conditions: diabetes, pancreatitis, liver disease, some antibiotics (cephalosporins) and steroids. Associated with hyperglycaemia, glucosuria usually (2+ or more Clinitest®) occurs. If glucosuria continues, it will lead to the development of osmotic diuresis, followed by hyperosmolar non-ketotic acidosis and possibly death. The patient should be watched carefully for glucose intolerance and if glucosuria, dry skin, oliguria, confusion or lethargy are noted, the nurse should be instructed to call the clinician. If hyperglycaemia persists due to continuing glucose intolerance, the blood glucose levels should be measured regularly and exogenous insulin may be infused or the flow rate decreased. Where insulin needs to be given, it is most economically given by a constant infusion for several reasons. If the patient is acutely sick (poor peripheral circulation), then intravenous infusion is the only way to ensure that injected insulin is available to the body. The intravenous route allows careful control of blood sugar in the unstable patient and the need for insulin by infusion is lower than with intermittent dosing.

Hypoglycaemia is less common, but may occur if hypertonic glucose is abruptly terminated or decreased. Symptoms include weakness, trembling, diaphoresis, headache, chills, rapid pulse and decreased consciousness. Attention to ensuring a constant flow of hypertonic glucose infusions will prevent hypoglycaemia from occurring. If the volume infused falls behind schedule, the rate should not be increased to 'catch up'. Instead it should be recalculated in order to infuse at a uniform rate the prescribed amount of solution over the remainder of the 24 h, provided this rate does not exceed the original drip rate by more than 10%.

Electrolyte imbalance due to deficiency of potassium, phosphorus and magnesium may occur. They are aggravated by active protein synthesis and cellular uptake of the above ions. Careful monitoring of laboratory values and the general condition of the patient, i.e. urine output, heart rate, etc., will help to detect deficiencies and excesses. These should be corrected immediately, usually through a change in the TPN prescription.

Trace element and vitamin deficiencies can be avoided by daily supplementation and should be added to the TPN, since stores are depleted in malnourished patients. Fat-soluble vitamins should be carefully controlled; excessive intake of vitamins A and D can cause toxic effects, especially hypercalcaemia. Hyperlipidaemia may occur as a result of overproduction of lipids from endogenous sources, over infusion of exogenous lipids, or reduced utilization. Combinations of these factors may also be observed. The overproduction of lipids causing hyperlipidaemia may result from infusing carbohydrates in excess of needs. Correspondingly, excessively high infusion rates of lipid emulsions may also cause hyperlipidaemia. Under these circumstances, reducing total caloric intake, both the carbohydrate and lipid moieties, can restore blood lipid levels to normal. Even with an appropriate caloric intake, however, a deficiency of lipoprotein lipase, as with the syndrome of Type I hyperlipoproteinaemia, may impair lipid clearance. This may occur also with severe protein deficiency and diabetes.

Hypercholesterolaemia may be seen when lipid emulsions are infused at high rates, i.e. in excess of 2 g/kg/day. The rise is temporary and the level of plasma cholesterol returns to normal within a few days of discontinuing the infusion.

Abnormalities of liver function, such as a slight rise in the level of alkaline phosphatase, are very common and generally return to normal without clinical consequences. Fatty liver is a common problem due to the infusion of carbohydrate in excess of caloric needs or in rare cases of essential fatty acid deficiency. Clinically the patient presents with a large tender liver and an elevation of serum glutamic-oxaloacetic transaminase.

The other hepatic clinical syndrome seen with TPN is cholestatic jaundice, with elevated serum bilirubin and alkaline phosphatase. This syndrome occurs commonly in children and bears a relation to the duration of TPN. However, it is not seen frequently in home TPN patients despite the fact that they have been receiving TPN for years. Hence the condition does not result simply from prolonged TPN, but is probably due to a combination of prolonged TPN and acute illness. This concept of a combination of factors causing cholestasis is supported by the observation that the condition is largely seen in sick hospital patients, rather than in relatively well patients receiving home TPN. One such factor may be sepsis since jaundice is most often seen clinically in adults who become septic or those with foci of infection. When pancreatitis is seen in association with TPN, potentially it may be due to either hypercalcaemia or hyperlipidaemia. However, in practice we have identified the former as being the main cause of pancreatitis.

Essential fatty acid deficiency is manifest by dry scaly skin and hair loss. This can be prevented or corrected with administration of an intravenous fat emulsion. When lipid is used as a source of calories, this deficiency is never seen.

ACKNOWLEDGMENTS

This work has been supported by the Fond National Suisse pour la Recherche Scientifique, Berne, Switzerland, and the Société pour l'Encouragement de la Recherche sur la Nutrition en Suisse, Lausanne, Switzerland.

REFERENCES

Abel RM, Beck CH, Abott WM 1973 Improved survival from acute renal failure after treatment with intravenous essential L-amino acids and glucose. New England Journal of Medicine 299: 685–699

Anderson GH, Patel DC, Jeejeebhoy KN 1974 Design and evaluation by nitrogen balance and blood aminograms of an amino acid mixture for total parenteral nutrition of adults with gastrointestinal disease. Journal of Clinical Investigation 53: 904–912

Askanazi J, Carpentier YA, Elwyn DH et al 1980a Influence of total parenteral nutrition on fuel utilization in injury and sepsis. Annals of Surgery 191: 40–46

Askanazi J, Elwyn DH, Silverberg BS et al 1980b Respiratory distress syndrome secondary to a high carbohydrate load: A case report. Surgery 87: 596–598

Aubin JP, Pomier-Layrargues G, Boris P 1983 Traitement de l'encéphalopathie hépatique du orrhotique par dessolutions conventionnelles ou modifiées d'acides aminés. Gastroenterologie Clinique et Biologique 7: 209–211

Baker JP, Detsky AS, Wessen DE et al 1982 Nutritional assessment: A comparison of clinical judgment and objective measurements. New England Journal of Medicine 306: 969–972

Baker JP, Detsky AS, Stewart S et al 1984 Randomized trial of total parenteral nutrition in critically ill patients: Metabolic effects of varying glucose–lipid ratios as the energy-source. Gastroenterology 87: 53–59

Bastow MD, Rawlings J, Allison SP 1983 Benefits of supplementary tube feeding after fractures of the neck of femur. British Medical Journal 287: 1589–1607

Bellinghieri G, Savica V, Mallamace A 1983 Correlation between increased serum and tissue L-carnitine levels and improved muscle symptoms in hemodialyzed patients. American Journal of Clinical Nutrition 38: 523–531

Bonau RA, Ang SD, Jeevanandam M, Daly JM 1984 Branched chain amino acid solutions: relationship to composition to efficacy. Journal of Parenteral and Enteral Nutrition 8: 622–627

Bozzetti F 1976 Parenteral nutrition in surgical patients. Surgery in Gynecology and Obstetrics 142: 16–20

Brennan MF 1979 Metabolic response to surgery in the cancer patient. Cancer 43: 2053–2064

Brough W, Horne G, Blount A, Irving MH, Jeejeebhoy KN 1986 Effects of nutrient intake, surgery, sepsis, trauma and long-term adminstration of steroid on muscle function. British Medical Journal 293: 983–986

Buse MG, Reid M 1975 Leucine, a possible regulator of protein turnover in muscle. Journal of Clinical Investigation 58: 1251–1261

Cahill GF, Aoki TT, Marliss EB 1972 In: Steiner DF, Freinkel N (eds) Handbook of physiology. American Physiological Society, Washington, DC, pp. 563–577

Calloway DH, Spector H 1954 Nitrogen balance as related to calorie and protein intake in active young men. American Journal of Clinical Nutrition 2: 405–415

Carpentier YA, Askanazi, J, Elwyn DH et al 1979 Effects of hypercaloric glucose infusion on lipid metabolism in injury and sepsis. Journal of Trauma 19: 649–654

Champault G, Patel JC 1979 Le risque infectieux en chirurgie digestive. Chirurgie 105: 751–768

Chan STF 1986 Muscle power after glucose–potassium loading in undernourished patients. British Medical Journal 293: 1055–1056

Clowes GHA, Georges BC, Villee CA Saravis CA 1983 Muscle proteolysis induced by a circulating peptide in patients with sepsis and trauma. New England Journal of Medicine 308: 545–552

Cuthbertson P 1932 Observations on disturbances of metabolism produced by injury to limbs. Quarterly Journal of Medicine 25: 233–246

Cuthbertson DP 1979 The metabolic response to injury and its nutritional implications: retrospect and prospect. Journal of Parenteral and Enteral Nutrition 3: 108–129

Daly JM, Mihranin MH, Kehoe JE, Brennan MF 1983 Effects of postoperative infusion of branched chain amino acids on nitrogen balance and forearm muscle substrate flux. Surgery 94: 151–158

Delany HM 1980 An improved technique for needle catheter jejunostomy. Annals of Surgery 115: 1235–1240

Detsky AS, McLaughin JR, Baker JP et al 1987 What is subjective global assessment of nutritional status? Journal of Parenteral and Enteral Nutrition 11: 8–13

Dickenson RJ, Ashton MG, Axon MTR et al 1980 Controlled trial of intravenous hyperalimentation and total bowel rest as an adjunct to routine therapy of acute colitis. Gastroenterology 79: 1199–1208

Duke JH, Jorgensen SB, Broell JR, Long CL, Kinney JM 1970 Contribution of protein to calorie energy expenditure following injury. Surgery 68: 168–174

Elwyn DH, Gump FE, Munro HN, Iles M, Kinney JM 1979 Changes in nitrogen balance of depleted patients with increasing infusions of glucose. American Journal of Clinical Nutrition 32: 1597–1611

Feinstein EI, Blumentanz MJ, Healer M 1981 Clinical and metabolic responses to parenteral nutrition in acute renal failure. Controlled double blind trial. Medicine 60: 124–137

Freeman JB 1977 Magnesium requirements are increased during total parenteral nutrition. Surgery Forum 28: 61–62

Freund H, Yoshimura N, Lunetta L, Fisher JE 1978 The role of the branched-chain aminio acids in decreasing muscle catabolism in vivo. Surgery 83: 611–618

Giordano C 1963 Use of exogenous and endogenous urea for protein synthesis in normal and uremic subjects Journal of Laboratory and Clinical Medicine 63: 231–245

Glynn MFX, Langer B, Jeejeebhoy KN 1980 Therapy for thrombotic occlusion of long-term intravenous alimentation catheters. Journal of Parenteral and Enteral Nutrition 4: 387–392

Golden MHN, Golden BE 1981 Trace elements: potential importance in human nutrition with particular reference to zinc and vanadium. British Medical Bulletin 37: 31–36

Goodgame JT, Lowry SF, Brennan MF 1978 Essential fatty acid deficiency in total parenteral nutrition: time course of development and suggestions for therapy. Surgery 84: 271–277

Greenberg GR, Marliss EB, Anderson GH et al 1976 Protein-sparing therapy in post-operative patients. Effects of added hypocaloric glucose and lipid. New England Journal of Medicine 294: 1411–1416

Greenberg GR, Jeejeebhoy K N 1979 Intravenous protein-sparing therapy in patients with gastrointestinal disease. Journal of Parenteral and Enteral Nutrition 3: 427–432

Greenberg GR, Fleming CR, Jeejeebhoy KN et al 1985 Controlled trial of bowel rest and nutritional support in the management of Crohn's desease. Gastroenterology 88: 1405 (Abstract)

Hammarqvist F, Wernerman J, Von der Decken Vinnars E 1988 The effects of branched chain amino acids upon postoperative muscle protein synthesis and nitrogen balance. Clinical Nutrition 7: 171–175

Harris JA, Benedict FG 1919 Standard basal metabolism constants for physiologists and clinicians. In: A biometric study of basal metabolism in man. Carnegie Institute of Washington, JB Lippincott, Philadelphia, pp. 233–250

Hill GL, King RFGJ, Smith RC et al 1979 Multi-element analysis of the living body by neutro-analysis. Application to critically ill patients receiving intravenous nutrition. British Journal of Surgery 66: 868–877

Jeejeebhoy KN, Zohrab WJ, Langer B, Philipps MJ, Kuksis A, Anderson GH 1973 Total parenteral nutrition at home for 23 months without complication and with good rehabilitation. A study of technical and metabolic features. Gastroenterology 65: 811–820

Jeejeebhoy KN, Anderson GH, Nakhooda AF, Greenberg GR, Sanderson I, Marliss EB 1976a Metabolic studies in TPN with lipid in man. Comparison with glucose. Journal of Clinical Investigation 57: 125–136

Jeejeebhoy KN, Marliss EB, Anderson GH, Greenberg GR, Kuksis A, Breckenridge C 1976b Fat emulsions in parenteral nutrition In: Meng HC, Wilmore DW (eds) Lipid in parenteral nutrition. American Medical Association, Chicago, pp. 45–54

Jéquier E 1987 Measurement of energy expenditure in clinical nutritional assessment. Journal of Parenteral and Enteral Nutrition. 11: 86–89

Keoane PP, Attrill H, Love M et al 1984 Relation between osmolality of diet and gastrointestinal side effects in enteral nutrition. British Medical Journal 288: 678–691

Kinney JM 1980 Assessment of energy metabolism in health and disease, Rep Ross Conf Med Res: 1st, 1978: 42–48

Kinney JM 1987 Indirect calorimetry in malnutrition: nutritional assessment or therapeutic reference? Journal of Parenteral and Enteral Nutrition 11: 90–94

Koretz RL 1984 What supports nutritional support? Digestive Disease Science 29: 577–590

Lennard-Jones JE 1992 A positive approach to nutrition as treatment. Report of a working party on enteral and parenteral nutrition. King's Fund Centre, London

Li J, Jefferson L 1978 Influence of amino acid availability on protein turnover in perfused skeletal muscle. Biochimica Biophysica Acta 544: 351–335

Long CL, Spencer JL, Kinney JM, Geiger JW 1971 Carbohydrate metabolism in man: effect of elective operations and major injury. Journal of Applied Physiology 31: 110–116

Long CL, Jeevanandam B, Kim BM, Kinney JM 1977 Whole body protein synthesis and catabolism in septic man. American Journal of Clinical Nutrition 30: 1340–1341

Lowe AHG 1982 Prolonged starvation. In: Extremes of nutrition. First British Society of Gastroenterology. Glaxo International Teaching Days

Lukaski HC, Mendez J, Buskirk ER, Cohn SH 1981 A comparison of methods of assessment of body composition including neutron activation analysis for total body nitrogen. Metabolism 30: 777–791

MacFie J, Smith RC, Hill GL 1981 Glucose or fat as a nonprotein energy source? A controlled clinical trial in gastroenterological patients requiring intravenous nutrition. Gastroenterology 81: 285–289

MacNeill KG, Harrison JE, Mernagh JR, Stewart S, Jeejeebhoy KN 1982 Changes in body protein, body potassium, and lean body mass during total parenteral nutrition. Journal of Parenteral and Enteral Nutrition 6: 106–112

Moore FD, Olsen KH, McMurray JD, Parker HV, Ball MR, Boyden C M 1968 The body cell mass and its supporting environment. Body composition in health and disease. W B Saunders, Philadelphia

Mullen JL, Buzby GP, Matthews DC, Smale BF, Rosato EF 1980 Reduction of postoperative morbidity and mortality by combined preoperative and postoperative nutritional support. Annals of Surgery 192: 604–613

Munro HN 1964 In: Munro HN, Allison JB (eds) Mammalian protein metabolism. Academic Press, New York, pp. 381–481

Nordenström J, Askanazi J, Elwyn DH et al 1983 Nitrogen balance during total parenteral nutrition: glucose vs fat. Annals of Surgery 197: 27–33

O'Morain C, Segal AW, Levi AJ 1984 Elemental diets as primary therapy for acute Crohn's disease. A controlled trial. British Medical Journal 288: 1859

Patel D, Anderson GH, Jeejeebhoy KN 1973 Amino acid adequacy of parenteral casein hydrolysate and oral cottage cheese in patients with gastrointestinal disease as measured by nitrogen balance and blood aminogram. Gastroenterology 65: 427–437

Perrot D, Bouletreau P, Seranne C 1982 Evaluation du degré de malnutrition chez les malades hospitalisés en chirurgie. Nouv Presse Méd 11: 1379–1383

Pichard C, Roulet M 1984 Constant rate enteral nutrition in bucco-pharyngeal cancer care. Otolaryngology 9: 209–214

Pichard C, Roulet M, Rössle C, Chiolero R, Jequier E, Fürst P 1988 Effects of L-carnitine supplemented total parenteral nutrition on lipid and energy metabolism in postoperative stress. Journal of Parenteral and Enteral Nutrition 12: 55–562

Pichard C, Roulet M, Schutz Y, Rössle C, Fürst P, Jequier E 1989 Clinical relevance of L-carnitine supplemented total parenteral nutrition in postoperative trauma. Metabolic effect of continuous or acute carnitine administration with special reference to fat oxidation and nitrogen utilization. American Journal of Clinical Nutrition 49: 283–289

Prasad AS, Meftah S, Abdallah J et al 1988 Serum thymulin in human zinc deficiency. Journal of Clinical Investigation 82: 1202–1210

Rombeau J, Barot LR, Williamson CE, Mullen JL 1982 Reduction of postoperative morbidity and mortality by combined preoperative total parenteral nutrition and surgical outcome in patients with inflammatory bowel disease. American Journal of Surgery 143: 139–143

Rosa AM, Shizgal HM 1984 The Harris–Benedict equation reevaluated: resting energy requirements and the body cell mass. American Journal of Clinical Nutrition 40: 168–183

Rose WC 1949 Amino acid requirements of man. Federal Proceedings 8: 546–552

Roulet M, Detsky AS, Marliss EB et al 1983 A controlled trial of the effect of parenteral nutritional support on patients with respiratory failure and sepsis. Clinical Nutrition 2: 97–105

Roulet M, Pichard C, Rössel C et al 1989 Adverse effects of high dose carnitine supplementation of TPN on protein and fat lipid oxidation in critically ill. Clinical Nutrition

Rudman D, Millikan WJ, Richardson TJ, Bixler TJ, Stackhouse WJ, McGarrity WC 1975 Elemental balances during intravenous hyperalimentation. Journal of Clinical Investigation 55: 94–104

Russell DMcR, Prendergast PJ, Darby PE et al 1983 A comparison between muscle function and body composition in anorexia nervosa: the effect of refeeding. American Journal of Nutrition 37: 229–237

Saba TM, Dillon BC, Lanser M E 1983 Fibronectin and phagocytic host defense: relationship to nutritional support. Journal of Parenteral and Enteral Nutrition 7: 62–68

Saverymuttu S, Hodgson HJF, Chadwick VS 1985 Controlled trial comparing prednisolone with an elemental diet plus non-absorbable antibiotics in active Crohn's disease. Gut 26: 994–1001

Sherwin RS 1978 Effect of starvation on the turnover and metabolic response to leucine. Journal of Clinical Investigation 61: 1471–1481

Shike M, Sturtridge WC, Tam CS et al 1981 A possible role of vitamin D in the genesis of parenteral nutrition-induced metabolic bone disease. Annals of Internal Medicine 95: 560–568

Shike M, Russel DMcR, Detsky AS et al 1984 Changes in body composition in patients with small-cell lung cancer. Annals of Internal Medicine 101: 303–311

Silwer H 1937 Die N-Ausscheidung im Harn bei Einschränkung des Kohlenhydategehaltes der Nahrung ohne wesentliche Veränderung des Energiengehaltes derselben. Acta Medica Scandinavica 79 (Suppl): 5–54

Starnes HF, Warren RS, Jeevanandam M et al 1988 Tumor necrosis factor and the acute metabolic response to tissue injury in man. Journal of Clinical Investigation 82: 1321–1325

Van Lanschot JJB, Feenstra BWA, Vermeij CG, Bruining HA 1986 Calculation versus measurement of total energy expenditure. Critical Care Medicine 14: 981–985

Walser M 1983 Rationale and indications for the use of alpha-keto analogues. Journal of Enteral and Parenteral Nutrition 8: 37–41

Walser M 1984 Therapeutic aspects of branched-chain amino acids. Clinical Science 66: 1–15

Waterlow JC, Jackson AA 1981 Nutrition and protein turnover in man. British Medical Bulletin 37: 5–10

Wahren J, Denis J, Desurmont P 1983 Is intravenous administration of BCAA effective in treatment of hepatic encephalopathy? A multicenter study. Hepatology 3: 475–480

Weinsier RL, Hunker EM, Krumdieck CL, Butterworth CE 1979 A prospective evaluation of general medical patients during the course of hospitalisation. American Journal of Nutrition 32: 418–426

Wene JD, Connor WE, DenBesten L 1975 The development of essential fatty acid deficiency in healthy men fed fat-free diets intravenously and orally. Journal of Clinical Investigation 56: 127–134

Whittaker JS, Jeejeebhoy KN 1989 Alimentation. In: Degroot LJ, Besser JM, Cahill GF et al (eds) Endocrinology, 2nd edn. WB Saunders, Philadelphia, pp. 2404–2423

Willard MD, Gilsdorf RB, Price RA 1980 Protein-malnutrition in a community hospital. JAMA 243: 1720–1722

Willicuts HD 1977 Nutritional assessment of 1000 surgical patients in an affluent suburban community hospital. Journal of Parenteral and Enteral Nutrition 1: 25A (Abstract)

Wolfe RR, Durkot MJ, Allsop JR, Burke JF 1979 Glucose metabolism in severely burned patients. Metabolism 28: 1031–1039

Wolman SL, Anderson GH, Marliss EB, Jeejeebhoy KN 1979 Zinc in total parenteral nutrition. Requirements and metabolic effects. Gastroenterology 76: 458–467

Young GA, Collins JP, Hill GL 1979 Plasma proteins in patients receiving intravenous amino acids or intravenous hyperalimentation after major surgery. American Journal of Clinical Nutrition 32: 1192–1119

30. Primary protein–energy malnutrition

B. E. Golden

Malnutrition is a clinical diagnosis which includes several overlapping syndromes. Common to these syndromes is growth failure in children and wasting in adults. They are due, primarily or secondarily, to inadequate supply, relative to demand, of energy or essential nutrients. This chapter deals mainly with primary malnutrition in children.

Primary malnutrition is associated with poverty. In Europe, until the late 19th century, it was common; now, it is rare except in the east, where war and political reorganization have caused large-scale deprivation. In the developing world, it continues to be the chief health problem in children.

The scientific basis of malnutrition was questioned in the early 20th century, as different terms were introduced to describe apparently different syndromes and different views as to their aetiology. Controversy has raged since the 1930s, when Cicely Williams (1935) first introduced the Ghanaian diagnosis kwashiorkor (the disease of the child deposed from the breast by the birth of the next one), to describe the often fatal syndrome characterized by initial growth failure and irritability, then skin lesions, oedema and fatty liver. In spite of much criticism at the time, the term kwashiorkor remains one of the most useful to describe that particular syndrome because it does not imply a cause. Over the next 20 years, around 50 alternative names were given to what was probably the same syndrome (Trowell et al 1954).

Most children with malnutrition do not, however, have the classic features of kwashiorkor. They are simply underweight, usually short for their age and sometimes thin. In 1959, Jelliffe proposed the term 'protein–calorie malnutrition' to include all the syndromes relating to inadequate feeding. This term has been largely replaced by 'protein–energy malnutrition' (PEM), or simply 'malnutrition'.

CLASSIFICATION

To plan appropriate health care, economic development and agriculture policies in individual communities, regions and countries, there is a need for simple, reliable methods of assessing nutritional status, particularly in children, and classifying the results in terms of severity. To choose the best available management regimen for a child, sensitive and specific methods of defining nutritional status are also required.

Childhood malnutrition is characterized by growth failure, resulting in a weight which is less than ideal for the child's age. Measuring weight and assessing age are therefore particularly important. They are generally easy and accurate to define except in communities where a child's age is known only in relation to principal events and season. When a child's age is totally unknown, the number of teeth erupted is a better indicator than height, head circumference or developmental milestones: tooth eruption is least delayed in malnourished children. Classifications of PEM based on weight and age are still the backbone of nutritional assessment methods for both population and individual assessments. Height, or length in children who are too young to stand, and oedema are more difficult to measure accurately but, for the individual, they discriminate well among the syndromes which require different management. The following definitions are useful:

weight-for-age (%) = 100 × child's wt/reference wt of a child of the same age
height-for-age (%) = 100 × child's ht/reference ht of a child of the same age
weight-for-height (%) = 100 × child's wt/reference wt of a child of the same ht.

The term 'reference' value is carefully chosen because few scientists can agree on what they consider to be 'ideal' weight or height. A 'standard' value also implies that a child should be on the 50th centile for ideal growth patterns in a healthy population, while 'normal' can be defined as any value between the 3rd and the 97th centile, i.e. approximately ± 2 SD of mean values (see Chapter 27). In practice, the 50th centile of the National Center for Health Statistics (NCHS) values collected from US children between birth and 18 years is used, but considered simply as a 'reference' value. Some nutritionists resent western-imposed standards which imply that different races are little different in size and shape. Those who insist on local reference figures often have to rely on inadequate data obtained from the affluent section of local society. Their data, expressed in this way, are then also difficult to compare with international data. In practice, most populations with short children have shown a secular increase in children's height and weight with increasing affluence. There is mounting evidence for the appropriateness of NCHS reference values. In India and many parts of Africa, South and Central America, where the growth patterns of well fed uninfected children have been studied, they are similar to the NCHS data.

For population samples, the Gomez Classification (Gomez et al 1956) (Table 30.1) is based on weight-for-age only. Estimating the proportions of children with grade II and grade III malnutrition has remained a widely used and efficient way of comparing different populations. However, the cut-off point of 90% may be too high, as many well nourished children are below this weight-for-age, yet fall within the range of the NCHS reference values. Oedema is also ignored in this classification: as this contributes to weight, a small but variable proportion of children will be classified as being 'better' than they really are. This affects the results of population surveys little, but is very important in terms of an individual's management.

In recent reports on the world nutrition situation (UN ACC/SCN 1987, 1989), nutritional status has been expressed simply as the proportion of malnourished children, defined as those below –2 SD of the mean of NCHS weight values. Depending on age, this cut-off point is equivalent to about 80% of the weight-for-age value taken as the 50th centile. By definition, only about 2.3% of reference children have weights below –2 SD of the mean.

The Wellcome Classification (Anonymous 1970) (Table 30.1) uses both weight-for-age and the clinical, qualitative assessment of the presence or absence of oedema. Oedema is probably the most consistent clinical feature of the 'kwashiorkor syndrome', which, as originally described (Williams 1935), was frequently fatal. This means that a prevalence of kwashiorkor of 1% in a single survey, i.e. the 'point' prevalence rate, underestimates the problem, since many children will have died before the survey. In many areas, oedema in a child is still a useful indicator of a poor short-term prognosis. In the Wellcome Classification, 'kwashiorkor' is used strictly to include only children with pitting oedema, while 'marasmus' only applies to children <60% weight-for-age.

The Waterlow Classification (Waterlow 1973) (Table 30.1) uses height-for-age and weight-for-height. Weight, height and age, but not oedema, need to be measured. Height-for-age estimates show how short or 'stunted' a child is compared with the reference height for his age, whereas weight-for-height estimates show how thin or 'wasted' he is in relation to a reference child of the same height. For the latter calculation, it is assumed that a stunted child (e.g. 2 years old) of the same height as a younger, reference child (e.g. 5 months old) should have the same weight as the reference child (of 5 months). This is not quite true, especially when older children are being compared with young infants, because they are different shapes. However, the Waterlow Classification is still useful in management. Wasted children

Table 30.1 Classifications of nutritional status

	% reference[1]	Nutritional class	
Gomez[2]			
Wt-for-age	90–109	'Normal'	
	75–89	Grade I or mild malnutrition	
	60–74	Grade II or moderate malnutrition	
	<60	Grade III or severe malnutrition	
Wellcome[3]		No oedema	Oedematous
Wt-for-age	60–79	Undernourished	Kwashiorkor
	<60	Marasmus	Marasmic-kwashiorkor
Waterlow[4]		Stunting:	
Ht-for-age	90–94	Mild	
	85–89	Moderate	
	<85	Severe	
Waterlow[4]		Wasting:	
Wt-for-ht	80–89	Mild	
	70–79	Moderate	
	<70	Severe	

[1] NCHS reference values (Hamill et al 1979) preferred
[2] Gomez et al (1956)
[3] Anonymous (1970)
[4] Waterlow (1973)

given short-term, vigorous treatment, will 'recover' within weeks, whereas stunted children require prolonged support over months or years if they are to recover their expected height. In practice, some children are both stunted and wasted and it is useful to know the extent of each.

It is advisable to use both the Wellcome and the Waterlow Classifications to choose the best available form of treatment for the individual malnourished child.

Other simple indices of PEM

In large-scale emergencies little apparatus is available, but it is useful to estimate wasting so that emergency action can be taken. Measures include mid-upper arm circumference (MUAC), MUAC in relation to height (using the so-called 'QUAC', Quaker Arm Circumference measuring stick), MUAC/head circumference (MUAC/HC), triceps skinfold (TF) and mid-upper arm muscle circumference (MUAC - πTF). The major problems with these measures are that skinfolds or circumferences do not show the same range of graded differences as that obtained from the weight of the whole body, i.e. the measure is a less 'sensitive' index of PEM. The other problem is that of the large differences between observers in their measurement techniques (Alleyne et al 1977). The somatic quotient (SQ) was introduced as a single all-embracing measure (like the developmental quotient, DQ) by McLaren & Kanawati (1972). SQ is the mean of weight, height, MUAC and HC, each expressed as percentage reference value for age. It has proved too complex and limited even for individual assessment. Weight/height$^{1.6}$ was introduced by Dugdale (1971) and is considered to be the best age-independent index of wasting, but again, it is less simple and therefore less popular than expressing weight-for-height as a percentage of the reference values. Chapter 27 provides the reference values for weight and height.

Adults

Malnourished adults also develop a weight deficit. However, unless they have also been malnourished in childhood, this is due to wasting alone, not stunting. Thus, for assessment of adult nutritional status and subsequent classification, the widely accepted index is the body mass index (BMI), i.e. weight/height^2 in metric units (Ferro-Luzzi et al 1992). The term chronic energy deficiency (CED) has also been introduced, based on BMI with different degrees of

CED (Table 30.2). The three degrees of CED parallel both the Gomez Classification for PEM in children and the grades of obesity (see Chapter 32). With a reduced body weight there are increasing risks of illness in both men and women; Indian studies show nearly a threefold increase in the mortality of men with a BMI below 16. Over 50% of babies born to mothers with a BMI below 16 after delivery are below 2.5 kg. This means that the ill health associated with underweight adults also potentially handicaps the next generation. Table 30.2 shows recent data on the prevalence of CED in different parts of the world. The reasons for the low BMI of adults are unclear, but could include chronic intestinal infections and selective nutrient deficiency with anorexia, as well as simple lack of food. Adult malnutrition has been neglected by nutritionists because children, pregnant and nursing mothers and the elderly are generally most at risk, but these new data suggest a major new area of nutritional concern.

WORLD PREVALENCE

Nutritional status may be regarded as a continuous variable. Thus, for most free-living groups of children with primary malnutrition, the 'iceberg phenomenon' applies: the majority of children in a community may have mild malnutrition, but far fewer have moderate malnutrition and only a very few, the 'tip of the iceberg', have severe malnutrition. This has been demonstrated repeatedly (Bengoa 1974, Ashworth & Picou 1976).

Table 30.2   The prevalence of adult chronic energy deficiency – females

	% population 20–60 years of age			
Country	Grade 0 BMI >18.5	I 18.4–17.0	II 16.9–16.0	III <16.0
Asia				
China	76	7	5	1
India	38	27	18	16
Africa				
Benin	50	23	17	8
Ethiopia	42	37	15	6
Zimbabwe	71	9	2	1
Togo	68	8	2	0
Tunisia	62	4	1	1
Americas				
Brazil	62	8	2	1

Based on data made available to FAO 1992 (Rowett Research Institute 1992)

Recent assessments have been made of children in Africa, Asia, the Americas and the Caribbean (UN ACC/SCN 1987, 1989). The prevalence levels of malnourished children under 5 years and general trends over the past 25 years are now available. By far the greatest problem of malnutrition is in south and southeast Asia, because not only is the population enormous, but also the prevalence of underweight children is two to three times higher than elsewhere (Table 30.3).

Up to 1980, the overall trend was one of improvement, with decreasing prevalence of malnutrition in Africa, Asia and the American regions, and decreasing numbers of malnourished children in the two latter regions. However, in the 1980s, the worldwide economic recession meant rapidly increasing prices, plummeting trade, increased national borrowing and therefore massive debts for the developing world to repay. There was also a relatively large number of natural disasters, e.g. droughts in Africa. In the second UN report (UN ACC/SCN 1989), the changing prevalence of malnourished children in individual countries was examined in relation to the economy and dietary pattern of the different countries. Although in general a gradual improvement had persisted, there were clear effects of season and of the regional crises. Seasonal effects were obvious in most African countries and in Chile, Thailand and Bangladesh: the prevalence of malnutrition increased during the rainy season just prior to a harvest and decreased just after a harvest. With each drought, harvest failure, earthquake, financial setback, measles epidemic, sudden food shortage or rapid price rise, there was an increase in the prevalence of malnutrition within a few months, and this could persist for several years.

During the 1980s natural disasters were mainly felt in Africa, while the debt problem was mainly felt in Latin America. Asian children appeared to be least affected by short-term crises and maintained their steady improvement in nutritional status. The UN report concluded that 'The nutritional status of young children is probably the most sensitive indicator of sudden changes in food security and health status, acting as an early signal of distress, ill health, famine and, eventually, death'.

More recently, the likely prevalence of malnourished children in 17 regions within Africa, Asia and the Americas has been forecast up to 2005 by Kelly (1991), based on a statistical model of each country. The model included previous prevalence rates of PEM, population densities, average per capita dietary energy supplies, infant mortality rates and various variables for particular countries. From this, it is predicted that the total numbers of malnourished children below 5 years will not change, but their prevalence will continue to fall slowly, from 54% in 1975 to 49% in 1990 to 46% in 2005. This world average is, of course, very high because of the dominant effect of south Asia, including India and Bangladesh (Table 30.3).

These studies have not distinguished oedematous malnutrition (kwashiorkor and marasmic kwashiorkor) from growth failure (undernutrition and marasmus). In the less developed world these conditions coexist in poor communities, often in the same family, and even in the same child at different stages. Thus, a child with oedematous malnutrition often loses his oedema to become a child with marasmus; the children at high risk of developing oedema are also those who are already malnourished, anthropometrically. In practice, there have been very few measurements of the relative prevalence of oedematous malnutrition. Kwashiorkor and marasmus kwashiorkor appear to vary widely in different communities and with time. In India in the 1960s, Gopalan estimated that there was roughly an 80% prevalence of growth failure but only a 1.0–1.5% point prevalence of frank kwashiorkor and 2–3% of marasmic (Gopalan 1975). From his own experience, McLaren (1974) observed that kwashiorkor was particularly common in Tanzania but rare in the Lebanon, where marasmus was common. Kwashiorkor tends to dominate in wet rather than dry regions in Africa, and in any specific country it tends also to occur during the wet season. Rural rather than urban communities are particularly affected. In most studies, the average age of those with kwashiorkor is greater than of those with marasmus. However, in different regions, the age of presentation varies. In Jamaica, for example, 4-month-old infants can present with the full kwashiorkor syndrome while marasmus,

Table 30.3 1990[1]. Estimated number and prevalence of malnourished[2] children <5 years, in selected regions

Region	Number (M)	Prevalence (%)
N America	0.3	2
S America	4.3	12
Caribbean	0.5	21
African continent	23.6	23
S Asia	91.0	69
E Asia	47.4	35

[1] Kelly (1991)
[2] <–2 SD NCHS reference weight-for-age

with marked stunting, can occur in 8-year-old children affected by the dysentery syndrome resulting from infection by the nematode parasite *Trichuris trichiura*.

GROWTH FAILURE

Malnutrition is more common and obvious in young children than in adults, as they require 'extra' food for growth. They also have little control over the supplies of food offered to them and have far smaller stores for coping with the setback of food shortage or infection. Growth failure means suboptimal rates of gain in skeletal and soft tissues. However, it is conveniently estimated as a slowing of linear growth, or stunting. A normal child's height velocity is maximal in the first 6 months (almost 3 cm/month), less in the second 6 months (about 1.5 cm/month) and less than 1 cm/month thereafter. Thus growth failure is particularly obvious in infancy. As this is also the time when weaning occurs, often with a fall in nutrient intake, it is not surprising that stunting in poor communities in the developing world is the most common outcome. For the individual child, it is rarely identified early enough. Complete catch-up in height rarely occurs, even in wards specializing in the treatment of malnutrition.

The determinants of growth in height are uncertain. Golden's (1985) analysis suggests that protein rather than energy intake is particularly important. Thus, selectively supplementing stunted children with milk protein can stimulate a spurt in height, whereas supplementing with energy, e.g. margarine, leads to an increase in weight but little or no spurt in height. These studies, conducted in Papua New Guinea (Malcolm 1970), are similar to studies conducted by Corey Mann in Britain in the 1920s. He found that protein-containing foods were particularly useful in allowing children to grow rapidly. This is in keeping with Millward's (1989) proposal that the 'anabolic' drive depends on sufficient protein to stimulate the complex interactions of growth hormone, insulin and other growth factors to allow a spurt in the growth of long bones.

The poor growth in height of children in less developed countries explains why so many children have a low weight-for-age when assessed by the Gomez Classification (Table 30.1). Most short or stunted children are of an appropriate weight for their height, so clearly the intake of nutrients is usually sufficient to allow the child's organs to grow proportionately to the skeletal length. Although children might be able to show a spurt in growth, particularly during puberty, the dietary and other conditions of adolescents in some countries are inadequate. Thus, stunted Afro-Jamaican and Indian children failed to catch up during puberty with 'normal', rapidly-growing North American teenagers (Ashcroft et al 1966). It is now widely agreed that a vast number of adults in the developing world are short because of growth failure in infancy (Martorell 1985).

The importance of stunting in childhood

A failure to grow in height might not itself seem important, but evidence worldwide increasingly suggests that it is a disadvantage. Although it is presumed that well fed children who are in the lower centile of the NCHS height standards are no less effective than their taller friends, there is now increasing evidence that stunting induced by environmental factors is linked to increased risks of infection, illness and even death (Waterlow et al 1980). Slower mental development is also found in stunted children (Grantham-McGregor et al 1991), but all these links could simply mean that poor children on a limited diet in an unhealthy environment have many handicaps and that stunting is simply the end result of a large number of bad environmental influences. Recently, however, Grantham-McGregor has shown that both mental development and growth in height can be improved by food supplementation alone. This means that dietary factors responsible for promoting bone growth are also helpful in allowing the mental development of the child. If this finding can be generalized, then the implications for child development are immense. The effective development of societies depends on the skills and ability of adults and children, so any long-term impairment of brain function by mild or moderate degrees of PEM in children is of immense worldwide significance.

If stunting persists into adulthood, people are also handicapped because small, short people have a lower capacity for physical work. Their lower body weight is physically a disadvantage and their lower maximal capacity for work, measured as the maximum oxygen uptake (VO_2max) means that the usual ability to sustain no more than 60% of the VO_2max output over long periods, e.g. by labouring in the field, is reduced. Thus the productivity of land workers is less in short, lightweight workers with a lower lean body mass (Spurr 1990) and short tea-pickers in India are also less productive.

On this basis, UN agencies are now recognizing that stunting can be a considerable disadvantage.

Thus, emergency measures to cope with malnourished children having a low weight-for-height must be matched by renewed efforts to promote children's growth for short-term and long-term societal reasons.

OEDEMATOUS MALNUTRITION

The distinction between growth failure (undernutrition and marasmus) and oedematous malnutrition (kwashiorkor and marasmic kwashiorkor), in terms of clinical features and pathology, is not clear-cut. Children who fail to gain weight normally are at increased risk of developing oedema and fatty liver. Fatty liver may well be a better distinguishing feature of the 'kwashiorkor syndrome' than oedema, but it is not a clinical feature. Pathological and ultrasound studies have shown that many malnourished children without oedema have excessive liver fat. Hair depigmentation and skin lesions are also not confined to children with oedematous malnutrition.

The causes of oedema, fatty liver, hair and skin lesions, mood abnormality and anorexia, are not yet resolved. The major hypotheses are shown in Table 30.4.

Pellagra was discounted early, as the clinical features were not similar and niacin supplements, the specific treatment for pellagra, had no effect on oedematous malnutrition. Shortly after, research groups in South Africa, the West Indies and India demonstrated that the livers of children who died from kwashiorkor contained excessive quantities of iron. Srikantia (1968) noted that serum ferritin concentrations were high in adults and children with nutritional oedema, and in monkeys who became oedematous when fed tapioca. He postulated that the ferritin stimulated antidiuretic hormone production, resulting in water retention and oedema. However, if this were the case, hyponatraemia would accompany the oedema, but it does not. Nor are the other features of the 'kwashiorkor syndrome' explained by his hypothesis.

Protein deficiency has persisted as a plausible hypothesis since the 1930s, and most research has

been on this subject. The main thrust of the hypothesis has been that protein deficiency limits albumin synthesis, resulting in low plasma albumin concentration and therefore low plasma oncotic pressure, which allows plasma fluid to leak from the capillary circulation into the interstitium. There is no doubt that children living in poverty are usually on a low-protein diet with a relatively low essential amino acid content (see Chapter 5).

In Jamaica, however, it was noted that resolution of oedema occurred on diets providing very little protein – 0.6 g/kg/day – of good quality but insufficient to allow any increase in plasma albumin concentration. This implied that oedema was not due to low plasma oncotic pressure. It was also observed that the rate of loss of oedema was closely related to the intake of energy, but not protein.

Oedematous malnutrition occurs in regions where cassava, yam, plantain, rice, maize and cruciferae are staple foods, but is not common in wheat-growing areas. This suggests that the amino acid balance, or protein quality, may be important. Dietary protein is also invariably associated with a variety of 'fellow travellers', essential macro- and micronutrients such as potassium, magnesium, zinc, sulphate, phosphate, B vitamins, etc. In many real-life and experimental conditions of 'protein deficiency', the limiting nutrient could be either a particular amino acid or one of the 'fellow travellers'. Deficiency of any one of these produces anorexia, experimentally. Also, potassium deficiency results in oedema whereas zinc deficiency results in skin lesions very similar to those of the kwashiorkor syndrome. When experimental animals are fed good-quality protein in inadequate amounts, together with adequate energy and other nutrients, the major effect is growth failure, not oedema. Thus, it is not yet clear what the role of protein and associated nutrients is in the aetiology of oedematous malnutrition.

Gopalan (1975) and others found no gross differences in protein intake between children who developed oedema and those who did not. Gopalan therefore concluded that kwashiorkor occurred in children who, because of an intrinsic difference, failed to adapt successfully to inadequate dietary intake by reducing their requirements, particularly by slowing growth. The mechanism of 'dysadaptation' was not explained. There is no evidence of an intrinsic metabolic difference in children who develop oedema: they usually recover successfully and show no obvious difference from children who never developed oedema.

Hendrickse et al (1982) produced evidence that, in several regions in Africa, oedematous children were

Table 30.4 Major hypotheses to explain the 'kwashiorkor syndrome'

Niacin deficiency – pellagra
Excess circulating ferritin
'Dysadaptation'
Aflatoxicosis
Protein deficiency
Free radical damage

suffering from aflatoxicosis: either their aflatoxin intake was higher than that of marasmic children or they could not metabolize and excrete it successfully. Aflatoxins can cause fatty liver in malnourished animals. They occur in mouldy crops, which are likely to be consumed by poor families, especially in wet climates and seasons when oedematous malnutrition is more common. However, high levels of serum aflatoxicol also occur in marasmus, so this is unlikely to be the only factor producing oedema. Aflatoxin is only one of many exo- and endotoxins to which children in less developed countries are exposed. Oedema commonly occurs during or just after an infection, a time when a child is exposed to increased toxins. Both toxins themselves and the body's mechanisms for clearing them result in an increased flux of free radicals. These damage cells, particularly lipid-based membranes, in their attempt to gain electrons. Normally, cells have several antioxidant mechanisms in place to prevent such damage; these protective mechanisms depend on the availability of many nutrients, including amino acids (especially S–containing), zinc, copper, magnesium, selenium, thiamin, riboflavin and vitamins C and E. Golden et al (1991) recently put forward a theory that deficiencies of some or all of these reduce a child's protection from free radical damage to such an extent that toxic insults from common infections, food toxins including aflatoxin, small bowel overgrowth, etc., result in cell membrane damage. This impairs homoeostasis in the vascular bed, the liver and the skin, etc. Data in support of this hypothesis include evidence of deficiency in most of the antioxidant protective mechanisms, and evidence of increased flux of free radicals in oedematous children. Excess hepatic iron has again been demonstrated. The plasma of oedematous children has very low transferrin concentrations, so iron is found in the free form and this aggravates free radical damage by initiating a chain reaction of radical formation. This new theory links with the old protein deficiency and aflatoxin theories, and it is still possible that Gopalan's dysadaptation in fact reflects poor free radical scavenging (see Chapter 13 on Vitamin E).

PATHOGENETIC FACTORS: THE DEVELOPMENT OF SEVERE MALNUTRITION

Children below 60% weight-for-age are usually also wasted, with weight-for-height below 80%. Stunting measures the cumulative history of episodes of stress whereas wasting signals a deteriorating condition at the time of measurement (Martorell 1985). Thus, being wasted is often the result of recent or acute weight loss associated with either a sudden fall in food supply, an increase in its demand, or abnormal losses of energy, nutrients or water. All of these occur in childhood infections.

Poverty, the common denominator of primary malnutrition in childhood, is associated with illiteracy, inadequate sanitation, poor personal hygiene, insufficient access to medical services, poor earning capacity, poor agricultural practices, overpopulation and inefficient and inappropriate use of resources. These factors operate at both a national and a family level, and their influence on the infant often begins before birth. Thus, a relatively high proportion of infants have low birthweights due to maternal undernutrition, infection, adolescent pregnancy, pre-eclamptic toxaemia of pregnancy and premature delivery. From birth, the child is reared in a dirty, overcrowded environment which is contaminated with high concentrations of pathogens from human and animal infections. While solely breastfed, the baby is relatively protected from gastrointestinal infections. Human milk tends to inhibit bacterial growth because it contains lysozyme, leucocytes, lactoferrin, interferon, complement and secretory IgA, as well as antibodies to specific pathogens in the environment that the child is exposed to. In contrast, when bottle-feeding starts, it is nearly impossible to keep the bottle clean. It costs too much in fuel and water to sterilize both bottles and teats. Cow's milk also lacks the anti-infective properties of human milk and is an excellent culture medium for many faecal bacteria. Thus, the child is often first infected during bottle feeding. Associated with infection, his 'supply' of feed tends to decrease because of anorexia. The problem is then made worse because the mother and her advisers or doctor limits food intake to reduce the diarrhoea, without realizing the benefit of feeding despite diarrhoea. Any vomiting during the acute stage and malabsorption will further exacerbate the problem at a time when the child's needs have increased because of the infection. Weight loss is therefore common when respiratory or intestinal infections occur in infancy. Following resolution of the infection, there is often a delay in returning to 'normal' feeds. Catch-up in weight is poor or absent.

At the same critical time of life, feeds are not only infected but monotonous, consisting of dilute porridges based on the staple crop. For the very young child the porridge is often strained, making it even more dilute and dirty. Commercial infant feeds are too expensive to use continuously and in some cultures are therefore used sparingly, like medicine.

Canned condensed and evaporated milks are sometimes used, often in very dilute form because of their expense. Infants are also fed 'bush teas' to assuage hunger as well as thirst, and medicinally, to treat infections, etc. Thus, the overall diet is inadequate in both quantity and quality.

When exclusive breastfeeding gives way to supplementary feeding, the growth rate of poor infants tends to fall and infections are frequent. With each infection, growth ceases and soft-tissue loss occurs: complete catch-up is unusual. As infections recur, inflammation and immune function also fail, so that the duration of each infection increases. As a result, the child experiences a progressive deficit in weight because there may be little or no increase in weight over many months, or even a year or two. This was clearly shown in longitudinal studies of children in Guatemalan villages (Mata et al 1977).

THE MALNOURISHED CHILD

Clinical characteristics

Children at particular risk of malnutrition are listed in Table 30.5. On this basis, people with relatively little training can identify such a child in the community. The most efficient quick 'tests' to assess nutritional status and decide on management include weight and age. Height measurement is more difficult but a brief examination, noting particularly the child's mood, appetite (if a feed can be offered), the presence of oedema and the condition of the eyes, is straightforward.

Obtaining a good history of the illness requires patience, tolerance and empathy. For obviously malnourished or ill children presented to the clinic or hospital service, clinicians in particular must be alert to the possibility of underlying disease.

Table 30.6 shows the main topics to be addressed in the history. In the developing world many children are born at home, so that brain damage and other congenital problems tend to go undiagnosed until the child presents with secondary malnutrition. In many regions, haemoglobinopathies such as sickle cell anaemia contribute to growth failure. A careful family

Table 30.5 Children at high risk of malnutrition

Home:	Very poor
Mother:	Adolescent; multiparous
Guardian:	Not a parent; low intelligence or knowledge; active or passive deprivation
Child:	<3 years old; birthweight <2.5 kg; congenital abnormality

Table 30.6 History: topics to be addressed

Present illness
Mother's pregnancy: birth, birthweight, perinatal events
Family history: parents' heights, causes of sibling illness/death
Socioeconomic history
Medical history: frequency of hospital visits, infections
Developmental milestones: ? regression
Past body weights with dates
Dietary history, before and since present illness
Appetite: vomiting, stools before and since present illness
Swelling, before and since present illness

history may reveal relatives with illness or early deaths. A child's local clinic card is helpful. An acute episode of malnutrition is often associated with mental regression, so a 1-year-old child who has started walking may stop completely. Health workers should remember that gross motor development in normal Caucasian children lags behind that of normal African children.

A dietary history often shows what the guardian feels is correct, rather than what the child received. For mobile children, a history of pica should be sought. The type, frequency and quantities of feed, other fluids and salt intake need to be obtained. In some cultures, various 'bush medicines', e.g. frankincense and myrrh, are widely used, but are highly toxic when given orally.

A child's appetite is one of the best guides to early prognosis. A recent decrease in appetite in a malnourished child is often the main evidence of infection: it is unlikely to improve while the infection remains. Force-feeding a child who is refusing to eat usually results in vomiting. Chronic vomiting, on the other hand, may be a symptom of underlying disease: it also accompanies rumination, which is fairly common in deprived children throughout the world. The signs of infection by the protozoan parasite *Giardia lamblia* and of small-bowel overgrowth are variable and rather nondescript; for both, they include anorexia and variable frequency and consistency of stools, which are usually foul-smelling with flatus. Intestinal parasites may be seen by the mother, and bloody stools accompany severe infections by *T. trichiura*. The mother or other guardian is often very aware of oedema, so its occurrence and duration should be checked with her.

Table 30.7 presents the major features of malnutrition on clinical examination. After estimating the child's nutritional status by anthropometric means (both Wellcome and Waterlow Classifications), other clinical features may be present which help differentiate between primary and secondary malnutrition, and which are characteristic of particular deficiencies. Severely malnourished children tend to have a characteristic mood abnormality, more pronounced if they have kwashiorkor. They are uninterested in their surroundings and in people, including their own mothers. They avoid eye contact. Often they do not respond to either comfort or pain and may cry continuously; they are hard children to love. However, this abnormal behaviour is one of the first signs to recover with successful treatment.

Oedema should 'pit', i.e. result in a lingering depression, on applying steady, moderate pressure for a timed 30 s. This is a 'controversial' sign, in that even experienced clinicians argue over borderline cases. Jowls are large, diffuse, symmetrical swellings, mainly over the lower cheeks and more common in oedematous children. Their cause, and even their anatomy, is not clear. Hepatomegaly, or enlarged liver, is variable in extent in malnourished children from different regions, and is much more common in children with oedema. It is associated with the accumulation of fat. In children with abdominal distension associated with small-bowel overgrowth, the liver may be pushed far upwards, which can limit respiratory capacity.

Skin lesions vary considerably, but usually evolve more rapidly in oedematous children. The basal epidermis thins while the keratin layer thickens. Areas exposed to trauma, insect bites and grazes, such as knees, skin creases and the areas around orifices, are affected first. Hyperpigmented layers of keratin and underlying superficial epidermis crack and strip when stretched due to trauma or when oedema is developing. The results are variously described as 'crazy pavement dermatosis', 'flaky paint desquamation', etc. Hypopigmented skin, with a very thin epidermis, is then exposed. This is easily breached, forming superficial and, soon, deep ulcers. Local signs of inflammation do not accompany infection via these ulcers. Severe oedema sometimes results in intraepidermal blisters. Palmar and plantar pallor implies anaemia or poor peripheral circulation: a cold periphery is then common. Purpura, or multiple miniature bruises, and jaundice implies liver failure, but this is a late feature. *Candida albicans* stomatitis (oral thrush) is very common. Herpes simplex stomatitis is far less common but characterized by local pain and refusal of feeds.

There is a wide variety of hair changes. In marasmic children, fine, silky, lanugo hair tends to reappear over the shoulders and periphery of the face; eyelashes are long, curved and silky. In both marasmic and oedematous children, scalp hair is often fine, straight, friable and poorly anchored, so that it can be plucked out painlessly, and bleached, sometimes white, sometimes red. This may give rise to a 'forest sign', or later a 'flag sign'. In the former, an African child's hair resembles a forest when viewed from the side: the original 'well nourished' hair is black curly 'foliage', whereas the more recent 'malnourished' hair is bleached, straight 'trunks'. The flag sign is a band of bleached hair grown when the child experienced a distinct period of malnutrition in the past. Some young children with oedematous malnutrition, particularly the so-called 'sugar babies' of Jamaica, present with apparently normal, very black hair; however, this tends to fall out within a few weeks.

In infants and young children, 'sunken' eyes commonly mean reduced circulating volume associated with dehydration. However, in malnourished children, sunken eyes may be present chronically due to tissue loss without hypovolaemia. This feature contributes to the 'old man look' of some marasmic children. Sunken eyes may also be a result of left ventricular failure (LVF) in grossly oedematous and therefore overhydrated children. Conjunctival pallor occurs in LVF and in anaemia. Severe anaemia is a bad prognostic sign. Jaundice is best seen in the sclera of the eyes. The most obvious signs of vitamin A deficiency are seen in the eyes. Initially, the

Table 30.7 Major clinical features in the malnourished child

Weight deficit	Stunting; general and local (buttocks, upper arm) wasting
Mood abnormality	Misery, irritability
Reduced activity	Milestone delay or regression
Oedema	Feet and lower legs; later, periorbital, hands
Jowls	
Hepatomegaly	Variable, often firm with sharp lower edge
Abdominal distension	Gaseous (ascites very rare)
Skin lesions	Hyper- and hypopigmentation and keratinization; 'flaky paint'/'crazy pavement'; delayed wound healing; pallor; purpura; jaundice
Mouth lesions	Smooth tongue; stomatitis, angular, general
Eye lesions	Sunken; conjunctival pallor; scleral jaundice; signs of vitamin A deficiency (Chapter 13)
Hair changes	Easily plucked out; thin, friable, straight, depigmented; 'forest sign'; 'flag sign'; persistent lanugo; long eyelashes
Bone changes	Signs of rickets, especially 'rosary' and 'bossing'

conjunctivae are injected, then they become wrinkled and dry (best seen from the side). Bitot's spots – foamy white thickenings lateral to the corneae – then develop. Later, corneal opacities appear and coalesce. Finally, the globe softens and ruptures (see Chapter 13).

Several specific deficiencies affect bone growth and, therefore, shape. Rickets (vitamin D deficiency) in very young, usually low birthweight, infants is associated with a soft, sometimes indentable skull. Later, bossing of the forehead, slow fontanelle closure and costochondral 'beading' – a 'ricketty rosary' – are the most prominent clinical signs. Walking is delayed, but this may be due to many reasons associated with primary malnutrition. When the child with rickets does get on his feet, bowing of the legs develops. Rickets can be confirmed radiologically. Scurvy (ascorbic acid deficiency) is characterized, in the young child, by inactivity and crying on being handled: testing for oedema appears to cause extreme pain. This is due to subperiosteal capillary haemorrhages. Petechial haemorrhages also occur in the skin and, after eruption of the teeth, periodontal bleeding occurs. Again, X-rays of the long bones show characteristic changes. Bone changes similar to those of scurvy also occur in copper deficiency. Hypochromic anaemia and neutropenia are associated. These features are uncommon but have been described in premature infants and in malnourished infants with prolonged diarrhoea or when fed large amounts of cow's milk, which is much lower in copper than human milk.

Pathophysiology

Growth failure and reduced physical activity are the child's responses to an inadequate dietary intake. Dietary requirements are further reduced by more subtle functional adaptations. Normally, body tissues and organs have functional reserves but these are energetically expensive to maintain. Children and adults adapt to inadequate intakes by reducing tissue weight and function.

An underweight non-oedematous child has a higher total body water when expressed as a percentage of body weight. Children with oedema have a larger proportion of their body water as extracellular fluid, but there are also variable increases in intracellular fluid volume. Total body protein, particularly the non-collagen proteins, are severely reduced. Total body potassium is also low, because the potassium-rich tissues, e.g. muscle, are reduced more than body weight and cell potassium concentration also falls. Total body sodium and cell sodium concentrations rise.

Most visceral organs, e.g. heart, brain, kidneys and gastrointestinal tract, are reduced in size but the liver remains relatively enlarged with fat, while the thymus atrophies excessively so that it may almost disappear. In children with marasmus and marasmic kwashiorkor, subcutaneous fat is almost absent; in both these conditions and in kwashiorkor muscle bulk is greatly reduced.

In muscle the fibre diameters are small and the remaining collagen is then prominent. Intracellular potassium, magnesium, zinc and copper concentrations are low, while sodium concentration is raised; zinc and copper levels relate to the fall in intracellular protein.

Children with oedematous malnutrition have considerably more fat in their liver – up to 50% of wet weight – than do children with marasmus. Fat starts to accumulate as droplets, mainly of triglyceride, in periportal hepatic cells. These enlarge, coalesce, distend the cells and then appear in cells farther afield. Eventually the fat is dispersed throughout the liver, which becomes yellow and greasy. The rate at which this occurs is unknown but, with recovery, the fat can almost disappear within a few weeks, leaving no apparent residual damage. Protein synthesis in the liver is reduced but other functions are relatively spared until malnutrition is severe. The usual biochemical tests of liver function do not correlate with liver size or fat content.

The stomach wall is thin and the mucosa atrophic. Resting and pentagastrin-stimulated acid secretion is markedly diminished. This facilitates small-bowel bacterial overgrowth. Different studies of the small-intestinal mucosa have revealed a variety of changes from mild to severe villous atrophy, with an intense lymphocyte and plasma-cell infiltrate in the mucosa and submucosa. Some of the variation may be due to different timing of biopsy samples. In most studies, more marked changes have been found in children with oedematous malnutrition than in those with marasmus. Structural improvement seems to occur quickly during rehabilitation.

Digestion and absorption of protein, fat and carbohydrate is generally depressed in malnutrition. Gastric acid and intestinal and pancreatic enzyme outputs are low, bile salt deconjugation occurs with small-bowel overgrowth, and mucosal atrophy is present. Overt gastrointestinal infection is common. However, provided only small quantities of feed are given, malabsorption is usually not a clinical problem. Thus, sufficient protein digestion occurs for over 70% of nitrogen intake to be absorbed. Urinary nitrogen output is low. Thus, the minimum protein requirement – that is, the intake that provides just enough nitrogen to counteract its loss from the body – is only 0.6 g/kg per child per day, a fraction of what is usually provided even in poor homes. At this stage, total body protein turnover, synthesis and breakdown are all low. This saves energy. Together with the reduced sodium pump activity in marasmic children, these adaptations result in a lower than normal resting metabolic rate. However, when circumstances demand an increase in metabolism, this cannot be met. For example, in a cold environment, thermogenesis does not increase in a severely malnourished child, so his core temperature falls.

Exocrine pancreatic deficiency and small-bowel overgrowth are the major factors underlying a relatively mild degree of fat malabsorption. Though faecal energy losses are usually not great, the supply of fat-soluble vitamins (A, D, E, K) may be limited by these problems.

The output of all the disaccharidases is reduced, lactase being the most severely affected and, apparently, the slowest to return to normal with rehabilitation. However, most severely malnourished children tolerate small amounts of lactose in milk and their tolerance usually increases quickly, as shown by their rapid rates of weight gain, without diarrhoea, on cow's milk formula.

Hormonal changes

The endocrine system is usually grossly atrophic but histologically fairly well preserved. Endocrine function, however, bears little relationship to the anatomical findings. There are marked changes in hormonal balance. It is not yet clear the extent to which they contribute to the different outcomes, or to which they are simply responses. Fasting plasma concentrations of somatomedin-C, insulin and glucagon are reduced. Total thyroxine (T_4), triiodothyronine (T_3) and free T_3 are also reduced. Tissue responsiveness to insulin and T_4 is reduced. These changes may be viewed as appropriate adaptations to an inadequate dietary intake. However, plasma thyroid-stimulating hormone, growth hormone, cortisol and aldosterone concentrations are usually raised, and, in several studies, more so in oedematous malnutrition. Aldosterone concentrations rise further during loss of oedema. Renin activity is generally elevated irrespective of the presence or absence of oedema. The reasons for these changes are not clear.

Glucose intolerance is a consistent feature of malnutrition. The reasons are complex and include low insulin production and high peripheral insulin resistance, high plasma cortisol and growth hormone

levels, and probably chromium and potassium deficiencies.

Mild to moderate anaemia (haemoglobin concentrations of 70–100 g/l) is common in malnutrition. The lifespan of erythrocytes is shortened and they vary widely in size and haemoglobin content. Serum concentrations of erythropoietin, erythropoiesis and reticulocyte counts are low. This appears to be due to deficiencies of several nutrients, including protein and folate. It is not due to simple iron deficiency, though many children in the developing world have clinical and biochemical evidence of iron-deficiency anaemia. In contrast, severely malnourished children have normal or high plasma ferritin concentrations, particularly those who subsequently die. Plasma iron concentrations are not low but transferrin concentrations are reduced, and so transferrin saturation tends to be high.

In some areas, malarial or hookworm infections and haemoglobinopathies contribute to more severe anaemia. Septicaemia causes haemolysis and profound anaemia. The total leucocyte count is usually normal in malnourished children. In septicaemic children, it tends to fall rather than rise (see below). Platelet counts are usually normal and, rarely, very low, even in severe malnutrition with purpura and prolonged bleeding time.

Malnutrition and infection

These two are synergistic, as noted earlier. As malnutrition increases, the susceptibility to invasion by microorganisms increases. Thus, the physical barriers, especially in the respiratory and gastrointestinal tracts and the skin, are thin and their protective secretions are reduced in quantity and quality, e.g. sweat output, gastric acid output and secretory IgA output are low, so the defences are easily breached. The duration of infection also increases. This results from impaired inflammatory and, particularly, cell-mediated immune responses. Local skin responses, swelling and pus formation are severely diminished and systemic infections are not associated with fever, tachycardia, leucocytosis or raised acute-phase proteins, so that underdiagnosis of infections is common in severe malnutrition. Also, neutrophil chemotaxis and bactericidal activities are reduced, as are virtually all of the components of complement. The cell-mediated immune response is particularly poor. Severe thymic atrophy is associated with depletion of small lymphocytes. Lymph node and splenic atrophy are associated with depletion of the thymus-dependent areas. The peripheral levels of

T-lymphocytes are decreased, lymphocyte transformation in response to phytohaemagglutinin is reduced, and their ability to form rosettes is impaired. Delayed hypersensitivity skin responses to a variety of antigens are reduced. In contrast, the humoral immune response seems to be relatively well preserved. Though secretory IgA is severely reduced, serum concentrations of immunoglobulins of all classes and peripheral levels of B-lymphocytes are increased in association with infection. In very ill children, the only signs of infection may be profound anorexia, hypothermia, hypoglycaemia and neutropenia.

Management

Most malnourished children are found in impoverished societies where medical care is poor and facilities are limited. So overwhelmed are many of the hospitals that it was widely recognized that malnourished children had a greater chance of survival at home than when admitted to a children's ward. Cross-infection, inappropriate treatment, an inability to cope with detailed nursing and infrequent feeding may all have contributed to the excess of deaths in hospital.

Wasted children can be managed at home successfully. For those who are stunted, recovery with catch-up to reference height-for-age values is uncommon, whether the child is kept in hospital or at home. It requires the concerted efforts of the family, the community and, usually, the continuing support of the welfare and medical services over several years.

Ideally, each child should be examined to exclude the possibility of underlying disease. When present, the child's treatment and prognosis may be different; this must be explained to the mother in order to gain her trust and cooperation. Primary malnutrition is also associated with frequent intercurrent infections, which should be treated as early and effectively as possible. Most virus infections, including HIV, cannot be treated effectively: they pose probably the greatest problem in management. However, small-bowel overgrowth and giardiasis, intestinal helminth infections, malaria, tuberculosis and local candidiasis are examples for which there are specific and fairly easily available treatments. Most acute respiratory infections are viral and, in malnourished children, they take longer to resolve and lead to greater weight faltering and risk of bacterial infection. The signs of pneumonia may be mild despite severe bacterial infection, so treatment must be given early.

The management of acute gastroenteritis, particularly in malnourished children, should be started early, with frequent closely supervised feeds of 'oral rehydration solution' (ORS) (2 volumes) to water (1 volume). A simple ORS can be made, with care, at home (Table 30.8). However, international agencies and aid and charity groups have combined to make convenient sachets of ORS powder easily available for reconstitution with boiled, cooled water. The most commonly used preparations in the less developed world contain relatively large amounts of sodium, whereas UK preparations contain less sodium and more glucose (Table 30.8). The combination of sugar and salt allows glucose-linked sodium absorption to occur while the enterotoxin-induced intestinal secretion continues. If possible, breastfeeding should continue ad libitum, and in non-breastfed children, bottle feeds of milk diluted from full strength if necessary, should be included. Feeds should be encouraged, not withheld: stopping the child feeding confers no advantage and often leads to unnecessary weight loss.

The management of the malnourished child at home also requires an improvement in the macro- and micro-environment of the child. Advice and help with the family's employment, income, knowledge of child care and the need for stimulating play are all important as well as improvements in hygiene, diet and feeding practice. One aim should be to increase energy intakes, at no extra cost, by substituting high-energy, low-cost foods for relatively expensive items, and by using food supplements. Food, vitamin and mineral supplements given for the child tend to be shared by the family, so more may need to be given to

Table 30.8 Oral rehydration solutions

	WHO[1]/ UNICEF	BNF[2]	Home
Method of preparation:	Dissolve sachets of powder in water		1 level teaspoon salt and 8 level teaspoons sugar to be dissolved together in 1 litre of water
Composition (mmol/l)			Approximately
Na+	90	35	85
Cl–	80	37	85
K+	20	20	0
HCO3	30	18	0
Glucose	110	200	117 (sucrose)

[1] World Health Organization (1984). A manual for the treatment of acute diarrhoea. Document WHO/CDD/SER/80.2 (rev 1)
[2] BNF Compound sodium chloride and oral glucose powder

help the child. These measures should be linked to a systematic community involvement in health promotion aimed at enhancing breastfeeding, improving hygiene, increasing rates of immunization and organizing special systems for child health care, with regular weight monitoring and, in many regions, greater efforts to help women with family planning. The whole issue of how best to develop and improve child care in rural and urban societies in poor, less-developed countries is immensely complicated and one of the principal concerns of many governments and other professionals. Nutritionists and doctors have a great deal to contribute in policy-making and implementation, so long as they are aware of other professional interests and skills (see Gopalan 1987).

Hospital management

Some children, particularly those with kwashiorkor, marasmic kwashiorkor and those with marasmus and severe wasting, benefit quickly from treatment in a specialized hospital ward, but this is rarely available. Indeed, to be able to apply this level of care suggests that funds are being spent disproportionately in tertiary level hospitals rather than on simple, community-based facilities. This distortion of the health services, widely evident in some parts of Africa, is a major issue of concern to WHO.

Hospital management is divided into three stages. In Stage 1, the child's acute problems are diagnosed and treated vigorously. Treatment includes antibiotic therapy, maintenance feeds and supplements. In Stage 2, 'high-quality' feeds are offered ad libitum in increasing amounts. This permits rapid catch-up to about the 50th centile weight-for-height. In Stage 3, the child is weaned to home feeds.

Stage 1. This should begin as soon as possible after admission. Many children endure long journeys to hospital only to die within hours of admission. After a clinical history has been taken and the child examined, the following investigations are helpful if routine treatment subsequently fails.

Blood analyses for:

1. Haemoglobin concentrations, erythrocytes, total and differential leucocyte counts and histology; where indicated, haemoglobin electrophoresis and blood grouping.
2. Serum electrolytes, urea and creatinine concentrations. A low serum sodium is ominous but does not mean sodium deficiency. A normal serum potassium does not mean that the child is not potassium-deficient. Urea and creatinine levels help estimate the extent of haemoconcentration and renal damage.
3. Culture, bacterial identification and sensitivities of samples and swabs taken for microscopy and culture from all sites likely to be infected.

Three samples of faeces should be examined for ova and cysts. Urine may be tested for sugars and protein, to exclude underlying diabetes mellitus and nephrotic syndrome, etc.

Chest X-ray is potentially useful, although a 'normal' result does not exclude chest infection; it helps to differentiate between rickets, scurvy and non-accidental injury.

Severely malnourished children should be assumed to be infected, probably septicaemic, with Gram-positive and Gram-negative organisms. In an ideal world, parenteral antibiotics are advised for most children, starting as soon as possible after specimens for culture have been taken. Antibiotic choice is best made by those familiar with the usual environmental pathogens and their sensitivities. Usually penicillin and gentamicin are efficient first-line antibiotics. They should be continued at recommended doses for 10 days if the child shows signs of improvement. If, however, the child's mood, appetite or oedema does not improve, if he becomes peripherally or centrally cold, or develops purpura or jaundice or a decrease in consciousness, then the infecting organisms are likely to be resistant to the antibiotics being given. A change to more appropriate antibiotics is then necessary. Useful second-line antibiotics include cloxacillin, cefotaxime and kanamycin and oral chloramphenicol. For small-bowel overgrowth (and/or *G. lamblia* infection), oral metronidazole is effective, though it tends to increase vomiting.

Every effort should be made to feed the ill, malnourished child sufficient energy ('maintenance energy') and protein to prevent further tissue catabolism, but it is important at this stage not to overfeed. About 400 kJ and 2.0 g protein/kg/day are recommended: that is, a protein/energy (P/E) ratio of approximately 5 g/MJ. The P/E ratio of most commercial infant feeds is higher than this (Table 30.9). However, by substituting vegetable oil and sugar for some of the water added to infant formula powder, one can devise a feed that supplies 400 kJ and 2.0 g protein/100 g prepared feed, which is not hyperosmolar or deficient in water (Feed A in Table 30.9). Such a feed is given at the rate of 100 g/kg per child per day, as frequent small feeds, e.g. 13 g Feed A/kg per child 3-hourly. Extra water or 4.3% dextrose/0.18 normal (N) saline may be given if the child is dehydrated or having excess fluid loss. When refusal or vomiting persists, the feed can be offered in smaller volumes more frequently, or at half strength, then increased in volume or strength as appropriate, at daily intervals. If that fails, a fine, soft nasogastric or nasojejunal tube can be inserted gently, and very frequent or continuous feeding commenced. Occasionally, however, a child can only tolerate continuous intrajejunal 'clear fluids' (Table 30.9) initially. Intravenous 'feeding' should be avoided, as a small mistake in rate or composition may be fatal. With enteral feeding, the intestinal mucosa acts as a barrier against such mistakes. Intravenous fluids may, however, be necessary when a child is significantly dehydrated or unable to tolerate any enteral fluid. The child's gastrointestinal and urine losses and body weight must then be closely monitored. The extremely ill child, unable to take feeds, may benefit from a small (10 ml/kg) intravenous infusion of fresh, cross-matched whole blood. With this, there is a high risk of circulatory overload and cardiac failure: a constant infusion pump is invaluable but rarely available.

When a marasmic child retains 'maintenance energy', he maintains his weight. When an oedematous child manages to retain this intake, he tends to lose weight as he loses oedema. In either case, success is heralded by improved mood and appetite.

Table 30.9 Composition of infant feeds

Product	Energy (kJ) (per 100 g prepared feed)	Protein (g)	P/E ratio (g/MJ)
4.3% dextrose/ 0.18 N saline	72	0	0
Commercial feeds[1]	260–330	2.0–3.6	6–14
Feed 'A'	400	2.0	5.0
Feed 'B'	554	3.1	5.6

Example recipes

Ingredients	1000 g prepared feed		
	Weight (g)	Energy (kJ)	Protein (g)
Feed 'A':			
Dry feed powder[2]	120	2064	19.6
Vegetable oil	20	756	0.0
Sucrose	70	1168	0.0
Water to	1000	0	0.0
Feed 'B':			
Dry feed powder[2]	190	3268	31.0
Vegetable oil	60	2268	0.0
Water to	1000	0	0.0

[1] Range of cow's milk and soy-based infant feeds
[2] In this case, Pelargon (Nestlé), but most infant feeds are appropriate

Table 30.10 Supplements

Product	Intake (ml/kg child/day)	Composition (per ml)
K/Mg supplement	2.0	1.0 mmol K 0.25 mmol Mg
Zn/Cu supplement	2.0	1.0 mg Zn 0.1 mg Cu

Recipes for supplements

Ingredients	K/Mg supplement (g/l)	Zn/Cu supplement (g/l)
KCl	37.3	
$MgCl_2$:$6H_2O$	50.8	
tri-K citrate	54.1	
Zn acetate:$2H_2O$		3.36
$CuCl_2$:$2H_2O$		0.25

Within a week of being on maintenance energy, most children are craving for more feed.

Malnourished children have intracellular deficits of potassium and magnesium. Both supplements should be given orally, if possible, as shown in Table 30.10. Ongoing diarrhoea increases these requirements. Severe skin lesions are associated with low plasma zinc (zinc status is particularly difficult to quantify in malnutrition): they heal more quickly when zinc supplements are given. Copper supplements should be given as well, even in the absence of overt copper deficiency (Table 30.10). An iodine supplement may be required in endemic goitre regions (Chapter 36). Large amounts of sodium, as in N or 0.5 N saline should be avoided, as most severely malnourished children have an excess of body sodium to eliminate. On prolonged ORS, oedema sometimes appears or increases. Severely malnourished children should not be given iron supplements until they reach Stage 2. All malnourished children should be given oral or nasogastric vitamin supplements, including vitamins A, B_1, B_2, B_6, nicotinamide, C, D, folic acid and, if possible, vitamin E. In areas where vitamin A deficiency is common, and in children with clinical signs, retinol palmitate and vitamin A should be given, as indicated in Chapter 13.

Common problems that occur during Stage 1 are shown in Table 30.11. Septicaemia is almost invariably fatal without the correct antibiotics in adequate dosage. Hypothermia results from both a cool environment, e.g. at night in the tropics, and because the malnourished child, without insulation and with a low metabolic rate from tissue loss and adaptation, is

Table 30.11 Problems during Stage 1 management of severe malnutrition

Persistent anorexia
Persistent oedema
Hypothermia
Hypoglycaemia
Persistent vomiting
Persistent diarrhoea
Congestive cardiac failure
Breathlessness
Paralytic ileus
Purpura, jaundice

unable to maintain his core temperature. Hypoglycaemia results from a 'fast' because of infrequent feeds or vomiting. Vomiting sometimes results from rumination, a chronic problem of deprived children, which can be treated by skilful feeding, affection and the patience of an experienced nurse. Persistent diarrhoea is rarely the result of primary or secondary lactose deficiency; continuing infection is common. Increasing oedema occurs with intravenous fluid therapy or transfusions, and occasionally when sodium-rich fluids are given orally. It also occurs in congestive cardiac failure with rapid, distressed breathing, anorexia and a weak pulse; tachycardia is uncommon. Treatment includes an immediate reduction in intake, diuretics and, in the longer term, cautious digitalization. Paralytic ileus is a rare cause of anorexia, vomiting and abdominal bloating in a very ill child. Purpura and jaundice are signs of liver failure.

Stage 2. After a few days, or when mood and appetite improve, Stage 2 management can begin by increasing daily the amounts of Feed A offered. Within a week, ad libitum feeding can start with eight 3-hourly feeds per day, and later, six 4-hourly feeds. During the early part of Stage 2, antibiotic therapy is discontinued but the child must be monitored. His potassium and magnesium, vitamin and trace element supplements should continue and oral iron, about 4 mg/kg/day, as ferrous sulphate, should be started.

Intake of Feed A usually increases by 50 ml/day to about 800 kJ/kg/day. Once oedema is lost, the rate of weight gain rises to 10–20 g/kg/day. By this stage, as feed volumes are now very large, children over 5 kg or 6 months may be offered 'high-energy feeds', such as Feed B (Table 30.9) supplying up to 40% more energy in the same volume. These are prepared by substituting a vegetable oil for some of the water. In so doing, the volume of feed should initially be reduced so that the jump in energy offered is not too great.

At this stage, the child requires increased mental stimulation, with play therapy as he becomes more active. The only common problems are now nosocomial infections, recurrent small-bowel overgrowth, or specific deficiencies due to consuming large quantities of a suboptimal diet. The major sign of all of these is weight faltering.

Stage 3. Once a child reaches the 50th centile of weight-for-height, his appetite and therefore intake decrease until intake is less than 500 kJ/kg/day. Weaning to an ad libitum mixed diet is then appropriate. The adjustment takes a few days before he returns to steady weight gain, after which he is ready for home.

This approach to hospital treatment is unusual because often children have to be sent home early to allow others to be treated. The benefits of ensuring very rapid recovery in Stage 2 are considerable, provided the guardians are also helped to improve their child care and knowledge of appropriate diets, and the children continue to be monitored in child welfare clinics. Breastfeeding, family planning and preventive measures, e.g. immunization, all need to be encouraged by integrating a preventive programme into the hospital management scheme. Many babies, rapidly discharged after surviving Stage 1 therapy, return to hospital or die within weeks. A sustained recovery programme and health promotion should become an essential of hospital management.

REFERENCES

Alleyne GAO, Hay RW, Picou DI et al 1977 Protein–energy malnutrition. Edward Arnold, London
Anonymous 1970 Classification of infantile malnutrition. Lancet 2: 302
Ashcroft MT, Heneage P, Lovell HG 1966 Heights and weights of Jamaican schoolchildren of various ethnic groups. American Journal of Physical Anthropology 24: 35–44
Ashworth A, Picou D 1976 Nutritional status in Jamaica (1968–74). West Indian Medical Journal 25: 23–34
Bengoa JM 1974 The problem of malnutrition. WHO Chronicle 28: 3–8

Dugdale AE 1971 An age-independent anthropometric index of nutritional status. American Journal of Clinical Nutrition 24: 174–176
Ferro-Luzzi A, Sette S, Franklin M, James WPT 1992 A simplified approach to assessing adult chronic energy deficiency. European Journal of Clinical Nutrition 46: 173–186
Golden M 1985 The consequences of protein deficiency in man and its relationship to the features of kwashiorkor. In: Blaxter K, Waterlow JC (eds) Nutritional adaptation in man. John Libbey, London, pp 169–185
Golden MHN, Ramdath DD, Golden B E 1991 Free radicals and malnutrition. In: Dreosti I E (ed) Trace

elements, micronutrients and free radicals. Humana Press, New Jersey, pp 199–221

Gomez F, Ramos-Galvan R, Frenk S et al 1956 Mortality in second- and third-degree malnutrition. Journal of Tropical Pediatrics 2: 77–83

Gopalan C 1975 Protein versus calories in the treatment of protein–calorie malnutrition: metabolic and population studies in India. In: Olson RE (ed) Protein–calorie malnutrition. Academic Press, New York, pp 329–341

Gopalan C 1987 Combating undernutrition. Basic issues and practical approaches. Nutrition Foundation of India

Grantham-McGregor SM, Powell CA, Walker SP, Himes JH 1991 Nutritional supplementation, psychosocial stimulation and mental development of stunted children: the Jamaican study. Lancet 338: 1–5

Hamill PVV, Dridz TA, Johnson CZ, Reed RB et al 1979 Physical growth: National Center for Health Statistics percentile. American Journal of Clinical Nutrition 32: 607–629

Hendrickse RG, Coulter JBS, Lamplugh SM et al 1982 Aflatoxins and kwashiorkor: a study in Sudanese children. British Medical Journal 285: 843–846

Jelliffe DB 1959 Protein–calorie malnutrition in tropical preschool children. Journal of Pediatrics 54: 227–256

Kelly AW 1991 Technical Working Paper for United Nations Administrative Committee on Coordination – Subcommittee on Nutrition (ACC/SCN)

McLaren DS 1974 The great protein fiasco. Lancet 2: 93–96

McLaren DS, Kanawati AA 1972 A somatic quotient. American Journal of Clinical Nutrition 25: 363–364

Malcolm LA 1970 Growth retardation in a New Guinea boarding school and its response to supplementary feeding. British Journal of Nutrition 24: 297–305

Martorell R 1985 Child growth retardation: a discussion of its causes and its relationship to health. In: Blaxter K, Waterlow JC (eds) Nutritional adaptation in man. John Libbey, London, pp 13–29

Mata LJ, Kromal RA, Urrutia JJ, Garcia B 1977 Effect of infection on food intake: perspectives as viewed from the village. American Journal of Clinical Nutrition 30: 1215–1227

Millward D , Rivers JPW 1989 The need for indispensible amino acids: the concept of the anabolic drive. Diabetes Metabolism Reviews 5: 191–212

Rowett Research Institute 1992 Body mass index: an objective measure for the estimation of chronic energy deficiency in adults. Report to FAO

Spurr GB 1990 The impact of chronic undernutrition on physical work capacity and daily energy expenditure. In: Harrison GA, Waterlow JC (eds) Diet and disease in traditional and developing societies. Cambridge University Press, Cambridge, pp 24–61

Srikantia SG 1968 The causes of oedema in protein–calorie malnutrition. In: McCance RA, Widdowson EM (eds) Calorie deficiencies and protein deficiencies. J & A Churchill, London, pp 203–211

Trowell HC, Davies JNP, Dean RFA 1954 Kwashiorkor. Edward Arnold, London

United Nations 1987 Administrative Committee on Coordination – Subcommittee on Nutrition (ACC/SCN). First Report on the World Nutrition Situation. WHO, Geneva

United Nations 1989 ACC/SCN Update on the Nutrition Situation. Recent trends in 33 countries. WHO, Geneva

Waterlow JC 1973 Note on the assessment and classification of protein–energy malnutrition in children. Lancet 2: 87–89

Waterlow JC, Ashworth A, Griffiths M 1980 Faltering in infant growth in less-developed countries. Lancet 2: 1176–1178

Williams CD 1935 Kwashiorkor. Lancet 2: 1151–1152

World Health Organization 1984 A manual for the treatment of acute diarrhoea. Document WHO/CDD/SER/802 (rev. 1)

31. Sepsis and trauma

J. Broom

Trauma has been known for almost 200 years to cause a generalized response in the body: John Hunter, in 1794, was the first to suggest that body tissues far removed from the site of injury are affected. Ninety years later, Claude Bernard showed experimentally that haemorrhagic shock in the dog led to an increase in blood glucose, but it was not until Cuthbertson's meticulous studies in the 1920s that the body's integrated physiological and metabolic response to trauma was first defined clearly. He showed that the environment affected the response, which was also influenced by the patient's nutritional state and dietary intake before, during and after the trauma. Francis Moore then extended these investigations but concentrated on surgical trauma, where injury is to some extent controlled. He was responsible for major advances in developing fluid and electrolyte therapy to maintain physiological homoeostasis in the immediate postoperative period. His treatise *Surgical metabolism* (Moore 1977) is the recognized text in this area. The tissue loss after trauma was also analysed by Kinney in New York, in collaboration with Cuthbertson in Glasgow, and thereby provided an in-depth study of the relation-ships between protein and energy metabolism (Cuthbertson 1982, Kinney 1989).

The metabolic response to trauma can be simply split into two main phases, as first suggested by Cuthbertson: the ebb phase and the flow phase (Fig. 31.1). Oxygen consumption falls in the first ebb phase, which may last up to 1–2 days. The oxygen uptake then rises and remains elevated until the stimulus to the hypermetabolism of tissues is reduced. The flow phase may last 3–10 days, depending on the severity of the response. The unclear distinction between the two phases may be shown more precisely by measuring changes in glucose flux: there is a switch from glycogenolysis to gluconeogenesis as patients move from the ebb to the flow phase. Fig. 31.1 shows that oxygen uptake may not recover from the ebb phase; a further decline in a 'necrobiotic phase' was considered by Cuthbertson as irreversible, with eventual death occurring. One of the features of this phase is a fall in blood glucose which, in clinical terms, is an extremely poor prognostic sign and generally heralds mortality. New approaches to treatment, however, now mean that death is not an inevitable outcome (see below).

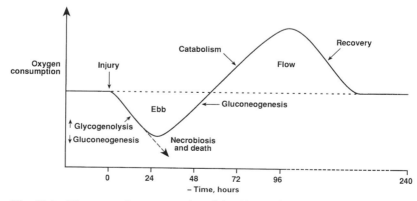

Fig. 31.1 Diagrammatic representation of the ebb and flow phases in the metabolic response to injury

EBB ('SHOCK') PHASE

The early phase in the response to trauma is primarily caused by a neuroendocrine response to the injury. There is a marked stimulation of the sympathetic nervous system, with a surge in adrenaline output from the adrenal medulla and a rise in cortisol production and secretion from the adrenal cortex in response to a rise in adrenocorticotrophic hormone (ACTH) output from the anterior pituitary. The posterior pituitary is also stimulated, so that there is a rise in antidiuretic hormone (ADH). This ADH increase may reflect the acute cardiovascular changes, which involve a marked sequestration of fluid in the extravascular space and a fall in the venous return, which then causes a fall in cardiac output. The parasympathetic output via the vagus is also stimulated, so there is not the expected compensatory increase in heart rate as venous return falls. As cardiac output declines tissue perfusion falls, with a reduction in oxygen uptake. The tissues themselves are not inhibited metabolically, so this period of very unstable physiology may not be associated with a low O_2 uptake if circulatory perfusion of the tissues is maintained.

The increase in sympathetic nervous system activity also stimulates glucagon and inhibits insulin secretion; these effects are seen within a few minutes of an incision during surgery, despite the patient being anaesthetized. In surgery or trauma the pain from the traumatized area and the release of tissue factors, e.g. cytokines, alter the central neuronal responses and hormonal secretion. Local anaesthesia of a painful peripheral injury or the use of subdural spinal anaesthetics can reduce the sympathetic and parasympathetic nervous system activity and the hormonal responses, but some response persists because of the tissue factors released. These factors also have direct effects on the vasculature, leading to peripheral vasodilatation and shock. Immediate fluid therapy with both electrolytes, e.g. 0.9% saline, and colloid, e.g. plasma, is very important to increase the patient's blood volume so that cardiac output can be boosted and tissue perfusion maintained. These resuscitative procedures are of extreme importance for the patient's survival; they prevent the development of Cuthbertson's necrobiotic phase. This phase is often termed the 'golden hour' because the effectiveness with which blood volume is restored and pain relieved makes a major difference to the chance of survival and then of a rapid recovery. Giving food, enteral or parenteral nutrition at this time is of little value compared with the urgent need for anaesthesia and blood volume expansion.

Metabolic alterations

The ADH response not only reduces urinary output but also has a direct effect on energy metabolism. Together with the depression of insulin and the increase in glucagon, catecholamine and cortisol production, it is responsible for stimulating ketogenesis. Surprisingly, ketogenesis at this early stage in very ill patients influences or predicts survival: patients with circulating ketone body concentrations above 2.0 mM have a lower morbidity and mortality. The development of ketosis at this stage is also associated with a lower loss of tissue protein and a less negative nitrogen balance. Women develop ketosis far better than men and survive major trauma better. This capacity for ketosis is independent of the fat content of the body and cannot be related to differences in body composition between males and females. Inducing and maintaining ketogenesis has therefore been used in therapy to reduce the loss of tissue protein after trauma (Blackburn et al 1973).

Several other alterations in energy metabolism are also seen in the ebb phase (Table 31.1). A rise in blood lactate concentrations is always found and seems to indicate tissue anoxia. Lactate production is stimulated as glucose is metabolized from stored glycogen in muscle and liver. Additional lactate can be produced from alanine released during proteolysis in muscle, but lactate production from alanine by the liver only occurs if the hepatic pH falls. This is a serious feature, which occurs when the blood flow to the liver itself is compromised. Gluconeogenesis in the early stages of the ebb phase is not stimulated until there is some recovery from the shock phase. Since

Table 31.1 The metabolic response to the ebb or shock phase of injury

Duration: Variable from 24–72 h after injury

Characteristics
O_2 consumption decreases
Blood glucose increases from hepatic glycogenolysis
Lactic acidaemia in proportion to tissue anoxia
Plasma alanine rises as peripheral protein catabolism increases. Hepatic gluconeogenesis starts to rise late in the phase
Peripheral lipolysis with increased plasma glycerol and free fatty acids
Ketogenesis rises markedly
Synthesis of acute phase proteins rises

Kinetic studies of substrate flux are difficult because of the unstable physiological state and the variety of injuries sustained by patients with this problem there is insufficient glycogen stored in the liver and muscle to maintain adequate blood glucose for longer than 24 hours, and gluconeogenesis cannot be stimulated soon after injury, then there will be inadequate glucose production and blood glucose concentrations will inevitably fall, unless glucose is given in modest amounts intravenously.

If blood glucose falls, then tissues such as the brain, red cells and renal medulla become dependent on adequate circulating concentrations of ketones. This may explain the great importance of early ketosis. Ketogenesis depends on an increased supply of free fatty acids (FFA) from lipolysis of adipose tissue (Newsholme & Start 1973). The glycerol released with FFA is also available to produce glucose in the liver. The FFA are available for direct use as an energy substrate, but this depends on the ability of the tissues to oxidize the FFA. Given the poor tissue perfusion and stimulated lipolysis in the ebb phase, it is therefore usual to find that the patient's serum contains very high levels of lipid after major injury or sepsis; the administration of extra fat intravenously at this stage may then be dangerous.

The ebb phase also sees the start of what is termed 'the acute-phase response'. Acute-phase proteins are derived from the liver and their synthesis is stimulated by the production of cytokines, such as interleukin-6 (IL6) (see below). As acute-phase hepatic production rises there is a marked fall in the plasma concentration of albumin, transferrin and other export proteins, such as retinol-binding protein (RBP). This change, described as the negative acute-phase response, is also cytokine-related but in this case depends less on a change in liver synthesis rates and more on the transfer of these proteins to the extravascular space;

membrane leakage may increase, but extracellular fluid return to the cardiovascular system drops dramatically. Membraneous changes are particularly dependent on another cytokine, interleukin-2 (IL2).

The early responses in muscle protein metabolism are also induced by a circulating protein, proteolysis-inducing factor, released from both macrophages and damaged tissue. As muscle breakdown is stimulated, the carbon skeletons of the branched-chain amino acids are used by the muscle as energy substrates. The keto acids derived from the branched-chain amino acids are released into the blood for use as ketogenetic substrates for the liver. Alanine is also released from proteolysis and serves as a nitrogen carrier because muscle takes up substantial amounts of pyruvate. This allows the transfer of nitrogen from the deamination and transamination of some of the amino acids released by muscle proteolysis for gluconeogenesis.

FLOW PHASE

Progression from the ebb to the flow phase of the response to injury is characterized by a gradual increase in oxygen uptake, with an associated switch from glycogenolysis to gluconeogenesis. The transition may depend on the severity of the injury and the effectiveness of the resuscitative measures taken during the early shock period. The flow phase itself can be split into two distinct parts, 'catabolism' and 'recovery' (Fig. 31.1).

The rate of O_2 uptake increases dramatically from the minimum seen in the ebb phase to a level well above the 'norm' for the non-injured state in the catabolic phase. It then gradually falls again to normal in the recovery phase. The maximum resting O_2

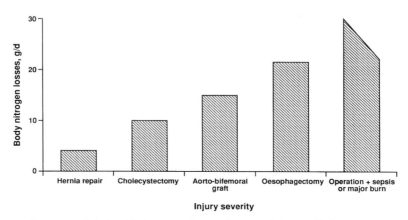

Fig. 31.2   Relationship between nitrogen losses and degree of injury stress

uptake and the time for its return to normal after injury depends on the extent of the trauma. The increases in O_2 uptake and in body protein losses with different degrees of trauma are shown in Fig. 31.2. This increase in O_2 uptake is related directly to the increased metabolic activity of tissues, except in major burn injury, where there is also a dramatic increase in energy expenditure to compensate for the large evaporative heat loss (see below). The extent of the injury is also mirrored in the protein metabolic response: the larger the injury the greater the loss of lean body mass, as demonstrated by the increase in urinary nitrogen excretion. This aspect of the metabolic response to trauma was first characterized by Cuthbertson & Zagreb (1979).

The increased metabolic activity affects all aspects of intermediary metabolism and all tissues (Table 31.2). The rise in blood glucose is proportional to the extent of the injury. Hepatic gluconeogenesis is markedly increased as a direct result of cytokine secretion. This drive to produce glucose from amino acids and glycerol is unaffected by giving oral or intravenous glucose. Therefore, infusing substantial amounts of glucose to these patients simply exaggerates the marked hyperglycaemia and produces additional fluid and electrolyte disturbances. This hyperglycaemic tendency is made worse by the development of a post-traumatic insulin-resistant state (Cahill 1984).

The basis for the negative nitrogen balance is complex, but it is now clear that nutritional input at

Table 31.2 Metabolic response to the flow phase of injury

Duration: From 1–3 days after injury, depending on the severity of the injury and measures taken to counteract the shock

Characteristics
Increased oxygen uptake
Increased gluconeogenesis and hepatic glucose output, independent of exogenous glucose input
Increased lipolysis and FFA utilization
Development of 'controlled' ketosis and increased ketone body utilization if not suppressed by exogenous glucose administration
Increased protein breakdown and increased urinary/nitrogen excretion
Protein synthesis variable depending on decreased circulating albumin and other hepatic export proteins
Acute-phase protein response with increased hepatic secretion of fibrinogen, ferritin, α-macroglobulin and many others

Summary: Loss of lean body mass

this stage has a marked effect on the mechanisms underlying it. Providing exogenous amino acids at this time stimulates protein synthesis and helps to limit the protein loss from the body. Urinary nitrogen losses, however, continue to be high because amino acid catabolism is sustained and protein breakdown rates are much less sensitive than normal to being inhibited by infused amino acids. As fluid exchange between the blood and the extravascular compartment returns to normal, extravascular albumin and other proteins return to the bloodstream. In addition, there is a rise in hepatic secretion of albumin which helps to compensate for plasma protein losses into the injured tissues or burn. In burned patients the protein loss into the burn itself can be enormous, so that, despite marked increases in hepatic protein synthesis and the provision of extra dietary protein or intravenous amino acids, the plasma concentrations of many proteins, including albumin, remain low.

METABOLIC RESPONSE TO SEPSIS

Sepsis is not simply an exaggerated response to trauma but has quite different effects on energy substrate metabolism. The overall differences between trauma, starvation and sepsis are illustrated in Fig. 31.3. There are differences in oxygen consumption, urinary nitrogen losses, circulating protein concentrations and in carbohydrate and fat metabolism.

Table 31.3 outlines the alterations seen in a patient with major sepsis. Depending upon the phase of sepsis, there may be a marked decrease or increase in resting O_2 uptake. When a patient has severe infection with a cavitating abscess, O_2 uptake is reduced, as in the ebb or shock phase. When the abscess is drained, however, the patient rapidly responds to the fall in toxin and cytokine leakage into the bloodstream, with an increase in O_2 uptake as in the normal flow phase of injury.

In sepsis, there may be a huge increase in glucose production by the liver, but this effect is variable and sometimes disputed. Poor tissue use of glucose and insulin resistance state during acute severe infection is combined with poor aerobic tissue metabolism. This explains the marked rise in blood glucose. One major difference between sepsis and trauma is the disappearance in sepsis of the ketotic response normally seen in the post-traumatic state. If ketone bodies increase in the circulation, this occurs for only a short period of time and defective ketogenesis seems the most likely explanation for this finding. The mitochondrial structure in the livers of septic patients is disrupted and swollen (Fig. 31.4). Experimentally

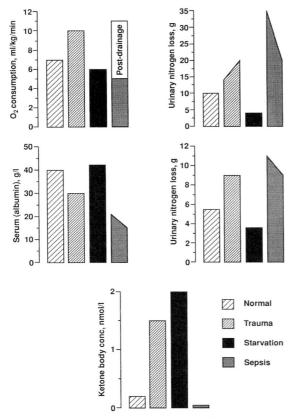

Fig. 31.3 Differences between the metabolic response to trauma, starvation and sepsis

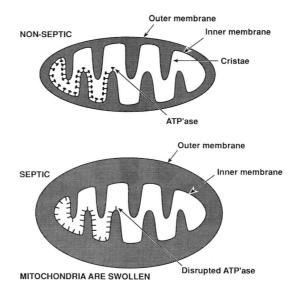

Fig. 31.4 Effect of septicaemia on mitochondrial membrane structure

the conformation of the adenosine triphosphatase (ATPase) proteins is also disrupted, with loss of the inner mitochondrial membrane structure and ATPase activity. Three specific sites in the energy transformation pathway are also blocked during sepsis:

Table 31.3 Metabolic responses to sepsis

Increase in glucose synthesis marked; poor peripheral glucose utilization; poor aerobic metabolism
Decreased plasma free fatty acids. Lipolysis changes unknown
No ketosis: ketone metabolism rates unknown
Marked rise in protein breakdown rates; large increases in urinary N
Increased visceral and acute-phase protein synthesis
Marked fall in plasma albumin concentration, with sequestration in the extravascular space
Probable glucose substrate or futile cycling accounting for ineffective use of high rates of protein breakdown
Variable effects on oxygen uptake

pyruvate dehydrogenase, citrate synthase and iso-citrate dehydrogenase. The overall effect of this is to reduce the aerobic metabolism of glucose and fatty acids. In this situation it is difficult to make efficient use of either infused lipid or glucose. The anaerobic metabolism of glucose via glycolysis therefore becomes more important, and helps to explain the huge increase in lactate production in septicaemia. Studies with liver biopsies in septic patients show an increase in phosphofructokinase-II activities in keeping with a marked stimulation of glycolysis, which seems to continue for some considerable time after sepsis begins. The control of glycolysis seems to depend on the increased production of fructose-2, 6-bisphosphate, which stimulates phosphofructokinase-I activity and therefore glycolysis. Glucose supply from gluconeogenesis is therefore essential; if gluconeogenesis is impaired, as it sometimes is, then marked hypoglycaemia develops and this, as in injury, is an indication of total system failure and impending death. Substrate cycles (see Chapter 8) may also be stimulated in septicaemia, with heat production and the inefficient use of glucose. This may explain the rapid loss of lean body mass in severe sepsis, as body protein is used for substantial glucose production which is then simply wasted as heat in the substrate or 'futile' cycles.

Once the source of infection in sepsis is isolated and drained, the body switches to use fat, which is to be the preferred fuel when insulin resistance limits peripheral glucose uptake. The respiratory exchange ratio drops to around 0.7 (see Chapter 3).

PROTEIN METABOLISM IN SEPSIS

The extremely rapid and large losses of protein and the conversion of amino acids to glucose for inefficient catabolism is not inevitable, but the protein catabolic responses involve the same processes as those seen in trauma. Thus the loss of protein is associated with an increase in the rate of muscle protein breakdown and an increase in circulating concentrations of plasma amino acids, especially alanine. The released amino acids are shunted to the liver for increased gluconeogenesis and visceral protein synthesis. They are almost certainly also redirected towards the immune system for specific host defence mechanisms. The acute-phase response to sepsis is exaggerated and the loss of albumin from the vascular compartment is also greatly increased.

Originally these changes were thought to depend on the infecting organism itself and its products, but it is now realized that the body's responses depend on its own production of a whole variety of prostaglandins and leukotrienes. These may be produced by macrophages and damaged tissues. The leukotrienes play a key role in inducing cytokine secretion. Thus leukotriene B4 can induce the secretion of the

Table 31.4   Signal-transduction pathways

Tyrosine kinase and protein phosphorylation
G-proteins and receptor–enzyme coupling
Adenylate cyclase and cyclic AMP
Phospholipases
Inositol phosphates
Prostaglandins/leukotrienes

cytokine interleukin-1 (IL1) by macrophages and of interferon-γ and IL2 by thymus-derived lymphocytes. Prostaglandin E2, however, suppresses the macrophage production of IL1 and immunosuppresses lymphocytes.

THE CYTOKINES

Cytokines are specialized, low-molecular-weight (15–30 KD) proteins produced by many cell types, but especially by activated macrophages. Such activation is provided by factors released from damaged tissue, or indeed by lipopolysaccharide (LPS) associated with the cell walls of bacteria invading host tissue. In general, cytokine release promotes recovery, certainly during sepsis but also in any traumatic situation or inflammatory process. Such cytokines released from macrophages and other tissues have powerful effects on a whole variety of body tissues (Fig. 31.5) and act as promoters and inhibitors of specific enzyme

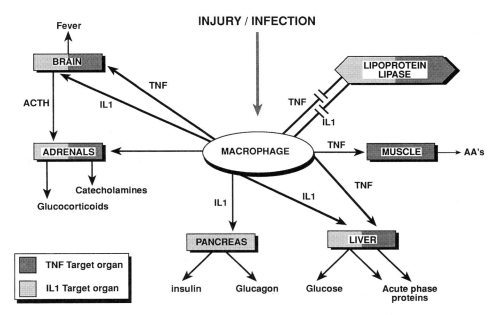

Fig. 31.5   Current understanding of macrophage-induced changes in nutrient metabolism in trauma and infection: AA, amino acids; ACTH, adrenocorticotrophic hormone: IL1, interleukin 1; TNF, tissue necrosis factor

Table 31.5 Classification of cytokines

I	Growth factors	Size of protein
	EGF	53AA
	PDGF	125AA (A chain)
		160AA (B chain)
	IGFI	70AA
	IGFII	67AA
II	Lymphokines (Interleukins)	
	IL1	α159AA
		β153AA
	IL2	133AA
	IL6	184AA
III	Colony-stimulating factors	
IV	Transforming growth factors	
V	Interferons	
VI	Tumour necrosis factors	

EGF = epidermal growth factor
PDGF = platelet-derived growth factor
IGF = insulin-like growth factor

pathways. Their mode of action is through specific protein receptors at the cell surface, and thereafter the cellular response is effected through various signal transduction pathways (Clemens 1991) (Table 31.4).

The list of cytokines continues to grow rapidly, with new additions being a regular feature. They can, however, be classified into distinct but related groups, with some amino acid sequence homology between groups. The distinction between groups is more for convenience than related to functional differences (Tables 31.5 and 31.6).

The interactions and balance between the various cytokines may be very important (Fig. 31.5) but are as yet poorly understood. Large amounts of interleukin-1 (IL1) and tumour necrosis factor (TNF) are produced, for example in the flow state of injury or sepsis, and this induces a hyperglycaemic response via gluconeogenic pathways in the liver, whereas TNF-α and IL2, produced particularly during the ebb or shock phase, tend to lead to hypoglycaemia.

TNF is a 17 KD protein whose metabolic effects have been extensively studied in animals. It has a very

Table 31.6 Physiological roles of cytokines

Control of cell proliferation
Control of phenotypic expression
Regulation of haematopoiesis
Regulation of immune response
Control of host defences against viruses and parasites
Regulation of inflammatory response and fever
Control of cytotoxic and phagocytic cells
Wound healing
Tissue remodelling and bone formation
Influences on cellular metabolism and control of nitrogen balance

Table 31.7 The effects of tumour necrosis factor (TNF)

Organ affected	Increased biological effect
Cardiovascular endothelium	Coagulation activity
	Macromolecule entry
	Interleukin-1 (IL1) synthesis
Leukocytes	Phagocytosis and free radical production
	Prostaglandin E2 release
	Further TNF and IL1 release
Lung	Capillary permeability
	PGE2 and leukotriene release
Liver	Acute-phase protein synthesis
	Gluconeogenesis
	Lipogenesis
Fat depots	Lipolysis, FFA and glycerol release
	Insulin resistance
Muscle	Protein breakdown and amino acid release
	Glycolysis with loss of glycogen
	Glucose transporter activity
Brain	Fever
	Anorexia
	Sympathetic nervous activity
	ACTH and ADH secretion

Many of these effects are promoted by interleukin-1

wide range of actions (Table 31.7) but also interacts with other cytokines and induces, for example, the release of prostaglandin E_2 (PGE$_2$) from the endothelial wall by stimulating the release of arachidonic acid from phospholipids of the membrane. Arachidonic acid is rapidly metabolized to produce PGE$_2$ which, depending on its site of synthesis, can produce varied effects, e.g. it induces fever if synthesized within the CNS specifically acting at the thermoregulatory centre in the hypothalamus; PGE$_2$ also induces hypotension by direct action at precapillary sphincters.

The fatty acid profile of endothelial membrane phospholipids and of their tissues seems to affect both the amount of prostaglandins released and their effects on the hormone system and on other tissues. The previous fatty acid and other nutrient content of the diet may therefore affect the patient's response to infection or trauma. It is now recognized that in the major sepsis syndrome there appears to be an exaggerated cytokine response and a disruption in the balance between the cytokines released, in particular TNF-α, with consequent multiple end-organ failure. Monoclonal antibodies to TNF-α are now being explored as a way of combating the major tissue effects of TNF-α and preventing the organ failure which remains a major problem in severely injured or septic patients (Billiau & Vandekerckhove 1991, Dinarello 1991).

In general in the future, and indeed currently with the introduction of anti-TNF drugs based on monoclonal antibody synthesis, it should be possible to promote host tissue responses that lead to wound healing and bactericidal action controlled by specific cytokines, but to repress those cytokines that are responsible for increased tissue destruction and unwanted host responses. Until this system of messenger molecules has been fully elucidated and understood, it still behoves the practising clinician to be able to support patients in terms of energy substrate metabolism and the provision of appropriate amino acids for tissue healing, immune system function and lean body mass synthesis.

NUTRITIONAL SUPPORT IN TRAUMA AND SEPSIS

This is dealt with in greater detail in Chapter 29 and the importance of nutritional support in hospitals, with special teams being formed to develop a coherent programme of monitoring and treatment, has been re-emphasized in a recent report on the role of enteral and parenteral feeding (Lennard-Jones 1992). Nutritional support is best given by the oral or by the enteral route with a nasogastric tube, or a tube specially inserted by surgery into the stomach or duodenum. Glucose supplied to the gut lumen is rapidly cleared and passed via the portal circulation to the liver as glucose. However, glucose presented to the intestine via the mesenteric arterial system is primarily metabolized to lactate. The pattern of amino acids used by the enterocyte is also different from that fed, so the pattern of amino acid normally passing to the liver is different. The intestinal route for providing the body with nutrients is therefore always to be preferred.

The acute management of trauma and sepsis requires the rapid restoration of the blood volume with saline, other electrolyte solutions, albumin and plasma. Without an adequate circulation, tissue perfusion falls and this then produces profound metabolic changes, as discussed above. Arteriolar vasoconstriction induced by a very active sympathetic nervous system can also reduce tissue perfusion. The body temperature may fall markedly as metabolism is inhibited. Anaesthesia is important in preventing the neurogenic part of the shock syndrome. Rapid and effective surgery limits tissue destruction and removes the tissue where blood supply has been cut off. The risk of infections is also minimized and progressive damage can be limited by splinting bones, stitching fascial layers and closing skin wounds. In sepsis it is important to localize the infection and identify the

organism, so that an appropriate antibiotic can be given. In all these circumstances there will be a loss of water, electrolytes and plasma proteins into both the damaged tissue and into the rest of the body. With the fall in tissue metabolism and peripheral circulation, the patient feels cold and his temperature progressively falls. Insulating the patient with blankets then helps to maintain body heat.

During this phase, as explained above, it is not advisable to force-feed the patient: treating the primary problem and restoring blood volume and circulatory output are far more important. High rates of glucose infusion can be hazardous at this time, leading to unnecessary hyperglycaemia; fat infusions also have limited usefulness because of the induced hypertriglyceridaemia.

Once the ebb phase has been dealt with, the patient then displays an increase in body temperature as metabolism rises and the flow phase is entered. It is at this stage that nutrient supply can be very important. Amino acid input is especially important in septic and severely traumatized patients, who also require modest amounts of glucose, e.g. 180 g/day. Fluid and electrolyte balance continues to be crucial, and in burned patients there can be remarkable losses. Losses are now being reduced by the use of artificial skin and skin grafting, but fluid and plasma protein losses can be huge. Nursing burned patients at 30°C is also important because the temperature of the burned skin is much higher than normal. If the room temperature is below the skin temperature, then the many litres of fluid leaking into the burned area derive their heat for evaporation from the body rather than from the air. This demand for heat is met by an increase in body metabolism. The relatively anoxic burned tissue also comes to depend almost entirely on glucose, so the demand for glucose may be substantial. Thus burned patients may need 6–10 litres of fluid daily and up to 30 MJ of energy. Some of this energy can be given as fat once the cytokine inhibition of lipoprotein lipase has passed. Different types of fat, e.g. medium-chain triglycerides and special fats developed with n-6 or n-3 fatty acids, are now being explored in an attempt to reduce nitrogen losses.

Numerous energy substrates in place of glucose have been tried in the past, but it is accepted that glucose is the best carbohydrate to use. Fructose, sorbitol or ethanol may be hazardous in the injured and shocked patient who already has an increased production of lactic acid.

With the exception of major burns patients, the energy requirements of traumatized and septic patients do not show the huge increases suggested in earlier assessments; O_2 uptake rises only minimally above the usual resting levels. It is therefore neither required nor advisable to provide such patients with more than 10–12 MJ per day. As the nitrogen requirement increases with the severity of the injury, the amino acids infused must represent a higher proportion of the energy. Thus the amino acid needs may double to 25% of total energy needs in severe injury. Special measures to replace continuing losses of protein must also be assessed individually in burned patients. The routes and general principles of feeding are dealt with in Chapter 29.

REFERENCES

Billiau A, Vandekerckhove F 1991 Cytokines and their interactions with other inflammatory mediators in the pathogenesis of sepsis and septic shock. European Journal of Clinical Investigation 21: 559–573

Blackburn GL, Flatt JP, Clowes GHA, O'Donnell TF 1973 Peripheral intravenous feeding with isotonic amino acid solutions. American Journal of Surgery 125: 447–454

Cahill GF Jr 1984 Insulin resistance in critically ill patients. Proceedings of 5th European Congress on Parenteral and Enteral Nutrition. Sir David Cuthbertson Lecture

Clemens MJ 1991 Cytokines. Medical Perspective Series. Read AP, Brown T (eds). Bios Scientific Publishers

Cuthbertson DP 1982 The metabolic response to injury and other related explorations in the field of protein metabolism: an autobiographical account. Scottish Medical Journal 27: 158–171

Cuthbertson DP, Zagreb HC 1979 The metabolic response to injury and its nutritional implications. Journal of Parenteral and Enteral Nutrition 3: 108–129

Dinarello CE 1991 Interleukin-1 and Interleukin-1 antagonism. Blood 77: 1627–1652

Kinney JM 1989 Weight loss, calorimetry and malnutrition. In: Kinney JM, Borum PR (eds) Perspectives in clinical nutrition. Pall Urban & Schwarzenberg, Baltimore, pp 3–22

Lennard-Jones JE 1992 A positive approach to nutrition as treatment. Report of a working party on the role of enteral and parenteral feeding in hospital and at home. King's Fund Centre, London

Moore FD 1977 Homeostasis: bodily changes in trauma and surgery. The responses to injury in man as the basis for clinical management. In: Sabiston DC (ed) David-Christopher Textbook of Surgery, 11th edn. Saunders, Philadelphia, pp 26–64

Newsholme EA, Start C 1973 Regulation in metabolism. J Wiley & Sons, Chichester, pp 315–323

32. Obesity

J. S. Garrow

OBESITY AS A PUBLIC HEALTH PROBLEM

An expert committee of the UK Department of Health and Medical Research Council identified obesity as 'one of the most important public health problems of our time' (James 1976), but in 1992 the prevalence of obesity is even higher, and the health hazards of obesity are being even better recognized in all the affluent countries of the world. The life insurance industry has known since the beginning of this century that people who are above a certain 'desirable' weight for height are liable to die young, and hence are less profitable to insure. No single disease accounts for all the excess mortality among obese people, but cardiovascular disease is the main cause of increased mortality, as it is the main cause of death among the general population. The mortality from coronary heart disease, congestive heart failure, stroke and hypertension all increase with age, but within any age group the mortality among obese individuals is greater than among lean ones. Other diseases associated with obesity are discussed below.

DEFINITION AND PREVALENCE OF OBESITY AND OVERWEIGHT

Life insurance companies publish tables of 'desirable weights', based on the mortality experience of people they have insured. As more data become available for analysis it emerges that this desirable range corresponds closely to the range of Quetelet's Index (QI, also known as body mass index, BMI) from 20–25. The index is calculated by dividing the individual's weight (kg) by the square of his or her height (m). Thus a person who weighs 65 kg and who is 1.73 m tall would have a QI of $65/(1.73 \times 1.73) = 21.7$, which is in the desirable range. In practice it is usually more convenient to use a chart such as that shown in Fig. 32.1 which shows the boundaries of QI 20, 25, 30 and 40.

It is arbitrary to choose a value for QI above which a person is deemed obese: mortality starts to increase significantly somewhere between 25 and 30, and increases rapidly at values of QI above 30. Very thin people also show decreased longevity, so that below 20 there is also increased mortality. Therefore there is an international consensus that 20–24.9 is a 'desirable range', 25–29.9 is overweight, over 30 is obese, and over 40 very obese. Garrow (1988) used the terms Grade O, Grade I, Grade II and Grade III for the ranges of desirable, overweight, obese and very obese respectively: this notation will be used hereafter in this chapter.

The prevalence of overweight and obesity in the adult population of the UK was determined in 1980 in a survey of a representative sample of 5000 men and 5000 women aged 16–64 years. At that time the proportion of men in Grades I, II and III was 34%, 6% and 0.1%, while for women it was 24%, 8% and

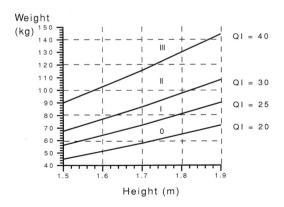

Fig. 32.1 Height–weight variation. The region 'O' indicates the desirable range of weight for height in adults. Below this is underweight, and grades of overweight are indicated by the bands I, II and III, which begin at Quetelet's Index values of 25, 30 and 40 respectively.

Table 32.1   Prevalence (%) of obesity (QI > 30) in a representative sample of men and women aged 16–64 years in the UK. Data for 1980 from Rosenbaum et al (1985) and for 1987 from Gregory et al (1990).

		Age (years)			
		16–24	25–34	35–49	50–64
Men	1980	2.5	4.5	8.0	7.7
	1987	3.0	6.0	11.0	9.0
Women	1980	3.5	4.5	9.9	14.3
	1987	6.0	11.0	10.0	18.0

0.3% respectively. The prevalence was higher among the older subjects. Another survey was done in 1987 using the same methodology, which showed an alarming increase in the prevalence of obesity (QI > 30), which overall had increased from 6% to 8% in men and from 8% to 12% in women. The increase occurred in all age groups, but particularly among women aged 25–34 years, in whom the prevalence appears to have doubled over the 7-year interval. This change is shown in Table 32.1.

It is difficult to make accurate comparisons of the prevalence of obesity in other countries, since the survey methodologies differ and, as shown above for the UK, the prevalence in a country may change greatly in a few years. A recent review of the prevalence of obesity (QI > 30) in different regions of Europe, among men and women aged 40–60 years, yields the average results in Fig. 32.2 (Siedell 1992).

In Third World countries which are liable to famine, obesity is in general rare, but the relatively affluent and urbanized parts of such countries show a rapidly increasing prevalence of obesity. Usually in affluent countries the prevalence of obesity is inversely related to social class, but there is no satisfactory explanation for this observed association. Although Grade I (QI 25–29.9) is usually more common among men than among women of the same age, obesity (QI > 30) is more common among women, and the preponderance of women increases with increasing severity of obesity. Men tend to reach the maximum prevalence of obesity at about age 45, but in women the prevalence increases to age 65 and then starts to decline. People who smoke cigarettes tend to be lighter than non-smokers, and ex-smokers tend to gain weight. It must be emphasized, however, that the fear of weight gain is not a good reason for continuing smoking: weight gain is not inevitable, and the person who stops smoking 20 cigarettes would have to gain about 20 kg in weight in order to lose the health benefit of stopping smoking. There are no marked regional differences in the prevalence of obesity in the UK when the effects of age, social class and smoking habit are allowed for.

HEALTH RISK OF OBESITY

The main cause of the premature death rate among obese people is heart disease: hypertension, coronary thrombosis and congestive heart failure are all significantly more common among obese people than among normal-weight controls. However the Seven Nations Study (Keys et al 1984) found that among men aged 45–60 years – if age, blood pressure, plasma cholesterol and smoking status were allowed for – obesity made no further contribution to predicting which men would suffer a heart attack. This finding was widely interpreted as meaning that obesity per se is not a risk factor. We now know that this is not the correct way to interpret these findings. Of course age and cigarette smoking are important contributors to the risk of heart disease in both obese and non-obese people, but obesity increases the risk (Manson et al 1990). High blood pressure, raised concentration of plasma low-density cholesterol and a low concentration of high-density cholesterol fractions are all important risk factors, but weight gain makes these factors worse and weight loss makes them better. A multivariate analysis of the data from the prospective community study from Framingham shows that obesity is related to the long-term risk of heart disease, even when the other major risk factors (age, blood pressure, plasma cholesterol, cigarettes smoked per day, glucose tolerance and left ventricular hypertrophy) have been

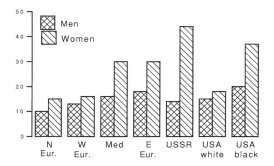

Fig. 32.2   The prevalence of obesity (QI > 30) among men and women aged 40–60 years in different geographical regions. (N Eur = Denmark, Finland, Iceland, Norway, Sweden; W Eur = Belgium, France, Germany, The Netherlands, United Kingdom; Med = Italy, Malta, Portugal, Spain, Yugoslavia; E Eur = Czechoslovakia, Germany (formerly DDR), Hungary, Poland; USSR = former Soviet republics). Data of Seidell et al 1992.

allowed for. Indeed, in women obesity was one of the best predictors of cardiovascular disease, following only age and blood pressure in relative importance (Hubert 1984). Longitudinal data from Framingham, and from the Veterans Administration Normative Aging Study (Borkan et al 1986) show that weight change in both men and women is significantly related to change in cardiovascular risk factors: weight gain in an individual was significantly associated with increased blood pressure, cholesterol, triglycerides, fasting glucose, postprandial glucose and uric acid, and with a decrease in forced vital capacity, whereas weight loss was significantly associated with an improvement of all these factors.

Fat distribution and health risk

A study in Gothenburg, Sweden, showed that people with a high waist–hip ratio (indicating that fat was largely in the abdominal cavity, rather than sub-cutaneously on the limbs) had a greater risk of heart disease and diabetes than people with a similar amount of fat distributed peripherally (Lapidus et al 1984). This probably relates to the insulin insensitivity which is caused by a high flux of free fatty acids in the portal circulation, because intra-abdominal fat cells can release fatty acids very rapidly. However, further studies have shown that the increased mortality among men was not significantly related to waist–hip ratio when the follow-up period was extended to 20 years (Larsson 1987), and the central distribution of fat is associated with both cigarette smoking and a high alcohol intake, which may have contributed to some of the observed excess mortality risk.

Obesity and insulin insensitivity

Non-insulin dependent diabetes mellitus (NIDDM) is not a major cause of death in normal-weight people, but it is an important contributor to morbidity and mortality in obese people. A man more than 140% of average weight is 5.2 times more likely to die of diabetes than a normal-weight man, and for women the mortality ratio is 7.9 times for a similar degree of overweight (Lew & Garfinkel 1979). A classic study of experimental obesity in Vermont has shown that the association between obesity and reduced insulin sen-sitivity (which is the primary problem in NIDDM) is a causal one. Young male volunteers, with no family history of diabetes or obesity, overate for 6 months and increased their weight by 21%, of which 73% was fat; they then showed significant changes in biochem-istry in the direction of diabetes. After weight loss to

normal values these changes reverted to normal (Sims et al 1973).

Other metabolic effects of obesity

Obesity is an important risk factor for gallstone formation, because the bile of obese people is super-saturated with cholesterol and hence liable to form gallstones. Excess adipose tissue contains a large amount of cholesterol. Adipose tissue is also a source of aromatase, the enzyme system which converts androgens to oestrogens. This probably explains the frequent menstrual problems of obese women. Obese men have an increased risk of cancers of the colon, rectum and prostate, whereas in women the increased risk involves the breast, ovary, endometrium and cervix; this may be associated with abnormal levels of sex hormones. Other penalties of obesity include osteoarthritis of the weight-bearing joints (especially back, hips and knees), problems with anaesthesia and surgery, and social discrimination (Garrow 1988).

All of these penalties of obesity decrease with weight loss, with the exception of the risk of gallstone formation. During weight loss in an obese person the cholesterol in adipose tissue is mobilized and the bile may become even more liable to form cholesterol stones.

Fig. 32.3 is an attempt to show how obesity and cigarette smoking, together with other factors which are discussed elsewhere in this book – such as a high intake of saturated fat, salt or alcohol, or lack of physical activity – can combine to increase the risk of

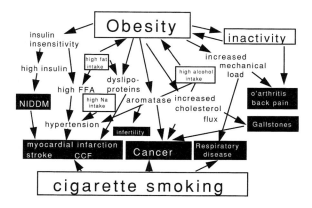

Fig. 32.3 Important diseases are shown in black boxes, and some alterable lifestyle factors which predispose to these diseases are shown in white boxes. Mechanisms that link lifestyle factors to disease risk are discussed in the text. (NIDDM = non-insulin dependent diabetes mellitus.)

many important diseases. This tendency of obesity to increase so many disease risks makes it a very important public health problem.

THERMODYNAMICS OF OBESITY AND WEIGHT LOSS

Methods for measuring body composition, and particularly the fat mass in living people, are described in Chapter 2. The excess weight in obese people comprises 75% fat and 25% fat-free tissue (which is about 75% water and 25% protein). Since fat has an energy value of 9000 kcal (37 MJ)/kg, and fat-free tissue about 1000 kcal (4 MJ)/kg, this mixture in adipose tissue has an energy value of 7000 kcal (29 MJ)/kg. We can therefore say with confidence that people who are, say, 20 kg overweight must, during their life, have had an energy intake which was 140 000 kcal greater than their energy expenditure.

Suppose this weight was gained over a period of 10 years, then the average energy imbalance is less than 40 kcal/day, but this does not mean that if a person who was previously in energy balance decides to eat an extra 40 kcal/day he will gain 20 kg in 10 years, for reasons which are explained in Chapter 9. Energy intake affects energy output in several ways. First, when the person started to eat more their dietary thermogenesis would increase, which would account for about 10% of the excess intake. Next, the energy stored would increase both the fat and the fat-free mass, and this would cause an increase in metabolic rate. Finally, there is some adaptive or regulatory change in metabolic rate which tends to oppose weight change: metabolic rate goes up with overfeeding and goes down with underfeeding, so that long before weight increased by 20 kg, energy expenditure would have increased by 40 kcal/day, and a new equilibrium would have been reached at a higher weight than previously.

The thermodynamics of weight loss is rather simpler than that of weight gain, because although there is a substantial metabolic cost involved in storing excess dietary energy as body fat, protein or glycogen, the mobilization of these energy stores is a process which has little metabolic cost. It is a common observation that dieters lose weight rapidly at first, and then more slowly, and this is often ascribed to some metabolic adaptation to the diet. In fact there are three reasons for the decreasing rate of weight loss: First, and most important, the initial weight loss includes a large proportion of glycogen, and 1 g glycogen binds about 3 g water, so the glycogen loss is accompanied by a corresponding loss of water and of

weight in excess of the amount expected on the basis of 1 kg being equivalent to 7000 kcal. Secondly, after the first few weeks the dieter becomes less conscientious about keeping to the diet. This can be demonstrated if dieters who have a weight 'plateau' are admitted to a metabolic ward where the diet is strictly calculated: weight loss immediately restarts (Garrow 1988). Thirdly, with substantial weight loss metabolic rate is reduced, so that on a given diet the energy deficit is reduced and weight loss becomes slower. It should be noted, however, that the average obese person has a metabolic rate which is higher than normal, and the decrease in metabolic rate on reduction to normal weight is the expected decrease from a high level to a normal one, and not to an abnormally low one (Dore et al 1982)

AETIOLOGY OF OBESITY

What is the cause of obesity? At a very simple level we can say, for the reasons given above, that a person who is 20 kg overweight has taken in about 140 000 kcal more than he or she required to maintain normal body composition. However, that is not a very satisfactory answer to the question. *Why* do some people take in much more energy than they require? To this simple question there is no simple answer, but some of the factors which predispose to obesity are briefly discussed below.

Genetic factors in human obesity

Obesity tends to run in families, but that does not prove that it is genetically determined. Transmission within a family may be cultural: for example obese dogs tend to have obese owners, but clearly this has nothing to do with genetics. Careful studies of parents and children, siblings, adoptees, and of identical and non-identical twins, have yielded estimates which range from about 5% to 70% concerning the extent to which genetic factors affect the risk of obesity. However, no-one is condemned inevitably to be obese because their parents were obese: it seems that the characteristic which is inherited is a tendency to overeat in some circumstances. If this tendency is resisted, obesity will not develop.

Age and sex

Table 32.1 shows that the prevalence of obesity increases with age in men up to age 50, and in women it continues to increase up to age 65. Fig. 32.2 shows that in every geographical region, in the age group

40–60 years, the prevalence is higher among women than among men.

Inactivity as a cause of obesity

Severely obese people are inactive, because they are too unfit to undertake much exercise. However, there is very little evidence that inactivity either in children or adults is a cause of obesity (Romanella et al 1991). Most people in affluent countries lead sedentary lives, and it is difficult to show that the average obese person is any more sedentary than his or her lean equivalent.

Childhood growth pattern as a predictor of later obesity

Severely obese people who come to hospital for investigation often were fat babies. This gave rise to the hypothesis that overfeeding in infancy caused an increase in the number of fat cells in the body, and hence the liability to obesity in adult life, but prospective studies have not supported this hypothesis. It is not possible to predict with useful accuracy which children will be overweight at age 7 years by analysing birthweight, or any aspect of rate of growth in infancy (Mellbin & Veuille 1973). Children from obese families who become overweight tend to grow taller and with an accelerated development; they tend to enter puberty earlier. There is also a significant relationship between the weight of a child in infancy, at age 7 and adult weight assessed at age 28 (Garn et al 1975, 1980).

Social factors as predictors of weight gain in adult life

In developed countries there is an inverse relationship between the prevalence of obesity and socioeconomic status. A study in Finland showed that the risk of rapid weight gain (>5 kg/5 years) was greatest for people with a low educational level, chronic disease, low physical activity during leisure hours, high alcohol consumption, and those who stopped smoking cigarettes (Rissanen et al 1991). Many attempts have been made to explain these associations on the basis that poorer and less well-educated people are more likely to eat fatty foods, rather than the more expensive fruit and vegetables, and to have many children, which also is associated with a high risk of weight gain. These explanations are unsatisfactory: in the study from Finland high parity was associated with high weight gain among women of low educational level, but with low weight gain in women of high

educational level. The only plausible explanation of these observations is that highly educated Finnish women who have many pregnancies are vigilant to prevent excessive weight gain, whereas those who are less well-educated are not.

TREATMENT OF OBESITY

A negative energy balance can be achieved by increasing energy output or decreasing energy intake, or a combination of both. The best strategy depends on the ability, inclinations and degree of obesity of the subject. It is useless to advise a severely obese person to make a significant increase in energy output by taking more physical exercise, because the exercise tolerance of such a person is very poor, and the level of exertion which will cause exhaustion will make only a trivial impact on overall energy balance. On the other hand, a relatively sedentary person who is only a few pounds overweight would do well to take more exercise, partly because that would help to restore weight to normal, and partly because exercise contributes to general fitness and confers other metabolic benefits, which are not completely understood.

It is important to remember that the obese person who seeks the help of a doctor or dietitian has almost certainly already tried to lose weight in some way, and is dissatisfied with the results obtained. It is useless to offer more advice until you have discovered what the patient has already tried, and why the outcome was regarded as unsatisfactory. Sometimes previous attempts have failed because the advice followed was unsound (e.g. 'it does not matter what you eat so long as you cut out all sugary foods') and sometimes because the expectations were quite unrealistic (e.g. 'you should lose 7 lb in the first week, and 20 lb in a month'). You will not carry much authority as an advisor unless you discover these misconceptions and expose the errors on which they are based. The following brief checklist should ensure that before starting to give advice to an obese patient you are aware of essential background facts: individual items are discussed more fully elsewhere (Garrow 1988).

Factors which influence the advice which is appropriate

1. *Age and weight-for-height of patient* (see Fig. 32.1). If the patient is in Grade O weight loss is not appropriate: the younger and more overweight the patient the greater is the benefit to be derived from weight loss.

2. *Patient's target weight and expected benefit from weight loss.* Beware the patient who is aiming for too low a target weight: it is reasonable to offer help to get the patient to QI = 25, but no lower. The benefits which can be expected from weight loss have been discussed above. Realistic rates of weight loss are discussed below.

3. *Previous attempts at weight loss.* What methods were tried, for how long, with what result, and why were they considered unsatisfactory?

4. *Domestic circumstances:* do these limit dietary options? Does the patient's employment involve catering or food handling, working night shifts, or business entertaining? Who does the shopping and cooking, and for whom else apart from the patient? Are other members of the household supportive concerning the patient's attempts at weight loss?

5. *Other diseases and medication.* Patients on medication for hypertension or diabetes should be aware that weight loss will affect the dosage required. Special considerations apply in pregnancy, epilepsy, gout, and with some psychotropic medication.

6. *A concealed agenda.* Sometimes it emerges from the above enquiries, or from the referring letter, that the patient has a particular objective in seeking help at this time: this may arise from a newspaper or television item about a new wonder treatment for obesity. If not, it may be helpful to ask if there is a particular form of treatment which the patient hoped to receive. Otherwise (from the patient's viewpoint) the real point of the visit may never be mentioned.

It only takes a few minutes to collect this information about each patient, and thus to obtain a basis on which appropriate advice can be given. Without this information it is likely that the interview will be a total waste of time for both patient and advisor. Before considering specific advice we need to beware of two common pitfalls in obesity treatment.

Appropriate rate of weight loss

In practice the range of rates of weight loss shown in Fig. 32.4 is best for most people: those who are younger, taller and more overweight may aim for the higher limit, while those who are older, shorter and less overweight should be satisfied with something near the lower limit. For the first month of dieting the rate of weight loss is more rapid due to the glycogen/water effect described above. Subsequently, the optimum rate of weight loss is 0.5–1.0 kg (1–2 lb)/week, which represents an average energy deficit of

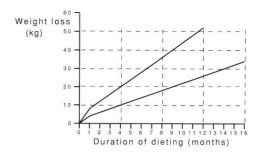

Fig. 32.4 Desirable rates of weight loss in overweight and obese people. An average energy deficit of 1000 kcal/day will cause weight loss at the upper limit of the zone, and 500 kcal/day at the lower limit. Younger, taller, male and more overweight patients should aim at the upper line, while the lower line is more appropriate for older, shorter, female and less overweight patients.

500–1000 kcal (2–4 MJ)/day. The disadvantage of energy deficits greater than 1000 kcal/day are that there may be excessive loss of lean tissue; it becomes difficult to provide the essential nutrients in such a restricted diet; it is unnecessarily unpleasant; and there will have to be further large adjustments when the target weight is achieved, to find a suitable weight-maintenance diet. The disadvantages of deficits less than 500 kcal/day are that it takes too long for the subject to reach the target weight, unless the initial excess weight was very small.

Dieting relationship trap

It is remarkable that hostility often arises between obese patients and the health care professional who is trying to assist with weight loss. It seems that both parties fall into what has been termed a 'dieting relationship trap' (Garrow 1992). The way in which it operates is as follows. Initially the patient comes for advice about losing weight, usually to obtain relief from some of the complications of obesity which have already been mentioned, and is pleased to find a doctor or dietitian who is willing and able to help with sensible dietary advice. If the patient is severely obese both parties may underestimate the time which it will take to achieve adequate weight loss, and the difficulty of sustaining dietary compliance over a period of many months.

On follow-up visits all goes well so long as satisfactory weight loss has been achieved since the last visit, but inevitably the time comes when the patient returns having not lost weight, or even having regained some weight. Obese patients usually suffer from low self-esteem, so when they perceive that they have failed both themselves and the health carer they are precipitated into an agony of self-reproach. They apologize profusely for their weakness, confess their unworthiness for any further help or consideration, and virtually invite the health carer to discharge them instantly, and with ignominy. Thus the trap is set.

Of course the correct response of the health carer at this point is to agree that it is disappointing that weight loss has temporarily ceased, to assure the patient that massive weight loss uninterrupted by setbacks is virtually unknown, and to get down to identifying the factors which precipitated the problem, and how they can best be avoided in the future: above all to provide encouragement, not criticism. The wrong response (into which it is all too easy to slip) is to agree that the patient is not worthy of further help or consideration, that weight loss is all a matter of discipline, and that in the absence of that discipline any attempt to help is a waste of the health carer's valuable time. Thus the blame for failure is fixed firmly on the patient, another attempt at dieting is destroyed, and the self-esteem of the patient is further reduced. If that is the best the health carer can do then it would be better not to undertake the care of obese patients.

On the other hand, it is possible to carry sympathy with the patient too far. There is little to be gained from regular monthly meetings between obese patient and carer at which the lack of any weight loss is noted, the difficulty of dieting is agreed, but nothing is done to increase the chance of success next time.

Summary: Objectives when treating obese patients

Obesity is worth treating because the obese patient is liable to severe physical and social handicaps, and it is the job of the health carer to help the patient to avoid these handicaps. This is achieved by giving the patient a realistic estimate of the health hazards associated with the condition in that patient, a realistic target weight and rate of weight loss, and advice and encouragement to follow the particular treatment strategy (of which the options are discussed below) which is most likely to achieve that target. We can endorse a statement which was made in the 5th edition of this book: 'Even if there were no other practical problems in human nutrition, the dietitian would more than justify her training and knowledge by the help she can give to fat people' (Davidson et al 1972). The statement is still true, but in the last 20 years we have learned a great deal more about why obesity increases the risk of disease, and what can be done about it.

TREATMENT BY DIET ALONE

Advice for reducing dietary energy intake

The rate of weight loss shown in Fig. 32.4 is achieved with an energy deficit of 500–1000 kcal/day. It may seem logical, therefore, to assess the present energy intake of the patient by means of a dietary history, and then prescribe a diet which provides 500–1000 kcal/day less than estimated habitual intake. In practice this is not useful, since it is so difficult to obtain a reliable estimate of habitual energy intake in obese patients (Garrow 1988). A rule of thumb is to start with a diet supplying 1000 kcal/day for an average obese woman (say age 30 years, weight 80 kg, height 1.6 m) and to increase this up to 1500 kcal/day for men or younger, taller or heavier women, or decrease to 800 kcal/day for older, shorter women. This estimate can be revised if the observed rate of weight loss is too high or too low. It is never necessary to prescribe a reducing diet outside the range of 800–1500 kcal/day.

The diet must provide the essential nutrients, so it is logical especially to seek to restrict those food items which provide energy but little else of nutritional importance, such as sucrose and alcohol. For reasons discussed elsewhere in this book it is desirable to restrict the intake of fat, and particularly saturated fat. This is partly because this policy is helpful in decreasing the risk of atheromatous heart disease, partly because fat is a concentrated energy source, and partly because there is some evidence that fat has a lower satiating capacity than isoenergetic quantities of carbohydrate or protein. The foods which are not restricted are fruit, vegetables and whole-grain cereals, since these are important sources of micronutrients and non-starch polysaccharides. It is important that protein intake should be adequate to avoid unnecessary loss of lean tissue, but extremely high-protein diets are expensive and have not been shown to be particularly effective or acceptable. Within these guidelines it is possible to construct an infinite variety of nutritionally sound reducing diets which can be adapted to the requirements of individual patients.

Very low-calorie diets (VLCD)

Commercial diets which provide the recommended daily amounts of micronutrients with minimal energy are heavily advertised, and are attractive to patients wishing to lose weight rapidly. The disadvantages are that the rapid weight loss may signify excessive loss of lean tissue, the commercial aspects may cause the product to be given to people for whom weight loss is not appropriate, and the prospects for maintaining weight loss are not good for people who have not learned the principles on which reducing diets should be based. Despite these anxieties some authorities believe that VLCD have a place in the treatment of severe obesity: others do not (Garrow 1989).

Acceptability of reducing diets

It is very difficult to predict which diet will prove most acceptable to a given obese patient. Presumably the diet the patient prefers is the one on which obesity developed, so a willingness to change from this is a necessary condition for successful weight loss. Some patients prefer exactly specified diets, whereas others prefer more flexibility. Patients may say that they find dieting difficult because they get hungry, but on closer questioning this may mean that they long for a particular forbidden item of food, such as chocolate. It is not clear if a small ration of chocolate (in this instance) is helpful or not: people differ. For some patients a monotonous bland diet (such as milk only) is easier to keep to than a varied diet, but for others it is intolerable.

Probably the factors which most help people to keep to a reducing diet are to have clear instructions about a diet appropriate for their weight, tastes and social circumstances, together with a realistic forecast of the rate of weight loss that this diet should produce. Good dietitians have the skill to provide this information: there is much more to it than simply handing out a standard diet sheet.

Frequency and timing of meals

Traditionally patients are advised to have small meals evenly spaced throughout the day, and this advice is probably sound, although there is no impressive evidence of efficacy based on randomized controlled trials. In a crossover protocol in a metabolic ward where obese patients were fed 800 kcal as either one or five meals per day, the patients were much hungrier, and lost more lean tissue, on the one-meal phase of the study than when they were receiving five meals per day (Garrow et al 1981). However, there is no evidence that meal frequency affects total energy output. It is probably useful for patients to establish a formal pattern of eating meals at specified times, since continuous snacking or 'grazing' makes it very difficult to establish any control over total energy intake (Booth et al 1970).

Behaviour therapy

In the last decade psychologists have greatly increased our understanding of dieting behaviour. Most of us eat more or less automatically. If a patient's eating behaviour is to be altered, it is first necessary to become aware of what is being eaten and the circumstances that tend to trigger inappropriate eating. The mere recording of a food diary is associated with some weight loss in most people, which suggests that we eat less when we are required to pay attention to what we eat, and such a food diary is also useful for the dietitian to assess the patient's habitual diet. There may be recurrent domestic situations which tend to precipitate binge eating: if these can be identified and avoided, it increases the chance of compliance with the diet. It is also very helpful if other members of the patient's household provide intelligent cooperation with dieting efforts: ignorant nagging or ridicule from other members of the family will defeat all but the most determined dieter.

The central premise of behavioural therapy for obesity is that eating behaviour is not instinctive, but learned. In obesity, eating behaviour is inappropriate so it should be relearned. This approach is very effective, and should be in the repertoire of every dietitian. However, it is a mistake to suppose that the treatment of obesity can be achieved by teaching the patient to eat 'normally': it is true that control of abnormal eating binges is necessary if worthwhile weight loss is to be achieved, but that alone will not cause the weight loss. Severely obese patients are being asked to eat *abnormally* over quite a long time: if they have excess energy stores amounting to (say) 140 000 kcal, they are being asked to eat 140 000 kcal less than their requirements over a period of several months. Certainly it is a mistake to imagine that behaviour therapy somehow avoids the need to restrict energy intake: what it does is to make that restriction of energy intake easier to achieve.

Weight-loss groups

It is probably useful for the obese patient to have an initial assessment one-to-one with a dietitian, so the necessary information described above can be collected. However, for follow-up sessions there are several advantages in working with groups of about 10–15 patients (Bush et al 1988). It is a more efficient use of the dietitian's time to talk to a group of patients than to repeat almost the same message many times to the members of the group individually. Provided that the group is skilfully and sensitively led, the patients benefit from associating with other people in a similar situation, and hearing answers to problems raised by other members of the group. This is particularly true for diffident patients who would not have had the courage to raise the problem themselves. However, group treatment is not a panacea, and may be disastrous if there is a particularly assertive or destructive personality within the group.

Long-term efficacy of dietary treatment

There are few good long-term controlled studies of the efficacy of purely dietary intervention in obesity, and the studies which have been published show rather poor results (Geppert & Splett 1991). Programmes which try to follow participants for 12 months always have high dropout rates, which is not surprising, because long before 12 months the participants have learned the essentials of dieting, and there is no great incentive to attend a clinic to be weighed when they could as easily weigh themselves at home. In one study which initially enrolled 95 women and 20 men, only 13 women and 4 men were still attending for monthly visits up to 1 year, but 80 women and 18 men were traced and weighed at home visits (Gilbert & Garrow 1983). In this study the patients were randomly assigned to one of three treatment methods: diet alone, diet with behaviour modification, or diet with an anorectic drug. Among the women traced after 1 year, in those on diet alone the weight loss (mean ± SD) was 1.6 ± 7.6 kg; in those on the anorectic drug 6.3 ± 8.3 kg; and in those as behaviour therapy, 7.6 ± 10.5 kg. A striking feature of the trial was the large variability in response within each treatment group. This underlines the point already made: that different obese patients have different requirements for treatment.

Effect of weight cycling on health and energy requirements

Epidemiological surveys have shown that people whose weight remains stable tend to live longer, and have less cardiovascular disease, than people who show large variations in weight (Wannamethee & Shaper 1990, Lissner et al 1991). It is not clear if the weight cycling causes the ill health: it might be that ill health, or a particular type of personality associated with heart disease, causes the weight cycling. However, on theoretical grounds alternating cycles of starvation and overeating are likely to be unhealthy. There is no good evidence that weight cycling has an

important effect on metabolic rate or body composition (Jebb et al 1991), but it is difficult to study people who undergo large cycles of weight change.

ADJUNCTS TO NUTRITIONAL THERAPY FOR OBESITY

Drug treatment

Anorectic drugs

The mechanisms which tend to maintain energy balance in man are discussed in Chapter 9. Hunger tends to make people on a low-energy diet eat more, so a drug which would abolish hunger should be useful. There are three types of medication which are intended to have this effect. Bulk fillers, such as guar gum, reduce food intake if taken in sufficient quantity, but the discomfort involved in taking quantities which have a significant effect is similar to the discomfort of the hunger they are designed to relieve, so they are not generally useful. Drugs related to amphetamine have a very significant anorectic effect on hunger, but they are also central nervous system stimulants, and hence liable to be abused. Large doses of amphetamine can produce a psychotic state similar to schizophrenia, so the prescription of these drugs is closely controlled.

Probably the most widely used anorectic drug is D-fenfluramine, which acts through the serotinergic system in the brain, and is sedative rather than stimulant. Its efficacy was tested in a large, long-term multicentre study in which the patients were prescribed a conventional energy-restricted diet and a tablet (15 mg D-fenfluramine bd. or placebo) for 12 months, with monthly assessments (Guy-Grand et al 1989). At 12 months 37% of the drug group and 45% of those on placebo had withdrawn for various reasons: the mean weight loss among those who completed the trial was 9.82 kg or 7.15 kg, for drug or placebo groups respectively: all the weight loss had occurred in the first 6 months. To achieve the desirable range of weight-for-height the average patient would have needed to lose about 36 kg, so at the end of the trial those who had taken the drug had about 26 kg still to lose, compared with the controls who had about 29 kg still to lose.

Similar results are reported for a long-term trial on fluoxetine in a dosage of 60 mg/day (Darga et al 1991). There were 45 patients who initially weighed 103 kg, so they had about 33 kg to lose. The dropout rate was 41% or 27% for drug or placebo group. After 1 year the mean weight losses in the completers on drug or placebo were 8.2 kg and 4.5 kg respectively, but the mean starting weight of the group on fluoxetine had been 5.8 kg greater than those on placebo. The maximum weight loss in the drug group was 12.4 kg at week 29, and thereafter they gained weight significantly, despite continuing to take the drug. Probably the benefits derived from the use of anorectic drugs do not outweigh the disadvantages. In the long term anorectic drugs have not proved very helpful to dieters, because although they decrease hunger in the short term they do nothing to help with the eventual problem of maintaining weight loss.

Thermogenic drugs

Thyroid hormone will increase the weight lost on a diet if given in higher dose than that which will replace the natural hormone, but the extra weight loss is mainly lean tissue. Recently there has been intense research to find a drug which will activate energy-wasting reactions in the body without adverse effects. Although several drugs are under development, none has yet proved useful in the treatment of obesity.

Drugs to inhibit digestion and absorption of food from the gut

Several substances will block the action of digestive enzymes in vitro, but are not effective in preventing the digestion of a meal when taken orally. If an effective drug is found it will be difficult to demonstrate its safety for long-term use, since the nutrients which are not absorbed in the small bowel will become available as a substrate for anaerobic metabolism by colonic bacteria. This will almost certainly cause flatulence, and may have more serious consequences as the bacteria in the colon adapt to the new energy supply. This class of drugs has not yet been shown to be useful in clinical practice.

Diuretics

Well known drugs increase urine output, and hence cause a temporary decrease in weight. These have no place in the treatment of obesity. Obese people often have some ankle oedema, since venous return from the legs is inefficient, but the correct management is to remove the excess fat which is overburdening the circulation, rather than giving diuretics to treat the swollen ankles.

Exercise as a treatment for obesity

Physical activity increases energy expenditure, physical fitness and sensitivity to the action of insulin, all of which are valuable effects for obese people. Although elite athletes can maintain very high levels of energy expenditure for sustained periods, the maximum rate of work of the average non-athlete is about 6 kcal (25 kJ)/min over 1 h. The average resting metabolism is about 1 kcal (4 kJ)/min, so after 1 h the jogger will have used about 360 kcal, while his twin who remained at rest used 60 kcal, so the net cost of an hour's jogging is about 300 kcal. This is probably the upper limit of the increase in energy expenditure that it is realistic to expect overweight people to achieve by exercise. At this level of exercise intensity there is no measurable elevation of metabolic rate when the exercise has stopped.

It is often claimed that physical training can selectively increase the fat-free mass of the body, so although the obese person may not experience weight loss, some fat is being replaced by an equal weight of muscle. A recent review of the evidence by Forbes (1992) did not find evidence to support this claim. Certainly obese patients should be encouraged to take exercise within the limitations of their tolerance, and they will benefit in physical fitness by doing so. However, exercise alone is not an effective method for achieving weight loss, nor of significantly altering the proportions of fat and lean issue in the body.

SURGICAL PROCEDURES

It is outside the scope of this book to give a detailed account of surgical procedures for the treatment of obesity, but general physicians and dietitians may be asked to give guidance to severely obese patients about surgery as an option 'instead of dieting'. The most important point is that surgical treatment of obesity (with one minor exception) is not an *alternative* to dieting, but a method for *trying to enforce* dieting. The minor exception is apronectomy: it is possible for the surgeon to cut away fat hanging in a fold of anterior abdominal wall, but this is really only applicable in severely obese patients, and preferably those who have already lost a considerable amount of their excess fat. Cutting or sucking fat from subcutaneous sites is advertised as a cosmetic procedure, but the amount of fat which can be removed is trivial in comparison with the total excess fat in a patient who has medically important obesity. In many cases the cosmetic result from an attempt to remove significant quantities of subcutaneous fat is very unsatisfactory.

Gastric bypass

This is an operation in which the gut is cut and rejoined to provide a relatively short exposure of the food to the action of digestive enzymes, while the majority of the bowel is short-circuited. The objective is to produce some degree of malabsorption, so that some of the energy in the food is not absorbed, and also so that a large energy intake provokes severe diarrhoea. The weight loss caused by operations of this kind depends more on the aversive consequences if the patient overeats, than on failure to absorb what is eaten.

Gastric stapling

In this operation a line of staples closes off all but a small pouch at the fundus, which empties through a small stoma into the main body of the stomach, so that only about 50 ml of food can be taken at a time. Typically patients lose about one-third of their excess weight in the year after operation, but there is then a tendency for weight regain. Weight loss is somewhat greater after the bypass than the stapling operation, but at the cost of greater metabolic complications, and a greater risk of nutrient deficiencies. Both operations are technically reversible, but weight gain after reversal is rapid and almost universal.

The relative advantages and disadvantages of these two operations have been reviewed in a Consensus Statement (1991): the main points which were agreed are set out below.

1. Patients seeking therapy for severe obesity for the first time should be considered for treatment in a non-surgical programme, with integrated components of a dietary regimen, appropriate exercise and behavioral modification and support.

2. Gastric restrictive or bypass procedures could be considered for well-informed and motivated patients with acceptable operative risks.

3. Patients who are candidates for surgical procedures should be selected carefully after evaluation by a multidisciplinary team with medical, surgical, psychiatric and nutritional expertise.

4. The operation should be performed by a surgeon substantially experienced in the appropriate procedures, and working in a clinical setting with adequate support for all aspects of management and assessment.

5. Lifetime medical surveillance after surgical therapy is a necessity.

There are views with which experts in the field would agree: the problem in real life is what to do with the severely obese patient who is not well motivated, or is not a good operative risk, or in whom the careful evaluation reveals some other reason why they are not ideally suited for surgery. The answer is that surgery is often selected because it seems to be the best choice at the time, but this decision may later be regretted by those who inherit the task of lifelong medical supervision.

Gastric balloon

Balloons have been inserted into the stomach to reduce gastric capacity without the hazards associated with abdominal operations in obese people. The results have been disappointing: weight loss is small and not sustained, and the risk of ulcerating the gastric mucosa is significant.

Jaw wiring

It is standard orthodontic practice to wire the upper and lower jaws together for the treatment of jaw fractures, or when it has been necessary to resect part of the lower jaw. With this procedure the patient can drink but not chew, and since liquid diets tend to have a low energy density they often lose weight. Advantage was taken of this effect in the treatment of obesity (Garrow 1974), but although weight loss of about 36 kg in 9 months was achieved it was not sustained when the wires were removed. The procedure is not justified unless it is combined with some method for helping the patient to maintain the weight loss (see below).

MAINTENANCE OF WEIGHT LOSS

If a patient manages to keep to a reducing diet for many months and achieves massive weight loss, it must not be assumed that the weight loss will be automatically maintained when the intense dieting effort is over. On the contrary, it should be assumed that a patient who reduces from, say, 100 kg to 70 kg will revert to 100 kg unless something is done to maintain the weight at 70 kg. After weight loss energy requirements are reduced (see Chapter 9), so if the patient goes back to eating 'normally' (that is, to the diet which previously supported a weight of 100 kg) then that is the weight which will be regained before equilibrium is re-established. We do not know what

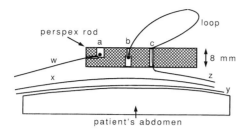

Fig. 32.5 A waist cord provides warning of unwanted weight regain in obese patients who have lost a substantial amount of weight. In this version a monofilament nylon fishing line (W) is secured to the end of a 35 mm long perspex rod by a knot in the hole (a). It is taken twice round the patient's waist (X and Y) and the third turn (Z) passes through the hole (c) and is secured by a knot in the hole (b), so the maximum circumference is fixed. Normally there is some slack in the cord, which is taken up as one or two loops around the right-hand end of the rod. These can be released to accommodate temporary periods of modest weight gain.

keeps people of desirable weight at their desirable weight, but whatever this characteristic may be it clearly is not possessed by the formerly obese person.

Most people in affluent countries control their weight at least in part by noting unacceptable increases in weight and altering energy intake (or output) to compensate. To a person who has never been more than 70 kg an increase to 80 kg is a new experience, which will cause some alarm, but this is not true of a person who was previously 100 kg. Reduced obese people benefit from a device which warns them of weight gain, which may be a spouse, a flatmate, or a favourite pair of jeans. Alternatively, this monitoring function can be performed by a nylon cord fixed round the waist which becomes tight if excessive weight is gained (Garrow 1988). A disadvantage with earlier versions of the waist cord was that it was either too loose to provide a sensitive monitor of unwanted weight gain, or else too tight to accommodate fluctuations in weight such as might occur premenstrually, or at an occasional celebratory meal. The version shown in Fig. 32.5 can be shortened by taking a turn or two round the perspex rod for normal use, but these can be released to accommodate temporary weight gain. The patient must remember to lose the weight and regain room for manoeuvre, before the next episode of temporary weight gain.

UNORTHODOX THERAPIES FOR OBESITY

Since there will always be many people hoping to lose weight without the inconvenience of dieting, there will

always be 'wonder cures' which contravene the laws of thermodynamics. These change all the time, but some typical examples will be briefly reviewed.

Slimming tea

Beverages originating in exotic oriental countries are on offer which are said to dissolve away fat. This is neither true nor possible. Volunteers taking a slimming tea achieved a weight loss which was 2.5 kg less than that achieved on a placebo treatment in a controlled trial in which subjects were recruited by a television programme (Sanders et al 1990).

Ornithine/arginine pill

Pills containing some products of intermediary metabolism are promoted on the grounds that they stimulate metabolism, and hence cause weight loss without dieting. Except for certain thermogenic drugs mentioned above, this is not true, and if it were true the disadvantages of thermogenic drugs have already been discussed. In the same television-inspired trial (Sanders et al 1990), volunteers on an arginine/ornithine pill did no better than those on placebo.

Hypnosis

It is plausible that hypnotic suggestion might make certain favourite fattening foods aversive. However, no good trial of hypnotherapy for obesity has shown significant weight loss. Since there are no foods which are uniquely fattening, and the subject must eat something, it seems to be too difficult to implant, by hypnosis, the quite complicated changes in eating behaviour which are required to achieve and sustain significant weight loss.

Human chorionic gonadotrophin

Many people associate obesity with hormonal dysfunction, and pregacy with weight change. This may account for the credence given to a treatment of obesity by intramuscular injections of the placental hormone chorionic gonadotrophin. However, several controlled trials have failed to show any superiority for this treatment over saline injections.

Food combination diets

Hay was probably the first to propound the view that certain macronutrients, such as protein and carbohydrate, could not be digested when taken together, since the digestive enzymes for protein worked in an acid medium whereas those for carbohydrate required an alkaline medium. (Although this is in general true, the digestion is achieved at different times and places: first the protein in the stomach, and then the carbohydrate in the small bowel.) This faulty understanding of gastrointestinal physiology was the basis for the Hay Diet (and many subsequent modifications) in which restrictions are placed on the types of food which can be eaten at one meal. These usually cause some weight loss, since the restrictions reduce total energy intake, but the weight loss is caused by the reduced energy intake and not by the separation of dietary macronutrients.

It is impossible and unnecessary to discuss all the bizarre treatments which are offered for obesity. It is hoped that the general principles set out in this book will enable the reader to explain to patients the flaws in treatments which are not based on sound nutritional principles.

REFRACTORY OBESITY

Hospital obesity clinics are often called upon to investigate the metabolism of an obese person who inexorably gains weight while apparently keeping rigorously to a diet supplying only 800 kcal/day. This implies that the energy expenditure of the patient must be less than 800 kcal/day, but when this is checked in those centres which are fortunate to have facilities for 24-hour calorimetry, the observed energy output is always far in excess of 800 kcal/day (Garrow 1988). The only conclusion compatible with thermodynamic principles which can be drawn from these observations is that the calculated diet was wrong: there may have been periods during which it was only 800 kcal/day, but on average it must have been much more, or prolonged weight gain would not have occurred. It should be emphasized that these patients are not deliberately lying about their dietary intake: they are reporting what they believe to be true. These unfortunate people may be driven to try all sorts of drastic treatments with starvation, drugs or abdominal surgery, because they believe that conventional diets are ineffective in their case, so it is important to establish the truth. In places where there are no facilities for calorimetry it may be useful to ask the patient to keep to a daily diet consisting solely of two pints of full-fat milk (or three of semi-skimmed) for 3 weeks (which provides 800 kcal/day), and to observe weight change over this period. If a weight loss of more than 2 kg is observed (as almost always happens) then an error in the calculation of the diet must be sought, but if no weight loss occurs and the degree of obesity warrants it, then the patient should be referred for calorimetry if possible.

SPECIAL GROUPS

Obese children

It is better not to try to get overweight children to lose weight, since weight loss is usually associated with a decrease in height growth. Ideally the child who is overweight at age 7 years should be managed so that weight gain is slowed while height continues to increase, with the objective of achieving a normal weight-for-height at age 12 years. This does not involve weight loss at any stage, and only a very modest restriction of energy intake such as may be achieved by substituting fruit for sweets, and low-energy drinks for sugary drinks, and by encouraging physical activity as much as possible. If the childhood obesity is not tackled until the teens are reached, the opportunity for this gentle physiological approach will have been lost. The general problems of dietary management of children are discussed further in Chapter 27.

Pregnancy and lactation

For similar reasons obese expectant and lactating mothers should not be asked to lose weight: the time for weight loss is between pregnancies. However, it is probably reasonable to aim for a constant weight during the pregnancy of a mother who starts obese, so that after childbirth she will weigh less than at the beginning of pregnancy. For discussion of nutrition in this group see Chapter 25.

Diabetes

Obese diabetics will usually be of the non-insulin dependent variety, in whom weight loss is a great advantage. However, caution is needed if diabetics are on insulin or hypoglycaemic drugs, since a change in diet or weight loss will affect the dosage required. Similar remarks apply to obese hypertensive patients, who will need reduced medication during and after weight loss. For dietary management of diabetes see Chapter 35, and for cardiovascular diseases see Chapter 41.

Ethnic minorities

The principles of management of obesity in ethnic minority groups are exactly the same as in anyone else, but of course the type of dietary advice given will need to take account of differences in national cuisine.

PREVENTION OF OBESITY

Since about one-third of the adult population in the UK is already overweight, the opportunities for primary prevention of obesity lie mainly with primary schoolchildren. The idea that fatness was determined in infancy by the number of fat cells is no longer tenable: fat babies often do not become fat children, and many fat children were not fat babies (Garrow 1988). However, fatness at age 13 years is quite a strong predictor of adult fatness, so the optimum time to prevent obesity is in the interval between 7 and 12 years, as described above.

Secondary prevention is also important: people who have lost weight are very liable to regain it if,

after a period of dieting, they 'eat normally'. This observation has led to the view that 'dieting makes you fat', and that it is not possible to maintain the weight lost by dieting. This view is wrong, but it does contain an element of truth. A detailed review of the effect on metabolic rate of dieting and weight loss is given by Garrow & Webster (1989). After weight loss there is a reduction in metabolic rate, because the weight which has been lost incurred some metabolic costs, and these costs are removed when the weight is lost. Therefore, if a person who was stable at a weight of 100 kg loses weight to 70 kg, but then goes back to his original diet, he will eventually stabilize again at 100 kg. To remain at 70 kg he will have to reduce his energy intake by about 15%, since that is the maintenance energy cost of the weight he has lost. It must be part of the task of community slimming clubs to offer advice and support to people who have achieved weight loss and need to prevent weight regain.

REFERENCES

Booth DA, Campbell HT, Chase A 1970 Temporal bounds of postingestive glucose-induced satiety in man. Nature 228: 1104

Borkan GA, Sparrow D, Wisniewski C, Vokonas PS 1986 Body weight and coronary heart disease risk: patterns of risk factor change associated with long-term weight change. American Journal of Epidemiology 124: 410–419

Bush A, Webster J, Chalmers G et al 1988 The Harrow Slimming Club: report on 1090 enrolments in 50 courses, 1977–1986. Journal of Human Nutrition and Dietetics 1: 429–436

Consensus Statement 1991 Gastrointestinal surgery for severe obesity. NIH Consensus Development Conference, March 25–27, 1991

Dagra LL, Carrol-Michals L, Borsford SJ, Lucas CP 1991 Fluoxetine's effect on weight loss in obese subjects. American Journal of Clinical Nutrition 54: 321–325

Davidson S, Passmore R, Brock JF 1972 Human nutrition and dietetics, 5th edn. Churchill Livingstone, Edinburgh

Dore C, Hesp R, Wilkins D, Garrow JS 1982 Prediction of energy requirements of obese patients after massive weight loss. Human Nutrition: Clinical Nutrition 36C: 41–48

Forbes GB 1992 Exercise and lean weight: the influence of body weight. Nutrition Reviews 50: 157–161

Garn SM, Bailey SM, Cole PE 1980 Continuities and changes in fatness and obesity. In: Schemmel R (ed) Nutrition, physiology and obesity. CRC Press, Florida, pp. 51–78

Garn SM, Clark DC, Guire KE 1975 Growth, body composition, and development of obese and lean children. In: Winick M (ed) Childhood obesity. John Wiley & Sons, London

Garrow JS 1974 Dental splinting in the treatment of hyperphagic obesity. Proceedings of the Nutrition Society 33: 29A

Garrow JS 1988 Obesity and related diseases. Churchill Livingstone, Edinburgh

Garrow JS 1989 Very low calorie diets should not be used. International Journal of Obesity 13 (Suppl 2): 145–147

Garrow JS 1992 Treatment of obesity. Lancet 340: 409–413

Garrow JS, Webster JD 1989 Effects on weight and metabolic rate of obese women on a 3.4 MJ (800 kcal) diet. Lancet i: 1429–1431

Garrow JS, Durrant ML, Blaza S, Wilkins D, Rayston P, Sunkin S 1981 The effect of meal frequency and protein concentration on the composition of the weight lost by obese subjects. British Journal of Nutrition 45:5–16

Geppert J, Splett PL 1991 Summary document of nutrition intervention in obesity. Journal of the American Dietetic Association Suppl: S31–35

Gilbert S, Garrow JS 1983 A prospective controlled trial of outpatient treatment for obesity. Human Nutrition: Clinical Nutrition 37C: 21–29

Gregory J, Foster K, Tyler H, Wiseman M 1990 The dietary and nutritional survey of British adults. HMSO, London

Guy-Grand B, Apfelbaum M, Crepaldi G, Gries A, Lefebvre P, Turner P 1989 International trial of long-term dexfenfluramine in obesity. Lancet ii: 1142–1145

Hubert HB 1984 The nature of the relationship between obesity and cardiovascular disease. International Journal of Cardiology 6: 268–274

James WPT 1976 Research on obesity: a report of the DHSS/MRC Group. HMSO, London

Jebb SA, Goldberg GR, Coward WA, Murgatroyd PR, Prentice AM 1991 Effects of weight cycling caused by intermittent dieting on metabolic rate and body composition in obese women. International Journal of Obesity 15: 367–374

Keys A, Menotti A, Blackburn et al 1984 The seven countries study: 2289 deaths in 15 years. Preventive Medicine 13: 141–154

Lapidus L, Bengtsson C, Larsson B, Pennert K, Rybo E, Sjostrom L 1984 Distribution of adipose tissue and risk of cardiovascular disease and death: a 12-year follow-up of participants in the population study of women in Gothenburg, Sweden. British Medical Journal 289:1257–1261

Larsson B 1987 Regional obesity as a health hazard in men – prospective studies. Acta Medica Scandinavica 723 (Suppl): 45–51

Lew EA, Garfinkel L 1979 Variations in mortality by weight among 750 000 men and women. Journal of Chronic Diseases 32: 563–576

Lissner L, Odell PM, D'Agostino RB et al 1991 Variability of body weight and health outcomes in the Framingham population. New England Journal of Medicine 324: 1839–1844

Manson JE, Colditz GA, Stamfer MJ et al 1990 A prospective study of obesity and risk of coronary heart disease in women. New England Journal of Medicine 322: 822–829

Mellbin T, Vuille JC 1973 Physical development at 7 years of age in relation to velocity of weight gain in infancy, with special reference to incidence of overweight. British Journal of Preventive and Social Medicine 27: 225–235

Rissanen AM, Heliovaara M, Knekt P, Reunanen A, Aromaa A 1991 Determinants of weight gain and overweight in adult Finns. European Journal of Clinical Nutrition 45: 419–430

Romanella NE, Wakat DK, Lloyd BH, Kelly LE 1991 Physical activity and attitudes in lean and obese children and their mothers. International Journal of Obesity 15: 407–414

Rosenbaum S, Skinner RK, Knight IB, Garrows JS 1985 A survey of heights and weights of adults in Great Britain. Annals of Human Biology 12: 115–127

Sanders TAB, Woolfe R, Rantzen E 1990 Controlled evaluation of slimming diets: use of television for recruitment. Lancet 336: 918–920

Seidell JC (ed) 1992 Obesity in Europe: prevalence and public health implications. WHO, Copenhagen

Siervogel RM, Roche AF, Guo S, Mukherjee D, Chumlea CC 1991 Patterns of change in weight/stature^2 from 2 to 18 years: findings from long-term serial data for children in the Fels longitudinal growth study. International Journal of Obesity 15: 479–485

Sims EAH, Danforth E Jr, Horton ES, Bray GA, Glennon JA, Salans LB 1973 Endocrine and metabolic effects of experimental obesity in man. Recent Progress in Hormone Research 29: 457–496

Wannamethee G, Shaper AG 1990 Weight change in middle-aged British men: implications for health. European Journal of Clinical Nutrition 44: 133–142

33. Nutritional management of diseases of the stomach and bowel

J. H. Cummings

EPIDEMIOLOGY

Mortality

The principal fatal gastrointestinal diseases are acute diarrhoea; cancer (of the large bowel, stomach, oesophagus, liver or pancreas); peptic ulcer; and liver disease (mainly hepatitis, alcohol-induced disease and cirrhosis). Worldwide, the major cause of death arising from the gut is acute diarrhoea due primarily to food poisoning or infection. Acute diarrhoea is common in every country of the world, but deaths associated with it occur primarily in the malnourished, those at the extremes of life or those whose health is compromised for other reasons (see Chapter 29). In industrialized countries cancer is the principal cause of gut-related deaths, and is responsible for 7% of all mortality in the UK (OPCS 1989). Of these cancers, that of the large bowel (colon and rectum) has the highest cumulative incidence worldwide, just ahead of the stomach. Twenty years ago stomach cancer was a more common problem but rates for this disorder have declined steadily since then (UICC/IARC 1966–87). By contrast, large-bowel cancer is increasing in countries such as Japan, where a transition is occurring from a traditional diet low in fat and high in starch to one containing more fat, meat and sugar (Bingham 1990). Diet has been implicated in the aetiology of both large-bowel and stomach cancer, but has little to offer in their management (see Chapter 45).

Morbidity

On the whole, most gut diseases are not fatal but are significant causes of poor health. The major gastro-intestinal causes of morbidity are:

1. Acute diarrhoea and vomiting
2. Peptic ulcer and dyspepsia (including heartburn and hiatus hernia)
3. Constipation and abdominal pain (including irritable bowel)
4. Haemorrhoids and anal fissure
5. Hernia
6. Gallstones
7. Appendicitis
8. Malabsorption syndromes (including coeliac disease and sprue)
9. Ulcerative colitis and Crohn's disease
10. Diverticular disease of the colon
11. Pancreatitis
12. Liver disease (mainly hepatitis, alcohol-induced disorders and cirrhosis)
13. Food intolerance

The list shows, in an appropriate order for the UK, those problems which occur most commonly as judged by hospital discharge statistics and consultations with physicians or primary care workers. Worldwide, acute diarrhoea and vomiting are the commonest. In the UK these conditions are responsible for 13% of all hospital discharges (DHSS/OPCS 1984) and 21% of persons consulting their family doctor (RCGP 1986). The main surgery to the gut includes repair of herniae, appendicectomy, treatment of haemorrhoids and anal fissure, removal of gallstones and surgery for peptic ulcer, although this latter is rapidly declining with the advent of new anti-secretory drugs.

Diet has a major role to play in the management of acute diarrhoea (through the use of oral rehydration therapy), in coeliac disease (gluten-free diets), malabsorption (low fat and nutritional supplements) and in constipation and diverticular disease (high non-starch polysaccharide and resistant starch diets). In the other conditions listed above diet and nutritional therapy may be useful adjuncts to treatment.

OESOPHAGEAL DISORDERS

Two common symptoms arise from the oesophagus: dysphagia and heartburn, either of which may be associated with chest pain.

480

Dysphagia

Dysphagia (difficulty in swallowing) is an important symptom because it is almost always accompanied by reduced food intake, leading rapidly to weight loss. It presents a major problem in managing a number of conditions, not all of which are oesophageal in origin.

Swallowing may conveniently be thought of as having two phases: oropharyngeal and oesophageal. In the oropharyngeal phase food is transferred from the mouth via the pharynx to the upper oesophagus. The oesophageal phase carries the food from pharynx to stomach.

Oropharyngeal dysphagia

Oral dysphagia, where the patient complains of inability to initiate swallowing by emptying the mouth, is usually due to neuromuscular disorders such as Parkinson's disease, motor neuron disease and muscular dystrophy. Table 33.1 shows the principal causes of dysphagia.

Pharyngeal dysphagia can be more problematic since it is associated with failure to coordinate closure of the entry to the trachea adequately, with the result that food is inhaled, causing choking and coughing immediately on swallowing. Fluids may be regurgitated through the nose. The major causes are stroke and head injury, but physical obstruction of the pharynx may occur with a pharyngeal pouch, an

Table 33.1 Principle causes of dysphagia

Oropharyngeal	
Neuromuscular	Stroke
	Head injury
	Muscular disorders
	Motor neuron disease
	Parkinson's disease
Physical obstruction	Pharyngeal pouch
	Goitre
Psychological	Globus hystericus
Infections	Acute tonsillitis
Oesophageal	
Neural	Achalasia
	Multiple sclerosis
	Diffuse oesophageal spasm
Muscular	Scleroderma
	Dystrophia myotonica
Physical obstruction	Stricture
	cancer
	chronic oesophagitis
	Diverticulum
	External compression
	(aortic aneurysm)
	Postoperative
Infections	Monilia

enlarged thyroid (goitre) or head and neck cancer. Another common cause is acute tonsillitis. Occasionally patients may complain of something permanently sticking in their throat, the so-called globus hystericus. No physical abnormality can be found and this is a psychological disorder.

Management of oropharyngeal dysphagia is difficult. There are no studies which show that a particular diet, e.g. soft or hard, is especially useful and patients need to be treated on their own merits. Proper assessment of the patient's swallowing ability is needed and, because this requires various medical skills, in some hospitals swallowing teams have been established. Attention must be paid to the state of alertness of the person, whether they can maintain an upright position during feeding, whether they have good oral and laryngeal function, a normal voice and a good cough reflex (Penington & Krutsch 1990). A major consideration is maintaining body weight, and to this end it is better to resort early to enteral feeding via a fine-bore nasogastric tube or gastrostomy, than wait for the patient to become emaciated, depressed and generally less able to cope.

Oesophageal dysphagia

Oesophageal dysphagia is usually due to a stricture, although neuromuscular disorders – notably achalasia and scleroderma – are not uncommon. The sensation of food sticking is usually referred to the retrosternal or xiphisternal region and occurs a few seconds after swallowing. Strictures of the oesophagus can be malignant and these are characterized by dysphagia for solid food, which gradually progresses. Benign strictures due to acid–pepsin disease are more chronic, and often preceded by a long history of heartburn. At first dysphagia is intermittent. Difficulty may be experienced with both solids and liquids, but can often be overcome by repeated swallowing or washing solid foods down with liquid. The oesophagus may be more cold-sensitive than usual.

Management of a malignant stricture is surgical. Benign strictures are more often treated conservatively with endoscopic dilatation and require attention to diet in order to maintain reasonable nutritional status. In addition to treating the cause of a benign stricture it is necessary to advise patients with oesophageal narrowing on how to maintain a range of food intake. If malnourished they may need protein or energy supplements in the form of liquid feeds. There are no absolute rules, and no well tested diets, but common sense dictates that the particle size of the diet be commensurate with the degree of oesophageal narrowing. Despite everyone's anxieties, patients with oesophageal stricture rarely choke, unlike those with pharyngeal disorders.

Heartburn

Heartburn is an irritating symptom which almost everyone experiences from time to time. Classically it is the occurrence of a hot or burning sensation retrosternally, which may be accompanied by the rise of acid into the mouth, and pain, which is often described as gripping, may radiate into the arms, throat and through to the back and thus be difficult to distinguish from angina. The burning sensation is due to reflux into the lower oesophagus of acid and pepsin from the stomach, often leading to inflammation (oesophagitis). The pain is probably the result of spasm of the circular muscle of the oesophagus, although the relationship between pain, motor changes, reflux, heartburn and symptoms is not exact and has spawned a vast literature in recent years.

The prime cause of heartburn is the reflux of gastric contents into the oesophagus. Normally this is prevented by an efficient valve mechanism at the gastro-oesophageal junction which comprises the lower oesophageal sphincter (LES), an intra-abdominal portion of oesophagus, the diaphragmatic hiatus, the angle of entry of the oesophagus into the stomach and gastric mucosal folds. In practice most reflux is due to lowering of the pressure in the LES, which may be just hypotonic (low pressure) in heartburn and, equally importantly, may relax inappropriately rather than just on swallowing. Efficient clearance of refluxed acid into the oesophagus by peristalsis is also defective in some patients with heartburn. Reflux is thought to occur mainly at night, when patients are recumbent, but recent studies using 24 hour oesophageal pH monitoring have shown that the period from 1700 to 2400 hours is when the oesophagus has most exposure to acid (Gudmundsson et al 1988). Pressure in the LES is raised by protein and lowered by fat, alcohol, smoking and coffee (Dennish & Castell 1971, Hogan et al 1972, Nebel & Castell 1973, Cohen 1980). LES pressure is also lower during pregnancy and may vary in response to oestrogen and progesterone levels during the normal menstrual cycle, giving greater tendency to heartburn during the luteal phase (Fisher et al 1978, Van Thiel et al 1979). Physical pressure on the abdomen, such as occurs during bending, especially in overweight people, and straining because of constipation, will aggravate reflux as may anatomical disruption of the gastro-oesophageal junction following surgery or in the presence of a hiatus hernia. Some drugs also lower LES.

Management

General measures are weight reduction, avoidance of tightly constricting clothing around the abdomen and cessation of smoking. The following is a checklist for the management of heartburn:

1. Reduce weight to ideal
2. Avoid constricting clothes and bending
3. Elevate head of bed or pillows
4. Stop smoking
5. Avoid alcohol, coffee and fatty foods, especially in the evening
6. Review drugs
7. Combat gastric acid
8. Consider surgery.

Sleeping position is also important. Elevation of the pillow on a 10 inch wedge is most beneficial in reducing acid exposure in the lower oesophagus (Hamilton et al 1988).

A variety of diets have been recommended for heartburn but none subjected to proper clinical trials. It is reasonable, however, in view of their effects on the LES, to ask patients to cut down on their fat intake, avoid alcohol and coffee and probably to avoid large meals late at night. These general measures are successful in the majority of cases.

Additional therapy, which can be very effective, is aimed at neutralizing or reducing gastric acid secretion using one of the powerful new anti-secretory drugs such as cimetidine, ranitidine or omeprazole, by giving simple antacids, and adding the prokinetic cisapride. In severe cases, especially where a large hiatus hernia is present, surgery is beneficial.

STOMACH AND DUODENUM

Peptic ulcer and dyspepsia

Gastric and duodenal ulceration remain amongst the commonest disorders of the gastrointestinal tract, with around 10% of the UK population affected during their lifetime. Duodenal ulcer is much more common than gastric ulcer and still kills significant numbers of people each year, largely through the complications of bleeding and perforation. Bleeding peptic ulcer is becoming more common because of the increased consumption of non-steroidal anti-inflammatory drugs (aspirin, indomethacin, diclofenac, ibuprofen, ketoprofen, naproxen, etc.) (Kurata & Corboy 1988).

The cause of peptic ulcer is unknown, but almost certainly involves acid secretion in the stomach. Other factors which are important include the integrity of the mucus layer, gastric emptying and duodenal motility, bicarbonate secretion in the stomach, gastric blood flow, prostaglandin production in the mucosa and infection with *Helicobacter pylori*. Modern treatments are targeted towards each of these. Diet has little proven role in either the cause or management of peptic ulcer.

Dyspepsia and indigestion

The cardinal symptom of peptic ulcer is pain. This is characteristically felt in the epigastrium, is burning or nagging in quality, occurs after meals, may wake the patient between 1 and 3 a.m. and is relieved by suppressing gastric acid. The pain of peptic ulcer is one of a number of gastroduodenal symptoms which are generally called dyspepsia. Dyspepsia is any sort of discomfort affecting the upper abdomen or lower chest and which is associated with meals. It is synonymous with indigestion. Dyspeptic symptoms include pain, heartburn, nausea, abdominal distension, discomfort, flatulence and regurgitation. The important point about dyspepsia, however, is that it is caused by a number of conditions, of which peptic ulcer is one. Other conditions include oesophagitis, gallbladder disease, pancreatitis, irritable bowel and other colonic disorders and hepatitis. The first step in the management of dyspepsia, therefore, is to make a diagnosis.

Management of peptic ulcer

This is focused on suppression of acid and elimination of secretion, strengthening mucosal resistance using drugs and elimination of *Helicobacter pylori*. Some general measures are useful. In young people with peptic ulcer a change in lifestyle is often called for. Stopping smoking is well established as a means of speeding up the healing of ulcers (Okada et al 1990), and a reduction in alcohol intake removes a known irritant of the gastric mucosa and a stimulant of gastric secretion. Coffee is also a secretogogue but dietary restrictions of alcohol and coffee are not of proven benefit and are not mandatory nowadays. Some studies even suggest that moderate alcohol intake may promote ulcer healing (Sonnenberg et al 1981). Avoidance of stress is thought to be helpful, although the bed rest once deemed essential is of only marginal benefit.

There are no sound data to suggest that any specific diet or frequency of meal consumption will aid in the healing of peptic ulcer. The early bland milk-based diets have fallen into disrepute because of their restrictive nature and lack of efficacy, and the fact that excessive milk intake promotes gastric secretion and may lead to hypercalcaemia. Neither is there sound evidence to avoid the eating of spicy foods, or 'acid' food such as citrus fruits. The use of dietary fibre has now appeared on the peptic ulcer scene and at least one clinical trial suggests a high-fibre diet may delay relapse after ulcer healing (Rydning et al 1982, Lancet Editorial 1987). This is an area for further study.

Peptic ulcer patients always expect dietary advice because they believe that their symptoms must in some way relate to what they eat. This provides the doctor or dietician with an opportunity to suggest a prudent diet to benefit their general health (see Chapter 51).

The most effective treatment for peptic ulcer is now drug therapy. A range of powerful medications is available which target different aspects of the potential cause of peptic ulcer. These include:

1. Drugs which inhibit gastric acid secretion by blocking H_2 receptors (e.g. cimetidine, ranitidine, famotidine, nizatidine)
2. Proton pump inhibitors (omeprazole) which block gastric acid secretion
3. Gastric acid neutralizers (antacids)
4. Anticholinergics, which inhibit acid and pepsin secretion (pirenzepine)
5. Drugs which increase the mucus defence (e.g. bismuth chelate and sucralfate)
6. Prostaglandin analogues which also inhibit gastric secretion (e.g. misoprostol)
7. Antibiotics and other compounds which eliminate *Helicobacter pylori* (bismuth chelate, metronidazole and amoxycillin).

So effective are these drugs that peptic ulcer patients can now expect ulcer healing while continuing to eat any sort of diet, smoke, drink and lead stressful lives. Never the less, the chance should be taken to modify these habits if only to prevent other problems in later life.

SEQUELAE OF GASTRIC SURGERY

Although the development of more effective drugs for the treatment of peptic ulcer has substantially reduced the number of patients who come to surgery, there remain in the population many people who had their operations in the 1950s–1970s, up to half of whom will experience some long-term side effect of their procedure. Moreover, surgery is still performed in peptic ulcer where prolonged medical treatment has failed, for bleeding and perforation, for pyloric stenosis and where there is a suspicion of malignancy in gastric ulcer.

The main types of operation are shown in Fig. 33.1. Selective (proximal) vagotomy is the most favoured since it is associated with a less than 10% complication rate. However, partial gastrectomy is still needed in some circumstances and is combined with various drainage procedures.

The normal stomach regulates the emptying of its contents carefully to ensure that material is delivered to the duodenum, which is not hypertonic, and at a rate which pancreatic and biliary secretions can work most effectively. Moreover, some breakdown and grinding of larger particles occurs in the gastric antrum. Gastric surgery disrupts these controls. Vagotomy will also bring alterations in motor activity in the small bowel. However, the absorptive capacity of the small bowel remains intact unless there is bacterial overgrowth in a blind loop, as in the Polya gastrectomy.

Major problems following gastric surgery are:

1. Early dumping
2. Diarrhoea
3. Bile vomiting
4. Small stomach syndrome
5. Weight loss
6. Anaemia
7. Rare sequelae: hypoglycaemia (late dumping), bone disease, B_{12} deficiency.

Almost all patients suffer some minor disturbance of gastrointestinal function following gastric surgery, but by 6 months postoperatively the major nutritional problems have begun to emerge. Partial gastrectomy causes more sequelae than truncal vagotomy and pyloroplasty, which in turn is more likely to cause problems than selective vagotomy.

Early dumping

This is the commonest post-surgical problem and is characterized by a feeling of fullness and abdominal distension within 30 minutes of starting a meal. It is usually accompanied by nausea, vomiting, sweating, faintness and palpitations. The pathophysiology was worked out many years ago (Machella 1950). Gastric surgery almost always leads to accelerated gastric emptying. This occurs for both solids and liquids after partial gastrectomy, and after truncal vagotomy with pyloroplasty. Selective vagotomy affects the emptying of liquids only. Accelerated gastric emptying leads to the 'dumping' into the duodenum of large amounts of hypertonic fluid which is normally held back by the intact stomach. The presence of this fluid causes secretion into the small bowel, distension and hypovolaemia, and may trigger autonomic reflexes with the release of vasoactive hormones such as serotonin, bradykinin and vasoactive intestinal polypeptide (VIP).

Management

The key to management lies in preventing hypertonic material from entering the upper gut. Principally this means cutting out sugary foods, including milk and anything containing low-molecular-weight carbo-

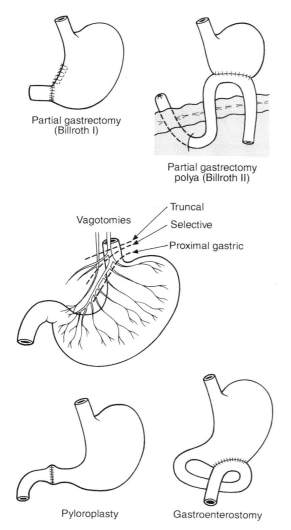

Partial gastrectomy
(Billroth I)

Partial gastrectomy
polya (Billroth II)

Vagotomies
Truncal
Selective
Proximal gastric

Pyloroplasty   Gastroenterostomy

Fig. 33.1 Operations for peptic ulcer.

hydrates. Patients should take their carbohydrates as starch, preferably in small frequent meals. Most alcoholic beverages are hypertonic. Soluble dietary fibre such as pectin may be helpful in slowing gastric emptying (Leeds et al 1981). Sugary drinks should not be taken with a meal, although the avoidance of all fluid with meals seems to be unnecessary. Some patients find it helpful to lie down for half an hour immediately after eating.

Bile vomiting

This is an unpleasant symptom associated mostly with partial gastrectomy and due to reflux into the stomach of bile-containing duodenal contents which disrupt the mucus layer protecting the gastric mucosa. The cause, again, is failure of the antroduodenal barrier which controls the movement of contents in this region. Patients will often have gastritis and may complain of persistent epigastric pain, relieved by vomiting bile-stained material. Management is difficult and there is no dietary advice of proven efficacy. Antacids are often used, together with cholestyramine which binds bile acids. Surprisingly, drugs which accelerate gastric emptying, such as metoclopromide and domperidone, may help.

Total gastrectomy

Substantial or total removal of the stomach is still occasionally performed and places the patient in an unenviable position. Eating almost always causes epigastic discomfort, fullness and nausea, and there may be dumping and bile vomiting. These patients are usually malnourished and require supportive dietary management. Meals must be frequent, 2-hourly, and not contain hypertonic foods (as for dumping). The patient should be warned to chew food thoroughly and not swallow indigestible material such as orange pith, which may obstruct the small bowel. Dietary supplements may be needed, especially in the early months, to maintain adequate calorie intake. Vitamin B_{12} and iron deficiency are common and must be treated.

Diarrhoea

Diarrhoea is a frequent complaint after gastric surgery and is said to be more common after vagotomy (post-vagotomy diarrhoea) than partial gastrectomy, but recent studies do not allow such a clear distinction to be drawn. Its cause is related to failure to control gastric emptying and denervation of the small bowel.

The result is rapid passage of food through the gut, increased bile acids in the colon and possibly mild malabsorption. Treatment should include a diet similar to that for early dumping, together with anti-diarrhoeal drugs (codeine and loperamide).

Late dumping

This condition is rare and comprises the onset of sweating, palpitations, weakness, confusion and occasionally loss of consciousness 2–3 hours after a meal. These symptoms will readily be recognized as those produced by hypoglycaemia. It is thought that the entry of hypertonic sugary foods into the duodenum leads to high levels of insulin secretion, which then cause the blood glucose to fall below fasting levels. Supernormal secretion of gastric inhibitory polypeptide (GIP) and loss of glucose into the large bowel may also be factors. Management of an acute attack is by giving glucose or sugar by mouth. Prevention requires the early dumping diet regimen.

Nutritional complications

Weight loss, iron-deficiency anaemia, B_{12} deficiency and osteomalacia may all occur after gastric surgery. Weight loss is very common and is due to reduced food intake because of the development of one of the many post-surgical syndromes. Frank malabsorption is rare. Many patients, however, start out overweight and provided their weight stabilizes after the initial loss and lies within the normal range for their height, age and sex, no specific therapy is required.

Iron-deficiency anaemia is usually mild, although it may be worse in menstruating women. It is due to a combination of reduced iron intake, poor absorption of food iron and increased losses from stomal ulcers and gastritis. It is best treated with a liquid iron preparation.

Vitamin B_{12} levels in blood tend to drift downwards over the years after partial gastrectomy. Frank deficiency occurs in up to 30% after a high gastrectomy, but can be readily managed with regular hydroxycobalamin injections.

Both osteoporosis and osteomalacia are more common in patients after gastric surgery. They are usually not evident for 6–10 years after operation (Eddy 1971). The cause is uncertain because no consistent evidence exists for low intakes or impaired absorption of either calcium or vitamin D. Furthermore, problems of metabolic bone disease after gastric surgery do not correlate with exposure to sunshine (Eddy 1971, Nilsson & Westlin 1971). Treatment, however, should be to encourage exercise and maintain vitamin D levels.

DIARRHOEA AND VOMITING

Causes of diarrhoea

Diarrhoea is the frequent passage of loose, watery stools. Acute diarrhoea is usually a short-lived, self-limiting condition. The major causes of acute diarrhoea are bacteria such as pathogenic *Escherichia coli*, *Campylobacter jejuni*, *Vibrio cholerae*, *Staphylococcus aureus*, *Clostridium perfringens*, *Bacillus cereus*, *Vibrio parahaemolyticus*, *Shigella* sp, *Salmonella* sp, *Yersinia* sp and a number of viruses. These give rise to the clinical syndromes of acute gastroenteritis, food poisoning and traveller's diarrhoea, which are not necessarily clearly distinguishable from each other, and to more specific conditions such as typhoid, dysentery and cholera.

Bacteria causing diarrhoea are usually classified according to whether they secrete an enterotoxin (toxigenic) or invade the bowel wall (invasive). Toxigenic diarrhoeas include cholera and enteropathogenic (or enterotoxigenic) *E. coli* (EPEC and ETEC), whilst the classic invasive organisms are *Shigella* (dysentery) and *Salmonella* (typhoid).

Chronic diarrhoea is found in a number of conditions, principally malabsorption syndromes (including coeliac disease, tropical sprue and pancreatic insufficiency), inflammatory bowel disease (ulcerative colitis and Crohn's disease), following gut resection, chronic parasitic and other infections (giardia and tuberculosis), drugs (including laxative abuse), irritable bowel and diverticular disease. It may also be idiopathic (of unknown cause).

Stool composition in diarrhoea

In chronic diarrhoea daily stool weights are usually in the range 200–1500 g/day, whereas in acute diarrhoea between 1 and 20 kg/day may be passed, the higher amounts being seen in conditions such as cholera (Watten et al 1959, Speelman et al 1986). Because there are massive faecal losses of water and electrolytes in acute diarrhoea, made worse if accompanied by vomiting and sweating, the essence of nutritional management is to replace these losses.

Fig. 33.2 shows the concentration of sodium and potassium in faeces in relation to stool output. Normal stool contains very little sodium and is high in potassium. As stool weight increases sodium concentration rises and potassium falls, so that at about

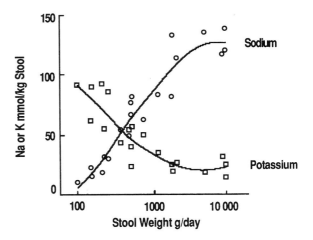

Fig. 33.2 Faecal electrolyte losses in relation to stool output. Data taken from Welch et al 1937, Lubran et al 1951, Watten et al 1959, Schnitka et al 1961, Matsumoto et al 1966, Speelman et al 1986, Vernia et al 1987, Cummings et al 1973, and Cummings, unpublished data. Total cases 272.

500 g of stool/day they are equimolar (55 mmol/kg) and thereafter approach plasma levels (130 mmol/l for sodium and 4 mmol/l for potassium) at stool outputs over 5 kg/day. Potassium concentrations never actually reach plasma levels, probably because of the cellular debris present in stool, which is rich in potassium. Table 33.2 shows daily losses computed from Fig. 33.2 and provides a ready reckoner for replacement if stool output can be measured. With stool weights of up to 1000 g/day, losses are not greater than dietary intakes found in westernized populations (i.e. about 150 mmol/day for sodium and 75 mmol/day for potassium) (Gleibermann 1973, Intersalt Cooperative Research Group 1988). Beyond this replacement therapy is essential and is advisable at much lower

Table 33.2   Electrolyte losses in adult faeces

Daily stool amount (g)	Losses (mmol/day)	
	Sodium	Potassium
<200	6	13
400	20	23
600	37	31
800	56	38
1000	76	45
2000	190	70
3000	316	88
4000	452	101
5000	595	111
6000 or more	130 mmol/kg	20 mmol/kg

stool outputs if there is accompanying fever, anorexia and vomiting. Special care must be taken with the young, elderly and chronically sick.

Management of acute diarrhoea

How can salt and water losses best be replaced? Acute diarrhoea, particularly in the very young, quickly gives rise to salt and water depletion. Symptoms are non-specific but include fatigue, irritability, drowsiness and muscle cramps, thirst, loss of appetite, nausea, headache and faintness. Urine volume decreases and salt depletion may itself lead to vomiting. Moderate dehydration is not easily recognized unless the patient is weighed daily. Postural hypotension is a useful sign.

Whereas severe diarrhoea may require rapid intravenous fluid and electrolyte replacement, the major advance in therapy in recent years has been the advent of oral rehydration therapy (ORT). First used to treat cholera in the Philippines (Phillips 1964), the principles and practice of such therapy apply to all causes of acute diarrhoea and all age groups. ORT makes use of the observation from research studies that the capacity of the gut to absorb salt and water, in the presence of glucose or amino acids, remains relatively intact despite pronounced sodium secretion induced by binding of enterotoxin to gut epithelial cells (Field et al 1972). In principle, therefore, ORT solutions combine the maximum tolerable amounts of salt within an absorbable carbohydrate.

Table 33.3 gives a list of available powders for formulating ORT and some ideas for home-made solutions. A variety of electrolyte concentrations are found, with the WHO-ORT the highest for sodium (except for Oxo). The WHO mixture is targeted at the mild to moderate diarrhoea of the tropics, whereas the other solutions are used more in non-tropical societies, where the wide variation in electrolyte content has been shown to be safe and effective in modestly dehydrated people (Cutting et al 1989). However, glucose-based ORTs are not without problems of their own. Good (microbiologically safe) water is needed and the high osmolarity may itself perpetuate the diarrhoea. Mixing errors may cause hypernatraemia. Stool output therefore remains high with ORT, and the duration of the diarrhoea is not shortened. This, together with practical problems in cost and distribution, has led to a decline in its use. An important recent advance, therefore, has been the use of soluble starch, such as found in rice or cereals, to replace part or all of the glucose (Patra et al 1982, Molla et al 1982). Rice-based solutions reduce the severity of diarrhoea, particularly in cholera (Gore et al 1992), are more palatable and reduce vomiting (Carpenter et al 1988, El-Mougi et al 1988, Molla et al 1989). Cereal starches are well digested in the gut and provide some protein as a further advantage.

Other therapy in acute diarrhoea includes rest, antibiotics where indicated, and antiemetics. Anti-diarrhoeals are not recommended. Supportive nutritional therapy in chronic diarrhoea is dealt with below.

MALABSORPTION

Malabsorption is a general term given to any condition in which there is impaired digestion and absorption of fat, protein or carbohydrate. Classically it is known as steatorrhoea, the passage of excessive amounts of fat in faeces, and is seen most commonly in pancreatic insufficiency, coeliac and Crohn's disease. However, in all these conditions there is also variable

Table 33.3 Electrolyte concentrations (mmol/1) of some oral rehydration therapy (ORT) solutions

Name	Sodium	Potassium	Glucose/sucrose	Made to recommended volume of (ml)
WHO-ORT[*]	90	20	111	1000
Dioralyte	35	20	200	200
Electrolade	50	20	111	200
Electrosol	35	20	200	200
Glucolyte	35	20	200	200
Paedialyte	75	20	139	250
Rehidrat	50	20	187[tt]	230
Oxo	140	5	0	200
Home brew[+]	34	14	280[+]	500

[*] WHO recommended solution
[+] Home brew recipe: dissolve $\frac{1}{4}$ teaspoonful salt and 4 heaped teaspoonfuls sugar in 150 ml boiling water. Add 150 ml fresh orange juice and make up to 500 ml with tap water. Sugar all present as sucrose
[tt] Glucose + sucrose

malabsorption of carbohydrate and protein in addition to fat. Specific disorders of carbohydrate absorption also occur, notably lactose, and, rarely, defects in monosaccharide transport are found. Isolated malabsorption of protein is effectively unknown although protein loss into the gut may occur in protein-losing enteropathy.

The causes of malabsorption most commonly encountered in clinical practice (Table 33.4) are coeliac disease and tropical sprue. Crohn's disease, following surgical resection of the stomach or small bowel, pancreatic insufficiency, infections and lactase deficiency. Patients with malabsorption usually present with the passage of stools which are bulky and porridgy, foul-smelling, greasy and difficult to flush away. There may be loss of appetite and weight, although in some forms of malabsorption such as pancreatic insufficiency appetite is increased. Other symptoms such as abdominal distension, increased gas, pain and general malaise occur. Late complications include anaemia and bone disease.

A wide variety of clinical tests for malabsorption is available. Initially the aim is to establish the presence of the malabsorption by measuring faecal fat, or otherwise assessing fat absorption, and screening the blood for specific nutritional deficiencies such as iron, B_{12} and folate. Breath hydrogen studies for carbo-hydrate malabsorption are qualitatively useful. Anatomical examination of the stomach and small bowel by X-ray is important, followed by mucosal biopsy. Specific tests to establish a particular diagnosis can then be used.

Nutritional management

The first essential is to make a diagnosis and treat the underlying disease. General strategies for coping with malabsorption are given below.

Weight loss

Weight loss is often the major problem. Although in theory it should be possible to maintain adequate energy intake with normal foods, patients often lose their appetite, lack the will to cook and may have stricturing lesions of the gut which cause pain on eating. Hence a large number of nutritional supplements have been developed (see below). Most of these are available on prescription in the UK, provided the patient has specific disorders, which include bowel fistula, disaccharidase intolerance, coeliac disease, cystic fibrosis, dysphagia, gastrectomy, other intestinal surgery and malabsorption. They are also available for a number of more general problems such as cancer cachexia, anorexia nervosa, liver disease, hypercholesterolaemia, and the rarer inherited disorders of metabolism. Details of all these are given in the current issue of the *British National Formulary* under Borderline Substances. In general they are much more expensive than normal food and patients should be encouraged to maintain some of their usual intake. Enteral or parenteral nutrition may be needed in severe cases (see Chapter 31 and Table 33.5).

Steatorrhoea

This diagnosis often leads to a request for a low-fat diet. Such diets are beneficial in the management of diarrhoea but can reduce energy intake significantly. To counteract steatorrhoea but keep energy intake high, nutritional supplement should be used (see above). Medium-chain triglycerides (MCT) are occasionally valuable because they are more readily hydrolysed by pancreatic enzymes than long-chain fat. Furthermore, they do not require micelle formation for their absorption, being taken up directly into the portal vein. They may enhance absorption of fat-soluble vitamins. However, they provide less energy per gram than long-chain fat (8.3 vs 9.0 kcal) and may undergo conversion to non-metabolizable dicar-

Table 33.4   Principal causes of malabsorption

Anatomical	Surgical resection (short bowel syndrome) Fistula Gastric surgery Blind loop and stricture Jejunal diverticulosis
Enzyme deficiencies	Pancreatic disease (see Chapter 35) Biliary obstruction Disaccharidase deficiencies
Mucosal defects	Coeliac disease Tropical sprue Crohn's disease Radiation
Systemic causes	Scleroderma Diabetes Lymphoma Thyroid disease Severe skin disorders
Drugs	Cholestyramine Antibiotics (especially neomycin) Excess laxatives
Infections	Giardia and parasitic infestation Tuberculosis Bacterial overgrowth Whipple's

Table 33.5 Nutritional management of malabsorption*

Problem	Nutritional management
Steatorrhoea	Low-fat diet Medium-chain triglycerides
Weight loss	Complete feeds: Clinifeed, Elemental 028, Enrich, Ensure, Flexical, Fortisip, Fortison, Fresubin, Isocal, Liquisorb, Osmolite, Pepti, Portagen, Pregestimil, Reabilan, Triosorbon, Vivonex Protein: Albumaid, Casilan, Duocal, Forceval-Protein, Maxipro Fat: Alembicol, Calogen, Liquigen, MCT Carbohydrate: Caloreen, Fortical, Hycal, Maxijul, Polycal
Abdominal distension and gas	Avoid sugars and low-molecular-weight carbohydrates. Take carbohydrate as readily digestible starch
Anaemia	Use iron, B_{12} or folate supplements as appropriate
Bone disease	Calcium tablets, vitamin D, sunlight, exercise
Minerals	Iron: ferrous sulphate, fumarate, gluconate, glycine sulphate and succinate available. Aim to give 100–200 mg of iron daily Zinc sulphate: aim to give about 100 mg of zinc daily Calcium: gluconate, lactate, carbonate, hydroxyapatite. Aim to give 1 g (25 mmol) daily
Vitamins	A - 25–50 000 units by mouth D - 30 000 units by injection K - 4–12 mg Folate - 1 mg B_{12} - 1000 µg 3-monthly

* In addition to treatment of underlying pathology

boxylic acids in the body, thereby reducing their calorie value further. They also cause diarrhoea. They are usually given in a dose of 15 ml four times a day and provide 350–400 kcal.

Gas and abdominal distension

Malabsorption leads to the entry into the large bowel of partly digested carbohydrate and protein, which will then be fermented by the colonic flora to produce carbon dioxide and hydrogen. Gas production is often a cause of complaint in patients with malabsorption and can be minimized by attention to the type of carbohydrate in the diet. In broad terms this means omitting food which contains non-absorbable sugars such as raffinose and stacchyose (beans and peas), avoiding lactose if there is any suggestion of lactase deficiency, and ensuring that any starch is in its readily digestible form (Englyst & Cummings 1987). Fermentation of non-starch polysaccharides (dietary fibre, NSP) is also a source of gas production in the colon. It is less of a problem with poorly digested NSP sources such as wheat bran. In general, rapidly fermented material gives rise to gas at such a rate that the colon cannot absorb it fast enough (Christl et al 1991), and it builds up within the lumen causing discomfort. The principles of a low-gas diet are outlined in Table 33.6.

Protein intake should not be restricted but meat and pulses should be well minced to ensure adequate digestion (Chacko & Cummings 1988).

Table 33.6 Diet to reduce gas formation

Sugars	Avoid non-absorbable sugars such as raffinose and stacchyose, mostly present in beans and peas. Lactose – avoid milk if evidence of lactase deficiency
Oligosaccharides	Fructans are not digested in small bowel. Present in artichokes, onions, leeks, chicory, salsify

Starch	Most starch should be freshly cooked and eaten hot, or as white bread. Rice starch is readily digestible.
	Avoid – unmilled grains and seeds
	         – unripe banana and incompletely cooked potato and maize
	         – cooked and cooled starches other than cereal starches

NSP (fibre)	Do not encourage consumption of high-fibre foods. Keep intake of fruit, vegetables and pulses to average or below average amounts. Soluble fibre is potentially worse than insoluble

Vitamins and minerals

These are often needed to treat anaemia and bone disease in malabsorption, or simply to avoid deficiency developing. It is best to provide supplements of individual vitamins and minerals rather than give mixed preparations. This allows the doses to be tailored to the patient's needs and monitored using conventional haematological and biochemical indices. Vitamins A and D are both toxic when taken in excess.

COELIAC DISEASE

Coeliac disease, a common cause of malabsorption, is a condition in which there is a morphologically abnormal jejunal mucosa, which improves when gluten is withdrawn from the diet and relapses on gluten challenge (Dawson & Kumar 1986, Davidson & Bridges 1987). The condition may affect all ages and has been known for many centuries, although the first clear description was by Samuel Gee in 1888 in the St. Bartholomew's Hospital Reports (Gee 1888) entitled 'On the coeliac affection'. He noted its frequent occurrence in young children and concluded that there must be a dietary cause. The crucial link with cereals was established by the Dutch paediatrician Dicke in 1950, and subsequently Dicke and his associates showed that it was the protein gluten which damages the intestine of these patients.

Coeliac disease, or more properly gluten-induced enteropathy, is most prevalent in Galway, Ireland (1 in 300) and occurs in all communities where wheat is a major staple. It is very rare in Africa, China and Japan. Both sexes are probably equally affected and there is evidence from twin studies of a genetic factor. Coeliac disease is associated with increased frequency of HLA B8 and HLA DR3 histocompatability antigens.

Aetiology

The cause of coeliac disease is sensitivity to a water-insoluble protein of cereals known as gluten. Gluten itself consists of an insoluble fraction, glutenin, and a soluble fraction containing a series of gliadins (α, β, γ and Ω). It is the gliadins that are toxic.

The way in which gliadin damages the mucosa is still unknown, but is probably through an immune mechanism. Coeliac mucosa contains increased numbers of immunocytes, secreting mainly IgM, IgA and IgG. Serum levels of IgA are raised and circulating antibodies to gluten fractions are found in blood (Levensen et al 1985), although levels of these do not correlate closely with disease severity. Other pointers to an immune mechanism include the association of coeliac disease with other autoimmune conditions such as thyroditis, diabetes and liver disease, the frequent presence of reticulin antibodies and the response of the coeliac patient to corticosteroids.

Pathology

The characteristic lesion of coeliac disease is the flat jejunal mucosa. Histologically villi are absent, there is crypt hypoplasia and the lamina propria is infiltrated with mononuclear cells. Mucosal enzyme activities, such as the disaccharidases, are decreased so there are both anatomical and functional reductions in digestive ability. The ileum is not usually involved except in severe disease. Gastritis and proctitis occasionally occur. Although the flat mucosa of coeliac disease is virtually pathognomonic of this condition, lesser degrees of mucosal abnormality, with the attendant nutritional consequences, occur in a variety of other conditions and should be borne in mind.

The causes of a flattened jejunal mucosa are:

1. Coeliac disease (gluten enteropathy)
2. Tropical spruce
3. Acute gastroenteris
4. Milk and soya protein intolerance (infants)
5. Kwashiorkor
6. Hypogammaglobulinaemia
7. Bacterial overgrowth
8. Dermatitis herpetiformis
9. Drugs, e.g. mefenamic acid.

Clinical features and diagnosis

In children, coeliac disease presents as failure to thrive, most commonly in the second year of life, with abdominal distension and wasting, notably around the buttocks. Children are typically miserable, lethargic, have no appetite and pass bulky, pale stools. Adult coeliac disease commonly presents in the third or fourth decades and is characterized by diarrhoea, anaemia and weight loss. However, gastrointestinal symptoms may be completely absent and the disease is often picked up during the investigation of anaemia. Rarely, an acute onset may occur with vomiting, abdominal distension, anorexia and diarrhoea.

The anaemia of coeliac disease is due to folate and iron deficiency. The diarrhoea is characteristically a steatorrhoea: coeliac disease was once known as idiopathic steatorrhoea. Weight loss occurs in about 60% of patients and abdominal pain, oral ulceration and anaemia occur in about 40%. Rarely, bone pain may occur with skin lesions, vitamin K deficiency, ankle oedema, amenorrhoea and depression as additional problems. Diagnosis is by jejunal biopsy. Supplementary assessment of the patient's condition may be made by haematological and biochemical tests, including faecal fat. Barium follow-through of the small bowel may show a characteristic dilated featureless bowel. The recently introduced intestinal permeability tests are a valuable adjunct in the diagnosis, and in monitoring the response to treatment in coeliac patients (Fotherby et al 1988). The condition must be distinguished from other forms of malabsorption, especially Crohn's disease, pancreatic insufficiency and Whipple's disease.

Nutritional management

Coeliac disease is perhaps the one disease above all other gut disorders where diet is the key to management. The toxic protein gluten is present in wheat, barley, rye and oats, so these must be excluded from the patient's diet for life. Rice and maize products are safe, as are soya products which are now more widely available. Doubt, however, remains about oats. Some patients are sensitive to oat gluten whereas others are not. In the initial management of the patient oats should be excluded, but may be introduced later and the patient's condition monitored using permeability tests.

Avoiding gluten is easier said than done. Although obvious foods such as breakfast cereals, bread, cakes, pastry, biscuits and pies can be omitted from the diet, hidden sources of gluten are more difficult. Wheat flour is added to many products. Fortunately this is usually made clear by food labelling, which patients must learn to look at. A simple home test kit for gluten in foods is available for coeliac patients (Skerritt & Hill 1991).

A diet without the major cereals is restricting, so a large number of gluten-free products have been developed. Many of these are available on prescription in the UK under the ACBS system (Advisory Committee on Borderline Substances). They are listed in Table 33.7.

Full information about diet for coeliac patients can be obtained in the UK from the Coeliac Society, PO Box 220, High Wycombe, Bucks HP11 2HY (telephone 0494 37278). The Society produces an excellent booklet listing brands of gluten-free foods, and a magazine which updates this list every 6 months. The Coeliac Society will also give helpful advice on holidays where gluten-free diets are available, life insurance

Table 33.7 Gluten-free products*

	Name	Supplier
Bread/bread mixes	Aproten	Ultrapharm
	Ener-G	General Designs
	Juvela	GF Dietary Supplies
	Rite-Diet	Welfare Foods
	Tritamyl	Procea
	Trufree	Cantassium
Pasta	Aglutella	GF Dietary Supplies
	Aproten	Ultrapharm
	Rite-Diet	Welfare Foods
Wafers/biscuits	Aglutella Azeta	GF Dietary Supplies
	Aproten	Ultrapharm
	Bi-Aglut	Ultrapharm
	Farley's	Farley
Cakes/cake mixes	Aproten	Ultrapharm
	Juvela	GF Dietary Supplies
Biscuits	GF Gluten-free	GF Dietary Supplies
	Glutenex	Cow & Gate
	Liga	Cow & Gate
	Nutricia	GF Dietary Supplies
	Polial	Ultrapharm
	Rite-Diet	Welfare Foods

* See *British National Formulary* (1992) and Thomas (1988) for more details.

companies, and many other aspects of the condition.

At the start of treatment it is useful to add iron and folate supplements. Recovery may take several months, although patients often say how much better they feel after only a week or two on the diet. Constipation can be a problem and coeliac patients may not, of course, take bran. Several bulk laxatives are available, based on ispaghula husk, methylcellulose and sterculia. In addition, some soya bran products are useful.

Once started, the gluten-free diet should be maintained for life. This applies to both children and adults. Long-term complications of coeliac disease occur, of which the most lethal is small-bowel lymphoma. There is now good evidence that a gluten-free diet reduces the risk of intestinal malignancy.

About 15% of patients do not respond to gluten withdrawal. These people often have more extensive disease and may become severely ill. They are managed with corticosteroids. However, the majority of coeliac patients when correctly managed have a normal life expectancy and can eat a wide variety of foods.

DERMATITIS HERPETIFORMIS

This is primarily a skin condition in which a blistering and irritating eruption occurs, most marked on the extensor surfaces. Many patients with dermatitis herpetiformis also have a flat jejunal mucosa, which is responsive to gluten withdrawal. The skin condition responds to the antileprosy drug Dapsone, but may also benefit from a gluten-free diet.

TROPICAL SPRUE

Tropical sprue has little in common with coeliac disease except the occurrence of similar morphological changes in the small-bowel mucosa. It is a chronic disorder of the intestine, acquired in tropical regions and characterized by partial villous atrophy leading to malabsorption of fat, vitamin B_{12} and folate, and which is cured by the administration of broad-spectrum antibiotics (Tomkins 1981).

It is important to understand that the morphology of the normal small-bowel mucosa is different in people from tropical countries from those in temperate climates. In the tropics normal finger-like villi are rarely present; instead, the mucosa appears flattened with leaves and ridges (Wood et al 1991). Tropical sprue, however, is a distinct entity in which there is progressive failure of bowel function which requires specific treatment and does not spontaneously resolve, as do the intestinal abnormalities of those who visit the tropics.

Tropical sprue occurs solely in those who have lived in, or have travelled to, India, southeast Asia, northern South America and parts of Africa. It presents as chronic diarrhoea, usually following an acute episode. Weight loss, anorexia, anaemia and oedema follow and the condition may be fatal if not treated. Both the jejunum and the ileum are involved in the pathology, which is probably due to a persistent enteric bacterial or viral infection. Patients have malabsorption of fat, B_{12}, folate and xylose, and may develop secondary lactose intolerance. Megaloblastic anaemia is common.

Specific treatment must include broad-spectrum antibiotics and folic acid. Diet therapy is supportive rather than therapeutic, although many patients will need to replace lost weight and may take several months to recover normal jejunal function.

SHORT BOWEL SYNDROME

Occasionally large amounts of the small bowel have to be removed surgically. The common reasons are following mesenteric embolism or thrombosis, intestinal strangulation, trauma, Crohn's disease and lymphoma. Although removal of 50–100 cm segments of small bowel is usually without any nutritional seque-

lae, unless it is the terminal ileum, larger resections which leave less than 1 m of bowel remaining result in severe, acute and long-term problems.

The outlook for, and management of, these patients depends on the amount of bowel resected, the site of resection, i.e. jejunum or ileum, the amount of any associated colonic resection, and the presence or absence of the ileocaecal valve. The worst scenario is a massive ileocolonic resection; the best is a mid-jejunal one. Survival is possible with as little as 30–60 cm of small bowel, once the patient is over the initial episode, because adaptation occurs in the residual small and large bowels.

During intestinal adaptation there is an increase in the mass of remaining bowel, hypertrophy of the mucosal surface and lengthening of the villi, resulting in a substantial increase in the absorptive surface (Weser 1979). This occurs as a result of the exposure of the remaining bowel to nutrients, bile and pancreatic enzymes, and the trophic effect of gut hormones and short-chain fatty acids (Polak et al 1982, Sakata 1987). The converse of this adaptation is the atrophy which occurs in starvation (Altmann 1972).

Pathophysiology and management

Ileal resection

The ileum is responsible for B_{12}, bile acid, salt and water absorption. Short resections of the terminal ileum (less than 100 cm), which often include the ileocaecal valve, result in bile malabsorption which leads to diarrhoea and mild steatorrhoea, and eventually B_{12} deficiency also occurs. Gallstones are more common. The key to management of these patients is the bile acid-binding resin cholestyramine. A single morning dose, when bile acid concentrations are highest in the duodenum, often suffices. B_{12} should be given prophylactically. A reduced-fat diet is not essential, but may help to reduce diarrhoea.

Ileal resection over 100 cm gives rise to substantial steatorrhoea, due to chronic bile acid deficiency. Diarrhoea and weight loss are common. A low-fat diet is effective at reducing the diarrhoea but may not help with weight maintenance. Vitamin B_{12} injections are essential. Often these patients have gastric hypersecretion which impairs pancreatic enzyme activity, and it may be useful to suppress this with H_2 blockers.

Massive resection

Massive resection of the jejunum and ileum presents an acute problem of watery diarrhoea, weight loss and malabsorption. Total parenteral nutrition (Chapter 29) must be instigated immediately and is life-saving until recovery has occurred. Oral feeding is introduced as soon as the patient can tolerate it, to encourage growth and adaptation of the remaining bowel mucosa. Initially this can be with complete enteral feeds but normal foods carry some advantages. Starchy foods are better than sugary ones because of their lower osmolarity, and are less likely to aggravate diarrhoea. A low-fat diet (30 g/day) is standard practice, although its use has been challenged (Simko et al 1980). Fat-soluble vitamin supplements are necessary and patients may require iron and zinc as well. Essential fatty acids can be given by rubbing a polyunsaturated oil into the skin. Intestinal adaptation usually takes about a year.

Patients who retain most of their large intestine following massive small-bowel loss may run into two rare complications: oxalate renal stones arise due to excess fat in the colon precipitating calcium salts and increasing oxalate solubility and secondly D-lactic acidosis arises as a result of microbial fermentation of excess carbohydrate reaching the caecum. These conditions can be treated with a low-fat, low-oxalate diet and antibiotics, respectively.

LACTOSE INTOLERANCE

Lactose, a disaccharide of glucose and galactose, is a sugar peculiar to milk and milk products. Its universal presence in milk means that all newborn mammalian species have the appropriate enzyme, lactase (B1-4 galactosidase) in the brush border to deal with this sugar. However, after weaning lactase activity declines rapidly in all species, including man. In the absence of lactase, milk drinking may produce diarrhoea, abdominal pain and distension. This is because unabsorbed lactose exerts an osmotic effect in the small bowel and results in large amounts of fluid and sugar entering the large bowel. There the sugar is rapidly fermented, producing gas, and if enough lactose is present osmotic diarrhoea ensues (Bayless et al 1975, Tandon et al 1981). Some human populations retain the ability to digest lactose. These are the traditional milk-drinking people who have their ancestors in the Aryan races of the Middle East and northern India. In practice this means that the majority of northern Europeans and peoples deriving from them, including North American whites and Australian and New Zealand whites, retain the ability to digest lactose, although even among these people 5–15% may be alactasic (Cook 1980, Neale 1968). In most areas of the world, including Asia, Africa, South America and the Mediterranean,

lactase activity is very low and milk drinking, with the exception of fermented milk, is uncommon.

Lactose intolerance may also be acquired as a result of gastrointestinal disease affecting the mucosa, the principal causes of which are listed in Table 33.8.

Practical management

Lactose intolerance may be diagnosed with certainty only by jejunal biopsy and assay of disaccharidase activity. However, two indirect tests are available. A blood glucose rise of less than 20 mg/100 ml of blood after a standard dose of 50 g of lactose (to adults) or a breath hydrogen increase over fasting of more than 20 ppm both indicate lactose intolerance. The breath hydrogen test however is subject to a number of potential errors.

In lactose intolerance secondary to other gastrointestinal disease, a low-lactose diet can be useful. This means a reduced intake of milk, ice-cream, made-up desserts containing milk, and many sauces. Most cheese is low in lactose, although milk is added back in the production of some soft cheeses which may then contain small amounts of lactose. Naturally made yoghurt is virtually lactose-free, but again milk and milk solids are added to many yoghurts today, giving them similar lactose levels to fresh milk (about 5 g/100 ml fresh whole milk). However, symptoms ascribed to lactose intolerance, secondary to gastrointestinal disease, are often due to intolerance of other components of the diet (see Chapter 44), and treatment of the primary condition is the key to management.

Most people with low lactase activity can, in practice, tolerate quite reasonable amounts of lactose in the diet – usually 10–15 g/day – provided it is taken in small amounts (Bayless et al 1975, Haverberg et al 1980). Lactose does not therefore need to be excluded from the diet, and in many parts of the world, such

---

Table 33.8 Causes of lactase deficiency (lactose intolerance)

Genetic	Absent at birth (rare)
	Declines after weaning (usual)
Acquired	Protein–energy malnutrition
	Coeliac disease
	Tropical sprue
	Small-bowel resection
	Crohn's disease
	Acute gastroenteritis
	Chronic alcoholism
	Immunodeficiency syndrome
	Cow's milk protein intolerance

as Finland, India and Africa, milk drinking is part of the culture despite low lactase levels. In fact, it is probably important to encourage the consumption of milk and milk products if available in populations with subsistence economies.

Other disaccharide deficiencies occur such as sucrase, isomaltase and trehalase, as well as isolated monosaccharide transport defects, particularly for glucose and galactose. These conditions are very rare and usually manifest themselves early in childhood. A number of inherited disorders of sugar metabolism, such as galactosaemia and fructose intolerance, also occur.

CROHN'S DISEASE

Crohn's disease is a chronic inflammation which may affect any part of the gut from mouth to anus. Characteristically it occurs in the ileocaecal region and colon and is discontinuous. It frequently recurs after surgical resection of the affected areas of gut. The involved bowel is thickened, with ulceration of the mucosa, stricturing and fistula formation. Histologically there is transmural inflammation, with mononuclear cells, lymphoid aggregates and granulomata.

The condition was first described in 1932 by Crohn and called regional ileitis (Crohn et al 1932). Before 1932 the disease may have been confused with tuberculosis because of its predilection for the ileocaecal area and the presence of granulomata. Crohn's disease probably occurs worldwide, although it is uncommon in Central and South America, Africa and Asia. The incidence in Europe is of the order of 1–5 cases/100 000 of the population per year (prevalence 10–70 cases/100 000). This has increased dramatically since 1950, although the rate is now levelling off. It is predominantly a disease of the young, with peak occurrence in the third and fourth decades, and a second peak of incidence in the elderly. It is commoner among whites than non-whites and among Jews. The cause at present is unknown (Mendeloff 1980) but a familial tendency exists.

The two major presenting complaints in Crohn's disease are abdominal pain and diarrhoea, which occur in 80–90% of cases. In the small-bowel form other clinical features include weight loss, anorexia, fever, nausea and vomiting, tiredness, intestinal obstruction and fistula. In the colonic form rectal bleeding is present in about 50% of cases, and perianal disease is common. Systemic manifestations of Crohn's disease include arthritis, iritis, and more rarely liver and skin

lesions. In children, retarded growth and sexual development are a problem but respond to adequate treatment.

Nutritional problems and their management

Nutritional problems, particularly anaemia and weight loss, are very common in Crohn's disease (Harries & Heatley 1986). The factors contributing to poor nutrition are multiple and are listed in Table 33.9.

The anaemia of Crohn's disease has many contributory causes but is usually due either to iron or folate deficiency or a combination of both. B_{12} deficiency is seen after ileal resection or in extensive ileal disease, and drugs, especially sulphasalazine, may cause haemolysis and aggravate folate deficiency. Blood examination for iron, ferritin, folate and B_{12} is essential to discover the cause of the anaemia. Treatment is first of the underlying problem and then by the prescription of appropriate haematinics.

Almost all patients with Crohn's disease lose weight, and it can be very difficult to maintain ideal weight in these patients. Management should be aimed at improving appetite and reducing malabsorption.

Appetite in Crohn's disease can be improved by the correction of micronutrient deficiencies, especially zinc, giving attention to drugs which may depress appetite, prescription of corticosteroids and encouraging consumption of as wide a range of foodstuffs as possible. Diets to control malabsorption have been dealt with earlier. Surgical resection of an isolated stricture or area of inflammation in the small bowel may also relieve symptoms and improve food intake.

Table 33.9 Contributory factors to malnutrition in Crohn's disease

Anorexia	Fear of provoking abdominal pain Effect of drugs Zinc deficiency (loss of taste) Salt deficiency (in severe diarrhoea)
Malabsorption	Mucosal inflammation Gut resection or bypass Blind loop syndrome Fistula
Enteric losses	Protein-losing enteropathy Bleeding into gut
Other factors	Psychological: depression Social: offensive stools Metabolic rate: changes in response to chronic infection, stress and drugs Self-imposed diets

Enteral and parenteral nutrition

In patients who do not respond to conventional treatment in Crohn's disease, various enteral and parenteral regimens providing 'bowel rest' have been used. The rationale for such treatments is that the absence of nutrients and potential antigens in the bowel lumen reduces motor and digestive activity and gives the mucosa a chance to heal itself. Parenteral regimens are designed to cope with nutritional deficiencies and ensure an adequate intake of protein and energy. Various options have been tried, including total parenteral nutrition (TPN), TPN plus some oral nutrition, and formula diets through nasogastric tubes. There has been a great deal of enthusiasm for these regimens since they were first tried about 20 years ago.

In acutely ill patients *intravenous feeding* may be life-saving by replenishing water and electrolyte losses and providing nutritional support until the disease remits. Bowel-rest regimens will induce remission in Crohn's disease, but no better than conventional treatment with corticosteroids. Moreover, there is no evidence as yet to suggest that bowel rest for a period of time influences the outcome of the disease over the ensuing year (Harries & Heatley 1986, Greenberg et al 1988). Full bowel-rest regimens are best reserved for patients who do not respond to conventional therapy, have inflammatory masses or high fistulas.

Enteral feeding with elemental diets (such as EO28) is less taxing for the patient and is as effective as conventional steroid treatment (O'Morain et al 1984) for inducing remission. It can be used as an alternative to steroids and thus offers the advantage of avoiding steroid-induced side effects. However it is not a realistic long-term strategy except in the severely ill. Elemental, not polymeric, diets must be used (Giaffer et al 1990). The suggestion that the benefit of elemental diet lies in the avoidance of dietary allergens (Jones et al 1985) awaits confirmation.

Sugar and refined carbohydrate

A number of studies have shown that at the time of diagnosis Crohn's disease patients have a high intake of sucrose (Heaton 1987). Such patients also have low intakes of dietary fibre. It is fashionable to blame high-sugar/low-fibre diets for a variety of conditions. However, it is very difficult to assess diet in Crohn's disease prior to the onset of the condition and there remains the possibility that patients have changed their diet to cope with their symptoms. Few patients with abdominal pain and diarrhoea would choose a diet rich in fruit, vegetables and cereals. A recent large multicentre trial in which a diet excluding sugars and rich in fibre was given did not result in any conclusive benefit in patient management (Ritchie et al 1987).

Other problems

Patients with Crohn's disease may develop osteomalacia and deficiencies of fat-soluble vitamins, magnesium and zinc. These should be dealt with by conventional therapy (see Malabsorption).

A problem almost pathognomonic of Crohn's disease is the frequent formation of strictures in the small bowel. These can be very narrow indeed and give rise to intestinal obstruction unless sensible precautions are taken with diet. Most foods can be tolerated if well chewed or comminuted before digestion. Particular care is needed in the chewing of whole segments of orange, nuts, raw and dried fruit, vegetables, large lumps of meat and, equally importantly, enteric-coated tablets.

THE LARGE INTESTINE

The large bowel has a role in digestion in that it provides a chamber where, through bacterial activity, energy is salvaged from carbohydrate which has not been digested in the small bowel.

The principal carbohydrates to reach the large intestine are resistant starch, non-starch polysaccharides (dietary fibre), dextrins, oligosaccharides (raffinose, stachyose, fructans), lactose in lactase-deficient people and, in addition, commercial preparations such as polydextrose, palatinit, lactulose and the bulk laxatives ispaghula and sterculia. It has been estimated that in people eating western-style diets between 10–60 g of carbohydrate enter the colon each day (Macfarlane & Cummings 1991). Substantially more may do so in communities where starchy foods provide the bulk of energy intake (see Chapter 4).

Some protein also escapes digestion in the small bowel, depending to some extent on its physical form. The amount is between 6 and 12 g/day from western diets.

Carbohydrate and protein are both broken down in the large bowel by the action of the anaerobic flora in a process known as fermentation (Macfarlane & Cummings 1991). The products of fermentation and their fate are listed in Table 33.10. Through fermentation, diet may play a part in the metabolism of colonic epithelial cells, liver, muscle and the microflora, and affect faecal output, breath gases and urine and blood composition. Diet thus has a significant part to play in the control of large-bowel function and in the management of the common colonic disorders.

Table 33.10 Principal products of fermentation and their fate

Substrate	Product	Main fate
Carbohydrate	Short-chain fatty acids	Absorbed —> blood
	Acetate	Metabolized by muscle
	Propionate	Cleared by liver
	Butyrate	Metabolized by colonic epithelial cells
	Lactate, ethanol	Absorbed —> liver
	Gases H_2, CO_2, CH_4	Expelled via breath or per rectum
	Bacterial growth	Faeces
Protein	Short-chain fatty acids	As above
	Branched-chain fatty acids	Absorbed —> liver
	Ammonia	Either absorbed or used by bacteria for protein synthesis
	Amines, phenols, carboxylic acids	Absorbed – metabolized in liver or mucosa; excreted in urine

CONSTIPATION

Constipation is a disorder of motor activity of the bowel and characterized by the infrequent and difficult passage of small amounts of hard faeces.

Although much has been written about the amount of faeces passed each day by individuals or populations, in fact few data exist. In the UK the median value is 106 g/day, with males 110 and females 89 g/day. Most people pass between 40 and 280 g/day, whilst 46% of the total population pass less than 100 g/day. Transit times, which correlate closely with stool weight and are a determinant of it, are 58 h for men and 70 h for women (Cummings et al 1992). Published average daily stool weights in other countries of the world are in the range 72–470 g. In the lowest quartile of the distribution (70–120 g/day) come Scotland, New York, Hawaiian whites and Japanese, New Zealand whites and Maori, and urban Swedes. In the highest quartile (220 g/day plus) are found rural Indians, Ugandans, Kenyans, Chile and Malay Chinese.

Constipation is a significant cause of morbidity. In both the UK and the USA 1% of the population consult their doctor annually because of constipation and overall 10–12% consider themselves to have symptoms of constipation. The prevalence is much greater in people over 60, with 20–30% constipated and taking laxatives from time to time (Connell et al 1965, Thompson & Heaton 1980).

Burkitt and colleagues have popularized the view that low stool weight is associated with an increased risk of certain western diseases, especially bowel cancer, diverticular disease, appendicitis and various anal conditions (Burkitt & Trowell 1981). In general, stool weights below about 150 g/day and slow transit (more than 4–5 days) are associated with greater risk of bowel disease. An association of low stool weight with an increased risk for bowel cancer has been shown in more recent studies (Cummings et al 1992). Experimentally induced constipation leads to irritable bowel-like symptoms (Marcus & Heaton 1987) and complaints of constipation are common in people on low-fibre diets.

Control of bowel habit

The principal factors known to control stool weight are transit time (probably an inherited characteristic) and diet (the major environmental variable). Although exercise, stress and hormones have been suggested as altering bowel habit there are few good data to support this. In well over 100 studies the property of NSP (dietary fibre) to increase the amount of stool passed, and to affect bowel habit in other ways, has been well established (Cummings 1986). Figure 33.3 shows the relationship between NSP intake and bowel habit over a range of 4–32 g NSP/day. NSP is not the only dietary component to affect bowel habit: any carbohydrate which reaches the colon will have a laxative effect, however small. This includes, most importantly, resistant starch, which is mildly laxative. Poorly absorbed ions such as sulphate will also increase stool weight if taken in sufficient quantities.

The way starch and fibre affect bowel habit is now well worked out. The old notion that fibre acted like an inert sponge in the colon has now been superseded by the knowledge that fibre and other carbohydrates are extensively metabolized by local bacteria. Faecal weight increases through a variety of mechanisms which include increased bacterial growth and excretion, unmetabolized NSP (such as bran) which will hold water and increase bulk, and stool volume increased by gas trapped in the matrix, which in turn will stimulate motor activity and result in faster transit, which allows less time for dehydration of the stool (Stephen & Cummings 1980, Cummings 1987).

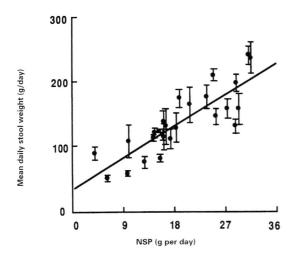

Fig. 33.3 Mean daily stool weight in 11 groups of healthy subjects (total n = 206) whilst eating controlled diets containing varying amounts of non-starch polysaccharides (NSP) (dietary fibre) (From Cummings et al 1992)

Management of constipation

There are many causes of constipation other than simply an inadequate fibre intake, and it is important to make a diagnosis first. Common causes include:

1. Diverticular disease
2. Irritable bowel syndrome
3. Megacolon
4. Central nervous system disorders (multiple sclerosis and Parkinson's disease)
5. Colorectal diseases (cancer, haemorrhoids and anal fissure)
6. Drugs (antacids, opiates, anticholinergics and many others)
7. Endocrine (hypothyroidism, diabetes)
8. Inactivity (due to travel or confinement to bed)
9. Self-imposed or therapeutic diets in slimmers and anorexia nervosa.

Pregnancy and the menstrual cycle also affect bowel habit.

General measures in management include allowing time for unhurried visits to the toilet. Neglecting the call to stool is a real cause of constipation. Patients are often advised to drink more fluid and take more exercise: neither are of proven value in constipation.

Laxatives are a valuable adjunct to the management of constipation. Bulk laxatives, which analytically are NSP, are most favoured at the moment and include

ispaghula, a seed mucilage from the Plantago family (Isogel, Fybogel, Regulan), sterculia, a plant gum (Normacol), methylcellulose (Celevac) and dephytenized bran (Trifyba). These laxatives are best taken with meals, starting with a dose of 3.5–7.0 g/day and increasing to 10.5–14.0 g if necessary. The aim is to produce one soft motion three or more times weekly.

Other British National Health Service–approved laxatives include stimulants (Senokot and Bisocodyl), salts (magnesium sulphate (Epsom salts) and sodium sulphate), faecal softeners (Docusate) and lactulose.

Diet

A diet high in NSP is of well established value in constipation. There is no universal dose: the amount required is that which will produce a satisfactory bowel habit. The aim should be to increase the patient's NSP intake from 12 to 18–24 g/day. Those who fail to respond to higher doses and whose constipation is of recent onset should be looked at carefully for organic disease. Patients with lifelong constipation of moderate severity respond only poorly to bulk stimulants. In choosing a diet it is worth remembering that wholegrain cereal sources are the most effective bulking foods (Cummings 1986). Rapidly fermented carbohydrates, such as low-molecular-weight sugars, oligosaccharides and soluble forms of dietary fibre, seem to be less effective. They also tend to give rise to excess gas. NSP intake can be increased by:

1. Increasing bread intake to 200 g/day and changing to 100% wholemeal
2. Eating a wholewheat breakfast cereal or one with added bran (50 g/day)
3. Increasing fruit and vegetable intake (to 400 g/day)
4. Eating more legumes such as beans and peas. However, this can produce problems with gas due to oligosaccharide fermentation
5. Bulk laxatives.

The dangers of a high NSP intake are very small. Patients who increase their NSP intake too quickly may experience abdominal distension, bloating, pain and increased flatus. A slow change in diet allows the gut to adjust to this. Other complications of NSP, such as intestinal obstruction and mineral malabsorption, are largely theoretical. However, because of the high phytic acid content of raw bran and bran products these should be avoided in patients whose mineral balance may be precarious, such as the elderly, young women and the unemployed (DHSS 1972, COMA 1989, Gregory et al 1990). High-fibre diets are not suitable for the treatment of constipation due to neurological disorders, or to obstructive lesions of the gut.

IRRITABLE BOWEL SYNDROME (IBS)

IBS is one of the commonest disorders seen in the hospital gastroenterology clinic, but it is poorly understood and has proved to be a graveyard for many good research intentions. IBS (or irritable colon, mucus colitis, spastic colon) is a disorder of motor activity of the whole bowel, although colonic symptoms usually predominate. It occurs very widely throughout the world and is commoner in women.

IBS has two main presenting features – abdominal pain and altered bowel habit. The pain may be anywhere in the abdomen but is usually in the left or right iliac fossa, and is related either to meals or defaecation. The bowel disturbance can be either diarrhoea or constipation or a mixture of both. Thus two general syndromes are recognized, abdominal pain and constipation (usual) and painless diarrhoea (less common). Other symptoms include abdominal distension, bloating, excess wind, passage of mucus, a sensation of incomplete rectal emptying and proctalgia fugax (fleeting rectal pain).

The cause of IBS is unknown, but motility studies have shown that IBS patients have a greater frequency of high-amplitude pressure waves during interdigestive periods, and these may be associated with abdominal pain. IBS patients also show exaggerated motility responses to meals and to pharmacological stimulation of the gut. IBS symptoms are common in the general population (Thompson & Heaton 1980) and the condition may simply reflect an increased sensitivity to normal gastrointestinal function. A major feature of the illness is the increased frequency of psychological disorders. Patients tend to be more anxious, depressed and generally neurotic than controls (Drossman et al 1988). Certainly stress is a major factor in precipitating symptoms. IBS is probably one feature of a general problem of smooth muscle dysfunction. Thus patients may also complain of urinary difficulties, dyspareunia and dysmenorrhoea. Some give a history of having had abdominal surgery without a major pathology being found. It is an essential feature of the diagnosis of IBS that physical examination and investigations reveal no significant organic abnormality.

Management

There is no specific remedy. Management must include reassuring the patient that there is no serious organic disease and supporting them while they come to terms with what is often a lifelong nuisance. A number of drug treatments have been tried, including antispasmodics, anticholinergics, antidepressants, bulk laxatives, dopamine antagonists, carminatives, opioids and tranquillizers, but none is of proven benefit. Properly designed clinical trials of treatment are few (Klein 1988). Antispasmodics and antidepressants are probably the most widely used and provide a psychological prop for the patient. Wheat bran and other bulk laxatives are frequently given, but results have been very variable. They may aggravate symptoms through gas production, although in patients who are predominantly constipated they are of benefit (Cann et al 1984).

Patients with IBS expect dietary advice, not least because they frequently volunteer that certain foods upset them. Great restraint should, however, be shown in restricting people from eating specific foods unless there is very good reason. Nothing is better designed to prejudice a patient's long-term nutrition than a blanket injunction not to eat certain foods, such as wheat or milk products, spicy foods, etc. without sound evidence. Often IBS patients are young and such advice is not a wise prescription for a lifetime's diet. If food intolerances are suspected (see Chapter 44), then an exclusion diet can be tried, but otherwise the opportunity should be taken to ensure that the patient is eating a prudent diet and has enough NSP and resistant starch to ensure a regular bowel habit.

DIVERTICULAR DISEASE

A diverticulum is a pouch which protrudes outwards from the wall of the bowel. Although diverticula may occur anywhere in the gut, the term diverticular disease is usually reserved for the condition when it affects the large intestine, particularly the sigmoid colon.

Diverticular disease is common and has emerged this century, mostly in industrialized societies. The prevalence is strikingly age-related, being rare in people under the age of 40 but affecting 30% or more over the age of 65. It is rare at present in developing countries, although beginning to emerge in some (Segal et al 1977), and appears fairly rapidly in those who migrate from low- to high-risk areas (Stemmerman & Yatani 1973).

The essential features of the pathology of diverticular disease are sigmoid muscular hypertrophy and diverticula. The wall of the bowel becomes greatly thickened due to changes in the circular muscle and taeni coli. This results in apparent shortening of the bowel, making the mucosa concertina up in folds over the hypertrophied muscle. The bowel lumen is narrowed. Diverticular disease almost always affects the sigmoid colon (95% of cases), involving more proximal bowel less commonly. The sigmoid alone is affected in 65% of patients. Fig. 33.4 shows the barium X-ray of a patient with multiple diverticula affecting almost all the bowel except the caecum. The barium-filled diverticula may be seen, together with marked narrowing of the descending and sigmoid colon.

Probably 80% of patients with diverticula never have any symptoms. Those who do have trouble complain of pain in the left iliac fossa, which may be colicky, and alteration in bowel habit. Complications occur in about 5% of patients and are principally the development of infection in a diverticulum (diverticulitis) which may proceed to perforation and abscess formation. Bleeding may also occur.

The cause of diverticula is unknown but its rise to prominence this century and pattern of distribution worldwide has led to the suggestion that it is due to lack of fibre in the diet (Painter 1975). It is commoner in omnivores than in vegetarians (Gear et al 1979), and

the cause of the muscular hypertrophy is thought to be the need to propel hardened bowel contents which result from diets low in fermentable carbohydrates such as fibre. Once the muscular thickening has occurred the bowel lumen becomes narrowed, thus closing off small chambers where high pressures build up and force herniation of diverticula through the bowel wall, a theory developed in the 1960s by Painter (1975). Certainly high intraluminal pressures are found in the sigmoid colon of diverticular disease patients. In fact, the motility pattern may be very similar to that seen in IBS and has led to the suggestion that diverticular disease is a later development of IBS. Currently, however, the two conditions are considered to be separate entities. The actual event initiating muscular hypertrophy in diverticular disease remains unknown. It may yet prove to be the production by bacteria in the lumen of an agent active on the neuromuscular components of the bowel wall.

Management

The treatment of diverticular disease was revolutionized in the late 1960s by Painter's work. Against the long-held belief that the bowel needed to be rested by a low-residue diet, free of roughage, seeds, pips, etc., he formulated his high-pressure theory of diverticular disease and said that lack of bulk was the cause of the condition. In an uncontrolled trial of wheat bran (Painter et al 1972), he managed to improve substantially the symptoms of most of his patients. Subsequently, controlled trials were carried out (Brodribb 1977) and Fig. 33.5 shows the results of a study in which patients were given a bran crispbread providing an additional 6.1 g of dietary fibre per day. This would have increased their fibre intake by about a third, and is equivalent to about 4 g of NSP. Wheat bran is more effective than other sources of NSP or bulk laxatives for diverticular disease, and coarse bran is better than fine (Kirwan et al 1974). Bran is not a panacea and may aggravate flatus production, feelings of abdominal distension and incomplete emptying of the rectum (Brodribb & Humphreys 1976). Other remedies include antispasmodics for the pain and, occasionally, antibiotics to control infection. Surgery is needed for life-threatening complications. Elective surgery has become much less common since the advent of treatment with fibre.

ULCERATIVE COLITIS

Ulcerative colitis is a chronic inflammation of the mucosa of the large intestine which causes bloody

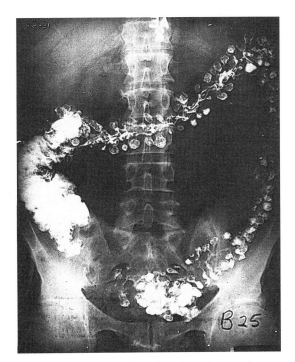

Fig. 33.4 An X-ray showing a large bowel containing barium. Numerous diverticula can be seen in almost all regions of the colon. The bowel lumen is narrowed, irregular and shows the typical pouches or diverticula.

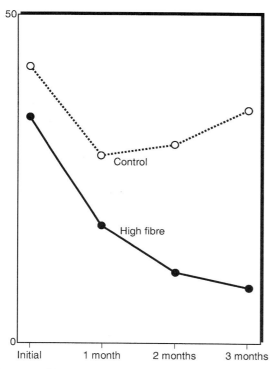

Total symptom
score

Fig. 33.5 Changes in mean symptom score over 3 months in 18 symptomatic diverticular disease patients who were given either bran crispbread (9 subjects) or a placebo (9 subjects) in addition to their usual diet (From Brodribb 1977).

diarrhoea. It is sometimes grouped together with Crohn's disease under the title 'inflammatory bowel disease', but the two diseases should be viewed as entirely separate conditions. In the present state of knowledge diet is not thought to have a role in the aetiology of ulcerative colitis, and is of very limited value in its management.

Ulcerative colitis is one of the diseases of modern civilization, being first described with certainty in 1909 (Fielding 1987) and predominantly affecting industrialized populations. It has an overall prevalence of 20–40 cases per 100 000 of the population in western people but is uncommon, although beginning to emerge, in Africa and India. It affects the sexes equally and usually presents between the ages of 20 and 40 years.

The cause of ulcerative colitis is unknown. Many people have sought an infectious aetiology but no agent has been found which satisfies Koch's postulates. There is some evidence of an inherited tendency in the disease, with Jewish people having a higher incidence, and with a high concordance in monozygotic twins. Certain HLA phenotypes (HLA-BW35) are more common in patients. Psychological and dietary factors have been implicated but largely discounted as causal.

The pathology of ulcerative colitis is one of inflammation affecting the mucosa only of the colon. The disease always involves the rectum and extends proximally towards the caecum in a continuous manner. The extent of disease is usually correlated with its severity and complication rate. Distal (sigmoid–rectal) disease is fairly benign, whereas involvement of the whole colon carries a cumulative risk of developing bowel cancer with time.

Clinically, patients present with diarrhoea and passing blood and mucus per rectum. The severity of an attack is gauged by the frequency of bowel actions, presence of fever, pulse rate, signs of complications such as anaemia, and toxic megacolon. An acute fulminating attack can be fatal, but mostly the condition runs a chronic relapsing course. Complications are either local – pseudopolyposis, strictures, toxic megacolon, perforations and cancer – or systemic – skin (pyoderma gangrenosum), eye lesions, arthritis (especially ankylosing spondylitis) and liver and biliary problems.

Management

Management is largely medical through the use of corticosteroids (either local or systemically), sulphasalazine or one of the more recently developed 5-amino-salicylic acid preparations. Surgery is required in severe or complicated cases. The operation of choice is total colectomy with either an ileostomy or ileorectal pouch construction. Diet has little influence on the disease, although many patients will ask for dietary advice. At one time low-residue diets were prescribed but these are not of proven benefit. Patients should be encouraged to eat as normal a diet as possible. Some patients' symptoms are aggravated by coexisting lactase deficiency, and improve on a diet free of cow's milk (Wright & Truelove 1965). Bowel-rest regimens have not proved beneficial in managing the inflammation in the colon.

ANAL CONDITIONS

Two common anal conditions, haemorrhoids and anal fissure, may benefit from dietary management.

Haemorrhoids

Haemorrhoids are vascular cushions of the anal canal which have prolapsed through the external sphincter and present as a tender swelling of the anal margin – the proverbial 'pile'. They are common in western countries and are thought to be due to constipation and straining at stool. However, recent epidemiological studies suggest that this may not be the case (Johanson & Sonnenberg 1990). They cause local pain and often bleed. Various surgical procedures have been devised to treat them, but avoidance of constipation is a valuable adjunct. Treatment with various bulking agents has been tried and the balance of trials is in favour of their being useful (Wood 1979, Moesgaard et al 1982).

Anal fissure

An anal fissure is a linear ulcer at the end of the anal canal. The cause is unknown but may be related to local trauma. They are common in the young and in women and can cause intense pain on defaecation. They often coexist with haemorrhoids. Management of chronic fissures is usually surgical, but bran given three times a day has been shown in one double-blind trial to be beneficial in preventing recurrence (Jensen 1987).

MANAGEMENT OF STOMA PATIENTS

Circumstances not infrequently demand that an opening is made into the gut in order either to feed the patient (gastrostomy, jejunostomy) or as part of the treatment for ulcerative colitis (ileostomy), Crohn's disease, cancer and, now more rarely, diverticular disease (colostomy).

Gastrostomy and jejunostomy

These are useful routes for the administration of enteral feeds in patients who have problems swallowing or require nutritional support in addition to their diet (see Chapter 29). Gastrostomy tubes may now be placed by percutaneous puncture, rendering this a simple and safe procedure. A wide variety of enteral feeds is available for both continuous and intermittent feeding. The major problems encountered include diarrhoea or constipation, nausea, vomiting and pulmonary aspiration, hyper- or hypoglycaemia, electrolyte abnormalities and trace element and vitamin deficiencies (Silk 1989). Nausea and vomiting may occur for many reasons, including delayed gastric emptying, fat intolerance, sudden large boluses of feed, drugs, psychological problems or systemic pathology such as infection. Diarrhoea occurs in up to 30% of patients and can be caused by intolerance of high osmolar load of feed, inappropriate gastrointestinal hormone release, antibiotic therapy, bacterial contamination of feeds, lactose intolerance and concomitant laxative therapy.

Complications tend to be more common with jejunostomy than gastrostomy, because the controlling benefits of the pyloric sphincter and gastric emptying on nutrient delivery to the small bowel are bypassed. The peak time for problems is in the early weeks of therapy, and a careful eye should be kept on patients for the first 10–14 days. Many patients with major gut or neurological problems are now managed successfully at home with enterostomy feeding regimens.

Ileostomy

An ileostomy is the end of the ileum brought out through the abdominal wall as a permanent fistula. It is made almost exclusively for patients who have had a total colectomy for ulcerative colitis or Crohn's disease. In general ileostomists can eat a normal diet and should be encouraged to do so. However, loss of the large intestine means that one important area of the gut for salt and water conservation has gone, as has the opportunity to salvage energy from unabsorbed carbohydrate through fermentation.

Salt and water balance

Adults in the UK pass around 100–120 g of faeces each day (see Fig. 33.3), whereas a person with an ileostomy will lose about 600 g (range 400–800 g). Ileostomy outputs are larger (800–1000 g) in those people who have had their operation for Crohn's disease, rather than ulcerative colitis, because there is usually some loss of small-bowel function as well. Most of the 600 g of material which passes each day into an ileostomy bag is water (about 560 ml), the only other important constituent being salt (sodium chloride) – about 4 g/day (range 2–6 g). Potassium (chloride) is also lost – usually less than 1.0 g – but is rarely physiologically significant. The amounts of other nutrients excreted in ileostomy effluent, such as calcium, magnesium, iron, zinc, vitamins, fat and protein, are no different from the amounts found in faeces, although additional losses are experienced by Crohn's disease patients and those with large outputs for other reasons. However, these losses of other nutrients are only occasionally a cause for concern (Cummings 1988).

Average water intake in the UK is about 2 litres and salt intakes are 10 g/day for men and 8 g/day for women. These are well above those needed to maintain normal health with an ileostomy. Most of the salt in western diets (75%) is added by manufacturers to processed foods such as bread, cereals, meats, sausages, cheese, tinned pasta, sauces, etc., whilst 10% is present naturally. A further 15% is added in cooking and at table. Potassium in ileostomy effluent (0.5 g/day) is more than compensated for by a daily intake of 2.5–3 g.

On the face of it, therefore, having an ileostomy does not pose any nutritional problems. In practice this is true most of the time, both for the standard ileostomy case and for patients with the new operation continent or pouch ileostomy, which does not need a bag. However, studies of ileostomy function have shown that the amount of salt and water lost each day is directly related to the total amount of effluent passed (McNeil et al 1982). If output exceeds 1000 g/day, there is then a danger that normal dietary intake of salt and water may be inadequate to keep up with losses.

Ileostomy outputs are likely to be excessive (over 1000 g/day) if the patient has Crohn's disease and has had a substantial ileal resection or a recurrence. *Ileostomy diarrhoea* may also occur acutely in any ileostomist, and is usually due to a viral infection, food poisoning, obstruction, abdominal infection or abscess. Ileostomy diarrhoea may quickly lead to salt and water depletion. This will occur much sooner if diarrhoea is accompanied by vomiting, fever and sweating. Salt and water deficiency usually go together. Common symptoms include excessive thirst, dry mouth, loss of appetite, nausea and vomiting, general fatigue, irritability, faintness, muscle cramps and headaches. One of the most useful warning signs is a decrease in urine volume.

Acute ileostomy diarrhoea can usually be managed conservatively. Maintaining an adequate water intake is easy. Excess water is excreted in urine and does not affect ileostomy output. A useful rule is to replace ileostomy losses by similar volumes of water, but water alone is not sufficient. Replacing salt (and potassium) losses requires more thought. Salt taken on its own increases ileostomy output and must therefore be mixed with some form of sugar or starch. Salt and water are therefore best replaced using the same oral rehydration therapy (ORT) as for acute diarrhoea (See Table 33.3).

People who have chronic ileostomy diarrhoea usually keep in balance by simply adding extra salt to food. In addition, drugs such as codeine phosphate and loperamide (Imodium) will reduce ileostomy output significantly. These drugs are not recommended in acute ileostomy diarrhoea. Bulking agents, such as ispaghula, thicken ileostomy output but also increase daily effluent volume.

General dietary advice

Most ileostomists eat a normal diet and do not suffer nutritional deficiencies (Bingham et al 1982). However, ileostomists experience digestive problems with some foods and in a survey of 79 ileostomists whose diets were compared to matched controls, more than 50% of patients had symptoms related to a variety of foods (Table 33.11). These either caused abdominal pain, an offensive odour, or were visible in the effluent. The ileostomists also ate diets containing less fibre than controls because they found it increased effluent volume. This meant lower intakes of fruit and vegetables. In general, therefore, ileostomists should:

Table 33.11   Summary of items of food reported to affect adversely more than 50% of ileostomy subjects who had tried them (From Bingham et al 1982)

Food items	Percentage affected	Main effects	Percentage avoiding or modifying intake as a result of effect
Nuts	60–90	Identifiable in effluent	70–90
Pips, pith, seeds, skin of fruit and tomatoes	50–90	Identifiable in effluent	50–85
Onions	50–80	Increased flow, flatus, odour-producing	50–75
Beetroot	70–80	Coloured flow, increased flow	30
Lettuce	60–70	Identifiable in effluent	50
Raw cabbage and carrot	50–60	Identifiable in effluent	50–75
Peas	50–60	Identifiable in effluent, flatus	50
Sweetcorn	50–60	Identifiable in effluent	75
Mushrooms	50–60	Identifiable in effluent, increased flow	60
Raisins, currants, sultanas	50–60	Identifiable in effluent	60–65

1. Eat a full and varied diet and should try everything
2. Be aware that certain foods, especially those high in fibre, will increase effluent output, and others may be visible in the effluent or cause occasional discomfort
3. Chew all food thoroughly, especially nuts
4. Beware of salt and water depletion when experiencing ileostomy diarrhoea (extra salt may be needed)
5. Be aware that some foods are more prone to cause odour than others, especially fish, onions, leeks and garlic. Excessive gas may be produced by peas and beans and fizzy drinks
6. Established ileostomists eat more in the morning and at midday and less in the evening to reduce the need to empty their bags at night
7. Subjects who find it difficult to gain weight after surgery, especially those with malabsorption, may prefer to eat refined carbohydrate and protein rather than fat and fibre.

Help for ileostomists may be obtained through The Ileostomy Association of Great Britain and Ireland, Central Office, Amblehurst House, Black Scotch Lane, Mansfield, Notts. NG18 4PF, Tel. 0623 28099.

COLOSTOMY

Colostomy, the opening of the large intestine as a fistula onto the anterior abdomen wall, is a much commoner operation than ileostomy. Temporary or loop colostomy is usually performed in adults to relieve more distal obstruction or abscess, after abdominal wounds, and in infants for anorectal anomalies. Permanent (end) colostomies may follow surgery for bowel cancer and diverticular disease. About 100 000 people have colostomies in the UK. Colostomies are usually either in the transverse or sigmoid colon.

The dietary and nutritional management of a colostomy is simpler than the ileostomy (Elcoat 1986). Constipation is more of a problem than diar-

rhoea, and patients are much more anxious about odour than of the stoma becoming obstructed. Left-sided colostomies can be managed very much in the same way as bowel habit. Transverse and right-sided colostomies are more likely to be loose and rapidly responsive to diet.

Constipation in a colostomy means very much the same as constipation in a person with an intact bowel, arises for mostly the same reasons and is managed similarly. The major causes are low intakes of non-starch polysaccharide and resistant starch, drugs or, more rarely, mechanical obstruction. Low fluid intake is wrongly cited as a cause of constipation except in countries where dehydration is common (i.e. hot, tropical and desert regions). Total immobility also slows bowel transit time. Treatment is the same as for normal constipation, except that suppositories and enemas are less easily retained.

Colostomy diarrhoea is more common in right-sided stomas and may be due to food poisoning, antibiotics, dietary causes or disease recurrence high up in the bowel. Colostomy output should always be measured to gauge the severity of the diarrhoea, and electrolyte replacement may be necessary if outputs exceed 1 kg/day. Otherwise bowel rest with a low-residues diet will reduce output, and antidiarrhoeal drugs may be useful in non-infectious cases.

FURTHER READING

Major texts which should be consulted for more detailed information about gastrointestinal disease are:

Misiewicz J J, Pounder R E, Venables C W (eds) 1987 Diseases of the gut and pancreas. Blackwell Scientific Publications, Oxford

Phillips S F, Pemberton S H, Shorter R G 1991 The large intestine: physiology, pathophysiology and disease. Raven Press, New York

Sleisenger M H, Fordthan J S 1989 Gastrointestinal disease: pathophysiology, diagnosis, management, 4th edn. W. B. Saunders, Philedelphia

REFERENCES

Altmann GG 1972 Influence of starvation and refeeding on mucosal size and epithelial renewal in rat small intestine. American Journal of Anatomy 133: 391–400

Bayless TM, Rothfield B, Massa C et al 1975 Lactose and milk intolerance: clinical implications. New England Journal of Medicine 292: 1156–1159

Bingham SA 1990 Mechanisms and experimental and epidemiological evidence relating dietary fibre (non-starch polysaccharides) and starch to protection against large

bowel cancer. Proceedings of the Nutrition Society 49: 35–53

Bingham S, Cummings JH, McNeil NI 1982 Diet and health of people with an ileostomy. I. Dietary assessment. British Journal of Nutrition 47: 399–406

British National Formulary No 23 April 1992. Joint publications of the British Medical Association and the Royal Pharmaceutical Society of Great Britain

Brodribb AJ 1977 Treatment of symptomatic diverticular disease with a high-fibre diet. Lancet i: 664–666

Brodribb AJ, Humphreys DM 1976 Diverticular disease: Part II – Treatment with bran. British Medical Journal 1: 425–428

Burkitt DP, Trowell H 1981 Western diseases. Arnold, London

Cann PA, Read N W, Holdsworth CD 1984 What is the benefit of coarse wheat bran in patients with the irritable bowel? Gut 25: 168–173

Carpenter CCJ, Greenough WB, Pierce NF 1988 Oral rehydration therapy – the role of polymeric substrates. New England Journal of Medicine 319: 1346–1348

Chacko A, Cummings JH 1988 Nitrogen losses from the human small bowel: obligatory losses and the effect of physical form of food. Gut 29: 809–815

Christl SU, Murgatroyd PR, Gibson GR, Cummings JH 1992 Production, metabolism and excretion of hydrogen in the large intestine. Gastroenterology 102: 1269–1277

Cohen S 1980 Pathogenesis of coffee-induced gastrointestinal symptoms. New England Journal of Medicine 303: 122–124

Committee on Medical Aspects of Food Policy. Sub-Committee on Nutritional Surveillance 1989. The diets of British schoolchildren. Department of Health. Report on Health and Social Subjects No 36. HMSO, London

Connell AM, Hilton C, Irvine G et al 1965 Variation of bowel habit in two population samples. British Medical Journal 2: 1095–1099

Cook GC 1980 Primary and secondary hypolactase (lactase deficiency). In: Tropical gastroenterology. Oxford University Press, Oxford, pp 325–339

Crohn BB, Ginzburg L, Oppenheimer GD 1932 Regional ileitis. A pathologic and clinical entity. Description of 14 cases. Journal of the American Medical Association 99: 1323–1329

Cummings JH 1986 The effect of dietary fiber on fecal weight and composition. In: Spiller GA (ed) CRC handbook of dietary fiber in human nutrition. CRC Press, Florida, pp 211–280

Cummings JH 1987 Constipation. In: Misiewicz JJ et al (eds) Diseases of the gut and pancreas. Blackwell Scientific, London, pp 59–70

Cummings JH 1988 Salt and water. In: Bosanko S, Penney C (eds) The ileostomy book The Ileostomy Association of Great Britain and Ireland, Mansfield, pp 23–27

Cummings JH, James WPT, Wiggins HS 1973 Role of the colon in ileal resection diarrhoea. Lancet i: 344–347

Cummings JH, Bingham SA, Heaton KW, Eastwood MA 1992 Faecal weight, colon cancer risk and dietary intake of non-starch polysaccharide (dietary fiber). Gastroenterology (in Press)

Cutting WAM, Belton MR, Brettle RP et al 1989 Safety and efficacy of three oral rehydration solutions for children with diarrhoea (Edinburgh 1984–85). Acta Paediatrica Scandinavia 78: 253–258

Davidson AGF, Bridges MA 1987 Coeliac disease: a critical review of aetiology and pathogenesis. Clinica Chimica Acta 163: 1–40

Dawson AM, Kumar P 1986 Coeliac disease. In: Booth CC, Neale G (eds) Disorders of the small intestine. Blackwell Scientific Publications, Oxford, pp 153–178

Dennish GW, Castell DO 1971 Inhibitory effect of smoking on the lower esophageal sphincter. New England Journal of Medicine 284: 1136–1137

DHSS 1972 A nutrition survey of the elderly. Report by the Panel on nutrition of the elderly. Report on Health and Social Subjects No 3. HMSO, London

DHSS/OPCS 1984 Hospital inpatient enquiry 1982. Series MB4 No 21, HMSO, London

Dicke WK 1950 Coeliac disease. Investigation of harmful effects of certain types of cereal on patients with coeliac disease. Doctoral thesis, University of Utrecht, The Netherlands

Drossman DA, McKee DC, Sandler RS et al 1988 Psychosocial factors in the irritable bowel syndrome. A multivariate study of patients and nonpatients with irritable bowel syndrome. Gastroenterology 95: 701–708

Eddy RL 1971 Metabolic bone disease after gastrectomy. American Journal of Medicine 50: 442–449

Editorial 1987 Diet and peptic ulcer. Lancet ii: 80–81

Elcoat C 1986 Stoma care nursing. Baillière Tindall, London

El-Mougi M, Hegazi E, Galal O et al 1988 Controlled clinical trial on the efficacy of rice powder-based oral rehydration solution on the outcome of acute diarrhoea in infants. Journal of Pediatric Gastroenterology and Nutrition 7: 572–576

Englyst HN, Cummings JH 1987 Resistant starch, a 'new' food component: a classification of starch for nutritional purposes. In: Morton ID (ed) Cereals in a European context. First European Conference on Food Science and Technology. Ellis Horwood, Chichester, pp 221–233

Field M, Fromm D, Al-Awqati Q, Greenough WB III 1972 Effect of cholera enterotoxin on ion transport across isolated ileal mucosa. Journal of Clinical Investigation 51: 796–804

Fielding JF 1987 Clinical features of ulcerative colitis. In: Misiewicz JJ et al (eds) Diseases of the gut and pancreas. Blackwell, Oxford, pp 725–744

Fisher RS, Roberts GS, Grabowski CJ, Cohen S 1978 Altered lower esophageal sphincter function during early pregnancy. Gastroenterology 74: 1233–1237

Fotherby KJ, Wraight EP, Neale G 1988 ^{51}[Cr]EDTA/^{14}C-mannitol intestinal permeability test. Clinical use in screening for coeliac disease. Scandinavian Journal of Gastroenterology 23: 171–177

Gear JSS, Ware A, Fursdon P et al 1979 Symptomless diverticular disease and intake of dietary fibre. Lancet i: 511–514

Gee SJ 1888 On the coeliac affection. St. Bartholomew's Hospital Reports 24: 17–20

Giaffer MH, North G, Holdsworth CD 1990 Controlled trial of polymeric versus elemental diet in treatment of active Crohn's disease. Lancet 335: 816–819

Gleibermann L 1973 Blood pressure and dietary salt in human populations. Ecology of Food and Nutrition 2: 143–156

Gore SM, Fontaine O, Pierce NF 1992 Impact of rice-based oral rehydration solution on stool output and duration of diarrhoea: meta-analysis of 13 clinical trials. British Medical Journal 304: 289–291

Greenberg GR, Fleming CR, Jeejeebhoy KN, et al 1988 Controlled trial of bowel rest and nutritional support in the management of Crohn's disease. Gut 29: 1309–1315

Gregory J, Foster K, Tyler H, Wiseman M 1990 The dietary and nutritional survey of British adults. OPCS Social Survey Division. HMSO, London

Gudmundsson K, Johnsson F, Joelsson B 1988 The time pattern of gastroesophageal reflux. Scandinavian Journal of Gastroenterology 23: 75–79

Hamilton JW, Boisen RJ, Yamamoto DT et al 1988 Sleeping on a wedge diminishes exposure of the esophagus to refluxed acid. Digestive Diseases Science 33: 518–522

Harries AD, Heatley RV 1986 Nutrition in inflammatory bowel disease. In: Heatley RV, Losowsky MS, Kelleher J (eds). Clinical nutrition in gastroenterology. Churchill Livingstone, Edinburgh, pp 146–160

Haverberg L, Kwon PH, Scrimshaw NS 1980 Comparative tolerance of adolescents of differing ethnic backgrounds to lactose-containing and lactose-free dairy drinks. I. Initial experience with a double-blind procedure. American Journal of Clinical Nutrition 33: 17–21

Heaton KW 1987 Dietary factors in the etiology of Crohn's disease. In: Jarnerot G (ed) Inflammatory bowel disease. Raven Press, New York, pp 109–117

Hogan WJ, Viegas de Andrade SRT, Winship DH 1972 Ethanol-induced acute esophageal motor dysfunction. Journal of Applied Physiology 32: 755–760

Intersalt Cooperative Research Group 1988 Intersalt: an international study of electrolyte excretion and blood pressure. Results from 24-hour urinary sodium and potassium excretion. British Medical Journal ii: 319–328

Jensen SL 1987 Maintenance therapy with unprocessed bran in the prevention of acute and fissure recurrence. Journal of the Royal Society of Medicine 80: 296–298

Johanson JF, Sonnenberg A 1990 The prevalence of haemorrhoids and chronic constipation: an epidemiologic study. Gastroenterology 98: 380–386

Jones VA, Dickinson RJ, Workman E et al 1985 Crohn's disease: maintenance of remission by diet. Lancet ii: 177–179

Kirwan WA, Smith AN, McConnell AA et al 1974 Action of different bran preparations on colonic function. British Medical Journal 4: 187–189

Klein KB 1988 Controlled treatment trials in the irritable bowel syndrome: a critique. Gastroenterology 95: 232–241

Kurata JH, Corboy ED 1988 Current peptic ulcer time trends: an epidemiological profile. Journal of Clinical Gastroenterology 10: 259–268

Leeds AR, Ebied F, Ralphs DN L et al 1981 Pectin in the dumping syndrome: reduction of symptoms and plasma volume changes. Lancet 1: 1075–1078

Levenson SD, Austin RK, Dietler MD et al 1985 Specificity of antigliadin and body in celiac disease. Gastroenterology 89: 1–5

Lubran M, McAllen PM 1951 Potassium deficiency in ulcerative colitis. Quarterly Journal of Medicine 79: 221–232

Macfarlane GT, Cummings JH 1991 The colonic flora, fermentation and large bowel digestive function. In: Phillips SF, Pemberton JH, Shorter RG (eds) The large intestine: physiology, pathophysiology and diseases. Raven Press, New York, pp 51–92

Machella TE 1950 Mechanism of post-gastrectomy dumping syndrome. Gastroenterology 14: 237–252

McNeil NI, Bingham S, Cole TJ et al 1982 Diet and health of people with an ileostomy. II. Ileostomy function and nutritional state. British Journal of Nutrition 47: 407–415

Marcus SN, Heaton K W 1987 Irritable bowel-type symptoms in spontaneous and induced constipation. Gut 28: 156–159

Matsumoto KK, Peter JB, Schultze RG et al 1966 Watery diarrhea and hypokalemia associated with pancreatic islet cell adenoma. Gastroenterology 50: 231–242

Mendeloff AI 1980 The epidemiology of inflammatory bowel disease. Clinical Gastroenterology 9: 259–270

Moesgaard F, Nielsen ML, Hansen JB, Knudsen JT 1982 High-fiber diet reduces bleeding and pain in patients with hemorrhoids. Diseases of the Colon and Rectum 25: 454–456

Molla AM, Sarkar SA, Hossain M et al 1982 Rice powder electrolyte solution as oral therapy in diarrhoea due to Vibrio cholerae and Escherichia coli. Lancet i: 1317–1319

Molla AM, Molla A, Rohide J, Greenough W B 1989 Turning off the diarrhea: the role of food and ORS. Journal of Pediatric Gastroenterology and Nutrition 8: 81–84

Neale G 1968 The diagnosis, incidence and significance of disaccharidase deficiency in adults. Proceedings of the Royal Society of Medicine 61: 1099–1102

Nebel OT, Castell DO 1973 Inhibition of the lower esophageal sphincter by fat – a mechanism for fatty food intolerance. Gut 14: 270–274

Nilsson BE, Westlin NE 1971 The fracture incidence after gastrectomy. Acta Chirurgica Scandinavica 137: 533–534

OPCS Mortality Statistics 1987 DH2 No 14. HMSO, London

Okada M, Yao T, Maeda K et al 1990 Predictors of duodenal ulcer healing during treatment with cimetidine. Gut 31: 758–762

O'Morain C, Segal AW, Levi AJ 1984 Elemental diet as primary treatment of acute Crohn's disease: a controlled trial. British Medical Journal 288: 1859–1862

Painter NS 1975 Diverticular disease of the colon – a deficiency disease of western civilization. William Heinemann Medical Books, London

Painter NS, Almeida AZ, Colebourne K W 1972 Unprocessed bran in treatment of diverticular disease of the colon. British Medical Journal 2: 137–140

Patra FC, Mahalanabis D, Jalan KN et al 1982 Is oral rice electrolyte solution superior to glucose electrolyte solution in infantile diarrhoea? Archives of Diseases in Children 57: 910–912

Penington GR, Krutsch JA 1990 Swallowing disorders: assessment and rehabilitation. British Journal of Hospital Medicine 44: 17–22

Phillips RA 1964 Water and electrolyte losses in cholera. Federation Proceedings 23: 705–712

Polak JM, Bloom SR, Wright NA, Daly MJ (eds) 1982 Basic science in gastroenterology: structure of the gut. Glaxo Group Research, Royal Postgraduate Medical School

Ritchie JK, Wadsworth J, Lennard-Jones JE, Rogers E 1987 Controlled multicentre therapeutic trial of an unrefined carbohydrate, fibre-rich diet in Crohn's disease. British Medical Journal 295: 517–520

Royal College of General Practitioners OPCS/DHSS 1986 Morbidity statistics from general practice. Third national study, 1981–1982. Series MB5 No 1, HMSO, London

Rydning A, Berstad A, Aadland E, Odegaard B 1982 Prophylactic effect of dietary fibre in duodenal ulcer disease. Lancet ii: 736–738

Sakata T 1987 Stimulatory effect of short-chain fatty acids on epithelial cell proliferation in the rat intestine: a possible explanation for trophic effects of fermentable fibre, gut microbes and luminal trophic factors. British Journal of Nutrition 58: 95–103

Segal I, Solomon A, Hunt JA 1977 Emergence of diverticular disease in the urban South African black. Gastroenterology 72: 215–219

Shnitka TK, Friedman MHW, Kidd EG, MacKenzie C 1961 Villous tumors of the rectum and colon characterized by severe fluid and electrolyte loss. Surgery, Gynecology and Obstetrics 112: 609–621

Silk DBA 1989 Hazards and problems in enteral feeding. In: Cummings J H (ed) The role of dietary fiber in enteral nutrition. Abbott International, Illinois, pp 96–111

Simko V, McCarrol AM, Goodman S et al 1980 High-fat diet in a short bowel syndrome: intestinal absorption and gastroentero-pancreatic hormone responses. Digestive Diseases Science 25: 333–339

Skerritt JH, Hill AS 1991 Self-management of dietary compliance in coeliac disease by means of ELISA 'home test' to detect gluten. Lancet 337: 379–382

Sonnenberg A, Muller-Lissner SA, Vogel E et al 1981 Predictors of duodenal ulcer healing and relapse. Gastroenterology 81: 1061–1067

Speelman P, Butler T, Kabir I et al 1986 Colonic dysfunction during cholera infection. Gastroenterology 91: 1164–1170

Stemmermann GN, Yatani R 1973 Diverticulosis and polyps of the large intestine: a necropsy study of Hawaii Japanese. Cancer 31: 1260–1270

Stephen AM, Cummings J H 1980 Mechanism of action of dietary fibre in the human colon. Nature 284: 283–284

Tandon RK, Joshi YK, Singh DS et al 1981 Lactose intolerance in North and South Indians. American Journal of Clinical Nutrition 34: 943–946

Thomas B (ed) 1988 Manual of dietetic practice. Blackwell Scientific Publications, Oxford, pp 188–192, 411–416

Thompson WG, Heaton KW 1980 Functional bowel disorders in apparently healthy people. Gastroenterology 79: 283–288

Tomkins AM 1981 Tropical malabsorption: recent concepts in pathogenesis and nutritional significance. Clinical Science 60: 131–137

UICC/IARC 1966–87 Cancer incidence in five continents, Vols I–V, 1966, 1970, 1976, 1981, 1987. IARC Scientific Publications, Lyon

Van Thiel DH, Gavaler JS, Stremple JF 1979 Lower esophageal sphincter pressure during the normal menstrual cycle. American Journal of Obstetrics and Gynecology 134: 64–67

Vernia P, Latella G, Breuer R I et al 1987 Electrolyte loss in stools of ulcerative colitis patients. Guidelines for replacement therapy. Italian Journal of Gastroenterology 19: 313–316

Watten RH, Morgan FM, Songhla YN et al 1959 Water and electrolyte studies in cholera. Journal of Clinical Investigation 38: 1879–1889

Welch CS, Adams M, Wakefield EG 1936 Metabolic studies on chronic ulcerative colitis. Journal of Clinical Investigation 16: 161–168

Weser E 1979 Nutritional aspects of malabsorption. Short gut adaptation. American Journal of Medicine 67: 1014–1020

Wood C (ed) 1979 Haemorrhoids – current concepts on causation and management. Royal Society of Medicine, Academic Press, London and Grune & Stratton, New York

Wood GM, Gearty JC, Cooper BT 1991 Small bowel morphology in British Indian and Afro-Caribbean subjects: evidence of tropical enteropathy. Gut 32: 256–259

Wright R, Truelove SC 1965 A controlled trial of various diets in ulcerative colitis. British Medical Journal 2: 138–141

34. Nutrition and the liver

M. H. N. Golden and K. W. Heaton

NUTRITIONAL EFFECTS OF LIVER DISEASE

The liver constitutes about 3% of the body weight in the adult and 5% in the infant. It receives about 28% of the total blood flow and consumes about 20% of the oxygen used by the body (Baldwin & Smith 1974). Its structure is adapted to its special function as a guardian interposed between the digestive tract and the rest of the body. Absorbed dietary components pass directly to the liver in the portal blood or, in the case of long-chain fat, indirectly by the lymphatic system. The liver handles large amounts of many nutrients: carbohydrates, amino acids, lipids, vitamins and trace minerals, as well as the pollutant xenobiotics, endotoxins, alkaloids and all the other non-nutrient and potentially harmful components of the diet. These are stored, metabolized or excreted by the liver into the blood or bile. The liver synthesizes most of the specialized transport proteins circulating in the plasma, as well as those proteins needed to maintain the integrity of the circulation, such as the clotting factors. The kidney is thought of as the primary organ of excretion, but this is only the case for small water-soluble, non-protein bound molecules. The liver is the primary site for removing and excreting lipid-soluble, protein-bound or large molecules that need to be converted into small water-soluble products prior to excretion. The liver thus serves to metabolize endogenous hormones, metabolic end-products such as bilirubin and urea, and tissue breakdown products as well as dietary pollutants. As the major guardian of the body, the liver's sinusoidal lining cells have considerable pinocytic and phagocytic capacity. The liver is quantitatively the most effective site for the removal of solid material, such as bacteria, from the circulation; it also removes virtually all the bacterial endotoxin that is absorbed from the intestine. The liver is the principal site for the coordination of the integrated metabolic changes that occur in response to infection, trauma or injury; collectively this is known as the acute-phase response.

It is apparent that the liver has a central role to play in almost every aspect of nutrition. The normal biochemical pathways of the fuels and nutrients, and their physiological modulation, are considered in other chapters. When the liver is diseased each of these functions is limited, but the extent differs with the various forms of disease. Normally there is a considerable reserve in the liver's capacity for most functions, therefore a particular liver disease has to cause a very marked reduction in a particular pathway before it becomes clinically obvious.

ABNORMALITIES OF LIVER DISEASE THAT AFFECT NUTRITIONAL STATUS

Carbohydrate metabolism

Fasting hypoglycaemia is surprisingly rare in liver disease. This is because normal glucose homoeostasis can be maintained with as little as 20% of the normal hepatic parenchymal mass, and the normal kidney can take over a considerable proportion of glucose production when liver production is impaired. Hypoglycaemia does occur, however, in fulminant hepatic failure or secondary to a toxic overdose with drugs such as acetaminophen or alcohol.

Glucose intolerance is more common in cirrhotics than in the normal population and is more marked after an oral than an intravenous load. Insulin levels are usually increased in advanced liver disease, perhaps because of reduced hepatic uptake. Fasting glucagon levels are also two to three times the normal level (Marco et al 1973). Glucagon levels do not decrease in response to glucose but rise excessively after alanine or arginine stimulation (Greco et al 1987). Growth hormone, 90% of which is cleared by the liver (Taylor et al 1972), is also markedly raised under basal conditions and fails to be suppressed by feeding (Panerai et al 1977). However, the liver is not stimulated by the high growth-hormone level to produce more insulin-like growth factors such as IGF-I; indeed, the IGF levels in liver disease are subnormal (Wu et al 1974). Basal somatostatin levels are raised and increase further with meals (Verrillo et al 1986).

Fasting blood gluconeogenic precursors and glycerol are usually increased in liver disease and the reduced capacity for gluconeogenesis leads readily to the development of lactic acidosis (Mulhausen et al 1967, Cohen 1976, Connor et al 1982) Sixty per cent of patients with lactic acidosis prove to have liver disease (Mulhausen et at 1967); lactic acidosis may be precipitated by feeding fructose, sorbitol or ethanol (Cohen 1976).

Other hormonal effects of liver disease

There is a modest increase in prolactin and sometimes in thyroid-stimulating hormone. The blood levels of the gonadotrophins, follicle-stimulating hormone and luteinizing hormone, are usually normal, as is adrenocorticotrophic hormone. In contrast to the pituitary hormones, there is an increase in T_4 and reverse T_3, with a decrease in the active hormone T_3 (Nomura et al 1975, Sheridan et al 1978, Chopra et al 1975). In man, circulating T_4 is converted to T_3 principally in the liver by the selenium-containing enzyme thyroxin 5′ deiodinase I. A decreased activity of this enzyme could account for the observed abnormalities.

There are gross changes in sex hormone level. Sex hormone-binding globulin is increased about eightfold (Van Thiel et al 1975), with a reduction in testosterone of about 50% and a universal reduction in free testosterone. Sex hormone-binding globulin seems to control the disposition of the sex hormones as well as their free levels. In liver disease, there is a markedly increased rate of conversion of the weak androgen androstenedione to oestrone and oestradiol by the liver.

Exogenous androgens, particularly 17α-alkylated androgens, lead to dilation of the biliary canaliculi, loss of canalicular villi, reduced excretion of bromo-sulphalein (BSP) and organic anions, benign hepatic tumours (adenomas), and occasionally hepatocarcinoma. These changes are less frequent with the non-17α-alkylated androgens (Lowdell & Murray-Lyon 1985). Nevertheless, these forms of toxic liver disease can occur in young athletes abusing anabolic steroids. This group is much more likely to consult a nutritionist than a physician, and is likely to be overlooked. The changes are reversible – even the adenomas – on stopping the steroids.

Salt and water metabolism

Impaired renal handling of sodium is one of the most frequent and florid manifestations of parenchymal hepatic disease. Although the important features of the condition have been described (Epstein 1992), its pathogenesis and rational management remain controversial. The abnormality is principally one of sodium, not water, metabolism. Most patients can excrete a urine of low osmolality when given excess water; however, when sodium is given it is quantitatively retained (Vaamonde 1983). There are two principal theories for this retention, with similarities to those used to account for the sodium retention in kwashiorkor. The first is that there is a reduced *effective* blood volume, with a reduced albumin concentration and diminished peripheral vascular resistance. The latter is characteristic of liver disease. The reduced resistance is due to both anatomic arteriovenous shunts and also to an undefined circulating vasodilator. Renal retention of sodium is thus seen as a secondary event. The second theory is the 'overflow' theory proposed by Lieberman et al (1970), with inappropriate sodium retention by the kidney and an increase in total plasma volume.

Blood coagulation

Most of the clotting factors and many of the inhibitors, such as antithrombin III, are synthesized in the liver. In patients with malabsorption of fat-soluble vitamins due to reduced bile salts, bleeding is a common problem. However, patients with hepatitis and cirrhosis may be unable to carboxylate the vitamin K-dependent clotting factors even after vitamin K is administered (Blanchard et al 1981). In liver disease, portal hypertension significantly affects platelet numbers and function. During the course of the disease a patient may manifest a number of coagulation abnormalities, such as decreased platelets, decreased clotting factors and enhanced fibrinolysis due to decreased clearance of plasminogen activators.

Liver disease and bone metabolism

Patients with a wide variety of liver diseases affecting the main hepatic cells, i.e. parenchymal liver disease (Mobarhan et al 1984), as well as obstructive cholestatic disease with jaundice (Kaplan 1987), develop an osteodystrophy. Histologically osteomalacia, osteoporosis and a lesion combining the features of both may be seen (Compston 1986). It usually develops insidiously in chronic liver disease, although

Table 34.1   Metabolic abnormalities in liver disease which affect bone metabolism

	Reference
Decreased vitamin D intake and less sun exposure	1
Decreased vitamin D absorption: bile acid deficiency: impaired mucosal absorption: sequestration by cholestyramine	2,3
Impaired hepatic 25-hydroxylation of vitamin D	4,5,6
Impaired intestinal absorption of calcium and phosphate: calcium soap formation with fatty acids: hyperparathyroidism	7,8,9
Decreased formation of 24,25–dihydroxycholecalciferol	10
Impaired hepatic production of vitamin D-binding protein	11
Increased urinary loss of vitamin D metabolites	12
Ineffective hepatic conversion of parathormone to active metabolites	13
Decreased production of somatomedin C (IGF-I)	14
Increased T_4, decreased T_3 and increased rT_3	15,16,17
Vitamin K malabsorption with decreased bone GLA protein-osteocalcin	
High corticosterol levels (liver responsible for A-ring reduction)	
High sex hormone binding globulin: very low free testosterone, increased oestrone, oestradiol and prolactin in men; women have ovarian atrophy	18,19,20
Marked decrease in activity	

(1) Davies et al 1983, (2) Krawitt et al 1977, (3) Malagelada et al 1974, (4) Hepner et al 1976, (5) Wagonfeld et al 1976, (6) Sonnenberg et al 1977, (7) Dibble et al 1981, (8) Whelton et al 1971, (9) Compston et al 1978, (10) Kaplan et al 1981, (11) Bikle et al 1986, (12) Bouillon et al 1984, (13) Martin et al 1979, (14) Wu et al 1974, (15) Nomura et al 1975, (16) Sheridan et al 1978, (17) Chopra et al 1975, (18) Gordon et al 1975, (19) Van Thiel et al 1981, (20) Van Thiel et al 1975

it can occur very rapidly; in infants, clinically significant disease can occur as early as 2 months of age (Spirer et al 1973). Children with liver disease have retarded growth. There are many interrelated abnormalities in liver disease that will adversely affect bone metabolism, and these are listed in Table 34.1. Which particular abnormality predominates is likely to determine which of the histological patterns develops in an individual patient.

In cholestatic disease bile salt deficiency with malabsorption of vitamin D, vitamin K and fat predominates. Fat, which is not absorbed, forms insoluble calcium soaps in the intestine, similar to the soap scum that occurs when washing in hard water. Indeed, the degree of calcium malabsorption is directly related to the degree of steatorrhoea (Whelton et al 1971). Many patients with these forms of liver disease have osteomalacia, which responds to vitamin D therapy (Kooh et al 1979). However, there are a number of patients with long-standing intrahepatic cholestasis who have an osteoporosis-like syndrome unresponsive to vitamin D (Kaplan 1987).

The liver converts vitamin D to its first major metabolite, 25-hydroxy cholecalciferol. This is the precursor for the second hydroxylation in the kidney, where the active hormone is produced. Experimentally, cholestasis or drugs such as cimetidine decrease the activity of the hepatic 25-hydroxylase. However, there is conflicting evidence as to whether patients with chronic liver disease can achieve normal levels of 25-hydroxy vitamin D; the consensus seems to be that clinically significant impairment is uncommon in cholestatic disease (Jung et al 1979), although it may occur in cirrhosis (Sonnenberg et al 1977). It is of interest that subnormal levels of 24,25-dihydroxy vitamin D, also produced by the kidney, have been found in patients with normal levels of 25-hydroxy vitamin D and 1,25-dihydroxy vitamin D, so the control of vitamin D metabolite formation may be abnormal in some forms of liver disease (Kaplan et al 1981). It should be emphasized, however, that bone disease may complicate liver disease in the absence of vitamin D deficiency and with adequate levels of 25-hydroxy vitamin D. The bone loss is frequently severe enough to produce spontaneous fractures, particularly of the axial skeleton.

Secondary hyperparathyroidism may be a factor in the skeletal abnormalities (Dibble et al 1981). The liver is also intimately involved in the peripheral metabolism of parathyroid hormone into biologically active metabolites (Martin et al 1979).

Table 34.2   Vitamin content of tissues (mg/kg wet weight) in relation to the recommended daily allowances of adults

	RNI Female (mg/day)	RNI Male (mg/day)	Liver (mg/kg)	Kidney (mg/kg)	Heart (mg/kg)	Muscle (mg/kg)	Brain (mg/kg)	Whole blood (mg/l)
Thiamin	0.4	0.4	2.2	2.8	3.6	1.2	1.6	0.02–0.08
Riboflavin	1.1	1.3	16.0	20.0	8.0	2.0	2.5	0.1–0.5
Nicotinic acid	13	17	58	37	41	47	20	3–7
B_6	1.4	1.2	2.5	1.1	0.8	0.9	0.7	0.03–0.08
B_{12} (μg)	1.5	1.5	500	200		8	10	0.2–0.8
Folate	0.2	0.2	9.5	2.1	1.0	0.8	1.1	0.005–0.020
Biotin	0.2	0.2	0.7	0.7	0.2	0.004	0.6	0.0002–0.0005
Pantothenic acid	3–7	3–7	43	19	16	12	15	0.15–0.50

RNI = UK recommended nutrient intake
– = not known

In children as well as adults, the decreased production of somatomedin (IGF-I) (Wu et al 1974) is likely to have a profound effect upon their growth as well as the maintenance of their skeletal mass (Bennett et al 1984).

Vitamin A and the liver

Normally over 90% of the body store of retinyl esters is in the liver. Two kinds of liver cell are involved in vitamin A metabolism (see Chapter 13). Chylomicron remnants and retinyl esters are taken up by parenchymal cells; these cells are also responsible for synthesizing retinol-binding protein (RBP) and hence for the mobilization of retinol from the liver. However, nearly all the vitamin A in the liver is transferred to specialized cells localized in the perisinusoidal space. Storage of vitamin A is the principal function of these cells, which are called either Ito cells, stellate cells or fat-storing cells. Once retinol, bound to RBP, is released from the liver the complex binds to transthyretin (prealbumin) which also binds the thyroid hormones. Patients with liver disease often have low levels of retinol, RBP and transthyretin. The patients with low retinol levels frequently show abnormal dark adaptation (Goodman 1984); however, the more florid manifestations of vitamin A deficiency are uncommon in liver disease unless associated with severe malnutrition.

Vitamin B group and the liver

The liver provides a store of riboflavin, nicotinic acid, folate, vitamin B_{12} and pantothenic acid. As the adult liver weighs about 2 kg, the data in Table 34.2 show that it contains between 10 and 200 times the RNI for these vitamins. On the other hand, thiamin and B_6 are not preferentially stored in the liver. One might expect that liver disease would be associated with vitamin deficiency where the liver forms the major repository in the body.

In an extensive study of patients with mild fatty liver, severe fatty liver and with cirrhosis, compared to normal biopsies as well as autopsy material, Baker et al (1964) showed that there were reduced levels of most of the vitamins in liver disease (Table 34.3).

Table 34.3   Hepatic levels of water-soluble vitamins in liver disease

		Normal biopsy	Normal autopsy	Steatosis Mild	Steatosis Severe	Cirrhosis
Vitamin B_{12}	μg/g	1.7	1.6	1.2	0.34	0.45
Folic acid	μg/g	11.2	9.8	6.7	3.0	3.1
Folinic acid	μg/g	3.9	3.8	3.2	1.8	1.7
Vitamin B_6	μg/g	12.4	9.7	4.6	1.6	3.7
Thiamin	μg/g	8.8	7.3	2.8	1.7	7.7
Nicotinic acid	μg/g	144	125	89	21	24
Biotin	ng/g	386	405	76	27	222
Pantothenic acid	μg/g	62	59	52	23	25

Data from Baker et al (1964)

Thiamin

Lack of dietary thiamin does not impair the capacity of the pentose phosphate pathway in the liver. Interestingly, patients with cirrhosis do not have a reduction in thiamin in the liver, although those with fatty liver do have a reduction (Frank et al 1971). Thiamin deficiency is frequently associated with alcoholic liver disease, but is uncommon in other forms of liver disease (Camilo et al 1981).

Riboflavin

In riboflavin deficiency, triglycerides accumulate in the liver (Sugioka et al 1969) and there is a reduced dehydrogenation of fatty acids, with diminished levels of arachadonic, linoleic and linoleic acids (Mookerjea & Hawkins 1960). There is frequently evidence of riboflavin deficiency in chronic alcoholism (Rosenthal et al 1973). The accumulation of liver fat in riboflavin deficiency resembles the changes found in alcoholics, and experimentally riboflavin administration to alcoholic rats reverses the accumulation of free fatty acids and esterified fat (Stanko et al 1978). There have so far been no trials of riboflavin supplementation in human fatty liver disease.

Nicotinic acid

There are no special hepatic stores of nicotinic acid. With alcoholism and cirrhosis there is a marked fall in the hepatic concentration of nicotinic acid. As with riboflavin, nicotinic acid treatment can prevent the increase in liver lipid caused by alcoholism (Baker et al 1976). This effect has been attributed to the inhibition of the peripheral release of free fatty acid as well as to the inhibitory action of nicotinic acid upon liver alcohol dehydrogenase. However, both riboflavin and nicotinic acid are essential for the maintenance of reduced glutathione in the liver, and thus for the protection of the liver against oxidative stress. The precise mechanism for these effects on fat accumulation is unknown.

Vitamin B_6

Although there is no store of vitamin B_6 in the liver, the liver is intimately involved in its metabolism. The liver plays a dominant role in the conversion of pyridoxine to pyridoxal and pyridoxal phosphate, the active forms of the vitamin used by other tissues. Intravenous pyridoxine normally substantially raises the plasma levels of pyridoxal phosphate, but there is little or no rise in patients with hepatitis, cirrhosis or cholestasis (Spannuth et al 1978). Unlike pyridoxal phosphate, plasma pyridoxal itself is often raised in cirrhotics (Henderson et al 1986). There seems to be a more rapid dephosphorylation of pyridoxal phosphate in liver disease. It has been suggested that 30–50% of alcoholics without liver damage, and 80–100% of those with liver damage, have vitamin B_6 undernutrition. This has not been focused upon by hepatologists and no trials of the effect of vitamin B_6 replacement seem to have been published.

Folic acid

There is about a 60% reduction in total liver folate content in cirrhosis (Leevy et al 1970). When folate is given to patients with liver disease they only deposit one-tenth of the amount of folate in their livers that normal subjects achieve. Healthy people given a folate-free diet develop megaloblastic changes in about 22 weeks; when chronic alcoholics are given a low-folate diet they develop similar changes in about 5 weeks (Eijhner & Hillman 1971). Ingestion of about 80 g alcohol per day is associated with low serum folate and megaloblastic changes in about 80% of subjects (Alpers et al 1983).

Although folate deficiency is common in alcoholics, it does occur in other forms of liver disease and the onset of viral hepatitis is associated with an excess urinary folate excretion (Retief & Huskisson 1969).

Vitamin B_{12}

Vitamin B_{12} deficiency is uncommon in liver disease unless it is complicated by gastric or ileal dysfunction. Acute liver damage causes a release of vitamin B_{12}; the increase in the serum B_{12} is directly proportional to the liver damage (Wiss & Weber 1964). In patients with acute hepatitis the free B_{12} is increased, whereas in chronic disease the bound B_{12} is increased. This is because, in chronic liver disease, there is an increase in the plasma concentration of the transcobalamins, particularly transcobalamin-I (Linnell 1975), so that vitamin B_{12} passes from the liver to the plasma. In healthy subjects, the major circulating form of vitamin B_{12} is methylcobalamin; in liver disease, 5-deoxyadenosylcobalamin may also appear in the plasma.

The liver and copper

Absorbed copper is taken up by the liver and stored in metallothionein in the liver. Excess copper is excreted in the bile. In diseases where there is an excessive copper absorption, or where there is a block in its excretion, copper accumulates in the liver. The levels

Table 34.4 Hepatic copper levels in various liver diseases

Condition	Liver copper (μg/g dry wt)
Normal	
Healthy adult	9–47
Fetus	80–146
Newborn baby	206–413
Pathological	
Wilson's disease	152–1828
Childhood cholestasis	52–1082
Primary biliary cirrhosis	29–1008
Extrahepatic biliary obstruction	111–226
India childhood cirrhosis	1367–4788
Idiopathic copper toxicosis	708–3255

can be very high (Table 34.4). Uncomplexed copper has a redox cycle between the cuprous and the cupric state when reducing equivalents are available; this one-electron oxidation–reduction cycle can be very damaging as each step generates a free radical. When copper accumulates to a level where it cannot be tightly bound to metallothionein, the resultant free radical damage gives rise to hepatic damage that leads to cirrhosis.

In Wilson's disease, the copper accumulation is secondary to a congenital defect in the export of copper from the liver to the plasma. In Indian childhood cirrhosis there is excessive absorption of copper mobilized from the brass jugs used to collect buffalo milk. In biliary disease there is an inability to excrete copper in the bile; it is possible that the accumulation of copper, in biliary disease, exacerbates the cirrhosis.

The liver and iron

About 10% of the total body content of iron is present in the liver iron stores, mainly in the storage protein ferritin. The liver also secretes the iron-transporting protein transferrin. Transferrin has a very high affinity for iron that both prevents it from undergoing redox cycling and also deprives invading organisms of iron. Iron is kept in the ferric state, and thus bound to transferrin, by the circulating ferroxidase, ceruloplasmin. Cells that require iron have specific receptors to which transferrin binds and makes the iron available.

The liver seems to be spared any serious ill-effects of iron deficiency. It is, however, particularly vulnerable to disorders characterized by iron overload, because iron, like copper, undergoes a redox cycle between the ferrous and the ferric states. It is to prevent radical injury that iron is tightly bound and kept in the ferric state. When the binding proteins are saturated or powerful reductants are available, free

radical damage can occur. Excess ascorbic acid, thought by many not to have any side effects, should not be given to patients with iron overload as it can exacerbate their condition. Iron overload occurs principally because of increased iron absorption or from multiple blood transfusions.

Haemochromatosis

Haemochromatosis is an inherited disease where there is an excessive absorption of iron in an haematologically normal person. The iron is deposited in the parenchyma of the liver.

Atransferrinaemia

Absence of transferrin is a rare disorder in which the liver takes up and does not release administered iron (Goya et al 1972).

Zellweger syndrome

This disease, once thought to be a variant of haemochromatosis, is characterized by widespread deposition of iron. This is caused by the absence of peroxisomes (Goldfischer 1979, Pfeifer & Sandhage 1979). The way in which peroxisomes are needed for normal iron metabolism is unknown. In kwashiorkor there is also an absence of peroxisomes (Doherty et al 1991) and an accumulation of iron in the liver (Golden & Ramdath 1987); whether the peroxisomal abnormality is related to the iron accumulation in kwashiorkor is unknown.

Alcoholic cirrhosis and porphyria

Hepatic iron overload in alcoholic cirrhosis is frequently encountered; in about 7% of patients severe siderosis is found which mimics haemochromatosis (Jakobitvits et al 1979). The mechanism driving iron accumulation in alcoholism is not understood.

Most patients with porphyria cutania tarda have hepatic siderosis with elevated serum iron 'levels (Grossman et al 1979); phlebotomy has a beneficial effect on the disease.

Transfusional overload

Patients with severe anaemia secondary to abnormal haemoglobin have an increased iron absorption and are frequently given blood transfusions, leading to iron overload. Unlike haemochromatosis, the iron accumulation is mainly in the Kupffer cells.

Bantu siderosis

Dietary iron overload is unusual except in particular circumstances. Amongst the South African Bantu, sorghum beer is brewed in empty iron kerosene drums, resulting in high levels of bioavailable iron that can lead to siderosis in those that drink it. The iron is largely reticuloendothelial in this form of siderosis, unlike experimental models of increased dietary iron overload where the iron is parenchymal. This suggests that the iron in Bantu siderosis is absorbed in a form which is not associated with transferrin transport to the liver parenchyma. Yeast siderophores in the beer are a possible explanation that has not been examined experimentally; alternatively, it has been suggested that concurrent ascorbate deficiency causes the abnormal iron distribution (Lynch et al 1967, Lipschitz et al 1971). The alcohol intake in Bantu beer drinkers will presumably exacerbate the siderosis in a similar fashion to that found in some western alcoholics.

GALLSTONES (CHOLELITHIASIS)

Gallstones or biliary calculi are by far the commonest biliary disease and the only one in which there is evidence for a role of diet. Calculi form within the gallbladder and usually stay there, in which case they generally cause no trouble. Why some stones cause symptoms and others do not is unknown: there is no relation to size, shape, density, number or composition. Most gallstones are multiple and up to 2 cm in diameter. Their rate of growth is usually 1-2 mm a year.

In developed countries, most gallstones are rich in cholesterol (>70%, w/w), present as monohydrate crystals. However, most gallstones also contain calcium salts, chiefly carbonate, phosphate, palmitate or bilirubinate, and about one-third of gallstones are composed mostly of such salts. The proportion of calcium-rich stones increases with age. Little is known of the aetiology of such stones but a good deal is known about cholesterol-rich stones.

Pathogenesis of cholesterol-rich gallstones

Physical and chemical factors interact in the pathogenesis of gallstones (Paumgartner & Sauerbruch 1991). The three major factors are supersaturation of the bile with cholesterol, imbalance of nucleating and antinucleating factors, and stasis within the gallbladder. Diet and nutritional state certainly affect the first and third factors, but it is not known whether they affect the second.

Bile is said to be supersaturated when its content of cholesterol exceeds its ability, at equilibrium, to suspend cholesterol in mixed micelles. Micelles are stable 4–8 nm particles in which discs of a phospholipid–cholesterol bilayer are surrounded by a ring of negatively charged bile acids. However, there are other cholesterol carriers in bile, namely, 40–80 nm unilamellar vesicles containing phospholipid and cholesterol. These vesicles are metastable; if their cholesterol content rises too high they fuse and form large, unstable, multilamellar vesicles which are also known as liquid crystals. It is these which, when time allows and nucleating factors are dominant, turn into crystals of cholesterol. For cholesterol crystals to turn into macroscopic stones requires the presence of mucus to trap the crystals and glue them together. An early stage in this process is biliary sludge. Sludge can disappear, stay the same, or turn into one or more stones.

Epidemiology

Gallstones are common in all industrialized countries. Women are affected twice as often as men and the prevalence rises with age to a peak of 30–60% in elderly women (Diehl 1991, Heaton et al 1991a). Among middle-aged people about one in 150 develop gallstones each year (Jensen & Jørgensen 1991).

As far as one can tell, gallstones are rare in rural areas of the third world. They have become much commoner in Europe in the last 100 years (Acalovschi et al 1987) but the incidence may now be falling, at least in western Europe (Hoogendoorn 1988, Teilum 1990). In Japan since the second world war there has been a sharp rise in cholesterol gallstones, especially in the cities (Nagase et al 1978). Although genetic factors are involved, as shown by family incidence and twin studies (Jørgenson 1988, Kesäniemi et al 1989), environmental factors seem to be preeminent. Good evidence for this is that, in the UK, gallstones are half as common as expected in vegetarians (Pixley et al 1985). Genetic susceptibility and unfavourable environment combine in the North American Indians to give them the highest prevalence of gallstones in the world – 70% of young Pima women have gallstones by the age of 30 (Sampliner et al 1970).

Conditions associated with gallstones

Table 34.5 lists the conditions and treatments which are associated with gallstones and the presumed nature of the link. The most important of these

Table 34.5   Conditions and treatments associated with gallstones

Condition	Probable mode of action
Obesity	Hypersecretion of cholesterol into bile
Hypertriglyceridaemia	Hypersecretion of cholesterol into bile
Constipation (slow colonic transit)	Altered composition of bile salt pool
Multiparity	Gallbladder stasis
Cirrhosis of liver	Hyposecretion of bile salts
Resection or disease of terminal ileum	Hyposecretion of bile salts (which are malabsorbed)
Abdominal surgery	Gallbladder stasis
Treatment with:	
total parenteral nutrition	Gallbladder stasis
octreotide (somatostatin)	Gallbladder stasis
oestrogens	Hypersecretion of cholesterol
progestogens	Hypersecretion of cholesterol
fibrates	Hypersecretion of cholesterol

numerically are obesity and hypertriglyceridaemia, which operate through increased secretion of biliary cholesterol, but there are other conditions which operate through hyposecretion of bile salts, altered composition of the bile salt pool and gallbladder stasis. All but the last of these mechanisms involve gallbladder bile becoming supersaturated with cholesterol as the main lithogenic process.

Obesity and fat distribution

Obesity has long been recognized as a risk factor for gallstones and it is the best documented one. A huge prospective study in American nurses showed a close association between weight gain since maturity and the risk of gallstones (MacLure et al 1989). In this study the line relating body mass index (kg/m²) to the risk of gallstones did not flatten out at the left-hand end, which implies that thinness protects against the disease. Teenage girls rarely develop gallstones but those who do are nearly always obese (Lee et al 1987).

Oddly, obesity is not a risk factor in older people (>50 years), nor in men, at least when it is expressed as body mass index (Scragg et al 1984a). On the other hand, abdominal obesity, measured as a raised waist–hip circumference ratio, is a risk factor in men (Heaton et al 1991b) and possibly in women too

(Hartz et al 1984). This fits with the idea that obesity operates through associated metabolic disturbances, especially insulin resistance and hyperinsulinaemia, since these disturbances are associated more with abdominal than with general obesity (see Chapter 32). Lack of physical exercise or loss of muscularity may also be a factor, since unfitness carries similar metabolic penalties to obesity (Houmard et al 1991) and men who develop a paunch are more likely to develop gallstones even if they do not gain weight (Heaton et al 1991b).

Insulin as a common factor

There are other reasons for suspecting that insulin is involved in the pathogenesis of cholesterol-rich gallstones besides the link with obesity and abdominal fat. Hypertriglyceridaemia is strongly associated with gallstones, independently of obesity (Thijs et al 1990), and with supersaturated bile (Alvaro et al 1986) and plasma triglycerides co-vary with plasma insulin (Laakso et al 1987). When late-onset diabetics are treated with insulin their bile becomes more saturated with cholesterol (Bennion & Grundy 1977, Kajiyama et al 1981). Insulin seems to promote the secretion of cholesterol into bile by activating the receptors on liver cells which enable low-density lipoprotein cholesterol to be transferred from blood into bile (Chait et al 1979). Furthermore, insulin activates the rate-limiting enzyme for cholesterol synthesis (Lakshmanan et al 1973). It is interesting, therefore, that plasma insulin tends to be high in people with gallstones, both in the fasting state and after a meal (Scragg et al 1984b, Heaton et al 1991b). A moderate intake of alcohol protects against gallstones (Scragg et al 1984a, La Vecchia et al 1991); it also makes people more sensitive to insulin so that their fasting level is lower (Razay et al 1992).

Thus, the insulin hypothesis can explain why gallstones are related to obesity, especially abdominal obesity, and to hypertriglyceridaemia, and can explain how alcohol protects. It may also explain some of the links between gallstones and diet (see below).

Colonic bacteria and colonic stasis

Cholesterol is not only excreted from the body via the biliary tract but a substantial amount of it – 300–500 mg/day, is metabolized to bile acids, which are also excreted into the bile and help to hold the cholesterol in solution. Whereas the biliary cholesterol, like dietary cholesterol, is poorly absorbed in the small intestine, the bile acids chenodeoxycholic and cholic acid are efficiently absorbed by passive diffusion throughout the small intestine and by specific transport mechanisms in the ileum. This recycling of the bile acid pool occurs up to 20 times per day. Bile salts escaping absorption enter the colon, where the taurine and glycine side chains are removed and the bile acids themselves are metabolized by anaerobic bacteria. Of the total circulating bile salt pool, about 80% consists of the primary cholate and chenodeoxycholate bile salts, the remainder consisting of secondary bile acids, i.e. those derived by bacteria, chiefly deoxycholate (DCA). In people whose colon has been removed there is no circulating DCA, only the primary bile salts.

Deoxycholate is formed in the caecum by the action of anaerobic bacteria on any cholate which has escaped reabsorption in the ileum. Unlike the ileum, the colon has no special transport system for absorbing bile salts, so DCA is absorbed slowly and incompletely. When colonic transit time is slowed down more DCA is absorbed and the circulating pool of DCA expands (Marcus & Heaton 1986). All this is relevant to gallstones because the more DCA there is in bile the more the bile is likely to precipitate cholesterol, and the greater is the risk of gallstones (Marcus & Heaton 1988). In the general population there is an association between gallstones and constipation, at least in non-obese people, whose gallstones are otherwise unexplained (Heaton et al 1991c). Thus anything, dietary or otherwise, which promotes colonic stasis is likely to increase the risk of gallstones.

The bacterial formation of deoxycholate is pH-dependent. If pH falls below 6.0, the enzyme 7-α-dehydroxylase which catalyses its formation, is inhibited. The pH in the right colon veers towards acid when bacteria ferment carbohydrate to short-chain fatty acids (see Chapter 4). Anything which increases the concentration of short-chain fatty acids in the colon might reduce the risk of gallstones by reducing biliary DCA levels.

Diet, eating habits and gallstones

There are several ways in which diet and eating habits could promote gallstones (Table 34.6).

Prolonged overnight fast

It has been reported that younger women with gallstones tend to have a longer overnight fast than controls matched for body mass index (Capron et al 1981). This could favour gallstone formation in two ways. First, fasting induces gallbladder stasis which allows time for crystals of cholesterol to form and grow. Secondly, as an overnight fast lengthens the bile in the gallbladder becomes more saturated with cholesterol (Bloch et al 1980).

Eating 'too much'

The strong links between obesity and gallstones encourage the belief that overeating is a key factor. Some case control studies have shown higher energy intakes in people with gallstones than in controls, but most have not (Sarles et al 1969, Scragg et al 1984a, Scragg 1986, Pixley & Mann 1988). Experimentally, raising the calorie intake increased the cholesterol content of bile in one study (Sarles et al 1971) but not

Table 34.6 Ways in which eating habits could promote gallstones and the strength of the evidence that they do so

Eating habit	Mechanism	Strength of evidence
Prolonged overnight fast/missing breakfast	Gallbladder stasis More saturated bile	Only one study
Eating 'too much'	Energy imbalance leading to obesity	Good for obesity Lacking for energy measurements
High intake of extrinsic sugars	Energy imbalance Amplifying insulin secretion	Moderate
Low fibre intake	Increased formation, absorption of deoxycholate	Good experimentally, weak epidemiologically
High cholesterol intake	Increased cholesterol absorption, secretion	Weak

in another (Werner et al 1984). In the best case–control study, high energy intake was associated with gallstones in women up to 49 years, but not in older women or in men (Scragg et al 1984a). All these studies used crude methods for assessing energy intake and none assessed energy output. It is possible that energy imbalance is a factor in men and women of all ages, but is due sometimes not to high energy intake but to low energy output, owing to physical inactivity or a thrifty genotype.

Extrinsic sugars and highly digestible starch

'Extrinsic' is the term recommended for sugars which have been extracted from their natural cellular matrix (Panel on Dietary Sugars 1989), otherwise known as added or refined sugars. They are often, and plausibly, blamed as promoting obesity and to the extent that they do this they must promote gallstones indirectly. Three case-control studies have specifically addressed the question whether people with gallstones eat excess extrinsic sugars. Two found they did and one did not (Scragg et al 1984a, Alessandrini et al 1982, Pixley & Mann 1988). Two further studies looked at table sugar consumption (Attili et al 1984, 1987). In one there was no difference and, in the other, people with gallstones ate less sugar. So the situation remains unclear with respect to epidemiological evidence for a role for sugars.

Experimentally, adding 100 g of sugars to the daily diet of people with gallstones raised their fasting plasma triglycerides (Werner et al 1984). This, together with the strong triglyceride–gallstones link, adds credence to the idea that sugars promote gallstones. So too do the facts that adding sugars to a meal enhances the plasma insulin response to that meal (Mazzaferri et al 1984) and that a high intake of sugars induces fasting hyperinsulinaemia in about 20% of healthy people (Reiser et al 1981).

If hyperinsulinaemia does indeed promote gallstones, then other rapidly digested carbohydrates such as the starch in finely ground flour and in cooked potatoes may be as important as sugar, or more so. In line with this idea, women with gallstones in Athens have been found to consume potatoes and cereal products more often than controls (Pastides et al 1990).

Dietary fibre (plant cell wall material)

The dietary fibre deficiency hypothesis for gallstones has achieved a certain currency because a plausible mechanism exists, via enhanced deoxycholate (DCA) absorption, and because it is consistent with animal models, in which stone-causing diets have generally been depleted of fibre (Heaton 1984). According to this hypothesis, lack of cell-wall material in ileal effluent entering the colon enhances DCA absorption in one or more ways:

1. Less carbohydrate (polysaccharide) is available for fermentation to short-chain fatty acids, so pH in the caecum rises and the bacterial enzymes forming DCA are more active.
2. Less particulate material is available to which DCA can bind hydrophobically, so more DCA is available for absorption.
3. The contents of the colon are less bulky and so are transported towards the anus more slowly, allowing more time for DCA to be absorbed.

Whatever the truth of these ideas, there is good evidence that adding wheat bran to a western diet reduces the DCA content of bile and makes it less saturated with cholesterol, at least, if it is initially supersaturated (Heaton 1987). Another reason for incriminating low dietary fibre is the connection between gallstones and slow intestinal transit (see above).

However, epidemiological evidence for a low intake of dietary fibre as a causative factor is lacking. Case–control studies are generally negative (Scragg et al 1984a, Pixley & Mann 1988, Jørgensen & Jørgensen 1989). Only one case–control study has included measurement of cereal fibre intake and it showed no difference (Alessandrini et al 1982). Further evidence against cereal fibre having an important role is the fact that adding bran to the diet of people whose gallstones had been dissolved medically did not prevent their stones from reforming (Hood et al 1988).

Unexpectedly, the evidence that vegetable fibre, or at least high vegetable intake, has a protective role is better. Three case–control studies which have attempted to measure vegetable intake have found it to be low in cases of gallstones (Alessandrini et al 1982, Attili et al 1987, Pastides et al 1990), as has a large prospective study (MacLure et al 1990). Only one study has been negative and that was a small one subject to type-2 error (Attili et al 1984).

There is some suggestion of a particular protective effect from beans (MacLure et al 1990, Thijs & Knipschild 1990), which is paradoxical because Mexicans, who eat a lot of beans, are particularly prone to gallstones, at least when they migrate to Texas (Diehl 1991). If vegetables and beans are protective their mode of action is obscure. A high intake of beans has been shown to *increase* the cholesterol saturation of bile (Nervi et al 1989).

Cholesterol

There is little evidence that a high intake of cholesterol promotes gallstones in man (Scragg 1986). In laboratory animals such as hamsters and prairie dogs it is easy to induce gallstones by feeding cholesterol, but these are not to be regarded as sensible models of the human disease. The animals in question develop severe hypercholesterolaemia (Heaton 1984), whereas in the human disease the plasma cholesterol level tends, if anything, to be lower than normal (Thijs et al 1990).

Alcohol

There is reasonably good evidence from case–control studies that drinking alcohol protects against gallstones (Scragg et al 1984a, Pastides et al 1990). A large prospective study in women showed a dose-related decrease in the risk of gallstones as alcohol intake increased, but as little as 5 g alcohol daily reduced the risk by 40% (MacLure et al 1989). The mechanism is probably via reduced secretion of cholesterol since, in an experiment, drinking half a bottle of white wine daily reduced the cholesterol saturation of bile (Thornton et al 1983).

Summary and conclusions

There is clear evidence that obesity promotes gallstones: in younger women it is the dominant factor. In men, and possibly women, it is abdominal fat distribution which matters. Obesity may operate through insulin resistance and hyperinsulinaemia. Evidence for specific eating habits or dietary components causing gallstones is inconclusive. However, there are some grounds for incriminating extrinsic sugars and rapidly digestible starch, again perhaps operating via hyperinsulinaemia. A low intake of dietary fibre 'ought' to be a cause of gallstones because of the links between the bacterially derived bile salt deoxycholate and gallstones, and between slow intestinal transit and the disease. However, epidemiological evidence is contradictory. Drinking alcohol in moderation is protective. A lifestyle which is healthy for other reasons is probably good for the gallbladder.

REFERENCES

Acalovschi M, Dumitrascu D, Caluser I, Ban A 1987 Comparative prevalence of gallstone disease at 100-year interval in a large Romanian town: a necropsy study. Digestive Diseases and Sciences 32: 354–357

Alessandrini A, Fusco MA, Gatti E, Rossi P A 1982 Dietary fibre and cholesterol gallstones: a case-control study. Italian Journal of Gastroenterology 14: 156–158

Alpers DH, Clouse RE, Stenson WF 1983 Manual of nutritional therapeutics. Little Brown, Boston

Alvaro D, Angelico F, Attili AF et al 1986 Plasma lipid lipoproteins and biliary lipid composition in female gallstone patients. Biomedica Biochemica Acta 45: 761–768

Attili AF and the GREPCO group 1984 Dietary habits and cholelithiasis. In: Capocaccia L, Ricci G, Angelico F et al (eds) Epidemiology and prevention of gallstone disease. MTP Press, Lancaster, pp 175–181

Attili AF and the Rome Group for the Epidemiology and Prevention of Cholelithiasis (GREPCO) 1987 Diet and gallstones: results of an epidemiologic study performed in male civil servants. In: Barbara L, Bianchi Porro G, Cheli R, Lipkin M (eds) Nutrition in gastrointestinal disease. Raven Press, New York, pp 225–231

Baker H, Frank O, Ziffer H et al 1964 Effects of hepatic disease on vitamin B complex vitamin titres. American Journal of Clinical Nutrition 14: 1–6

Baker H, Frank O, Sorrell MF 1976 Nicotinic acid and alcoholism. Bibliotheca Nutritio et Diet 24: 32–39

Baldwin RL, Smith NE 1974 Molecular control of energy metabolism. In: Sink JD (ed) The control of metabolism. Pennsylvania State University Press, University Park, pp 17–30

Bennett AE, Wahner HW, Riggs BL, Hintz RL 1984 Insulin-like growth factors I and II: aging and bone density in women. Journal of Clinical Endocrinology and Metabolism 59: 701–704

Bennion LJ, Grundy SM 1977 Effects of diabetes mellitus on cholesterol metabolism in man. New England Journal of Medicine 296: 1365–1371

Bikle DD, Halloran BP, Gee E et al 1986 Free 25-hydroxyvitamin D levels are normal in subjects with liver disease and reduced total 25–hydroxyvitamin D levels. Journal of Clinical Investigation 78: 748–752

Blanchard RA, Furie BC, Jorgensen MJ et al 1981 Acquired vitamin K-dependent carboxylation deficiency in liver disease. New England Journal of Medicine 305: 242–248

Bloch HM, Thornton JR, Heaton KW 1980 Effects of fasting on the composition of gallbladder bile. Gut 21: 1087–1089

Bouillon R, Auwerx J, Dekeyser L et al 1984 Serum vitamin D metabolites and their binding protein in patients with liver disease. Journal of Clinical Endocrinology and Metabolism 59: 86–89

Camilo ME, Morgan MY, Sherlock S 1981 Erythrocyte transketolase activity in alcoholic liver disease. Scandinavian Journal of Gastroenterology 16: 273–279

Capron JP, Delamarre J, Herve MA et al 1981 Meal frequency and duration of overnight fast: a role in gallstone formation? British Medical Journal 283: 1435

Chait A, Bierman EL, Albers JJ 1979 Low-density lipoprotein receptor activity in cultured human skin fibroblasts – mechanisms of insulin-induced stimulation. Journal of Clinical Investigation 64: 1309–1319

Chopra IL, Chopra U, Smith SR et al 1975 Reciprocal changes in serum concentrations of 3,3',5-triiodothyronine (reverse T_3) and 3',3,5-triiodothyronine (T_3) in systemic illness. Journal of Clinical Endocrinology and Metabolism 41: 1043–1049

Cohen RD 1976 Disorders of lactate metabolism. Journal of Clinical Endocrinology and Metabolism 5: 613–625

Compston JE 1986 Hepatic osteodystrophy: vitamin D metabolism in patients with liver disease. Gut 27:1073–1090

Compston JE, Horton LWL, Thompson RPH 1978 Treatment of osteomalacia associated with primary biliary cirrhosis with parenteral vitamin D_2 or oral 25-hydroxyvitamin D_3. Gut 20: 133–136

Connor H, Woods HF, Murray JD, Ledingham JG 1982 The utilisation of L(+) lactate in patients with liver disease. Annals of Nutrition and Metabolism 26: 308–314

Davies M, Mawer EB, Klass HA et al 1983 Vitamin D deficiency, osteomalacia and primary biliary cirrhosis. Digestive Diseases Science 28: 145–153

Dibble JB, Sheridan P, Hampshire R et al 1981 Evidence for secondary hyperparathyroidism in the osteomalacia associated with chronic liver disease. Clinical Endocrinology 15: 373–383

Diehl AK 1991 Epidemiology and natural history of gallstone disease. Gastroenterologic Clinics of North America 20: 1–20

Doherty F, Golden MHN, Brooks SEH 1991 Peroxisomes and the fatty liver of kwashiorkor – an hypothesis. American Journal of Clinical Nutrition 54: 674–677

Eijhner ER, Hillman RS 1971 The evolution of anaemia in alcoholic patients. American Journal of Medicine 50: 218–232

Epstein M 1992 The kidney in liver disease. Elsevier, New York, pp 35–53

Frank O, Luisada-Opper A, Sorrell MF et al 1971 Vitamin deficits in severe alcohol fatty liver of man calculated from multiple reference points. Experimental and Molecular Pathology 15: 191–197

Golden MHN, Ramdath DD 1987 Free radicals in the pathogenesis of kwashiorkor. Proceedings of the Nutrition Society 46: 53–68

Goldfischer S 1979 Peroxisomes in disease. Journal of Histochemistry and Cytochemistry 27: 1371–1373

Goodman DS 1984 Plasma retinol binding protein. In: Sporn MB, Roberts AB, Goodman DS (eds) The retinoids, Vol 2. Academic Press, New York, pp 41–88

Gordon GG, Olivo J, Rafii F, Southern L 1975 Conversion of androgens to estrogens in cirrhosis of the liver. Journal of Clinical Endocrinology and Metabolism 40: 1018–1026

Goya N, Miyazaki S, Kodate S, Ushio B 1972 A family of congenital atransferrinemia. Blood 40: 239–245

Greco AV, Crucitti F, Ghirlanda G et al 1987 Insulin and glucagon concentrations in portal and peripheral veins in hepatic cirrhosis. Diabetologia 17: 23–28

Grossman ME, Bickers DR, Poh-Fitzpatrick MB et al 1979 Porphyria cutania tarda: clinical features and laboratory findings in 40 patients. American Journal of Medicine 67: 277–286

Hartz AJ, Rupley DC, Rimm AA 1984. The association of girth measurements with disease in 32 856 women. American Journal of Epidemiology 119: 71–80

Heaton KW 1984 The role of diet in the aetiology of cholelithiasis. Reviews in Clinical Nutrition 54: 549–560

Heaton KW 1987 Effect of dietary fiber on biliary lipids. In: Barbara L, Bianchi Porro G, Cheli R, Lipkin M (eds) Nutrition in gastrointestinal disease. Raven Press, New York, pp 213–222

Heaton KW, Braddon FEM, Mountford RA et al 1991a Symptomatic and silent gallstones in the community. Gut 32: 316–320

Heaton KW, Braddon FEM, Emmett PM et al 1991b Why do men get gallstones? Roles of abdominal fat and hyperinsulinaemia. European Journal of Gastroenterology and Hepatology 3: 745–751

Heaton KW, Emmett PM, Symes CL et al 1991c Gallstones in people who are not obese may be explained by slow colonic transit. Gut 32: A1210

Henderson JM, Codner MA, Hollins B et al 1986 The fasting B_6 vitamin profile and response to a pyridoxin load in normal and cirrhotic subjects. Hepatology 6: 464–471

Hepner GW, Roginsky M, Moo HF 1976 Abnormal vitamin D metabolism in patients with cirrhosis. Digestive Diseases 21: 527–532

Hood K, Gleeson D, Ruppin D, Dowling H 1988 Can gallstone recurrence be prevented? The British/Belgian post–dissolution trial. Gastroenterology 94: A548

Hoogendoorn D 1988 Opmerkelijke verschuivingen in het epidemiologische patroon van galsteenziekte en van kanker van de galblaas. Nederlandische Tijdschrift Geneeskunde 27: 1243–1248

Houmard JA, Wheeler WS, McCammon MR et al 1991 Effects of fitness level and the regional distribution of fat on carbohydrate metabolism and plasma lipids in middle- to older-aged men. Metabolism 40: 714–719

Jakobivits AW, Morgan MY, Sherlock S 1979 Hepatic siderosis in alcoholics. Digestive Diseases Science 24: 305–310

Jensen KH, Jørgensen T 1991 Incidence of gallstones in a Danish population. Gastroenterology 100: 790–794

Jørgensen T 1988 Gallstones in a Danish population: familial occurrence and social factors. Journal of Biosocial Science 20: 111–120

Jørgensen T, Jørgensen LM 1989 Gallstones and diet in a Danish population. Scandinavian Journal of Gastroenterology 24: 821–826

Jung RT, Davie M, Siklos P et al 1979 Vitamin D metabolism in acute and chronic cholestasis. Gut 20: 840–847

Kajiyama G, Oyamada K, Nakao S, Miyoshi A 1981 The effect of diabetes mellitus and its treatment on the lithogenicity of bile in man. Hiroshima Journal of Medical Sciences 30: 221–227

Kaplan MM 1987 Primary biliary cirrhosis. New England Journal of Medicine 316: 521–528

Kaplan MM, Goldberg MJ, Matloff DS et al 1981 Effect of 25-hydroxyvitamin D_3 on vitamin D metabolites in primary biliary cirrhosis. Gastroenterology 81: 681–685

Kesäniemi YA, Koskenvuo M, Vuoristo M, Miettinen TA 1989 Biliary lipid composition in monozygotic and dizygotic pairs of twins. Gut 30: 1750–1756

Kooh SW, Jones G, Reilly BJ 1979 Pathogenesis of rickets in chronic hepatobiliary disease in children. Journal of Pediatrics 94: 870–874

Krawitt E, Grundman MJ, Mawer EB 1977 Absorption, hydroxylation and excretion of vitamin D_3 in primary biliary cirrhosis. Lancet 2: 1246–1249

Laakso M, Pyörälä K, Voutilainen E, Marniemi J 1987
Plasma insulin and serum lipids and lipoproteins in
middle-aged non-insulin-dependent diabetic and non-
diabetic subjects. American Journal of Epidemiology 125:
611–621

Lakshmanan MR, Hepokroeff CM, Ness GC et al 1973.
Stimulation by insulin of rat liver hydroxymethylglutaryl
coenzyme A reductase and cholesterol-synthesizing
activities. Biochemical and Biophysical Research
Communications 50: 704–710

La Vecchia C, Negri E, D'Avanzo B et al 1991 Risk factors
for gallstone disease requiring surgery. International
Journal of Epidemiology 20: 209–215

Lee SS, Wasiljew BK, Lee MJ 1987 Gallstones in women
younger than thirty. Journal of Clinical Gastroenterology
9: 65–69

Leevy CM, Thompson A, Baker H 1970 Vitamins and liver
injury. American Journal of Clinical Nutrition 23: 493–499

Lieberman FL, Denison EK, Reynolds TB 1970 The
relation of plasma volume, portal hypertension, ascites
and renal sodium retention in cirrhosis: the overflow
theory of ascites formation. Annals of the New York
Academy of Science 170: 202–212

Linnell J 1975 The fate of cobalamins in vivo. In: Babior
BM (ed) Cobalamin biochemistry and pathophysiology.
Wiley, New York, pp 287–333

Lipschitz DA, Bothwell TH, Seftel HC et al 1971 The role
of ascorbic acid in the metabolism of storage iron. British
Journal of Haematology 20: 155–163

Lowdell CP, Murray-Lyon IM 1985 Reversal of liver
damage due to long-term methyltestosterone and safety of
non-17α-alkylated androgens. British Medical Journal
291: 637

Lynch SR, Seftel HC, Torrance JD et al 1967 Accelerated
oxidative catabolism of ascorbic acid in siderotic Bantu.
American Journal of Clinical Nutrition 20: 641–647

MacLure KM, Hayes KC, Colditz GA et al 1989 Weight,
diet and the risk of symptomatic gallstones in middle-
aged women. New England Journal of Medicine 321:
563–569

MacLure KM, Hayes KC, Colditz GA et al 1990 Dietary
predictors of symptom-associated gallstones in middle-
aged women. American Journal of Clinical Nutrition 52:
916–922

Malagelada JR, Pihl O, Linscheer WG 1974 Impaired
absorption of micellar long-chain fatty acid in patients
with alcoholic cirrhosis. American Journal of Digestive
Diseases 19: 1016–1020

Marco J, Diego J, Villaneuva ML et al 1973 Elevated plasma
glucagon levels in cirrhosis of the liver. New England
Journal of Medicine 289: 1107–1111

Marcus SN, Heaton KW 1986 Intestinal transit, deoxycholic
acid and the cholesterol saturation of bile – three
interrelated factors. Gut 27: 550–558

Marcus SN, Heaton KW 1988 Deoxycholic acid and the
pathogenesis of gallstones. Gut 29: 522–533

Martin KJ, Hruska KA, Freitag JJ et al 1979 The peripheral
metabolism of parathyroid hormone. New England
Journal of Medicine 301: 1092–1098

Mazzaferri EL, Starich GH, St Jeor ST 1984 Augmented
gastric inhibitory polypeptide and insulin response to a
meal after an increase in carbohydrate (sucrose) intake.
Journal of Clinical Endocrinology and Metabolism 58:
640–645

Mobarhan SA, Russell RM, Recker RR et al 1984 Metabolic
bone disease in alcoholic cirrhosis: a comparison of the
effect of vitamin D_2, 25-hydroxy vitamin D or supportive
treatment. Hepatology 4: 266–273

Mookerjea S, Hawkins WW 1960 Some anabolic aspects of
protein metabolism in riboflavin deficiency in the rat.
British Journal of Nutrition 14: 231–238

Mulhausen R, Eichenholz A, Blumentals A 1967 Acid–base
disturbances in patients with cirrhosis of the liver.
Medicine 46: 185–189

Nagase M, Tanimura H, Setoyama M, Hikasa V 1978
Present features of gallstones in Japan. A collective review
of 2144 cases. American Journal of Surgery 135: 788–790

Nervi F, Covarrubias C, Bravo P et al 1989 Influence of
legume intake on biliary lipids and cholesterol saturation
in young Chilean men. Identification of a dietary risk
factor for cholesterol gallstone formation in a highly
prevalent area. Gastroenterology 96: 825–830

Nomura S, Pittman CS, Cambers JB et al 1975 Reduced
peripheral conversion of thyroxine to triiodothyronine in
patients with hepatic cirrhosis. Journal of Clinical
Investigation 56: 643–652

Panerai AE, Salemo P, Menneschi M et al 1977 Growth
hormone and prolactin responses to thyrotrophin-
releasing hormone in patients with severe liver disease.
Journal of Clinical Endocrinology and Metabolism 45:
134–140

Panel on Dietary Sugars 1989 Dietary sugars and human
disease. DHSS Special Report No. 37. HMSO, London

Pastides H, Tzonou A, Trichopoulos D et al 1990 A case-
control study of the relationship between smoking, diet
and gallbladder disease. Archives of Internal Medicine
150: 1409–1412

Paumgartner G, Sauerbruch T 1991 Gallstones:
pathogenesis. Lancet 338: 1117–1121

Pfeifer U, Sandhage K 1979 Licht- und elektronen-
mikroskopische laberbefende beim cerebo-hepato-ranalen
syndrom nach Zellweger (peroxisomendefizienz). Virchow
Archiv [Pathologie und Anatomie] 384: 269–284

Pixley F, Mann J 1988 Dietary factors in the aetiology of
gallstones: a case control study. Gut 29: 1511–1515

Pixley F, Wilson D, McPherson K, Mann J 1985 Effect of
vegetarianism on development of gall stones in women.
British Medical Journal 291: 11–12

Razay G, Heaton KW, Bolton CH, Hughes AO 1992
Alcohol consumption and its relationship to
cardiovascular risk factors in British women. British
Medical Journal 304: 80–83

Reiser S, Bohn E, Hallfrisch J et al 1981 Serum insulin and
glucose in hyperinsulinemic subjects fed three different
levels of sucrose. American Journal of Clinical Nutrition
34: 2348–2358

Retief FP, Huskisson YJ 1969 Serum and urinary folate in
liver disease. British Medical Journal 2: 150–153

Rosenthal WS, Adham NF, Lopez R, Cooperman JM 1973
Riboflavin deficiency in complicated chronic alcoholism.
American Journal of Clinical Nutrition 26: 858–860

Sampliner RE, Bennett PH, Comess LJ et al 1970
Gallbladder disease in Pima Indians. Demonstration of
high prevalence and early onset by cholecystography. New
England Journal of Medicine 283: 1358–1364

Sarles H, Chabert C, Pommeau Y et al 1969 Diet and
cholesterol gallstones. American Journal of Digestive
Diseases 14: 531–537

Sarles H, Crotte C, Gerolami A et al 1971 The influence of calorie intake and of dietary protein on the bile lipids. Scandinavian Journal of Gastroenterology 6: 189–191

Scragg RKR 1986 Aetiology of cholesterol gallstones. In: Bateson MC (ed) Gallstone disease and its management. MTP Press, Lancaster, pp 25–55

Scragg RKR, McMichael AJ, Baghurst PA 1984a Diet, alcohol and relative weight in gallstone disease: a case-control study. British Medical Journal 288: 1113–1119

Scragg RKR, Calvert GD, Oliver JR 1984b Plasma lipids and insulin in gallstone disease: a case-control study. British Medical Journal 289: 521–525

Sheridan P, Chapman C, Losowsky MS 1978 Interpretation of laboratory tests of thyroid function in chronic active hepatitis. Clinica Chimica Acta 86: 73–80

Sonnenberg A, Lilienfeld-Toal HV, Sonnenberg GE et al 1977 Serum 25-hydroxy vitamin D_3 levels in patients with liver disease. Acta Hepato-Gastroenterologica 24: 256–258

Spannuth CL, Mitchell D, Stone J et al 1978 Vitamin B_6 nutriture in patients with uremia and liver disease. In: Human vitamin B_6 requirements. National Academy of Sciences, Washington, pp 180–192

Spirer Z, Heiman I, Shorr S et al 1973 Rickets and protracted neonatal obstructive jaundice. Helvetica Paediatrica Acta 28: 437–442

Stanko RT, Medelow H, Shinozuka H, Adibi SA 1978 Prevention of alcohol-induced fatty liver by natural metabolites and riboflavin. Journal of Laboratory and Clinical Medicine 91: 228–235

Sugioka S, Porta EA, Corey PN, Hartroft WS 1969 The liver of rats fed riboflavin at two levels of protein. American Journal of Pathology 54: 1–19

Taylor AL, Lipman RL, Salman A, Mintz DH 1972 Hepatic clearance of human growth hormone. Journal of Clinical Endocrinology 34: 395–399

Teilum D 1990 Prevalence of gallstones at autopsy at the Institutes of Forensic Medicine in Aarhus and Copenhagen, Denmark, in 1944–1985. Scandinavian Journal of Gastroenterology 25: 901–904

Thijs C, Knipschild P 1990 Legume intake and gallstone risk: results from a case-control study. International Journal of Epidemiology 19: 660–663

Thijs C, Knipschild P, Brombacher P 1990 Serum lipids and gallstones; a case-control study. Gastroenterology 99: 843–849

Thornton J, Symes C, Heaton K 1983 Moderate alcohol intake reduces bile cholesterol saturation and raises HDL cholesterol. Lancet 2: 819–822

Vaamonde CA 1983 Renal water handling in liver disease. In: Epstein M (ed) The kidney in liver disease, 2nd edn. Elsevier, New York, pp 55–86

Van Thiel DH, Gavaler JS, Lester R et al 1975 Plasma estrone, prolactin, neurophysin and sex steroid-binding globulin in chronic alcoholic men. Metabolism 24: 1015–1019

Van Thiel DH, Gavaler JS, Spero JA et al 1981 Patterns of hypothalamic–pituitary–gonadal dysfunction in men with liver disease due to differing etiologies. Hepatology 1: 39–46

Verrillo A, de Teresa A, Martino C et al 1986 Circulating somatostatin concentrations in healthy and cirrhotic subjects. Metabolism 35: 130–135

Wagonfeld JB, Nemchausky BA, Bolt M et al 1976 Comparison of vitamin D and 25-hydroxy vitamin D in primary biliary cirrhosis. Lancet 2: 391–394

Werner D, Emmett PM, Heaton KW 1984 The effects of dietary sucrose on factors influencing cholesterol gallstone formation. Gut 25: 269–274

Whelton MJ, Kehayoglou AK, Agnew JE et al 1971 Calcium absorption in parenchymatous and biliary liver disease. Gut 12: 978–983

Wiss O, Weber F 1964 The liver and vitamins. In: Rouiller CH (ed) The liver: morphology, biochemistry, physiology. Volume 2. Academic Press, New York, pp 145–162

Wu A, Grant DB, Hambley J, Levi AJ 1974 Reduced somatomedin activity in patients with chronic liver disease. Clinical Science 47: 359–366

35. Diabetes

W. P. T. James and D. W. M. Pearson

There are several forms of diabetes (Table 35.1), all characterized by a failure to maintain the concentration of blood glucose within the normal range. The old terms of 'juvenile onset' and 'maturity onset' diabetes have been replaced by 'Type I' and 'Type II' because the age of onset is not the initial determinant of the form of diabetes. A classification of diabetes is presented in Table 35.1. Borderline forms of high blood glucose are now defined by the World Health Organization as 'impaired glucose tolerance' (IGT), formerly known as chemical diabetes: 2–5% of these patients each year progress to have higher glucose levels characteristic of diabetes. IGT is variable with a quarter of the subjects responding normally 5 years later to a further test challenge of 75 g glucose. This oral glucose tolerance test is the standard way of assessing the ability of the pancreas to produce insulin and for the tissues to respond to the circulating insulin. Doctors and dietitians need to recognize that the principles that underlie the management of diabetes have changed markedly in the last 30 years. Therefore there remains a great deal of confusion. This confusion needs to be resolved if a rational and practical programme is to be developed for patients with diabetes mellitus.

TYPE I DIABETES

Type I diabetes mellitus or insulin dependent diabetes mellitus (IDDM) presents with acute symptoms induced by a high blood glucose. Although the clinical symptoms may be present for only days or weeks, the pathophysiological processes which result in Type I diabetes may have been emerging for years. It is recognized that individuals of HLA tissue type DR3 and DR4 have increased susceptibility to diabetes and β cell damage in such individuals may be triggered by environmental causes such as viral infections or chemicals. An ongoing autoimmune process results in β cell failure, and eventually the clinical symptoms of diabetes. Hyperglycaemia develops because the glucose in the blood fails to be taken up into tissues as the blood insulin levels fall. Antibodies to the pancreatic islet β cells, which

Table 35.1 The different forms of diabetes mellitus

Type I: Usually arising in childhood or young adults, associated with pancreatic damage linked to viral infection; autoimmune damage. More likely in those who were bottle- rather than breastfed. Susceptibility linked to specific blood group subtypes, e.g. HLA type DR3 and DR4 on chromosome 6. A condition of insulin deficiency.

Type II: Occurring usually in middle or old age and associated with insulin resistance and a high insulin output insufficient to cope with the demand for effective insulin action. Usually precipitated by weight gain in genetically susceptible subjects. Associated with high secretion of proinsulin (the precursor of insulin secretion) and amylin output.

Type II MODY (maturity onset diabetes of the young) : A subgroup with distinct genetic characteristics presenting with modest diabetes (see text).

Tropical diabetes mellitus: A condition linked to low-grade pancreatitis with pancreatic exocrine duct damage often accompanied by pancreatic calculi. Linked to the long-term effects of malnutrition.

Pancreatic insufficiency: Unusual disorders relating to pancreatic islet cell damage, e.g. from pancreatitis associated with alcoholism or from haemochromatosis. A condition of insulin deficiency.

Hormonal diabetes, e.g. Cushing's disease or in association with corticosteriod therapy which induces insulin resistance; acromegaly or glucagonomas or phaeochromocytomas.

Genetic disease, e.g. receptor abnormalities, glycogen storage disease.

produce insulin, are found in the blood before and for 1–2 years after diagnosis. In 20% of patients antibodies persist and other autoimmune diseases are also found. Some patients who are moderately overweight have autoantibodies but are misclassified as having NIDDM because they can be maintained on a diet and sulphonylureas (see below) for a time before the autoimmune pancreatic damage and insulin dependence signifies their IDDM condition. The classic symptoms of IDDM at presentation are thirst, frequency of micturition and weight loss and can be explained on a biochemical basis. The patients become dehydrated because of the marked water loss as water is excreted with glucose by the kidney once the kidney's threshold for glucose absorption is exceeded. Glucagon secretion is high and insulin output low. These patients may also present with extreme ketosis because of excess acetone, acetoacetate and β-hydroxybutyrate production. This leads to ketogenesis which, when severe, also dehydrates the patient because ketones as organic acids as well as glucose leak into the urine and require water and cations such as potassium to be excreted. The patient may therefore present in a very ill, dehydrated and semi-comotose state with a sweet breath from the volatile acetone being excreted via the lungs. Rehydration, electrolyte replacement and insulin therapy is then required. In clinical practice the diagnosis is usually made before patients become seriously unwell and therapy can commence with subcutaneous insulin and oral fluids. In such patients education with regard to insulin therapy, diet and modification of lifestyle are the major considerations.

TYPE II DIABETES

This condition, also known as non insulin dependent diabetes mellitis (NIDDM), was previously known as maturity onset diabetes and characterized by the development of progressive insulin resistance. About 2–3% of the population has Type II diabetes but the rate is increasing as adults become more overweight and live longer; the prevalence of diabetes rises to 7% in those over 80 years of age and the prevalence of diabetes in a country can be predicted from the proportion of adults who are overweight and particularly in those with a trunkal distribution of fat and a high waist/hip circumference ratio (see Chapter 32). The risk of developing diabetes in adults with a body mass index (BMI) of >30 is five times that of adults with a BMI of <25. Individuals who are physically active, e.g. those who jog, swim, dance or engage in similar exercises for 20 min three times weekly, have only a 40% chance of developing diabetes compared with inactive individuals (Helmrich et al 1991).

The cause of Type II diabetes is unclear, but seems to involve both an impaired pancreatic secretion of insulin and the development of tissue resistance to insulin. The early phase of glucose intolerance, whether in normal weight or obese subjects, is characterized by an abnormal early plasma glucose rise in response to carbohydrate intake: the early secretion of insulin is impaired and glucagon secretion is not suppressed. The rate of endogenous production and release of glucose by the liver therefore continues despite the inflow of dietary glucose. Blood glucose rises excessively and this finally stimulates a prolonged surge in insulin secretion (Mitrakou et al 1992). Those mechanisms in the tissues which respond to higher glucose and insulin levels then seem to adjust so that the usual activation of the insulin receptor by insulin becomes less effective and 'insulin resistance' develops. This insensitivity to insulin's action means that glucose levels in the blood tend to rise further after a meal and this in turn stimulates insulin secretion. As subjects gain weight their insulin resistance increases, so the demand for insulin secretion also increases. Physical activity rapidly improves the sensitivity of tissues to insulin independent of any effect on body weight. With the usual steady decline in physical activity and progressive weight gain with age, insulin resistance usually rises as adults age. There is therefore an ever increasing demand for more insulin. Eventually the pancreatic capacity for insulin output proves inadequate to maintain blood glucose levels at their usual levels, so both fasting blood glucose and postprandial glucose levels increase excessively and diabetes results. The individual is unaware of the problem until he develops blood glucose levels which exceed the kidney's capacity to reabsorb the filtered load in the renal tubules. There is then a spill-over of glucose into the urine. The glucose imposes an osmotic load which leads to high urinary water losses and therefore thirst. Urinary frequency and thirst are therefore early symptoms of diabetes. The person may present with other symptoms such as pruritis vulvae, blurring of vision or symptoms attributable to complications associated with diabetes, e.g. retinopathy, cataract, foot problems and vascular disease. The diagnosis may be made at a screening examination. The presence of complications at diagnosis suggests a prolonged asymptomatic period and health professionals should have a level of awareness of undiagnosed diabetes so that optimal management can be started as soon as possible and thereby reduce the burden of diabetic complications. There is no such condition as 'mild diabetes', asymtomatic patients are at risk of micro- and macrovascular complications and need effective dietetic advice.

The pancreatic capacity for insulin production varies from person to person; this capacity may be reduced in those with low birth weight suggesting an effect of fetal nutrition on early pancreatic cellularity and development (Hales et al 1991). Type II diabetes also has a strong familial element. One genetic basis for individual susceptibility to this disorder is emerging with a subtype of Type II diabetes with autosomal dominant inheritance showing a link to an abnormal glucokinase gene on chromosome 7p (Hattersley et al 1992). This subtype of maturity-onset diabetes of the young (MODY) presents from the second decade and can usually be treated by diet or diet and sulphonylurea tablets. The glucokinase gene is expressed in both the pancreatic β cells and the liver and, since it plays a key role in the regulation of glucose metabolism in these tissues, the glucokinase enzyme has been termed the 'pancreatic glucose sensor'. All MODY is characterized by a subnormal β cell secretion in response to glucose loading as in the other forms of Type II diabetes.

Type II diabetes also involves abnormalities in the secretion of a newly described protein, amylin, from the same pancreatic β cells that secrete insulin. Amylin is a protein of 37 amino acids which is secreted, like insulin, in excess in those with glucose intolerance (Koda et al 1992). It is absent from the plasma in Type I diabetes. Amylin can itself act as a potent stimulus for glycogenolysis and it reduces the peripheral uptake of glucose by muscle. With long-term pancreatic overstimulation, not only does peripheral insulin resistance increase, further exacerbating the diabetes, but the amylin polymerizes and accumulates between the β cells of the pancreas. These amyloid-like collections progressively replace the damaged β cells. This may explain why patients with Type II diabetes deteriorate progressively with time as their pancreatic islet cell damage worsens and the capacity for insulin secretion falls.

CARDIOVASCULAR DISEASE IN DIABETES MELLITUS

Patients with diabetes are particularly likely to develop vascular disease (Table 35.2). This is of two forms — microvascular and macrovascular disease. In microvascular disease there is not only a thickening of

Table 35.2 The causes of death (%) in subjects wth and without diabetes. From Kleinman et al (1988)

	Diabetes		No Diabetes	
	Men	Women	Men	Women
Cardiovascular disease of which	65	57	53	53
Coronary artery disease	46	35	35	28
Diabetes, e.g. coma	7	21		
Other causes	28	22	47	46

the capillary basement membrane but increased capillary permeability which leads to the formation of haemorrhages, the leakage of exudates of fibrin and oedema from the vessel walls; these vessels then become thickened and blocked. In the eye these changes can lead to blindness and in the kidney to renal failure. These microvascular complications seem to be proportional to the degree and duration to which blood glucose has been raised and out of control. Blindness and kidney failure are particular problems in the long-term management of Type I diabetes. Cataracts can also form very rapidly in poorly controlled patients and are thought to reflect the excessive synthesis of the sugar alcohol, sorbitol, produced from glucose by the hexose-6-phosphate pathway within the lens which then becomes damaged. The high blood glucose levels are also considered to promote the development of cataracts because of the diffusion of polyols into the lens.

Macrovascular disease, involving the coronary, cerebral and peripheral arteries as well as the aorta, seems to be a more severe form of the common atherosclerotic disease observed in Western societies (see Chapter 41). The peripheral form of arterial disease is a particular problem, perhaps because of the occlusion of the small vessels supplying the arterial wall itself. The combination of vascular disease and sensory neuropathy results in the dramatically increased susceptibility to serious foot ulceration, infection and ischaemic damage. Table 35.2 shows that the major cause of death in both Types I and II diabetes is cardiovascular disease. This new recognition has led to a very different approach to dietary management.

Basis for accelerated cardiovascular disease in diabetes

The chronically elevated blood glucose levels in diabetes lead to the glycosylation of a great variety of proteins which, if including those of endothelial

Table 35.3 Balancing the diet in diabetes

	Advantages	Disadvantages
Vegetables	Rich in: — Soluble fibre — Insoluble fibre — Antioxidants	
Fruit	Rich in: — Soluble fibre — Antioxidants	High simple sugar content
Fish	Rich in n-3 fatty acids	(? Heavy metal contamination)
Fat	Slows gastric emotying	Promotes thrombosis and atherosclerosis depending on fatty acid
Protein	— Modest glucose stimulating effect — Satiating	— ? Amplifies tendency to deterioration in renal function — In meat or dairy products, often associated with dietary fat, especially saturated fatty acids
Alcohol	Moderate intakes reduce cardiovascular mortality and morbidity	— Induces weight gain — Metabolized in preference to glucose

surfaces and lipoproteins, may induce the scavenger receptor mediated uptake of low density lipoproteins by the macrophages lying on and within the endothelium. These macrophages are now linked to the stimulation of the atherosclerotic process (see Chapter 41).

An additional cause of macrovascular disease may relate to the poor conversion of n-6 and n-3 essential fatty acids to their longer-chain metabolites via the insulin-dependent desaturation step. The prostaglandins, in appropriate balance, are responsible for normal platelet function and the clearance of clots from arterial walls, so increasing attention is now being paid to the possible use of γ-linolenic acid to bypass the desaturation step in the metabolism of linoleic acid (see Chapter 6). In addition, the use of substantial amounts of fish in the diet provides pre-existing n-3 long-chain fatty acids as well as the α-linolenic acid precursor: this higher intake of fish may be important in the long-term management of diabetes. The thrombotic tendency in diabetes will be amplified by a high fat, low carbohydrate diet. Thus the emphasis on controlling carbohydrate intake and allowing a high fat diet, seen in the 1950s and 1960s, may explain why atherosclerosis and cardiovascular diseases have become the principal cause of death in both Type I and Type II diabetes. Free radical and antioxidant mechanisms may also be involved; see Chapter 41.

HISTORICAL ASPECTS OF THE DIETARY MANAGEMENT OF DIABETES

There have been several revolutions in dietary management over the last 30 years but there are continuing dilemmas (Table 35.3). But prescribing the right amount of energy has always been a central issue.

Originally, before insulin was regularly available, starvation therapy was frequently used for Type I diabetes in the hope of keeping the patient alive, but with the discovery of insulin by Banting, Best and Macleod it was possible to give food and control the blood glucose at reasonable levels by choosing the dose and timing for subcutaneous injections of insulin. The problem then was how to meet the patient's energy needs but also prescribe small precise amounts of carbohydrate. Balancing the amount of carbohydrate fed with the insulin given was considered to be the key to controlling the immediate post-prandial rise in blood glucose. This then led to a whole series of tests based on monitoring the response to food and prescribing the correct amount of carbohydrate at different times of the day. Once the amount of dietary carbohydrate had been specified carefully, then enough fat and protein was prescribed to meet the patient's energy needs. This, in practice, led to the use of relatively low carbohydrate, high fat diets. These unfortunately promoted the atherosclerosis and thrombosis to which patients with diabetes are so prone. The emphasis on simplicity also led to a system of carbohydrate exchanges with little regard to the type of carbohydrate used, i.e. a rapidly digested or slowly digested starch. Counting carbohydrate units in the diet was useful for improving short-term control. This management system was then assessed to see whether it helped to minimize the microvascular disease and rapid cataract formation which were known to develop rapidly in patients who were poorly controlled and therefore had high blood glucose levels. Now the emphasis has swung to ensuring control of both glucose and lipid levels so that microvascular and macrovascular disease can be prevented (Table 35.4).

Table 35.4 Different approaches to evaluating diabetic diets

Short term*	Longer term
Glucose responses to a meal	Changes in body weight and compostion
Diurinal glucose responses to meals throughout the day	Blood HbA$_{lc}$ levels for monitoring glycosylated haemoglobin levels
Fasting blood and urinary glucose levels after a special day's feeding	Monitoring blood lipid levels
24-hour urinary glucose output on first day	Repeated tests of retinal permeability or renal function, e.g. creatinine clearance, microalbuminuria

*Each of these options is also used as a testing after feeding the patient a liquid formula or a normal diet over several weeks before testing.

In practice, three approaches to dietary management have evolved based on first assessing energy needs. First, there was a pragmatic attempt to assess a patient's diet which, with many techniques such as 24-hour recall or simple dietary histories administered in the clinic, led to an underestimation of intake. Secondly, the dietary prescription was based on a crude assumption about the patient's energy needs, the figures being taken from tables based on age and sex but without regard to the patient's weight. Thus a crude value was chosen, e.g. 2000 kcal or 1500 kcal, for energy needs but the diet was then adjusted if the patient became too hungry, changed weight or became more difficult to control. Thirdly, with the recognition in 1973 by FAO that approximate energy needs could be expressed for adults simply on a weight basis, a new scheme evolved in the best clinics of prescribing, e.g. 46 kcal/kg for a moderate activity male and 40 kcal/kg for a moderate activity female with subsequent adjustments for individual needs and daily variations in exercise patterns.

EVALUATING THE MOST APPROPRIATE DIETS FOR DIABETES

People with diabetes vary so much that it is not surprising that progress in evaluating the most appropriate diet has been slow and complicated. As well as major differences in insulin resistance, body size and insulin secretion from the pancreas, there are whole variety of different dietary manipulations, e.g. with fish, soluble fibre or special dietary carbohydrates, such as sorbitol, to be tested. All of

these combinations may need to be evaluated in many different ways but the techniques for evaluation also vary: they are either short term, i.e. hours, days or weeks, and relate predominantly to glucose control, or longer term over months or years and relate to the development of microvascular and macrovascular disease (Table 35.4). Interactions between dietary factors also have to be recognized. Thus fat delays gastric emptying so it may itself modify the blood glucose response to a meal. Fat, once absorbed, is also involved in an interplay in the Randle cycle with glucose metabolism (Randle 1986). If patients with diabetes are overfed, then the dietary fat will be preferentially deposited despite a high blood glucose level. As fat depots increase basal lipolysis rises, particularly during insulin insufficiency, and free fatty acids rise to compete as a metabolic fuel with glucose. This further exacerbates the problem of diabetes. Thus weight changes are important and can have a marked effect on diabetic control.

CURRENT METHODS IN THE DIETARY MANAGEMENT OF TYPE I DIABETES MELLITUS (IDDM)

Education is the cornerstone of modern diabetic management and people with diabetes need to be taught the practical skills of insulin administration and blood testing and have the knowledge to deal with different day-to-day situations and activities. The education package must try to promote a healthy lifestyle to minimise the immediate and longer term impact of diabetes on health. Dietary counselling must complement the advice from the other members of the diabetic team and the advice should be tailored to individual needs.

In normal weight individuals the person has to receive daily injections of insulin. The amount of injectable insulin that they require depends on four principal factors:

1. The extent of islet cell damage;
2. The amount of exercise taken;
3. Whether the cellular response to insulin is normal or poor leading to insulin 'resistance';
4. The amount, type, absorption and metabolism of food eaten.

The energy equivalence of the food needs to match the person's energy needs. These are in turn determined by the person's metabolic rate and the level of physical activity (See Chapter 3).

Different types of injectable insulin act over different time scales. Thus a subcutaneous injection of 'soluble' insulin will last for 6–8 hours but have a maximum impact at 2–4 hours (Table 35.5). It should be emphasized that these figures are only guidelines and that there will be considerable individual variability. An insulin regimen should be selected to suit a particular individual's needs.

The immediate aim of dietary management is to ensure that when a dose of insulin is injected, the blood glucose does not fall too fast or too low. In Type I diabetes, soluble insulin is usually given 2–3 times daily, so this means that within 30 min of a subcutaneous injection of insulin the blood glucose level may be falling as the insulin passes around the body. Insulin is therefore usually given 30 min before meals. The brain is dependent on glucose metabolism unless the patient is ketotic with elevated blood ketone levels. Therefore it is important to avoid blood glucose concentrations falling too rapidly and to a low level. Mental impairment occurs in patients when glucose levels fall rapidly even if the absolute level is not particularly low. The varying susceptibility of different patients to hypoglycaemia may reflect adaptive changes in cerebral glucose transporters responsible for controlling the uptake of glucose into the brain. Most subjects have some warning of hypoglycaemia because of the reflex increase in sympathetic nervous system activity with a rise in pulse rate, pallor, sweating, fine muscle tremor and sometimes an acute sense of hunger. Patients with Type I diabetes learn to recognize these symptoms and compensate by taking rapidly absorbed carbohydrate, e.g. dextrose tablets of 3 g dextrose each. Two tablets are usually sufficient for limiting an hypoglycaemia episode. Anxious patients tend to overcompensate and this is a mistake because, by taking a larger dose of carbohydrate, hyperglycaemia develops which may then be misinterpreted as a need for more insulin. Dietary education programmes for people with diabetes and their relatives must include information about the recognition and management of hypoglycaemia. Suitable carbohydrate for immediate ingestion should be carried together with a diabetic identity card. Recognizing the problems of infection, alcohol drinking, delayed meal times and exercise is part of the initial education needed. Legal requirements in relation to driving licences must also be met. Multiple injections of insulin are now popular with a dose of quick-acting, highly purified insulin before each of three meals together with an additional dose of intermediate insulin or long-acting insulin before the evening meal. This system is helped by the availability of portable multi-dose 'pen injectors' for handling the insulin injections.

MANAGEMENT OF TYPE II DIABETES (NIDDM)

The education and management of people with NIDDM depends on their individual needs. The approach will differ for a middle-aged overweight smoker from that for a very elderly subject with IGT. The aim in all patients is to relieve the symptoms of diabetes and to minimise its impact on micro- and macrovascular disease. All patients will need dietary assessment and almost all need to modify their diet.

Table 35.5   Examples of insulin preparations used in the UK

	Species	Purity*	Retarding agent	Action hours		
				Initial	Maximum	Total
Short acting						
Neutral soluble	Beef	3	–	0.5	2–4	6–8
Human Actrapid (Novo)	Human	1	–	0.5	2–4	6–8
Intermediate						
Isophane	Beef	3	Protamine	1.2	5–8	18
Humulin I (Lilly)	Human	1	Protamine	0.5–2	2–8	14–18
Long Acting						
Humulin Zn	Human	3	Protamine + zinc	3	8–12	30–40
Hypurin protamine zunc (Weddell)	Beef	2	Protamine + zinc	3	8–12	30–40
Mixed Preparations						
Human Mixtard (Novo/nordisk) Human1.						

*1 = highly purified; 2 = purified; 3 = conventional.

All will need long-term ongoing education and screening for complications.

Traditionally a sequence of treatment is tried in Type II diabetes. First, dietary methods are used to reduce weight and the intake of quickly absorbed carbohydrates. Diet should also aim to limit the saturated fat intake and thereby the excessive cardiovascular disease characteristic of Type II diabetes. If dietary measures (Table 35.10) fail to control glycaemia after a period of reasonable compliance, drug therapy is prescribed in addition to diet. There are two groups of oral hypoglycaemic drugs. Sulphonylurea therapy is useful in normal weight Type II diabetes but can result in hypoglycaemia if dosage is inappropriate. Biguanide and sulphonylurea drugs can be combined for maximum effect but 30% of patients eventually are transferred to insulin within 4 years of therapy.

This feature may be explained in terms of continuing amylin production in some patients who present with insulin resistance or Type II diabetes but then become dependent on insulin as their pancreatic insulin secretory capacity fails. Whatever the additional treatment, diet is central to management in people with Type II diabetes.

PLANNING DIETS

The planning of a diabetic diet can proceed in five stages (Table 35.6). The energy needs of the patient can be estimated from their sex, age, body weight and general level of physical activity as explained in Chapter 3. The energy needs of children less than 10 years of age are calculated on the basis of moderate activity but in affluent societies many children now spend too much time watching television. Energy needs may therefore, for this group, be 5–10% less than predicted (see Table 3.6). Differences between individual children in their energy requirement are important and can have a range which is about ±25% of the average values shown. A very active child will need 20–30% more than the average needs calculated from Table 3.6: the increased need will become obvious within 48 hours because the child will be hungry and when exercising may become hypoglycaemic. Fasting blood glucose measurements (see below) will also be low, e.g. <4.5 mmol/l, or the child may complain of early morning headaches or have ketones in the urine on waking because of some hypoglycaemia during the night. These features may not develop, however, if the child is on a relatively low carbohydrate, high fat diet; this is dealt with in the next section. Individual adjustments must therefore be made to the prescribed diet based on the child's appetite — this is the best guide to energy needs and will usually automatically set the intake at an appropriate level for the growth and physical activity of the child. The system for predicting intake is therefore a guide to the individual negotiation with a child of how best to manage their diabetes.

ADOLESCENT ENERGY REQUIREMENTS

In those aged 10 years and over energy needs are based on first estimating the basal metabolic rate (BMR) from the equations set out in Table 3.7. These equations relate to the sex and body weight of the adolescent. The BMR value in MJ or kcal per day is then multiplied by the physical activity level (PAL) of the individual which can be judged from a simple

Table 35.6 The sequence used when developing a diabetic diet

1. Estimating the average daily energy need

2. Calculating the absolute intake of carbohydrate

3. Specifying the type of dietary carbohydrate

4. Adjusting the pattern of intake to account for the timing and type of insulin injected, the patient's work schedule, leisure activities and for the diurinal variation in insulin sensitivity

5. Specifying intakes of n-3 fatty acids, vegetables and fruit for metabolic, antioxidant and non-starch polysaccharide (fibre) needs

Table 35.7 Exercise patterns and acute carbohydrate needs in diabetes

Adolescent boy playing 90 min in competitive football using $6 \times$ BMR on average during sport

BMR = in MJ/day for 10–17 year olds
$= 0.074 \times 60$ kg weight $+ 2.754$ MJ

24-hour BMR = 7.2 MJ or 300 kJ/hour

Increment of activity $= 5 \times$ BMR for 1.5 hours $= 2.25$ MJ

Extra carbohydrate use at 35% of energy = 788 kJ
or approximately 49 g carbohydrate

If sport includes repeated anaerobic exercise, perhaps 50% energy needs were met by carbohydrate

Therefore extra acute carbohydrate demand = 70 g

assessment of their activity patterns. Since adolescents go through their pubertal growth spurt at different ages and at different rates it is important to take account of their weight and to adjust to the changing body weight as puberty proceeds. Insulin requirements increase significantly during the rapid growth phase and regular discussion between teenager, dietitian and physician helps to achieve some degree of control at this difficult physiological and emotional time. After the rapid growth phase insulin requirements may reduce and this is a particular feature in teenage girls. If their dosage is not appropriately decreased their insulin-driven appetite can lead to problems of obesity. Dietetic advice needs to take account of peer group pressure and the lifestyle of teenagers. A confrontational approach is unlikely to be successful and may limit future cooperation for other health care professionals. Advice needs to be relevant and should address issues such as smoking, 'junk food', sports and exercise. The actual energy cost of pubertal growth is, however, modest and far outweighed by the cost of sports and general physical activity undertaken particularly by boys. The issue of how to time insulin and dietary carbohydrate to cope with sports is dealt with below.

ADULT ENERGY NEEDS

Table 3.7 sets out the equations, and the principles are dealt with more extensively in Chapter 3. The estimated BMR of the patient is estimated from the age as well as by sex and weight. A suitable multiplier is then chosen corresponding to the patient's estimated PAL. Again this is a preliminary guide but is likely to be much more accurate than the estimation of energy needs from a simple dietary history or 24-hour recall. The adult will make it clear if their energy needs are being exceeded because they will complain of having to eat too much or they will begin to gain weight. Hunger with weight loss will become clear within 3–5 days.

CARBOHYDRATE NEEDS

Ideas on this issue have been transformed in the last 10 years: the older concepts are considered in a separate section dealing with the history of dietetic therapy and the confusion that resulted from early approaches to the problem. It is now recognized that the disposal of absorbed carbohydrate is under immediate metabolic control provided insulin is available, whereas dietary fat is absorbed by different mechanisms, transported

from the intestine via the lymph rather than the portal blood stream and readily deposited in adipose tissue by a pathway involving the non-insulin sensitive enzyme, lipoprotein lipase. Thus feeding a high fat diet to a patient with diabetes not only bypasses the fine control of metabolism by insulin, but readily leads to fat storage and other unfortunate side effects on lipoprotein metabolism and cardiovascular diseases. Since these diseases are the commonest complication leading to premature death in both Type I and Type II diabetes, it is clearly vital to ensure that the amount as well as the type of fat eaten is controlled (see below). Therefore current advice to patients with diabetes is to have 50–55% of dietary energy as carbohydrate in a diabetic so that total dietary fat is limited to 30–35% of energy. This high carbohydrate diet allows carbohydrate balance to be linked more readily with energy balance and insulin needs.

The conversion of the 55% value of carbohydrate energy needs to absolute carbohydrate allowances in grams per day is simple since 16 kJ/g (4 kcal/g) is the conversion factor used. This conversion can also be put in diagrammatic form (Lean & James 1986).

TYPE OF CARBOHYDRATE

Carbohydrates are absorbed at very different speeds and so have very different effects on the blood glucose response to a meal. There is now increasing interest in establishing what effect the carbohydrate from a particular food has on the blood glucose response. The smaller the response the more favourable the food is considered to be. The response is expressed as a glycaemic index, i.e. the increase in blood glucose after a 50 g load of the food compared with the increase seen after a bolus of 50 g glucose. The two areas under the response curves are compared, with the response of the test food being expressed as a percentage of the standard glucose value. Table 35.8 gives a few examples of the glycaemic response of different foods.

A dose of pure glucose is absorbed very rapidly in the fasting state with a clear rise in blood glucose occuring within 5 min. Another monosaccharide, galactose, is absorbed quickly but then has to be transformed into glucose within the liver before glucose levels rise. Fructose, however, is absorbed more slowly, is metabolized via an insulin independent pathway to acetyl CoA and therefore can be used as a fuel in many tissues without producing a rise in blood glucose and without needing insulin for its transport into tissues. This has led to the popularity in Europe of fructose-containing

Table 35.8 The glycaemic response of different foods expressed as a glycaemic index, i.e. as a percentage of the response to an equivalent (50 g) weight of pure glucose in solution

Fruit–derived foods	
Apple	39
Bananas	62
Orange juice	46
Pulses	
Lentils	29
Kidney beans	29
Haricot beans	31
Soya beans	15
Cereals	
White bread	69
Wholemeal bread	72
Oatmeal biscuits	54
Ryvita	69
Cornflakes	80
Porridge oats	49
All Bran	51

foods for diabetes management, because it is then possible to meet the energy requirements of patients without rapid fluctuations in blood glucose or an increase in insulin requirements. Its use can, however, increase plasma triglycerides. Disaccharides are usually absorbed as rapidly as glucose but their effects on blood glucose depend on the metabolic route of the different constituent sugars. Thus sucrose, the disaccharide of glucose and fructose, provides half its energy in the form of fructose. Glucose syrups, manufactured by hydrolysing starches such as maize starch, are polymers of glucose which are being introduced into foods because they are sweet and relatively non-cariogenic. In the management of diabetes, however, they can be considered as simple refined sugars which are rapidly absorbed into the circulating pool of glucose. The glucose from starchy foods tends to be absorbed more slowly, but Table 35.8 shows that there are marked variations between different starches. In general fruits, such as apples, contain their sugars and starch encased within the physical structure of the plant cell wall and this seems to determine the speed with which the carbohydrate can be digested and absorbed. Some foods, such as bananas, vary substantially in the nature of their carbohydrate content. Thus the starch in green bananas is almost totally unavailable to digestion and passes into the colon where it is fermented to produce acetate, propionate and butyrate as well as gas. Only

absorbed propionate is glucogenic, so the glycaemic response to green bananas is very low. In an over-ripe banana, however, the starches have been converted to sucrose, or even fructose and glucose, and these are not only sweet but rapidly absorbed leading to a high glycaemic value. Thus the glycaemic index may vary with the ripeness of the fruit.

Cereals have a lower glycaemic index, probably because their starches are less readily hydrolysed by the intestine's digestive enzymes. The complex structure of starches is also affected by all their closely associated non-starch polysaccharides (NSP). Thus the pectins, galactomannans and other hemicelluloses in the soluble NSP fractions found in fruit, vegetables, cereals and pulses restrict starch hydrolysis as well as producing gels in the intestine which retard the diffusion of glucose to the intestinal wall and therefore reduce the glycaemic index further. The soluble NSPs in pulses seem particularly effective in slowing glucose uptake, so pulses are a useful source of slowly absorbed glucose. The different glycaemic values of different types of food therefore need to be remembered when trying to organize the meal and insulin schedule. A readily absorbed carbohydrate is appropriate if soluble insulin is being injected before breakfast, but the snack taken 2 hours after breakfast would best have a low glycaemic index to allow the buffering of the longer-term effect of the soluble insulin.

PATTERN OF EATING

Patients with Type I diabetes in the first few months of their illness have some residual pancreatic function, but as islet damage progresses they should be assumed to have no control over their tissue glucose uptake other than by the use of insulin injections. It is therefore clear that the current trend in the Western world to eat one large meal a day is quite inappropriate for a patient with diabetes. A standard approach of devising three meals plus three snacks a day has now evolved to try to reduce the daily fluctuations in blood glucose. If soluble insulin is injected first in the morning, then breakfast is needed 30 minutes later. A small breakfast, for example of cereals with low fat milk and some fruit is suitable. Within 2 hours, however, the surge in absorbed glucose will be slowing but the soluble insulin will be entering the blood stream at a high rate from its injected subcutaneous site. Therefore a further mid-morning snack, e.g. wholemeal bread sandwiches with a tuna fish filling low in fat, is appropriate if the patient's energy needs are substantial. Following this pattern two further doses of soluble insulin may be injected with two more meals plus snacks to match the time of action of insulin. Nocturnal hypoglycaemia is a well recognised problem with many insulin regimens and a suitable bed-time snack may help.

Physical activity

The doses of insulin and the amount of food may then need to be adjusted in anticipation of exercise. Exercise promotes glucose uptake into muscle even with only modest levels of circulating insulin. This adjustment is usually based on individual clinical experience of whether the child or adult becomes hypoglycaemic when exercising: patients soon recognize the importance of taking small carbohydrate snacks with them to the sport's field to avoid a sudden hypoglycaemic episode. It is recommended that extra carbohydrate be taken in anticipation of the exercise. The energy cost of the exercise can be estimated from Tables, e.g. Annex 3, Department of Health (1991), with about 35% of the energy used being derived from carbohydrate (Ahlborg et al 1974). Thus a boy engaged in a game of football may, over a 90-min match, play at an average of $6 \times BMR$. For a 60 kg boy this amounts to 788 kJ extra of which about 49 g will be carbohydrate (Table 35.7). The type of carbohydrate supplement can be varied depending on the type and time of exercise, e.g. with an aerobic class in the evening, the extra before, to avoid hypos during the class, and the extra after, to avoid hypos during the night.

Adjustments to the dose of insulin used or to dietary carbohydrate can also be made in the light of experience with multiple measures of blood glucose taken at intervals throughout the day. This is increasingly seen as part of the normal assessment of the effectiveness of diabetic control; the effect of a day's physical activity can then be monitored as part of the scheme for adjusting diets and insulin therapy.

There is a recognized diurnal variation in the body's sensitivity to insulin for reasons that are not very clear. Two to 3 hours before waking insulin resistance rises so that blood glucose rises around dawn. There is a recognized diurnal variation in the body's sensitivity to insulin for reasons that are not very clear. Other physiological or pathological processes, such as infections of other intercurrent illness may influence insulin requirement. It is important that insulin dosage is tailored to individual needs and people with diabetes understand the factors which can affect blood glucose control.

Meal frequency

Ellis (1934) showed that, in insulin-dependent diabetics, nourishment taken as hourly doses of 10–30 g of glucose (day and night), matched by frequent small doses of insulin, decreased the 24-hour insulin requirements. This is clearly a very artificial regimen. In normal subjects, Gwinup et al (1963) also showed an improvement in oral glucose tolerance on the morning after 10 meals had been taken the previous day (from 8.00 am to 8.00 pm) compared with an isocaloric intake via three meals. Increasing meal frequency also reduces the plasma concentrations of total and low density lipoprotein cholesterol and phospholipids (Irwin & Feeley 1967), with a reduced demand for insulin in Type II diabetes (Jenkins et al 1989).

All this favours a daily regimen of six small meals daily rather than two or three larger meals only. The three meals, three snacks regimen would seem appropriate for the insulin-dependent diabetic who has settled into a steady way of life, but during the difficult teenage years and early twenties, food intake is bound to vary because of social forces. In those liable to obesity, the exposure to food six times daily may be too much of a temptation. For the diabetic treated by diet alone, or a combination of diet and oral hypoglycaemic agents, large meals should be avoided and four episodes of eating daily may be a suitable compromise.

CONSUMPTION OF FISH

Red meat is often surrounded by saturated fat, as well as containing droplets of such fat, intimately with the muscles fibres, both outside and inside. The polyunsaturated nature of many fish oils is probably the main reason for the beneficial levels of plasma lipids in those eating diets rich in fish. This raises questions as to whether the emphasis should be on the consumption of lean or oily fish. Fish oils, such as Maxepa, are active in reducing plasma triglyceride concentrations, but do not lower total serum cholesterol. Indeed, they may increase LDL cholesterol if taken as 6 g of n-3 fatty acids daily, by comparisons with an olive oil regimen. In other studies, either 1.7 g or 3 g daily of these acids have been associated with increased total and LDL cholesterol. The seemingly beneficial traditional Eskimo diet not only has a high intake of long chain, highly unsaturated fish fatty acids, but also 50% less saturated fatty acids than the average mainland European diet. A Dutch study in rats suggests that the prothrombotic effect of saturated fatty acids may overwhelm the antithrombotic effect of marine polyenes more readily than that of the terrestrial polyunsaturated fatty acids (Bang et al 1980, Hornstra 1989).

In a study of overall cardiac mortality in relation to fish oils, the lowered mortality was not associated with a reduction in ischaemic heart disease events; the beneficial effects on the risk of death may have been due to a change in the liability to post-infarction ventricular fibrillation (VF). It seems likely that the main benefit of the *n*-3 fatty acids (such as docosahexaenoic acid (22:6) and eicosapentaenoic acid (20:5)) is to limit heart arrhythmias, as shown in experimental studies. The saturated animal fatty acids seem experimentally to promote cardiac arrhythmias after coronary occlusion. The cardiovascular effects of the *n*-3 fatty acids have been well reviewed (Leaf & Weber 1988).

USE OF VERY LOW CALORIE DIETS (VLCD) IN DIABETIC REGIMENS

These diets are effective in producing marked metabolic improvement in non-insulin dependent diabetes (NIDD). They should not be used by diabetics unless they are also markedly obese. If they are treated with insulin then a marked reduction in the insulin dose used is essential. Sulphonylurea doses should be reduced. These diets can be helpful temporarily in NIDDM patients: when body weight falls over a month, fasting glucose may halve. Total plasma cholesterol also falls by 30–40% and fasting plasma triglyceride levels become normal (Hanefield & Weck 1989, Henry et al 1986). A more prolonged experience suggests that beyond 2 months on a VLCD, patients no longer comply with the diet and the difficulty becomes one of restabilizing the patient on a normal diet which they can control without simply regaining the weight that they lost (James 1984). The UK Government, concerned about the use of VLCD at low energy levels, e.g. <330 kcal/day, imposed a limit of 400 kcal/day for women and 500 kcal/day for men on these regimens. The expert group also indicated that only under clear medical supervision should these diets be prolonged for more than a month (Department of Health 1987). In obese patients, unsupervised dieting is endemic to Western societies, but patients with diabetes would normally be expected to be medically supervised. This reduces the risk but without care unadjusted drug and insulin therapy can have catastrophic results with profound hypoglycaemia; hypotension and dehydration with pre-renal failure can also occur. These regimens, though popular, have not yet been shown to be advantageous in diabetes on a long-term basis. There is no reason to believe that the weight loss is sustained longer by using VLCD and a beneficial fall in blood pressure in hypertensive diabetics may be no greater than with a similar weight reduction achieved by other means.

DIETARY ADHERENCE

Failure to follow dietary advice is widespread although most patients do change their eating habits. Turnbridge & Wetherill (1970) found that fewer than one-third of patients actually eat within 10% of their prescribed total carbohydrate allowance, and only about two-thirds managed to eat within 30% of the intended consumption! When specific amounts of carbohydrate are prescribed it is not easy to assess in practice the patient's fat intake, so weight change is unpredictable, particularly if a diet is used together with a hypoglycaemic drug. Thus the UK prospective study of Type II onset diabetes has shown those randomly allocated to receive only dietary management had a greater weight loss in the first year than those also given a hypoglycaemic drug. Nevertheless the patients on diet alone ended the year with higher blood glucose levels.

Too often doctors have prescribed diets crudely and attempted, unsuccessfully, to persuade patients to follow the diets by threatening them with the diabetic complications or with the need for insulin injections if the patient does not comply with the diet. The failure of this approach has led to the recognition that a more sensitive behavioural approach is needed (Wing & Jeffrey 1979). Methods are used which reinforce compliance by a system of self-monitoring: the patient documents his or her own behaviour. Habits are then shaped or modified towards the desired goal by 'tailoring' the diet to the individual patient and may be helped by developing a scheme of rewards for successful change. For example, one reward system was developed where there was a financial down-payment but the patients could reclaim the money if they lost 8 kg over a 16-week period with weekly visits to the clinics. The money being paid out as weight was lost was also dependent on whether they had the required blood test. A second group received the same attention but without the financial incentives, and a third, control group was simply provided with the dietary advice and asked to attend monthly. The results showed no extra benefit from the financial arrangement but the two groups attending weekly initially did better during the 4 month test than those seen monthly. However, at 1 year there was little

Table 35.9   Optimal management of diabetes

	Type I (IDDM)	Type II (NIDDM)
Insulin therapy	Multiple insulin injections to mimic endogenous secretion	Not needed if dietary management effective; oral hypoglycaemic drugs often used before insulin therapy
Diet	High >55% carbohydrate; Low fat <30%; Increased polyunsaturated fat with P:S ratio >1.0 and n–3 fatty acids >30% of PUFA intake; Fibre rich especially soluble fibre intake; Low free glucose, sucrose or other readily absorbed and metabolized sugar; 6 meals daily	
Exercise	Walking half an hour, 4 days weekly	
Alcohol	<2 units /day normally; <4 units/day on special events	
Therapeutic effects desired	Avoidance of hypoglycaemia	
Blood glucose	Fasting level <6 mmol; 2 hour postprandial <8 mmol/l — self-monitoring	
Urinary glucose	Nil	
Glycosylated glucose	Keep within normal range of local laboratory	
Blood cholesterol	<6.5 mmol/l	
Triglyceride (fasting)	<2 mM	
Blood pressure limit	<150/85 mmHg for <60 years	
Body mass index	<25.0 kg/m^2	

difference in weight loss between the groups. Blood glucose and other indices of control were better in those who lost most weight, but no simple scheme emerged for helping with the desired weight loss. When challenged, diabetics who fail to lose much weight claim they are hungry, tired, depressed or cold when attempting to slim. This raises the fundamental issue of both short- and long-term weight control. This issue is considered in Chapter 32.

The best management of the different forms of diabetics is shown in Table 35.9, which includes a scheme for monitoring blood glucose using a simple system where the patient is taught to do their own tests of blood glucose during the day. A finger-prick is used to collect a drop of blood on to special enzyme impregnated strips of paper which respond by changing colour in a way dependent on the glucose concentration in the drops of collected blood. By monitoring diurnal fluctuations in glucose, a patient is able to adjust their regimen even if they show little change in their urinary glucose output because their renal threshold for glucose reabsorption is too high. The normal renal threshold for glucose varies between 7 and 12 mmol/l and if urinary glucose is present it usually means that blood glucose levels are at least twice the normal level. Therefore blood glucose monitoring undertaken at home is the best way of assessing the degree of control during the day. Prolonged increases in blood glucose lead to the glycosylation of haemoglobin A at the terminal valine of the β chain. This produces HbA$_{1c}$. This, with two other minor forms of glycosylated haemoglobin, are

measured together and provide another longer-term index of overall control of the diabetes.

THE FUTURE OF DIABETIC DIETS

Although the optimum system set out in Table 35.10 includes the latest British Diabetic Association recommendations (Lean et al 1991), it is recognized that there is more than one diet composition that can be used. For example, saturated fatty acids can be replaced by either complex carbohydrate or with poly- or monounsaturated fatty acids in different

Table 35.10   UK dietary recomendations for people with diabetes (Lean et al 1991)

Energy	to maintain BMI = 22 kg/m^2
Carbohydrate (% energy)	50–55
Sucrose or fructose (added)	<25 g/day
Dietary fibre	>30 g/day
Total fat (% energy)	30–35
Saturated fat	<10%
Monounsaturated fat	10–15%
Polyunsaturated fat	<10%
Protein (% energy)	10–15
Salt	<6 g/day
If hypertensive	<3 g/day
'Diabetic foods'	Avoid

Note: These proposed fat intakes reflect the concern in the UK to advise diets which are considered practical. In countries with pre-existing lower fat intakes there should be no advice to increase them to these UK proposed levels. The dietary fibre is measured by the old methods and 30 g corresponds to 18 g non-starch polysaccharides.

proportions, to suit individual or local eating habits. It should also be noted that the advice summarized in Table 35.10 should not be pushed to extremes. For example, an intake of 15 g/day of soluble fibre will produce about 10% improvement fasting plasma glucose, glycosylated haemoglobin and cholesterol, but huge doses up to 100 g/day achieve little further improvement. Artificially high intakes of poly-unsaturated fatty acids are not advised: about 8% of energy is appropriate. Although there are benefits for the diabetic patient of about 0.2 g/day of eicosapentaenoic acid from fish, intakes as high as 4 g/day may aggravate hyperglycaemia and serum LDL concentration.

Changes in dietary management can be expected as more rigorous methods are developed for assessing what in practice patients eat and how these diets affect particularly the processes which account for the eye, renal and cardiovascular changes in patients with diabetes.

Recently the problem of managing diabetes has been reassessed by a European group for the World Health Organization, and the International Diabetes Federation. Five-year targets to reduce diabetic complications were developed, e.g. to reduce blindness and end-stage diabetic renal failure by a third or more and to halve the rate of limb amputations for diabetic gangrene. This new St Vincent declaration presents the diabetic team and dietitians in particular with immense demands and will require new and more vigorous approaches to clinical care and preventive work.

REFERENCES

Ahlborg G, Felig P, Hagenfeldt L, Hendler R, Wahren J 1974 Substrate turnover during prolonged exercise in man. Journal of Clinical Investigation 53: 1080–1090

Bang HO, Dyerberg J, Sinclair HM 1980 The composition of the Eskimo food in North-Western Greenland. American Journal of Clinical Nutrition 33: 2657–2661

Department of Health 1987 Committee on Medical Aspects of Food Policy. The use of very-low-calorie diets in obesity. HMSO, London

Department of Health 1991 Committee on Medical Aspects of Food Policy. Report on Health and Social Subjects No.41. Dietary Reference Values for Food Energy and Nutrients for the United Kingdom. HMSO, London

Ellis A 1934 Increased carbohydrate tolerance in diabetics following the hourly administration of glucose and insulin over long periods. Quarterly Journal of Medicine NS3: 137–153

FAO 1973 Energy and protein requirements. Report of a Joint FAO/WHO Expert Committee. FAO, Rome

Gwinup G, Bryon RC, Rousch W, Kruger F, Hamwig GJ 1963 Effect of nibbling versus gorging on serum lipids in man. Lancet 2: 165–167

Hales CN, Barker DJP, Clark PMS et al 1991 Fetal and infant growth and impaired glucose tolerance at age 64. British Medical Journal 303: 1019–1022

Hanefield M, Weck M 1989 Very low calorie diet therapy in obese non insulin dependent diabetes patients. Internal Journal of Obesity 13 (Suppl 2): 23–37

Hattersley AJ, Turner RC, Permutt MA et al 1992 Linkage of type 2 diabetes to glucokinase gene. Lancet 339: 1307–1310

Helmrich SP, Ragland DR, Leung RW, Paffenbarger RS 1991 Physical activity and reduced ocurrence of non-insulin-dependent diabetes mellitus. New England Journal of Medicine 325: 147–152

Henry RR, Wallace O, Olefsky JM 1986 Effects of weight loss on mechanism of hyperglycaemia in obese non insulin dependent diabetes mellitus. Diabetes 35: 990–998

Hornstra G 1989 Fish and the heart. Lancet ii: 1450–1451

Irwin MI, Feeley RM 1967 Frequency and size of meals and serum lipids, nitrogen and mineral retention, fat digestibility and urinary thiamine and riboflavin in young women. American Journal of Clinical Nutrition 20: 816–824

James WPT 1984 Treatment of obesity: the constraints on success. Clinics in Endocrinology and Metabolism 13: 635–663

Jenkins DJA, Wolever TMS, Vuksan V 1989 Nibbling versus gorging: metabolic advantages of increased meal frequency. New England Journal of Medicine 321: 929–934

Kleinman JC, Donahue RP, Harris MI, Finucane FF, Madans JH, Brock DB 1988 Mortality among diabetics in national sample. American Journal of Epidemiology 128: 389–401

Koda JE, Fineman M, Rink TJ, Dailey GE, Muchmore DB, Linarell LG 1992 Amylin concentrations and glucose control. Lancet 339: 1179–1180

Leaf A, Weber PC 1988 Cardiovascular effects of n–3 fatty acids. New England Journal of Medicine 318: 549–557

Lean MEJ, James WPT 1986 Diabetes: Prescription of diabetic diets in the 1980s. Lancet 1: 723–725

Lean MEJ, Brenchley S, Connor H et al 1991 Dietary recommendations for people with diabetes: an update for the 1990s. Journal of Human Nutrition and Dietetics 4: 393–412

Mitrakou A, Kelley D, Mokan M et al 1992 Role of reduced suppression of glucose production and diminished early insulin release in impaired glucose tolerance. New England Journal of Medicine 326: 22–29

Randle PJ 1986 Fuel selection in animals. Biochemical Society Transactions 14: 799–806

Tunbridge R, Wetherill J H 1970 Reliability and cost of diabetic diets. British Medical Journal ii: 78

Wing RR, Jeffrey RW 1979 Outpatient treatments of obesity: a comparison of methodology and clinical results. International Journal of Obesity 3: 261–279

36. Iodine-deficiency disorders

B. S. Hetzel

The importance of iodine as an essential element arises from the fact that it is a constituent of the thyroid hormones thyroxine (T_4) and triiodothyronine (T_3). These hormones are essential for normal growth and physical and mental development in animals and man.

The most familiar iodine deficiency disorder is goitre – swelling of the thyroid gland in the neck. Goitre has been noted and commented on since ancient times. In the Renaissance period, goitre was a common feature of paintings of the Madonna in Italy. Indeed, Thomas Wharton in 1656 suggested that the larger thyroid in the female had the function of beautifying the neck (Langer 1960). However, the understanding of iodine deficiency has now gone far beyond goitre to all the effects of iodine deficiency on growth and development, including brain development, now denoted by the term 'iodine-deficiency disorders' (IDD). The adoption of this term reflects the new dimension of understanding of the full spectrum of the effects of iodine deficiency, on the fetus, the neonate, the child and adolescent, and the adult (Hetzel 1983).

The studies in man have been complemented by recent studies in animal models which have established the effects of iodine deficiency on brain development and fetal survival, and have confirmed that these effects are mediated through the thyroid-gland secretion of the thyroid hormones.

The definition of the problem of IDD as one concerned with brain development, and not just enlargement of the thyroid gland as 'goitre', and the recognition of the large populations at risk (see below) has led to acceptance of IDD as one of major priority in international health and nutrition. A resolution was passed by the World Health Assembly in Geneva in 1986, which pointed to the feasibility of substantial progress in the prevention and control of IDD within the following 5–10 years. More detailed discussion of these various aspects can be found elsewhere for the nature and pathogenesis of IDD (see Stanbury & Hetzel 1980 and Hetzel et al 1990, and for public health, Dunn et al 1986 and Hetzel 1987). A more general account of the problem of IDD, with reference to its global distribution, is also available (Hetzel 1989).

ECOLOGY AND DEMOGRAPHY OF IODINE DEFICIENCY

There is a cycle of iodine in nature (Fig. 36.1). Most of the iodine resides in the ocean; it was present during the primordial development of the earth, but large amounts were leached from the surface soil by glaciation, snow or rain, and were carried by wind, rivers and floods into the sea. Iodine occurs in the deeper layers of the soil and is found in oil-wells and

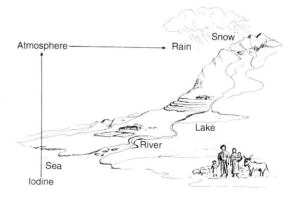

Fig. 36.1   The iodine cycle in nature. The atmosphere absorbs iodine from the sea which then returns through the rain and snow to the mountainous regions. It is then carried by rivers to the lower hills and plains, eventually returning to the sea. High rainfall, snow and flooding, increase the loss of soil iodine, which has often already been denuded by past glaciation. This causes low iodine content of food for man and animals. (Reproduced with permission from Hetzel 1989.)

natural gas effluents. Water from such deep wells can provide a major source of iodine. In general, the older an exposed soil surface the more likely it is to be leached of iodine. The mountainous areas of the world are particularly affected: the most severely deficient areas are those of the Himalayas, the Andes, the European Alps and the vast mountains of China, but iodine deficiency is likely to occur in all elevated regions subject to glaciation and higher rainfall, with run-off into rivers. However, it also occurs in flooded river valleys such as the Ganges in India.

Iodine occurs in soil and the sea as iodide. Iodide ions are oxidized by sunlight to elemental iodine, which is volatile, so that every year some 400 000 tons of iodine escape from the surface of the sea. The concentration of iodide in seawater is about 50–60 μg/l; in the air it is approximately 0.7 μg/m^3. The iodine in the atmosphere is returned to the soil by the rain, which has concentrations in the range 1.8–8.5 μg/l. In this way the cycle is completed.

However, the return of soil iodine is slow and small compared with the original loss, and repeated flooding ensures persistent iodine deficiency in the soil. The crops become iodine-deficient, so those human and animal populations which are totally dependent on food grown in such soil become iodine-deficient. The iodine content of plants may be as low as 10 μg/kg, compared with 1 mg/kg dry weight in plants in a non-iodine deficient soil. Vast iodine-deficient populations in Asia subsist in flooded river valleys in, for example, India, Bangladesh and Burma.

An indication of the iodine content of the soil can be given by the local drinking-water concentration. In general, iodine-deficient areas have water iodine levels below 2 μg/l, as in Nepal and India (0.1–1.2 μg/l) compared with levels of 9.0 μg/l in the city of Delhi, which is not iodine-deficient.

Iodine intake and bioavailability

Table 36.1 provides an indication of the likely iodine content of different foods, but plant foods are especially likely to show a reduced iodine content in deficient soils. Milk and meat are richer sources and the best natural sources are seafoods. Cooking reduces the iodine content of foods, with over half of the iodine escaping during boiling, whereas only about a fifth is lost in frying or grilling.

Iodine is readily absorbed, but only a half of other organic iodine compounds, or the thyroid hormones themselves, in animal foods are absorbed. Since a population's mean requirement amounts to 100–150 μg/day, it is clear that food sources rather than water intake are the important contributors to iodine intake. Where iodine deficiency occurs this will persist unless a supplement is given or the diet made more varied with foods drawn from non-deficient areas.

European diets became more varied in origin during the 19th century, but substantial areas of iodine deficiency remain in Germany, Italy and Spain, as well as in other more localized areas. In developing countries globally (Fig. 36.2) about 1 billion are at risk of IDD, of which 200 million are suffering from goitre; over 5 million are gross cretins with mental retardation, according to a recent World Health Organization Report (WHO 1990) and 15 million suffer from lesser degrees of mental defect (Table 36.2).

PHYSIOLOGY OF IODINE DEFICIENCY

The healthy human adult body contains 15–20 mg of iodine, of which about 70–80% is in the thyroid gland. The thyroid weighs only 15–25 g, so its concentrating power is remarkable. The presence of iodine in the thyroid was first demonstrated by Baumann in 1895.

Table 36.1   The average iodine content of foods (μg I/g) (From Koutras 1986)

	Fresh basis		Dry basis	
	Mean	Range	Mean	Range
Fish (freshwater)	30	17–40	116	68–194
Fish (marine)	832	163–3180	3715	471–1591
Shellfish	798	308–1300	3866	1292–4987
Meat	50	27–97		
Milk	47	35–56		
Eggs	93			
Cereal grains	47	22–72	65	34–92
Fruits	18	10–29	154	62–277
Legumes	30	23–36	234	223–245
Vegetables	29	12–201	385	204–1636

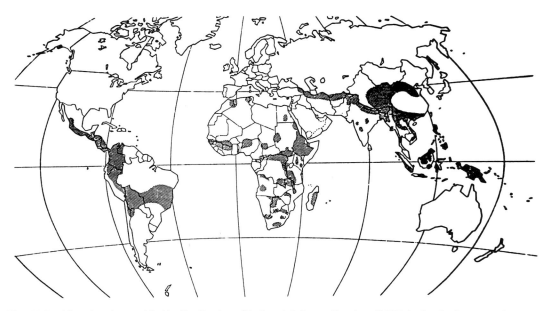

Fig. 36.2   Map showing worldwide distribution of iodine deficiency disorders (IDD) in developing countries. (Reproduced with permission from World Health Organization 1990)

Iodide is rapidly absorbed through the gut. Once the need for thyroidal iodine has been met, excess iodine is excreted by the kidney so the urinary iodine output then reflects the iodine intake. Iodine in milk, present only as iodide, also responds to iodine intake. Iodophors used widely in the western world in the dairy industry increase the iodide content of cow's milk.

The very active iodide trapping mechanism in the thyroid maintains a gradient of 100:1 between the thyroid cell and the extracellular fluid. In dietary iodine deficiency this gradient may exceed 400:1 in order to maintain the uptake of 60 µg of iodine per day needed for the output of thyroxine. This increased gradient was first shown in the field with radioiodine in Mendoza, Argentina, by Stanbury in 1951. As urinary iodine excretion fell there was a rise in ^{131}I uptake by the thyroid (Stanbury et al 1954). Despite adaptive increases in trapping, the amount of iodine in the gland is closely related to intake and may be reduced to below 1 mg in the iodine-deficient enlarged thyroid (goitre).

Iodine exists in the thyroid as inorganic iodine and the iodine-containing amino acids monoiodotyronine (MIT), diiodotyronine (DIT), thyroxine (T_4), triiodothyronine (T_3), polypeptides containing thyroxine, and thyroglobulin. Thyroglobulin is a glycoprotein (mol wt 650 000) with iodinated amino acids in a peptide linkage. It is the chief constituent of the colloid that fills the thyroid follicle and serves as the storage form of the thyroid hormones and contains 90% of the total iodine in the gland.

Iodine exists in the blood as thyroxine (T_4), triiodothyronine (T_3) (Fig. 36.3) and inorganic iodine. The level of inorganic iodine falls in iodine deficiency and rises with increased intake. T_4 and T_3 are mainly bound to the plasma proteins – only about 0.5% is free in human serum. The level of free T_4 determines tissue levels of thyroid hormone so measuring free T_4 is the best way to assess thyroid status and diagnose reduced thyroid function (hypothyroidism) or increased thyroid function (hyperthyroidism). In the past, total blood organic iodine

Table 36.2   Estimated prevalence of iodine deficiency disorders in developing countries, by region and numbers of persons at risk (in millions) (From World Health Organization 1990)

	At risk	Goitre	Overt cretinism
Africa	227	39	0.5
Latin America	60	30	0.3
Southeast Asia	280	100	4.0
Asia (other countries including China)	400	30	0.9
Eastern Mediterranean	33	12	—
Total	1000	211	5.7

(mainly thyroxine) was measured with the plasma protein-bound iodine (PBI) method and gave satisfactory but less specific results than the free T_4 measurement. T_3 and diiodotyrosine are included in the PBI measurement but are less than 10% of the total organic iodine. Plasma T_3 increases in iodine deficiency, and the plasma precursor iodotyrosines rise in hyperthyroidism or after thyroid stimulation. Automated systems with radioimmunoassay and data handling for thyroidal hormone assays in large numbers are now available, and help in public health monitoring.

Production and regulation of the thyroid hormones

An active transport mechanism which requires energy traps iodide in the thyroid. This 'iodine pump' is regulated by the thyroid-stimulating hormone (TSH) from the pituitary. Other ions can act as competitors of iodine trapping, e.g. thiocyanate. Thiocyanate is derived from the metabolism of hydrogen cyanide (HCN), which is found in foods such as cassava, the dietary staple in Zaire and many other countries. This explains the occurrence of goitre and severe hypothyroidism in Zaire.

The iodide is released into the colloid between the thyroid cells, where it is oxidized by hydrogen peroxide derived from the thyroid peroxidase system (Fig. 36.4). It then combines with tyrosine in the thyroglobulin to form MIT and DIT. The oxidation process then continues with the coupling of MIT and DIT to form the iodotyrosines. This oxidation process can be readily blocked by various drugs, including

propylthiouracil and carbimazole, which are widely used for the treatment of hyperthyroidism There may also be a congenital defect in biosynthesis so that iodide cannot be bound to tyrosine – this is a cause of congenital goitre and hypothyroidism which may run in families, but defects of this nature do not explain why some iodine-deficient individuals develop goitre when others do not.

The iodinated thyroglobulin, with its iodinated amino acids, is taken up by the thyroid cells by a process called 'pinocytosis'. Proteolytic enzymes then break it down to release the T_4 and T_3 into the blood (Fig. 36.4). The unused iodotyrosines are conserved and recycled back into thyroglobulin, but when the thyroid output is high, recycling may not keep pace with the production of free MIT and DIT, which then leak into the blood but have no biological effect.

The complex regulation of thyroid hormones involves not only the thyroid, but the pituitary, the brain and the peripheral tissues.

The thyroid secretion is under the control of the pituitary gland through the thyroid-stimulating hormone (TSH). TSH is a glycoprotein (mol wt 28 000), with two subunits. The X subunit has virtually the same structure as other pituitary hormones but the B subunit is specific for TSH, and essentially the same across different species.

TSH secretion is controlled through a 'feedback' mechanism by the level of T_4 in the blood. As T_4 falls, TSH secretion is increased and stimulates thyroid activity, including T_4 secretion, thereby helping to maintain T_4 levels. This stimulation is ineffective in severe iodine deficiency, so blood levels of T_4 remain low and TSH high. A low T_4 and high TSH are

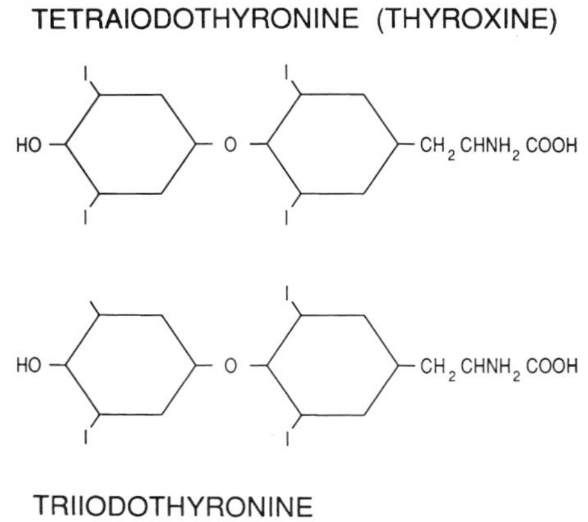

TETRAIODOTHYRONINE (THYROXINE)

HO —⬡— O —⬡— CH_2 $CHNH_2$ COOH

HO —⬡— O —⬡— CH_2 $CHNH_2$ COOH

TRIIODOTHYRONINE

Fig. 36.3 Chemical formulae of thyroxine tetraiodothyronine (T_4) and triiodothyronine (T_3).

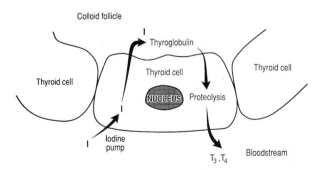

Fig. 36.4 Diagram showing pumping of iodine by the thyroid cell and then passive diffusion into the colloid follicle, where it is bound within the protein molecule of thyroglobulin into organic form as the thyroid hormone. The thyroglobulin is then reabsorbed by the cell. It is then broken down to liberate the thyroid hormones which pass into the bloodstream. (Reproduced with permission from Hetzel 1989.)

diagnostic of hypothyroidism due to iodine deficiency at various stages in life, but particularly in the neonate. In many western countries every newborn child is now checked for the level of thyroid hormones soon after birth (usually by a heel-prick sample of blood on the 4th or 5th day), so that if there is deficiency thyroxine treatment can be given rapidly.

Thyroid activity during pregnancy

In the human, the thyroid and pituitary have developed by the end of the first 12 weeks of gestation and the hypothalamus develops from the 10th to the 30th weeks. Maturation of neuroendocrine control occurs after the 20th week. Between 18 and 22 weeks TSH can be detected in the blood so the pituitary can stimulate the thyroid: there is then a rise in T_4. T_3 remains low because the 5-deiodinase enzyme removes the inner-ring 5 iodine atom to form reverse T_3 which has no hormonal activity. Just before birth, there is a decline in this enzyme with a rise in the 5-deiodinase enzyme acting on the outer ring, so the biologically active T_3 rises rapidly and reverse T_3 falls. This change prepares the organism for the transition from intrauterine to extrauterine life. Failure of this conversion to produce sufficient T_3 in iodine deficiency may be a factor in the stillbirths that occur as part of the spectrum of severe IDD.

Role of the thyroid in growth and development

Thyroid function is essential for normal growth and development. Thyroid hormone deficiency from an absent thyroid, congenital thyroid defect or severe iodine deficiency, leads to severe retardation of growth and maturation of almost all organ systems. Body weight does not increase and there is retardation of bone growth. Estimates of cellular growth from DNA measurements show that retardation is most apparent in tissues that are rapidly proliferating. Thus the sensitivity of different organs to thyroid deficiency varies. The brain is particularly susceptible to damage during the fetal and early postnatal periods. At birth, the child's brain is very immature and less than a third of its mature weight. Despite generally satisfactory results, some residual mental deficiency occurs in neonatal hypothyroidism even with optimal thyroxine treatment. Later intelligence testing, however shows a sharp decline if thyroxine therapy is delayed after the age of 3 months. This shows that thyroidal control of neonatal brain development is even more important than fetal development.

Development of goitre

Understanding the physiology of thyroid hormone production helps explain the development of goitre in iodine deficiency, which is the primary cause of goitre. Other factors known as 'goitrogens', e.g. thiocyanates, enhance the effect of iodine deficiency and are called 'secondary factors'. As iodine deficiency interferes with thyroid hormone synthesis, blood T_4 levels fall but T_3 rises, because the less iodinated hormone is produced preferentially. The fall in T_4 stimulates TSH output which increases thyroidal iodide uptake and hormonal turnover, and cells of the thyroid follicles enlarge and then multiply. The colloid reserves of thyroglobulin are gradually used up, so that the gland has a much more cellular appearance than normal (Fig. 36.5). Clinically, 'goitre' is regarded as significant when the size of the lateral thyroid lobes is greater than the terminal phalanx of the examiner's thumb. More precise measurements can now be made using ultrasound.

EXPERIMENTAL IODINE DEFICIENCY

Most observations on naturally occurring iodine deficiency have been made on farm animals, in which reproductive failure and thyroid insufficiency have been well reported in the older literature (see Hetzel & Maberly 1986). In areas of iodine deficiency, fetal development is retarded or arrested at some stage in gestation, with early embryo death or resorption, abortion, stillbirth, or the birth of weak, hairless offspring after a prolonged pregnancy and delivery, when placental membranes are often retained. Subnormal thyroid hormone levels in cattle lead to a high incidence of aborted, stillborn and weak calves.

Thyroidectomy of ewes before conception reduces the prenatal and postnatal viability of their lambs, even though the lambs' thyroids appear to be normal. Feeding ewes goitrogenic kale also increases lamb mortality, but this responds to iodine administration during pregnancy.

Morphological and biochemical changes seen in the hyperplastic goitre of man are also observed in experimental iodine deficiency in animals. More recently, the effects of iodine deficiency on development, particularly that relating to the fetus, have been investigated. These studies on the sheep, marmoset (new world primate, *Callithrix jacchus jacchus*) and the rat have been particularly concerned with fetal brain development, because of its relevance to the human problem of endemic cretinism and brain damage resulting from fetal iodine deficiency.

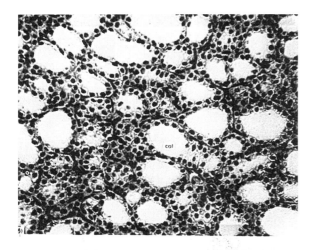

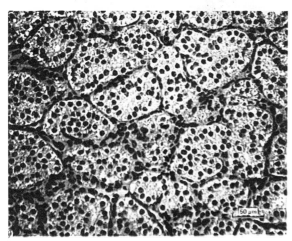

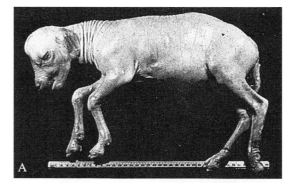

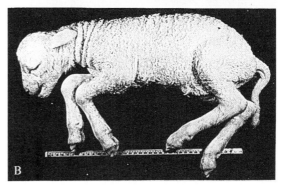

Fig. 36.5 Thyroid tissue from newborn marmosets showing the presence of colloid material in the follicles of the normal control gland (top) compared to its absence in the iodine-deficient gland (bottom) with great increase in size and number of the thyroid cells. (Reproduced with permission from Mano et al 1985.)

Fig. 36.6 Effect of severe iodine deficiency during pregnancy on lamb development. A 140-day old lamb fetus (normal gestation period 150 days) was subjected to severe iodine deficiency (A) through feeding the mother an iodine-deficient diet (5–8 µg day) for 6 months prior to and during pregnancy, compared to a control lamb of the same age fed the same diet with the addition of an iodine supplement (B). The iodine-deficient lamb shows absence of wool coat, subluxation of the leg joints and a dome-like appearance of the head due to skeletal retardation. The brain was smaller and contained a lower number of cells, compared to the control. (Reproduced with permission from Hetzel & Potter 1983.)

Iodine deficiency in the sheep

The sheep is a good model for studying iodine deficiency because maternal–fetal relationships are readily monitored. One example is given to demonstrate the usefulness of animal experiments in understanding major issues of public health importance. Severe iodine deficiency can be produced in sheep by feeding a low-iodine diet providing only 5–8 µg of iodine per day. After 5 months, although body weights are maintained, a goitre develops, plasma T_4 and T_3 values fall, TSH rises and urinary iodine output is low. When deficient and iodine-supplemented ewes serving as a control were mated with normal fertile rams, the deficient ewes had an abortion and stillbirth rate of 21% compared with the normal group of 4.3%. This shows the specific effect of iodine deficiency on fetal survival.

The iodine-deficient fetuses in late pregnancy had a very abnormal appearance. They weighed less and there was a notable absence of wool growth. Goitre, partial dislocation of the foot joints and deformation of the skull were also present. Bone maturation was slowed, as shown by the delayed appearance of the epiphyses in the limbs (Fig. 36.6) Lowered brain

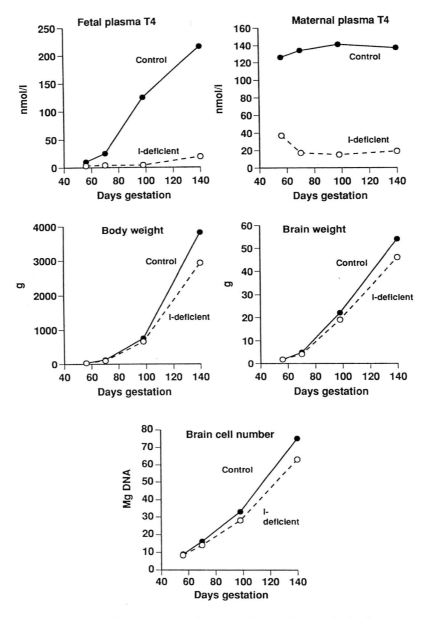

Fig. 36.7   Effect of severe iodine deficiency on fetal development in the sheep. Number of observations varied in each group from two to seven animals. (Modified from Potter et al 1982.)

weight and brain DNA were noticed as early as 70 days, indicating a reduction in cell number probably due to slowed neuroblast multiplication, which normally occurs from 40–80 days in the sheep (Fig. 36.7). A greater density of cells, a reduced migration of brain cells and an increased water content of the brain, all indicators of delayed maturation, were observed in the cerebellum and cerebral hemispheres at 140 days (normal gestation is 150 days). Myelination in the cerebral hemispheres and brainstem was also slowed, as shown by their lowered cholesterol DNA/ratios.

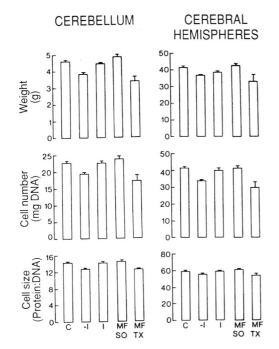

CEREBELLUM   CEREBRAL
                    HEMISPHERES

Fig. 36.8   Comparison of brains of sheep fetuses at 140 days' gestation. C = control; -I = iodine-deficient; I = iodine at 100 days; MFSO = mother + fetus sham operated; MFTX = mother + fetus thyroidectomized. (Reproduced with permission from Hetzel 1983.)

Giving the pregnant ewes an injection of iodized oil at 100 days of pregnancy restored the maternal and fetal plasma T_4 values to normal, and improved the physical appearance of the fetuses. Brain growth, DNA and cholesterol/DNA ratios all increased to normal, suggesting that a catch-up in neuroblast development had occurred during pregnancy. Histological examination, however, revealed that the density of synapses in the cerebral cortex was still less than those of the control fetal brains, despite the iodide injection. The effects of iodine deficiency and iodized oil administration on the cerebellum and cerebral hemispheres are compared with those of the control brains in Fig. 36.8.

Removing the thyroids from fetal sheep at 50–60 days of pregnancy produces profound but similar changes to iodine deficiency, but fetal thyroidectomy at 98 days causes less severe effects. This improvement is not seen if the ewe was thyroidectomized before conception (McIntosh et al 1983).

These observations suggested that normal brain development relies on the availability of both maternal and fetal thyroid hormones. It has become clear (Obregon et al 1984a, Woods et al 1984) that embryonic tissues in the rat are provided with T_4 and T_3 only 4 days after uterine implantation, and well before the onset of fetal thyroid function at 17 days. In the human, there is also now evidence of maternal thyroxine transfer across the placenta barrier late in pregnancy (Vulsma et al 1989), so the old concept of early mammalian development being independent of thyroid hormones is clearly wrong (Hetzel & Potter 1983).

Similar changes in thyroidal state, brain development and histology are observed in non-human primates such as the marmoset when pregnant animals are iodine-deficient. The effects are worse in the second than the first pregnancy (Mano et al 1987).

Maternal iodine deficiency in the rat has also been shown to reduce the number of viable embryos and their individual body weights. Maternal thyroidectomy has a similar but more severe effect (Morreale de Escobar et al 1985). Extensive studies have also been made in rats fed the diet consumed by the people of Jixian village (near Jamusi) in the Northern Heilongjiang Province of China (Li et al 1985). The village had an endemic cretin rate of 11% and the diet included main crops (maize, wheat), vegetables and water from the area, with an iodine content of only 4.5 µg/kg. After the rats had eaten the diet for 4 months goitre was obvious in the newborn rats, which had T_4 levels of 3.6 µg/100 ml, compared with the control of 10.4 µg/100 ml. Thyroidal uptake of ^{125}I was higher and brain weight was reduced. Cerebral cell density was increased and in the cerebellum there was delayed disappearance of the external granular layer, with reduced incorporation of ^3H leucine compared with the control group. Similar data in a rice-eating area of south China (Zhong et al 1983) have been reported.

These experimental findings in three different species of animals (rat, sheep and monkey) are important because they prove that severe lack of dietary iodine does cause reproductive failure and retardation in both fetal brain and somatic development.

IODINE-DEFICIENCY DISORDERS IN MAN

Extensive reviews of the global geographic prevalence of endemic goitre (Fig. 36.9) have been published, notably by Kelly & Sneddon (1960) and more recently by Stanbury & Hetzel (1980) and by Hetzel (1989).

Goitrogens in general are of secondary importance to iodine deficiency as aetiological factors in endemic goitre (Karmarker et al 1974). More recent research

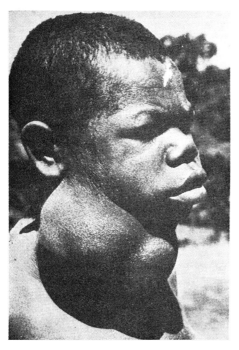

Fig. 36.9   Young New Guinean woman with a large goitre. (Reproduced with permission from Hetzel 1970.)

(Bourdoux et al 1980) has shown that staple foods from the third world, such as cassava, maize, bamboo shoots, sweet potatoes, lima beans and millet, contain cyanogenic glucosides which are capable of liberating large quantities of cyanide by hydrolysis. Not only is the cyanide toxic, but the predominant metabolite is the goitrogen thiocyanate. With the exception of cassava, these glycosides are located in the inedible portions of the plants, or occur in the edible portion in such small quantities that they do not cause a major problem. Cassava, on the other hand, is cultivated extensively in developing countries and represents an essential dietary source of energy for more than 200 million people living in the tropics (Delange et al 1982). The additional effect of cassava on iodine deficiency in the aetiology of endemic goitre and endemic cretinism has now been demonstrated in non-mountainous Zaire (Delange et al 1982), and in Sarawak, Malaysia (Maberly et al 1983).

Apart from goitre, recent work now reveals a great variety of effects of iodine deficiency on human growth and development. These iodine-deficiency disorders (IDD) are best described in relation to four different phases of life (Table 36.3).

Iodine deficiency in the fetus

Iodine deficiency in the fetus due to maternal iodine deficiency leads to a greater incidence of stillbirths, abortions and congenital abnormalities, which can be reduced by iodization as in the experimental studies just described. The effects are similar to those observed with maternal hypothyroidism, which can be reduced by thyroid hormone replacement therapy (McMichael et al 1980).

Endemic cretinism occurs when the iodine intake of the population falls below 25 µg/day. Cretinism is still widely prevalent, affecting for example up to 10% of the populations living in severely iodine-deficient areas in India (Kochupillai & Pandav 1987), Indonesia (Djokomoeljanto et al 1983) and China (Ma Tai et al 1982). In its most common form it is characterized by mental deficiency, deaf-mutism and spastic diplegia, which is referred to as the 'nervous' or neurological type, in contrast to the less common 'myxoedematous' type characterized by hypothyroidism with dwarfism.

These two conditions were first described in modern medical literature by McCarrison (1908) and the differences are summarized in Table 36.4. The condition still exists in the same areas of the Karakoram Mountains and in the Himalayas (Kochupillai &

Table 36.3   The spectrum of iodine deficiency disorders (From Hetzel 1987)

Fetus	Abortions
	Stillbirths
	Congenital anomalies
	Increased perinatal mortality
	Increased infant mortality
	Neurological cretinism
	mental deficiency
	deaf–mutism
	spastic diplegia
	squint
	Myxoedematous cretinism
	dwarfism
	mental deficiency
	Psychomotor defects
Neonate	Neonatal goitre
	Neonatal hypothyroidism
Child and adolescent	Goitre
	Juvenile hypothyroidism
	Impaired mental function
	Retarded physical development
Adult	Goitre with its complications
	Hypothyroidism
	Impaired mental function
	Iodine-induced hyperthyroidism

Increased susceptibility to radiation hazard is another effect of iodine deficiency, particularly in Europe

Table 36.4 Comparative clinical features in neurological and hypothyroid cretinism (From Hetzel & Potter 1983)

	Neurological cretin	Hypothyroid cretin
Mental retardation	Present, often severe	Present, less severe
Deaf–mutism	Usually present	Absent
Cerebral diplegia	Often present	Absent
Stature	Usually normal	Severe growth retardation usual
General features	No physical signs of hypothyroidism	Coarse dry skin, husky voice
Reflexes	Excessively brisk	Delayed relaxation
ECG	Normal	Small voltage QRS complexes and other abnormalities of hypothyroidism
X-ray limbs	Normal	Epiphyseal dysgenesis
Effect of thyroid hormones	No effect	Improvement

Pandav 1987). Neurological, myxoedematous and mixed types still occur in the Hetian District of Sinkiang, China, some 300 km east of Gilgit, where McCarrison made his original observations (Fig. 36.10) (Ma Tai et al 1982). More recent studies have been reported from western China by Boyages et al (1988). In both China and India, the condition occurs most frequently below the mountain slopes in the fertile silt plains that have been leached of iodine by snow waters and glaciation.

Cretinism is also prevalent in Oceania (Papua New Guinea), Africa, e.g. Zaire, and in South America in the Andean region involving regions of Ecuador, Peru, Bolivia and Argentina (Pharoah et al 1980). In all these situations, with the exception of Zaire, neurological features are predominant. In Zaire the myxoedematous form is more common, probably due to the high intake of cassava (Delange et al 1982). However, there is considerable variation in the clinical manifestations of neurological cretinism, which include isolated deaf-mutism and mental defects of varying degrees. In China the term 'cretinoid' is used to describe these individuals.

The common form of endemic cretinism is not usually associated with severe clinical hypothyroidism, as in the case of the so-called sporadic cretinism, although mixed forms with both the neurological and myxoedematous features do occur. The neurological features are not reversed by the administration of thyroid hormones, unlike the hypothyroidism (Fierro-Benitez et al 1970). This poor response, once brain development has failed, is not surprising (see experimental section).

Endemic cretinism spontaneously disappeared in southern Europe without iodization, as noted by Costa et al (1964) in northern Italy and by Konig & Veraguth (1961) in Switzerland, so its relationship to iodine deficiency was in doubt. Whether a greater variety of foods available from outside the region was responsible, whether goitrogen intake changed or selenium status improved (see Chapter 12) was unknown.

The prevention of endemic cretinism

In order to resolve the doubt about the relation of iodine deficiency to cretinism, a controlled trial using

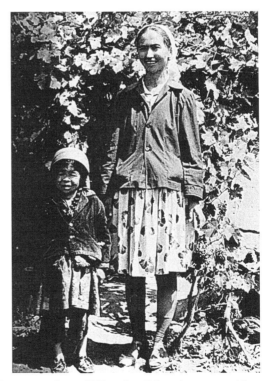

Fig. 36.10 Severe IDD: a dwarfed cretin woman with a barefoot doctor of the same age from the Hetian district, Xinjiang, China. (Courtesy of Dr Ma Tai of Tianjin, with permission.)

iodised oil (2.15 g iodine in 4 ml) given by intramuscular injection to alternate families was carried out in Papua New Guinea. The other families received saline injections. Each child born subsequently was examined for evidence of motor retardation, as assessed by the usual milestones of sitting, standing or walking, and for evidence of deafness. Examination was carried out without knowledge as to whether the mother had received iodized oil injection or saline. Infants presenting with a full syndrome of hearing and speech abnormalities, together with abnormalities of motor development with or without squint, were classified as suffering from endemic cretinism. Later follow-up confirmed the diagnosis of cretinism in these cases (Pharoah et al 1971, Pharoah & Connolly 1987). There was a significant reduction in recorded fetal and neonatal deaths in the treated group (Table 36.5). This is consistent with other evidence indicating the effect of iodine deficiency on fetal survival.

Of the seven cretins born to women who had received iodized oil, six were conceived before the injection and in the seventh case the timing was unclear. The ages of all the cretins born between 1966 and 1972 in relation to the injection of iodized oil are shown in Fig. 36.11. This trial therefore showed that an injection of iodized oil given prior to pregnancy could prevent the occurrence of the neurological syndrome of endemic cretinism in the infant. The occurrence of the cretinism syndrome in those who were pregnant at the time of oil injection indicated that the damage had probably occurred during the first half of pregnancy.

The level of maternal thyroxine was also found to affect the mortality and the occurrence of cretinism of current and recent past pregnancies in Papua New Guinea. Mothers with biochemical evidence of iodine deficiency but without clinical evidence of hypothyroidism had more stillbirths, cretins and neonatal deaths in their surviving babies.

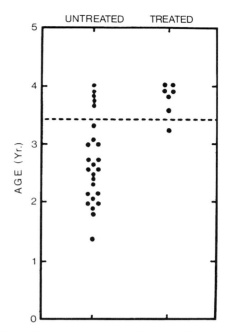

Fig. 36.11   The results of a controlled trial of iodized oil injection in the Jimi River District of the highlands of Papua New Guinea. Alternate mothers were given an injection of iodized oil and saline in September 1966. All newborn children were followed up for the next 5 years. Each dot represents a cretin child. The figure shows that mothers given iodized oil injections do not have subsequent cretin children, in comparison with their persistence in the untreated group. (Reproduced with permission from Pharoah et al 1971.)

Table 36.5   Controlled trials of iodized oil in iodine-deficient pregnant women

	Papua New Guinea			Zaire	
	Untreated	Treated		Untreated	Treated
Total no. of children	406	412			
Normal	380	405	Birthweight (g)	2634	2837†
Stillborn	97	66†	Perinatal mortality/1000	188	98†
Cretins	26	7*†	Infant mortality/1000	250	167†
			Development quotient	104	115†

* At least six of the seven mothers were pregnant when treated
† $p < 0.05$ or more
Data from Zaire were made on a variable number (66–263) of children in each group (Thilly 1981); Papua New Guinea data from Pharoah et al 1971

The value of iodized oil injection in the prevention of endemic cretinism has been confirmed in Zaire and in South America. Mass injection programmes have been carried out in New Guinea in 1971–1972 and in Zaire, Indonesia and China. Recent evaluations of these mass programmes in Indonesia and China indicate that endemic cretinism has been prevented where correction of iodine deficiency has been achieved (Ma et al 1982, Dulberg et al 1983). The effects of iodine deficiency on the fetus therefore seem to be mediated by maternal thyroxine before the onset of fetal thyroid function, and are not due to fetal deficiency of elemental iodine as originally suggested (Pharoah et al 1971). The placental transfer of thyroxine lends credibility to this view.

Iodine deficiency in the neonate

An increased perinatal mortality due to iodine deficiency has been shown in Zaire from the results of a controlled trial of iodized oil injections given in the latter half of pregnancy (Thilly 1981) (Table 36.5). There is a substantial fall in perinatal and infant mortality, with improved birthweight. Low birthweight of whatever cause is associated with a higher rate of congenital anomalies and higher risk throughout childhood.

In Table 36.6 a comparison is made between the incidence of permanent and transient neonatal hypothyroidism in Europe and North America. The rates of permanent hypothyroidism are similar, but the rate for transient hypothyroidism is greater in Europe (Delange et al 1986) than in North America by a factor of more than 7. Transient hypothyroidism has been previously reported in Europe, mainly from areas with a borderline or clearly deficient iodine supply. It has also been shown that this condition can be corrected by iodine supplementation; without supplementation normal neonatal brain growth and development are threatened. The importance of correcting low thyroxine levels was emphasized with the recognition that the major determinant of brain (and

pituitary) triiodothyronine (T_3) is serum thyroxine (T_4) and not T_3 (as is true of the liver, kidney and muscle)(Crantz & Larsen 1980). Low levels of brain T_3 have been demonstrated in the iodine-deficient rat in association with reduced levels of serum T_4, and these have been restored to normal with correction of iodine deficiency (Obregon et al 1984b).

Neonatal urinary iodine excretion has been used as an index of the intake of milk iodine from the mother in an international study in Europe and Canada. Transient hypothyroidism was much commoner in Freiburg (Germany), where the lowest level of urine iodine excretion was observed, than in Stockholm (Sweden). Intermediate levels were found in Rome (Italy) and Brussels (Belgium). Other epidemiological data indicate persistent IDD in former East Germany, the former West Germany, Italy and Spain, as well as in other more localized regions (European Thyroid Association 1985). These data indicate the urgent need for correction of iodine deficiency in many parts of Europe.

In developing countries there is a much higher rate of neonatal hypothyroidism shown in blood taken from the umbilical vein just after birth (Table 36.7). The incidence of neonatal hypothyroidism was related to the severity of the iodine deficiency, as indicated by the prevalence of goitre and cretinism and the level of excretion of iodine in the urine. Neonatal observations in Zaire also showed rates of 10% of chemical hypothyroidism (Ermans et al 1980). Here the hypothyroidism persists into infancy and childhood if the deficiency is not corrected, and retardation of physical and mental development results.

These results emphasize that many more children are likely to suffer from mental deficiency in a severely iodine-deficient population than those who are clinically obvious cases of cretinism.

Iodine deficiency in infancy and childhood

Iodine deficiency in children is characteristically associated with goitre, the classification of which has been standardized by the World Health Organization (see below). The goitre rate increases with age, so that it reaches a maximum with adolescence. Girls have a higher prevalence than boys. Assessing goitre rates in schoolchildren over the period 8–14 years is convenient because they are available in schools and the rates will indicate iodine deficiency within a community. Casual samples of urine for measuring urinary iodine can also be conveniently used. Urine iodine data will be discussed later.

Table 36.6 Comparison of the incidence of permanent and transient primary hypothydroidism in North America and Europe (From Delange et al 1986)

Regions	Number of infants screened	Incidence per 100 000 of primary hypothyroidism	
		Permanent	Transient
North America	1 238 247	22	1.6
Europe	1 276 307	25	12.1

Table 36.7 Iodine deficiency and incidence of neonatal chemical hypothyroidism (NCH) (From Kochupillai & Pandav 1987)

Area of study	Goitre prevalence (%)	Cretinism prevalence (%)	Urinary iodine group*	Incidence of NCH (per 1000 births)
Bhutan	60	2–13	V	115
Deoria (India)	80	3–5	V	133
Corakhpur (India)	70	0–4	V	85
Gonda (India)	60	0–4	V	75
Kathmandu (Nepal)†			II	15
Delhi (India)	29	Nil	II	6
Kerala (India)	1.3	Nil	–	1

† In Nepal ongoing iodized salt prophylaxis is only partially successful
* Group II: None of the population studied had urinary iodines less than 25 µg/g creatinine; in Group V, urinary iodine in over half the population was less than 25 µg/g
NCH was defined as a neonatal umbilical vein blood T_4 level below 3 µg/dl and TSH > 50 µl/ml
Kerala is recognized as an area without goitre

Schoolchildren living in iodine-deficient areas have impaired school performance and lower IQs than children from non-iodine deficient areas. Obtaining suitable controls and assessing other causes of poor school performance is difficult. Thus populations in iodine-deficient areas are often remote, socially deprived, with poor school facilities, a lower socioeconomic status and poorer general nutrition. All these factors have to be taken into account as well as developing suitable mental ability tests appropriate for use in Third World countries. Nevertheless, tests of psychomotor development, e.g. motor coordination, can be regarded as independent of educational status. Thus differences in bimanual dexterity in threading beads and putting pegs into a pegboard were tested in New Guinea and related to the mother's iodine status. Low maternal thyroxine levels during pregnancy significantly affected the children's dexterity, even when tested at the age of 10–12 years (Connolly et al 1979, Pharoah et al 1981, Pharoah & Connolly 1987). Now, however, a wide range of psychological tests applied in Indonesia and a deficient area of Spain show that children's mental development lags behind that of children from non-iodine deficient areas and the differences in psychomotor development become apparent only after the age of 2.5 years (Bleichrodt et al 1987).

In Chile and China, children with goitre perform less well in IQ tests (Muzzo et al 1986, Boyages et al 1989). These differences can be affected by correcting the iodine deficiency. Fierro Benitez et al (1986) compared the long-term effects of iodized oil injections in two highland villages from Ecuador in 1966. In children aged 8–15 of mothers from one village receiving iodized oil prior to the second trimester of pregnancy, it was found that 'Scholastic achievement was better in the children of treated mothers when measured in terms of school year reached, for age,

school dropout rate, failure rate, years repeated and school marks. There was no difference between the two groups by certain tests (Terman–Merrill, Wechsler or Goddenough). However, both groups were impaired in school performance – in reading, writing and mathematics, but more notably the children of untreated mothers'. These results indicate the significant role of iodine deficiency, but other factors could also be important in the school performance of these Ecuadorean children because of their social deprivation and general poor nutritional state. Similar findings were seen in Bolivia with children given oral iodized oil directly. Mental performance improved particularly in those whose goitres became smaller, and the effect was greater in the girls.

Iodization programmes have also led to increases in the levels of circulating thyroid hormones in children in India (Sooch et al 1973) and in China (Zhu 1983). These changes occur whether or not the child is goitrous and indicate a mild degree of hypothyroidism without any apparent symptoms.

The rationale for correcting the deficiency of children and adults with endemic goitre and lowered serum T_4 levels is the improvement of T_4 supply to the brain for local T_3 production and action. Thus cerebral function can be expected to improve once iodine deficiency is corrected, provided fetal damage has not occurred.

Iodine deficiency in the adult

The common effect of iodine deficiency in adults is goitre. Characteristically there is an absence of classic clinical hypothyroidism in adults with endemic goitre. However, laboratory evidence of hypothyroidism with reduced T_4 levels is common. This is often accompanied by normal T₃ levels and raised TSH levels (Hetzel 1987, Zhu 1983).

Iodine administration in the form of iodized salt (Zhu 1983), iodized bread (Clements et al 1960) or iodized oil (Buttfield & Hetzel 1967) have all been demonstrated to be effective in the prevention of goitre in adults. Iodine programmes readily increase serum T₄ levels and may also reduce existing goitre in adults. This is particularly true of iodized oil injections (Buttfield & Hetzel 1967). The visual improvement in the swelling of the neck leads to ready acceptance of the measure by people living in iodine-deficient communities.

In northern India a high degree of apathy has been noted in populations living in iodine-deficient areas. This may even affect domestic animals such as dogs! It is apparent that reduced mental function is widely prevalent in iodine-deficient communities, with impairment in their capacity for initiative and decision-making. This means that iodine deficiency is a major block to the human and social development of communities living in an iodine-deficient environment. Correcting iodine deficiency can therefore make a major contribution to development.

An instructive example of the value of an iodized salt programme comes from the northern Chinese village of Jixian in Heilongjiang Province (Li & Wang 1987). In 1978 there was a goitre rate of 65% with 11.4% cretins, many of whom were severely affected; the village was known locally as 'the village of idiots'. Children aged 10 had a mental development equivalent to those aged 7 elsewhere. Girls from other villages did not want to marry and live there. Economic development was retarded, with no truck driver or teacher available in the village.

Iodized salt was then introduced in 1978 and within 4 years the goitre rate had dropped to 4%. No cretins were born after 1978. People's attitude changed greatly and they became much more positive. Their average income increased from 43 yuan in 1981 to 223 yuan in 1982 and 414 yuan in 1984; by then, income was higher than the average income per capita in the district. In 1983 cereals were exported for the first time. Before iodization no family had a radio, but after 55 families acquired a TV set. Ten years later 44 girls had come from other villages to marry boys in Jixian. Seven men had joined the People's Liberation Army, whereas before they had been rejected for goitre. These effects can be largely attributed to the correction of community hypothyroidism by iodized salt, and indicate the important social and economic benefits that can result from the correction of severe iodine deficiency.

Iodine-induced hyperthyroidism

The main hazard of iodization is transient hyperthyroidism, seen mainly in those over the age of 40 (Connolly et al 1970, Stewart et al 1971). It is caused by autonomous thyroid function resulting from long-standing iodine deficiency (Vidor et al 1973). It can be reduced by minimizing iodization in those over the age of 40 (Stanbury et al 1974). In the long term, as IDD is prevented, this therapeutic hyperthyroidism will disappear.

Requirements for iodine

Given the data obtained on prevalence, data on IDD in relation to iodine intakes and the effects of therapy, it is possible to develop recommendations for the prevention of these disorders. The usual recommended level for the population's mean intake of iodine is 100–150 µg/day. This level is adequate to maintain the normal thyroid function that is essential for growth and development. In the presence of goitrogens in the diet, intake should increase to 200–300 µg/day. This higher intake should therefore apply to those areas where a high intake of goitrogen can be expected, e.g. in those populations with a heavy reliance on cassava, maize, bamboo shoots, sweet potatoes, lima beans and millets. The US RDAs in 1989 are shown in Table 36.8; these are endorsed by WHO (Appendix 2). The recent UK reference values are included, showing similar values but set out to encompass the range from the lowest to the highest requirement value. The US RDA values in childhood are in general equivalent to the lower RNI in the UK, but neither country has seen it necessary to make allowances for substantial goitrogen intake.

METHODS FOR CORRECTING IODINE DEFICIENCY

Iodized salt has been the method favoured since the 1920s, when it was first successfully used in Switzerland (Burgi et al 1990). Since then, successful programmes have been reported (Dunn et al 1986) from many countries, e.g. in Central and South America, Guatemala, Colombia, in Europe (Finland) and in Asia (China and Taiwan).

The difficulties in producing and maintaining enough high-quality iodized salt for millions of people are vividly demonstrated in India, where there has been a breakdown in supply. The Indian government aimed to adopt universal salt iodization by 1992. In Asia, the cost of iodized salt production and

Table 36.8 Recommended intakes of iodine

	Population requirements (μg/day)			
	US RDA intake		UK reference nutrient intakes	
Age		Age	Lower	Upper
0–6 months	40	0–3 months	40	50
		3–6 months	40	60
6–12 months	50	6–12 months	40	60
		1–3 years	40	70
1–10 years	70–120	4–6 years	50	100
		7–10 years	55	110
11 years to adulthood	120–150	11–14 years	65	130
		15–18 years	70	140
		Adults	70	140
Pregnancy	175	} No increments for either		
Lactation	175			

distribution at present is of the order of 3–5 cents per person per year (Hetzel et al 1987). This must be considered cheap in relation to the social benefits, but there is still the problem of the salt reaching the people in need. Distribution is difficult and the iodine content will fall if the salt is left uncovered or exposed to heat. People may also not be told that the salt should be added after cooking, to reduce the iodine loss. Cooking reduces the iodine content of foods – with frying and grilling by about 20–25%, but boiling may involve losses of up to 60%.

Finally there is the difficulty of making sure the salt is eaten when distributed. Although there is no difference in taste, the introduction of a new variety of salt when the old type is appreciated and familiar is likely to be resisted. For example, in the Chinese Provinces of Sinjiang and Inner Mongolia, so strong was the preference for desert salt of very low iodine content that a mass programme to inject iodized oil was needed before cretinism could be prevented (Ma et al 1982).

Iodized oil by injection

Controlled trials in New Guinea established the value of injected iodized oil in the prevention of goitre and cretinism (Pharoah et al 1971). The injections can be administered through local health services where they exist, or by special teams. In New Guinea the injection of a population in excess of 100 000 was carried out by public health teams, along with immunization with triple antigen. Iodized oil Lipiodol, a poppyseed oil in which 1 ml contains 480 mg iodine (Guerbet, Paris, France) is suitable for use in a mass programme. Injections, together with the massive distribution of iodized salt, have been effective in Indonesia (Hetzel et al 1987, Dunn 1987), and in China injec-

tions are given by barefoot doctors (Ma et al 1982). Iodized walnut oil and iodized soya bean oil are new preparations developed in China since 1980 (Dunn 1987). The oil should be administered to all females up to the age of 40 years, and all males up to the age of 20 years. A repeat of the injection would be required in 3–5 years, depending on the dose given and the age (Buttfield & Hetzel 1967). In children the need is greater than in adults, and the recommended dose should be repeated in 3 years if severe iodine deficiency persists. Iodized oil is singularly appropriate for isolated village communities characteristic of mountainous endemic goitre areas such as Nepal. The striking regression of goitre following iodized oil injection ensures general acceptance of the measure (Hetzel 1987). There are advantages to the use of injections because people link them with the benefit of the recent successful smallpox eradication campaign. The disadvantages are the immediate discomfort produced and the risk of transmission of infection such as hepatitis B and AIDS. Sensitivity phenomena have not been reported.

However, the major problem of injections is their cost, although this has been reduced with mass packaging to a cost not far in excess of that of iodized salt, especially if the population to be injected is restricted to women of reproductive age and children, and the primary health care team is already available to undertake the injections (Dunn et al 1986, Hetzel et al 1987).

Iodized oil by mouth

A single oral dose of iodized oil may be effective for 1–2 years, and has been used in South America and in Burma. Oral administration of iodized oil to women and children could be carried out through maternal and child health centres and schools – a 1 ml dose is effective in Tanzania for 12 months. Recent studies in India and China reveal that oral iodized oil lasts only half as long as a similar dose given by injection, so more extensive studies are needed to assess the effectiveness of this approach (Dunn 1987).

Iodized bread and iodized water have also been used for special problem areas, but the two real alternatives for mass use are iodized salt and iodized oil (Dunn 1987).

ASSESSING IODINE-DEFICIENCY DISORDERS FOR PUBLIC HEALTH PROGRAMMES

In public health programmes carrying out iodine supplementation, the problem is to assess a population or group living in an area or region that is suspected of being iodine-deficient. Comprehensive studies on methods are available (e.g. Stanbury & Hetzel 1980, Dunn et al 1986, Hetzel et al 1987) but, briefly, one needs:

1. Population statistics, including the number of children under 15 years of age in whom the effects of iodine deficiency are so important;
2. The goitre rate, including the prevalences of palpable or visible goitre classified according to accepted criteria;
3. The rates of cretinism and 'cretinoidism' in the population;
4. Urinary iodine excretion;
5. The level of iodine in the drinking water;
6. The level of serum thyroxine (T_4) in various age groups. Particular attention is now focused on the levels in the neonate because of the importance of the T_4 level for early brain development.

Basic population data are usually available and must be used to develop comprehensive iodization programmes. There are difficulties in reaching the whole iodine-deficient population, especially because of the remoteness of many of these communities. Observing schoolchildren is one method, with advantages of access and convenience, and this has been used extensively in most surveys.

A classification of goitre severity has been adopted by the World Health Organization (Thilly et al 1980). There are still minor differences in technique among different observers. In general, visible goitre is more readily verified than the palpable type. The most recent authoritative review of the classification of goitre and cretinism was carried out at the PAHO/WHO meeting in Lima, November 1983 (Dunn et al 1986).

Definition of goitre

The normal thyroid gland is not usually palpable. The generally accepted definition of the normal thyroid is that of Perez et al (1960): 'A thyroid gland whose lateral lobes have a volume greater than the terminal phalanges of the thumbs of the person examined will be considered goitrous'. Table 36.9 describes the different stages or grades of goitre.

A surface outline technique for the assessment of goitre has been introduced (McLennan & Gaitan 1974), while more recently sonography has been described (Wachter et al 1987). The latter holds promise for increasing the objectivity of surveys, as there is a large subjective element in the assessment.

An area is arbitrarily defined as having a public health problem if more than 10% of the population or of children aged 6–12 are found to be goitrous. This figure is chosen because a prevalence below this level is not uncommon, even when all known environmental factors are apparently controlled.

Definition of endemic cretinism

Cretinism is endemic when:

1. *Epidemiological assessment* shows it to be associated with endemic goitre and severe iodine deficiency.
2. *Clinical manifestations* comprise mental deficiency, together with either a) a predominant neurological syndrome including defects of hearing and speech, squint, and characteristic disorders of stance and gait of varying degree; or b) predominant hypothyroidism and stunted growth. Although in some regions one of the two types may predominate, in other areas a combination of the two syndromes will occur.
3. Prevention is demonstrated by adequate correction of iodine deficiency.

It is now clear that endemic cretinism represents only the extreme end of a broad spectrum of develop-

Table 36.9 Description of different stages of goitre (From Dunn et al 1986)

Stage 0	No goitre
Stage Ia	Goitre detectable only by palpation and not visible even when the neck is fully extended
Stage Ib	Goitre palpable and visible only when the neck is fully extended. This stage also includes nodular glands, even if not goitrous
Stage II	Goitre visible with the neck in normal position; palpation is not needed for diagnosis
Stage III	Very large goitre that can be recognized at a considerable distance

mental abnormalities, including decreased intellectual and delayed psychomotor performance such as a delay in motor milestones and the age of walking. These abnormalities are also prevented by correcting iodine deficiency.

Survey methods are reviewed by Thilly et al (1980) and are still valid. Schoolchildren should be examined as a first step because of their availability and susceptibility to goitre. If the goitre prevalence in a representative sample exceeds 10% then the total population should be studied more intensively.

The level of iodine in drinking water indicates the level of iodine in the soil, which in turn determines the level of iodine in the crops and animals in the area. Iodine levels of water in iodine-deficient areas are usually below 2 µg/l (2 ppm).

Urine iodine excretion should also be carried out by a reliable laboratory. Measurements of 24-hour excretion are desirable but difficult to implement in the field. The range of iodine excretion in casual samples of approximately 30–40 children provides a good indication of the level of iodine nutrition as originally proposed by Follis (1964). In the past the level has usually been expressed as a ratio to the creatinine content, i.e. in micrograms of iodine per gram creatinine, to correct for urinary volume changes. However, the level of creatinine may also be affected by severe malnutrition or a failure to preserve the urine. The simple concentration of iodine for a sample of 40 subjects is now considered to be satisfactory (Thilly et al 1987).

The level of serum thyroxine (T_4) provides an indirect measure of iodine nutritional status. Radioimmunoassay methods with automated equipment have greatly assisted this approach. Particular attention should be given to levels of T_4 in the neonate; levels below 4 µg% must be regarded as prejudicial to brain development (Burrow 1980).

Neonatal hypothyroid screening has been initiated in several less developed and iodine-deficient regions. Within an iodine-deficient population, serum T_4 levels are lowest at birth and lower in children than in the adult population. In addition, goitrogens such as cassava seem to be much more potent at reducing serum T_4 levels in neonates and children than in adults (Delange et al 1982). This may be a critical factor, since T_4 levels are then lowest at the most crucial time of development, especially brain development. There is thus a strong argument for extending neonatal hypothyroid screening beyond the developed countries to regions where iodine deficiency may be a problem, to assess the severity of iodine deficiency for public health purposes by suitable population sampling.

Experience over the past 2 years now indicates that TSH is more stable under tropical conditions and is now the generally preferred determination both for the developed world and for developing countries.

Further special investigations of intellectual status and psychomotor activity may be carried out for research purposes (Bleichrodt et al 1987). The type of test has to be considered carefully because of cultural bias. Data on children's school performance may also be useful.

Data indicating the socioeconomic impact of IDD and its control are of great importance in providing justification for public health programmes. A recent review has provided guidelines for such studies (Levin 1987).

To summarize, the most critical evidence is that obtained from measuring urinary iodine and from measuring TSH levels in the population, including the neonate. The results of these two determinations indicate the severity of the problem. They can also be used to assess the effectiveness of remedial measures.

NATIONAL PROGRAMMES FOR CONTROL OF IODINE-DEFICIENCY DISORDERS

A global strategy should be based on national and regional iodization programmes. The particular methods to be adopted to correct iodine deficiency will vary by region and by nation. This may depend on the availability of salt, its pattern of consumption, and the acceptability of iodized salt. Iodized oil, both on a small scale in isolated mountainous regions and on a large scale, has provided a major alternative to iodized salt in many countries such as Zaire, where using iodized salt is not feasible.

The gradations of severity of IDD provide the indications for an iodization programme. The classifications based on urinary iodine may be extended to the following general recommendations (Hetzel 1987):

1. Mild IDD (Grade 1): with urinary iodine, median values in the range 50–10 µg/dl, requires iodized salt (or possibly economic development alone) for the correction and the prevention of goitre.
2. Moderate IDD (Grade 2): with median urinary iodine in the range 2–5.0 µg/dl requires an effective iodized salt programme; often iodized oil may be necessary in addition, to produce a quantitative correction for the more severely iodine-deficient groups.
3. Severe IDD (Grade 3): with median urinary iodine values below 2.0 µg/dl, iodized oil is required for quantitative correction. Iodized salt might be used

as a follow-up measure if economic development permits; but if subsistence agriculture continues, administration of iodized oil needs to be continued.

The availability of suitable technology is a basic need, but is only one element in an effective iodization programme. Political, social and economic factors are all relevant to the success or failure (Clugston et al 1987) of these programmes.

Fig. 36.12 provides a convenient representation of the relations among these various elements. The steps listed below could be considered as a series of objectives in an iodization programme (Hetzel 1987).

1. Assessment (collect data and assess situation)
2. Communication (i.e. disseminate the findings of step 1)
3. Planning (develop or update plan of action)
4. Political decision (achieve political support)
5. Implementation
6. Monitoring and evaluation

The process then begins a further cycle with new data, dissemination of the results of the first programme, and development of an improved programme to correct the deficiencies of the first.

It should be emphasized that prevention and eradication of IDD require constant vigilance, with regular

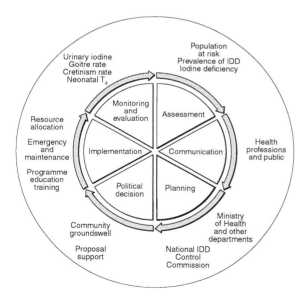

Fig. 36.12 A model showing the social process involved in a National IDD Control Programme. The successful achievement of this process requires the establishment of a National IDD Control Commission, with full political and legislative authority to carry it out. (Reproduced with permission from Hetzel 1987.)

feedback of epidemiological data including estimates of the iodine content of salt, the iodine content of urine in the vulnerable population (especially school-children, who are readily accessible through school attendance), goitre prevalence and levels of TSH, including neonates if possible.

Assessment

Multiple regional measurements are usually necessary. Urinary iodine and neonatal levels of serum TSH are desirable in samples from total populations living in an iodine-deficient area. Laboratories with suitable equipment for determining urinary and water iodine (and salt iodine) are essential. The determination of TSH can now be conveniently carried out by radioimmunoassay from spots of blood on filter paper. These samples can be sent by post to central laboratories for processing. Automated equipment permits large numbers of samples to be tested cheaply (Hetzel & Maberly 1986, Burrow 1980). Goitre surveys of selected samples of the population at the highest risk are now preferred to time-consuming goitre surveys of the whole population.

Communication

The results of the surveys must be disseminated among administrators, politicians, health professionals and the public. Recent findings on the impact of iodine deficiency on human growth and development are not well known among health professionals and health administrators in developing countries, so there is a real need to educate them. The key message to be 'marketed' through all the means available is that the terrible consequence of iodine deficiency are totally preventable. This message must be stated in a way that is easily understood by the communities at risk and by their leaders.

Planning

Recent experience indicates the need for appropriate national IDD Control Commissions with legislative and political support to be responsible for control programmes. These commissions should have representatives from various government departments (health, education, industry) as well as the salt industry, the pharmaceutical industry, the university system and the media.

The distribution of iodized salt remains the major approach for most programmes, but its limitations have now become apparent. In areas of severe iodine deficiency in China, for example, effective iodized salt production and distribution has not always been possible for the huge populations affected. In these circumstances mass administration of iodized oil by injection or orally is feasible through the primary health care system.

Political decision

The resources required for major iodization programmes have to be provided by political decision-making. To obtain the attention of politicians it is often important to have evidence of support within the community. Before a 'ground swell' of opinion can be fostered, it is necessary to ensure that the information on the disabilities caused by IDD are widely publicized. The loss of productivity and the poor quality of life need to be emphasized in schools, clinics and other centres, as well as through the media. Thus marketing strategies must be developed (Hetzel et al 1987).

Implementation

Implementing an iodization programme can follow once the necessary political support has been obtained and allocation of resources made.

Implementation involves discussion, planning and coordination by various government departments such as nutrition, family planning and mental health. Training programmes will be required for staff from these sections, as well as for the personnel actually carrying out the programme.

Monitoring and evaluation

The most direct method of assessing success or failure in correcting iodine deficiency is by determining urinary iodine. Evidence of regression of goitre rates and the prevention of cretinism will then emerge. If laboratory services permit, measuring blood TSH in adults or neonatal TSH in cord blood samples will also indicate whether iodine deficiency has been corrected.

Monitoring and evaluation are essential for iodization programmes, particularly because there is a need to ensure that the iodine deficiency is quantitatively corrected in order to reduce fetal damage and impaired mental function in children (Fig. 36.13). Priority must be given to areas and regions with severe IDD. This means that resources and technology must be focused. Both injection or oral administration of iodized oil should be available. The teams and organization already

developed in many countries for the extended programme immunization (EPI) programmes can be of great value to an iodized oil injection programme in a region with severe IDD, with population targets and costs specified.

Such a transition has taken place in Nepal, where some 2 million injections of iodized oil have been given in 28 remote northern districts where iodized salt could not be distributed. A single injection of the oil (1 ml) provided an adequate supply for prevention of IDD for about 4 years (Acharya 1987).

National plans need to be made, specifying sequential population targets and the costs. Severe IDD should have particular attention.

INTERNATIONAL ACTION

The gap between our new knowledge of IDD and the application of control programmes in developing coun-

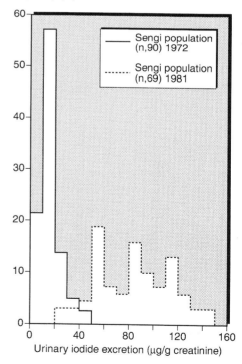

Fig. 36.13 Effect of iodized salt and iodized oil programme in Central Java. Several iodine deficiency was indicated by low urine excretion in 1972, with a 7% rate of cretinism. In 1981 an evaluation indicated that a normal urine iodine (interrupted line) was associated with total prevention of cretinism since 1974 when the programme began. (Reproduced with permission from Hetzel 1987.)

tries has led to the formation of the International Council for the Control of Iodine Deficiency Disorders (ICCIDD). The inaugural meeting of this multidisciplinary group of epidemiologists, nutritionists, endocrinologists, chemists, planners and economists was held in Kathmandu, Nepal, in March 1986. All aspects of IDD control programmes were presented in a monograph (Hetzel et al 1987). The ICCIDD has established a global multidisciplinary network of some 300 people with expertise relevant to IDD and IDD control programmes. It works closely with WHO, UNICEF and national governments within the UN system in the development of national programmes. The feasibility of substantial progress in the prevention and control of IDD in the next 5–10 years was endorsed in a World Health Assembly Resolution in 1986, and this was reinforced in 1990.

A Global Strategy for a Ten-Year Programme for the elimination of IDD as a public health problem by the year 2000 has now been adopted by the UN agencies, and in September 1990 the World Summit for Children, held at the United Nations in New York, was attended by 71 heads of state and 80 other government representatives. The World Summit signed a declaration and approved a plan of action which included the elimination of IDD as a public health problem by the year 2000. This was followed in October 1991 by a conference entitled 'Ending hidden hunger'. This was a policy and promotional meeting on micronutrients including iodine, vitamin A, and iron, attended by multidisciplinary delegations from 55 countries with major IDD problems. There was a firm commitment at this meeting to the goal of eliminating IDD and vitamin A deficiency and to reducing iron deficiency by one-third of the level in 1990.

These objectives were accepted following the previous triumphs of smallpox eradication and the success of the expanded programme of immunization which was celebrated at the United Nations in October 1990.

These various developments encourage the hope that very significant progress can be made towards the elimination of IDD within the next decade. This should bring great benefits to the quality of life of the many millions of people affected by this preventable disorder (Hetzel 1989).

REFERENCES

Acharya S 1987 Monitoring and evaluation of an IDD control program in Nepal. In: Hetzel BS, Dunn JT, Stanbury JB (eds) The prevention and control of iodine deficiency disorders. Elsevier, Amsterdam, pp 213–216

Bleichrodt N, Garcia I, Rubio C et al 1987 Development disorders associated with severe iodine deficiency. In: Hetzel BS, Dunn JT, Stanbury JB (eds) The prevention and control of iodine disorders. Elsevier, Amsterdam, pp 65–84

Bourdoux P, Mafuta A, Hanson A, Ermans AM 1980 Cassava toxicity: the role of linamarin. In: Ermans A (ed) Role of cassava in the etiology of endemic goiter and cretinism. International Development Research Center, Canada, pp 15–27

Boyages SC, Halpern J-P, Maberly GF et al 1988 A comparative study of neurological and myxedematous endemic cretinism in Western China. Journal of Clinical Endocrinology and Metabolism 67: 1261–1271

Boyages SC, Collins JK, Maberly GF et al 1988 Iodine deficiency impairs intellectual and neuromotor development in apparently normal people: a study of rural inhabitants from North Central China. Medical Journal of Australia 150: 676–682

Burgi H, Supersaxo Z, Selz B 1990 Iodine deficiency diseases in Switzerland one hundred years after Theodor Kocher's survey. A historical review with some new goitre prevalence data. Acta Endocrinologica 123: 577–590

Burrow GN 1980 Neonatal thyroid screening. Raven Press, New York

Buttfield IH, Hetzel BS 1967 Endemic goitre in Eastern New Guinea with special reference to the use of iodized oil in prophylaxis and treatment. Bulletin of the World Health Organization 36: 243–262

Clugston GA, Dulberg EM, Pandav CS, Tilden R L 1987 Iodine deficiency disorders in South East Asia. In: Hetzel BS, Dunn JT, Stanbury JB (eds) The prevention and control of iodine deficiency disorders. Elsevier, Amsterdam, pp 273–308

Connolly KJ, Pharoah POD, Hetzel BS 1979 Fetal iodine deficiency and motor performance during childhood. Lancet 2: 1149–1151

Connolly RJ, Vidor GI, Stewart JC 1970 Increase in thyrotoxicosis in endemic goiter area after iodation of bread. Lancet 1: 500–502

Costa A, Cottino F, Mortara M, Vogliazzo U 1964 Endemic cretinism in Piedmont. Panminerva Medicine 6: 250–259

Crantz FR, Larsen PR 1980 Rapid thyroxine to 3,5,3'-triiodothyronine conversion and nuclear 3,5,3'-triiodothyronine binding in rat cerebral cortex and cerebellum. Journal of Clinical Investigation 65: 935–938

Delange F, Iteke FB, Ermans AM (eds) 1982 Nutritional factors involved in the goitrogenic action of cassava. International Development Research Center, Canada

Delange F, Heidemann P, Bourdoux P et al 1986 Regional variations of iodine nutrition and thyroid function during the neonatal period in Europe. Biology of the Neonate 49: 322–330

Djokomoeljanto R, Tarwotjo I, Maspaitella F 1983 Goitre control program in Indonesia. In: Ui N, Torizuka K, Nagataki S, Miyai K (eds) Current problems in thyroid research. Excerpta Medica, Amsterdam 605: 394–397

Dulberg EM, Widjaja K, Djokomoeljanto R, Hetzel BS, Belmont L 1983 Evaluation of the iodinization programme in Central Java with reference to the prevention of endemic cretinism and motor coordination defects. In: Ui N, Torizuka K, Nagataki S, Miyai K (eds)

Current problems in thyroid research. Excerpta Medica, Amsterdam, pp 19–22

Dunn JT 1987 Iodized oil in the treatment and prophylaxis of IDD. In: Hetzel BS, Dunn JT, Stanbury JB (eds) The prevention and control of iodine deficiency disorders. Elsevier, Amsterdam, pp 127–134

Dunn JT, Pretell EA, Daza CH, Viteri FE (eds) 1986 Towards the eradiction of endemic goitre, cretinism, and iodine deficiency. Scientific Publication No 502, PAHO, Washington

Ermans AM, Bourdoux P, Lagasse R et al 1980 Congenital hypothyroidism in developing countries. In: Burrow G (ed) Neonatal thyroid screening. Raven Press, New York, pp 61–73

European Thyroid Association 1985 Goitre and iodine deficiency in Europe. Lancet 2: 1289–1292

Feirro-Benitez R, Stanbury JB, Querido A et al 1970 Endemic cretinism in the Andean region of Ecuador. Journal of Clinical Endocrinology and Metabolism 30: 228–236

Fierro-Benitez R, Cazar D, Stanbury JB et al 1986 Long-term effect of correction of iodine deficiency on psychomotor and intellectual development. In: Dunn JT, Pretell EA, Daza CH, Viteri FE (eds) Towards the eradication of endemic goiter, cretinism, and iodine deficiency. PAHO, Washington, pp 182–200

Follis RH 1964 Recent studies in iodine malnutrition and endemic goitre. Medical Clinics of North America 48: 1919–1924

Hetzel BS 1970 The control of iodine deficiency. Medical Journal of Australia 2: 615

Hetzel BS 1983 Iodine deficiency disorders (IDD) and their eradication. Lancet 2: 1126–1129

Hetzel BS 1987 An overview of the prevention and control of iodine deficiency disorders. In: Hetzel BS, Dunn JT, Stanbury JB (eds) The prevention and control of iodine deficiency disorders. Elsevier, Amsterdam, pp 7–31

Hetzel BS 1989 The story of iodine deficiency: an international challenge in nutrition. Oxford University Press, Oxford

Hetzel BS, Maberly GF 1986 Iodine. In: Mertz W (ed) Trace elements in human and animal nutrition, 5th edn. Academic Press, San Diego, pp 139–208

Hetzel BS, Potter BJ 1983 Iodine deficiency and the role of thyroid hormones in brain development. In: Dreosti I, Smith RM (eds) Neurobiology of the trace elements. Humana Press, New Jersey, pp 83–133

Hetzel BS, Dunn JT, Stanbury JB (eds) 1987 The prevention and control of iodine deficiency disorders. Elsevier, Amsterdam

Hetzel BS, Potter BJ, Dulberg EM 1990 The iodine deficiency disorders: nature, pathogenesis and epidemiology. In: Bourne G H (ed) World review of nutrition and dietetics, Vol 62. S Karger, Basel, pp 59–119

Karmarkar MG, Deo MG, Kochupillai N, Ramalingaswami V 1974 Pathophysiology of Himalayan endemic goitre. American Journal of Clinical Nutrition 27: 96–103

Kelly FC, Snedden WW 1960 Prevalence and geographical distribution of endemic goitre. In: Clements FW, de Moerloose J, de Smet MP et al (eds) Endemic goitre. Monograph series no. 44 World Health Organization, Geneva, pp 27–333

Kochupillai N, Pandav CS 1987 Neonatal chemical hypothyroidism in iodine deficient environments. In:

Hetzel BS, Dunn JT, Stanbury JB (eds) The prevention and control of iodine deficiency disorders. Elsevier, Amsterdam, pp 85–93

Konig MP, Veraguth P 1961 Studies of thyroid function in endemic cretins. In: Pitt-Rivers R (ed) Advances in thyroid research. Pergamon Press, London, pp 294–298

Koutras DA 1986 Iodine: distribution, availability and effects of deficiency on the thyroid. In: Towards the eradication of endemic goitre, cretinism and iodine deficiency. Pan American Health Organization, Washington DC, pp 15–27

Langer P 1960 History of goitre. In: Endemic goitre. World Health Organization, Geneva, pp 9–25

Levin HM 1987 Economic dimensions of iodine deficiency disorders. In: Hetzel BS, Dunn JT, Stanbury JB (eds) The prevention and control of iodine deficiency disorders. Elsevier, Amsterdam, pp 195–208

Li Jianqun, Wang Xin 1987 Jixian: a success story in IDD control. IDD Newsletter 3: 4–5

Li Jianqun, Wang Xin, Yan Yugin et al 1985 The effects of a severely iodine-deficient diet derived from an endemic area on fetal brain development in the rat – observations in the first generation. Neuropathology and Applied Neurobiology 12: 261–276

Ma Tai, Lu Tizhang, Tan Uybin, Chen Bingshong, Zhu HI 1982 The present status of endemic goiter and endemic cretinism in China. Food and Nutrition Bulletin 4: 13–19

Maberly GF, Eastman G, Waite KV et al 1983 The role of cassava. In: Ui N, Torizuka K, Nagataki S, Miyai K (eds) Current problems in thyroid research. Excerpta Medica, Amsterdam, pp 341–344

McCarrison R 1908 Observations on endemic cretinism in the Chitral and Gilgit Valleys. Lancet 2: 1275–1280

McIntosh GH, Potter BJ, Mano MT et al 1983 The effect of maternal and fetal thyroidectomy on fetal brain development in the sheep. Neuropathology and Applied Neurobiology 9: 215–223

MacLennan R, Gaitan E 1974 Measurement of thyroid size in epidemiological surveys. In: Dunn JT, Medeiros-Neto GA (eds) Endemic goitre and cretinism: continuing threats to world health. Scientific Publication 292, PAHO, Washington, pp 195–197

McMichael AJ, Potter JD, Hetzel BS 1980 Iodine deficiency, thyroid function, and reproductive failure. In: Stanbury JB, Hetzel BS (eds) Endemic goitre and endemic cretinism. Wiley, New York, pp 445–460

Mano MT, Potter BJ, Belling GB, Hetzel BS 1985 Low-iodine diet for the production of severe I deficiency in marmosets (Callithrix jacchus jacchus). British Journal of Nutrition 54: 367–372

Mano MT, Potter BJ, Belling GB et al 1987 Fetal brain development in response to iodine deficiency in a primate model (Callithrix jacchus jacchus). Journal of Neurological Sciences 79: 287–300

Morreale de Escobar G, Pastor R, Obregon MJ, Escobar Del Rey F 1985 Effects of maternal hypothyroidism on weight and thyroid hormone content of rat embryonic tissues, before and after onset of fetal thyroid function. Endocrinology 117: 1890–1900

Muzzo S, Leiva L, Carrasco D 1986 Influence of a moderate iodine deficiency upon intellectual coefficient of school age children. In: Medeiros-Neto GA, Maciel R, Halpern A (eds) Iodine deficiency disorders and congenital hypothyroidism. Ache, Sao Paulo, pp 40–45

Obregon J, Mallol R, Pastor G et al 1984a L-thyroxine and 3,5,3′ Triiodo-L-thyronine in rat embryos before onset of fetal thyroid function. Endocrinology 114: 305–307

Obregon MJ, Santisteban P, Rodriguez-pena A et al 1984b Cerebral hypothyroidism in rats with adult-onset iodine deficiency. Endocrinology 115: 614–624

Perez C, Scrimshaw NS, Munoz JA 1960 Technique of endemic goitre surveys. In: Endemic goitre. World Health Organization, Geneva, pp 369–383

Pharoah POD, Connolly DC 1987 A controlled trial of iodinated oil for the prevention of endemic cretinism: a long-term follow-up. International Journal of Epidemiology 16: 68–73

Pharoah POD, Buttfield IH, Hetzel BS 1971 Neurological damage to the fetus resulting from severe iodine deficiency during pregnancy. Lancet 1: 308–310

Pharoah POD, Delange F, Fierro-Benitez R, Stanbury JB 1980 Endemic cretinism. In: Stanbury JB, Hetzel BS (eds) Endemic goitre and endemic cretinism. Wiley, New York, pp 395–421

Pharoah POD, Connolly KJ, Hetzel BS, Ekins RP 1981 Maternal thyroid function and motor competence in the child. Developmental Medicine and Child Neurology 23: 76–82

Potter BJ, Mano MT, Belling GB et al 1982 Retarded fetal brain development resulting from severe dietary iodine deficiency in sheep. Neuropathology and Applied Neurobiology 8: 303–313

Sooch SS, Deo MG, Karmarkar MG et al 1973 Prevention of endemic goitre with iodized salt. Bulletin WHO 49: 307–312

Stanbury JB, Hetzel BS (eds) 1980 Endemic goitre and endemic cretinism: Iodine nutrition in health and disease. Wiley, New York

Stanbury JB, Brownell GL, Riggs DS et al (eds) 1954 The adaptation of man to iodine deficiency. Harvard University Press, Cambridge, pp 11–209

Stanbury JB, Ermans AM, Hetzel BS et al 1974 Endemic goitre and cretinism: public health significance and prevention. World Health Organization Chronicle 28: 220–228

Stewart JC, Vidor GI, Buttfield IH, Hetzel BS 1971 Epidemic thyrotoxicosis in Northern Tasmania: studies of clinical features and iodine nutrition. Australian and New Zealand Journal of Medicine 1: 203–211

Thilly CH 1981 Goitre et crétinisme endémiques: role étiologique de la consommation de manioc et stratégie d'éradication. Bulletin of Belgian Academy of Medicine 136: 389–412

Thilly CH, Delange F, Stanbury JB 1980 Epidemiologic surveys in endemic goitre and cretinism. In: Stanbury JB, Hetzel BS (eds) Endemic goitre and endemic cretinism: iodine nutrition in health and disease. Wiley, New York, pp 157–184

Thilly CH, Bourdoux P, Swennen B et al 1987 Assessment and planning for IDD control programs. In: Hetzel BS, Dunn JT, Stanbury JB (eds) The prevention and control of iodine deficiency disorders. Elsevier, Amsterdam, pp 181–194

Vidor GI, Stewart JC, Wall JR et al 1973 Pathogenesis of iodine-induced thyrotoxicosis: studies in Northern Tasmania. Journal of Clinical Endocrinology and Metabolism 37: 901–909

Vulsma T, Gons MH, de Vijlder JJM 1989 Maternal–fetal transfer of thyroxine in congenital hypothyroidism due to a total organification defect or thyroid agenesis. New England Journal of Medicine 321: 13–16

Wachter W, Pickhardt CR, Gutekunst R et al 1987 Use of ultrasonography for goitre assessment in IDD. Studies in Tanzania. In: Hetzel BS, Dunn JT, Stanbury JB (eds) The prevention and control of iodine deficiency disorders. Elsevier, Amsterdam, pp 95–108

Woods RJ, Sinha AK, Ekins RP 1984 Uptake and metabolism of thyroid hormones by the rat fetus in early pregnancy. Clinical Science 67: 359–363

World Health Organization 1990 Report to the 43rd World Health Assembly, Geneva

Zhong Fu-guang, Cao Xu-mao, Liu Jia-liu 1983 Experimental study on influence of iodine deficiency on fetal brain in rats. Chinese Journal of Pathology 12: 205–208

Zhu XY 1983 The present status of endemic goitre and endemic cretinism in China, with special reference to studies in Gui-Zhou on the changes of iodine metabolism and pituitary thyroid functional status two years after iodine prophylaxis. In: Ui N, Torizuka K, Nagataki S, Miyai K (eds) Current problems in thyroid research. Excerpta Medica, Amsterdam, pp 13–20

37. Clinical nutrition and bone disease

R. Smith

Bone disease may result from nutritional deficiency or nutritional excess (Table 37.1). Although it is difficult to demonstrate that calcium deficiency alone causes bone disease in man, there is some evidence to relate peak bone mass and subsequent bone loss to calcium intake. For this reason, osteoporosis is included in this chapter as a nutrition-related disease. The bone disorders most clearly related to nutrition are rickets (in childhood) and osteomalacia (in adult life), both due to a deficiency of vitamin D or a disturbance of its metabolism. In the UK (but not in other westernized countries) vitamin D deficiency in the Asian populations of northern cities is the most frequent cause of rickets and osteomalacia. Of the main other causes, some have nutritional relevance.

Table 37.1 Clinical nutrition and bone disease

Nutritional deficiency	Vitamin D	Rickets/osteomalacia
	Vitamin C	Scurvy
	Copper	Fractures (premature infants; parenteral nutrition)
	Pyridoxine	Homocystinuria
Nutritional excess	Vitamin A	Hyperostosis Ligamentous ossification
	Vitamin D	Idiopathic hypercalcaemia in infancy
	Aluminium	Aluminium osteodystrophy (dialysis and parenteral nutrition)
	Fluoride	Endemic Iatrogenic
	Cadmium	Fanconi syndrome Rickets/osteomalacia
Nutrition-related	Calcium	Osteoporosis

In contrast, scurvy due to lack of vitamin C is a very uncommon nutritional disorder in the western world, but it has scientific features which serve to remind us of the importance of the major component of the organic matrix of bone, i.e. collagen (see Chapter 14). In a similar way, lack of copper, especially in small babies or in those on parenteral nutrition, can give rise to bone disease attributable to defective function of the copper-dependent amino acid oxidases, which leads to failure of the collagen cross-link formation.

Bone disease due to nutritional excess is unusual. It can occur in the idiopathic hypercalcaemia of infancy, supposedly related to vitamin D excess in early life, and with hypervitaminosis A, causing generalized cortical hyperostosis in children. Interestingly, treatment of skin disease such as ichthyosis with vitamin A analogues can cause widespread ligamentous calcification. Excess ingestion of fluoride, either in the diet (endemic fluorosis) or as a treatment for osteoporosis, produces marked hyperostotic changes in parts of the skeleton and the ligaments attached to it. The increased use of haemodialysis in chronic renal failure produces a situation which allows the normal selective mechanism of intestinal absorption to be overcome; this can lead to the accumulation of aluminium derived from tap water in dialysis fluid, which produces a variety of bone diseases collectively known as aluminium osteodystrophy. A similar vitamin D-resistant bone disease in patients treated with prolonged parenteral nutrition may be due to aluminium excess. Finally, cadmium excess can also produce bone disease but in a more indirect way. It causes multiple renal tubular abnormalities and generalized aminoaciduria (the Fanconi syndrome), leading to osteomalacia or rickets. (Concise reviews of some of these metabolic bone diseases are provided by Smith 1987, Stevenson 1988, Lindsay 1988, Eisman 1988 and Thakker & O'Riordan 1988.)

SPECIFIC NUTRITIONAL DEFICIENCIES

Osteomalacia and rickets

Osteomalacia in adults and rickets in childhood result from a deficiency of vitamin D or a disturbance of its metabolism (Table 37.2). The physiology of vitamin D has been extensively reviewed (Reichel et al 1989). The relative frequency of these causes differs according to movements of populations and geographical and dietary differences. Thus so-called nutritional or privational rickets became common 30 years ago in Asian immigrants, particularly in Glasgow, which reflected the rickets endemic in the populations of industrial Victorian cities, and had the same main causes (Stamp et al 1980, Stephens et al 1982, Dunnigan et al 1982, Henderson et al 1987). After nutritional vitamin D deficiency coeliac disease is probably the next most frequent cause of rickets or osteomalacia. Many of the other causes (Table 37.2) are very rare (Table 37.3) and do not require further consideration here (Stamp 1982). Inherited hypophosphataemia ('vitamin D-resistant rickets') still provides a difficult clinical problem and is a significant cause of bone disease. The causes of rickets are best understood against the background of our knowledge of

Table 37.2 The main causes of rickets and osteomalacia

Vitamin D deficiency
    Asian immigrants
    Elderly

Malabsorption
    Coeliac disease
    Post-gastrectomy
    Intestinal bypass surgery

Renal disease
    Tubular: Inherited hypophosphataemia
                Fanconi syndrome
    Glomerular: Osteodystrophy
                Dialysis bone disease (Aluminium excess)

Rare
    Vitamin D-dependent rickets:
        Type 1 – 1α-hydroxylase lack
        Type 2 – Vitamin D receptor deficiency
    Oncogenous rickets:
        Mainly mesenchymal tumours

(Aluminium excess and bisphosphonate (EHDP) overdose lead to excess of osteoid, simulating osteomalacia

For an alternative classification, based on the changes in vitamin D metabolites see Tam et al (1989)
For further details see Table 37.3

Table 37.3 Causes and features of some forms of osteomalacia and rickets

Cause	Clinical features	Biochemistry (plasma)	Comments
Renal tubular			
Inherited hypophosphataemia	Short stature No myopathy	Low P only	Usually X-linked dominant Other forms exist
Renal tubular acidosis	Bone disease and nephrocalcinosis	Low P plus acidosis	Treatable by bicarbonate alone
Multiple defects (Fanconi syndrome)			
Cystinosis	Dehydration Deposition of cystine crystals	Low P Severe acidosis	Recessive. Untreated die in late childhood
Oculocerebro-renal, syndrome (Lowe's syndrome)	Cataracts Mental retardation	Low P plus acidosis	X-linked
Acquired (many causes including myeloma)	Rickets/OM plus underlying disorder	For rickets plus cause	Unusual complication of gammopathy
Vitamin D-dependent			
Type I Defective 1α-hydroxylation	Severe rickets plus myopathy	Ca↓P↓P'ase↑	Low 1,25 (OH)$_2$D
Type II Receptor defect	Severe rickets plus alopecia and loss of teeth	Ca↓P↓P'ase↑	High 1,25 (OH)$_2$D
Oncogenous			
Many causes	Adult-onset osteomalacia	Low P	Low 1,25 (OH)$_2$D

OM = osteomalacia

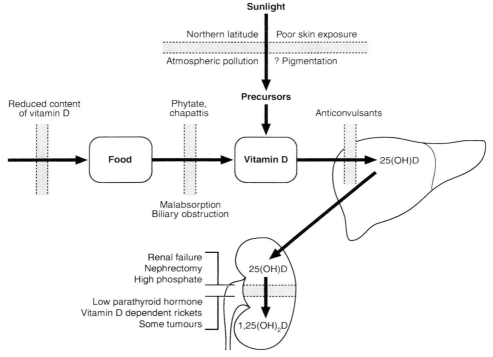

Fig. 37.1   The known main causes of osteomalacia and rickets in relation to the sources and metabolic pathways of vitamin D (see also Fig. 11.3) (from Smith (1987) with permission).
The shaded bars indicate factors which reduce the amount of vitamin D in the body (rectangle) or its subsequent conversion to 1,25 $(OH)_2D$.

vitamin D metabolism (Fig. 37.1). Recent work re-emphasizes the importance of ultraviolet light in vitamin D economy, and the widespread effect of this vitamin/hormone throughout the body (Holick 1987, Webb & Holick 1988).

Diagnosis

The signs and symptoms of rickets/osteomalacia are well described in current paediatric and adult texts (Forfar & Arneil 1984, Behrman & Vaughan 1987). The shared clinical features are deformity, bone pain and tenderness, and proximal muscle weakness. In rickets the enlarged epiphyses and costochondral junctions emphasize that the abnormalities occur at the growing ends of the long bones. The biochemical changes include low plasma calcium, a reduction in plasma phosphate, an increase in the plasma alkaline phosphatase and a reduction in urine calcium excretion. However, the biochemistry of rickets and osteomalacia depends on its cause (Table 37.4). One or other of the biochemical changes may be used to detect osteomalacia; in addition, the measurement of

25-hydroxy vitamin D levels in the plasma can be used to detect vitamin D deficiency. Patients with nutritional osteomalacia will have very low levels of 25-OHD; but not all patients with subnormal 25-OHD develop bone disease. In rickets radiographs show a widened, jagged and cupped metaphysis, and in osteomalacia, Looser zones. These are often bilateral and symmetrical and typically occur in the pubic rami, around the borders of the scapulae and the long bones, but can be seen virtually anywhere in the skeleton. The appearance is of a linear area of failure of mineralization resembling a partial fracture (it is therefore sometimes called a pseudo-fracture). Where necessary, the diagnosis of osteomalacia is confirmed by transiliac bone biopsy.

Examination of the undecalcified sections show an excessive thickness of osteoid and an increased coverage of the mineralized surfaces with unmineralized osteoid. A similar appearance may be seen in hypos-phosphatasia (Eisman 1988) and bisphosphonate overdosage (with disodium etidronate, EHDP), but in these conditions the other features of osteomalacia are not present.

Table 37.4 Biochemical changes in osteomalacia and rickets

Cause	Plasma	Urine	Comments
Nutritional (Vitamin D deficiency)	Ca N or↓P↓P'ase↑	Ca↓	25-OHD↓ 1,25-(OH)$_2$D usually N Also biochemistry of underlying diseases
Malabsorption	Ca N or↓P↓P'ase↑	Ca↓	As for nutritional
Renal Tubular (see also Table 37.3)	Ca N or↓P↓P'ase↑	Ca↓ or N	Those with Fanconi syndrome have systemic acidosis
Glomerular	Ca↓P↑P'ase↑	Ca↓	Biochem of renal failure. 1,25 (OH)$_2$D reduced
Vitamin D deficiency Type I	Ca↓P↓P'ase↑	Ca↓	1,25 (OH)$_2$ low
Type II	Ca↓P↓P'ase	Ca↓	1,25 (OH)$_2$D high
Oncogenous rickets/osteomalacia	Ca N P↓P'ase↑	Ca↓ or N	1,25 (OH)$_2$D low

P'ase = Plasma alkaline phosphatase   N = normal

Special forms of rickets

'Nutritional rickets' This occurs particularly in Asian immigrants in northern cities, but may also be a problem in elderly people who are housebound. Studies in the Asian population have shown that the incidence of osteomalacia is related to reduced exposure to ultraviolet light; where ultraviolet light is limited, dietary factors also become important. Thus in a recent survey of patients with so-called nutritional rickets from UK cities at different latitudes (Coventry, Bradford, and Glasgow) the prevalence increased from south to north. In Glasgow, where estimated ultraviolet exposure is low, dietary factors became increasingly important (Henderson et al 1987). Previous work on rickets and osteomalacia among the Asian population has stressed the contribution of a vegetarian diet and the high consumption of chapattis to these disorders. The possible relationship between dietary calcium deficiency and osteomalacia or rickets has always been a mystery. However, Clements et al (1987) suggest that calcium lack and the ensuing hypocalcaemia which increases the circulating concentration of 1,25 (OH)$_2$D$_3$ increases the breakdown of 25 (OH)D$_3$. Although in theory vitamin D deficiency in Asians could be corrected by exposure to sunlight, this is difficult to achieve in practice.

However, a striking reduction in Asian rickets in Glasgow occurred when free vitamin D supplements became available to children up to 18 years of age in that city (Dunnigan et al 1985).

Although the frequency and importance of vitamin D deficiency is now well established in the Asian immigrant population, it is less well recognized in the Caucasian geriatric patient. In the elderly, especially those in institutions, plasma 25-OH levels are consistently lower throughout the year than in young controls; Bouillon et al (1987) also found that in the elderly group there was a seasonal variation in 1,25 (OH)$_2$D which was absent in the controls. It was suggested that this was due to substrate 25-OHD deficiency. A significant number of elderly persons with femoral neck fracture have osteomalacia as well as osteoporosis, but the exact percentage of those with such fractures is controversial, since it can depend on the investigator's interpretation of bone biopsy findings. Since most patients with proximal femoral fractures do not have bone histology, the presence of osteomalacia is then assessed from biochemical and, in the minority, radiological grounds.

The detection of osteomalacia in the elderly is difficult unless there are clear radiological, biochemical and clinical abnormalities. Bone biopsies suggest a prevalence of some 4% in geriatric units, which increases with age and is more common is women (Campbell et al 1984). Identification of borderline osteomalacia may be helped by a therapeutic trial with vitamin D (Hosking et al 1983).

As for the Asian immigrants, it may be that osteomalacia in the elderly at risk is best prevented by the widespread administration of vitamin D, either as a daily small dose (25 μg) or as a single larger injection (15 mg), or in short courses of relatively large oral doses (for instance, 1.25 mg daily for 2 weeks) (Lancet 1987a). Where larger doses are given, biochemical monitoring is necessary.

Malabsorption

Although the malabsorptive causes of osteomalacia vary with surgical practice, coeliac disease is probably still the most common in this group. With the decline in classic partial gastrectomy, osteomalacia following gastric operations is now rare (Nilas & Christiansen 1987), but it is a predictable problem following bypass surgery for extreme obesity. The skeleton may also be affected in Crohn's disease and ulcerative colitis, but these diseases produce osteoporosis rather than osteomalacia. Such patients are often also taking corticosteroids. The skeleton is rarely affected in liver disease unless this is prolonged. Again, osteoporosis is the most frequent change.

Renal causes

There are many causes of osteomalacia associated with renal disease, and some of these are influenced by nutritional factors (Tables 37.2 and 37.3). They may be divided according to tubular and glomerular causes. The major renal tubular cause of rickets is inherited hypophosphataemia, which is transmitted as an X-linked dominant characteristic, in which the main abnormality is a persistently low plasma phosphate (Thakker & O'Riordan 1988). In contradistinction to phosphate deficiency occurring from overdosage of aluminium hydroxide or other phosphate binders, nuclear magnetic resonance studies suggest that the intracellular phosphate concentration is probably normal (Smith et al 1984). This suggests that there is an inborn abnormality in the exchange of phosphate between intra- and extracellular compartments.

Renal glomerular failure produces a condition known as renal glomerular osteodystrophy, in which defective intestinal absorption of calcium due to a reduction in the production of 1,25-dihydroxy vitamin D is associated with an increase in bone resorption due to an excess of parathyroid hormone. The

stimulation of parathyroid hormone secretion results from hypocalcaemia, itself due to a progressive increase in plasma phosphate as renal insufficiency progresses. The combination of defective mineralization and increased bone resorption produces catastrophic bone disease, particularly in children.

A wide range of bony changes occurs in patients with renal glomerular failure, including osteomalacia, osteoporosis, osteosclerosis and osteitis fibrosa cystica. The exact relationship between these diseases (Kanis et al 1988) and their natural history is not clear, although defective 1-α hydroxylation of 25-hydroxy vitamin D is a common theme (Palma et al 1983). Successful renal transplantation will improve the bony disorders, but they will progress during dialysis. One form of 'dialysis bone disease' in these patients is related to aluminium poisoning (see below). The progression of renal glomerular osteodystrophy may be delayed by preventing the steady increase in plasma phosphate (as the glomerular filtration rate falls); this can be done by reducing dietary phosphate and giving oral phosphate binders.

Other rare forms of rickets

These include vitamin D-dependent rickets and the rickets often associated with mesenchymal non-malignant tumours. Neither of these are nutritional in origin but both provide insights into vitamin D metabolism.

Vitamin D-dependent rickets This is a very rare and heterogeneous syndrome in which the clinical, biochemical and radiological features of vitamin D-deficiency rickets occur without demonstrable lack of vitamin D (Thakker & O'Riordan 1988, Liberman & Marx 1989). For this reason the term 'pseudo vitamin D-deficiency rickets' was originally used. There are two distinct inherited disorders, Type I and Type II. In Type I vitamin D-dependent rickets, 1-α hydroxylation of 25-hydroxy vitamin D is defective and circulating 1,25 $(OH)_2D_3$ levels are very low. In the Type II disorder there is end-organ resistance to 1,25 $(OH)_2D_3$ and the circulating concentrations are high. Type II vitamin D dependency is inherited as a recessive trait (consanguinity is frequent) and, in addition to the features of severe rickets, the infant may have alopecia and abnormal dentition. Recently it has been shown that in these patients there are single base mutations in the gene coding for the 1,25 $(OH)_2D$ receptors which lead to changes in the amino acid sequence in the DNA binding region at the tips of the zinc 'fingers'. The mutations, which are different for each family, presumably account for the end-organ resistance to 1,25 $(OH)_2D_3$ (Hughes et al 1988).

Oncogenous rickets and osteomalacia

Certain mesenchymal tumours (such as fibrosing haemangiomas and haemangiopericytomas) are associated with acquired hypophosphataemic rickets or osteomalacia. The bone disease is cured by their removal, and the initially very low levels of $1,25 (OH)_2D_3$ return to normal. This form of rickets has been described in numerous similar mesenchymal tumours at many different sites. Rickets and osteomalacia may also be associated with osteosarcoma, fibrous dysplasia, neurofibromatosis and linear sebaceous naevus syndrome, and the underlying mechanisms may be similar, although they are largely unknown. There is some evidence that such tumours inhibit 1-α hydroxylation of 25-OHD (Miyauchi et al 1988).

Vitamin C deficiency

Ascorbic acid is essential for the proper synthesis of collagen; in its absence the proline residues in collagen are insufficiently hydroxylated and the collagen is not formed into fibres. The main clinical manifestation of vitamin C deficiency is scurvy. The clinical features in infants are described in paediatric texts (Behrman & Vaughan 1987). An infant with scurvy and periosteal haemorrhage has swollen and tender legs, and lies in a position likened to that of a frog. There is a widespread subperiosteal haemorrhage in the long bones, with cupped and fractured metaphyseal plates. Other changes described in the metaphysis include an opaque line, on the diaphyseal side of which is a zone of bone destruction. There may be evidence of initial calcification of the subperiosteal haemorrhage. During healing the subperiosteal haematomas continue to calcify and may become very clear on X-ray; the scorbutic band in the metaphysis and the ringed appearance of the epiphyses become more obvious. In adults, vitamin C deficiency does not appear to affect the skeleton.

Copper deficiency

Copper is vital for a number of biochemical reactions and particularly for the function of amino acid oxidases. Lysyl oxidase is essential for the synthesis of the lysine aldehydes, which are intermediates in the cross-linking of collagen. Copper deficiency thus leads to bone disease. In addition, copper-related bone disease occurs in an X-linked recessive disorder of copper metabolism, Menkes' syndrome. Copper-related bone disease is also seen in Wilson's disease, but in this instance it is rickets or osteomalacia secondary to the Fanconi syndrome, which in its turn results from the effect of the copper abnormality on the renal tubule.

The bone disease of copper deficiency occurs in premature infants and in those who have been on prolonged parenteral nutrition. It is not described in full-term or breastfed infants. Its features have been reviewed based on 52 cases in the paediatric literature (Shaw 1988). The syndrome in infants includes psychomotor retardation, hypopigmentation, sideroblastic anaemia, neutropenia, hepatosplenomegaly and bone changes; there can be osteoporosis, blurring and cupping of the metaphyses, sickle-shaped metaphyseal spur formation, subperiosteal bleeding and new bone formation and fractures. The plasma copper concentration is normally less than 40 µg/dl, and caeruloplasmin less than 13 mg/dl.

The predisposing factors for this copper deficiency syndrome are low birthweight and a dietary lack of copper, either in parenteral solutions or in copper-deficient (cow's) milk. Antecedent malnutrition due to starvation or malabsorption may contribute in some cases (Chapter 12).

The types of bone disease produced by copper deficiency are important because of their similarity to those of non-accidental injury, and because they may be confused with rickets or scurvy (Shaw 1988). Non-accidental injury usually produces asymmetrical injuries at different stages of healing, and may be associated with signs of neglect.

Pyridoxine: vitamin B_6

Pyridoxine is essential for the function of cystathionine synthase, and inherited homocystinuria is often a vitamin B_6-dependent disease. In this condition there are skeletal abnormalities: the bones appear osteoporotic, the vertebrae are abnormal in shape and the femoral heads appear too large for the acetabuli (Mudd & Levy 1978).

Phosphate deficiency

Hypophosphataemia and whole-body phosphate deficiency may result from persistent treatment with phosphate-binding antacids such as aluminium hydroxide. This is an acquired cause of hypophosphataemic osteomalacia. Bone disease and proximal myopathy is associated with an increase in plasma $1,25 (OH)_2D_3$ secondary to the low phosphate. Hypophosphataemia occurs as an inherited disease, and is one of the causes of apparently vitamin D-resistant rickets (p.559). Myopathy is absent and $1,25 (OH)_2D_3$ not increased. Premature infants may suffer from a lack of phosphate, which is said to contribute to rickets (Lancet 1987b).

SPECIFIC NUTRITIONAL EXCESS

A number of conditions associated with excessive intake of nutrients produce specific disorders of the skeleton (Table 37.1).

Vitamin A excess

Retinoic acid and its derivatives have profound effects on osteoblastic function both in vitro and in vivo (Boyd 1988). There are two main skeletal abnormalities resulting from an excess of vitamin A. The first of these is cortical hyperostosis (seen particularly well in children), and the second is ectopic ossification of the ligaments, seen in adults. In children, prolonged overdosage with vitamin A increases cortical density, particularly of the long bones, but the bones are abnormally fragile and likely to fracture. Other signs of vitamin A intoxication may be present.

The prolonged use of retinoic acid derivatives for skin disease, particularly psoriasis and ichthyosis, can lead to calcification of the ligaments, especially around the spine, where there is also new bone formation, with stiffness and reduced mobility.

Vitamin D excess

Acute intoxication with vitamin D continues to occur either with native vitamin D or with 1,25-dihydroxy vitamin D, or 1-α-hydroxy vitamin D used therapeutically (Davies & Adams 1978). Such acute events do not produce skeletal abnormalities. In the past, it was considered that idiopathic hypercalcaemia of infancy was related to excessive intake of vitamin D in early life. In the severe forms of this disease there is a characteristic appearance (elfin face syndrome), mental simplicity, and sometimes congenital heart disease (William's syndrome). Further study of this disorder suggests an abnormal regulation of 25-OHD levels. The 25-OHD concentration may be increased when the patients are hypercalcaemic (Stern & Bell 1989). Radiographs of the long bones show increased metaphyseal density.

Aluminium excess

In certain conditions aluminium accumulates in the skeleton, producing so-called aluminium osteodystrophy (Alfrey 1984, Nebecker & Coburn 1986). This was first described in patients who were on prolonged haemodialysis: the aluminium accumulated

from the dialysis fluid. It appears to produce two types of bone disease, in the first of which there is excessive deposition of osteoid, with the histological appearance of osteomalacia. In the second condition, the bone appears to be aplastic, with little increase in osteoid but reduced osteoblastic activity (Andress et al 1987). In aluminium-related osteodystrophy it seems likely that the different histological features are related to the amount of aluminium within the bones. It is proposed that the higher rate of aluminium accumulation produces a profound suppression of mineralization. In aplastic bone disease with a supposedly lower body aluminium, the amount of osteoid is normal. In both forms the reduction in osteoblastic activity and bone formation is likely to be a direct effect of aluminium on the cells (Andress et al 1987). Aluminium bone disease may also occur in subjects on prolonged parenteral nutrition (Salusky & Coburn 1988).

Fluoride excess

The skeleton is affected by an increase in ingested fluoride. This may occur as part of the high fluoride intake in the form of endemic fluorosis, or when fluoride is given as treatment for osteoporisis. In endemic fluorosis, reported from particular geographical areas, progressive hyperostosis and ligamentous calcification leads to reduced mobility and spinal cord and root compression. Fluoride is also given therapeutically for osteoporosis, where it may produce a considerable increase in vertebral trabecular bone density, but this increase is not reflected throughout the whole of the skeleton, and some evidence suggests that the increase in trabecular bone at the spine is at the expense of the cortical bone in the periphery. Administration of sodium fluoride is also associated with gastrointestinal problems and with pain around the ends of the long bones, which may or may not be areas of compression fractures.

Cadmium excess

An example of industrial pollution causing osteomalacia and rickets was that of cadmium poisoning reported from Japan. Cadmium damages the renal tubules, producing a Fanconi syndrome which may lead to osteomalacia or rickets.

NUTRITION-RELATED BONE DISEASE

Osteoporosis

Osteoporosis is mentioned here because of its possible relationship to dietary calcium, which remains controversial and has also been discussed with other aspects in Chapter 11. Osteoporosis is possibly best thought of as a nutrition-related bone disease. This leaves open the question of calcium, and it also takes note of the fact that peak bone mass may be determined by other nutritional factors, particularly of protein and energy during growth.

Osteoporosis and calcium intake

It is impossible to summarize even a fraction of the work on the relationship between calcium and osteoporosis, and the reader should concentrate on the extensive reviews of Heaney et al (1982), Heaney (1986), the work of Nordin (1989), and Nordin & Polley (1987) and the recent review of Kanis & Passmore (1989) and the ensuing correspondence. Both Heaney and Nordin emphasize the importance of calcium intake to bone health, particularly in the elderly, and conclude that calcium supplementation of the diet is necessary in many situations. Kanis & Passmore (1989), on the contrary, assemble evidence which suggests that such supplementation is neither necessary nor justified in otherwise healthy people.

Heaney's (1986) review emphasizes the importance of the transmenopausal changes in the efficiency of utilization of dietary calcium, described by Heaney et al in 1978, and of the findings of Matkovic et al in 1979, describing the apparent effect of calcium intake and fracture incidence in two Yugoslav villages. In the first it was established that to maintain calcium balance it was necessary for postmenopausal women to take at least 1500 mg daily, compared with 1000 mg around and before the menopause. In the second, the bone mass was greater and the fracture rate less in subjects who had grown up in the village with the highest calcium intake (Matkovic et al 1979). Heaney (1986) realizes that the basis for the NIH calcium intake recommendations of 1000 mg/day for oestrogen-replete perimenopausal women and 1500 mg/day for oestrogen-deficient postmenopausal women is by no means solid. He proposes that the nutritional (predominantly calcium) and endocrine environment has a permissive role, whereas mechanical loading is considered to modulate the expression of genetic potential (Fig. 37.2). It follows that the ability to see a relationship between calcium intake and bone mass will depend entirely upon where the threshold falls with respect to intake in the groups being studied. For instance, with a calcium intake above the permissive threshold there will be no clear relationship between this intake and bone mass; with an intake below the threshold, such a relationship should exist. This will naturally be complicated by individual variation in the

threshold. Heaney (1986) reviews the data which show that the average woman in the USA consumes an amount of calcium well below the recommended daily allowance, and that 25% of such women from the age of 30 onwards consume less than 300 mg daily on average. (Apart from any direct effect of calcium, this low calcium intake is associated with reduced energy intake and expenditure and less mechanical loading of the skeleton, which will reduce its mass.) Such low intakes of calcium are not necessarily important for the skeleton if the body can compensate by increasing the efficiency of its absorption. In contrast, where this efficiency is low very large calcium intakes are necessary to increase net absorption. Since one of the main determinants of intestinal calcium absorption is 1,25 $(OH)_2D$, it is important to investigate the possible changes in vitamin D metabolism with age.

However, as already seen, vitamin D deficiency in man produces osteomalacia and not osteoporosis, and it is only in experimental animals that it can be convincingly shown that calcium deficiency causes osteoporosis. The possibility that in man malabsorption of calcium produces sufficient parathyroid overactivity to cause osteoporotic bone disease has not been proved. The reverse, that the malabsorption of calcium is secondary to osteoporosis, is an alternative which is attractive and has many proponents. In this case, the rate of bone loss in osteoporosis would be independent of the calcium intake.

Such investigations and theories have been at the centre of differences about the cause of osteoporosis for many years. They began at a time when research in bone disease was largely confined to calcium metabolism and the hormones which control it, to the detriment of work on the mechanical and genetic

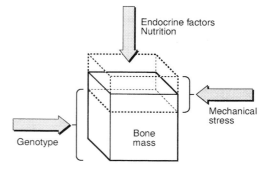

Fig. 37.2 The main factors controlling bone mass. It is proposed that mechanical stress is responsible for the full development of the genetic potential of bone mass, and that nutritional and endocrine factors are permissive, i. e. they allow the full expression of bone mass only when they are not deficient. (From Heaney (1986) with permission.)

effects on the skeleton and on its non-mineral components. It is now realized that bone cannot be dealt with in calcium terms alone, and indeed Kanis & Passmore (1989) find much of the evidence relating calcium intake to bone health untenable. In brief, they find that many conclusions derived from calcium balance data are erroneous, because of well known faults such as abrupt changes of intake and failure to allow for adaptation to low intakes; they consider that there is no convincing evidence to relate calcium intake to bone mass, and that any effect of supplemental dietary calcium in preventing bone loss is temporary and occurs only in the elderly. Since osteoporosis, especially in the elderly, is such an important disorder because of the structural failure and ensuing immobility and mortality it produces, it is important to settle the calcium problem as soon as possible, although the likelihood of doing so seems remote.

Causes

There are many causes of osteoporosis (Smith 1987, Riggs & Melton 1988, Stevenson 1988) (Table 37.5). Unlike osteomalacia, in osteoporosis there is a reduction in the amount of bone per given volume, but without any change in its composition. In particular, there is no defect in mineralization and no excess of osteoid. Important in the definition of osteoporosis is that the amount of bone is sufficient to predispose to fracture.

A more precise mathematical definition, which has a relationship to fractures defines osteoporosis as a condition where the bone mineral density is more than 2 SD below the mean for young adults. The strict definition of osteoporosis excludes those bone disorders associated, for instance, with metastatic deposits and also parathyroid bone disease (osteitis fibrosa cystica), where the composition is abnormal.

Postmenopausal osteoporosis Osteoporosis is most common in postmenopausal females. The reasons for this are discussed elsewhere (see Chapter 11). Compared with men, women have a lower peak bone mass and a more rapid loss of bone related to the postmenopausal decline in oestrogens. In addition, there are well recognized risk factors for osteoporosis, some of which operate in both sexes. These include a strong family history of osteoporosis, short stature and small bones, early menopause, white or Asian race, inactivity, cigarette smoking, leanness, nulliparity, excessive alcohol consumption, and possibly a low calcium intake. A number of these factors are related to each other.

The symptoms and signs of osteoporosis are those associated with fractures, since bone loss itself is

Table 37.5 Osteoporosis classified according to frequency and cause

Common	Old age
	Menopause
	Immobility
Less common	Endocrine
	Corticosteroid excess
	Hypogonadism
	Hypopituitarism
	Thyrotoxicosis
	Coeliac disease (with osteomalacia)
Rare	Mastocytosis
	Anorexia nervosa
Topical	Space travel
	Obsessional exercise
Inherited	Osteogenesis imperfecta
	(Brittle bone syndrome)
Chromosomal	Turner's syndrome
Idiopathic	Juvenile
	Pregnancy
	Young adult

symptomless. The main features are pain, deformity and fracture. Fractures affect the forearm, vertebrae and femoral necks. The physical signs are related to the site of fracture. Vertebral fractures are the most frequent and the earliest manifestation of osteoporosis, producing kyphosis and pain in the back with loss of height. In osteoporosis, routine biochemistry is often normal and any biochemical or haematological abnormality should suggest another diagnosis. Radiographs show loss of density and bony trabeculae and thinning of the cortex. In addition there is often evidence of structural collapse, such as wedging of the vertebrae. Various measurements of bone mass show a significant reduction in density. There are many ways of assessing the amount of bone present. Although single-photon densitometry of the forearm is relatively cheap and reproducible, it does not necessarily indicate what is happening in the rest of the skeleton, particularly the spine and femoral neck, for which instruments with a dual source (photon or X-ray) are necessary.

Other causes Of the rarer causes of osteoporosis (Table 37.4) three have a clear relationship to nutrition, namely coeliac disease, anorexia nervosa and obsessional exercise.

Coeliac disease is common and may cause osteomalacia (or rickets), osteoporosis, or a combination of both. It may be present at any age and in numerous ways, such as recurrent iron-deficiency anaemia, delayed puberty and bone disease. Steatorrhoea is not a common presentation. Diagnosis is by small-intestinal biopsy, which shows the atrophic mucosa. In other gastrointestinal disorders such as Crohn's disease and ulcerative colitis, osteoporosis may occur. This is often related to treatment with corticosteroids.

Anorexia nervosa is not a new disorder but its skeletal manifestations were largely neglected until it became possible to measure spinal bone density, which demonstrated how often it is associated with osteoporosis. Fractures of the spine and long bones are increased in frequency in anorexia nervosa, which may be regarded as an example of extreme starvation. It is likely that the osteoporosis is mainly due to the associated oestrogen deficiency (and possible cortisol excess). Reduced spinal bone density also occurs in female marathon runners and those who take excessive exercise. Thus recent studies in American female athletes have shown that the spinal density is related to oestrogen levels, which are lowest in those amenorrheic athletes running the greatest distances.

The other causes of osteoporosis emphasize the effect of hormones on the skeleton, and also show that there are patients who develop osteoporosis during physiological changes such as growth and pregnancy. In neither of these is the cause known, though it could be related to deficiency of the calciotrophic hormones normally responsible for protecting the skeleton.

Finally, the cause of osteoporosis in young adults may remain quite undiscovered, even when the bone changes are very severe. One very rare example is provided by mastocytosis, where bone biopsy will demonstrate the widespread deposition of mast cells throughout the skeletal tissue.

Controversies in osteoporosis

The reader should be aware of the current controversies which exist concerning the management of osteoporosis, which is the most common metabolic bone disease. As seen above, there is divergent opinion on the role of calcium in prevention and treatment. For peri- and postmenopausal women hormone replacement therapy (HRT) with combined oestrogen (and progestogen) is increasingly prescribed, since it has been convincingly demonstrated that oestrogen prevents subsequent bone loss in such women. Such treatment also appears to decrease overall mortality, although it may be associated with a slightly increased risk of breast carcinoma (Barrett-Connor 1989). Except in certain circumstances it remains impossible to identify those women who will develop osteoporosis and structural failure with fracture. Until this is done, the use of HRT is likely to be limited.

SUMMARY

The growth, composition and amount of the skeleton and its subsequent decline depends on many factors, of which nutrition is only one. In some instances, particularly those associated with specific vitamin deficiency and excess, the nutritional component is clear. In others, such as osteoporosis, the changes in the skeleton depend as much on genetic, mechanical and endocrine factors as they do on nutrition. In future it will be important to define the relative importance of these factors more precisely, in order to be able to prevent and treat common bone disorders.

REFERENCES

Alfrey AC 1984 Aluminium intoxication. New England Journal of Medicine 310:1113–1115
Andress DL, Maloney NA, Coburn JW et al 1987 Osteomalacia and aplastic bone disease in aluminium-related osteodystrophy. Journal of Clinical Endocrinology and Metabolism 65:11–15
Barrett-Connor E 1989 Postmenopausal oestrogen replacement and breast cancer. New England Journal of Medicine 321:319–320
Behrman RE, Vaughan VC 1987 Nelson Textbook of Paediatrics, 13th edn. WB Saunders, Philadelphia
Bouillon RA, Auwerx JR, Lissens WD, Pelemans WK 1987 Vitamin D status in the elderly: seasonal substrate deficiency causes 1,25-dihydroxycholecalciferol deficiency. American Journal of Clinical Nutrition 45:755–763
Boyd AS 1988 An overview of the retinoids. American Journal of Medicine 86: 568–574
Campbell GA, Hosking DJ, Kemm JR, Boyd RV 1984 How common is osteomalacia in the elderly? Lancet ii:386–388
Clements MR, Johnson L, Fraser DR 1987 A new mechanism for induced vitamin D deficiency in calcium deprivation. Nature 325:62–65
Davies M, Adams PH 1978 The continuing risk of vitamin D intoxication. Lancet ii:621–623
Dunnigan MG, McIntosh WB, Ford JA, Robertson I 1982 Acquired disorders of vitamin D metabolism. In: Heath D, Marx SJ (eds) Butterworths International Medical Reviews. Clinical Endocrinology 2, Calcium disorders. Butterworths, London 125–150
Dunnigan MG, Glekin BM, Henderson JB et al 1985 Prevention of rickets in Asian children: assessment of the Glasgow campaign. British Medical Journal 291:239–242
Eisman JA 1988 Osteomalacia. In: Martin TJ (ed) Baillière's clinical endocrinology and metabolism, Vol 2 No 1. Baillière Tindall, London, 125–155
Forfar JO, Arneil GC 1984 Textbook of paediatrics, 3rd edn. Churchill Livingstone, Edinburgh, 1298–1306

Heaney RP 1986 Calcium, bone health and osteoporosis. In Peck WA Bone and mineral research, Vol 4. Elsevier, Amsterdam 255–301

Heaney RP, Recker RR, Saville PD 1978 Menopausal changes in calcium balance performance. Journal of Laboratory and Clinical Medicine 92:953–963

Heaney RP, Gallagher JC, Johnson CC et al 1982 Calcium nutrition and bone health in the elderly. American Journal of Clinical Nutrition 36:986–1013

Henderson JB, Dunnigan MG, McIntosh WB et al 1987 The importance of limited exposure to ultraviolet radiation and dietary factors in the aetiology of Asian rickets: a risk-factor model. Quarterly Journal of Medicine 63:413–425

Holick MF Photosynthesis of vitamin D in the skin: effect of environment and lifestyle variables. Federation Proceedings 46:1876–1882

Hosking DJ, Kemm JR, Knight ME et al 1983 Screening for subclinical osteomalacia in the elderly: normal ranges or pragmatism? Lancet ii:1290–1292

Hughes MR, Malloy PJ, Kieback DG et al 1988 Point mutations in the vitamin D receptor associated with hypocalcaemic rickets. Science 242:1702–1705

Kanis JA, Passmore R 1989 Calcium supplementation of the diet. British Medical Journal 298:137–140, 205–208

Kanis JA, Cundy TF, Hamdy NAT 1988 Renal osteodystrophy. In: Martin TJ (ed) Baillière's Endocrinology and metabolism, Vol 2 No 1. Metabolic bone disease. Baillière Tindall, London 193–241

Lancet 1987a Vitamin D supplements in the elderly. Lancet i:306–307

Lancet 1987b Metabolic bone disease of prematurity. Lancet i:200

Liberman VA, Marx SJ 1989 Disorders of vitamin D metabolism deficiency and resistance. In: Tam CS, Heersche JNM, Murray TM (eds) Metabolic bone disease: cellular and tissue mechanisms. CRC Press, Boca Raton, 173–202

Lindsay R 1988 Management for osteoporosis. In: Martin TJ (ed) Baillière's Clinical endocrinology and metabolism, Vol 2 No 1. Metabolic bone disease. Baillière Tindall, London, 103–124

Matkovic V, Kostial K, Simonovic I et al 1979 Bone status and fracture rates in two regions of Yugoslavia. American Journal of Clinical Nutrition 32:540–549

Miyauchi A, Fukase M, Tsutsumi M, Fujita T 1988 Haemangiopericytoma-induced osteomalacia: tumour transplantaiton in nude mice causes hypophosphataemia and tumour extracts inhibit renal 25-hydroxy vitamin D 1-hydroxylase activity. Journal of Clinical Endocrinology and Metabolism 67: 46–53

Mudd SH, Levy HL 1978 Disorders of transulfuration. In: Stanbury JB, Wyngaarden JB, Fredrickson DS (eds) The metabolic basis of inherited disease, 4th edn. McGraw Hill, New York 459–503

Nebeker HG, Coburn JW 1986 Aluminium and renal osteodystrophy. Annual Review of Medicine 37:79–95

Nilas L, Christiansen C 1987 Vitamin D deficiency after highly selective vagotomy. Acta Medica Scandinavica 221:303–306

Nordin BEC 1984 Metabolic bone and stone disease, 2nd edn. Churchill Livingstone, Edinbiurgh, 71–111

Nordin BEC 1989 The calcium deficiency model for osteoporosis. Nutrition Reviews 47:65–72

Nordin BEC, Polley KJ 1987 Metabolic consequences of the menopause. Calcified Tissue International 41, Suppl. 1:1–59

Palma FJM, Ellis HA, Cook DB et al 1983 Osteomalacia in patients with chronic renal failure before dialysis or transplantation. Quarterly Journal of Medicine 207:332–348

Reichel H, Koeffler HP, Norman AW 1989 The role of the vitamin D endocrine system in health and disease. New England Journal of Medicine 320:980–991

Riggs BL, Melton LJ 1988 Osteoporosis. Aetiology, diagnosis and management. Raven Press, New York

Salusky IB, Coburn JW 1988 Bone disease with renal insufficiency during total parenteral nutrition. In: Manolagas SC, Olefsky, JM (eds) Metabolic bone disease and mineral disorders. Contemporary Issues in Endocrinology and Metabolism 5:193–221

Shaw JCL 1988 Copper deficiency and non-accidental injury. Archives of Disease in Childhood 63:448–455

Smith R 1987 Disorders of the skeleton. In: Weatherall DJ, Ledingham JGG, Warrell DA (eds) Oxford textbook of medicine, 2nd edn. Oxford University Press, Oxford, 17.1–17.38

Smith R, Newman RJ, Radda GK et al 1984 Hypophosphataemic osteomalacia and myopathy: studies with nuclear magnetic resonance spectroscopy. Clinical Science 67:505–509

Stamp TCB 1982 The clinical endocrinology of vitamin D. In: Parsons JA (ed) Endocrinology of calcium metabolism. Raven Press, New York, 363–422

Stamp TCB, Walker PG, Perry W, Jenkins MV 1980 Nutritional osteomalacia and late rickets in Greater London 1974–1979. Clinical and metabolic studies in 45 patient. In: Avioli L V, Raisz L G (eds) Clinics in endocrinology and metabolism, Vol 9 No 1. WB Saunders Co, London, 81–105

Stephens WP, Klimiuk PS, Warrington S et al 1982 Observation on the natural history of vitamin D deficiency amongst Asian immigrants. Quarterly Journal of Medicine 51:171–188

Stern PH, Bell NH 1989 Disorders of vitamin D metabolism – toxicity and hypersensitivity. In: Tam CS, Heersche JNM, Murray TM (eds) Metabolic bone disease: cellular and tissue mechanisms. CRC Press, Boca Raton, 203–213

Stevenson JC 1988 Osteoporosis: pathogenesis and risk factors. In: Martin TJ (ed) Baillière's Clinical endocrinology and metabolism, Vol 2 No 1. Metabolic bone disease. Baillière Tindall, London, 87–101

Tam CS, Heersche JNM, Murray TM (eds) 1989 Metabolic bone disease: cellular and tissue mechanisms. CRC Press, Boca Raton

Thakker RV, O'Riordan JLH 1988 Inherited forms of rickets and osteomalacia. In: Martin TJ (ed) Baillère's Clinical endocrinology and metabolism, Vol 2 No 1. Metabolic bone disease. Baillère Tindall, London, 157–189

Webb AR, Holick MF 1988 The role of sunlight in the cutaneous production of vitamin D_3. Annual Review of Nutrition 8:375–399

38. Dietary factors in dental diseases

A. J. Rugg-Gunn

Attitudes to teeth have changed considerably over the centuries, and differ between countries. In the past, man could not have survived without teeth, which were essential both for eating and as a tool; infection from dental abscesses was a potential killer. Advances in medicine have ensured that, in affluent societies, few people die from dental causes. The ability of food manufacturers and cooks to provide soft diets and the advances in prosthetic dentistry have ensured that people can be adequately nourished without their natural teeth. So, why worry about teeth? The answer is that people value their natural teeth, which usually feel, look and function better than artificial teeth.

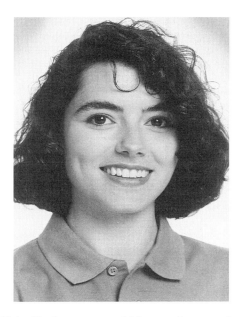

Fig. 38.1 Teeth are an essential feature of an attractive face. (This illustration is kindly provided by Reach® toothbrushes, dental floss and Dentotape®. Reproduced by kind permission of Oxford University Press.)

Glamour magazines display smiling faces (Fig. 38.1) and reveal that an essential component of any film star's face is a row of attractive teeth which are pearly white in colour, well aligned and surrounded by pink, healthy gums, firm jaws, cheeks and lips. Teeth are important, not only in eating and speaking, but also in enhancing appearance and raising a person's social acceptability. Because people value their teeth, but their teeth and gums are ravaged by disease, the cost of dental services is very high. In the UK in 1991 the cost of the NHS dental services was over £1000 million sterling. The provision of dental services in Britain is very efficient, and this sum is low by international standards.

This chapter describes the diseases of the teeth, the role of diet in their aetiology, and how dietary advice might be given to improve dental health. Emphasis is placed on the evidence that sugar plays an important role in dental disease because doctors, nutritionists and dietitians are often confused by conflicting evaluations and the desire of industrial interests to maintain sugar intakes. It is therefore important to know the arguments, so that patients and the community are not misled.

DISEASES OF THE HUMAN DENTITION

Man has two dentitions. The deciduous dentition begins to appear in the mouth at about 6 months of age, consists of 20 teeth and is shed by early adolescence; the permanent dentition consists of 32 teeth and supplements, and replaces the deciduous dentition between the ages of about 6 and 21 years.

The calcification of the deciduous teeth begins in utero and enamel formation is completed during the first year of life. The first teeth erupt at about 6 months of age and the dentition is complete by about 2½ years. At about 6 years the first permanent molars erupt behind the deciduous molars and the permanent incisors begin to replace the deciduous incisors.

The second permanent molars erupt at about 12 years, and by this age all the deciduous teeth will normally have been shed and replaced by permanent teeth. The third permanent molars erupt between 18 and 24 years. The eruption times of all teeth, but especially the third molars, vary considerably.

Teeth consist of three mineralized tissues: enamel, dentine and cementum. The bulk of a tooth consists of dentine, which is mesodermal in origin. The dentine forming the roots of the tooth is covered by a thin layer of bone-like material called cementum, while the outer layer of the crown of the tooth consists of enamel – a hard substance of ectodermal origin. In a young person, only enamel is exposed to the oral environment, although in older people some of the root cementum may become exposed as the tooth's supporting tissues recede. These supporting tissues consist of the alveolar bone of the maxilla or mandible, covered by epithelium. The epithelium around the necks of the teeth is called the gingivae (or gums). The teeth are held in the alveolar bone by the periodontal ligament, which allows the teeth to move slightly. Although enamel contains no cells, nerves or blood vessels and is insensitive, dentine is very sensitive to many stimuli. The nerves and blood vessels supplying the dentine come from the pulp that forms the soft centre of a tooth and is in turn supplied by nerves and blood vessels from the alveolar bone via the apical foramen of the tooth.

Teeth tend to form into a regular curve in both the upper (maxillary) and lower (mandibular) jaws, due, in part, to pressure from the tongue on the inner surface, and the cheeks and lips on the outer surface (Fig. 38.2). When the jaws are closed, the upper and lower teeth come together enabling food to be bitten (by the incisors and canine teeth) or chewed (by the premolar and molar teeth). With age, teeth become worn down by eating (attrition), become grooved or polished by abrasion (e.g. by the over-zealous use of toothbrush and abrasive toothpaste) or eroded by dietary (or occasionally gastric) acids.

The two most common diseases of the teeth are dental caries (decay) and periodontal (gum) disease. Dental caries begins on the tooth surface, usually in the enamel, but can begin in the cementum or dentine of tooth roots in older people, and then progressively destroys the hard tissues of the teeth. When the dentine is involved the tooth may be sensitive, particularly to cold drinks or foods, and if caries reaches the pulp, the resulting pulpitis is likely to be painful. Infection can then spread into the alveolar bone, leading to an alveolar abscess.

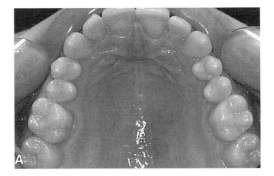

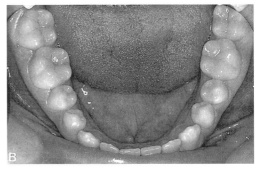

Fig. 38.2 Maxillary (a) and mandibular (b) teeth in a person aged 17 years. Each jaw has, on each side, two incisors, one canine, two premolars and two molars.

Periodontal disease is more insidious and less likely to cause discomfort or pain. The periodontal ligament and adjacent bone are slowly destroyed, so that the tooth becomes more and more mobile and may eventually fall out. The precursor of periodontal disease is inflammation of the gingivae, which lose their pink colour and firm stippled appearance, and become swollen and red and tend to bleed if pressed or brushed. This is called gingivitis, and can either reverse (if the conditions are favourable) to a healthy state or progress to periodontal disease. The exact mechanism as to how gingivitis progresses to periodontal disease is still unclear, but there is no doubt that gingivitis is an essential precursor of periodontal disease.

An essential factor in the aetiology of dental caries and gingivitis is dental plaque. This is a white, slightly glutinous layer, which builds up on the surfaces of teeth when they are not cleaned. Seventy percent of plaque is microorganisms, while water and polysaccharides (principally polyglucans) and the occasional shed epithelial cell occupy the space between the microorganisms. Dental plaque can usually be found in areas around the teeth which are least easily cleaned, mainly in the pits and fissures of the occlusal (or chewing) surfaces, between adjacent teeth (on the approximal surfaces), or along the gingival margin of the tooth on the buccal (outer) or lingual (inner) surfaces of the teeth. Gingivitis is basically caused by irritants from the dental plaque which permeate through the thin non-keratinized epithelium adjacent to the tooth surface.

The aetiology of caries is also simple in outline. Dietary sugars diffuse into dental plaque, where they are metabolized by plaque microorganisms to acids. Most of the acid produced is lactic, with some acetic, formic and propionic acids also being produced. With acid production, the pH of dental plaque falls from a resting value of about 6.8 to values as low as 4.5. Dental enamel consists of crystals of hydroxyapatite arranged in a characteristic way in a thinly dispersed organic matrix: 96% of enamel is inorganic mineral. This mineral phase of the enamel is dissolved by the plaque acids, and the caries process has begun. It is usually reckoned that 5.5 is the 'critical pH' below which the enamel hydroxyapatite will dissolve. When the pH rises above this value remineralization (or healing of the carious lesion) can occur. Thus a carious cavity in the tooth occurs when plaque pH is constantly being lowered, so that demineralization is greater than any remineralization. This aspect of the frequency of ingestion of sugars keeping plaque pH low and preventing any remineralization is important, and will be considered in more detail later. Another relevant point is the amount of calcium and phosphate in the plaque, since high levels of these minerals in the plaque fluid will help to resist the dissolution of the tooth.

The caries process is not a simple dissolution of the surface of dental enamel. For various reasons, dissolution occurs fastest just below the tooth surface: this has the appearance of a chalky white spot (Fig. 38.3). Eventually this white spot (or precavitation carious lesion) loses so much mineral that it breaks down and a carious cavity is formed. Once this stage is reached, it is usual to fill or restore the tooth as remineralization will not occur, although cavities can arrest if the local conditions are very favourable. If precavitation lesions are seen, it is important that they are given every chance to remineralize by removing the overlying plaque and decreasing the amount and frequency of sugar ingestion. In addition, fluorides (e.g. in toothpastes, mouthrinses or in water) aid remineralization.

It must also be appreciated that factors other than the ingestion of sugars and the presence of dental plaque influence the occurrence of dental caries. One

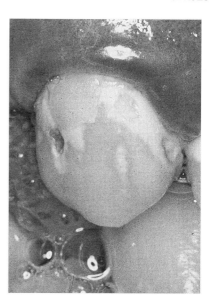

Fig. 38.3 Dental caries. A small cavity has recently formed within the chalky white area (which is known as a precavitation carious lesion). The gingivae are inflamed due to the persistent presence of dental plaque.

important factor is the quantity and quality of saliva. Some foods are better than others at stimulating salivary flow, and this also will be discussed later. Relevant aspects of the quality of saliva are its buffering power and calcium and phosphate content. The structure of tooth enamel may be of some importance and can be altered by the diet while the teeth are forming. It is also possible that antibodies reaching dental plaque via the gingival crevice or via the saliva may reduce the virulence of plaque microorganisms. Saliva contains amylase, which breaks down dietary starch if in an available form. The resultant maltose or glucose can then be used by plaque microorganisms and plaque acids produced. The relative cariogenicity of dietary starch and sugars will be discussed later.

One further unfavourable property of dental plaque is that it can become mineralized by the deposition of calcium and phosphate in saliva to form dental calculus, or tartar, around the necks of teeth. This calculus does no harm per se, but makes it impossible to remove plaque effectively, so that it is an important factor in the aetiology of gingivitis and periodontal disease. It is removed by scaling of the teeth by a dental hygienist or dentist. Diet appears to have little influence on the occurrence of dental calculus.

Sometimes teeth do not fit into a nice regular arch and the upper and lower teeth do not come together in an attractive and functional way. This is called malocclusion. In years past it was thought that eating soft diets and insufficient chewing could be a cause of narrow dental arches and malocclusion. There is really no evidence for this, and current views are that diet is unimportant in the cause of dental malocclusion.

Of the two most important diseases of teeth – dental caries and periodontal disease – diet is very much more important in the cause and prevention of caries than in periodontal disease.

DENTAL CARIES

Diet can affect the teeth while they are forming, before they erupt into the mouth (a pre-eruptive effect) and, once erupted, by a local direct effect. Much research was undertaken in the 1920s and 1930s on the pre-eruptive effect of diet on tooth structure (see below). Over the past 50 years, opinion on the relative importance of the pre- and posteruptive influences of diet has changed. The posteruptive effect is now considered much more important.

The evidence relating diet to dental caries is vast (see Rugg-Gunn 1989, 1993), with overwhelming evidence that sugars are the most cariogenic (caries-inducing) item in the diet. The frequency of eating sugar, the amount eaten and the cariogenicity of different dietary sugars have all to be considered. The cariogenicity of starch, the relative cariogenicity of naturally occurring and 'free' sugars (sometimes called 'added' sugars), the possible effect of factors in foods which may protect teeth against caries, and the effect on teeth of alternative sweeteners, are important issues for nutritionists and dentists.

There are six main sources of evidence relating diet to dental caries. These are:

1. Human observational studies (epidemiology)
2. Human interventional studies (clinical trials)
3. Animal experiments
4. Enamel slab experiments
5. Plaque pH studies
6. In vitro laboratory experiments.

It is important to consider evidence from all these sources in order to make sensible conclusions and offer effective advice.

Sugar and dental caries

Human observational studies

The epidemiological evidence relating diet to dental caries is of several types. At its crudest level, sugar

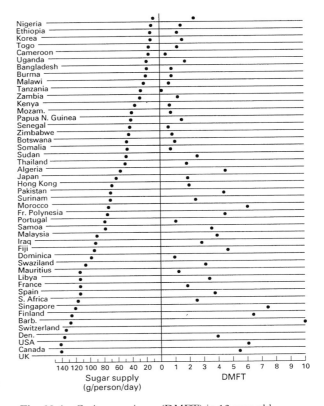

Fig. 38.4 Caries experience (DMFT) in 12-year-old children and sugar supplies in 47 countries. Data from Sreebny (1982). (Reproduced by kind permission of Oxford University Press.)

intake and caries can be compared on an inter-country basis. Fig. 38.4 represents data for 47 countries (Sreebny 1982). The correlation between sugar supply and caries experience in 12-year-olds is +0.7. On a linear regression, for each rise in sugar supply of 20 g/person/day, caries increased by 1 DMFT (the number of *d*ecayed, *m*issing or *f*illed *t*eeth per person). For the 21 nations with a sugar supply less than 50 g/person/day, caries experience was consistently below 3 DMFT.

The consumption of refined sugar – i.e. sugar other than that intrinsically present in foods, such as fruits – is a fairly recent phenomenon in many areas of the world. With increases in trade, many isolated communities such as Eskimos, have adopted a westernized diet. Caries in Eskimos was very low before the introduction of a high-sugar diet (Zitzow 1979) but dental disease subsequently increased rapidly (Moller et al 1972). For example, in the Anaktuvuk community in

Alaska, the mean number of cariously affected deciduous teeth in young children increased from four to ten over a 9-year period (Bang & Kristoffersen 1972). In Greenland, which has the largest group of people of Eskimo descent, caries was virtually unknown (Pederson 1938) but by 1977, the number of cariously affected tooth surfaces in 7-year-olds was 20, and in 14-year-olds was 19 permanent tooth surfaces. These figures are among the highest in the world (Jakobsen 1979). In many developing countries, caries experience is increasing in parallel with sugar consumption. The World Health Organization has collected caries data from many countries, and of the 20 underdeveloped countries where surveys on the dental health of 12-year-olds have been conducted, 15 have recorded marked increases in dental caries. In all countries where caries experience has increased, per capita sugar consumption has also increased (Sheiham 1984).

One of the best examples of an increase in caries occurring after a change to a high-sugar diet was recorded in the island of Tristan da Cunha. This isolated island in the south Atlantic has a population of about 200. Prior to 1940, their diet was very low in sugar but, since 1940, when a wireless station was installed, sugar has been imported and sold. Sugar consumption rose between 1938 and 1966 from 2 to 150 g/person/day, while the percentage of teeth affected by caries rose, over the same period of time, from 4% to 42% in young children, from 1% to 33% in adolescents, and from 9% to 38% in adults (Fisher 1968).

Other epidemiological studies have looked at caries experience in special groups of people habitually eating low amounts of sugar. One example is Hopewood House in Australia, where children received a lacto-vegetarian diet with virtually no sugar or white flour. Annual dental examinations and dietary surveys from 1947 to 1962 showed that 46% of 12-year-olds were free of caries, compared with only 1% in similarly aged schoolchildren living nearby (Harris 1963). A very low caries rate is also found in patients with hereditary fructose intolerance who avoid eating fructose or sucrose (Newbrun 1978).

A country at war usually experiences a reduction in the availability of sugar. Sognnaes (1948) reviewed 27 wartime studies from 11 European countries covering 750 000 children: a reduction in caries was observed in all these studies. Sugar restriction was particularly severe in Japan, where sugar consumption fell from 15 kg/person/year before the second world war to 0.2 kg/person/year in 1946. The close relation between annual sugar consumption and annual caries inci-

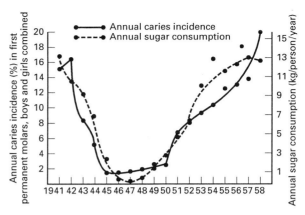

Fig. 38.5 The relation between the annual caries incidence in first permanent molar teeth in 7894 Japanese children and annual sugar consumption in Japan. Data from Takahashi (1961). (Reproduced by kind permission of Oxford University Press.)

dence in the first permanent molars can be seen in Fig. 38.5.

Fifty-five cross-sectional observational studies correlating an individual's sugar consumption with their caries experience (Rugg-Gunn 1989) showed that statistically significant correlations are usually found in young, rather than older, children. In older children the dental assessment measured the lifetime experience of caries, but diet was only assessed at the end. Better designed but difficult studies require a longitudinal analysis of diet and caries incidence together. One such English study lasting 2 years showed that the weight of daily sugar intake was positively correlated with the incidence of caries in 12–14-year-old children (Rugg-Gunn et al 1984). The statistically significant correlation was, however, low (+ 0.14) but the 31 (of 405) children eating the most sugar developed nearly one carious tooth surface per year more than the 31 children who had the lowest sugar intake. The study showed that the sugar–caries relation was independent of toothbrushing frequency or the effectiveness of toothcleaning.

Human interventional studies

There have been two human interventional studies of importance. First the Vipeholm Study (Gustaffson et al 1954), which is probably the biggest single study in the field of dental caries ever undertaken. The Vipeholm Hospital near Lund in southern Sweden, in 1951, contained 964 mentally deficient patients, 80%

of whom were male. The patients were divided, by wards, into one control group and six test groups. Groups were given high sucrose intakes at meals only, or at and between meals, in non-sticky or sticky forms. The study was complicated, but from the results it is reasonable to conclude that consumption of sugars even at high levels is associated with only a small increase in caries increment if taken up to four times a day as part of meals, and that consumption of sugar between meals as well as at meals is associated with a marked increase in caries increment.

The second important human interventional study took place in Turku, Finland, between 1972 and 1974 (Scheinin & Makinen 1975). The aim of this 2-year clinical trial was to study the effect on dental caries of nearly total substitution of the sucrose in a normal diet with either fructose or xylitol. Because full cooperation in adhering to the diet was essential, and because it was planned to carry out a wide range of biochemical and microbiological tests, the study was restricted to adults. The number of new carious lesions developing during the 2 years was 7.2 in the sucrose group, 3.8 in the fructose group and 0.0 in the xylitol group. These figures, which are widely quoted, include precavitation carious lesions as well as actual carious cavities. When only cavities were counted, the results showed 56% fewer cavities in the xylitol group than in the sucrose group, but a similar number of cavities formed in the sucrose and fructose groups. Thus, the xylitol diet was less cariogenic than the sucrose or fructose diets, but fructose was no less cariogenic than sucrose. The persistent inability of plaque microorganisms to metabolize xylitol to acids probably explains this cariostatic effect. Xylitol seems a suitable substitute for sucrose from the dental point of view, with little evidence of osmotic diarrhoea even at daily intakes up to 200 g xylitol; no undesirable metabolic effects are reported.

Animal experiments

The local effects of sugars and the frequency and amount, concentration and type of sugar, have all been tested. Kite et al (1950) fed two groups of rats the same high-sugar cariogenic diet. One group ate their diet in the normal way; the other received their diet via stomach tube, thus bypassing the mouth. No caries was observed in the rats fed by stomach tube, whereas the conventionally fed animals developed an average of seven carious lesions. Thus the sugar has to be present in the mouth for caries to occur.

The strong correlation between the frequency of consumption of a high-sugar diet and caries develop-

Table 38.1 The mean number of carious fissure surfaces and daily food intake in four groups of rats fed at different frequencies per day; six animals per group (Konig et al 1968)

Group	Eating frequency per day	No. of carious fissures	Daily food intake (g)
1	12	0.7	6.0
2	18	2.2	6.0
3	24	4.0	6.0
4	30	4.7	6.0

ment is clearly seen in many rat studies (see Table 38.1). The relationship to total sugar intake is not always simple. Huxley (1977) found that whereas caries increased linearly with sugar concentration (0, 15, 30 and 56%) in rats receiving one type of basic diet, no linear increase was observed in those fed a different basic diet. Fig. 38.6 shows the results of Hefti & Schmid (1979), where caries severity increased with increasing sugar concentration but the

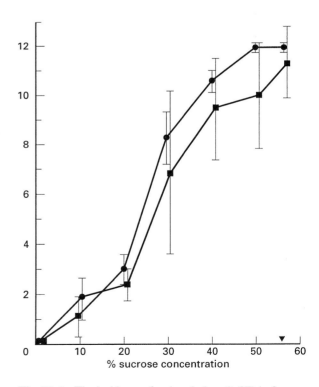

Fig. 38.6 The incidence of carious lesions (± SE) in fissures (●) and smooth surfaces (■) in rats fed diets containing 0, 10, 20, 30, 40, 50 and 56% sucrose. (Reproduced from Hefti & Schmid (1979) with kind permission of the editor, *Caries Research*.)

increase in severity declined when sugar concentrations exceeded about 40%. The frequency of sugar intake was similar in the groups of rats in these studies, so the weight and concentration of sugar eaten related to the severity of caries.

All the common dietary sugars (glucose, fructose, galactose, lactose, maltose and sucrose) are cariogenic in rat experiments. There is some difference of opinion as to whether sucrose is the most cariogenic dietary sugar. Some studies (Guggenheim et al 1966) have shown this to be so, but this may be due to the superinfection or monoinfection of the rats with streptococci, some strains of which utilize sucrose preferentially and do not thrive in its absence. No studies have shown sucrose to be less cariogenic than other sugars.

Enamel slab experiments

A further method of studying the cariogenicity of foods in humans is to use intraoral appliances which carry small slabs of tooth enamel. Several designs of appliance and methods of measuring the caries process have been used. Appliances can be dipped into test foods or sugars and then placed in the mouth, with the enamel slabs being examined for the earliest signs of caries. This human study is then ethically acceptable. Sucrose, glucose and fructose induce caries-like lesions in the enamel slabs; lactose, sorbitol and mannitol induce significantly fewer lesions than sucrose, and xylitol had no effect (Koulourides et al 1976). Increasing the concentration of sugars or the frequency of exposure to sugars increased the demineralization of the enamel slabs (Tehrani et al 1983).

Plaque pH studies

Many studies have measured the pH of dental plaque before, during and after eating or drinking. Before a meal plaque pH is usually about 6.8, but falls when sugars are eaten. The extent and duration of the fall indicates the amount and rate of acid production, rather than the development of caries.

Plaque pH can be measured on samples of plaque removed at various times, or a miniature glass electrode can be inserted into the plaque and worn in a special appliance within the mouth of volunteers. Comparing the results from measuring samples of removed plaque (Figs 38.7 and 38.8) with those from an indwelling glass electrode (Fig. 38.9) shows that the pH levels are higher in the removed samples. However, in general the ranking of foods is similar

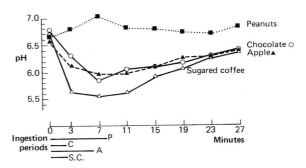

Fig. 38.7 Measurements of plaque pH after eating four foods, obtained using the 'sampling method'. (Reproduced by kind permission of the editor, *British Dental Journal*.)

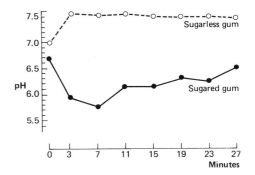

Fig. 38.8 Measurements of plaque pH during chewing of sugared or sugarless (sorbitol-containing) chewing gum. (Reproduced by kind permission of the editor, *British Dental Journal*.)

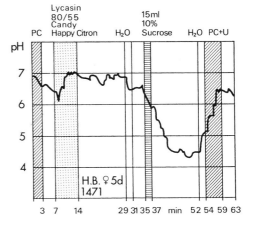

Fig. 38.9 Measurements of plaque pH during eating of a sugarless (Lycasin-containing) sweet or use of a sucrose rinse. (Reproduced from Imfeld (1977) by kind permission of the editor, *Helvetica Odontologica Acta*.)

and this is the relevant practical issue. There is no doubt that sugar-containing foods produce larger depressions in plaque pH than non-sugary foods. It is also fairly clear that lactose and galactose give a smaller pH drop than sucrose, glucose, fructose or maltose. Many studies have shown that the sugar alcohols (xylitol, sorbitol and mannitol) and related sweeteners (hydrogenated glucose syrup and isomalt) do not depress plaque pH. Indeed, chewing sugarless chewing gum (Fig. 38.8) actually raises plaque pH, because chewing increases salivary flow and fast-flowing saliva is alkaline.

Incubation experiments

The final type of study providing evidence on diet and dental caries is the in vitro experiment which tests the ability of plaque microorganisms to metabolize a test food to acid. In general, sugar-containing foods are rapidly metabolized to acid, whereas starchy foods are metabolized more slowly. Xylitol is not metabolized at all and sorbitol, mannitol and hydrogenated glucose syrup are broken down only slightly. These tests show that 5.5 is about the 'critical pH' below which dental enamel dissolves in saliva or, more importantly, in plaque fluid. Foods can also be tested for factors which protect the enamel (see below).

These different types of study allow the following conclusions to be drawn. First, evidence from all sources indicates that sucrose is very cariogenic. Some evidence, notably from animal experiments, indicates that glucose, fructose and maltose may be less cariogenic than sucrose, but this view is not supported by incubation experiments and plaque pH experiments. The few human clinical trials are rather equivocal on this point. If there are any differences in the cariogenicity of sucrose, glucose, fructose and maltose, they are small and unlikely to be of practical importance. From several types of evidence it is reasonable to conclude that lactose and galactose are less cariogenic than the other common dietary mono- and disaccharides.

A second aspect to consider is the relative importance of the frequency of eating sugars, the mass of sugars consumed and the concentration of sugar in foods. There is no doubt that frequency of eating is a very important variable. This is evident from plaque pH studies and clearly demonstrated in the Vipeholm study and numerous animal experiments. The mass of sugar eaten and its concentration in food are closely linked, so it is difficult to separate the two. Both concentration and mass are important in animal and in human enamel slab experiments. Epidemiologically,

many studies have shown correlations between the mass of sugars eaten and the prevalence of dental caries, and between the frequency of eating sugars and caries. Since the frequency of eating and the weight of foods eaten are highly correlated, it may not matter whether the dietary advice is to reduce the frequency or the quantity of sugar eaten.

Starch and dental caries

It has been suggested that all carbohydrate foods, sugars and starches should be considered cariogenic (Biscuit, Cake, Chocolate and Confectionery Alliance 1987). Because authorities in many developed countries recommend that starch consumption should increase as the consumption of sugar and fats falls, it is important that this assertion is examined. A fuller review of this subject has been published by the British Health Education Authority (Rugg-Gunn 1988).

Sreebny (1982, 1983) correlated epidemiologically the caries status of 12-year-olds in 47 countries with the availability of sugar and cereals in those countries. Cereal availability was quantified as (a) energy from cereal per day, and (b) energy from cereal as a percentage of energy intake. It can be seen from Table 38.2 that the bivariate correlations between cereal availability and caries varied between −0.45 and +0.45 (left-hand column), but were low and mainly negative when the data were controlled, by partial correlation,

Table 38.2 Correlations and partial correlations between caries experience (DMFT) (for 12-year-olds) and sugar or cereal availability in 47 countries. (Raw data taken from Sreebny 1982, 1983)

		Bivariate correlation	Partial correlation, controlling for sugar availability
Total cereals	cal/day	−0.25	−0.03
	% of energy	−0.45[*]	−0.13
Wheat	cal/day	+0.45[*]	+0.05
	% of energy	+0.29	−0.03
Rice	cal/day	−0.07	+0.10
	% of energy	−0.09	+0.10
Maize	cal/day	−0.37[+]	−0.24
	% of energy	−0.40[++]	−0.26
Sugar	(g/day)	+0.70[*]	
controlling for total cereal (cal/day)			+0.67[*]
controlling for wheat (cal/day)			+0.60[*]

[*] $p < 0.005$
[++] $p < 0.02$
[+] $p < 0.05$

for sugar availability (right-hand column). In contrast, the bivariate correlation between the sugar availability and caries was +0.70 and fell to only +0.67 and +0.60 when the data were controlled for total cereal and wheat availability, respectively. These findings suggest a much closer relationship between caries and sugar availability than between caries and the availability of starchy cereal foods on a worldwide basis.

Many countries throughout the world have traditionally eaten high-starch low-sugar diets, and these people have had a very low caries experience. Deterioration of their dental health has coincided with the introduction of free (or refined) sugars into their diet. The islanders of Tristan da Cunha (see above) are an example of these changes occurring in a defined community.

The recognized extremely low caries experience in people with hereditary fructose intolerance (Table 38.3) occurs in patients with a normal starch consumption (Newbrun et al 1980), so starchy foods are not cariogenic. This is supported by the Turku study on the use of xylitol: caries rates dropped profoundly, despite the persistent starch intake. No clear correlations between starch intake and caries experience have been reported (Martinsson 1972, Hankin et al 1973, Kleemola-Kujala & Rasanen 1979).

In rats, bread was shown to cause caries (Konig 1969, Bowen et al 1980), but it was less cariogenic than sucrose. Human studies with the enamel slab test compared the effects of two biscuits, one sugar-rich, the other sugar-free, with the effect of a 5% sucrose solution. Demineralization of the enamel slabs was substantially greater with sucrose than with either biscuit (Thompson & Pearce 1982) – sugar rather than starch was the real problem.

Table 38.3 Caries experience (DMFS = number of decayed, missing or filled tooth surfaces) and diet of people with hereditary fructose intolerance (HFI) and controls (Newbrun et al 1980)

	HFI	Controls
Number	17	14
Age (years)	29	27
DMFS	3	36
Sugar (g/day)	3	48
Starch (g/day)	160	140
Energy Protein Fat Vitamin Minerals	} similar	

Plaque pH experiments have given inconsistent results. Samples of plaque measured after eating cooked starch or starchy foods are less acidic than after sugar meals, but an indwelling glass electrode records very low pH values after both starchy foods and sugar. Indwelling glass electrodes may be 'hyperresponsive' (Newbrun 1984) and produce an 'all or none' response (Edgar 1985).

From all this evidence we can conclude that: (a) cooked staple starchy foods such as rice, potatoes and bread, are of very low cariogenicity in man and (b) if finely ground, heat-treated and eaten frequently, starch can cause caries but the impact is less than that caused by sucrose. The addition of sucrose increases the cariogenicity of cooked starchy foods, so that foods containing baked starch and substantial amounts of sucrose appear to be as cariogenic as a similar amount of sucrose on its own.

Protective factors in foods

Osborn & Noriskin (1937) suggested about 50 years ago that foods within the mouth provided substances which protected teeth against dental caries, and direct effects in the mouth of food components such as phosphates are now recognized. Other substances, e.g. fluoride, are incorporated into teeth while they are forming, and also help to protect teeth (see below). Inorganic phosphates protect against dental caries by increasing the availability of phosphate in plaque, so that demineralization is resisted and remineralization encouraged. Sodium phosphates are more effective than calcium salts, probably because of the lower solubility of the calcium phosphates. Organic phosphates act mainly by binding to the tooth surface and reducing enamel dissolution. Phytates are the most effective of these compounds.

Although phosphates have looked very promising as anti-caries substances in incubation and animal experiments, they have been very much less effective in human experiments. One reason may be the higher salivary phosphate levels in humans than in rats, so that there is less scope for a preventive effect in man. Phytates also reduce the absorption in the gut of some micronutrients, e.g. zinc, and are therefore unsuitable as food additives.

Honey is often promoted as a health food, and does contain esters and cations which could theoretically reduce caries development (Edgar & Jenkins 1974). However, evidence from rat experiments indicates that honey is as cariogenic as sucrose or a mixture of fructose, glucose and sucrose in the same proportions (45%, 35% and 5%) as in honey (Shannon et al 1979).

In the Vipeholm study (see above), patients in the chocolate group developed less caries than other groups receiving similar sugar levels and frequency of eating. This led to speculation that chocolate might contain protective factors. Animal experiments also suggested that cocoa might have a caries-protective effect (Stralfors 1966). The active ingredient has been isolated ('s-Gravenmade & Jenkins 1986), but extraction is expensive and as a method of caries prevention it is likely to be much less effective than fluoride. Glycyrrhizinic acid, a major constituent of liquorice, also has caries-preventive properties, but it is unlikely to be used as an additive because of a number of undesirable properties.

Intrinsic sugars versus free sugars

Table 38.4 lists the sources of free and intrinsic sugars in the diets of Northumberland schoolchildren aged 12–14 years (Rugg-Gunn et al 1986). Sixty-nine percent of all sugars were free sugars and most of these came from three sources – confectionery, table sugar and soft drinks. The only important sources of intrinsic sugars were milk and fruit. Whether sugars present intrinsically in milk and fruit are a serious threat to dental health is therefore also an important question.

Lactose, present in cow's milk at about 4%, can be fermented to acid but proves to be the least cariogenic of the common dietary sugars (see above). Milk also contains protective factors, e.g. calcium and phosphate: their high levels prevent the dissolution of

Table 38.4 Grams weight and percentage contribution of various groups of foods to the free and intrinsic sugars intake of 405 11–14-year-old Northumbrian children; 69% of total sugars were free sugars. (Rugg-Gunn et al 1986)

Groups of foods	Sugars			
	Free		Intrinsic	
	g	%	g	%
Confectionery	23	28	1	4
Table sugar	20	24	0	0
Soft drinks	14	17	2	6
Biscuits and cakes	10	12	3	8
Sweet puddings	7	9	6	15
Syrups and preserves	3	3	2	4
Breakfast cereals	2	3	1	1
Milk, butter, cheese		0	12	32
Fruit		0	6	15
Other	3	3	6	15
	81	100	37	100

(Free column: Confectionery, Table sugar, Soft drinks braced together = 69%)

enamel. Proteins in milk also tend to be absorbed on to the enamel surface, preventing dissolution (Jenkins & Ferguson 1966) and casein may have a specific anti-caries effect. Enamel slab (Bibby et al 1980, Thompson et al 1984) and rat (Reynolds & Johnson 1981) experiments have all indicated that milk is not cariogenic and may even be protective against caries.

There have been a few reports of caries developing in infants receiving 'on demand' breastfeeding (Hackett et al 1984). Human milk contains higher levels of lactose (7 g/100 ml) and lower levels of calcium, phosphorus and protein than cow's milk. All these factors would increase cariogenic potential and lessen the caries-protective effect of human milk compared with cow's milk. Given the importance of breastfeeding 'on demand' (see Ch. 26) and the very few reported cases of infantile caries, this potential problem should not discourage breastfeeding.

The caries-protective effect of cheese is well established from plaque pH studies (Rugg-Gunn et al 1975), enamel slab experiments (de A Silva et al 1986) and rat experiments (Edgar et al 1982). Many fruits contain sugars which can be fermented to acid by plaque bacteria, but apples have commonly featured in dental health programmes as a symbol of dental health. They were advocated mainly as a cleansing food at the end of a meal, due to their crisp texture and fibre content, but the evidence for their effectiveness is slight. There have been two clinical trials investigating apple-eating and caries (Slack & Martin 1958, Averill & Averill 1968) and one assessing carrots (Reece & Swallow 1970). One of two trials (Slack & Martin 1958) showed a very slightly lower caries incidence with apple eating; the other trial with carrots showed no effect. There is only one report (Bibby 1983) in the dental literature of caries being associated with fruit-eating in man, so fruits must be considered to be of low cariogenicity but not caries-preventive.

Fruits must be clearly distinguished from fruit juices. Fruit juices are cariogenic (Winter 1980), but it is not clear whether this depends on any added sugar, on the absence of salivary stimuli from the fibre-associated components of fruit, or whether the normal enveloping of sugars within the fruit's cell walls is crucial. Nevertheless, sweetened fruit juices induce caries, particularly in young children, whereas fresh fruits do not.

Alternative sweeteners

Many substances apart from sugars taste sweet, but relatively few are permitted for use in foods. They can be classified as either bulk sweeteners or intense sweeteners. The bulk sweeteners provide the same energy and sweetness as sugars, whereas the intense sweeteners provide little or no energy. The list of permitted sweeteners in the UK was revised in 1983 (Ministry of Agriculture, Fisheries and Food 1982) and includes the bulk sweeteners sorbitol, mannitol, xylitol, hydrogenated glucose syrup and isomalt, and the intense sweeteners saccharin, aspartame, acesulfame K and thaumatin. Cyclamate is widely used in Europe but not permitted in the UK or the USA. The bulk sweetener lactitol was approved and added in 1988. The cariogenicity of these sweeteners has been reviewed (Rugg-Gunn & Edgar 1985). Because of their composition, intense sweeteners are very unlikely to promote caries and research has been directed towards their potential caries-inhibiting properties, so far with little success.

The effect on teeth of bulk sweeteners is predictable from the tests noted above. Sorbitol and mannitol are fermented slowly, but xylitol is hardly fermented at all; these three sugar alcohols have a low cariogenicity.

There is some evidence that chewing confectionery (principally chewing gum) made with non-sugar sweeteners can aid the remineralization of precavitation carious lesions. This caries-preventive action is because chewing a non-sugar flavoursome food increases salivary flow, and fast-flowing saliva is alkaline and contains adequate mineral levels to help mineralization. Cheese has a similar effect, but has the added advantage of providing additional calcium and phosphate. Increasing salivary flow in this way may be especially useful in patients with low salivary flow due to disease, radiation, old age or drugs.

Polyols (sugar alcohols) have the disadvantage of inducing diarrhoea because of the osmotic effect of unabsorbed sugars in the lower small intestine. However, this problem seems to have been exaggerated. In the Turku study, on average 50 g/day of xylitol was taken for 2 years, and only one of the 52 participants withdrew because of unacceptable levels of intestinal disturbance.

DIET AND PERIODONTAL DISEASE

Periodontal disease is widespread in the world, with almost every adult affected to a greater or lesser degree. Progressive destruction of the supporting alveolar bone and periodontal membrane results in tooth mobility and loss of function. Periodontal disease progresses from gingivitis, and by far the most important cause of these diseases is the persistent presence of plaque on teeth adjacent to the gingivae.

Dental calculus helps the retention of plaque and these can be considered as most important extrinsic causes of periodontal disease. Intrinsic factors, which modify an individual's response to these extrinsic factors, can be nutritional as well as hormonal (e.g. pregnancy) or related to a wide variety of diseases (e.g. diabetes, blood dyscrasias).

On a population basis, there is very little evidence that the general nutritional status of a population modifies the progression of periodontal disease (Russell 1963). The most important determinant of periodontal disease is age – tooth support is gradually lost with age. The second most important determinant is the quantity of plaque and calculus on the teeth. Thus, periodontal disease was 40% worse in Ceylonese than Norwegian adults, but so was oral cleanliness (Waerhaug 1967). When the data were standardized for the state of oral hygiene, no difference in the severity of periodontal disease was seen between Norway and Sri Lanka. Assessing the importance of specific deficiencies may be difficult in population studies because periodontal disease develops very slowly, and nutritional evaluation rarely reflects lifelong nutritional conditions. Individual nutritional deficiencies which may be strongly related to periodontal disease may affect only a few individuals; the problem is hidden in a large epidemiological survey. Thus, vitamin C deficiency leads to bleeding and red, swollen gums. These changes are not caused by the deficiency itself but by the abnormal gingival response to local irritation. The gingivitis does not occur without local irritants, such as dental plaque, so in the absence of teeth there are few gum changes in vitamin C deficiency. When present, the gum changes readily respond to vitamin C therapy.

Animal experiments have shown that a number of nutritional deficiencies can cause gingivitis and/or periodontal disease. Vitamin A deficiency causes gingival hyperkeratosis, destruction of the periodontal membrane and resorption of alveolar bone. Gingivitis is commonly seen in vitamin B complex-deficient animals as a non-specific inflammatory change in response to local irritants. Vitamin D deficiency or an imbalance in the Ca/P intake results in disturbance in the formation and calcification of alveolar bone and teeth, whereas protein deficiency is related to osteoporosis of the alveolar bone and an increased inflammatory response to irritants. Other deficiencies appear to have no effect on periodontal tissues, but many deficiency diseases frequently have oral signs, for example angular cheilosis, and tongue changes in deficiencies of the B vitamins (see Ch. 14).

The local dietary effects on the mouth have little effect on periodontal health. It is claimed that a hard fibrous diet toughens the gums but evidence that it prevents gingivitis and periodontal disease in man is lacking. Six studies in the UK, Scandinavia and the USA have investigated the effect of apple-eating on gingivitis, but none demonstrated any effect. Sugar encourages the development of some plaque organisms, but there is no evidence that this leads to increased levels of gingivitis or periodontal disease.

DIET AND THE STRUCTURE OF TEETH

Sixty years ago, dental caries was considered to be a deficiency disease. This was the age of the vitamins and it was the belief of dental scientists in Britain that vitamin D deficiency led to imperfectly formed and caries-susceptible dental enamel. Mellanby (1923, 1937) observed that vitamin D deficiency in puppies resulted in hypoplastic (pitted or otherwise imperfectly formed) teeth. She also observed that many children had hypoplastic teeth and that these tended to have more carious cavities than teeth with well formed enamel. Subsequently, Mellanby (1937) and Young (1937) carried out a clinical trial in which three groups of Birmingham children were given dietary supplements of either cod-liver oil (rich in vitamin D), olive oil (low in vitamin D) or treacle. Children receiving cod-liver oil developed statistically significantly less caries in their newly erupted teeth than those in the olive oil or treacle groups.

By the 1940s opinion was changing, and the posteruptive effect of dietary sugar became accepted as the most important dietary factor in caries aetiology. Mellanby's neglected hypothesis may still have relevance in less developed countries, where dietary deficiency and illness lead to a high prevalence of hypoplastic teeth. These may be more caries-susceptible when there is a rapid increase in sugar availability. Hypocalcaemia in the neonate (due for example to vitamin D deficiency, prematurity or neonatal tetany) is a recognized cause of enamel hypoplasia (Nikiforuk & Fraser 1981).

Vitamin A deficiency in animals has been shown to result in enamel hypoplasia. Protein deficiency in rats also leads to dental hypoplasia and to impaired salivary gland development, with a reduced salivary flow. The importance of these deficiencies in man is undetermined.

Despite the obvious importance of calcium in tooth development, there is very little evidence that dietary calcium influences caries susceptibility or resistance, probably because the plasma calcium levels are normally tightly controlled. Teeth are very much less susceptible to calcium deficiency than bone. Caries tends to be lower in areas with hard water (Dean et al 1942, Ockerse 1944), but the fluoride content of the water is a much more important determinant of caries severity than water hardness.

The inverse relation between the fluoride concentration in drinking water and caries development is well known (Fig. 38.10) (Murray et al 1991). The effectiveness and safety of water fluoridation are clearly established: by 1981, 210 million people in 35 countries were receiving artificially fluoridated water, while another 103 million received water where the optimum fluoride level occurred naturally (Murray 1986). In temperate climates, including the UK, the optimum level of fluoride is 1.0 mg/l, while in warmer climates it might be nearer 0.6 mg/l. If the fluoride level in drinking water increases above the optimum level, dental enamel may be imperfectly formed. These defects, known as enamel opacities or dental fluorosis, range from small white diffuse opacities to severe pitting and staining of the enamel. It is important to realize that fluoride is not the only cause of opacities in teeth, and other causes can be general (affecting many teeth) or local (e.g. infection or trauma to the deciduous predecessor) (Pindborg 1982). The optimum level of fluoride is the level where a substantial caries reduction is observed with a negligible prevalence of enamel opacities.

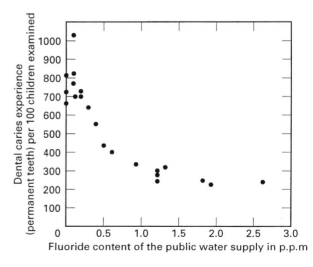

Fig. 38.10   The relation between the dental caries experience of 12–14-year-old children in 21 cities of the USA, and the fluoride content of the water supplies. (From Dean et al 1942.)

Fluoride prevents dental caries by being incorporated into the teeth while they are forming – the systemic effect – and also by local action in the mouth after teeth have erupted (the topical action). Fluoride in toothpastes and mouthrinses provides a topical effect, and these are not supposed to be swallowed. On the other hand, fluoride-containing tablets are to be swallowed so that the forming teeth benefit. It is useful if fluoride tablets dissolve slowly in the mouth to provide a topical effect on erupted teeth first, before the ingested fluoride gives a systemic effect on the developing teeth. Water fluoridation also acts both systemically and topically. This means that for maximum caries-preventive effect, a person should receive fluoridated water from birth. However, a worthwhile topical effect does occur if a person moves into a fluoridated area in childhood, and, possibly in adulthood. Other vehicles for systemic fluoride administration are salt and milk, but neither of these are used extensively. The only other worthwhile dietary sources of fluoride are tea and fish (if the bones are eaten). There have been some reports of tea drinking being related to lower caries experience (Mann et al 1985) but the relation is not clear cut, perhaps because of the common habit of adding sugar to tea. The preventive role of fluoride is dealt with extensively by Murray et al (1991).

Trace elements other than fluoride influence caries experience. Dietary molybdenum, strontium, boron and lithium are related to a lower caries experience in man, while higher selenium intakes are associated with a higher caries prevalence. Foods, e.g. vegetables, are the main sources of trace elements, but strontium, like fluoride, has water as its main dietary source (Curzon & Cutress 1983). Fluoride has a much greater influence on caries experience than other trace elements.

DIET AND STAINING OF TEETH

The surface of teeth can become stained by foods or drinks. Those blamed most frequently are tea, coffee, curries, liquorice and iron tonics. Tooth-coloured filling materials, often used to restore front teeth, and areas of enamel roughened by early caries or hypoplasia, become stained more readily than sound enamel. Dental calculus and the exposed roots of teeth also readily become stained. This is purely an aesthetic problem and such stains can usually be removed by polishing by a dentist or dental hygienist. There is a curious interaction between chlorhexidine, which is widely available as an anti-plaque mouthwash, and tea, which makes staining more

likely. If this is a problem, the avoidance of tea while using chlorhexidine mouthwashes is a sensible precaution.

EROSION OF TEETH

The definition of dental erosion as the progressive loss of tooth substance by a chemical process not involving bacterial action, distinguishes it from dental caries. It tends to occur in tooth surfaces not commonly covered by dental plaque. Of the three recognized causes – dietary, gastric and industrial – dietary acids are the most important (Asher & Read 1987). Dental erosion can occur at any age, for example, when acid fruit juices are given frequently to young children (Smith & Shaw 1987). Acid-flavoured drinks, which are often carbonated, also produce problems in children and adolescents. Sucking citrus fruits, vinegar use and iron tonics are also responsible (Eccles 1982). Erosion occurs most commonly in adolescence, with loss of the tooth substance predominantly on the palatal surface of the upper front teeth. The tooth surface retains its shiny appearance but the loss of enamel and dentine can occur so rapidly that the pulp of the tooth is exposed. Gastric regurgitation also tends to occur in young children, occasionally unnoticed by patient or parent, and in later life is sometimes associated with anorexia nervosa. Workers in the car battery industry used to have dental erosions, but this is now rare due to improved factory hygiene. Preventing further erosion in children and adults depends on finding the cause (which is often difficult) and providing good dietary advice. Dentists can usually replace the missing tooth tissue.

DIETARY ADVICE FOR DENTAL HEALTH

By far the most important dietary advice for dental health is to restrict the consumption of free (added) sugars. This is simple to say but difficult to achieve in practice, because of the very strong pressure from manufacturers of sugar and sugar-containing foods and drinks, who extol the virtues of sugar. An excellent summary of dietary advice for dental health is published by the Health Education Authority (1986).

Changing diet requires more than just giving advice (see Chapter 51): it involves promoting healthy eating at several levels. For a country, these levels might be central (e.g. government), local or district, and individual. The action required at each of these will be discussed.

Dietary advice during pregnancy

No specific dietary advice is required for the future dental health of a fetus, other than that included in advice for the general wellbeing of the child. In developed countries, diets are usually adequate to ensure that developing teeth are well formed, but in underdeveloped countries hypocalcaemia-induced linear dental hypoplasia may commonly be due to dietary deficiencies. Such teeth are more prone to caries if sugar intakes are high after tooth eruption.

Dietary fluoride supplements are no longer recommended during pregnancy: they do no harm (at the recommended dose) but the advantage to the future child is small and not considered worth the effort.

The dental health of the mother-to-be should not be ignored, but dietary advice for her is no different from that for any adult (see below). Pregnancy gingivitis is sometimes a problem but is hormonal, not dietary, in origin. There is no truth in the belief that the fetus removes calcium from a mother's teeth, making them softer and more likely to decay.

Infant

The first teeth erupt at about 6 months, but this is very variable. Avoiding unnecessary intakes of free sugars is sensible from an early age, since dietary habits begin early. Bottle feeds require no further addition of sugar. Adding sugar to milk feeds, and particularly to fruit drinks, is strongly linked to extensive dental caries in young children (Winter 1980). This should only be done in very exceptional circumstances. Comforter bottles containing sweetened drinks have an especially bad reputation as a cause of extensive caries in infants and young children. The habit of giving infants dummies smeared with jam or honey is now, thankfully, dying out. Very rarely, on-demand breastfeeding has been associated with caries in infants. This occurs so rarely and breastfeeding is too important to be discouraged for this small risk.

A small group of infants and young children have to take oral medicines daily for a long time. To ensure they are taken they are often sweetened, usually with sugars. Their use is associated with high caries experience in children who may already be medically compromised. A number of alternative non-sugar sweeteners are now available, and medicines formulated with these dentally safe sweeteners should be recommended whenever possible (Hobson 1985).

Some manufacturers of infant foods have made great efforts to remove free sugars from their

Table 38.5 Fluoride dietary supplements – age-related dosages (mg/day) (Murray et al 1991)

Age	Concentration of fluoride in drinking water (ppm F)		
	< 0.3	0.3–0.7	> 0.7
2 weeks–2 years	0.25	0	0
2–4 years	0.50	0.25	0
4–16 years	1.00	0.50	0

products. Concentrated fruit juices should not be substituted for more obvious free sugars; fruit juices are important sources of water and vitamin C, but it is essential to restrict their use to no more than necessary and not use them as a comforter: plain safe water is an under-used drink. The consumption of confectionery causes caries in infants and children and should be seen as an exception dietary item, rather than a regular part of daily intake.

An adequate intake of fluoride is desirable. If the fluoride level of the water supply is less than optimal, dietary fluoride supplements may be recommended. These can be purchased in pharmacies, prescribed by a general practitioner or issued at community dental clinics. The current recommended dosage in the UK is given in Table 38.5. The District Dental Officer can supply further information on local water fluoride levels and recommendations on daily fluoride supplements.

Children and adolescents

The most important sources of dietary sugars are confectionery, table sugar and soft drinks (see Table 38.4). These three sources provide over two-thirds of the intake of free sugars, which in turn account for over two-thirds of the intake of all sugars. Restricting the intake of these three sources would do much to reduce the quantity of sugars eaten and the frequency of sugar consumption, and so reduce the high increment of caries which occurs in childhood. The method by which each person or each household brings about a reduction in their consumption of free sugars is an individual matter. Some families may decide to restrict confectionery consumption to one day a week, e.g. Saturday lunchtimes, or soft drinks to no more than once a day. Soft drinks with non-sugar sweeteners can be a useful occasional alternative. Sugar added to tea or coffee may be particularly harmful to teeth, and encouraging people to omit sugar from these drinks is likely to be well worth while. It is important to give positive advice, with suggestions for healthier snack foods.

Dietary fluoride supplements can be recommended if the public water supply contains insufficient fluoride (Table 38.5).

Adults and the elderly

The incidence of dental caries is highest in young children, adolescents and the elderly, and seems to be lowest in younger adults. Caries does occur in adults, especially around old fillings and in the roots of teeth. Confectionery, table sugar, soft drinks, biscuits, cakes and puddings are important sources of sugar, and should be the main target for dietary advice.

As dental services and dental health improve, more elderly people retain their natural teeth. The main advice for this group of people is still restriction of their sugar intake. This may also be desirable to improve the nutrient density of the diet of these people with declining energy requirements. The elderly may have greater difficulty in eating – their natural teeth may be mobile due to periodontal disease, and their artificial teeth may be a poor fit or difficult to manage. It is important that such people seek dental advice regularly in order to make eating as efficient and comfortable as possible. Mincing foods is sometimes necessary to ensure that a nutritious diet is eaten.

Saliva has many important functions in aiding eating, swallowing, speaking, and in preventing dental caries and other oral infections. Salivary flow decreases in old age due to atrophy, and can be markedly reduced by some diseases, e.g. Sjøgren's syndrome, after radiotherapy to head and neck, and as a response to a number of drugs. Rampant caries can follow destruction or removal of the salivary glands, and its control may require severe sugar restriction together with intensive topical fluoride therapy. Salivary substitutes are available (Rugg-Gunn 1985) and are useful to many patients.

Special groups

High-carbohydrate diets are required for some patients (e.g. with phenylketonuria and cystic fibrosis) and dietitians may well feel that it is essential for the patient's wellbeing that much of this carbohydrate is taken as sugars. The patient's dentist must accept this, and it will require cooperation between the dietitian, dentist and family to ensure that caries is prevented as much as possible by means other than sugar restriction.

The mentally handicapped often have difficulty in feeding, and a dentist can often help by adapting eating utensils so that they are easier to grip (Hunter 1987). One slight advantage in the dental care of hospitalized or mentally handicapped persons is that dietary control of dental caries is, in theory, easier. It is important that people who provide the diet for such people appreciate the need to restrict the provision of high-sugar foods and drinks.

Action required at national, local and individual levels to promote dental health by dietary means

A government can do much to promote dental health. For example, the introduction of water fluoridation may require legal action which can only be undertaken centrally. In Ireland and Singapore, water fluoridation is mandatory. Labelling of foods should be uniform, allowing informed consumer choice: sugar labelling is an essential part of this. Restriction of the use of sugar in medicines requires a governmental decision. Health service rules need to be geared to prevention: for example, encouraging dentists to give good dietary advice is better than paying them to restore diseased teeth. Agricultural policy needs to be compatible with national health goals: at present, sugar production is heavily subsidized in the EC. Perhaps most important of all, changes in the nation's diet required for greater health need to be agreed by all professional groups and accepted by the public. The advice to be given to the public is best coordinated by one central agency, such as the Health Education Authority.

The objectives agreed at a national level will then need to be implemented at a local level. The district food policy and the message for healthy eating need to be agreed and implemented by all professional groups, including dentists. Cooperation between dietitians and dentists can assist in the care of many individual patients. Half the population of the UK attend a dentist regularly (approximately once a year). Dietitians should be aware of the potential this provides for dietary advice, and ensure that dentists are kept adequately informed on general dietary matters.

REFERENCES

Asher C, Read MJF 1987 Early enamel erosion in children associated with excessive consumption of citric acid. British Dental Journal 162: 384–387

Averill HM, Averill JE 1968 The effect of daily apple consumption on dental caries experience, oral hygiene status and upper respiratory infection. New York State Dental Journal 34: 403–409

Bang G, Kristoffersen T 1972 Dental caries and diet in an

Alaskan Eskimo population. Scandinavian Journal of Dental Research 80: 440–444

Bibby BG 1983 Fruits and vegetables and dental caries. Clinical Preventive Dentistry 5: 3–11

Bibby BG, Huang CT, Zero D, Mundorff SA, Little MF 1980 Protective effect of milk against 'in vitro' caries. Journal of Dental Research 59: 1565–1570

Biscuit, Cake, Chocolate and Confectionery Alliance 1987 Submission to the COMA panel on sugars, London

Bowen WH, Amsbaugh SM, Monell-Torrens S, Brunelle J, Kuzmiak-Jones H, Cole MF 1980 A method to assess cariogenic potential of foodstuffs. Journal of American Dental Association 100: 677–681

Curzon MEJ, Cutress TW 1983 Trace elements and dental disease. John Wright, Boston

de A Silva MF, Jenkins GN, Burgess RC, Sandham HJ 1986 Effects of cheese on experimental caries in human subjects. Caries Research 20: 263–269

Dean HT, Arnold FA, Elvolve E 1942 Domestic water and dental caries V. Public Health Report 57: 1155–1179

Eccles JD 1982 Erosion affecting the palatal surfaces of upper anterior teeth in young people. British Dental Journal 152: 375–378

Edger WM 1985 Prediction of the cariogenicity of various foods. International Dental Journal 35: 190–194

Edgar WM, Jenkins GN 1974 Solubility-reducing agents in honey and partially refined crystalline sugar. British Dental Journal 136: 7–14

Edgar WM, Bowen WH, Amsbaugh S, Monell-Torrens S, Brunelle J 1982 Effects of different eating patterns on dental caries in the rat. Caries Research 16: 384–389

Fisher FJ 1968 A field study of dental caries, periodontal disease and enamel defects in Tristan da Cunha. British Dental Journal 125: 447–453

Glickman I 1964 Clinical periodontology, 3rd edn. Saunders, Philadelphia

Guggenheim B, Konig KG, Herzog E, Muhlemann HR 1966 The cariogenicity of different dietary carbohydrates tested on rats in relative gnotobiosis with a Streptococcus producing extracellular polysaccharide. Helvetica Odontologica Acta 10: 101–113

Gustaffson BE, Quensel CE, Lanke LS et al 1954 The Vipeholm dental caries study. The effect of different levels of carbohydrate intake on caries activity in 436 individuals observed for five years. Acta Odontologica Scandinavica 11: 232–364

Hackett AF, Rugg-Gunn AJ, Murray JJ, Roberts GJ 1984 Can breast feeding cause dental caries? Human Nutrition: Applied Nutrition 38A: 23–28

Hankin JH, Chung CS, Kau MCW 1973 Genetic and epidemiologic studies of oral characteristics in Hawaii's schoolchildren: diet patterns and caries prevalence. Journal of Dental Research 52: 1079–1086

Harris R 1963 Biology of the children of Hopewood House, Bowral, Australia. 4. Observations on dental caries experience extending over 5 years (1957–61). Journal of Dental Research 42: 1387–1399

Health Education Authority 1986 The scientific basis of dental health education; a policy statement. HEA, London

Hefti A, Schmid R 1979 Effect on caries incidence in rats of increasing dietary sucrose levels. Caries Research 13: 298–300

Hobson P 1985 Sugar-based medicines and dental disease. Community Dental Health 2: 57–62

Hunter B 1987 Dental care for handicapped patients. John Wright, Bristol

Huxley HG 1977 The cariogenicity of dietary sucrose at various levels in two strains of rat under unrestricted and controlled frequency feeding condition. Caries Research 11: 237–242

Jakobsen J 1979 Recent reorganisation of the public dental health service in Greenland in favour of caries prevention. Community Dentistry: Oral Epidemiology 7: 75–81

Jenkins GN, Ferguson DB 1966 Milk and dental caries. British Dental Journal 120: 472–477

Kite OW, Shaw JH, Sognnaes RF 1950 The prevention of experimental tooth decay by tube-feeding. Journal of Nutrition 42: 89–103

Kleemola-Kujala E, Rasanen L 1979 Dietary pattern of Finnish children with low and high caries experience. Community Dentistry: Oral Epidemiology 7: 199–205

Konig KG 1969 Caries activity induced by frequency-controlled feeding of diets containing sucrose or bread to Osborne-Mendel rats. Archives of Oral Biology 14: 991–993

Konig KG, Schmid P, Schmid R 1968 An apparatus for frequency-controlled feeding of small rodents and its use in dental caries experiments. Archives of Oral Biology 13: 13–26

Koulourides T, Bodden R, Keller S, Manson-Hing L, Lastra J, Housch T 1976 Cariogenicity of nine sugars tested with an intraoral device in man. Caries Research 10: 427–441

Lindhe J 1983 Textbook of clinical periodontology. Munksgaard, Copenhagen

Mann J, Sgan-Cohen HD, Dakuar A, Gedalia I 1985 Teadrinking, caries prevalence, and fluorosis among northern Israeli Arab youth. Clinical Preventive Dentistry 7: 23–26

Martinsson T 1972 Socioeconomic investigation of schoolchildren with high and low caries frequency. III. A dietary study based on information given by the children. Odontologica Rev 23: 93–114

Mellanby M 1923 The relation of caries to the structure of teeth. British Dental Journal 44: 1–13

Mellanby M 1937 The role of nutrition as a factor in resistance to dental caries. British Dental Journal 62: 241–252

Ministry of Agriculture, Fisheries and Food 1982 Food additives and contaminants committee report on the review of sweeteners in food. FAC/REP/34. HMSO, London

Moller IJ, Poulson S, Orholm Nielsen V 1972 The prevalence of dental caries in Godhavn and Scoresbysund districts, Greenland. Scandinavian Journal of Dental Research 80: 168–180

Murray JJ 1986 Appropriate use of fluorides for human health. World Health Organization, Geneva

Murray JJ, Rugg-Gunn AJ, Jenkins GN 1991 Fluorides in caries prevention, 3rd edn. Butterworth-Heinemann, Oxford

Newbrun E 1978 Cariology. Williams and Wilkins, Baltimore

Newbrun E 1984 Diet and dental caries. In: Guggenheim B (ed) Cariology today. Karger, Basel, pp 340–52

Newbrun E, Hoover C, Mettraux G, Graf H 1980 Comparison of dietary habits and dental health of subjects with hereditary fructose intolerance and control subjects. Journal of American Dental Association 101: 619–626

Nikiforuk G, Fraser D 1981 The etiology of enamel

hypoplasia: a unifying concept. Journal of Pediatrics 98: 888–893

Ockerse T 1944 Relation of fluoride content, hardness and pH values of drinking water and incidence of dental caries. South African Medical Journal 18: 255–258

Osborn TWB, Noriskin JN 1937 The relationship between diet and dental caries in South African Bantu. Journal of Dental Research 16: 431–441

Pederson PO 1938 Investigations into dental conditions of about 3000 ancient and modern Greenlanders. Dental Record 58: 191–198

Pindborg JJ 1982 Aetiology of developmental enamel defects not related to fluorosis. International Dental Journal 32: 123–131

Reece JA, Swallow JN 1970 Carrots and dental health. British Dental Journal 128: 535–539

Reynolds EC, Johnson IH 1981 Effect of milk on caries incidence and bacterial composition of dental plaque in the rat. Archives of Oral Biology 26: 445–451

Rugg-Gunn AJ 1985 Practical aspects of diet and dental caries in the elderly. In: Derrick D (ed) The dental annual. John Wright, Bristol, pp 159–165

Rugg-Gunn AJ 1988 Starchy foods and fresh fruits: their relative importance as a source of dental caries in Britain. A review of the literature. Occasional paper No. 3. Health Education Authority, London

Rugg-Gunn AJ 1989 Diet and dental caries. In: Murray JJ (ed) The prevention of dental disease, 2nd edn. Oxford University Press. Oxford, pp 4–114

Rugg-Gunn AJ 1993 Nutrition and dental health. Oxford University Press, Oxford

Rugg-Gunn AJ, Edgar WM 1985 Sweeteners and dental health. Community Dental Health 2: 213–223

Rugg-Gunn AJ, Edgar WM, Geddes DAM, Jenkins GN 1975 The effect of different meal patterns upon plaque pH in human subjects. British Dental Journal 139: 351–356

Rugg-Gunn AJ, Hackett AF, Appleton DR, Jenkins GN, Eastoe JE 1984 Relationship between dietary habits and caries increment assessed over two years in 405 English adolescent schoolchildren. Archives of Oral Biology 29: 983–992

Rugg-Gunn AJ, Hackett AF, Appleton DR, Moynihan PJ 1986 The dietary intake of added and natural sugars in 405 English adolescents. Human Nutrition: Applied Nutrition 40A: 115–124

Russell AL 1963 International nutrition surveys, a summary of preliminary dental findings. Journal of Dental Research 42: 233–244

Scheinin A, Makinen KK 1975 Turku sugar studies. I-XXI.

Acta Odontologica Scandinavica 33 (Suppl 70), 1–349

's-Gravenmade EJ, Jenkins GN 1986 Isolation, purification and some properties of a potential cariostatic factor in cocoa that lowers enamel solubility. Caries Research 20: 433–436

Shannon IL, Edmonds EJ, Madsen KO 1979 Honey: sugar content and cariogenicity. Journal of Dentistry for Children 46: 29–33

Sheiham A 1984 Changing trends in dental caries. International Dental Journal 13: 142–147

Slack GL, Martin WJ 1958 Apples and dental health. British Dental Journal 105: 366–371

Smith AJ, Shaw L 1987 Baby fruit juices and tooth erosion. British Dental Journal 162: 65–67

Sognnaes RF 1948 Analysis of wartime reduction of dental caries in European children. American Journal of Diseases of Children 75: 792–821

Sreebny LM 1982 Sugar availability, sugar consumption and dental caries. Community Dentistry: Oral Epidemiology 10: 1–7

Sreebny LM 1983 Cereal availability and dental caries. Community Dentistry: Oral Epidemiology 11: 148–155

Stralfors A 1966 Inhibition of hamster caries by cocoa. Archives of Oral Biology 11: 323–328

Takahashi K 1961 Statistical study on caries incidence in the first molar in relation to the amount of sugar consumption. Bulletin of the Tokyo Dental College 2: 44–57

Tehrani A, Brudevold F, Attarzadeh F, van Houte J, Russo J 1983 Enamel demineralization by mouthrinses containing different concentrations of sucrose. Journal of Dental Research 62: 1216–1217

Thompson ME, Pearce EIF 1982 The cariogenicity of experimental biscuits containing wheatgerm and rolled oats, and the effect of supplementation with milk powder. New Zealand Dental Journal 78: 3–6

Thompson ME, Dever JG, Pearce EIF 1984 Intraoral testing of flavoured sweetened milk. New Zealand Dental Journal 80: 44–46

Waerhaug J 1967 Prevalence of periodontal disease in Ceylon. Associations with age, sex, oral hygiene, socioeconomic factors, vitamin deficiencies, malnutrition, betel and tobacco consumption and ethnic group. Acta Odontologica Scandinavica 25: 205–231

Winter GB 1980 Problems involved with the use of comforters. International Dental Journal 30: 28–38

Young M 1937 The role of nutrition as a factor in resistance to dental caries. British Dental Journal 62: 252–259

Zitzow RE 1979 The relationship of diet and dental caries in the Alaskan eskimo population. Alaska Medicine 21: 10–14

39. Nutritional management of diseases of the blood

I. Chanarin

Haemopoietic cells have the same requirements for nutrients as all other growing cells. The rate of renewal of blood cells, however, is greater than that of any other tissue in the mammalian body and this makes the haemopoietic system particularly vulnerable to deficiencies of folate and cobalamin (Cbl), which have an important role in nucleotide synthesis. Further, the requirement for iron, an essential component of the haemoglobin molecule, makes iron supply an important limiting factor in red blood cell production. Thus deficiencies of iron, folate and Cbl are relatively common. It is rare for deficiencies of other nutrients to affect haemopoiesis but this can occur in relation to ascorbic acid, vitamin E, vitamin A, riboflavin and copper.

A vegetarian diet is associated with adverse effects on haemopoiesis. First, Cbl is entirely absent from the vegetable kingdom and a strictly vegetarian diet does not contain Cbl other than that arising by contamination from a water supply or bacteria. Secondly, iron is only poorly available for intestinal absorption from a vegetarian diet and nutritional iron deficiency is common.

IRON

The metabolism of iron is considered in detail in Chapter 12. Factors relating to blood disorders are briefly recapitulated here.

Physiological considerations

Body iron totals some 3–4 g in adults. Most of the iron is present in circulating haemoglobin in red blood cells, with far smaller amounts in myoglobin and various haem and non–haem enzymes, including cytochromes concerned with the oxidative production of energy. The remaining iron is a reserve (storage iron) linked to ferritin and haemosiderin (degraded ferritin) in liver, spleen and bone marrow.

Clinical signs and symptoms of iron deficiency

Iron deficiency of modest degree may come to light as the result of blood tests in asymptomatic subjects. More usually, the patient shows the symptoms and signs of anaemia and the severity increases as the level of haemoglobin falls. Lack of energy, tiring easily, shortness of breath, palpitations, headache, weakness, dizziness and irritability may occur. Occasionally patients complain of paraesthesiae of hands and feet. Long–standing anaemia is accompanied by considerable adaptation to the reduced haemoglobin level, and in such patients tiredness may be the only complaint. Effects on epithelial surfaces may result in a sore mouth and tongue, angular stomatitis and a sensation of a lump in the throat with difficulty in swallowing. Nails break easily and may be misshapen. Pica or eating of materials such as ice, clay, paper, dirt etc., occurs particularly in children.

Examination shows pallor, particularly of the mucous membranes. There may be a smooth, shiny, atrophic tongue mucosa. Red cracks may be present at the angles of the mouth. Nails may be irregular, broken and classically spoon-shaped (koilonychia). Long-standing severe anaemia may be accompanied by splenomegaly.

Radiography may show a postcricoid web and atrophic gastritis. There is impairment of cell-mediated (T-lymphocyte) immunity and impairment of neutrophil killing of phagocytosed bacteria by cells from iron-deficient subjects. However, iron therapy can precipitate or activate latent infection such as pyelonephritis or falciparum malaria. In the tropics iron therapy should probably be given with anti-malarial prophylaxis.

Laboratory findings

Iron deficiency is manifested by a fall in haemoglobin below the level that is normal in that individual and, in time, below 13 g/dl in men and 12 g/dl in women. There is a fall in the size of the red cells to below 80 fl and the smaller red cells will have less haemoglobin so that the mean corpuscular haemoglobin (MCH) falls below 27 pg. Initially the small red cells may appear fully haemoglobinized in the stained blood film but, in time, iron deficiency reduces the haemoglobin content so that hypochromia is evident. In severe anaemia the red blood cell appears as a thin pink ring.

Neutrophil nuclei tend to become hypersegmented and the platelet count tends to rise, in part as a response to blood loss but also due to lack of iron.

The serum iron level (normal 11–28 μmol/l) is below 11 and the iron-binding capacity (normal 47–70 μmol/l) increases above 70. Transferrin saturation is below 16% (normal 16–60%). The serum ferritin level falls below 11 μg/l and stainable iron is absent from aspirated marrow particles.

Anaemia with small red blood cells also occurs in thalassaemia syndromes and in the anaemia of chronic disorders. These must be differentiated from iron-deficiency anaemia. The thalassaemias are a heterogeneous group of disorders of haemoglobin synthesis, all of which result from a reduced rate of production of one or more of the globin chains of haemoglobin. Thalassaemia syndromes are characterized by relatively high red-cell counts, often exceeding 6 million/μl. The serum iron and ferritin levels are normal in uncomplicated thalassaemia trait. Beta thalassaemia trait is characterized by a raised haemoglobin A2 level.

Anaemia of chronic disorders may closely resemble iron deficiency, but unlike iron deficiency the iron-binding capacity is either normal or low. Ferritin, being an acute-phase protein, may give misleading results in infections etc., and values between 50 and 100 μg/l may be found in the absence of iron stores. If there is still doubt about the diagnosis, marrow aspiration will show that iron is present in marrow fragments taken from patients with the anaemia of chronic disorders, unless there is accompanying iron deficiency as may occur in patients with rheumatoid arthritis treated with non-steroidal analgesics, which tend to induce blood loss.

Some authors include sideroblastic anaemia as needing to be differentiated from iron deficiency. The blood film in sideroblastic anaemia shows a mixture of normochromic and hypochromic red cells, but the MCV is invariably raised and not low, as in iron deficiency, thalassaemia and usually anaemia of chronic disorders.

Microcytosis is the norm in infants and young children, and adult values in a blood count are not attained until the mid-teens. Iron deficiency is common in infants and a serum iron and iron-binding capacity is needed whenever there is doubt, or a response to oral iron can be tried.

Diagnosis

A firm diagnosis of iron deficiency requires a blood count showing the features described above, and either a low serum iron level with an increase in iron-binding capacity or a low serum ferritin level. In some circumstances a therapeutic trial of oral iron may be useful.

To establish that iron deficiency is due to nutritional deficiency requires an assessment of the subject's diet and the exclusion of blood loss, mainly via menstruation and the gastrointestinal tract. In some patients intestinal malabsorption due to gluten sensitivity, gut resection or post gastrectomy, may be the cause. A careful history must be taken and samples of faeces must be examined for hookworm ova and occult blood. Gastrointestinal blood loss is often intermittent, and endoscopy or a barium series may be required to exclude bleeding lesions in the upper and large gut. The ingestion of aspirin and non-steroidal analgesics must be excluded. A diet likely to lead to iron deficiency is a strictly vegetarian one from which foods of animal origin are excluded. Milk, often taken as tea, occasional cheese and eggs are often insufficient to improve iron bioavailability in such a diet. An accompanying low serum cobalamin level will confirm the inadequate intake of animal products.

Treatment

Treatment of iron deficiency is by oral iron salts, of which ferrous sulphate, usually available as a tablet supplying 200 mg of iron, is the most satisfactory. The tablets are best taken without food. Ascorbate, such as in orange juice, enhances iron absorption, and in overt iron deficiency ferrous sulphate is given three times a day. Some patients have gastrointestinal discomfort with the medication and these should start with one tablet daily.

Response is accompanied by clinical benefit and a rise in the haemoglobin level of about 1 g/dl week. Treatment should aim to replenish iron stores as well as to correct the anaemia, and this may require 6 months of therapy. It should be added that the large unphysiological amounts of iron used in treatment quite overwhelm the subtle mechanisms regulating physiological iron absorption, and the iron enters the enterocyte by passive diffusion. A more balanced diet, where this is possible, is desirable, but economic, traditional or religious situations may make this difficult.

COBALAMIN

Cbl originates from bacterial synthesis. Herbivores have active Cbl synthesis via the bacterial flora in their foregut, and this is their source of Cbl. Animals grazed on cobalt-deficient pastures exhibit a variety of disorders as a result of Cbl deficiency and due to inadequate Cbl synthesis in their foregut. Carnivores obtain Cbl from animal products in their diets.

Cbl is absent from the plant kingdom and reports of its demonstration in one or other fruit, root or leaf is due to contamination by soil bacteria or from water. A clean, strictly vegetarian diet supplies no Cbl. Fruit bats normally obtain Cbl by inadvertently eating insects on the outside of fruit. Fruit bats fed washed fruit develop a neuropathy and die of Cbl deficiency in about 9 months.

Dietary intake of cobalamin

Individuals consuming mixed diets such as those in Europe, North and South America generally take between 3 and 7 µg Cbl in 24 hours. Calculations based on food intake in tropical Africa suggest an intake of 0.49–2.8 µg Cbl/24 h. Elsewhere, 24-hour Cbl intake has been assessed as 0.46 µg (India), 0.3 µg (Bangladesh), 1.36 µg (Pakistan), 0.72 µg (Indonesia), 1.02 µg (Burma) and 1.24 µg (China).

Direct assay of the Cbl contents of diets by the duplicate food preparation method in Sweden showed a mean 24-hour intake of 5 µg (Borgström et al 1975).

Cbl is stable to heat such as that involved in cooking, other than when the pH exceeds 12, but some is leached into cooking liquids and may be lost in this way. Dietary Cbl is protein–linked as part of holoenzymes and there is no free Cbl. Cbl is readily freed from the enzyme in the stomach and upper gut by proteolytic enzymes.

Requirement for cobalamin

The FAO/WHO (1988) recommendation for a safe level of intake is shown in Table 39.1. These data indicate that western diets supply more Cbl than is required, and vegetarian diets less than is 'safe'.

Dietary assay in South India showed a 24-hour intake of 0.25–0.5 µg (Baker & Mathan 1981) and in Caucasian vegetarians in Australia a daily intake of 0.26 ± 0.23 µg (SD). Despite this low intake the

Table 39.1 Dietary requirements for cobalamin

Group	Safe level of intake (µg/24 h)
Adults	1.0
Pregnancy	1.4
Lactation	1.3
Infants	0.1
Children 1–10 years	0.04 µg/kg
Children 11–16	1.0

majority of subjects remain healthy. Only 21 of 431 (4.8%) Australian vegetarians had serum Cbl levels below 100 pg/ml. However, a much higher frequency of low serum Cbl levels has been found in Indian vegetarians. Mehta et al (1964) found that the mean serum Cbl level among a group of vegetarian medical students was 121 pg/ml, as compared to a mean of 366 pg/ml in a group on a mixed diet. In London, serum Cbl in 1000 consecutive samples from Indians who were largely vegetarian, showed a mean level of 198 pg/ml, as compared to 334 pg/ml in an age-matched Caucasian group taking a mixed diet; 54% of the Indian subjects had low serum Cbl levels (Chanarin & Stephenson 1988).

Assessment of the daily Cbl intake of vegetarians who developed nutritional Cbl deficiency shows values no different from those consumed by the bulk of the vegetarian population (Chanarin 1990). It must be concluded that a Cbl intake of up to 0.5 µg/24 h is not 'safe', in so far as it will not protect a small minority from developing evidence of a deficiency state. Perhaps a minimum safe level of Cbl intake is one that maintains the serum Cbl level above the range associated with megaloblastic anaemia, that is, above 170 pg/ml, and this is somewhere between 0.5 and 1.0 µg/24 h.

Absolutely strict vegetarians are rare: most take some form of animal produce, the commonest of which is cow's milk (whole, pasteurized) which contains 3.6 µg Cbl/l. Among Indians it is often boiled and taken in tea. Yoghurt has about 0.8 µg Cbl/l and is often mixed into food. Cheese may be taken occasionally: Cheddar has about 10 µg Cbl/kg and cottage cheese about 6 µg Cbl/kg. Whole eggs supply about 30 µg Cbl/kg. Packaged cereals and other foods frequently have Cbl added and this is a significant and acceptable source of dietary Cbl to many vegetarians. Nevertheless, many patients in whom nutritional Cbl deficiency has developed have indicated that they do take cow's milk most days and cheese once or more weekly, and even occasional eggs.

Signs and symptoms of nutritional cobalamin deficiency

These observations are based on a study of 95 patients with nutritional Cbl deficiency seen among Hindu Indian patients who were lifelong vegetarians (Chanarin et al 1985). There were 43 men and 52 women and their age at diagnosis ranged from 13 to over 80 years. Their symptoms were tiredness (33%), shortness of breath (25%), loss of appetite (23%), loss of weight (22%), generalized aches (19%) due to associated osteomalacia, calcium and vitamin D deficiency, vomiting (19%), paraesthesiae (11%), change in skin pigmentation (8%), sore mouth and/or tongue (7%), diarrhoea (6%) and headache (5%). Five per cent of the patients had attended the infertility clinic and in 6% macrocytosis in a blood count was an unexpected finding. Loss of hair colour was present in a 19-year-old male with a haemoglobin level of 3.6 g/dl. Oral Cbl therapy restored the normal jet black colour of his hair.

The physical findings reflected the degree of anaemia. Apart from pallor of the mucous membranes, a smooth tongue was common. One severely anaemic patient had a 3 cm splenomegaly which disappeared after Cbl therapy. Fourteen had jaundice. None had neuropathy.

Haematology

The haemoglobin level at diagnosis ranged from 3.0 to 16 g/dl. In 26 patients the haemoglobin level was above 13 g/dl, but all were macrocytic. Fifteen patients, however, had either a normal or a low MCV, the lowest being 60 fl. In all these patients the marrow was megaloblastic, which was the basis of diagnosis. The explanation for the normal or low MCV was accompanying iron deficiency in eight, beta-thalassaemia trait in five and alpha-thalassaemia trait in the remaining two.

Serum Cbl levels were low in all. Red-cell folate was low in 31 out of 78 patients, but no patient required folate to achieve a response. This is the expected finding in Cbl deficiency.

Cbl absorption was tested in 85 patients and was normal in 80 and impaired in five. Three of the latter were retested after several months of Cbl therapy and in all three the test had returned to normal. Transient Cbl malabsorption is well known in long-standing Cbl deficiency.

Sixteen of 47 patients excreted more than 5 g of faecal fat per 24 hours on a 100 g/24 h fat intake. Faecal fat excretion was retested after Cbl therapy in three patients who had had daily fat excretions of 20.7, 7.1 and 10.3 g. In these the faecal fat excretion declined to 4.3, 2.3 and 4.3 g respectively, which are normal values. A reduced urinary xylose after 5 g orally was present in 16 out of 43 patients, this being further evidence of intestinal malabsorption due to Cbl deficiency.

Jejunal biopsies were available in 42 patients; these were normal in 37. Three showed partial villous atrophy, one moderate and one severe atrophy. All but one had severe anaemia and faecal fat excretion was increased in four. Clinically these patients were indistinguishable from the remaining 90 patients. The abnormal biopsies were interpreted as being secondary to Cbl deficiency.

Fifteen patients had associated osteomalacia. Serum calcium was low in 28 out of 90 patients and alkaline phosphatase was raised in 23. Serum albumin was normal in all but one 80-year-old. Serum bilirubin was raised in 40 patients.

Thirteen of the 95 patients had active tuberculosis, either in the past or currently, involving mainly the lymph glands, lungs and bone. In the UK a very high frequency of tuberculosis has been noted in Asiatic Indians (MRC tuberculosis survey 1980). When the incidence of tuberculosis in Caucasians was given a value of 1, that in Indians was 38, and in West Indians of African origin, 3. The Indian population is largely vegetarian and an impairment in bacterial killing by phagocytes from Cbl-deficient subjects, as well as from iron-deficient subjects, has been noted (Kaplan & Basford 1976, Skacel & Chanarin 1983). A nutritional survey among 1187 Indian subjects to see if there was any relationship between diet and tuberculosis showed that the incidence of tuberculosis in vegetarians was 133 per 1000, and in those on mixed diets 48 per 1000. This difference was highly significant, suggesting that Cbl and iron deficiency in vegetarians may have a role in determining susceptibility to tuberculosis. The high frequency of iron deficiency has been discussed.

Diagnosis of nutritional cobalamin deficiency

Nutritional Cbl deficiency can be suspected in a vegetarian patient with a macrocytic blood picture, bearing in mind the possibility that the macrocytosis may be absent when the patient has thalassaemia trait or iron deficiency. In the latter case iron therapy will bring out macrocytosis. Unless the peripheral blood changes are characteristic of megaloblastic anaemia, a marrow examination is necessary for diagnosis and this will show megaloblastic haemopoiesis.

A low serum Cbl level was found in 54% of 1000 sera from Indian subjects, but only ten new patients each year were seen with megaloblastic anaemia. Thus measurement of the serum Cbl level is not helpful in distinguishing those who have a megaloblastic anaemia, but a normal level excludes such deficiency.

Other causes of megaloblastic anaemia must be excluded. Of 129 Indians with megaloblastic anaemia, 20 had pernicious anaemia, one carcinoma of the stomach, four megaloblastic anaemia in pregnancy, four had megaloblastic anaemia due to nutritional folate deficiency generally associated with alcoholism, and the remaining 100 had nutritional Cbl deficiency (Chanarin et al 1985).

Elsewhere the situation is more complex. In Sri Lanka Senewirante et al (1974) reported on 47 patients, all but two being women. Fifteen responded to 4 µg oral Cbl daily, indicating that they had nutritional Cbl deficiency; ten had a second response when 50 µg of oral folate was added to the Cbl, indicating a dual deficiency; and 22 responded only to folate, indicating a folate deficiency. Caucasians who adopt a vegetarian diet rarely develop a megaloblastic anaemia.

To establish that the nutritional megaloblastic anaemia is due to Cbl deficiency it is necessary to show that the patient responds fully to Cbl taken by mouth in an amount present in a mixed diet – about 5 µg daily. Such responses are not as dramatic as those seen with a large injection of Cbl. There is only a modest reticulocyte rise, or even none at all, but a steady rise in the haemoglobin level to the normal range and a fall in the MCV to normal. A fall in the MCV below 80 fl generally indicates that iron deficiency has supervened and oral iron has to be added to achieve a full response.

In older patients where pernicious anaemia is the common alternative diagnosis, it may be more sensible to carry out a Cbl absorption test at an early stage. The usual way is the urinary excretion method, which entails an injection of 1000 µg of cyanoCbl. This will restore a normal blood picture. Nutritional Cbl deficiency is diagnosed if the Cbl absorption test is normal and the patient responds to Cbl. As indicated, transient Cbl malabsorption can occur as a result of long-standing Cbl deficiency (5 out of 85 patients) and in these further steps to exclude pernicious anaemia are necessary. These will entail the study of gastric function, such as the presence of acid and intrinsic factor in gastric juice, serum gastrin level and gastric biopsy. Normal gastric function excludes pernicious anaemia. Rarely, Cbl deficiency can be due to abnormalities of the small gut such as strictures, diverticuli, etc. These will be suspected if Cbl malabsorption persists and is not corrected when intrinsic factor is given with $^{57}CoB_{12}$ in the test.

Nutritional management

In the short term, treatment with either oral or parenteral Cbl will restore the blood to normal. Even those patients treated initially with oral Cbl will benefit in the long term by one or more injections of hydroxoCbl to restore Cbl stores.

Some 11% of 100 patients with nutritional Cbl deficiency relapsed and were seen on a second occasion with the same diagnosis. Ideally, patients should be persuaded to include foods of animal origin, dairy produce, fish, poultry, etc. in their diets. Young patients are quite amenable, but older patients are far less likely to change their customs. Food supplementation is a successful way of providing Cbl, and this is available in relation to various prepacked cereal products. Cbl supplements are available such as cytocon (50 µg Cbl per tablet) or in liquid form as a multivitamin preparation. A 50 µg dose will allow some 2 µg to be absorbed, which is the maximum amount taken up from a single dose by a physiological mechanism. With a very large dose of oral Cbl about 1% is absorbed by passive diffusion. Strict vegetarians should take a daily dose of oral Cbl to meet their normal requirements.

Nutritional Cbl deficiency in infants

Severe nutritional Cbl deficiency is usually associated with infertility, and needs to be considered as a diagnosis in vegetarian women attending an infertility clinic. However, pregnancy can occur and may be successful. Under these circumstances only minimal Cbl stores are passed on to the fetus and the infant can present with megaloblastic anaemia due to Cbl deficiency. Cbl stores are normally transferred to the fetus in utero in the last few weeks of pregnancy, when there is avid accumulation of Cbl in the placenta. At term, cord blood Cbl levels average 572 pg/ml, whereas maternal serum Cbl levels average 290 (Ek 1982). In animals the bulk of a dose of labelled Cbl given in late pregnancy is recovered from the placenta and offspring. Cbl deficiency in the mother, either nutritional or due to undiagnosed pernicious anaemia, results in low fetal Cbl stores.

The Cbl level in breast milk is the same as that in maternal plasma. A low maternal plasma Cbl level is accompanied by a low Cbl level in breast milk, and Cbl deficiency develops in the neonate.

In India a disorder has been described in the breastfed infants of Cbl-deficient mothers. The infants have retarded development, abnormal skin pigmentation and a megaloblastic anaemia (Jadhav et al 1962). The mothers were vegetarian and the infants responded to Cbl therapy. Giving Cbl to the mother will restore the level in breast milk and provide Cbl for the infant.

There are at least six reports of a similar disorder in the offspring of Caucasian mothers who had been strict vegetarians for between 5 and 12 years. The mothers were all well. The infants developed normally for the first 4 months of life and presented clinically between 6 and 12 months of age. They were lethargic and hyperirritable. They were weak and could not support their heads, nor turn over. They stopped smiling and became inactive and withdrawn. One infant had marked hypotonia, exaggerated reflexes, positive extensor plantar responses, partial optic atrophy and diffuse brain atrophy, and was in coma on presentation. Most affected infants were underweight, and increased pigmentation on the backs of the hands, particularly over the knuckles, and feet, may occur. One child was in cardiac failure. The haemoglobin level ranged from 2.2 to 7.3 g/dl in five infants and was 13 g/dl in the sixth. Most had a raised MCV, all had low serum Cbl levels and marrows were severely megaloblastic. Increased methylmalonic acid and homocysteine in the urine was noted in one infant. All responded dramatically and completely to Cbl injections.

Similarly untreated and undiagnosed pernicious anaemia in younger women can be associated with a normal pregnancy and development of megaloblastic anaemia in the infant at between 4 and 14 months of age. The mothers, although clinically well, all had evidence of pernicious anaemia and one had attended an infertility clinic for 10 years. The subject has been reviewed by Chanarin (1990).

FOLATE

Composition of dietary folate

All fresh foods contain a variety of folate analogues. Virtually all are reduced, that is, they are tetrahydrofolates and the analogues differ from each other in glutamic acid chain length and whether they carry a substituent, which, if present, is either a formyl or a methyl. Because natural folates are reduced, reducing agents are required to prevent oxidation during collection, storage and assay. This has usually been achieved by adding fresh ascorbate. Under these circumstances 98% of dietary folates were reduced,

63% carried a methyl group, 27% a formyl group and 9% was unsubstituted folate (Perry 1971). In fresh foods 5- and 6- chain polyglutamates predominate but within days endogenous folate conjugases convert these into monoglutamates (Bird et al 1965). This is not prevented by freezing but only by heat in the presence of ascorbate, which inactivates the enzyme.

Natural folates are labile and are lost by heating unless protected by reducing agents, by exposure to UV light and by leaching into water during cooking. Exposure to atmospheric oxygen can cause oxidation, which is followed by cleavage of the molecule at the 9–10 bond between the pteridine and the PABA-glutamate moieties. Cooking results in a variable folate loss, but about 40–50% loss is common (Chanarin 1979, 1990). Data for dietary folate intake are compiled on cooked foods. The distribution of folates throughout a 24 hour diet is shown in Table 39.2. All foods contribute some folate although some, like liver, have relatively high levels.

Daily folate intake

Good data are available from Canada, Sweden, the UK and the USA. In Canada the mean daily intake is 205 µg/24h for men and 149 µg/24h for women (Department of Health and Welfare 1977). In the UK the average daily intake assessed annually over 3 years was 210–213 µg. In Sweden, males had daily folate intake of 361 µg and females 129 µg (Jägerstad et al 1979). In the USA a low-income diet supplied 184 µg/24h and a high-income diet 250 µg/24h (Bailey & Wagner 1982). Tables listing folate content of foods are published by the US Department of Agriculture (1976) with regular updated supplements and in the UK by Holland et al (1991).

Physiological folate analogues, i.e. reduced forms, with one glutamic acid residue are virtually completely absorbed from the gut. There is uncertainty

Table 39.2 Distribution of folate analogues in different foodstuffs over 24 hours (Chanarin 1990)

Foodstuff	Folate (µg)
Meat	13.9
Liver	26.6
Milk	34.0
Eggs, cheese, yoghurt	18.3
Vegetables	64.1
Fruit	24.6
Bread	19.5
Cereal, cake, sweets, beer	24.1

concerning the absorption of folate polyglutamates, as these have Glu residues in excess of one removed. Probably about 70% are absorbed. All resulting folate monoglutamates are converted to 5–methylH$_4$ folate in the enterocyte and this analogue appears in portal blood.

Detection of folate deficiency

The detection of folate deficiency, either subclinical or clinically overt, depends on the assay of folate levels in appropriate tissue samples. The clinical aspects of deficiency are dealt with in Chapter 14.

Red-cell folate levels

This is the most satisfactory means of measuring tissue folate stores. Assay is microbiological with *Lactobacillus casei* or an isotope dilution method of whole blood haemolysed in 1% fresh ascorbate. The result is expressed in terms of folate per unit of packed red cells, so that the packed red-cell volume is required for calculation. Healthy subjects have red-cell folates ranging from 145 to 400 ng/ml red cells. Folate is incorporated into red cells during erythropoiesis. A young red-cell population, as indicated by a raised reticulocyte count, has a higher red-cell folate level than mature red cells and this implies some loss of folate from young red cells shortly after their release from marrow to the circulation. Thereafter the folate is locked in the red cell until its demise after about 110 days. Change in red-cell folate is slow, since it requires the addition of a significant amount of new red cells with a different folate content to the circulation. A low red-cell folate is unequivocal evidence of folate deficiency.

Serum folate

The serum folate level is less satisfactory as a test for folate deficiency as the level falls even after a few days of low intake. It is low in one-third of all hospital admissions, although few of these will have tissue depletion of folate. A low serum folate is best looked upon as indicative of a negative folate balance, but this will have to be continued for several months to deplete folate stores. The normal range is usually between 3 and 20 ng of folate/ml.

Liver folate

A liver sample may occasionally be available following a percutaneous biopsy or after laparotomy. The normal range is probably 4–17 µg/g of wet liver with a mean of 7.0.

Urinary formiminoglutamic acid excretion

The metabolism of formiminoglutamic acid requires the transfer of the formimino- (–CH=NH) group derived from histidine catabolism to H$_4$folate. The formimino- group is then converted to –CH$_2$– or methylene. In the absence of a folate acceptor, as in folate deficiency, formiminoglutamic acid accumulates particularly after a loading dose of its precursor, histidine, and is excreted in the urine. Although the excretion is generally increased in folate deficiency some of the other enzymes in the histidine breakdown pathway are also affected, and often its precursor, urocanic acid, appears in urine in large amounts instead of formiminoglutamic acid. This test is often abnormal in many patients probably not suffering from folate deficiency, and is rarely used.

Recommended daily allowance for folate

This is set out in Table 39.3. The RDA recommended by FAO/WHO is the same as the Canadian and USA recommendation of 3.1µg folate/kg body weight/24 h (see also Appendix 2).

Basal folate requirements have been estimated at about 50–70 µg/24 h. These are based on the daily loss of folate, partly as assessed by liver biopsy. Thus the total folate content of a normal human liver ranges from 7.5 to 22.5 mg and falls to 1.5 mg in patients with folate-deficient megaloblastic anaemia. On this basis the folate loss over the period before megaloblastic anaemia appears ranges from 48 to 158 µg/24 h (Chanarin 1979). On the other hand, an optimal haematological response in a folate-deficient patient with megaloblastic anaemia requires 200 µg

Table 39.3 Dietary requirements for folate

Group		Safe level of intake (µg/24h)
Adult males		200
Adult females		170
Pregnancy		370–470
Lactation		270
Children	1–6 years	50
	7–12 years	102
	13–16 years	170
Infants	0–0.25 years	16
	0.26–0.5 years	24
	0.6–1 year	32

folate daily. Further dietary folate intakes have been correlated with folate status, largely red-cell folate. Populations having a mean folate intake of 150–200 μg/24 h generally have about 8% of the population showing subclinical evidence of folate deficiency. Thus it appears that folate intake on a western-type diet just meets the requirements of almost 95% of the population and a recommendation of 3.1 μg of folate/kg/24 h reflects these observations.

Frequency of nutritional folate deficiency

Folate deficiency due only to inadequate dietary intake is frequent in developing countries, but unusual in developed countries. More often, inadequate folate intake shows itself in subjects with an increased requirement for folate, either short-term as in pregnancy, or permanent as in some haemoglobin disorders such as sickle-cell anaemia. Under these circumstances folate deficiency and its clinical consequences may result.

The frequency of folate deficiency in pregnancy is probably the best test for this deficiency in any population. Folate is required for the synthesis of the basic components of DNA, and hence an increase in cell division, as is present in the developing fetus, results in an increased folate requirement which is likely to be fairly similar in all pregnant women with singleton pregnancies. The capacity of a woman to cope with the increased folate requirement in pregnancy depends on folate stores on the one hand and folate intake during pregnancy on the other. At term, between 24 and 32% of women on mixed diets in London had low red-cell folates, indicating folate deficiency (Chanarin 1990). In Nigeria 85% of primigravidae had low red-cell folates at term (Fleming et al 1968). Another way to assess the frequency of folate deficiency in pregnancy is to examine the bone marrow. Folate deficiency will be shown by the presence of megaloblasts. In London, Montreal, Johannesburg and Texas one-quarter of all marrows were megaloblastic; in Ireland and Nigeria the frequency was 30% and in South India reached 60%. This is the frequency of manifest folate deficiency in these populations during pregnancy.

Apart from pregnancy a National Health and Nutrition survey in the USA found low red-cell folates in 8% of adult males over the age of 20, in 13% of women aged 20–44, but in only 4% of women above 45 years of age. A similar frequency of low red-cell folates (8%) was found among the elderly in Wales and in the USA, although this was higher (18%) for institutionalized elderly subjects.

Good data from developing countries are not available, although the high frequency of megaloblastic anaemia in pregnancy indicates that folate deficiency and iron deficiency are probably the most common deficiency states encountered clinically.

Clinical effects of folate deficiency

The usual effect of folate deficiency is to cause a megaloblastic anaemia and the presenting features are similar to those found in patients with Cbl deficiency. Depression and weakness are not uncommon in folate-deficient megaloblastic anaemia, but neuropathy as found in Cbl deficiency is rare (Shorvon et al 1980).

Haematology of folate deficiency

As with Cbl deficiency, patients are generally anaemic and have abnormally large red blood cells, that is, a raised MCV. Exceptions have been discussed in relation to Cbl deficiency. In more anaemic patients, total white cells and platelets are both low. In a moderately anaemic patient the blood film shows macrocytosis with variable anisocytosis (variation in size of red cells), occasional pear-shaped red cells, and increased numbers of neutrophils with 4–6 nuclear lobes. Marrows are megaloblastic. The serum and red-cell folate levels are low.

Differentiation from Cbl deficiency depends on additional investigations. Thus if the serum Cbl level is normal in a patient with a megaloblastic anaemia, the diagnosis is folate deficiency. However, a low serum Cbl level does not necessarily mean Cbl deficiency. Thirty per cent of patients with primary folate deficiency have low serum Cbl levels, which rise into the normal range after 1 week of folate therapy. The explanation for this is not known.

Normal Cbl absorption in those on mixed diets excludes Cbl deficiency. Raised urinary excretion of methylmalonic acid indicates Cbl deficiency but a normal level in mild anaemia is not conclusive as excluding Cbl deficiency.

Folate and growth

Folate deficiency can cause marked growth retardation and delay the onset of puberty. This was shown among subjects with sickle-cell anaemia, which further increases folate requirement. Folate therapy was followed by dramatic growth spurts and women over 20 years of age who had been amenorrhoeic started regular menses thereafter (Watson-Williams 1962).

Folate and neural tube defects

In 1981 two studies reported a reduction in the incidence of neural tube defects when either folate or multivitamins including folate were given before and after conception to women who had previously given birth to an affected child (Smithells et al 1981, Laurence et al 1981). These reports were confirmed by a large study involving 1817 women with a history of neural tube defect. In the groups given 4 mg of folate daily, six neonates had a neural tube defect as compared to 21 in the women not receiving folate. This difference was highly significant (MRC Vitamin Study Research Group 1991). Earlier studies had shown that women giving birth to affected infants usually had normal red-cell folates, thus neural tube defects may not be the result of simple maternal folate deficiency. It is more likely that there is a relatively high folate requirement by the fetus at a stage of development when vascularization is such that nutrients may not reach the developing cells in adequate amounts. Abnormally high plasma folate levels may overcome this physiological failure by allowing folate to diffuse in to reverse this localized deficiency. Perhaps a higher folate supplement, such as 10–20 mg daily, may be even more efficacious, but see Chapter 25.

Simple nutritional deficiency

In western countries, groups at risk of nutritional folate deficiency are premature infants, pregnant women and the elderly. Low red-cell folate values have been found in 12% of elderly patients admitted to hospital, among 10% of elderly in residential homes in Norway, and in 8% of the elderly living at home in Wales. A value based on 14 reports in the USA suggested 8.7% folate deficiency in the elderly at home and 18% among the elderly in institutions. The cause is either poverty or disability, including depression. The relatively high frequency of low red-cell folate in the elderly, however, does not necessarily translate into large numbers of patients with folate-deficient megaloblastic anaemia. The deficiency is generally subclinical, and relatively rarely does it appear as megaloblastic anaemia unless associated with other factors, including alcoholism. Diagnosis requires the exclusion of other causes of megaloblastic anaemia, in particular pernicious anaemia.

In developing countries clinically overt deficiencies are far more common, but there are no reliable figures. The frequency of low red-cell folate levels in Africa range from 26 to 37%.

Premature infants

There is active transfer of 5-methyl-H_4folate to the fetus in the last weeks of pregnancy. In paired maternal and cord blood samples the serum and red-cell folate levels were 3.2 and 149 ng/ml for the mother and 17.1 and 325 ng/ml for the fetus (Ek 1982). Prematurity has an adverse effect on the amount of folate stored by the fetus, and the red-cell folate is significantly lower in premature infants of 25–37 weeks gestation (270 ng/ml) as compared to full-term infants (340 ng/ml). Folate levels decline rapidly in neonates, reaching their nadir at 7–10 weeks postnatally in prematures and in 11–12 weeks in full-term infants. Even in full-term infants folate stores may be exhausted by the 12th week, after which the newborn is dependent on dietary sources.

A further factor adversely affecting folate levels is the heating and reheating of milk feeds, as well as the effects of storage. Stored frozen or old human milk shows a fall from 45 µg/l to 30 µg at 4 weeks, 25 µg at 8 weeks and 19 µg at 12 weeks. The pasteurization of milk largely destroys the ascorbate present and reheating such a milk sample causes a fall in folate from 54 to 10 µg/l. The supplementation of powdered milk with folate has addressed this problem.

The effect of folate deficiency in premature infants is anaemia that is not corrected by oral iron, and a failure to gain weight. A folate supplement should be given to premature infants (see Table 39.3).

Goat's milk anaemia

A macrocytic anaemia in children reared on goat's milk was described more than 70 years ago and case reports continue to appear. The kid eats grass, etc. within days of birth, and is not dependent on maternal milk for either folate or Cbl. The folate and Cbl contents of goat and human milk are 6 and 52 µg/l for folate and 0.1 and 4 µg/l for Cbl respectively. The very low folate content of goat's milk ensures that human infants receiving mainly goat's milk as their diet will develop a folate-deficient megaloblastic anaemia at 3–5 months of age. A folate supplement must be given if goat's milk is to be used (Chanarin 1969).

Pregnancy

The cause of megaloblastic anaemia in pregnancy is an increased folate requirement that is not met from the diet. Folate in pregnancy is required for the increase in cell division that accompanies expansion of the maternal red cell mass, development of the placenta, growth of the uterus and fetus and, finally, supplying fetal stores of folate in the last weeks of pregnancy.

Increased folate requirement is evident by the 20th week of pregnancy, when there is a faster clearance of i.v. folate from plasma and, subsequently, by a decline in serum and red-cell folate levels. There is an altered renal threshold for folate in pregnancy so that the average urinary folate loss is 14 µg/24 h as compared to 4.2 µg/24 h in the non-pregnant state. In some, the 24-hour folate loss in urine during pregnancy reaches 50 µg (Landon & Hytten 1971).

The serum Cbl level falls in pregnancy, due in part to dilution by the physiological increase in plasma volume but also in the last few weeks to active transfer of most of the dietary Cbl to the fetus. However, pregnancy does not produce maternal Cbl deficiency. Maternal Cbl stores in those on mixed diets are some 3000 µg and that of a full-term fetus is only 50 µg. Thus the loss of Cbl to the fetus in pregnancy makes little impact on maternal Cbl stores. Unlike folate, there is no evidence of increased Cbl requirement with increased cell division. Thus megaloblastic anaemia in pregnancy is always due to folate deficiency, and low serum Cbl levels, unless they persist well after pregnancy, can be ignored.

Low red-cell folates have been found on first attendance at an antenatal clinic in 16% of women in New York (Herbert et al 1975) and in Brazil (Regina et al 1984), 10% in London (Chanarin et al 1968) and 31% in Nigeria (Fleming et al 1968). At term, low red-cell folates were present in 24–32% of women in London and in 85% of Nigerian primigravidae. On the other hand, red-cell folates were maintained during pregnancy in Danish and Australian women. Megaloblastic marrow changes in pregnancy indicating manifest folate deficiency range from 25 to 60% of all women near term.

Iron deficiency is the major cause of anaemia in pregnancy. It is difficult to recognize early evidence of folate deficiency because of the dominance of iron deficiency on the blood picture. Macrocytes among an otherwise microcytic hypochromic red cell population might suggest the onset of megaloblastic anaemia. Hypersegmented neutrophils in the blood film also suggest megaloblastic change, although this can occur in simple iron deficiency. Failure to respond to oral iron raises a suspicion of additional folate deficiency.

When megaloblastic anaemia is more pronounced the diagnosis is easier, although it must not be forgotten than an increase in the MCV is one of the physiological changes in pregnancy and by itself should not suggest a megaloblastic anaemia. This increase in MCV averages 4fl, but in some women reaches 20 fl and is not influenced by oral folate (Chanarin et al 1977). The confirmation of megaloblastic anaemia is made by marrow aspiration. Diagnosis is almost always made either in the last weeks of pregnancy or, in half the women, in the puerperium.

A seasonal incidence of megaloblastic anaemia in pregnancy has been noted in various countries, the peak frequency being at the end of the part of the year when fresh vegetables and fruits are least available. In some women megaloblastic anaemia recurs in further pregnancies, suggesting continued folate deficiency. The frequency of megaloblastic anaemia is ten times greater in twin pregnancies indicating a much higher folate requirement with twins.

The role of nutritional factors was highlighted by studies in which the haematological outcome was correlated with serum and red-cell folate levels measured throughout pregnancy. The women having megaloblastic marrows near term had the lowest serum and red-cell folate levels at first presentation in early pregnancy (Chanarin et al 1968, Temperly et al 1968), indicating probable pre-pregnancy nutritional folate deficiency.

Prophylaxis The provision of once-daily oral iron and folate supplements throughout pregnancy is one of the most successful health measures taken in the last 25 years. Megaloblastic anaemia in pregnancy is now a rarity in countries where such prophylaxis is practised, and is only seen in women who have had no medical supervision throughout pregnancy. Indeed, a generation of obstetricians has appeared who have never seen megaloblastic anaemia or even severe iron deficiency in pregnancy, and hence have questioned the need for this prophylaxis.

There has been debate about the amount of folate supplement required during pregnancy. One approach has been to determine the amount of additional folate needed to maintain the red-cell folate level during pregnancy; the second has been to determine the amount of folate needed to prevent the appearance of megaloblastic anaemia. Fifty µg of folate/24 h had no significant effect on the red-cell folate level, 100 µg/24 h produced a rise in red-cell folate in the first half of pregnancy, followed by a plateau in the second half. Higher doses of folate were accompanied by a marked elevation of red-cell folate which continued throughout pregnancy (Hansen & Rybo 1967, Chanarin et al 1968). These data led to the recommendation of a total daily folate intake of 370 µg/24 h (see Table 39.3). The supplement should be 200 µg of pteroylglutamic acid per 24 hours, so that even those on a poor diet will receive adequate folate while those on a reasonable or good diet will probably get more than they need. Excess folate will be excreted in the urine or degraded with breakdown products appearing in the urine.

Assessment of folate requirement by the amount needed to prevent the emergence of megaloblastic anaemia has proved less satisfactory because of the difficulty of recognizing the blood changes, and even the interpretation of marrow aspirates can be difficult when there is accompanying iron deficiency.

It is sensible to combine folate with iron in a single tablet, and it is desirable to give the least amount of iron that is effective, since the side effects of iron, such as gastrointestinal upsets, increase with the amount taken. 30 mg of iron (present in 90 mg ferrous fumarate) once daily both prevents anaemia and maintains the serum iron level throughout pregnancy (Chanarin & Rothman 1971). Nevertheless, most iron and folate preparations contain more iron than this. Apart from avoiding excess iron, which leads to poor compliance, attractive packaging such as a once-daily pop-out tablet, and enquiries about compliance at antenatal clinics, encourage women to maintain their prophylaxis.

Prematurity and folate deficiency

Apart from neural tube defects, which are reduced in frequency by folate supplements at the time of conception and in early pregnancy, only prematurity has been shown to be related to folate deficiency. A high frequency of low-birthweight infants is found among South African Bantu women on a staple diet of boiled maize. In this study the effects of supplements of iron alone, iron and folate, and iron, folate and Cbl, in both African and Caucasian women were compared. The Caucasian group consumed a mixed western diet. Iron was given at a dose of 200 mg/24 h, folate as 5 mg/24 h and Cbl as 50 µg/24 h. The supplements produced no effect on birthweight or duration of pregnancy in the Caucasian group. In the African group given only iron, 19 out of 63 neonates weighed less than 2270 g and this fell to four out of 65 in the folate-supplemented group. Cbl made no difference. Folate was associated with an increase in birthweight from 2466 g to 2798 g (Baumslag et al 1970). These observations have been widely confirmed (Chanarin 1985). In addition, folate supplementation prolonged the duration of gestation by 1 week and increased placental size from 456 g to 517 g (Chanarin 1985).

Other factors

Nutritional folate deficiency can complicate alcoholism when alcohol is substituted for food (Chanarin 1990). It may complicate the anticonvulsant treatment of epilepsy as well as disorders with an increased requirement for folate, such as haemolytic anaemia and some exfoliative skin disorders.

OTHER NUTRITIONAL DEFICIENCIES AFFECTING HAEMOPOIESIS

Vitamin A (retinol)

The main clinical manifestations of vitamin A deficiency are xerophthalmia and corneal damage leading to blindness (see Chapter 13). Chronic vitamin A deficiency is accompanied by an anaemia, sometimes severe, that resembles the anaemia of chronic disorders. It has the features of iron deficiency, including a low serum iron level, but the iron-binding capacity is normal or low and storage iron is present. Anaemia develops in experimentally induced vitamin A deficiency in man, with haemoglobin levels falling from 15 to 12 g/dl (Majia et al 1977).

Riboflavin deficiency

Volunteers on riboflavin-deficient diets and given a riboflavin antagonist develop pure red-cell aplasia (Lane & Alfrey 1963). This is occasionally seen in nutritional deficiencies accompanying alcoholism, when a smooth, cherry-red tongue is said to be one of the manifestations.

Ascorbic acid (vitamin C) deficiency

Vitamin C deficiency leads to clinical scurvy and about 80% of such patients are anaemic. The relationship of this anaemia to that of folate deficiency has caused much interest. Ascorbate and folate are both water-soluble vitamins present in similar foodstuffs. Both are labile and susceptible to oxidative destruction. A diet low in ascorbate is most likely to be low in folate as well.

When anaemia is normocytic and the marrow is normoblastic, a haematological response is obtained only with oral ascorbate. In many patients the marrow is megaloblastic and most of these also respond only to ascorbate, although there is some evidence that such a response will not occur if the diet lacks folate (Zalusky & Herbert 1961). Other patients with scurvy and megaloblastic marrow respond very well to folate alone, and there may be a second response when ascorbate is added (Chanarin 1969, 1979).

The data are best explained on the basis that nutritional deficiencies of folate and ascorbate tend to coincide, since a diet lacking the one will certainly lack the other. Despite suggestions that the reducing properties of ascorbate are required for maintaining folate analogues in a reduced state, this applies only to the in-vitro situation and there is no evidence that ascorbate is required for folate metabolism in vivo.

Vitamin E (α-tocopherol) deficiency

This compound serves as an antioxidant in man. Deficiency is rare but can occur in low-birthweight infants at about 4–6 weeks of age. Anaemia develops, with a raised reticulocyte count, a raised platelet count and oedema of the dorsum of the feet and pretibial area (Ritchie et al 1968). It responds to vitamin E medication. Deficiency may occur in association with steatorrhoea, such as that in cystic fibrosis.

Copper deficiency

The rare anaemia due to copper deficiency may occur in malnourished children. These children show radiological changes with osteoporosis, spontaneous rib fractures and abnormal metaphyses (Graham & Cordano 1969). The anaemia is microcytic and unresponsive to iron. Anaemia due to copper deficiency has also been described in adults on parenteral nutrition, and may be macrocytic (Oppenheimer et al 1987). Diagnosis requires the demonstration of low serum copper levels. The response to oral copper is prompt. Copper is present in a variety of enzymes in man.

REFERENCES

Bailey LB, Wagner PB 1982 Quoted by: Rosenberg IH, Bowman BB, Cooper BA, Halsted CH, Lindenbaum J. Folate nutrition in the elderly. American Journal of Clinical Nutrition 36: 1060–1066

Baker SJ, Mathan IV 1981 Evidence regarding the minimal daily requirement of dietary vitamin B_{12}. American Journal of Clinical Nutrition 15: 77–84

Baumslag N, Edelstein T, Metz J 1970 Reduction of incidence of prematurity by folic acid supplementation in pregnancy. British Medical Journal 1: 1161–1117

Bird OD, McGlohon VM, Vaitkus JW 1965 Naturally occuring folates in the blood and liver of the rat. Analytical Biochemistry 12: 18–35

Borgström B, Norden A, Åkesson B, Jägerstad M 1975 A study of food. Consumption by the duplicate-portion technique in a sample of the Dalby population. Scandinavian Journal of Social Medicine. Supplement 10: 75–77

Chanarin I 1969 The megaloblastic anaemias. Blackwell, Oxford

Chanarin I 1979 The megaloblastic anaemias, 2nd edn. Blackwell, Oxford

Chanarin I 1985 Folates and cobalamins. Clinics in Haematology 14: 629–641

Chanarin I 1990 The megaloblastic anaemias, 3rd edn. Blackwell, Oxford

Chanarin I, Rothman D 1971 Further observations on the relation between iron and folate status in pregnancy. British Medical Journal ii: 81–84

Chanarin I, Stephenson E 1988 Vegetarian diet and cobalamin deficiency: their association with tuberculosis. Journal of Clinical Pathology 41: 759–762

Chanarin I, McFadyen I, Kyle R 1977 The physiological macrocytosis of pregnancy. British Journal of Obstetrics and Gynaecology 84: 504–508

Chanarin I, Rothman D, Ward A, Perry J 1968 Folate status and requirement in pregnancy. British Medical Journal ii: 390–394

Chanarin I, Deacon R, Lumb M, Muir M, Perry J 1985 Cobalamin folate interrelations: a critical review. Blood 66: 479–489

Chanarin I, Malkowska V, O'Hea A-M, Rinsler MG, Price AB 1985 Megaloblastic anaemia in a vegetarian Hindu community. Lancet ii: 1168–1172

Deacon R, Perry J, Lumb M, Chanarin I 1990a Formate metabolism in the cobalamin-inactivated rat. British Journal of Haematology 74: 354–359

Deacon R, Bottiglieri T, Chanarin I, Lumb M, Perry J 1990b Methylthioadenosine serves as a single carbon source to the folate coenzyme pool in rat bone marrow cells. Biochimica et Biophysica Acta 1034: 342–346

Department of National Health and Welfare 1977 Canada Food Consumption Patterns Report, Ottawa, DNHW

Ek J 1980 Plasma and red cell folate values in newborn infants and their mothers in relation to gestational age. Journal of Paediatrics 97: 288–292

Ek J 1982 Plasma and red cell folate in mothers and infants in normal pregnancies. Relation to birth weight. Acta Obstetrica et Gynaecologica Scandinavica 61: 17–20

FAO/WHO Expert Consultation 1988 Requirements of Vitamin A, Iron, Folate and Vitamin B_{12}. Food and Agriculture Organization of the United Nations, Rome

Fleming AF, Hendriks JD de V, Allan NC 1968 The prevention of megaloblastic anaemia in pregnancy in Nigeria. Journal of Obstetrics and Gynaecology of the British Commonwealth 75: 425–432

Graham GG, Cordano A 1969 Copper depletion and deficiency in the malnourished infant. Johns Hopkins Medical Journal 124: 139–150

Hansen H, Rybo G 1967 Folic acid dosage in prophylactic treatment during pregnancy. Acta Obstetrica et Gynaecologica Scandinavica 46 Supplement 7: 107–112

Herbert V, Zalusky R 1962 Interrelation of vitamin B_{12} and folic acid: folic acid clearance studies. Journal of Clinical Investigation 41: 1263–1276

Holland B, Welch AA, Unwin ID, Buss DH, Paul AA,

Southgate DAT 1991 McCance and Widdowson's The composition of foods. The Royal Society of Chemistry, Cambridge, and MAFF, London

Jadhav M, Webb JKG, Vashaava S, Baker S 1962 Vitamin B_{12} deficiency in Indian infants, a clinical syndrome. Lancet ii: 903–907

Jägerstad M, Norden Å, Åkesson B 1979 Relation between dietary intake and parameters of health status. In: Borgström B, Nordén Å, Åkesson B, Abdulla H, Jägerstad M (eds) Nutrition and old age. Universitets Forleget, Oslo, pp 236–264

Kaplan SS, Basford RE 1976 Effect of vitamin B and folic acid deficiencies on neutrophil function. Blood 47: 801–805

Landon MJ, Hytten FE 1971 The excretion of folate in pregnancy. Journal of Obstetrics and Gynaecology of the British Commonwealth 78: 769–775

Lane M, Alfrey CP 1963 The anaemia of human riboflavin deficiency. Blood 22: 811

Laurence KM, James N, Miller MH, Tennant GB, Campbell H 1981. Double-blind randomized controlled trial of folate treatment before conception to prevent recurrence of neural tube defects. British Medical Journal 282: 1509–1511

Majia LA, Hodges RE, Arroyave G, Viteri F, Torún B 1977 Vitamin A deficiency and anemia in Central American children. American Journal of Clinical Nutrition 30: 1175–1184

Mehta BM, Rege DV, Satoskar RS 1964 Serum vitamin B_{12} and folic acid activity in lactovegetarians and non-vegetarian healthy adult Indians. American Journal of Clinical Nutrition 15: 77–84

MRC Tuberculosis and Chest Diseases Unit National Survey of Tuberculosis Notification in England and Wales 1978–79 1980 British Medical Journal 281: 895–898

MRC Vitamin Study Research Group 1991 Prevention of neural tube defect: results of the Medical Research Council Vitamin Study. Lancet 338: 131–137

Oppenheimer SM, Hoffbrand BI, Dormandy TL, Parker N, Wickens DG 1987 Macrocytic anaemia due to copper deficiency in a patient with late-onset hypogammaglobulinaemia. Postgraduate Medical Journal 63: 205–207

Perry J 1971 Folate analogues in a normal mixed diet. British Journal of Haematology 21: 435–441

Regina E, Guigliani J, Jorge SM, Goncalves AL 1984 Folate and vitamin B_{12} deficiency among parturients from Porto Alegre, Brazil. Revista de Investigation Clinica (Mexico City) 36: 133–136

Ritchie JH, Fish MB, McMasters V, Grossman M 1968 Edema and hemolytic anemia in premature infants. A Vitamin E deficiency syndrome. New England Journal of Medicine 279: 1185–1190

Senewirante B, Hettirachchi J, Senewirante K 1974 Vitamin B_{12} absorption in megaloblastic anaemia. British Journal of Nutrition 32: 491–501

Shorvon SD, Carney MWP, Chanarin I, Reynolds EH 1980 The neuropsychiatry of megaloblastic anaemia. British Medical Journal 281: 1036–1038

Skacel PO, Chanarin I (1983) Impaired chemiluminescence and bacterial killing by neutrophils from patients with severe cobalamin deficiency. British Journal of Haematology 55: 203–215

Smithells RW, Sheppard S, Schoralo CJ et al 1981. Apparent prevention of neural tube defects by periconceptional vitamin supplementation. Archives of Diseases in Childhood 56: 911–918

Temperley IJ, Meehan MJM, Gatenby PBB 1968 Serum folic acid levels in pregnancy and their relationship to megaloblastic marrow change. British Journal of Haematology 14: 13–19

US Department of Agriculture 1976 Composition of foods. Agriculture Handbook no. 8–1. US Department of Agriculture, Washington

Watson-Williams EJ 1962 Folic acid deficiency in sickle-cell anaemia. East African Medical Journal 39: 213–220

40. Diseases of the kidneys and urinary tract

I. H. Khan, P. Richmond and A. M. MacLeod

Dietary management forms an important aspect of the care of patients with a variety of renal diseases. Many patients presenting with acute renal failure from a variety of causes may also require temporary dialysis. A second group of patients with end-stage renal failure (ESRF) require renal replacement therapy (RRT), either in the form of dialysis or as renal transplantation, for survival, and their day-to-day care relies on an integrated team of nephrologists, nursing and technical staff, social workers, and dietitians with an interest in renal disease. The number of patients in Europe now offered RRT has increased nearly twofold over the past decade, and is now more than 150 000 (Geerlings et al 1991). This reflects the acceptance for RRT of increasing numbers of older patients (>60 years), and patients with diabetes or other morbid conditions, e.g. coronary heart or obstructive airways disease (Khan et al 1993). A substantial number of patients with the nephritic and nephrotic syndromes, with renal calculi or with chronic renal failure not yet requiring RRT also need special dietary attention.

The principal aims of the dietary management of patients with renal disease are: the prevention of symptoms and complications of uraemia (the symptom complex of renal failure); the possible slowing of progressive chronic renal failure; the prevention and treatment of undernutrition and the management of hyperlipidaemia.

RENAL PHYSIOLOGY

The management of patients with renal diseases is firmly based on understanding renal pathophysiology. The kidneys are each composed of approximately one million similar functional units called nephrons. Each nephron consists of a glomerulus, which is a tuft of capillaries invaginated into an epithelial sac (Bowman's capsule), from which arises a tubule. The blood flow through the kidneys is large, amounting to about one-quarter of the cardiac output at rest, i.e. 1300 ml/min. Branches of the renal arteries give rise to afferent arterioles which divide to form the glomerular capillaries. These unite to form the efferent arterioles, which supply blood to the renal tubules.

The hydrostatic pressure within the glomerular capillaries results in the filtration of fluid into Bowman's capsule. This fluid is similar in composition to plasma, except that it normally contains no fat and very little protein.

The filtrate, formed in the glomerulus at a rate of approximately 125 ml/min, passes first into the proximal convoluted tubule and from there through the loop of Henle and distal convoluted tubule to the collecting ducts. The filtrate is modified according to the needs of the body by the selective reabsorption of its constituents and of water, and by tubular secretion. Of the 180 000 ml of water and 22 500 mmol of sodium filtered through the glomerular capillaries during the course of each day, only about 1500 ml of water and 100–200 mmol of sodium are excreted in the urine.

The kidneys are essential for maintaining many aspects of the internal chemical environment of the body. Their main functions are indicated in Table 40.1. As excretory organs they remove such waste products of nitrogen metabolism as urea, uric acid and creatinine, as well as hydrogen ions and sulphates which arise from the degradation of sulphur-containing amino acids. They also excrete surplus quantities of water, sodium, potassium, phosphate, magnesium and other ions.

By modifying the composition of urine the kidneys maintain not only the volume of the body fluids but also their electrolyte composition within narrow limits. In the healthy adult, for example, extreme responses to dehydration and overhydration are produced by a change in either direction of only 2% in the water content of the body. The daily urinary volume can be reduced from the usual 1500 ml to

Table 40.1   Functions of the kidneys

	Daily load in adults	Effects in renal failure
Excretion		
Nitrogenous metabolites		Increased plasma concentration (azotaemia)
Urea	(dietary protein × 1/3)g	
Uric acid	4 mmol	
Creatinine	10 mmol	
Other metabolites		
Sulphates	25–40 mmol	Acidosis
Hydrogen ions	40–80 mmol	Acidosis
Drug metabolites		Drug toxicity
Surplus nutrients		
Water	1500–5000 ml	Fluid overload and oedema
Sodium	100–200 mmol	
Potassium	60–80 mmol	Hyperkalaemia
Calcium	2–7 mmol	Hypocalcaemia
Chloride	100–200 mmol	
Phosphate	20–40 mmol	Hyperphosphataemia
Endocrine		
Vitamin D-1-α-hydroxylation		Bone disease
Erythropoietin synthesis		Anaemia
Renin secretion		?
Hormone degradation		?

only 500 ml following water deprivation, and increased to approximately 20 litres following the ingestion of very large quantities of water.

The kidneys also have important endocrine functions. They are the site of activation of vitamin D. 25-hydroxy vitamin D formed in the liver is converted in the tubular cells of the kidney to 1,25-dihydroxy vitamin D, the most active metabolite of the vitamin. The activated vitamin acts on the intestine to increase calcium absorption, and maintains the normal mineralization of bone. The kidneys also produce erythropoietin and renin. Erythropoietin, a glycoprotein hormone, is essential for the production of red blood cells by the bone marrow. Renal failure is almost always accompanied by anaemia, and insufficient erythropoietin production is now known to be the major factor leading to the anaemia of renal failure. Certain renal diseases, for example polycystic kidney disease and renal tumours, produce excess erythropoietin and this results in greater erythropoiesis and polycythaemia (an excess of red blood cells).

Renin is released by the kidneys in response to a low blood pressure or lack of adequate blood flow (ischaemia) to the kidneys. It converts the liver-derived angiotensinogen to angiotensin 1, which is further activated in the lungs to angiotensin 2. This substance has potent vasoconstrictor properties and directly increases the systemic blood pressure. It also stimulates aldosterone release from the adrenal glands, which leads to salt and water conservation. Several polypeptide hormones, including parathyroid hormone, calcitonin, insulin and gastrin, are also degraded in the kidneys.

ASSESSMENT OF RENAL FUNCTION

Both clinical observation and biochemical analyses of plasma and urine should be used to provide a reliable assessment of renal function; any test used in isolation can be misleading. Many symptoms and signs are non-specific, but are often valuable guides to therapy. Thirst, polyuria and polydipsia – features of diabetes mellitus and diabetes insipidus, as well as of chronic renal failure – indicate that the kidneys are unable to conserve water, so the patient has an increased requirement for water which must be satisfied if fluid balance is to be maintained. Peripheral and pulmonary oedema indicate that the extracellular fluid volume and total body sodium are both increased. A failure in the renal regulation of sodium metabolism leads to water and sodium overload; this can result from cardiac failure as well as from intrinsic renal disease. Whatever the cause, the patient benefits from measures designed to promote the loss of body sodium. The absence of oedema, hypertension and polyuria in a patient with biochemical signs of advanced renal failure sometimes indicates the presence of excessive renal sodium loss due to defective tubular reabsorption of sodium. This condition often responds to judicious sodium supplementation with a restoration of total body sodium, extracellular fluid and plasma volumes, an improvement in renal blood flow and glomerular filtration rate (GFR), and improved overall renal function.

Inexpensive and convenient biochemical indices of renal function are blood haemoglobin concentration, and plasma levels of urea, creatinine, sodium, potassium, bicarbonate, calcium, inorganic phosphate, albumin and alkaline phosphatase. These used to be monitored serially.

Changes in renal excretory function alter plasma concentrations of urea and creatinine, so these metabolites are assayed to assess the progression of renal insufficiency. Serum creatinine concentration is affected by a patient's muscle mass, meat intake and GFR. Muscle-wasting diseases and a low meat intake may result in low serum creatinine concentrations, which then do not correlate with the actual GFR. Creatinine is also secreted to a variable extent by the renal tubules and from the gut; creatinine clearance measurements overestimate the actual GFR. A rise in creatinine levels does not occur until the GFR has fallen considerably but, as renal failure advances, creatinine clearance becomes less reliable as an indicator of GFR.

New radionuclide markers are now commonly used for estimating GFR, e.g. ^{51}Cr edetic acid, ^{125}I iothalamate or ^{99}Tc DTPA. The normal GFR in adults is around 125 ml/min. There is a large glomerular reserve, so that renal failure rarely produces symptoms until the GFR falls below 30 ml/min. Renal replacement therapy is usually required when the GFR falls below about 5 ml/min.

Diagnostic radiological and radionucleotide imaging tests are important tools in assessing renal function. Ultrasound scanning is a non-invasive and virtually risk-free investigation that allows rapid assessment of renal size, and is useful for excluding urinary tract obstruction.

The serum concentration of potassium and phosphate ions increases as the GFR falls, and failure of the renal tubules to conserve bicarbonate ions results in metabolic acidosis. The secondary effects of renal dysfunction on vitamin D and bone metabolism are often indicated by changes in plasma calcium and alkaline phosphatase concentrations. The plasma sodium concentration reflects a change in body water as often as a change in sodium balance; it is increased in dehydration and decreased in overhydration or in water intoxication. Since sodium is an important determinant of extracellular and plasma volumes, changes in body sodium are more reliably assessed clinically by the presence or absence of peripheral oedema, and by measuring the blood pressure.

The excretory capacity of the kidney varies at different stages of acute and chronic renal failure and with different types of renal diseases: in tubulo-interstitial diseases urinary volumes are larger than in glomerulonephritis. Other sensible and insensible water losses must be taken into account when assessing the fluid requirements of a patient. Since 1 litre of water weights 1 kg, weighing the patient at the same time each day or at each clinic visit under standard conditions provides an invaluable guide to changes in body water.

Abnormal urinary constituents such as blood and protein do not always indicate the presence of renal disease, but do call for further investigation. In glomerulonephritis both the activity of the disease process and the response to treatment can be followed by measuring the quantity of protein excreted in a 24-hour urine collection. The excretion rates of sodium and potassium can also be measured, to assess either the response to diuretic therapy or requirements for dietary supplements.

PRINCIPLES OF DIETETICS IN RENAL DISEASE

In the management of patients with renal disease, dietetics is of greatest value when renal function is impaired. There is little or no need to interfere with the eating habits and way of life of patients when the kidneys continue to preserve ionic balance and sodium excretion, as they usually do in urinary tract infections, asymptomatic glomerulonephritis, mild proteinuria and hypertension. Tubular disorders, such as the Fanconi syndrome, which can result in abnormal losses of phosphate, sodium, potassium and magnesium, can in most cases be treated by giving supplements of the appropriate salts, in addition to a normal food intake.

Dietary intervention in renal disease has an important role in promoting the general wellbeing of the patient. By monitoring protein intake and controlling fluid, sodium, potassium and phosphate intake, plasma urea and electrolyte levels can be maintained within normal limits, thus reducing the risk of symptoms. Patients should not, however, have to comply with severely restricted diets, e.g. very low-protein diets, which may minimize changes in plasma urea concentration but lead to severe muscle wasting. The nutritional status of the patient must be considered and adequate energy, minerals and vitamins provided. This is of particular importance with children, where it is essential to promote their growth.

Although the kidneys are affected by many different diseases, the ways in which renal function can be impaired are relatively few, and disorders requiring the specialized help of a dietitian are encompassed in four clinical syndromes: acute glomerulonephritis, the nephrotic syndrome, acute renal failure, and chronic renal failure and end-stage renal disease.

GLOMERULAR DISEASE

Acute glomerulonephritis

Acute glomerulonephritis (GN) is characterized by acute inflammation of the glomeruli, with congestion, cellular proliferation and infiltration of polymorphonuclear leucocytes and other cells associated with inflammation. The 'acute nephritic syndrome' may result from a variety of pathological types of glomerulonephritides. Clinically, hypertension, oliguria, haematuria and often peripheral and pulmonary oedema occur. Acute renal failure may then develop and, rarely, dialysis is required. The nephritic syndrome may arise as a result of the following types of glomerular diseases.

Acute post-infectious glomerulonephritis

The classic nephritic syndrome commonly follows an infection, which may be bacterial, viral or parasitic. The most frequently described form of post-infectious GN follows infection of the upper respiratory tract with β-haemolytic streptococci. A few weeks after an infection the patient presents with signs and symptoms of acute nephritic syndrome. Pathologically there is deposition of immune complexes (streptococcal antigens with antibody formed against them) in the glomerular basement membrane.

Antiglomerular basement membrane disease

Antibodies directed against the basement membrane of the glomeruli may result in rapidly progressive GN and acute renal failure. When antibodies are directed against the basement membranes of the lungs, as well as that of the glomeruli, then alveolar haemorrhage with haemoptysis also develops. This rare condition is known as Goodpasture's syndrome.

Crescentic glomerulonephritis

This is a pathological term used when there is proliferation of the epithelial cells of Bowman's capsule, leading to obliteration of the Bowman's space. It may result from a variety of causes of acute GN. Usually the presence of crescent formation implies a severe nephritis, with gross reduction of the GFR and rapidly developing renal failure.

Renal vasculitis

A group of diseases characterized by inflammation of medium and small blood vessels comprise the vasculitides, which may affect almost any organ in the body. Wegener's granulomatosis and microscopic polyarteritis usually involve the kidneys, and can result in acute nephritis and renal failure. These two diseases are now being increasingly diagnosed with the use of the antineutrophil cytoplasmic antibody test (ANCA), which is usually positive.

Other forms of acute GN

Henoch–Schönlein purpura, bacterial endocarditis, systemic lupus erythematosus and membranoproliferative glomerulonephritis can all cause acute nephritic syndrome.

Medical treatment of acute GN

The treatment of post-infectious GN is mainly aimed at dealing with the symptoms rather than the cause, but antimicrobial drugs should be given to clear the infection. The use of salt and water restriction and diuretics forms the main treatment of acute nephritis. Immunosuppressive drugs such as steroids and cyclophosphamide are useful specific treatments in renal vasculitis, and plasma exchange is used in Goodpasture's syndrome to remove circulating antiglomerular basement membrane antibody.

Dietary management of acute GN

The dietary treatment of acute GN depends on the patient's response to the disease. Protein restriction is not usually necessary unless the patient is uraemic. It is more likely that their protein intake will be low, and protein supplements may be necessary. Salt and fluid restriction will depend on the level of fluid retention. Oliguric patients should have their intake restricted to 500 ml plus the volume of the previous day's urine output, and sodium intake is restricted to 80–100 mmol daily.

Nephrotic syndrome

The nephrotic syndrome is characterized by heavy proteinuria (>3.5 g/1.73 m^2 body surface area per 24 hours), oedema and hypoalbuminaemia. Patients with heavy proteinuria but who are not oedematous or hypoalbuminaemic are said to have 'nephrotic range' proteinuria.

It has been shown that hepatic albumin synthesis increases in nephrotic syndrome (Ballmer et al 1992), and there is a hypothesis that synthesis of high molecular weight proteins is also increased since the absolute plasma concentration of such proteins rises in this condition (Cameron 1992). The liver compensates by overproducing its export proteins. The majority of clinical abnormalities of the nephrotic syndrome, such as hyperlipidaemia and hypercoagulability, can be explained by the increased hepatic secretion of lipoproteins and coagulation factors; there is also an increased susceptibility to infection.

When the plasma albumin level falls, the balance of hydrostatic and colloid osmotic pressures across capillaries throughout the body is altered, favouring the movement of water and solute from the circulating blood plasma to the interstitial fluid. The plasma volume falls and, in compensation, sodium is reabsorbed avidly from the renal tubules. Sodium is retained in the body and the plasma volume restored at the expense of a greatly increased extracellular volume, which manifests clinically as peripheral oedema.

The nephrotic syndrome results from a wide variety of renal and systemic disorders. A common cause, seen mainly in children, is called minimal change disease, because on light microscopy the glomeruli appear normal. Electron microscopy reveals a loss of foot processes in the glomerular epithelial cells. Minimal change disease is usually benign, and only rarely leads to renal impairment or hypertension. Focal sclerosing glomerulonephritis is another cause of nephrotic syndrome. This usually results in renal impairment leading to end-stage renal failure. In membranous glomerulonephritis – characterized by subepithelial deposits – there is thickening of the basement membrane. It is mediated through immunological mechanisms and may be primary or secondary to other diseases such as cancer, viral infections and drugs such as gold and penicillamine, which are used in rheumatoid arthritis.

Other renal conditions resulting in the nephrotic syndrome include membranoproliferative GN, analgesic nephropathy, renal artery stenosis (rare), immunoglobulin A disease and, occasionally, acute glomerulonephritis. Diabetes mellitus, systemic lupus erythematosus, amyloidosis and sarcoidosis are recognized systemic causes of the nephrotic syndrome. Renal vein thrombosis was for a long time considered to be a cause of the nephrotic syndrome, but is now believed to be a consequence rather than a cause.

The prognosis in nephrotic syndrome depends on the underlying cause. Some patients, especially those with minimal change disease, may undergo spontaneous or drug-induced remission, whereas others progress to renal impairment which may lead to end-stage renal failure.

Medical treatment

Any underlying non-renal cause should be sought and treated appropriately. Patients with minimal change disease usually respond to steroids with or without other immunosuppressive agents, such as cyclophosphamide or cyclosporin A. The role of immunosuppression in other causes of nephrotic syndromes is controversial. Various drug therapies, such as the use of anticoagulants and antiplatelet agents, are largely experimental. The management of the patient with nephrotic syndrome is thus mainly directed towards the removal of salt and water, and the avoidance and treatment of complications such as thrombosis and hyperlipidaemia. Salt and water restriction and the appropriate use of diuretics are the mainstay of treatment. In severely hypoalbuminaemic patients with gross fluid overload, the use of salt-poor albumin intravenously may promote and augment diuresis. Nephrotic patients are at risk of intravascular volume depletion as a result of over-enthusiastic diuretic therapy. This may lead to renal hypoperfusion and acute renal failure. As a general rule daily fluid loss should not exceed 1 kg, lest hypovolaemia becomes a problem. A useful indicator of volume depletion is the presence of postural hypotension.

Dietary management of nephrotic syndrome

Because of the heavy proteinuria and the resulting fall in serum albumin levels, a high-protein diet con-

Table 40.2   The composition of some dietary supplements commonly used in renal disease

Product name	Unit	Energy (kcal/100 g or 100 ml)	Protein	Fat	CHO	Na	K
			(g/100 g or 100 ml)			(mmol/100 g or 100 ml)	
Powders (may be added to liquids)							
Maxijul	100 g	375	0	0	96	2	0.1
Maxipro	100 g	390	88	0	0	14	11.5
Duocal super soluble	100 g	470	0	22	72	<0.2	<0.1
Liquids							
Provide	250 ml	60	3.6	<1	11.2	<1–3	<1–4
Protein Forte	200 ml	100	10	1.6	9.5	1.9	3.8
Fortimel	200 ml	100	9.7	2.1	10	2.2	15.1
Fortical	200 ml	123	0	0	30	0.15	0.1
Fortisip	200 ml	150	5	6.5	18	3.5	3.9
Ensure Plus	100 ml	150	6.25	6	20	5.1	4.7
Maxijul liquid	200 ml	187	0	0	50	<1	<0.1
Nepro	237 ml	200	7	9.3	21.5	3.5	2.7
TwoCal HN	237 ml	200	8.4	8.9	21.5	5.7	5.9
Duocal	100 ml	150	0	7.1	23	0.9	0.8

taining 80–100 g of protein was prescribed for these patients in the past. However, clinical trials have failed to show any benefits of such a high-protein diet (Kaysen et al 1989), and indeed they may even have a detrimental effect on the hepatic synthesis of albumin (Lee 1980). Furthermore, the consumption of large amounts of protein by patients with glomerulonephritis may promote the progression of renal insufficiency (Brenner et al 1982, El Nahas et al 1984). As patients are frequently anorexic they may have difficulty in complying with a high-protein diet. At present, a protein intake of 1 g of protein/kg ideal body weight (IBW) is recommended in many habitual diets.

Energy intake needs to be adequate for correct utilization of protein to maintain the patient's nitrogen balance. Approximately 200 kcal (840 kJ)/g of dietary nitrogen is usually sufficient, although there are variations in individual requirements (see Appendix 2). Sodium restriction to an intake of 80–100 mmol/day is useful if oedema has not been controlled successfully with diuretics. Most of the dietary salt intake is derived from salt already added to manufactured food, and not adding salt to a habitual diet will only reduce intake by 15% (James et al 1987). Hence a low-salt diet should be prescribed, and the patient instructed not to add further salt. At this stage fluid restriction may also be necessary.

The dietitian should calculate the patient's daily intake in the first few days of admission to assess whether the dietary recommendations of 1 g protein/kg IBW and an adequate energy intake are being achieved. In many patients with nephrotic syndrome appetite is poor, and a protein supplement may be required. The choice of this is governed by individual patient preference and the degree of fluid and salt restriction (Table 40.2). On discharge, some patients may need to continue with a supplement until their appetite improves.

Elevations in serum lipid concentrations are a feature of the nephrotic syndrome (D'Amico & Gentile 1991). Increased serum concentration of total cholesterol, low-density lipoprotein (LDL) cholesterol and very low-density lipoprotein (VLDL) cholesterol are the most frequent abnormalities reported in nephrotic patients. These abnormalities have been shown to reverse once patients achieve remission (Joven et al 1990). There is evidence for increased conversion of VLDL to LDL, and decreased LDL clearance due to downregulation of LDL receptors (Warwick et al 1990). The data on high-density lipoprotein (HDL) cholesterol have been less consistent, with both high and low levels being reported. Recent well controlled studies have shown increased levels of total, LDL and VLDL cholesterol, but normal levels of HDL cholesterol in the majority of patients with nephrotic syndrome. A possible explanation may be that the low molecular weight of HDL apoproteins allows them to be lost in the urine, accounting for the lipiduria in such patients (Appel 1991).

Some studies have suggested an increase in ischaemic heart disease in patients with nephrotic syndrome (Berlyne & Mallick 1969), whereas others showed no such increase (Wass & Cameron 1981). Since the majority of patients with nephrotic syndrome go into remission there is no consensus on the importance of treating hyperlipidaemia in nephrotic syndrome. The risk to the individual patient will depend on many other factors, such as genetic predisposition, the duration of unremitting nephrotic syndrome and hyperlipidaemia, concurrent hypertension, diabetes and the use of steroids. Dietary intervention, such as the substitution of polyunsaturated fats for some of the saturated fat in the diet, the reduction of total fat intake and weight reduction in the obese, would be appropriate. In the minority of patients with unremitting nephrotic syndrome and hyperlipidaemia, lipid-lowering drugs may be prescribed. Bile-acid sequestrants such as cholestyramine, fibric acid derivatives such as gemfibrozil, and HMG-CoA reductase inhibitors have been effectively used in the nephrotic syndrome, and their use has recently been reviewed (Appel & Appel 1990).

ACUTE RENAL FAILURE

Acute renal failure results from a wide variety of insults to the kidneys. It may present while the patient is in hospital for a primarily non-renal illness, or in the community when he or she may present with uraemia. The estimated incidence of acute renal failure requiring dialysis in Europe is 30 per million of the population per year. Failure of other organs in addition to the kidneys is common, and poses special problems in management. Often, the care of patients with acute renal failure requires a multidisciplinary approach involving anaesthetists, surgeons, nephrologists and urologists, and many patients are cared for in intensive therapy units. The prevailing high mortality in acute renal failure, despite modern RRT, is mainly attributable to the underlying precipitating causes of renal failure, and multiorgan involvement. As a result, the mortality from acute renal failure remains greater than 50% in surgical and post-traumatic cases. Many cases of acute renal failure seen in hospitals may be avoidable if attention is given to fluid balance, avoiding nephrotoxic agents and prolonged hypotension, and if urinary tract obstruction is detected and treated early.

The causes of acute renal failure are conventionally divided into pre-renal, renal and post-renal (Table 40.3). Patients with underlying chronic renal impairment may present with acute-on-chronic renal failure. The clinical features of acute renal failure are those due to the precipitating underlying disorder, in addition to those of uraemia.

Table 40.3   Causes of acute renal failure

Type	Cause
Pre-renal	Fluid loss
	Diarrhoea and vomiting
	Heat injury
	Burns
	Excessive diuresis
	Blood loss
	Gastrointestinal
	External bleeding
	Surgery
	Hypotensive states
	Cardiogenic shock
	Heart failure
	Sepsis
Renal	Acute glomerulonephritis
	Vasculitis
	Disseminated intravascular coagulation
	Nephrotoxic agents
	Sepsis
	Untreated pre-renal causes
	Bilateral renal infarction
	Obstetric complications, e.g. eclampsia
	Hypercalcaemia
Post-renal	Prostatic enlargement
	Bilateral ureteric stones
	Urethral strictures
	Postoperative bladder dysfunction
	Carcinoma of the cervix

Acute renal failure classically starts with a phase of very low urinary output (oliguria), which is followed by a recovery phase characterized by a diuresis. During the oliguric phase the body accumulates nitrogenous waste products, water, potassium, sodium, inorganic acids and phosphate. The life-threatening features of acute renal failure comprise pulmonary oedema, hyperkalaemia and acidosis on top of the underlying disorder, and this is often further complicated by septicaemia and the failure of other organs, e.g. the liver, heart or lungs. Nitrogenous waste products may accumulate at a rapid rate as a result of tissue breakdown with the catabolic response to trauma and infection. The recovery (diuretic) phase of acute renal failure may be delayed for several weeks. The renal tubules then cannot concentrate urine effectively and there is a risk of fluid and electrolyte depletion during the diuresis. Hypokalaemia and hyponatraemia are common; the latter is common following relief of urinary tract obstruction. The urinary output may be 3–5 litres/day.

Oliguria is not a universal feature of acute renal failure. Urinary output may cease (anuria) and alter-

Table 40.4 Biochemical features for differentiating pre-renal and renal acute failure

Parameter	Pre-renal	Renal
Urinary sodium	<20 mmol/l	>20 mmol/l
U_{osm}/P_{osm} ratio	>1.5	<1.5
U_c/P_c ratio	>40	<20

U=urine, P=plasma, Osm=osmolality, C=creatinine

nate with high outputs, i.e. polyuria in obstruction of the urinary tract. High-output renal failure occurs when urinary water losses are substantial but nitrogenous compounds are poorly excreted and still accumulate in blood. In evaluating the cause of renal failure, measuring plasma and urine sodium, creatinine and osmolality may help distinguish between pre-renal and renal causes (Table 40.4). However, if diuretics have been administered too much reliance should not be placed on these tests.

Radiological investigations are invaluable in evaluating the patient with acute renal failure. A plain abdominal X-ray may reveal calculi causing obstruction to both ureters, and ultrasonography is useful for demonstrating obstruction and for determining the size of the kidneys. If the cause of acute renal failure is not obvious, then provided there are two normal-sized kidneys and no clotting defect or urinary infection, a renal biopsy may be indicated.

Medical treatment of acute renal failure

The extra-renal causes of acute renal failure, e.g. infection and trauma, must be treated as well as the uraemia. Loss of body fluids can lead to so-called 'pre-renal' acute renal failure. This should be treated promptly by appropriate fluid replacement, because this helps to prevent the development of tubular necrosis. During the oliguric phase the patient should be given a daily volume of fluid equalling the previous 24-hour urine output plus extra-renal fluid losses from the gut, drains and fistulae. An estimated 500 ml should be added for the insensible fluid losses from the skin and respiratory tract. Many patients with acute renal failure are pyrexial and require assisted ventilation; insensible water losses may rise to 1 litre/day. Renal replacement therapy should be instituted early rather than late, especially in patients who are catabolic. The indications for dialysis include fluid overload, hyperkalaemia and severe acidosis. Haemodialysis is employed, usually on a daily basis,

to remove toxic waste products and to remove fluid prior to infusing blood products or parenteral nutrients (details of dialysis are discussed in the section on chronic renal failure). In patients with cardiovascular instability, haemofiltration (a continuous blood purification method involving the removal of large quantities of plasma water, with fluid replacement) may be tolerated much better than intermittent daily haemodialysis.

Renal replacement therapy with peritoneal dialysis is now seldom used for treating acute renal failure unless haemodialysis facilities are unavailable, or when therapy is used as a 'holding procedure' while arrangements are made to transfer patients to a haemodialysis centre. Despite appropriate treatment not all patients with acute renal failure recover renal function completely, and some may either require permanent renal replacement treatment, or be left with residual renal insufficiency. This is especially true for ischaemic renal damage, e.g. in patients who undergo prolonged ischaemia during surgery for abdominal aortic aneurysms.

Dietary management of acute renal failure

Renal replacement therapy has improved the prognosis of patients with acute renal failure. Before this facility was available many patients died of uraemia; now, there is a greater risk of death from infection and poor wound healing if there is inadequate nutritional support. The dietitian's role in monitoring the nutritional status of these patients is thus important. Patients with acute renal failure are usually divided into three groups, according to their underlying diagnosis and degree of catabolism (Lee 1980): non-catabolic, which usually results from non-traumatic medical causes, e.g. drug overdose; moderately catabolic, which usually develops after surgery; and severely catabolic, occurring with major trauma, burns or where there is significant sepsis. These three groups have different nutritional requirements.

Non-catabolic

The dietary needs of non-catabolic patients are determined by serum biochemistry, which should be assessed daily. If serum creatinine concentration is less than 400 µmol/l, dietary protein restriction is not usually necessary. Some centres prefer to provide a high biological value (HBV) protein intake of 0.6 g/kg ideal body weight (IBW).

Unfortunately, the provision of adequate protein and energy to these patients is often difficult because their debilitated state induces anorexia. Food should therefore be given in a form which will be acceptable, which may mean the use of protein supplements, the choice being determined by the electrolyte status and fluid needs (see Table 40.2). A minimum energy intake of 1.4 × BMR (basal metabolic rate) is required. BMR varies with sex, age and weight, as explained in Chapter 3, so the requirement must be worked out for each patient or read off from a table (Department of Health 1991) or a graph. The provision of adequate intake may be difficult in the anorexic patient, and usually requires the addition of glucose or glucose polymers such as Maxijul or Fortical, to the diet. A combined fat and carbohydrate source, e.g. Duocal, may be added to drinks, puddings, etc.

Daily recording of the patient's weight is important, and the institution of food intake charts is useful. In this way the dietitian can assess daily food consumption and make any necessary changes. In some instances tube feeding may be required, either on a 24-hour basis or as an overnight supplement if oral intake is possible during the day. Again, fluid and electrolyte restriction must be taken into account. Nepro, which is relatively low in electrolytes but high in energy per unit volume, may be useful in these circumstances (see Table 40.2).

In the oedematous anuric or oliguric patient sodium restriction is generally required. Foods with a high sodium content may cause thirst and should be avoided. Normally a diet containing 80–100 mmol of sodium is recommended, but occasionally a lower salt consumption (40 mmol sodium) is necessary if the degree of fluid restriction is severe.

An elevated plasma potassium may be controlled by restricting dietary potassium intake. Intervention is needed at a plasma level of 5 mmol/l, and a restriction of 0.6–0.7 mmol/kg IBW is usually adequate. Severe hyperkalaemia is controlled by the administration of cation exchange resins, e.g. calcium resonium given either orally or rectally. These resins bind the potassium in the intestinal secretions in exchange for the less well absorbed calcium ions. Glucose and insulin given intravenously can rapidly reduce serum potassium concentration, and is a useful short-term measure for dangerously high potassium levels while dialysis is being arranged. Insulin acts by stimulating potassium entry from the plasma into the cells, but controls hyperkalaemia for only a few hours. A dose of 12 units of soluble insulin can be given in 50 ml of 50% glucose over a period of 30 min. Constant monitoring of blood glucose after the infusion is necessary, to assess the possible development of hypoglycaemia.

Moderately catabolic and highly catabolic

Dietary treatment must be aggressive and feeding should be started early and not delayed. Protein, potassium and fluid intake used to be restricted, but now the policy is to feed the patient and then dialyse as necessary. This helps reduce the severe muscle wasting due to catabolism and inadequate nutrition. Moderately catabolic patients require 9–14 g of nitrogen daily (60–90 g of protein); severely hypercatabolic patients need 14–18 g of nitrogen (90–115 g of protein). Nitrogen loss can be up to 30–50 g daily. The liver in these patients may have a limited ability to deaminate amino acids, so 20 g of nitrogen daily should be the maximum amount prescribed. Requirements for sodium and potassium are calculated on an individual basis, depending on serum electrolyte concentrations. If patients with catabolic renal failure are fed orally, the protein intake should be 1–1.2 g/kg/day. The optimal energy intake varies according to the underlying disease. Acute renal failure causes little increase in energy expenditure, but in patients with septicaemia the energy expenditure increases by up to 25%. The BMR can be estimated from the Schofield equations (Department of Health 1991), and as set out in Chapter 3, e.g. for males aged 30–59 years:

$$BMR \ (MJ/day) = 0.048 \times wt \ (kg) + 3.653$$

for females aged 30–59 years:

$$BMR \ (MJ/day) = 0.34 \times wt \ (kg) + 3.538$$

The daily energy requirement in a given patient can be based on the estimated BMR, as described earlier, multiplied by an adjustment factor for the underlying disease, e.g. 1.25. The adjustment factor for severe infections is 1.4–1.6, and for severe burns covering more than 40% of the surface of the body is 1.85–2.05. This multiple of BMR then has to be multiplied by an activity/feeding factor which, for hospitalized patients confined to bed, may be taken as 1.2. The fluid volume required to administer such energy levels is around 2.5 litres/day. In practice there is a limit to the amount of fluid that can be removed during a single dialysis session, and fluid for administering nutrients is often restricted to 1–1.5 litres. The remaining fluid allowance is required for the continuous infusion of crystalloid fluid to maintain the patency of catheters for monitoring central venous and pulmonary arterial pressures, and for administrating sedative drugs, muscle relaxants and inotropic agents; bolus intravenous injections of antibiotics and other drugs may also be necessary.

Feeding should be via the gut where possible, but when enteral feeding is not tolerated due to diarrhoea or vomiting, or when there is the risk of lung aspiration, then parenteral nutrition should be considered via a central venous catheter.

Patient requirements for parenteral nutrition are estimated using the same criteria as enteral feeding (Forrest & Hartley 1991). The preferred source of nitrogen for total parenteral nutrition (TPN) is a solution of pure crystalline L-amino acids. These are available in a wide variety of concentrations and volumes. Where fluid restriction is necessary, a more concentrated solution such as Aminoplex 24 can be useful. Some solutions contain large amounts of electrolytes, whereas others are electrolyte-free. The latter are the usual choice in acute renal failure, where electrolyte restriction is usually required.

Patient requirements for electrolytes and minerals vary greatly. Potassium, phosphate and magnesium restrictions are often required, and these can simply be omitted from the TPN formulation and then added in small quantities according to individual needs. Daily biochemical monitoring is essential to ensure that requirements are being met.

Vitamins and trace elements are often given in standard doses from special ready-to-use vials. One or two vials daily of, for example, Solivito (Kabi-Vitrium) will provide adequate amounts of water-soluble vitamins, and one vial of Addamel or Additrace (Kabi-Vitrium) daily provides a reasonable range of trace elements. Extra quantities of individual trace elements such as zinc may be given as required.

As dialysis treatment is phased out and the patient's plasma biochemistry returns to normal, all dietary restrictions can cease. At this stage the patient should be encouraged to eat normally, with dietary supplementation where necessary. Some loss of appetite and taste sensation will remain a problem, and the dietitian will need considerable skill to keep the patient hydrated and in positive nitrogen balance.

CHRONIC RENAL FAILURE

It has been estimated that around 80 new patients per million of the population each year in the UK suffer from advanced chronic renal insufficiency (serum creatinine concentration persistently >500 μmol/l) (Feest et al 1990). The number of patients with less severe renal failure is likely to be greater than this, and the prevalence of patients with renal failure sufficient to require RRT in Britain is 360 per million of the population. This figure includes patients on dialysis and those with a functioning renal transplant.

The conditions leading to end-stage renal failure as a result of chronic renal failure vary with geographical area. In Europe the commonest causes are glomerulonephritis (24.1%), interstitial nephritis (17.3%), diabetes mellitus (12%), renovascular disease (10.3%) and cystic disease (8.3%). Chronic renal failure of uncertain aetiology comprises 14.8% of all patients with end-stage renal failure (Brunner et al 1989). The remainder of cases are secondary to multisystem diseases such as systemic lupus erythematosus, and rare congenital disorders such as oxalosis. In North America diabetes mellitus is the commonest known cause of renal failure (30%) followed by hypertension (26%) and glomerulonephritis (14%) (USRD Report 1989). The causes of chronic renal failure also vary with age, with reflux nephropathy, renal hypoplasia and congenital cystic diseases being more common in children.

Clinical features

The clinical features of chronic renal failure depend upon the degree of renal insufficiency. Patients may be asymptomatic, and are often diagnosed incidentally when serum urea and creatinine concentrations are requested. Often the patient with chronic renal failure presents to the non-nephrologist in the first instance. Investigations for anaemia, dyspnoea, pruritis, bone pain and neuropathy may all lead to a diagnosis. Because the kidneys have large functional reserves, symptoms may not occur until the GFR falls below 20 ml/min. When the GFR falls below 10 ml/min, symptoms of uraemia are almost always present (Fig. 40.1), and patients with a GFR below 5 ml/min usually require renal replacement therapy. However, these are general guidelines and patients with some conditions, such as diabetic nephropathy, or those with cardiac failure, may be symptomatic at higher levels of GFR.

Anaemia is almost invariable in chronic renal failure because erythropoietin production is insufficient. Uraemic inhibitors of erythropoiesis may be involved, and the red blood cells have a shortened lifespan. Bleeding from the gastrointestinal tract is also common in renal failure and may lead to iron deficiency, which may further aggravate the anaemic state.

As the GFR declines serum phosphate concentration rises. Due to the lack of active vitamin D, the intestinal absorption of calcium is impaired and

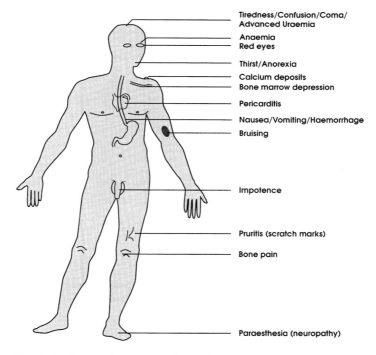

Tiredness/Confusion/Coma/
Advanced Uraemia

Anaemia
Red eyes

Thirst/Anorexia

Calcium deposits
Bone marrow depression

Pericarditis

Nausea/Vomiting/Haemorrhage

Bruising

Impotence

Pruritis (scratch marks)

Bone pain

Paraesthesia (neuropathy)

Fig. 40.1   Signs and symptoms of uraemia.

hypocalcaemia ensues. The high phosphate and low serum calcium concentrations stimulate the secretion of parathyroid hormone, which results in demineralization of bone. These changes in calcium and phosphate metabolism, and the secondary hyperparathyroid activity, result in renal bone disease, which comprises a spectrum of bone disorders including osteoporosis, osteomalacia and osteitis fibrosa. Failure to control hyperphosphataemia may result in bone pains and fractures. Occasionally a high calcium and phosphate product leads to soft-tissue calcification in the eyes, skin and muscles.

Some clinical features of chronic renal failure may be specific for the underlying renal disorders, e.g. rash and arthropathy in systemic lupus erythematosus, and lung symptoms in sarcoidosis and the vasculitides. As renal function declines, nocturia and polyuria develop. These are secondary to a loss of the kidney's concentrating ability, and are due to the high concentration of urea in the tubules of the remaining functioning nephrons producing an osmotic effect on fluid output. The loss of concentrating ability may result in an acute exacerbation of chronic renal failure if there are abnormal fluid losses, for example following gastroenteritis or infection.

The uraemic state is associated with various defects of both the cellular and the humoral components of the immune system. This may explain the increased susceptibility of patients to infections.

Medical management of chronic renal failure

The course of chronic renal insufficiency cannot be predicted with certainty. Some patients remain in a state of chronic 'stable' renal failure for many years, whereas others progress steadily towards end-stage disease. Because of the variable and unpredictable course of chronic renal failure it has been very difficult to evaluate suggested therapeutic interventions.

The patient with chronic renal insufficiency has a reduced renal reserve, and therefore is susceptible to acute deterioration of renal function as a result of fluid depletion from gastroenteritis or blood loss, but hypotensive episodes, e.g. myocardial infarction and catabolic states such as infections and trauma, are also important. Urinary tract obstruction is a common reversible cause of deterioration of renal function in stable chronic renal failure, and should be sought in all acute-on-chronic cases. Nephrotoxic drugs, such

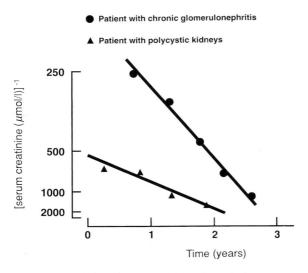

Fig. 40.2   Relationship between the reciprocal of serum creatinine concentration and time in two patients with chronic renal failure. (From Catto & Power 1988, with permission)

as non-steroidal anti-inflammatory drugs and aminoglycosides, should be avoided if possible.

Uncontrolled hypertension accelerates the progression of chronic renal failure. It is important, therefore, to follow the patient regularly, with special attention being paid to the control of high blood pressure, the treatment of urinary tract infection and the monitoring of serum electrolytes and creatinine concentration. By plotting the inverse of serum creatinine concentration against time, the approximate rate of progression can be assessed and a general impression of when replacement therapy will be required may be gained (Fig. 40.2). In practice, most nephrologists measure serum creatinine concentration and initiate dialysis when it approaches 1000 μmol/1, or earlier if the patient develops severe acidosis, marked fluid retention, hyperkalaemia or uraemic symptoms.

When the serum phosphate concentration rises above 2.0 mmol/1, dietary phosphate restriction should be introduced. Because intestinal phosphate absorption is not decreased in renal failure and a phosphate-free diet is impractical, efforts are made to bind the phosphate in the diet. In the past aluminium hydroxide was used, but because aluminium was absorbed and proved to be toxic, calcium carbonate is now given with meals routinely to bind the phosphate (Coburn & Salusky 1989). Aluminium toxicity was serious and caused anaemia, osteomalacia and encephalopathy. Patients who are hypocalcaemic,

however, benefit from a rise in serum calcium when calcium carbonate is given between meals. 1-Hydroxy vitamin D or 1,25-dihydroxy vitamin D is given to hypocalcaemic patients to suppress parathyroid overactivity; the latter is the activated form of vitamin D, while the former preparation requires hepatic hydroxylation at the 25C position for conversion to the active metabolite.

As renal failure advances anaemia almost invariably occurs, and any iron deficiency should be treated with supplementary iron. The role of recombinant human erythropoietin in the pre-dialysis patient is not well established, but early studies indicate that treatment of such patients with erythropoietin does not adversely affect the progression of renal failure. The use of erythropoietin in dialysis patients is discussed later.

Conservative dietary management of chronic renal failure

Measures to retard progression of disease

Once there has been a critical loss of renal function, renal failure progresses inexorably in the majority of cases. This has led to a search for measures to retard this progression. In partially nephrectomized rats, dietary protein restriction, antihypertensive agents, and limiting hyperlipidaemia and phosphorus intake all reduce progressive renal failure experimentally, but the relevance of these observations to humans is unclear. El Nahas & Coles (1986) and Giovannetti (1986) have highlighted the difficulties in designing and carrying out studies to assess the role of dietary protein restriction. A recent study (Locatelli et al 1991) based on a prospective randomized multicentre trial concludes that protein restriction does not retard the progression of chronic renal insufficiency. However, the authors admit that compliance was poor for the group which was assigned the low-protein diet, and that the difference in protein intake between the two groups was significantly less than that which was required by the study protocol. A North American multicentre trial is in progress (Klahr 1989).

Protein   In practice, many specialist renal units assess the patient's protein intake when their serum creatinine rises above 300 μmol/1. At this stage, if protein intake exceeds 1 g/kg body weight/day, a reduction to that level is suggested. Restriction to 0.6 g of protein/kg IBW when the patient becomes symptomatic is commonly suggested, e.g. for a 60 kg person this would provide 36 g of protein daily. It is recommended that 70% of the protein intake in a

Table 40.5   Foods with a high potassium content

Food group	Foods high in potassium
Wholegrain cereals	These may be included in the diet and require careful monitoring
Meat and meat products	All meat
Fish and fish products	All fish
Dairy products	Milk, eggs, yoghurt
Nuts	All nuts
Fruit and vegetables	Dried pulses, baked beans, sweetcorn, mushrooms, spinach, instant potatoes, potato waffles, crisps, bananas, figs, vegetable juice
Beverages	Build up, Horlicks, Ovaltine, drinking chocolate, cocoa, coffee, wine, sherry
Sugar and confectionery	Chocolates, liquorice, toffees, molasses, black treacle, syrup, dried fruit
Miscellaneous	Yeast extracts (Marmite), beef extracts (Oxo, Bovril), stock cubes, bottled sauces, ketchups, pickles, chutneys, instant puddings, Gram flour, cream of tartar
Herbs and spices	Salt substitutes (Ruthmol, Selera), curry powder, chilli, ginger

(Reproduced from Thomas 1988, with permission)

restricted diet should be of high biological value. The use of high-energy low-protein products and other dietary supplements is important in patients with a poor appetite, and there is a wide variety of bread, biscuits, pastas, etc. available on prescription. These sources of carbohydrate are of special importance to the diabetic patient, who must maintain an intake of 150–350 g of carbohydrate daily. An energy supplement such as Maxijul (powder or liquid), Duocal or Fortical is usually necessary; originally cream and other fatty foods were used to maintain energy intake until it was recognized that a high-fat diet should be avoided, to prevent hyperlipidaemia in renal patients.

Reduction of protein intake in both diabetic and non-diabetic individuals to below 0.6 g of protein/kg IBW is not advisable, because the intake of essential amino acids may become insufficient to maintain nitrogen balance (Mitch 1991); a further reduction in total protein intake requires the addition of essential amino acids or ketoacids to the basic diet (Mitch et al 1984). It is important to assess protein and energy intake regularly, and to take particular care that malnutrition and muscle wasting do not occur.

Potassium   Hyperkalaemia can follow blood transfusions, treatment with certain drugs, e.g. angiotensin-converting enzyme inhibitors, and may be precipitated by infection, trauma or surgery, and is found in severely acidotic patients when renal function is only moderately impaired. A normal potassium intake is 80 mmol/day for a typical western diet. Intakes vary according to different cultures and food habits; vegetarians and vegans have particular problems with potassium control, as many foods which constitute their diet, i.e. pulses, nuts and fruits, are rich dietary sources of potassium. When serum levels reach the upper limit of normal (5.0 mmol/1) a

restriction to 50 mmol/day by removing food with a particularly high potassium content (Table 40.5) is usually adequate. Further restriction to 30–40 mmol/day may be necessary if renal function deteriorates further to end-stage failure.

Phosphate   As plasma phosphate rises oral calcium carbonate or magnesium carbonate is introduced to reduce phosphate absorption and maintain plasma levels within the normal range (0.7–1.2 mmol/1). Dietary phosphate is also controlled at 600–700 mg/day. If the patient is already on potassium and protein restriction then only a few extra dietary restrictions are required, e.g. dairy products and cereals, particularly bran. The phosphate binders must be taken at the correct time, i.e. just before meals and snacks, so that they can bind in the stomach with the phosphate in the food (Coburn & Salusky 1989).

Sodium   Salt restriction is usually more of a concern when the patient starts dialysis. The patient with chronic renal failure loses 60–100 mmol/day, even when salt intake is restricted, and dehydration occurs if sodium losses become excessive. A moderate salt intake (80–100 mmol of sodium) is needed in cases of severe hypertension and oedema.

Fluid   Fluid restriction is introduced when urinary volume drops or there is fluid overload. An intake of 500 ml plus the equivalent of the previous day's output from urine, fistulae, etc. is recommended.

RENAL REPLACEMENT THERAPY

Dialysis

Patients with end-stage renal failure depend upon maintenance dialysis in order to survive. Dialysis therapy cannot substitute for healthy normally functioning kidneys, but it allows patients to avoid the life-threatening features of uraemia. Not all symptoms are relieved by dialysis, and patients still have to observe dietary and, in most cases, fluid restrictions. Haemodialysis and peritoneal dialysis are the two options, and most patients are offered a choice of therapy. The principles are the same for both types. A semipermeable membrane acts as a filter which separates the blood from the dialysate compartment. Diffusion of solutes across the dialyser membrane results in removal of uraemic toxins from the blood compartment, while high molecular weight substances such as proteins are retained in the blood. The dialysate concentration of electrolytes is controlled to allow diffusion of excess electrolytes and urea from the blood. Either acetate or bicarbonate is used in the dialysate to correct acidosis. Water is removed by ultrafiltration; this is achieved in haemodialysis by generating hydrostatic pressure across the dialysate membrane, and in peritoneal dialysis by osmosis, using various concentrations of glucose in the dialysate fluid.

Haemodialysis

Haemodialysis requires blood and dialysate circuits. Blood and dialysate are brought into the dialyser, which has an artificial membrane made of cellulose or other material. The dialyser is either 'flat-bed', with sheets of membrane to separate blood and dialysate, or 'hollow fibre'. In the latter type blood flows through microscopic lumina in a bundle of thousands of hollow fibres, while dialysate circulates around the fibre. The flow of blood needed for adequate dialysis is high – usually 200–300 ml/min – and the dialysate flows at 500 ml/min. Such high blood flow rates can only be obtained by creating a system giving access to a substantial blood vessel. This usually takes the form of an arteriovenous fistula, which is created surgically by anastomosing an artery (usually in the forearm) to an adjacent vein. The high arterial pressure results in 'arterialization', or thickening of the wall of the veins, in about 4–6 weeks. The vein can then be repeatedly cannulated to provide an adequate blood flow into the dialysis machine before being returned to the same vein. Before the blood passes into the dialyser, the anticoagulant heparin is added to prevent clotting. The blood then passes through the dialyser while the dialysate flows in the opposite direction. The dialysate drains out and the purified blood is returned to the vein. This procedure continues for a total of 3–6 hours. Various monitors in the haemodialysis machine

ensure that there is no leakage of blood, air or dialysate during the process. The machine also has a proportioning system which dilutes the concentrated dialysate with water. The hydrostatic pressure across the dialyser membrane is also regulated to allow the net removal of water from the blood.

The pressure difference across the membrane can be increased by switching off the dialysate flow. In this way water can be removed rapidly, although solute removal is negligible. This technique is particularly useful for patients whose serum biochemistry (particularly potassium, bicarbonate, urea and creatinine) is satisfactory but who have excess intra- and extravascular fluid, resulting in hypertension, peripheral and particularly pulmonary oedema. Usually the dialyser surface area is $1 \, m^2$, but a large variety of sizes with varying permeability is available.

For emergency haemodialysis, for example in acute renal failure, an arteriovenous shunt has to be constructed by cannulating adjacent arteries and veins. After the dialysis is completed a permanent shunt can then be constructed. Alternatively, rapid vascular access can be achieved by cannulating a large central vein such as the subclavian or internal jugular.

Most patients with end-stage disease on haemodialysis are given 12 hours of dialysis weekly in two or three 4–6 hourly sessions. Haemodialysis may also be carried out at home, provided the patient is helped by a relative who has learnt the technique.

Peritoneal dialysis

According to the European Renal Registry, in 1990 there were a total of 91 383 patients in Europe on haemodialysis, and 11 862 on continuous ambulatory peritoneal dialysis (CAPD) (Geerlings et al 1991).

Peritoneal dialysis makes use of the human peritoneal membrane for blood purification. In man this is about $1 \, m^2$ in surface area, and the peritoneal cavity is normally only a potential space containing virtually no fluid. The peritoneal membrane is vascular and consists of mesothelial cells. In peritoneal dialysis dialysate is poured from a collapsible bag and tubing into the peritoneal cavity via a peritoneal catheter and allowed to equilibrate for 6–8 hours. The dialysate is then drained out and fresh dialysate fluid is instilled. Fluid removal in peritoneal dialysis relies on creating an osmotic gradient across the peritoneal membrane, whereas haemodialysis relies on hydrostatic pressure.

For ultrafiltration in peritoneal dialysis, glucose is used as an osmotic agent, various concentrations being used to vary the amount of ultrafiltration. Acetate or lactate is used as a buffer instead of bicarbonate, which cannot be used as precipitation of bicarbonates of divalent ions will occur. Lactate is preferred because the presence of acetate causes glucose to caramelize during the autoclaving process. Long-term peritoneal dialysis usually takes the form of CAPD, self-administered by the patient and usually undertaken three or four times every 24 hours. Usually 1500–2000 ml of dialysate are used in each exchange.

CAPD is especially useful in patients who have difficulty with vascular access, such as diabetics or those who suffer from heart failure and cannot tolerate the haemodynamic changes of haemodialysis. Infection is the main problem with CAPD, and the patient must be meticulous in using totally aseptic techniques during the handling of the fluids and catheters. The dialysate removed from the peritoneum should be clear; if it is turbid this suggests that peritonitis has begun. This should be treated with appropriate antibiotics, given usually into the peritoneum.

Peritoneal dialysis can also be carried out on an intermittent basis (IPD), for 36–48 hours each week split into three or four 12-hourly periods. A machine is needed and the process is usually carried out at night while the patient is asleep. Intermittent peritoneal dialysis can also be carried out in hospital.

Diet in dialysis

Haemodialysis

Because of the technical advances in dialysis dietary restrictions have become less severe, so the quality of a patient's life has improved substantially. Nevertheless, some dietary guidelines are still necessary. An adequate protein intake is essential as dialysis is a catabolic process. During haemodialysis catabolic hormones such as glucagon, glucocorticoids and adrenaline are released. There is also loss of as much as 7 g of amino acids and 2–3 g of peptides into the dialysate (Wolfson et al 1982). Complement activation also occurs as a result of blood contact with synthetic membranes. Each dialysis session leads to a loss of amino acids which need to be replaced. The prescription of dialysis remains empirical, and has largely been determined by the clinician's judgement. During dialysis blood urea nitrogen concentration decreases as a function of three parameters: dialyser urea clearance (K), treatment time (T) and the volume of distribution of urea (V). On the other hand, the increase in urea during the interdialytic period depends on the rate of generation of urea (a

function of the protein catabolic rate (PCR), which in stable non-catabolic patients reflects dietary protein intake), the volume of distribution of urea and the residual renal function. In the national Cooperative Dialysis Study (NCDS) a KT/V value of 1–1.4 was associated with less morbidity provided the PCR was 1 g/kg/day (Parker et al 1983). An intake of 1–1.2 g/protein/kg IBW is recommended, with 70% in the form of animal protein because the loss of essential amino acids in the dialysis fluid is proportional to the plasma concentrations and not limited by adapted and restricted catabolism. In the anorexic or elderly patient this can be difficult to achieve without the use of a protein supplement, e.g. Fortisip, Fortimel, Provide and Protein Forte (see Table 40.2). Regular assessment of protein intake is important.

A high-fibre, low-fat and low-sugar diet should be used when possible to limit the risk of hyperlipidaemia. Weight loss in obese patients may be achieved by carefully restricting their intake to a level of 500 kcal below their current needs, which will change as they lose weight. An intake of about 35 kcal/kg/day is generally recommended. However, the overweight dialysis patient should be advised to lose weight. The majority who are underweight may need an energy supplement such as Maxijul or Fortical. Particular care is required for children who are anorexic.

The maintenance of serum potassium levels within normal limits (3.5–4.9 mmol/1) following a dialysis session should be the aim, with sufficiently frequent and effective dialysis to limit pre-dialysis potassium to <5.5 mmol/1. An intake of 30–60 mmol is recommended. However, other factors influence serum potassium levels and must be considered, e.g. constipation (the faeces are the main route of potassium excretion in end-stage renal failure), the potassium content of the dialysis fluid, acidosis, infection, tissue damage and drugs. In acidotic states there is a release of potassium from the intracellular to the extracellular space which cannot be excreted in renal failure. Correction of acidosis improves hyperkalaemia. Potassium intake can be reduced by restricting the foods mentioned in Table 40.5. All fruits and vegetables contain some potassium, and the daily intake of these foods should be restricted to one portion of fresh fruit or two servings of tinned fruit without the juice, and two small servings of vegetables or salad. A further reduction in potassium can be achieved by boiling vegetables and potatoes in a large volume of water for 30 min (Bower 1989).

Hyperphosphataemia can lead to secondary hyperparathyroidism and bone disease, i.e. renal osteodystrophy. This can be prevented by restricting the

Table 40.6   Foods with a high phosphate content

Food group	Foods high in phosphate
Dairy	Hard cheese (Cheddar), soft cheese (Brie), cheese spreads, eggs, milk (including evaporated and condensed)
Protein	Liver, kidney, sweetbreads, veal, pigeon and other game, herring, kippers, mackerel, sardines, salmon, trout, whitebait, prawns, scampi, crab
Cereals	Muesli, All Bran, wholemeal bread, oatcakes
Nuts	All
Beverages	Malted milk drinks (Horlicks, Ovaltine), drinking chocolate, cocoa
Miscellaneous	Yeast extracts (Marmite), beef extracts (Oxo, Bovril), chocolate, toffee, fudge, marzipan, baking powder

(Reproduced from Thomas 1988, with permission)

intake of phosphate to 0.8–1.1 g/day, by reducing the consumption of foods high in phosphate (Table 40.6), and using oral phosphate binders. Many patients find these difficult to swallow with the imposed fluid restriction, so they often refuse or forget to take them just before food as prescribed.

In general urinary output diminishes the longer a patient remains on dialysis. This fact should be emphasized when they commence replacement therapy so that the patient can anticipate a change in urinary output. Around 500 ml/day is allowed in addition to the equivalent volume of any urine passed. Fluid accumulation is measured by weighing the patient (1 kg weight = 1 litre of body water) and a maximum of 2 litres of fluid may be gained between dialysis – less if cardiac failure is present. The dietitian and nursing staff must teach the patient to measure their urinary volume. Teaching patients to keep their own fluid charts on the ward is a useful exercise and helps prepare for future restrictions, which many find very difficult to comply with.

A dietary sodium restriction of 80–100 mmol/day is normal. An excessive salt intake will result in increased thirst and make adherence to fluid restriction even more difficult. Control of hypertension is also more effective if salt intake is restricted.

Dialysis patients require supplementation with water-soluble vitamins, which are removed from the diet by prolonged cooking to remove potassium and by dialysis itself. B-complex vitamins, folic acid and vitamin C should be prescribed. Excessive vitamin C intake can, however, lead to accumulation of oxalic acid, which may lead to calcium oxalate being deposited in the soft tissues and bones (Yamauchi et al 1986). Vitamin A is bound to retinol, which is a protein of high molecular weight and is not dialysable. Supplementary vitamin A is therefore not necessary and should not be prescribed, as toxic accumulation

in bone may occur. Iron supplements are given to make up for blood losses during haemodialysis, which may amount to 5 litres/year. Patients receiving erythropoietin treatment also need iron supplements. Iron overload can occur in patients who have received multiple blood transfusions. 1-α-hydroxy vitamin D or 1,25-dihydroxy vitamin D are useful for preventing bone disease. Calcium and phosphate are regularly monitored in all patients on dialysis.

Peritoneal dialysis

Because dialysis is continuous, fluid and dietary restrictions are usually less severe. Nitrogen balance may be neutral, with a protein intake of 0.98 g/kg/day, and positive with a protein intake of 1.4 g/kg/day. The recommended protein intake for CAPD patients is at least 1.1 g/kg/day. During episodes of peritonitis protein loss from CAPD fluid may be as high as 15–20 g/day, and supplementation may be necessary, particularly as the patient is likely to be anorexic.

The consumption of the recommended quantity of protein can be difficult if the patient's appetite is poor. A low-phosphate, low-electrolyte protein supplement may be necessary in these circumstances, e.g. Protein Forte. This can be discontinued if appetite improves. However, many CAPD patients require continuous supplementation to maintain health. The protein intake should be evenly distributed throughout the day when possible, to avoid uraemic symptoms.

A large energy intake is not necessary in CAPD, as 70% of the glucose in the CAPD bags is absorbed through the peritoneum. Patients should therefore be discouraged from eating foods of low nutritional value, i.e. those that are high in fat and sugar. A low-fat diet is also advisable, both to reduce the risk of hyperlipidaemia and to maintain IBW.

Obesity can be a major problem in the CAPD patient because of absorption of sugar from the dialysate. Between 400 and 900 kcal are gained per day, depending upon the glucose concentration of the dialysate. Diabetics in particular are at risk, and need careful guidance and regular monitoring. A high-fibre diet to prevent constipation is advisable. Patients should be aware of those foods which are particularly high in potassium, but actual restriction is not usually necessary. Consistently high potassium levels will need investigation and perhaps stricter dietary control.

Dietary phosphate restriction similar to that of patients on haemodialysis is usual. However, because CAPD patients consume larger quantities of protein at both meal times and snacks, larger doses of phosphate binders may need to be prescribed. Normally a fluid intake of 1000 ml plus the equivalent of the previous day's urinary output is recommended, although more accurate guidance can be obtained by monitoring net fluid loss from each dialysis cycle and the patient's weight. Most patients are anuric, and an increase in weight usually indicates fluid retention.

Hyperlipidaemia in dialysis patients

Patients on haemodialysis and peritoneal dialysis have a high incidence of ischaemic heart disease and accelerated atherosclerosis, and cardiovascular death remains the leading cause of mortality. Many factors undoubtedly contribute to accelerated atherosclerosis, and hyperlipidaemia is suggested as a major cause. Hypertriglyceridaemia is the most common abnormality in patients with renal failure and those on dialysis; hypercholesterolaemia is rare. Studies have documented the efficacy of low-saturated-fat diets in patients treated with dialysis, but the long-term benefits of such intervention remain to be defined. Therapy such as dietary restriction, exercise programmes and correction of other risk factors such as smoking, is advisable. There is little experience with lipid-lowering drugs in dialysis patients.

Nutritional status of patients on dialysis

Anthropometric measurements

Anthropometry is recognized as an important method in the assessment of nutritional status. Measurements of height, weight and body proportions provide useful data in the initial assessment of a patient with end-stage renal failure. For those starting dialysis, baseline measurements of body mass index (BMI) will indicate the presence of obesity or undernutrition. Mid-upper arm circumference (MUAC) and triceps skin fold (TSF) are useful measurements for monitoring changes in body composition and response to any dietary supplementation which may be necessary. The mid-arm muscle circumference (MAMC) can be calculated using the formula:

$$\text{MAMC (cm)} = \text{MUAC (cm)} - 3.14 \times \text{TSF (cm)}$$

The measurement should be recorded post-dialysis and in the non-fistula arm. This is useful for assessing the body protein stores and hence the degree of undernutrition.

Dietary assessment

An estimation of dietary intake needs to be calculated at regular intervals by the dietitian to ensure that patients are eating within the recommended guidelines. The simplest method is to take a dietary history, remembering to include both dialysis and non-dialysis days, as eating habits vary considerably during a typical week.

ERYTHROPOIETIN TREATMENT

The advent of recombinant human erythropoietin therapy has revolutionized the treatment of anaemia in renal failure, and most dialysis patients nowadays should no longer require blood transfusions for anaemia. Numerous trials have now shown that erythropoietin is safe and effective if used carefully. Many symptoms of chronic renal failure previously thought to be due to uraemia are reversed by correcting anaemia. Erythropoietin is administered either intravenously or subcutaneously, twice or thrice weekly. The dose varies with individuals and the response is dose-dependent. Usually patients with a haemoglobin below 80 g/l should be treated, and a target of 100 g/l should be met. Treatment with erythropoietin leads to increased utilization of iron as a rapid erythrocytosis occurs, and iron supplements are therefore required in most cases. The most frequently encountered side effect is hypertension (Winearls et al 1986). The cause of this is unclear, although reactive vasoconstriction following relief of chronic hypoxaemia and an increase in blood viscosity have been suggested as possible mechanisms (Neff et al 1971). Occasionally it may produce a clotting tendency, perhaps due to increased platelet stickiness, resulting in an increased need for heparin in haemodialysis patients (Bommer et al 1987). When anaemia is corrected with erythropoietin the patient often feels much better and appetite improves, but with subsequent increases in plasma potassium and phosphate which need anticipatory management. A lack of response to erythropoietin may occur in patients with iron deficiency, continuing blood loss, aluminium intoxication, infection and malignancy.

RENAL TRANSPLANTATION

A transplant is the optimum treatment for end-stage renal failure. The transplanted kidney may be obtained from a cadaver or from a living relative. Most patients on dialysis are now offered a place on a renal transplant waiting list. In 1990 a total of 1889 transplants were carried out in the UK, 1776 of which were from cadavers and 113 from live relatives (Geerlings et al 1991). The donor's and recipient's blood groups must be compatible; some patients, such as those who have received transplants in the past or those who have been given multiple blood transfusions, may develop antibodies to HLA antigens, which make them highly sensitized to antigens from a broad spectrum of donors. Before the transplant is carried out the recipient's serum is cross-matched with cells from the prospective donor, to ensure compatibility.

Following a successful transplant operation the patient requires immunosuppressive drugs to prevent rejection. The most commonly used of these are prednisolone, azathioprine and cyclosporin A. These drugs may produce unwanted side effects, including leucopenia, susceptibility to infection, weight gain, renal dysfunction, hypertension, osteoporosis and hyperlipidaemia; a renal transplant patient therefore requires regular follow-up. Transplanted patients may develop episodes of transplant rejection which require treatment with high doses of steroids or monoclonal antibodies. Sometimes there is recurrence of the primary renal disease, or the development of new renal disease. Focal glomerulosclerosis, membranoproliferative glomerulonephritis, Goodpasture's disease and immunoglobulin A disease may recur in the transplanted kidney, and such disease recurrence, as well as irreversible rejection, may lead to the patient requiring dialysis again. The patient with a renal transplant therefore poses unique medical and nutritional problems.

Dietary management of the transplant patient

After the dietary and fluid restrictions of renal replacement therapy the newly transplanted patient needs encouragement to increase his fluid and nutritional intake. Later, a steroid-induced increase in appetite may lead to excessive weight gain and hyperlipidaemia. Some patients will remain hypertensive and will be advised to continue salt restriction. Others may develop diabetes mellitus, as a result of steroid therapy. Occasionally cyclosporin A causes hyperkalaemia on a long-term basis. Hyperlipidaemia is a common problem in the transplanted patient, and has many causes. Immunosuppressive drugs, diabetes, the use of beta-blockers and obesity following transplantation all contribute. Transplant patients should therefore be encouraged to eat a diet low in fat and sugar and high in non-starch polysaccharides, and to maintain their ideal body weight. Lipid-lowering drugs must be used with care in these patients, as many produce side effects in conjunction with immunosuppression.

STONES IN THE URINARY TRACT

Chemistry of renal calculi

At least 95% of stones are made up of calcium salts. About 3% are uric acid salts and about 1% are cystine. Most stones contain a mixture of mainly calcium oxalate, calcium phosphate and magnesium ammonium phosphate, but about one-third are pure calcium oxalate. Stones form more readily in infected urine in which bacteria have converted urea into ammonia, so making the urine more alkaline.

The solubility of a salt in urine depends on the product of its ionic activities. These are difficult to measure, and are determined in part by the presence of other ions in the urine. Salts in urine can become supersaturated, and the crystals of calcium oxalate present in all urines probably result from their being precipitated from a supersaturated solution of calcium oxalate. The crystals, however, are small and normally washed out when the urine is voided.

Crystal growth is determined by other chemical constituents of the urine, and is affected by disease and diet. Substances which inhibit crystal growth are also present in urine. These include citrate, pyrophosphate, nephrocalin and glycosoaminoglycans, which vary in urinary concentration for unknown reasons.

Bladder calculi

Bladder stones usually occur in males; in adults they are generally associated with prostatic obstruction or other causes of urinary stagnation. Stagnation and infection of urine and prolonged confinement to bed each predispose to stone formation. Bladder stones used to be common in young boys in Britain, and are still prevalent in tropical regions. There has been a decline in childhood bladder stones throughout Europe and North America, for unknown reasons, although children from working-class families on poorer diets were more affected. Epidemiological evidence suggests that a single-cereal diet (wheat, rice or millet) may be a significant causative factor of endemic bladder calculi (Halstead 1981). This theory may explain the so-called 'bladder stone belt' extending from the Middle East across India and the Far East from Thailand to Indonesia. Maize, the staple food in much of Africa, does not seem to be associated with bladder stones. Milk consumption may have a protective role against bladder stone formation, and in one Thai community where infants are weaned early, often on the first day after birth, bladder stones are hyperendemic (Valyasevi et al 1967).

Renal calculi

Renal colic, the excruciating pain caused by a stone passing down the urinary tract, is well known in all countries. The pain stops when the stone is passed naturally or removed by a surgeon. A patient may never have another attack, or attacks may recur at irregular and sometimes long intervals. Some patients have frequent attacks, when they pass many small stones or 'gravel'.

Most stones remain in the kidney, where they often produce no symptoms and are known as 'silent stones'. There they may grow, sometimes to a very large size. Repeated infection may lead to chronic pyelonephritis, a common cause of chronic renal failure.

Factors predisposing to stone formation

Increased urinary calcium

Hypercalciuria implies that the 24-hour urinary calcium on a free diet is higher than normal. The normal range of urinary calcium, however, varies according to geographical region, and a particular definition of normality therefore applies only to specific population groups. An accepted definition of hypercalciuria is the excretion of >7.5 mmol/day in women and 10 mmol/day in men, or >0.1 mmol/kg/day of calcium in either sex when the patient is screened on a defined 50 mmol/day calcium intake (a typical western diet) (Sharman 1988). Idiopathic hypercalciuria has been classified into absorptive, renal and resorptive. Secondary hypercalciuria occurs with primary hyperparathyroidism, sarcoidosis, vita-

min D excess, immobilization and medullary sponge kidneys. These are associated with an increased incidence of stone formation. Dietary hypercalciuria is not common and almost always disappears when the patient is evaluated on a controlled diet. A daily urinary excretion of calcium above 300 mg in men and 250 mg in women has been called 'hypercalciuria', and is present in about 8% of the healthy British population. Idiopathic hypercalciuria tends to run in families, and the absorptive type has been classified into two forms. In both there is a normal or low parathormone level, fasting urinary calcium levels below 0.11 mg/dl creatinine clearance, and excess calcium absorption with a rise in the urinary value to over 0.2 mg/dl after a 1 g oral calcium load in a synthetic meal. Persistent hypercalciuria, i.e. >200 mg after a week on a 400 mg calcium diet is indicative of type 1 absorptive hypercalciuria, whereas a calcium excretion of <200 mg/day indicates type 2. Type 1 may be managed by the use of a calcium-binding resin such as sodium cellulose phosphate, as well as dietary changes, whereas type 2 is controllable by dietary means alone. However, the role of the cellulose resin remains controversial.

Less than half of the patients who form calcium stones have measurable hypercalciuria. In these there is increasing evidence that a low urinary citrate output may occur, particularly in women, and citrate therapy is now being assessed (Coe et al 1992) Hypercalciuria with increased risk of stone formation occurs in hyperparathyroidism, which is the cause of 5–10% of all calcium stones.

It seems sensible for a patient who has passed a calcium stone to reduce the risk of a recurrence by going on a low-calcium diet. This entails limiting the consumption of milk, yoghurt and cheese (see Table 40.8).

Increased urinary oxalate

Along with calcium, urinary oxalate, forms about 70% of stones seen in the western world. About 10% of urinary oxalates are dietary in origin. The greater part of the oxalate excreted in the urine is of endogenous origin and often comes from tissue metabolism of glycine.

The commonest cause of hyperoxaluria is gastrointestinal malabsorption, which paradoxically causes increased absorption of dietary oxalates. Fatty acid malabsorption leads to calcium binding in the gut, to produce calcium soaps of the fatty acids. This leaves the oxalates free and unbound to be absorbed. Enteric hyperoxaluria is also exaggerated by a diet low in calcium. Treatment therefore is aimed at reducing dietary oxalate and encouraging a high calcium intake, to ensure the precipitation of calcium oxalates in the intestinal lumen. Cholestyramine can also be given to absorb some of the malabsorbed bile salts, and thereby improve diarrhoea.

Primary hyperoxaluria arises from rare inherited (autosomal recessive) errors of metabolism. Two errors depend on separate enzyme defects in the metabolism of glycine. Stone formation occurs in childhood, recurrences are common and often damage the kidneys and lead to chronic renal failure.

A typical English diet contains about 120 mg of oxalic acid, of which 75 mg comes from five cups of tea. It is sensible for anyone who has passed a stone containing oxalate to avoid tea, and also rhubarb and spinach, which contain a high amount of oxalic acid (250–800 mg/100 g). A low-oxalate diet, e.g. 30 mg/day is very restrictive and should be tried only in patients who have formed stones repeatedly at short intervals and have marked hyperoxaluria, which is then shown after an oral oxalate load to be of exogenous origin.

Increased urinary uric acid

About a quarter of patients with uric acid stones have hyperuricosuria, and in most cases excessive dietary intake of purines is found to be the cause. Such sources include liver, kidneys, sweetbreads, anchovies, sardines and brains. There are three correctable factors that lead to pure uric acid stone formation: the volume, pH and uric acid concentration of the volume, and the pH of urine. At low urinary pH the uric acid is less soluble. When the pH is raised to 6.5, five-sixths of the uric acid is dissolved. Therefore patients should be given alkalis such as potassium citrate daily, and encouraged to drink an adequate fluid intake.

Increased urinary cystine

Cystinuria is due to an inborn error of metabolism. The renal tubules fail to reabsorb the amino acids cystine, lysine, arginine and ornithine. These pass in large amounts into the urine, where cystine, the least-soluble amino acid, tends to precipitate out and form stones.

Prevention of stone formation

Fluid intake

This is by far the most important measure to be used against all forms of stone. A good flow of urine washes out particles of gravel. Normally urine flow is at its lowest during the night, and so water should be drunk before going to bed. All patients who have suffered from stones should drink sufficient to produce at least 2.5 litres of urine daily – the occasional measurement of urinary output is a useful reminder of this necessity. The fluid intake is especially important for those who live in the tropics or work in a hot environment, as urinary output is diminished by the amount of water lost in sweating.

Drugs

Bendrofluazide reduces urinary calcium by about 30%, by an unknown but probably renal tubular mechanism. Pyridoxine may be given to patients who form oxalate stones in the hope of diverting glycine metabolism towards serine and away from oxalate. Penicillamine given by mouth is useful in cystinuria, as it combines with cystine which is then excreted in a more soluble form. Patients who take drugs for long periods should be under medical supervision.

Diet

Particular emphasis should be directed at the calcium and oxalate content of the diet, as an excess of both these nutrients has been associated with the formation of stones (Tables 40.7 and 40.8). Since phytic acid present in cereal fibre binds calcium in the gut, a high-fibre diet should be encouraged to reduce calcium absorption.

Table 40.7   Foods rich in oxalate

Food	Oxalate (mg/100 g)
Beetroot	500
Chocolate	117
Rhubarb	600
Peanuts	187
Tea infusion	55–78 mg/100 ml

Table 40.8   Foods rich in calcium (>200 mg/100 g)

Food group	Foods rich in calcium
Dairy products	Dried skimmed milk, Cheddar cheese, yoghurt
Cereals	Muesli
Meat and fish	Pilchards, sardines

The avoidance of high purine-containing foods (coffee, sardines, anchovies, meat and fish), from the diet in those with a tendency to form uric acid stones was the usual mode of treatment in the past, but now the xanthine oxidase inhibitor allopurinol is used to prevent the formation of uric acid from purines. Its success has made severe dietary restriction of purine-rich foods unnecessary. A high fluid intake and measures to increase the pH of the urine are also recommended.

REFERENCES

Appel G 1991 Lipid abnormalities in renal disease. Kidney International 39: 169–183

Appel GB, Appel AS 1990 Lipid lowering agents in proteinuric disease. American Journal of Nephrology 10 (Suppl 1): 110–115

Ballmer PE, Weber BA, Roy–Chaudhury PB et al 1992 Elevation of albumin synthesis rates in nephrotic patients measured with [I^{13}C]leucine. Kidney International 41: 132–138

Berlyne GM, Mallick NP 1969 Ischaemic heart disease as a complication of nephrotic syndrome. Lancet ii: 399–400

Bommer J, Alexiou C, Muller–Buhl U, Eidfert J, Ritz E 1987 Recombinant human erythropoietin therapy in haemodialysis patients – dose determination and clinical experience. Nephrology Dialysis and Transplantation 2: 238–42

Bower J 1989 Cooking for restricted potassium diets in dietary treatment of renal patients. Journal of Human Nutrition and Dietetics 21: 31–38

Brenner BM, Meyer TW, Hostetter TH 1982 Dietary protein intake and the progressive nature of kidney disease. New England Journal of Medicine 307: 652–659

Brunner FP, Wing AJ, Dykes SR, Brynger HOA, Fassbinder W, Selwood NH 1989 International review of renal replacement therapy: strategy and results. In: Maher JF (ed) Replacement of renal function by dialysis. Kluwer, Dortrecht pp. 697–720

Cameron JS 1992 Clinical consequences of the nephrotic syndrome. In: Cameron JS, Davison AM, Grunfeld JP, Kerr D, Ritz E (eds) Oxford textbook of clinical nephrology. Oxford Textbook of Clinical Nephrology. Oxford University Press, Oxford, pp. 276–292

Catto GRD, Power DA (eds) 1988 Nephrology in clinical practice. Edward Arnold, London

Coburn JW, Salusky IB 1989 Control of serum phosphorus in uremia. New England Journal of Medicine 320: 1140–1142

Coe FL, Parks JH, Asplin JR 1992 The pathogenesis and treatment of kidney stones. New England Journal of Medicine 327: 1141–1152

D'Amico G, Gentile MG 1991 Pharmacological and dietary treatment of lipid abnormalities in nephrotic patients. Kidney International 39 (Suppl): 65–69

Department of Health 1991 Dietary reference values for food energy and nutrients for the United Kingdom. Report on Health and Social Subjects 41. HMSO, London

El Nahas AM, Coles GA 1986 Dietary treatment of chronic renal failure: ten unanswered questions. Lancet i: 597–600

El-Nahas AM, Masters-Thomas A, Brady SA et al 1984 Selective effect of low protein diets in chronic renal diseases. British Medical Journal 289: 1337–1341

Feest TG, Mistry CD, Grimes DS, Mallick NP 1990 Incidence of advanced chronic renal failure and the need for end-stage renal replacement therapy. British Medical Journal 301: 897–900

Forrest CE, Hartley GH 1991 Parenteral nutrition in acute renal failure. Journal of Human Nutrition and Dietetics 4: 361–367

Geerlings W, Tufveson F, Brunner FP et al 1991 Combined report on regular dialysis and transplantation in Europe, XXI, 1990. Nephrology Dialysis Transplantation 6 (Suppl 4): 5–29

Giovannetti S 1986 Answers to ten questions on the dietary treatment of chronic renal failure. Lancet ii: 1140–1142

Halstead SB 1981 Cause of bladder stones in England: a retrospective epidemiological study. In: Smith LH, Robertson WG, Finlayson PB (eds) Urolithiasis. Clinical and basic research. Plenum, London, pp. 325–328

James WPT, Ralph A, Sanchez-Castillo CP 1987 The dominance of salt in manufactured food in the sodium intake of affluent societies. Lancet i: 426–428

Joven J, Villabona C, Vilella E 1990 Abnormalities of lipoprotein metabolism in patients with the nephrotic syndrome. New England Journal of Medicine 323: 579–584

Kaysen GA, Davies RW, Hutchison FN 1989 Effect of dietary protein intake and angiotensin-converting enzyme inhibition in Heyman nephritis. Kidney International 36 (Suppl 27): 154–162

Khan IH, Catto GRD, Edward N, Fleming LW, Henderson IS, MacLeod AM 1993 Influence of co-existing disease on survival on renal-replacement therapy. Lancet 341: 415–418

Klahr S 1989 The modification of diet in renal disease study. New England Journal of Medicine 320: 864–866

Lee HA 1980 Nutritional support in renal and hepatic failure. In: Karran SJ, Alberti KGM (eds) Practical nutritional support. Pitman Medical, London, pp. 275–282

Locatelli F, Alberti D, Graziani G et al 1991 Prospective, randomized, multicentre trial of effect of protein restriction on progression of chronic renal insufficiency. Lancet 337: 1299–1304

Mitch WE 1991 Dietary protein restriction in patients with chronic renal failure. Kidney International 40: 326–341

Mitch WE, Walser M, Steinman TI, Hill S, Zeger S, Tungsanga K 1984 The effect of a ketoacid–amino acid supplement to a restricted diet on the progression of chronic renal failure. New England Journal of Medicine 311: 623–629

Neff MS, Kim KE, Persoff M, Oneseti G, Swartz C 1971 Hemodynamics of uremic anemia. Circulation 43: 876–883

Parker TF, Laird NM, Lowrie EG 1983 Comparison of the study groups in the National Cooperative Dialysis Study. A description of morbidity, mortality, and patient survival. Kidney International 23 (Suppl 13): s42–9

Sharman VL 1988 Hypercalciuria. In: Catto GRD (ed) New clinical applications in nephrology–calculus disease. Kluwer Academic, Lancaster, pp. 35–58

Thomas B 1988 Manual of dietetic practice. Blackwell, Oxford

United States Renal Data Report 1989 The National Institutes of Health, The National Institutes of Diabetes and Digestive and Kidney Diseases, Division of Kidney, Urologic and Hematologic Diseases, Bethesda, MD

Valyasevi A, Halstead SB, Dhanamita S 1967 Studies in bladder stone disease in Thailand. 6. Urinary studies in children, 2–10 years old, resident in a hypo- and hyperendemic area. American Journal of Clinical Nutrition 20: 1362–1368

Warwick GL, Caslake MJ, Boulton Jones JM, Dagen M, Packard CJ, Shepherd J 1990 Low-density lipoprotein metabolism in the nephrotic syndrome. Metabolism 39: 187–192

Wass VJ, Cameron JS 1981 Cardiovascular disease and the nephrotic syndrome. The other side of the coin. Nephron 27: 58–61

Winearls CG, Oliver DO, Pippard MJ, Reid C, Downing MR, Cotes PM 1986 Effect of human erythropoietin derived from recombinant DNA on the anaemia of patients maintained by chronic haemodialysis. Lancet ii: 1175–1178

Wolfson M, Jones MR, Kopple JD 1982 Amino acid losses during haemodialysis with infusion of amino acids and glucose. Kidney International 21: 500–506

Yamauchi A, Fujii M, Shirai D et al 1986 Plasma concentration and peritoneal clearance of oxalate in patients on continuous ambulatory peritoneal dialysis (CAPD). Clinical Nephrology 25: 181–185

41. Diseases of the heart and circulation: the role of dietary factors in aetiology and management

J. Mann

Diseases of the circulatory system account for an appreciable proportion of total morbidity and mortality in adults throughout the world. The different conditions assume varying degrees of importance in developing and affluent countries. For example, in developing countries rheumatic heart disease is common, but new cases of this disease are relatively infrequent in most affluent societies, where coronary heart disease (CHD) has assumed epidemic proportions. This chapter describes those diseases of the heart and circulation in which nutritional factors play an important role in aetiology and management.

CORONARY HEART DISEASE

The basic pathological lesion underlying CHD is the atheromatous plaque, which occludes one or more of the coronary arteries to a varying extent. In addition, a superimposed thrombus or clot may further occlude the artery. A variety of cells and lipids are involved in the pathogenesis of the atherosclerotic plaque and the arterial thrombus, including lipoproteins, cholesterol, triglycerides, platelets, monocytes, endothelial cells, fibroblasts and smooth-muscle cells. Nutrition may influence the development of CHD by modifying one or more of these factors. Two major clinical conditions are associated with these processes: angina pectoris is characterized by pain or discomfort in the chest which is brought on by exertion or stress, and which may also radiate down the left arm and to the neck. It results from a reduction or temporary block to the blood flow through the coronary artery to the myocardium. The pain usually passes with rest and seldom lasts for more than 15 minutes. A coronary thrombosis or myocardial infarction results from prolonged total occlusion of the artery, which causes infarction or death of some of the heart muscle and is associated with prolonged and usually excruciating central chest pain. The terms coronary thrombosis and myocardial infarction are used to describe the

same clinical condition, although they really describe two pathological processes. A detailed description of the pathology and clinical features may be found in any textbook of medicine (Weatherall et al 1987).

Epidemiology

In most industrialized countries CHD is the commonest single cause of death. In England and Wales about 27% of all deaths are the result of CHD. In recent years, in addition to the approximately 180 000 deaths every year in England and Wales, there have been on average 115 000 hospital discharges. This is still an appreciable underestimate of the total morbidity resulting from CHD. Many cases of myocardial infarction, especially in older people, are not admitted to hospital and there are no statistics regarding the far greater number of people who are debilitated by angina pectoris even though they may not have suffered an acute myocardial infarction. It should be noted that in 60% of all fatal myocardial infarctions, death occurs in the first hour after the attack. Most CHD deaths, therefore, occur too rapidly for treatment to influence the prognosis. In Britain roughly £500 m per annum is spent on patients suffering from CHD, which accounts for 10% of all working days lost due to illness, and sickness benefits amount to more than £250 m (Elkan et al 1988).

There are marked international differences in the rate of occurrence of CHD. For example, in one study among men aged 40–59 initially free of CHD, the annual incidence rate (occurrence of new cases) varied from 15 per 100 000 in Japan to 198 per 100 000 in Finland (Keys 1980). Table 41.1 shows that even among industrialized countries, mortality rates also vary considerably. Some of the variation between countries is undoubtedly due to differences in diagnostic practice and coding of death certificates, but numerous studies using comparable methods have confirmed that real differences do exist in the

Table 41.1 Age-standardized mortality from coronary heart disease in 1985 in selected countries, based on the population of Europe (Rates per 100 000 aged 30–69 years)

Country	Males	Females	Country
N Ireland	406	142	Scotland
Scotland	398	130	N Ireland
Finland	390	125	USSR
USSR	349	105	Hungary
Czechoslovakia	346	104	Ireland
Ireland	339	101	Czechoslovakia
Hungary	326	94	New Zealand
England and Wales	318	94	England and Wales
New Zealand	296	80	USA
Norway	266	79	Finland
Australia	247	76	Australia
Sweden	243	56	Sweden
USA	235	55	Norway
Canada	230	54	Poland
Federal Republic of Germany	204	52	Federal Republic of Germany
Switzerland	140	33	Italy
Italy	136	30	Switzerland
Spain	104	24	Spain
France	94	20	France
Japan	38	13	Japan

frequency of the disease. In Europe there is an approximately fourfold difference between France, Italy and Spain on the one hand and such countries as Finland, Scotland and Northern Ireland on the other (Uemura & Pisa 1988).

These international comparisons have played an important part in the search for causes. The experience of migrants suggests that these variations between countries are likely to be the result chiefly of environmental and behavioural differences. People who have migrated from a low-risk country (e.g. Japan) to a high-risk country (e.g. the USA) tend to have rates of CHD approaching that of the host country. There is also some evidence for the reverse: Finns living in Sweden have appreciably lower rates than those in their country of origin. In the UK, where CHD rates are appreciably higher in Scotland and Northern Ireland than in England, CHD risk depends upon country of residence at the time of death rather than country of birth (Stamler 1979).

There have been major changes in the CHD rates of many countries (Table 41.2). Among men these include the increase in many European countries, Australia and New Zealand during the period 1952–1967, and the continuing increase in eastern Europe during the later period (1970–1985), whereas in nearly all western European countries, North

Table 41.2 Percentage change in age-standardized death rates from coronary heart disease in selected countries (ages 30–69 years)

Country	Males 1952–1967 %	Males 1970–1985 %	Females 1952–1967 %	Females 1970–1985 %
N America				
Canada	+7	−41	−12	−43
USA	+4	−49	−9	−48
Eastern Europe				
Czechoslovakia	+10	+10	−41	+2
Hungary	+64	+39	+17	+15
Poland	–	+72	–	+59
Western & northern Europe				
France	+60	−9	+21	−29
Switzerland	+6	−11	−37	−20
Finland	+24	−23	−8	−31
Norway	+99	−14	+27	−23
England & Wales	+24	−11	−6	−2
N Ireland	+24	−9	−9	−16
Scotland	+17	−11	−11	−5
Oceania				
Australia	+19	−46	+9	−51
New Zealand	+39	−32	+15	−30

American and Oceania rates have shown an appreciable decline. In most countries except for eastern Europe the rates in women have been declining. In general the decline has been most marked in countries where the attempt to reduce cardiovascular risk factors has been most effective. This change over a relatively short period of time encourages the belief that the disease is preventable if the causes can be found and modified. The hope is to reduce morbidity and mortality from CHD in those who are in the prime of life. The data which relate dietary factors directly to CHD are relatively sparse, and will be considered here. There is much indirect evidence for the relationship between diet and CHD and this will be considered in the section describing risk factors.

CORRELATIONS BETWEEN CHD RATES AND FOOD INTAKE

Most of the early attempts to study dietary determinants of CHD rates were based on national food consumption data, the balance sheets of the Food and Agriculture Organization, (or, in the UK, more reliably on household food surveys) and on the national mortality statistics before 1970, during which time CHD was increasing (at least in men) in most affluent societies. The studies have either been cross-cultural comparisons at a single point in time, or an examination of increasing trends in relation to changing food consumption data in one or more countries. Positive associations with saturated fat, sucrose, animal protein and coffee, and negative correlations with flour (and other complex carbohydrates) and vegetables are some of the best described. However, population food consumption data are notoriously unreliable (they are usually derived from local production figures, imports and exports, often with an incomplete account of quantities not utilized as food), and the accuracy with which mortality is recorded varies from country to country. Consequently, such data do not provide direct evidence concerning aetiology, only clues for further research (Armstrong et al 1975).

Perhaps more interesting are recent studies from the USA, the UK, Australia, New Zealand and Iceland, which have examined the downward trend of CHD rates in relation to dietary change. There are certainly associations between falling CHD rates apparent in these countries and changes in some foods and nutrients, but in view of the strong correlations (positive and negative) among different dietary constituents it is difficult to be sure which dietary factor is principally involved, or indeed whether dietary change is simply occurring in parallel with some other more important environmental factor (e.g. increasing physical activity and reduction in cigarette smoking) (Sytkowski et al 1990, Dwyer & Hetzel 1980, Beaglehole et al 1981, Sigfusson et al 1991).

PROSPECTIVE OBSERVATION OF SUBJECTS FOR WHOM DIET HISTORIES ARE AVAILABLE

Measured food consumption by people in 16 defined cohorts in seven countries, and 10-year incidence rates of CHD deaths, form the rather more reliable basis for the correlations tested by Keys and co-workers (The Seven Country Study) (Keys 1980, Keys et al 1986). The strongest correlation was noted between CHD and the percentage of energy derived from saturated fat (Fig. 41.1). Weaker inverse associations were found between percentages of energy derived from mono-unsaturated and polyunsaturated fat and CHD. Total fat was not significantly correlated with CHD death. Of the other well known risk factors for CHD investigated in this study (see below), only cholesterol and blood pressure appeared to explain the geographical variation, leading to the suggestion that it is principally the nutrition-related factors which determine whether countries are likely to have high CHD rates. This study also provides evidence that the degree of risk conferred by factors not specifically related to nutrition is strongly influenced by nutrition-related factors. This is well illustrated by the more powerful relationship between cigarette smoking and CHD in the USA and Europe, where saturated fat intake and mean cholesterol levels are higher in the north than in southern Europe (Fig. 41.2).

Relatively few studies have been able to show a relationship between the dietary intake of individuals within a country and subsequent risk of CHD. In one, male bank staff, bus drivers and bus conductors in London completed at least one 7-day weighed dietary record. Those with a high intake of dietary fibre from cereals had a lower rate of CHD subsequently than the rest. A high energy intake (apparently reflecting physical activity) and, to a lesser extent, a high ratio of polyunsaturated to saturated fatty acids in the diet were also features of men who subsequently remained free of CHD (Morris et al 1977). In another prospective investigation – employees of the Western Electric Company in Chicago – the most striking finding was an inverse association between CHD mortality and the consumption of polyunsaturated fatty acids. A positive association was also noted between CHD

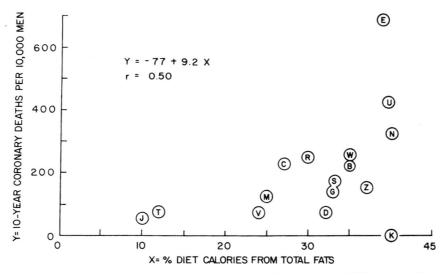

Fig. 41.1 Data from the original Seven Country Study showing the association between CHD and the dietary saturated fat content. (B=Belgrade, C=Crevalcore, D=Dalmatia, E=East Finland, G=Corfu, J=Ushibuka, K=Crete, M=Montegiorgio, N=Zutphen, R=Rome, S=Slavonia, T=Tanushimaru, U=USA, V=Velika Kisna, W=West Finland, A=Zregnjamin).

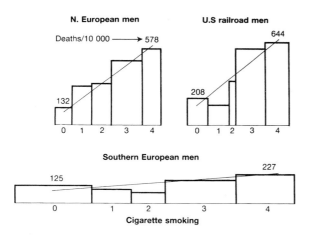

Fig. 41.2 The different risks of smoking for CHD in countries with different diets. The width of the bars is proportional to the number of men in each smoking class. Scales are the same for all three populations. The numbers above each bar indicate the number of CHD deaths per 10 000. The regression lines of death rate on smoking, are shown.
0 = never smoked, 1 = ex-smoker, 2 = 2–10 cigarettes per day, 3 = 10–19 cigarettes per day, 4 = >20 cigarettes per day.

mortality and dietary cholesterol and with the Keys score (see Chapter 41). No association was found between CHD and saturated fat intake considered in isolation (Shekelle et al 1981). In the Dutch cohort of the Seven Country Study a relationship was observed between fish intake and CHD (Kromhout et al 1985). In these studies dietary assessment was carried out very carefully; failure to find similar associations in other prospective studies could be due to insensitivity of their dietary survey techniques. It should also be emphasized that in these studies a single point estimate of dietary intake is assumed to be characteristic of the individual, and is being related to CHD occurrence many years later.

Prospective studies of Seventh Day Adventists and people shopping in health food stores suggest an appreciable reduction of CHD risk in vegetarians, when taking into account possible confounding factors such as cigarette smoking, but in these studies it is not possible to determine which aspects of the vegetarian diet might be protective, or indeed whether the protective effect is explained by some associated but unstudied factor (Phillips et al 1980, Burr & Butland 1988).

Low levels of long-chain polyunsaturated fatty acids of both the *n*-3 and the *n*-6 series in the blood and adipose tissue are associated with an increased risk of subsequent CHD (Miettinen et al 1982, Riemersma et al 1986). The composition of tissue lipid reflects the type of fat eaten and such studies provide reinforcement for the importance of the nature on dietary fat in the aetiology of CHD. However, dietary fat can

Table 41.3 Risk factors for coronary heart disease

Irreversible

Masculine gender
Increasing age
Genetic traits, including monogenic and polygenic disorders
  of lipid metabolism
Body build

Potentially reversible

Cigarette smoking
Hyperlipidaemia: increased levels of cholesterol and
  triglyceride
Low levels of high-density lipoprotein (HDL)
Obesity
Hypertension
Physical inactivity
Hyperglycaemia and diabetes
Increased thrombosis: increased haemostatic factors and
  enhanced platelet aggregation

Psychosocial

Low socioeconomic class
Stressful situations
Coronary-prone behaviour patterns: type A behaviour

Geographic

Climate and season: cold weather
Soft drinking water

clearly not be the only epidemiological determinant and recent reviews have focused on the potential important protective effects of antioxidants and certain trace elements. Fruit and vegetables are major sources of these essential micronutrients, and high intakes characterize populations (e.g. those living in the Mediterranean countries) and subgroups within populations (e.g. those of high socioeconomic status) which have low CHD rates (Duthie et al 1989). Even sophisticated epidemiological studies cannot fully explain the relationships between foods, nutrients and CHD, and further information comes from the study of nutritional determinants of cardiovascular risk factors.

CARDIOVASCULAR RISK FACTORS AND THEIR NUTRITIONAL DETERMINANTS

Attempts to explain the pathological process underlying CHD and to identify individuals at risk suggest that there is no single cause of the disease. An understanding of the characteristics which put individuals at particular risk of developing CHD provides a useful background against which to examine in more detail the role of diet in the aetiology. The term 'risk factor' tends to be used rather loosely to describe features of lifestyle and behaviour, as well as physical and chemical attributes which predict the likelihood of developing CHD. Potential risk factors are often identified when comparisons are made of people who have developed CHD with healthy controls (case-control studies) and confirmed by cohort studies in which these factors are measured in a large group of apparently healthy people who are followed prospectively; the presence, absence or degree of each factor can then be related to the risk of developing CHD. Table 41.3 lists most of the important risk factors for CHD which have been identified in this way. The irreversible psychosocial and geographic factors, as well as cigarette smoking and physical activity, are reviewed in textbooks of medicine and epidemiology (Weatherall et al 1987). This review deals principally with potentially reversible factors which have been shown to be influenced by dietary factors and which are not discussed in other chapters.

Hyperlipidaemia

Raised levels of blood lipids found in lipoproteins (cholesterol and triglyceride) may place individuals at increased risk of CHD in two ways. A relatively small proportion of people have an exceptionally high risk because of a clearly inherited disorder of lipid metabolism. A large number of people (probably around half the adult population in high-risk countries) have a slight to moderately increased risk because their blood lipids are higher than desirable. This probably results from an interaction between polygenic and environmental (largely dietary) factors.

Hypercholesterolaemia in the population at large

No other blood constituent varies so much between different people as cholesterol. From New Guinea to east Finland, the mean serum cholesterol ranges from 2.6 to 7.0 mmol/l (100–270 mg/100 ml) when estimated by the same method in the same age and sex group (Truswell & Mann 1972). Of the known risk factors for CHD, total serum cholesterol appears to be the most important determinant of the geographic variation in the distribution of the disease. In the Seven Country Study, median cholesterol values were highly correlated with CHD death (r=0.8, Fig. 41.3), accounting for 64% of the variance in the CHD death rates among the cohorts (Keys 1980). Among individuals within a population the association is equally strong: in over 20 prospective studies in different countries, total plasma cholesterol has been shown to be related to the rate of development of

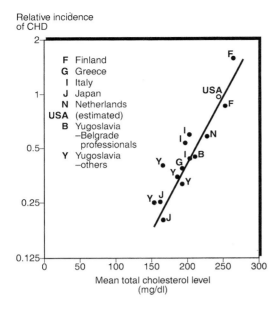

Relative incidence of CHD

F Finland
G Greece
I Italy
J Japan
N Netherlands
USA (estimated)
B Yugoslavia
  –Belgrade
  professionals
Y Yugoslavia
  –others

Mean total cholesterol level (mg/dl)

Fig. 41.3 Serum cholesterol level and incidence of new coronary heart disease in different populations and subgroups. Calculated from Keys (1980), adapted by P Peto, and redrawn with permission.

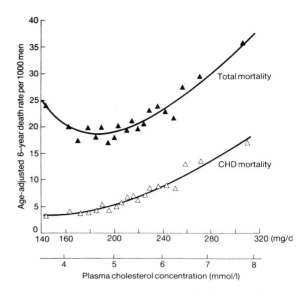

Fig. 41.4 Within-population relationship between plasma cholesterol and coronary heart disease and total mortality – MRFIT Study (Martin et al 1986).

CHD, the association being 'dose'-related, occurring in both sexes and being independent of all other measured risk factors. The association between cholesterol and CHD and total mortality in the largest prospective study carried out thus far is shown in Fig. 41.4. The risk of CHD varies over an approximately fivefold range in relation to the plasma cholesterol levels found in an average American population (Martin et al 1986). There is no discernible critical value: the risk tends to increase throughout the range. Although the absolute risk associated with any given cholesterol level varies in different parts of the world, within almost every population sampled the risk is greater in people with higher than with lower values. The association of total cholesterol with CHD mortality appears to derive chiefly if not entirely from the low-density lipoprotein (LDL) fraction, with which it is highly correlated. Oxidized LDL can be taken up by macrophages and deposited in the atheromatous plaque. Inhibition of oxidation, resulting from adequate dietary intakes of antioxidants, vitamins C and E and carotenoids, may protect LDL cholesterol against oxidation and help to slow the progression of the atherosclerotic lesions (Duthie et al 1989, Parthasarathy et al 1990). In research, as well as in clinical practice, confusion may arise if cholesterol is measured soon after a myocardial infarction, since levels tend to fall and readings may be falsely low for up to 3 months after this acute event.

Low levels of total or LDL cholesterol appear to be associated with an increased risk of non-cardiovascular death – chiefly cancer – but studies in a number of populations indicate that this inverse association is confined to deaths in the very early years of follow-up. A low cholesterol may thus be a metabolic consequence of cancer, present but unsuspected at the time of the initial examination (Broitman 1988). In addition, most of the studies were small, so that the findings were shown only for lung cancer, the commonest cancer which is primarily related to cigarette smoking, with inconsistent associations in the few patients who developed colon and breast cancer (Isles et al 1989). In the largest studies, of more than 92 000 people in Sweden and California, cholesterol was either positively but weakly, or not at all, related to large-bowel cancer risk (Tornberg et al 1986, Klatsky et al 1988).

Limited data from the USA, Finland and Iceland concerning changes in population cholesterol levels suggest a decrease in parallel with the decline in CHD mortality rates in those countries. In Britain there appears to have been little change (Sytkowski et al 1990, Dwyer & Hetzel 1980, Beaglehole et al 1981, Sigfusson et al 1991).

Mean cholesterol levels tend to be similar in adult men and women, but this similarity hides the strikingly different age trends observed in cross-sectional studies (Fig. 41.5). Hormonal factors have been implicated, but there is neither a single convincing explanation for these sex differences nor is it clear to what extent they account for the differences in CHD rates in men and women (Mann et al 1988).

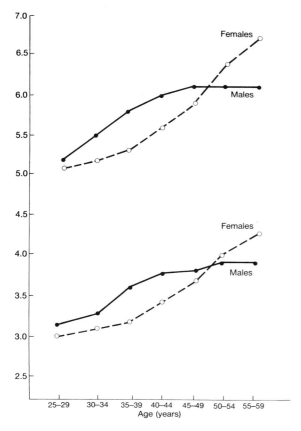

Fig. 41.5 Relationship between total and LDL cholesterol, gender and age. Upper panel: total cholesterol (mmol/l). Lower panel: LDL cholesterol (mmol/l).

Diet and cholesterol levels

Although there is no doubt that polygenic factors play an important role in the metabolism of cholesterol, levels of total and LDL cholesterol may also be profoundly influenced by a number of dietary factors. In healthy individuals, and in most types of hyperlipidaemia, a very high proportion of total cholesterol

occurs in LDL. Dietary factors which determine total cholesterol are in fact principally doing so via an effect on LDL. Overweight and obesity are strikingly related to total and LDL cholesterol: there is graded increase in cholesterol with increasing body mass index. In the Seven Country Study, mean concentrations of cholesterol of each group were highly correlated with percentage of energy derived from saturated fatty acids, and even more strikingly related to a formula which also took into account the intake of polyunsaturated fatty acids (Fig. 41.6) (Keys 1980). In the 1950s and 1960s many experiments were carried out to determine the effects of different dietary fats on plasma lipids of individuals. These careful feeding studies confirmed that plasma cholesterol was raised by saturated fatty acids (SFA) and lowered by polyunsaturated fatty acids (PUFA). Various formulae were developed to calculate the change in cholesterol which might be expected from changing the proportions of saturated and polyunsaturated fatty acids in the diet. The simplest and best known is that developed by Keys and colleagues, which suggests that saturated fatty acids raise plasma cholesterol twice as much as polyunsaturated ones lower it (Keys et al 1977). The Keys formula may be simplified as follows:

$$\Delta \text{ plasma cholesterol in mmol/l} = 0.035 \ (2\Delta S - \Delta P)$$

where ΔS and ΔP represent the changes in percentages of dietary energy derived from saturated and polyunsaturated fatty acids. In practice, the formula provides only a rough prediction of the changes that occur. This may be because genetic factors may, at least in part, explain variations in response, because free-living human beings participating in a trial may not always fully comply with dietary instructions and because the effects of saturated fatty acids with different chain lengths and of the various unsaturated fatty acids are not identical.

Early experiments suggested that palmitic acid (C16:0), myristic acid (C14:0) and lauric acid (C12:0) raised plasma cholesterol more than those with either shorter or longer chains (Horlick 1959, Hegsted et al 1965, Keys et al 1965a). Bonanome and Grundy have recently re-established that stearic acid (C18:0) consumption is associated with lower levels of total and LDL cholesterol than those found on similar intakes of palmitic acid (C16:0). Indeed, the cholesterol-lowering effect was similar to that seen on oleic acid (Bonanome & Grundy 1988). This observation was based on formula-feeding studies and the practical application is discussed below.

The effects of unsaturated fatty acids on total and LDL cholesterol are also rather more complex than

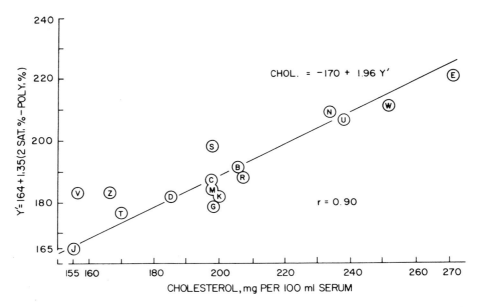

Fig. 41.6 Relationship of mean serum cholesterol concentration of the cohorts in the Seven Country Study to fat composition of the diet expressed in the multiple regression equation, including intake of saturated and polyunsaturated fatty acids. Cohorts as in Fig. 41.1.

were suggested by the early experiments. Monounsa-turated fatty acids (MUFA – the experiments have involved principally oleic acid, C18:1) appear to have the ability to lower cholesterol to roughly the same extent as the *n*-6 polyunsaturated fatty acids from plant sources (predominantly linoleic acid, C18:2) (Shepherd et al 1978, Mattson & Grundy 1985, Grundy 1986). The *n*-3 polyunsaturated fatty acids predominating in marine oils (eicosapentaenoic acid, C20:5 and docosahexaenoic acid, C22:6) have a variable effect on the LDL cholesterol of healthy individuals. Large quantities reduce LDL as a result of a reduction in very low-density lipoprotein (VLDL), which in turn may be due to a reduction in the rate of synthesis of apolipoprotein B (Lancet Editorial 1988).

Most unsaturated fatty acids exist naturally with the double bonds in the *cis* form, but a small proportion of the fatty acids in meat and dairy products exist in the *trans* form and sometimes *cis* unsaturated fatty acids shift to the *trans* form during processing. The shift to *trans* configuration makes an oil more solid by raising the melting point. *Trans* fatty acids appear mostly as monounsaturated fatty acids. It appears that *trans* isomers of oleic acid (the main *trans* fatty acids of manufactured food such as margarine) raise LDL to the same extent as saturated fatty acids (Mensink & Katan 1990).

The ratio of polyunsaturated to saturated fatty acids (P/S) was widely used to indicate the cholesterol-lowering potential of the diet. Low P/S ratios (around 0.2) are generally associated with high cholesterol levels and a high population risk of CHD. Higher ratios (around 0.8) are found in Mediterranean countries and are believed to be associated with more favourable levels of cholesterol and reduced CHD risk. However, in the light of the recent data summarized above it seems that the P/S ratio may be an unacceptable oversimplification. Ulbricht and Southgate have suggested that this ratio should be replaced by an index of atherogenicity (IA) (Ulbricht & Southgate 1991). Their proposed index involves an inversion of the P/S ratio, so that the IA would be highest for the most atherogenic dietary components. The lower-chain-length saturated fatty acids and stearic acid are omitted from S, and P is considered to include monounsaturated fatty acids, so that their proposed ratio becomes:

$$\frac{aS' + bS'' + cS'''}{dP + eM + fM'}$$

where S' = C12:0, S'' = C14:0 and S''' = C16.0; P = sum of *n*-6 and *n*-3 PUFA, M = oleic acid (C18:1) and M' = sum of other MUFA. a–f are empirical constants, with b set at 4 because C14:0 appears to have the most

Table 41.4 Indices of atherogenicity and thrombogenicity for some foods and diets

	Index of atherogenicity (IA)	Index of thrombogenicity (IT)
Coconut oil	13.63	6.18
Milk, butter, cheese	2.03	2.07
Palm oil	0.88	1.74
Lamb:		
roast breast, lean and fat	1.00	1.58
chop, lean only	1.00	1.33
Beef:		
topside roast, lean	0.72	1.06
raw mince	0.72	1.27
grilled sausages	0.74	1.39
Pork:		
roast leg, lean	0.60	1.37
grilled sausages	0.58	1.35
fried streaky bacon, lean and fat	0.69	1.66
Hard margarine (vegetable oils only)	0.56	1.26
Stewed ox liver	0.41	0.82
Chicken, roast, meat and skin	0.50	0.95
PUFA margarine	0.35	0.53
Olive oil	0.14	0.32
Sunflower oil	0.07	0.28
Raw mackerel	0.28	0.16
Eskimo diet	0.39	0.28
Danish diet	1.29	1.51
British diet	0.93	1.21

powerful effect in elevating LDL, and a, c, d, e, and f set at unity in the absence of firm evidence to assign other values. Indices of atherogenicity for some foods and diets are shown in Table 41.4. This is an interesting proposal but does not take into account the effects of *trans* monounsaturated fatty acids, nor the facts that *n*-3 and *n*-6 fatty acids do not have comparable effects on LDL. Furthermore, a detailed breakdown of the fat composition of foods is not routinely available in the food composition tables of many countries. Until further consideration has been given to this concept it may be helpful to discontinue use of the P/S ratio and to offer recommendations in terms of the reference values given in Table 41.10.

The effects of various dietary fatty acids on cholesterol levels are summarized in Table 41.5. Plasma and total LDL cholesterols will also fall if the percentage of dietary energy provided by all fats is reduced. It is not clear whether this is entirely accounted for by a reduction in the saturated fatty acid intake.

More controversy surrounds the importance of dietary cholesterol as a determinant of plasma cholesterol. There is no doubt that contrasting extreme cholesterol intakes (e.g. 800 mg and 100 mg/day) in the context of a diet relatively high in saturated fatty acids can produce an appreciable effect on plasma cholesterols, and the Keys formula has been modified to include changes in dietary cholesterol:

$$\Delta \text{cholesterol in mmol/l} = 0.035\,(2\Delta S - \Delta P) + 0.08\Delta \sqrt{\text{chol/MJ}}, \text{ where chol/MJ is the cholesterol intake in mg/MJ}$$

It has also been suggested that some individuals are consistent 'hyperresponders' to dietary cholesterol, i.e. they show an exaggerated increase in plasma cholesterol when dietary cholesterol is increased, whereas others ('hyporesponders') show little or no response. Very high intakes of dietary cholesterol have been shown to down-regulate LDL receptors which are necessary for LDL to be internalized and broken down in cells. All this implies that dietary cholesterol has an important influence on levels in the blood. However, the great majority of the experiments upon which the above conclusions are based have involved extreme contrasts rather than comparisons within the usual range of intakes, when increased intake may be more readily balanced by inhibited endogenous production. There is less evidence that a 'dose'–response gradient occurs over the usual range of intakes seen in relatively affluent societies (200–500 mg cholesterol per day). Furthermore, recent studies have shown that when saturated fatty acid intake is reduced, the effects of dietary cholesterol on plasma cholesterol are minimal and there is little evidence for the phenomenon of hyperresponse. Thus, provided average intakes (around 300 mg) are not exceeded it appears that dietary cholesterol is much less important than dietary fat in determining total plasma and LDL cholesterol (Keys et al 1965b, Edington et al 1987, 1989).

Carbohydrates per se have little direct effect on total and LDL cholesterol levels, although increasing carbohydrate enables a reduction of saturated fatty acids which in turn will be associated with a reduction in this lipoprotein fraction. It has been suggested that soluble dietary fibre (non-starch polysaccharide) results in a reduction in total and LDL cholesterol. Much early research involved the use of guar gum, but recent attention has centred around oat bran and dried beans (Jenkins et al 1986, Anderson et al 1990). However, there is no evidence that these foods have any particular merits over other foods high in soluble fibre (barley and rye products, lentils, chickpeas, and

Table 41.5 Dietary determinants of plasma lipids

'Unfavourable' or 'possibly unfavourable' effects	
Saturated fatty acids SFA (especially C12:0, C14:0, C16:0)	↑↑↑LDL cholesterol
Trans monounsaturated fatty acids, MUFA	↑↑LDL cholesterol, ↓ HDL cholesterol
Dietary cholesterol	↑LDL cholesterol when fed in large amounts with high SFA intake
*Fibre-depleted complex carbohydrates	↑VLDL and triglyceride, ↓ HDL if carbohydrate comprises 60% or more total energy
*Sucrose	↑VLDL and triglycerides if taken in large amounts (>140 g/day) and with high SFA
'Beneficial' effects	
Cis monounsaturated fatty acids MUFA (C18:1)	↓↓ LDL cholesterol
Soluble dietary fibre	↓ LDL cholesterol
'Beneficial ' as well as 'possibly unfavourable' effects	
n-6 polyunsaturated fatty acids (C18:2)	↓↓ LDL cholesterol, ↓ HDL if taken in large amounts
n-3 polyunsaturated fatty acids (C20:5, C22:6)	↓↓ VLDL ↑LDL especially in hyperlipidaemia

* effect probably transient

↓↓↓ or ↑↑↑ appreciable change
↓↓ or ↑↑ modest change
↓ or ↑ some change

fruits high in pectin). The results of the studies have not been entirely consistent: some have shown no effect of feeding foods high in soluble fibre. A number of factors may account for the apparently conflicting results. It seems that very high intakes of soluble fibre may be required to produce an effect on LDL cholesterol. It may be that soluble fibre only exerts its effect when the fat composition of the diet has also been changed. The soluble fibre component of apparently similar foods can vary appreciably. Some researchers have even suggested that soluble fibre may exert its effects by enhancing satiety and reducing the intake of saturated fatty acids and possibly other energy-dense nutrients (Swain et al 1990). However, on balance it does seem as if, at least under certain circumstances, soluble fibre does have an effect on total and LDL cholesterol, but it is important to emphasize that the effect is almost certainly less than that of dietary fat. There is evidence, at least in normal subjects, that the effects of fibre and fat modification are additive (Leadbetter et al 1991). The mechanism of LDL lowering has not been established, but soluble fibre may act like the lipid-lowering drug cholestyramine, and promote sterol excretion as well as LDL-receptor mediated removal. Insoluble fibre does not influence lipid metabolism to any appreciable extent (Judd & Truswell 1985).

The effects of dietary protein on lipids and lipoproteins have been less well studied. In one set of studies complete replacement of mixed animal proteins by a soybean protein preparation led to a large fall in plasma cholesterol in normal and hypercholesterolaemic subjects (Descovich et al 1980). Other experiments have shown smaller effects on LDL cholesterol (van Raaij et al 1982), so that widespread recommendations concerning the use of vegetable proteins to reduce LDL cholesterol is not justified.

Despite the ability to profoundly influence total and LDL cholesterol by the dietary manipulations described here, and the correlations between dietary variables and cholesterol in cross-cultural comparisons, it has not usually been possible to show a relationship between reported intake of macronutrients and dietary fibre and plasma cholesterol level within a population. This has usually been ascribed to the crude methods available for assessing dietary intake, and to the fact that within the relatively narrow range of dietary intakes seen in affluent societies, polygenic determinants of lipid metabolism are more important than dietary factors. Vegetarians and vegans have, as groups, been shown to have lower total and LDL cholesterols than non-vegetarians (Thorogood et al 1987). In addition, a recent study of vegetarians, vegans, fish eaters (who do not eat meat) and omnivores in Britain has enabled lipid levels to be examined over a wide range of intakes within a single population, and revealed an association between total and LDL cholesterol and intakes of saturated fatty acids and cholesterol, and an inverse association between these lipid measurements and polyunsaturated fatty acids and dietary fibre (Thorogood et al 1990).

Hypertriglyceridaemia

People who have had myocardial infarctions tend to have higher levels of triglycerides and very low-density lipoprotein (VLDL) than controls. Prospective studies have confirmed this increased risk, but there has been considerable controversy as to whether it is independent of other factors known to be associated with both raised levels of triglycerides and cardiovascular risk (e.g. obesity, hyperglycaemia, hypercholesterolaemia, hypertension). A recent analysis of data from the large Framingham prospective study suggests that raised levels of triglycerides are associated with increased CHD risk only in the presence of reduced HDL cholesterol, i.e. <1 mmol/l (Fig. 41.7) (Castelli 1986). Raised levels of triglyceride appear to be particularly important in determining cardiovascular risk in people with diabetes (West et al 1983). Triglyceride levels show less cross-cultural variation than cholesterol levels but similar trends for age and sex, though at all ages men have higher levels than women (Fig. 41.8). Increased physical activity is associated with a reduction in triglyceride levels.

Diet and triglycerides

The most important dietary factors influencing triglyceride levels are obesity and intake of alcohol. While alcohol-associated hypertriglyceridaemia is usually associated with very high intakes, susceptible individuals may develop appreciably raised triglyceride levels even with modest intakes. An excessive intake of alcohol is one of the commonest causes of hypertri-

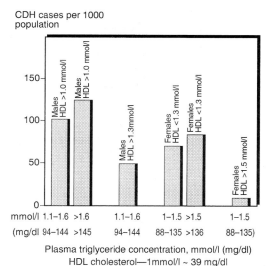

Fig. 41.7 Plasma triglyceride concentration, HDL and CHD.

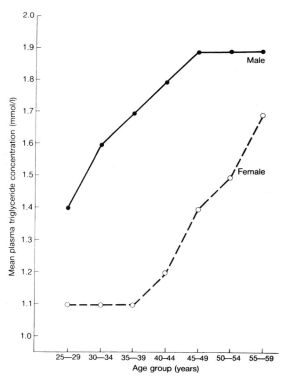

NOTE: S.D. varies between 0.6 and 1.5

Fig. 41.8 Fasting plasma triglyceride concentration according to age and gender. (Data from Mann et al 1988.)

Table 41.6 'Genetic–metabolic' classification of hyperlipidaemia. The WHO (Fredrickson) type is also indicated ($\uparrow$ = raised; $\uparrow\uparrow$ = markedly raised; N = normal; + = uncommon; ++++ = extremely common)

	Atherosclerosis risk	Xanthomas	Inheritance	Relative prevalence	Lipid abnormalities	WHO type
Familial hypercholest-erolaemia	+++	Tendon	Autosomal dominant	++	Cholesterol & LDL$\uparrow\uparrow$ triglyceride N or slightly$\uparrow$	IIa occasionally IIb
Familial combined hyperlipid-aemia	++	-	Uncertain	+++	Cholesterol & LDL$\uparrow$ Triglyceride & VLDL$\uparrow$	IIb occasionally IIa and IV
Remnant hyperlipopro-teinaemia	++	Tuboeruptive and palmar	Apo EIII deficiency and other factors	+	Cholesterol $\uparrow\uparrow$ Triglyceride $\uparrow\uparrow$ Intermediate density lipoprotein $\uparrow$	III
Familial hypertrigly-ceridaemia Excessive synthesis	Uncertain	Eruptive	Probably auto-somal dominant	+	Triglyceride & VLDL $\uparrow\uparrow$ Chylomicrons $\uparrow$	IV
Lipoprotein lipase/apo CII deficiency	Uncertain	Eruptive	Probably recessive	Rare	Triglyceride $\uparrow\uparrow$ Chylomicrons $\uparrow\uparrow$ VLDL $\uparrow$	IV, V
Common hypercholest-erolaemia	+	-	Polygenic	++++	Cholesterol and LDL $\uparrow$	IIa

Adapted from Lewis (1987)

glyceridaemia in patients referred to a lipid clinic. Alcohol results in hypertriglyceridaemia by providing an increased energy intake, and also by stimulating hepatic synthesis (Banaona & Lieber 1975).

Fasting triglycerides increase when either starch or sugar is added to an experimental diet (probably largely associated with the increased energy intake), when an appreciable proportion of usual fat intake is isoenergetically replaced by fibre-depleted carbohydrate, or when sucrose or fructose are given in substantial quantities to replace energy previously provided by complex carbohydrates. The mechanism in each of these situations is thought to be increased hepatic synthesis. The hypertriglyceridaemic effect of sucrose is only seen when substantial quantities (around 140 g or greater) are consumed, and when a relatively high proportion of dietary fat is derived from saturated fatty acids. There is some evidence to suggest that adaptation may occur and that the effect of these manipulations of dietary carbohydrate may not persist much longer than 6 weeks (Department of

Health 1989). Eicosapentaenoic and docosahexaenoic acids can produce appreciable reductions in triglyceride levels (Editorial 1988).

Inherited disorders of lipid metabolism

There are a number of genetically determined clearly defined disorders of lipid metabolism, characterized by raised levels of cholesterol and/or triglyceride, which must be distinguished from the polygenic form of hyperlipidaemia described above and sometimes referred to as 'common hypercholesterolaemia'. The characteristics of the most important of the inherited disorders are described in Table 41.6 and in more detail elsewhere (Lewis 1987). *Familial hypercholesterolaemia* is the most clearly described. The condition is characterized by marked elevation of total and LDL cholesterol, resulting from a reduction in LDL receptors on the surfaces of cells, autosomal dominant inheritance, often cholesterol-filled xanthomas in extensor tendons (particularly on the hands) and a very high risk of premature CHD. Untreated, 85% of males with this condition will have had a myocardial infarction before the age of 60 years. The metabolic abnormality and clinical consequences result from impaired removal of LDL from the circulation. On the other hand, *familial combined hyperlipidaemia*, which is characterized by increased LDL and VLDL, results from increased production of these lipoproteins. The mode of inheritance is not quite so clearly understood but the condition is associated with an equally great risk of cardiovascular disease. Remnant hyper-lipoproteinaemia and familial hypertriglyceridaemia are rather less common. Although drug treatment is often necessary, dietary modification (see later) remains extremely important in the management of these conditions. There is some evidence that, even in these clearly inherited disorders, environmental factors may influence the pretreatment lipid levels. Familial hypercholesterolaemia has been clearly documented in China, but levels of total and LDL cholesterol in those with heterozygous familial hypercholesterolaemia is lower than in people with the condition in affluent western countries. Dietary factors would seem to be the most likely explanation for this difference, although of course there are many differences other than diet when comparing China with such countries (Junshi et al 1983).

Reduced levels of high-density lipoproteins

There has been much interest in high-density lipopro-tein (HDL) as a protective factor against CHD. Women have higher HDL levels than men and a lower CHD risk. The data in Table 41.7, taken from the Framingham Study, show that those with high levels of HDL had an appreciably lower rate of CHD over the 10 years of follow-up than those with lower levels, and there is evidence of a gradient effect (Gordon et al 1981). Some prospective studies have found that this protective effect is not sustained when controlling for the effects of other risk factors, but a recent analysis of four large American prospective studies in which HDL measurements were available suggests than an in-crement of 0.026 mmol/l (1 mg/100 ml) is associated with a 2–3% reduction in CHD (Gordon et al 1989). HDL levels do not differ markedly with age, are favourably influenced by physical activity, and are reduced in heavy cigarette smokers.

Dietary factors do not profoundly influence HDL levels, although regular fish eaters (who do not also eat meat) have been shown to have significantly higher levels than vegetarians, vegans and regular meat eaters (who may or may not eat fish as well) (Thorogood et

Table 41.7 Levels of high-density lipoprotein (HDL) cholesterol and subsequent incidence of coronary heart disease

HDL cholesterol		CHD rate/1000 population
mg/dl	mmol/l	
All levels		77
<25	<0.65	177
25–44	0.65–1.38	103
45–64	1.40–1.64	54
65–74	1.64–1.90	25

al 1987). Increasing carbohydrate to around 60% of total energy from more usual levels in affluent societies (around 45%) is associated with small but significant decreases in HDL (Grundy 1986). This effect has been demonstrated in relatively short-term studies, and it is not known whether it is sustained with prolonged intakes in this range. Further, it appears that this HDL-lowering effect of high-carbohydrate diets may be reduced or prevented if the carbohydrate is high in soluble fibre (Mann 1984). Very high intakes of polyunsaturated fatty acids (e.g. when associated with P/S > 1.0) have also been shown to result in reduced levels of HDL (Mattson & Grundy 1985). The effect is not seen in diets high in *cis* monounsaturated fatty acids, but monounsaturated fatty acids with a *trans* configuration are associated with a reduction of HDL (Mensink & Katan 1990). Most dietary studies have not included measurement of the subfractions of HDL. HDL_2 is the subfraction which is inversely related to CHD, and it has been suggested that dietary modification principally influences HDL_3, which is not believed to be related to CHD. This issue requires further research. Much has been made of the positive association between moderate levels of alcohol intake and HDL (Haskell et al 1984). Given the undesirable consequences of excessive intakes of alcohol, this observation should not be used as an indication of possible health benefits from drinking alcohol.

Apoproteins and lipoprotein (a)

Apoproteins are the protein components of the plasma lipoproteins. They are involved in maintaining the structural integrity of the lipoprotein particles and have a role in receptor recognition and enzyme regulation. They are classed A, B, C, D and E, with subclasses. Apoprotein B constitutes 90% of the protein component of LDL and is also a major protein of chylomicrons and VLDL. It is thought to have a vital function in the metabolism of LDL, VLDL and IDL. Apoprotein B levels are predictive of subsequent CHD, an effect which appears to be independent of total cholesterol levels. The interaction between diet and apoprotein B is complex. Dietary factors which influence LDL will clearly have an effect on apoprotein B levels. However, apoB is believed to explain some of the genetic variations in LDL response to changes in dietary fat. A similar situation prevails with regard to apoA, the major protein in HDL and which determines HDL production and metabolism. ApoA is very strongly correlated with HDL cholesterol measured on a stable diet, and also explains the variation in HDL response when changing from a high- to a low-fat diet. Less is known about the effects of dietary factors on other apoproteins, and there is clearly much more to be learned about the interactive effects between diet and apoproteins (Ball & Mann 1986).

There has been a recent upsurge of interest in lipoprotein (a), Lp(a), which is assembled from LDL and apolipoprotein (a). Concentrations may vary from near zero to over 1000 mg/l, and there is now convincing evidence of a strong independent association with CHD (Rosengren et al 1990). Plasma levels are genetically determined, and evidence to date suggests that modifying diet does not lower serum lipoprotein (a) concentrations (Maserei et al 1984).

Factors determining thrombogenesis

It has long been clear that clinical CHD could not entirely be explained in terms of atheroma, but much less attention has been given to the study of thrombogenesis and its determinants. There is no doubt that platelets are intimately involved in the pathogenesis of arterial thrombosis. However, there has been no standardized assessment of platelet function in large-scale epidemiological studies. The lack of international standardization and the time required for measurement of platelet function have made such surveys prohibitive. Most of the evidence supporting a relationship between diet, platelets and heart disease is derived from small-scale epidemiological studies, as well as clinical and basic nutrition research. Interest in the role of diet and platelet function was renewed in the mid-1970s, when a group of Danish researchers pursued the observation that in Greenland the death rate from CHD was low, despite the fact that the population consumed a diet which was high in cholesterol and total fat. The fat in the diet of the Greenland Eskimo is derived almost exclusively from marine foods, which contain large quantities of the n-3 fatty acids eicosopentaenoate (EPA C20:5) and docosahexaenoate (DHA 22:6). There is now a substantial body of evidence to suggest that the low CHD incidence in the Eskimo is at least in part attributable to their high intake of n-3 fatty acids (Bang et al 1980, Fisher et al 1986). However, the effects of fatty acids on thrombosis is complex.

When considering this issue it is necessary to remember that there are three series of prostanoids and thromboxanes which have profound and different effects on platelet function and vascular tone. Each series of prostanoids is derived from a different fatty acid: the 1 series from dihomogammalinolenic acid (DHLA); the 2 series from arachidonic acid (AA); and the 3 series from eicosapentaenoic acid (Fig. 41.9). In most diets little DHLA and AA is consumed. However, significant quantities of these fatty acids, particularly AA, are produced in the body from linolenic acid. In a state of normal health, vasodilation must be balanced with vasoconstriction and platelet adhesion and aggregation to healthy and uninjured arterial wall should be minimized. When injury does occur to the vessel wall, platelets are stimulated to release AA from their membrane phospholipids and this fatty acid is immediately converted to thromboxane A_2 (T_xA_2), a potent

Fig. 41.9 Prostanoids formed from different fatty acids (Ulbricht & Southgate 1991)

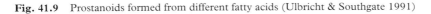
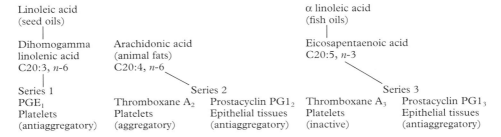

Linoleic acid (seed oils)			α linoleic acid (fish oils)	
Dihomogamma linolenic acid C20:3, n-6	Arachidonic acid (animal fats) C20:4, n-6		Eicosapentaenoic acid C20:5, n-3	
Series 1 PGE$_1$ Platelets (antiaggregatory)	Series 2 Thromboxane A_2 Platelets (aggregatory)	Prostacyclin PG1$_2$ Epithelial tissues (antiaggregatory)	Series 3 Thromboxane A_3 Platelets (inactive)	Prostacyclin PG1$_3$ Epithelial tissues (antiaggregatory)

proaggregatory and vasoconstrictive compound. Simultaneously the endothelial cells of the arterial wall metabolize significant quantities of AA to prostacyclin (PGI$_2$), a compound which exerts strong antiaggregatory and vasodilatory activity. It is believed that a proper balance of T$_x$A$_2$ to PGI$_2$ production is essential for normal arterial health. However, an overproduction of T$_x$A$_2$ is associated with an increased risk of thrombogenesis (Sinclair 1984). Fatty acids of the n-3 series (eicosapentaenoate and docosahexaenoate) have a particularly powerful antithrombogenic effect (Editorial 1988). They act by inhibiting conversion of AA to thromboxane A$_2$ and by facilitating the production of prostacyclin PGI$_3$, a potent inhibitor aggregation (Rao et al 1983, Lagarde 1990). These effects are seen with purified forms of fish oil fed in capsules as well as on diets containing appreciable quantities of oily fish. Fatty acids of the n-6 series also reduce platelet aggregation and do so by providing series 1 prostanoids as well as by increasing the fluidity of platelet membranes (MacIntyre et al 1984). The antithrombogenic effects of monounsaturated fatty acids have been less studied, but there is some evidence that *cis* oleic acid acts as an inhibitor of platelet aggregation, though the effect is less than for polyunsaturated fatty acids (Lagarde et al 1981, Crawford 1987).

Although there have been many studies of the antithrombogenic effect of polyunsaturated fatty acids in humans, the thrombogenic effect of saturated fatty acids has been more studied in laboratory animals. The findings are nevertheless quite consistent: the longer-chain saturated fatty acids (C14:0, C16:0 and C18:0) all appear to accelerate thrombosis formation. One possible mechanism may be via the inhibition of antiaggregatory prostacyclin (Hornstra & Lessenberg 1975, McGregor et al 1980, Renaud et al 1986, O'Dea et al 1988). Of particular interest is the fact that stearic acid (C18:0) which appears not to have adverse effects on LDL, has thrombogenic properties. In the past the P/S ratio was regarded as an indicator of thrombogenicity as well as of atherogenicity (Hornstra 1989). As has been indicated, this represents an oversimplification to the extent of being misleading. For example, sunflower oil would be more antithrombotic than oily fish. Ulbricht and Southgate have also developed an index of thrombogenicity (IT) which appears even more complex than their index of atherogenicity:

$$IT = \frac{mS^{iv}}{nM + 0M^1 + p(n-6) + q(n-3) + \dfrac{n-3}{n-6}}$$

where S^{iv} = sum of C14:0, C16:0 and C18:0; n-6 = n-6 PUFA; n-3 = n-3 PUFA; M and M^1 are as defined for IA and m, n, o, p and q are empirical unknown constants; m has arbitrarily been set at unity; n, o and p have been assigned the value of 0.5 because MUFA and n-6 PUFA are less antithrombogenic than n-3 PUFA; q has been given the value 3. The denominator was devised in order to give fish (which is high in MUFA as well as n-3 PUFA) the lowest IT and to take into account the effects of the various fatty acids described above. The IT of selected foods and diets are shown in Table 41.4.

This is a fascinating new concept which warrants further research, but one which is not yet appropriate for routine use since there is insufficient evidence to set accurate values for the constants, possible different effects of *trans* MUFA are not taken into account, detailed fatty acid composition of many foods is not available, and since the fatty acid composition of many foods (e.g. lean meats) has changed appreciably, with up-to-date information not yet being available in food tables.

Dietary factors may also influence thrombogenesis via an effect on the coagulation system. The physiological function of this system is to secure haemostasis after an injury by promoting the production of thrombin which enables the conversion of soluble fibrinogen to insoluble fibrin. Several prospective epidemiological studies have now suggested that a number of factors involved in the coagulation system (most notably factor VII and fibrinogen) are important predictors of CHD, suggesting that an inappropriately high level of coagulability might predispose to accelerated thrombogenesis (Meade et al 1980). Determinants of these clotting factors are summarized in Table 41.8 (Meade et al 1985).

Table 41.8 Characteristics associated with high or lower than usual levels of Factor VIIc activity and fibrinogen

Factor VIIc	Fibrinogen
High levels	
Increasing age	Increasing age
Obesity	Obesity
Oral contraceptive use	Oral contraceptive use
Menopause	Menopause
Diabetes	Diabetes
High-fat diet	Smoking
	Low employment grade
Low levels	
Black ethnic group	Moderate alcohol intake
Vegetarians	

High levels of fibrinogen are most strongly associated with obesity and cigarette smoking. Factor VII is associated to a greater extent with dietary factors: increasing dietary fat can cause an elevation of factor VII within 24 hours (Miller et al 1989). This suggests that raised levels of blood cholesterol, which are strikingly correlated with factor VII, are not responsible for this coagulation factor elevation; the hypercholesterolaemic effect of saturated fatty acids would not manifest so rapidly. Rather, raised levels of both factor VII and blood cholesterol may be a parallel consequence of a higher intake of total and saturated fatty acids. Levels of a range of clotting factors, including factor VII, are lower in populations and groups eating a low-fat, high-P/S ratio, high-fibre diet, and individuals changing to such a diet show a reduction in these factors (Meade & North 1977). It is thus not fully established which dietary factors are the main determinants of blood coagulation, although total fat intake does seem to be particularly important.

Hyperglycaemia and diabetes

Several studies have shown that people with diabetes and impaired glucose tolerance have an appreciably increased risk of CHD. Despite strong genetic influences dietary factors play an important role in the aetiology of non-insulin dependent (type 2) diabetes. Appreciable obesity (body mass index >30) is associated with a considerable increase in risk of diabetes, and there is some evidence that lesser degrees of obesity may also confer some risk. However, the obesity-mediated risk is most marked in those with truncal obesity, confirming the complexity of the genetic–nutritional interaction in the aetiology of diabetes. There is less evidence for the role of specific dietary factors. Type 2 diabetes is certainly uncommon in populations eating a high-fibre, high-carbohydrate, low-fat diet but there is no definitive evidence that any of these dietary factors are protective, nor that fibre depletion or a high intake of fat or sucrose are in themselves predisposing. These factors may influence the risk of diabetes indirectly by encouraging increased energy intake. The relationship between dietary factors, obesity and diabetes, as well as the dietary treatment of diabetes, is discussed in Chapters 32 and 35.

Hypertension

There is a striking relationship between systolic and diastolic blood pressure and CHD. There is no doubt that obesity and an excessive alcohol intake are related to blood pressure, and weight reduction and alcohol restriction can lower blood pressure levels (Reisin et al 1978, Cox et al 1990). The precise role of other dietary factors – excessive sodium, saturated fat, coffee, meat and low potassium and calcium – is less well established. The role of dietary sodium in particular has been the subject of a great deal of debate.

About 50 years ago Dahl suggested that differences in salt intake were a major cause of population differences in blood pressure. This conclusion was largely based on the near-linear correlation between population salt intake and prevalence of hypertension. Glieberman undertook a more critical review of 27 published studies (Glieberman 1973). She concluded that there was a relation between salt intake and blood pressure, but that since increased dietary salt is usually found with greater acculturation, it could not be concluded whether salt or other cultural changes or both were responsible for the increase in blood pressure. However, in the majority of studies reviewed, methods for assessing dietary sodium and blood pressure were inadequate. Twenty-four-hour urinary sodium excretion provides the best available method of assessing sodium intake, and this method together with standardized blood pressure measurements has been used in the Intersalt study, which collected data on over 10 000 people aged 20–59 years from 52 centres in 32 countries (Intersalt Cooperative Research Group 1988). Sodium excretion ranged from 0.2 mmol/24 h among the Yanomamo Indians of Brazil, through around 150 mmol in typical western populations to 242 mmol/24 h in north China. The populations with very low sodium excretion (≤50 mmol/24 h) had low median blood pressures, a low prevalence of hypertension and virtually no increase in blood pressure with age. In the remaining centres sodium was related to blood pressure levels in individuals, and influenced the extent to which blood pressure increased with age. The overall association between sodium and median blood pressure or prevalence of hypertension was less striking, and was not statistically significant when excluding the four centres with very low sodium intakes.

On the basis of these findings it could be calculated that a 100 mmol/day reduction in dietary sodium might reduce systolic blood pressure by 3.5 mmHg, and diastolic pressure by 1.5 mmHg, though adjustment for potassium excretion, body mass index and alcohol reduces these estimates to 2.2 and 0.1 mmHg respectively. A number of explanations have been put forward to explain why even meticulous studies such as Intersalt may underestimate the relationship between dietary sodium and blood pressure, especially when considering the population association.

The reasons are similar to those used to explain the lack of association within populations between dietary fat and cholesterol, i.e. unreliability of assessing dietary intake or even a single measurement of urinary sodium; a narrow range of intakes in most populations, genetic variability; a threshold intake at about 60–70 mmol, above which the amount taken may not matter; current intake may have little significance, assuming a long timeframe for the development of hypertension; inability to take into account other factors influencing blood pressure, including obesity and alcohol. It is also conceivable that in high-risk populations the most important role for dietary sodium is an enabling factor which sets the scene for other factors to operate.

In the light of these observations the results of recent meta-analyses of observational data among and within populations are of particular interest. Law and colleagues analysed data from published reports of blood pressure and sodium intake for 24 different communities throughout the world and 14 published studies that correlated blood pressure recordings in individuals against measurements of their 24-hour sodium intake (Law et al 1991). These analyses suggest that the Intersalt study may have appreciably underestimated the association of blood pressure with sodium intake, and that the association increases with age and initial blood pressure. For example, at age 60–69 years the estimated systolic blood pressure reduction in response to a 100 mmol/24 h reduction in sodium intake was on average 10 mmHg, but varied from 6 mmHg for those on the 5th blood pressure centile to 15 mmHg for those on the 95th centile.

The results of the intervention trials involving sodium restriction are equally interesting. Examination of the individual studies suggests rather inconsistent results, but once again Law and collaborators have aggregated the results of 68 crossover trials and ten randomized controlled trials of dietary salt reduction. In people aged 50–59 years, a reduction of daily sodium intake of 50 mmol (about 3 g of salt), attainable by moderate dietary salt reduction, would, after a few weeks, lower systolic blood pressure by an average of 5 mmHg and by 7 mmHg in those with high blood pressure; diastolic blood pressure would be lowered by half as much. It is estimated that such a reduction in salt intake by a whole western population would reduce the incidence of stroke by 26%, and of CHD by 15%. Reduction also in the amount of salt added to processed foods would lower blood pressure by twice as much and could prevent as many as 70 000 deaths per year in Britain (Law et al 1991).

With regard to clinical practice, it is also important to know whether salt restriction will allow smaller doses of antihypertensive drugs to be used than might otherwise have been the case. There seems little doubt that most antihypertensive drugs (thiazides, beta blockers and angiotensin-converting enzyme inhibitors) are more effective with reduced sodium intake. This may not apply to calcium antagonists and it should be noted that very low sodium intakes (less than 50 mmol/day) with high doses of thiazide can cause postural hypotension (Ritz et al 1988).

The heterogeneity in the response of individuals to sodium restriction suggests the possibility of the existence of a group of hyperresponders. There is as yet no firm confirmation of this phenomenon, nor any suggestion as to how such individuals might be defined.

Of the other dietary factors which have been considered in the aetiology of hypertension, most attention has been given to potassium. In the Intersalt study urinary potassium excretion, an assumed indicator of intake, was negatively related to blood pressure, as was the urinary sodium/potassium concentration ratio (Intersalt Cooperative Research Group 1988). The trials have reached conflicting conclusions, but a pooled analysis suggests that potassium supplementation reduces blood pressure in normotensive and hypertensive subjects by an average of 5.9–3.4 mmHg (Cappucio & MacGregor 1991).

The relationship between saturated fat, coffee, calcium and blood pressure has been less well studied, or the effect does not appear to be sustained when controlling for other variables. However, there is an increasing body of evidence concerning the effect of a vegetarian diet (Beilin et al 1988). Vegetarians have long been known to have lower blood pressure than meat eaters. A series of carefully controlled studies from Perth, Western Australia, have shown that significant reductions in both systolic and diastolic pressures occur when subjects are changed from a typical western diet to a vegetarian diet (Fig. 41.10). In addition to excluding meat and fish, vegetarian diets have less saturated fat and cholesterol, more dietary fibre and complex carbohydrates and various differences with regard to micronutrients when compared with a usual diet, and more research will be required to disentangle which aspects are particularly relevant in the effect on blood pressure.

In the light of all this, what practical nutritional guidance may be offered in the prevention and management of hypertension? The importance of avoiding (and reducing when necessary) obesity and excessive alcohol intake has been established beyond

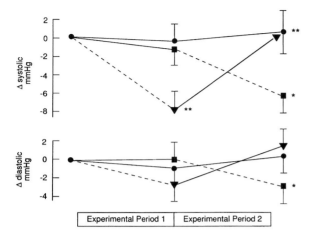

Fig. 41.10   Changes (Δ) in systolic and diastolic blood in control groups who made no dietary changes throughout the study (●—●), and groups randomized to receive either a control or vegetarian diet and then crossed over to the alternative dietary regimen. Broken line (----) represents the period in the vegetarian diet and unbroken line (——) the control period.

doubt. Dietary sodium undoubtedly plays a role in hypertension. The data of Law and colleagues suggest that salt restriction is much more important than has previously been recognized by many authorities. Even moderate salt restriction by the population at large could confer substantial public health benefits, and for patients with diagnosed hypertension an appreciable reduction of dietary sodium should be regarded as one of the cornerstones of therapy. The practical application may vary from country to country. For example, in the UK a relatively small proportion (15%) of salt is derived from cooking or table sources, whereas in Italy 36% is derived from these sources. An increase in potassium may also confer significant benefit, but should be achieved through a diet rich in fruit and vegetables rather than by increasing high potassium salt substitutes (Swales 1991). There is as yet insufficient evidence regarding the other dietary factors, but further studies attempting to discover which characteristics of the vegetarian diet account for the lower blood pressure in vegetarians than omnivores may produce further clues.

CLINICAL TRIALS OF CHOLESTEROL LOWERING

There is considerable epidemiological evidence to suggest that dietary change will reduce CHD risk, and irrefutable data concerning the ability of dietary modification to favourably influence risk factors for CHD. However, the most direct evidence for the benefits of dietary change should come from clinical trials which include a sufficient number of subjects to be able to examine whether a particular change is able to reduce morbidity and mortality from CHD, and by doing so influence total mortality. The early studies were single-factor intervention trials where an attempt was made to modify only one risk factor – cholesterol – and the dietary manipulation was principally that of increasing the P/S ratio. More recent studies have adopted a multifactorial approach. In these, various dietary changes were made in order to achieve maximum cholesterol lowering. Such changes will of course also influence risk factors other than cholesterol. In addition, there has usually been an attempt to also modify risk factors which are not diet-related (e.g. cigarette smoking). Much of the confusion in interpreting these clinical trials has resulted from the fact that none was specifically designed to examine the effect of diet on total mortality. The trials have been reviewed in detail elsewhere (Holme 1990). This review will consider only a selection of the trials most relevant to current dietary recommendations and give a brief overview of the remaining primary (i.e. those carried out on people who have no evidence of pre-existing CHD) and secondary trials (i.e. those carried out on people with pre-existing CHD).

Los Angeles Veterans Administration Study (Dayton et al 1969)

This was the first of the major intervention studies, in which 846 male volunteers (ages 55–89 years) were randomly allocated to 'experimental' and 'control' diets taken in different dining rooms. The control diet was intended to be typical of the North American diet (40% energy from fat, mostly saturated). The experimental diet contained half as much cholesterol, and predominantly polyunsaturated vegetable oils (n-6 PUFA) replaced approximately two-thirds of the animal fat, achieving a P/S ratio of 2. As a result of skilled food technology, the study was conducted under double-blind conditions. During the 8 years of follow-up, cholesterol in the experimental group was 13% lower, and coronary events as well as deaths due solely to atherosclerotic events appreciably reduced, as compared with the controls (Table 41.9). The beneficial effect of the cholesterol-lowering diet was most evident in those with high cholesterol levels at the outset of the study. Deaths due to other and uncertain causes occurred more frequently in the experimental group, though no single other cause predominated. The increase in non-cardiovascular mortality in the experimental group raised for the first time the suggestion that cholesterol lowering might be harmful in some respects, despite the reduction in CHD. This will be discussed in more detail later in the chapter.

Oslo Trial (Hjermann et al 1981, 1986)

In the Oslo trial men at high risk of CHD (as a result of smoking or having a cholesterol level in the range of 7.5–9.8 mmol/l) were divided into two groups; half received intensive dietary education and advice to stop smoking, the other half served as a control group. An impressive reduction in total coronary events was observed (Table 41.9) in association with a 13% fall in cholesterol and a 65% reduction in tobacco consumption. The beneficial effect of intervention was reflected also in a significant improvement in total mortality; there were no significant differences between the two groups with regard to non-cardiac causes of death. Detailed statistical analysis suggests that approximately 60% of the CHD reduction can be attributed to serum cholesterol change and 25% to smoking reduction. The composition of the experimental diet was quite different from that used in the Veterans Administration trial: total and saturated fat were markedly reduced without any appreciable increase in n-6 PUFA, and fibre-rich carbohydrate was increased. These differences could have accounted for the different results with regard to non-cardiovascular diseases.

Diet and Reinfarction Trial (DART) (Burr et al 1989)

Only one trial has examined the effects of diets high in n-3 PUFA. Burr et al randomized 2033 men who had survived myocardial infarction to receive or not to receive advice on each of three dietary factors: a reduction in fat intake and an increase in the ratio of polyunsaturated to saturated fat; an increase in fatty fish intake; and an increase in cereal fibre. Within the short (2 years) follow-up period the subjects advised to eat fatty fish had a 29% reduction in all causes of mortality compared with those not so advised. The other two diets were not associated with significant differences in mortality, but in view of the fact that fat modification only achieved a 3–4% reduction in serum cholesterol, it is conceivable that compliance with the fat-modified and fibre diets may have been less than that on the fist diet. Furthermore, diets aimed to reduce atherogenicity are likely to take longer to show a beneficial effect than those aimed to reduce thrombogenicity. These results are of particular interest since they are the first to show that very simple advice aimed to reduce thrombogenicity (at least two weekly portions, 200–400 g, of fatty fish) can appreciably reduce mortality.

Lifestyle Heart Trial (Ornish et al 1990)

This prospective randomized controlled trial attempted to determine the effect of lifestyle change on coronary atherosclerosis rather than morbidity or mortality. Subjects randomized to a strict low-fat vegetarian diet were also advised to stop smoking, to increase physical activity and were given stress-management training. They showed a striking trend towards regression of coronary narrowing compared with the control group. The diets were extremely low in fat (6.8% of dietary energy) and as such not appropriate to dietary recommendations. Nevertheless, the findings are of considerable interest since they provide evidence that lifestyle changes can result in regression of atherosclerosis.

Table 41.9 Number of deaths and cases of CHD, odds ratios (OR) and percentage differences in cholesterol between treated (T) and control (C) groups in selected trials

Study	Number of subjects (T/C)	Total deaths (T/C)	CHD (T/C)	Odds Ratios Death	Odds Ratios CHD	% Δ chol
VA diet Study (Dayton et al 1969)	424/422	174/177	60/88	0.98	0.68	13%
Oslo (Hjermann et al 1981, 1986)	604/628	16/24	19/36	0.69	0.53	10%
DART (Burr et al 1989) (fish advice)	1015/1018	94/130	127/149	0.71	0.84	Negligible
MRFIT (Multiple Risk Factor Intervention Trial Research Group 1982)	6428/6438	265/260	277/280	1.02	0.99	2%
WHO Collaborative (1983)	24 615/25 169	997/924	773/756	1.10	1.04	Negligible

Overall perspective of the trials

Attention has been given to the fact that at least two large multifactorial intervention trials (the multiple risk factor intervention trial (Multiple Risk Factor Intervention Trial Research Group 1982) and the WHO collaborative trial (World Health Organization Collaborative Group 1983)) found no differences between treated and control groups. This should not be regarded as surprising, since in both studies intervention achieved a negligible difference in cholesterol. Furthermore, the two countries participating in the WHO study that did achieve risk factor reduction (Italy and Belgium) showed reductions in all cause mortality as well as coronary heart disease. A helpful perspective of the trials has been provided by Peto et al, who have pointed out that in all studies, especially the smaller ones, the final results are subject to a considerable margin of error (Peto et al 1987). Consequently they have fitted confidence intervals to the differences in CHD rates between control and experimental groups in the randomized diet and drug cholesterol-lowering trials. In Figure 41.11 the percentage differences in the odds of CHD are plotted in relation to the achieved cholesterol lowering. The latter is presented as strength of intervention, calculated by multiplying the cholesterol difference between experimental and control groups by duration of trial in years. The best regression line through the origin is indicated. The wide confidence intervals resulting from the small number of subjects in some studies explains some of the apparently conflicting findings, but the calculated confidence limits of each study include the regression line. The association between the strength of intervention and reduction in CHD risk is impressive, providing strong confirmatory evidence for the aetiological importance of cholesterol in CHD as well as suggesting that cholesterol reduction, even in middle-aged individuals, may be of benefit in reducing coronary events. The data are particularly striking when considering patients with elevated cholesterol (such as those included in the Oslo study) among whom benefit was even more marked than among those with average cholesterol levels.

Much has been made of the fact that several studies have shown an increase in some non-cardiac causes of mortality, and that as a result total mortality has not been significantly reduced (Oliver 1991). The pos-

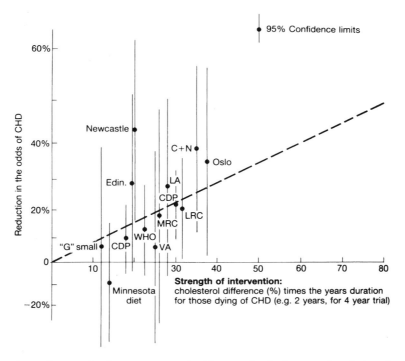

Fig. 41.11   Coronary heart disease reduction versus strength of intervention in the unconfounded randomized trials (Peto et al 1987, reproduced with permission).

sibility that cholesterol-lowering diets (and in particular those high in polyunsaturated fatty acids) might increase the risk of cancer first came from the Los Angeles study. PUFA are liable to peroxidation and the paradox exists that diets very high in those fatty acids might actually initiate cancer or CHD. Clearly the latter does not occur, and a meta-analysis of several primary prevention trials found no convincing evidence of increased cancer risk (Ederer et al 1971, Muldoon et al 1990). Nevertheless, it should be emphasized that there are no populations that consume high amounts of *n*-6 PUFA such as have been used in some clinical trials. Furthermore, there is evidence for an increased risk of gallstones in people taking a diet high in polyunsaturated fat (P/S ratio of 1.5 or greater), so intakes in this range would not be recommended. Lewis (1991) has reviewed the safety aspects of cholesterol lowering and pointed out that there is no evidence for a causal association between low cholesterol levels and non-cardiac mortality. The inconsistency of the findings, the absence of a graded continuous relationship and the fact that several studies suggest that appreciable cholesterol lowering (at least 8–9%) is associated with an improvement in total mortality led most authorities to accept that the diets now recommended for reducing CHD risk are not associated with an appreciable risk of non-cardiac mortality. However, a small minority still believe that because of possible risks cholesterol-lowering diets should be reserved for those with particularly high cholesterol levels who are likely to benefit most from cholesterol reduction, and not for the population at large (Oliver 1991).

NUTRITIONAL STRATEGIES FOR HIGH-RISK POPULATIONS

There is now widespread acceptance in most countries with high CHD rates of the need for strategies to reduce the frequency and extent of CHD risk factors. The nutritional approach aims principally to reduce atherogenic as well as thrombogenic risk by reducing obesity, lowering total and LDL cholesterol and triglycerides, increasing HDL cholesterol, lowering blood pressure levels and reducing platelet aggregation. As has been indicated above, the dietary changes required to modify risk factors are more complex than had been previously believed to be in case, but it is nevertheless possible to recommend a range of dietary principles which are likely to facilitate one or more of these changes. Two principal approaches are used to achieve these changes: a population strategy and an individual strategy (Lewis et al 1986).

The need for a population strategy

The population strategy hinges on the observation that in communities with high CHD incidence the distribution of many risk factors is at a higher level than in populations with low CHD rates. Of all the risk factors for CHD, cholesterol is probably the most powerful and has certainly been the most studied. Figure 41.12 compares the distribution of cholesterol levels in south Japan, which has a very low CHD incidence, and east Finland, where CHD rates are exceptionally high. It is hypothesized that this upward displacement of risk factor distribution, which is believed to account for the striking difference in CHD incidence, may be largely explained by environmental factors and be amenable to change as a result of alterations in lifestyle.

Figure 41.13 is based on calculations by Rose on data derived from the Framingham study, and has been widely used to demonstrate the need for a population strategy (World Health Organization Expert Committee 1982). It shows clearly within a high-risk population how CHD risk to the individual increases steadily with increasing levels of cholesterol. However, because there are relatively few people with levels at the upper end of the distribution, only a small number of all CHD cases in the community arise in these high-risk echelons. On the other hand, large numbers of people are at modestly increased risk of CHD because of average or only slightly above average (though still untoward) levels of cholesterol. Although the risk to individuals in this category (i.e.

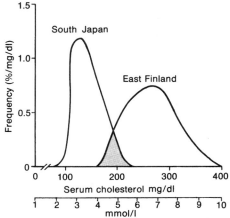

Fig. 1. Cultural differences in serum cholesterol levels.

Fig. 41.12 Cultural differences in serum cholesterol levels.

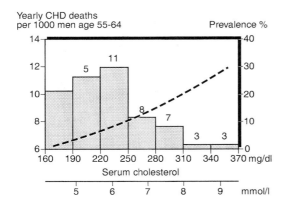

Fig. 41.13 Prevalence distribution (histogram) of serum cholesterol concentrations related to coronary heart disease mortality (broken line) in men aged 55–64 years. The number above each column represents an estimate of attributable deaths per 1000 population per 10-year period. (Derived from the Framingham Study)

the 'relative risk') is not so great, the majority of all CHD cases are drawn from this section of the population.

Clearly a 'high-risk' preventive strategy aimed solely at those at greatest risk of CHD (e.g. those with cholesterol levels >7 mmol/l) will have little impact on the epidemic proportions CHD has reached in many countries. In order to make an impact on the problem overall, it is essential to shift the entire distribution of cholesterol (and other risk factors) to a range where overall risk is low. The principal disadvantage of such an approach is that many individuals are being asked to make changes that are likely to produce a relatively small reduction in their personal CHD risk, while those at much greater risk are unaware that they require more radical lifestyle changes or preventive medical care, including drug therapy (Lewis et al 1986).

Desirable cholesterol levels

There has been much debate about which cholesterol levels are likely to be associated with the lowest achievable levels of lipoprotein-mediated risk of CHD.

In 1979, a multidisciplinary workshop suggested that the mean serum cholesterol of an adult population should not exceed 4.7 mmol/l. The 1982 World Health Organization Expert Committee suggested that mean levels of total cholesterol in adults should be below 5.2 mmol/l (200 mg/dl) (World Health

Organization Expert Committee 1982). The principal justifications for this level are that populations with high CHD rates have higher levels, that CHD is relatively infrequent in countries with lower mean levels, and that, within single populations, subgroups with the lowest levels have the lowest risk of CHD. A National Institutes of Health Consensus Development Conference regarded this level as an attainable goal for *individuals* as well as populations and suggested a lower level of 4.7 mmol/l as an appropriate target for younger adults. These levels are, of course, appreciably lower than the reference ranges quoted by many laboratories. Such reference ranges are based on a statistical concept of normality, rather than comprising desirable levels as defined above, and are derived from observed levels in populations with a high incidence of CHD. Before considering what might be achieved in practice by a population strategy, it is necessary to consider what, in theory, might be achieved by different sets of dietary recommendations aimed at reducing CHD risk.

Nutritional recommendations for high-risk populations

Many earlier sets of recommendations gave particular emphasis to the intake of total dietary fat and dietary cholesterol, and concentrated almost exclusively on the need for dietary advice to achieve lowering of blood cholesterol. Current recommendations acknowledge the importance of thrombogenesis and other cardiovascular risk factors, and also that lipoprotein-mediated risk and its determinants involve more than a simple consideration of blood cholesterol. Table 41.10 shows the recently published dietary reference values for fat and carbohydrate in the UK (Department of Health 1991). Emphasis has moved away from total fat which, it is suggested, should be calculated from the sum of fatty acid intakes and glycerol, though restriction of total fat is clearly important for those who are obese. The reduction in saturated fatty acids to 10% of total dietary energy is much greater than previously recommended (Department of Health 1984) and is more in line with North American and WHO recommendations. This acknowledges the particular importance of SFA in atherogenesis as well as thrombogenesis, and represents a very considerable reduction from present levels of intake. It has been suggested that stearic acid is not associated with an elevation of LDL, as is the case with SFA of shorter chain length. However, it is impractical to distinguish between the different saturated fatty acids and, given the fact that stearic

Table 41.10   Dietary reference values for fat and carbohydrate for adults as a percentage of daily total energy intake (percentage of food energy) (Department of Health 1991)

	Individual minimum	Population average	Individual maximum
Saturated fatty acids		10(11)	
Cis polyunsaturated fatty acids		6(6.5)	10
	n-3:0.2		
	n-6:1.0		
Cis monounsaturated fatty acids		12(13)	
Trans fatty acids		2(2)	
Total fatty acids		30(32.5)	
Total fat		33(35)	
Non-milk extrinsic sugars	0	10(11)	
Intrinsic and milk sugars and starch		37(39)	
Total carbohydrate		47(50)	
Non-starch polysaccharide (g/day)	12	18	24

The average percentage contribution to total energy does not total 100% because figures for protein and alcohol are excluded. Protein intakes average 15% of total energy, which is above the RNI. It is recognized that many individuals will derive some energy from alcohol, and this has been assumed to average 5% approximating to current intakes. However, the Panel allowed some groups not to drink alcohol and that for some purposes nutrient intakes as a proportion of food energy (without alcohol) might be useful. Therefore average figures are given as percentages both of total energy and, in parenthesis, of food energy.

acid is probably thrombogenic even though it may not be atherogenic, such distinctions may be of academic rather than practical significance. It is recommended that *cis* MUFA should continue to provide on average 12% of dietary energy, though a greater proportion than at present might be expected to be derived from vegetable rather than animal sources. Although an increase in MUFA has not been suggested in the British recommendations, some increase would seem to be perfectly acceptable in the light of the evidence summarized above, and this has been incorporated into recent recommendations in New Zealand (Nutrition Task Force 1991). It is suggested that *cis* polyunsaturated fatty acids should continue to provide an average of 6% of total dietary energy and that this should be derived from a mixture of *n*-6 and *n*-3 PUFA. It is not possible on the basis of present evidence to recommend a precise ratio of *n*-6 to *n*-3. Dietary intake of PUFA should not exceed 10% of total energy. A slightly higher average intake (up to 8%) has been recommended in some countries (Nutrition Task Force 1991), but there seems to be a consensus that, at least at present, an upper limit of around 10% is appropriate. *Trans* fatty acid intake should not exceed the current estimated average of 5 g/day or 2% of dietary energy. Total fatty acid intake

should therefore average 30% and total fat (i.e. including glycerol) 33% of total dietary energy including alcohol, or 35% of energy derived from food. Little emphasis is given to dietary cholesterol, but it should be noted that average dietary cholesterol intake in Britain is relatively low, and most other sets of recommendations suggest that populations' mean intake should be below 300 mg/day.

Dietary reference values are given for carbohydrates and non-starch polysaccharides. These are not specifically aimed at reducing cardiovascular risk and it is of interest that, whereas an increase of non-starch polysaccharide is recommended, there is no specific advice to increase soluble forms, as has been suggested in other recommendations. There is also no specific advice regarding antioxidant intake in relation to cardiovascular disease, although a high intake of fruit and vegetables, which is suggested in all dietary guidelines, should ensure adequate intakes. It is beyond the scope of this review to attempt a detailed translation of recommendations and reference values into guidelines for the population, although a few general comments are offered. A reduction of dairy products and red meat has formed the cornerstone of some guidelines in the past. Dairy products contribute over 40% of dietary saturated fatty acids and reduction of butter, full-fat milk and cheese, as well as hard margarine, is an important means of reducing intakes of SFA. Skimmed or semi-skimmed milk, reduced-fat cheeses and predominantly unsaturated margarines, particularly those high in oleic acid, are suitable alternatives. However, a change in the composition of many red meats so that lean meat now has less SFA and more MUFA and PUFA than previously has meant that moderate amounts (up to 180 g/day) can be safely incorporated into dietary advice aimed at achieving optimal lipoprotein profiles (Watts et al 1988). The findings of the Diet and Reinfarction Trial also provide reinforcement of the epidemiological findings, which suggest that eating fish (especially oily fish) several times a week may confer additional benefit.

On the basis of the Keys formula plus an additional effect from other dietary modifications, it might be expected that dietary change along the lines suggested here would reduce cholesterol levels by at least 16%, which would mean a reduction in the mean adult population cholesterol levels in countries such as Britain from the present level of around 5.9 mmol/l to 5.0 mmol/l or less. However, this would involve full compliance with dietary recommendations. There is little information to suggest what might be achieved in practice, but in two countries (Finland and the USA) intervention programmes which have included dietary advice along the lines suggested here, together with other lifestyle changes, have been evaluated (Farquhar et al 1977, Tuomilehto et al 1986). In both North Karelia, Finland (Tuomilehto et al 1986) and Stamford on the west coast of the USA (Farquhar et al 1977) the most impressive results were seen in the reduction of cigarette smoking. In both countries the reductions in cholesterol (around 3%) and blood pressure were much lower than expected, suggesting that for some reason compliance with the dietary advice was much less than expected. Inappropriate information and education programmes, lack of availability of appropriate foods and unsatisfactory food labelling are some possible explanations for the rather disappointing results.

Mean change and individual change in practice: Limitations of the population strategy

It could be argued that a more favourable climate for the implementation of dietary guidelines exists in the 1990s than was the case in the early 1970s. However, an 8% reduction in cholesterol might be regarded as an optimistic assessment as to what might be achieved in practice – that is, half of what would be predicted

from full compliance with the recommendations. If this assumption of an 8% change is correct, the mean level in Britain would be expected to fall from 5.9 to about 5.5 mmol/l, still well above the WHO target, and an appreciable number of individuals would continue to have cholesterol levels above those representing the upper end of the desirable range. Table 41.11, once again based on cholesterol levels in Britain, shows that with full compliance with the WHO or British recommendations only about 5% of the population, as compared with around 25% at present, would remain at appreciable risk of CHD as a result of hypercholesterolaemia (cholesterol >6.5 mmol/l) and 15% of the population would be at some risk as compared with just under 50% at present. However, with a more realistic expectation of an 8% reduction in serum cholesterol, around 13% of the population would remain at considerable risk. In countries with a higher mean level than in Britain, this figure would of course be appreciably greater. This group would include virtually all those with familial hyperlipidaemia, who have a very high incidence of CHD.

A number of conclusions may be drawn from these observations. First, attempts to achieve population change should be as energetic as possible, and should include educational measures aimed at the population as well as legislative measures to facilitate change (e.g. a high tax on cigarettes and widespread availability of appropriate, relatively low-cost foods). The greater the reduction in mean cholesterol, the fewer the number that will remain at high risk. Secondly, a strategy that aims to reduce risk in such individuals is

Table 41.11 Percentage of population in Britain aged 25–59 years with cholesterol levels exceeding 6.5 and 5.2 mmol/l, and percentage predicted to exceed these limits following adoption of dietary recommendations

	Serum cholesterol level	
	>6.5 mmol/l	>5.2 mmol/l
Prevalence Study 1984–1985 (Mann et al 1988)	25	47
Mean cholesterol reduction 16.5% (World Health Organization (1982) British dietary reference values) (Department of Health 1991)	4.5	15
Mean cholesterol reduction 8% (optimistic estimate of what might be achieved in practice)	13	31

an essential complement to the population strategy, at least for the foreseeable future and until such a time as high-risk populations are prepared to make major lifestyle changes. Finally, it would seem to be essential for the various population strategies to be evaluated with regard to the risk reduction achieved. Programmes suitable for one community might not necessarily be appropriate for others.

DIETARY ADVICE FOR HIGH-RISK INDIVIDUALS

The principles of dietary advice for individuals are similar to those which aim to reduce lipid levels in high-risk populations, but the targets are more strict. The ability to give advice to individuals known to be at particular risk results in appreciably greater cholesterol reductions. One large general practice-based study achieved an average 15% reduction in cholesterol levels, but reductions in cholesterol of up to 25%, and in triglyceride of 20–40%, are frequently reported from lipid clinics where patients receive individual advice from dietitians. There is, of course, individual variation in response and few patients with familial hypercholesterolaemia will respond adequately without drug therapy in addition. All those who tend to have cholesterol levels greater than

6.5 mmol/l and/or triglycerides greater than 3 mmol/l should ideally receive such individual advice from a dietitian or a nutritionist skilled in dietary counselling. There are fewer sets of international and national recommendations, but some principles of diet for high-risk people are indicated in Table 41.12. In addition to food lists (see Table 41.13) individuals require advice about methods of preparation and recipes, especially if present cooking habits differ appreciably from those recommended. Demonstrations and sample meal tasting can be particularly useful approaches. In the past, widely differing diets have been recommended for those with different forms of hyperlipidaemia. It has now been clearly established that this was unnecessary and the guidelines indicated in Table 41.12 permit a much simpler approach.

There has been debate concerning whether older people with cardiovascular risk factors, and those who have established cardiovascular disease but no obvious risk factors, should receive dietary advice along the lines suggested here (Agner 1984). The relative risk of cardiovascular disease associated with recognized risk factors does appear to decrease with increasing age, and there have been few clinical trials which have shown benefits of risk reduction in the elderly. No doubt there is an age beyond which there are minimal

Table 41.12   Principles of diet modification for individuals with hyperlipidaemia

	Initial advice for hypercholesterolaemia and endogenous hypertriglyceridaemia	Advice for resistant hypercholesterolaemia	Advice for chylomicronaemia syndrome
Total fatty acids (% total energy)	<30	≈25	15**
saturated fatty acids and *trans* unsaturated fatty acids	<10 (range 6–10)	6–8	
polyunsaturated fatty acids	≈8 (range 6–10)	6–8	
monounsaturated fatty acids	up to 18 (range 10–18)	10–15	
Dietary cholesterol (mg/day)	<300	<200	<200
Dietary fibre (g/day)*	35	45	35
Protein (% total energy)	12	12	20

*   Special emphasis given to soluble dietary fibre
** This usually involves reducing total fat to below 25 g per day. Medium-chain triglycerides which are not transported in chylomicrons may be added if liver function is normal
Supplementary fat-soluble vitamins may be required

Table 41.13   Guidelines for a lipid-lowering diet

	Advisable	May be eaten in moderation	Should be avoided
Fats	All fats should be limited to a minimum unless otherwise directed	Equivalent to 5 g of fat: 1 tsp of polyunsaturated margarine, monounsaturated margarine; 1 tsp of the following oils: safflower, soyabean, sunflower, corn, wheatgerm, grapeseed, sesame, walnut, olive, rapeseed, peanut; 2 tsp of low fat polyunsaturated spreads	Butter, dripping, suet, lard, palm oil, coconut oil. Margarines *not* labelled poly- or monounsaturated. Cooking or vegetable oils of unknown origin. Hydrogenated fats and oils
Meats	Average serving 150–200 g Mixed light and dark poultry meat (skinned), turkey, veal, rabbit, game	Not more than 100–250 g (cooked weight) 3–5 times a week: Lean beef, lamb, pork, steak mince. Average serving of liver or kidneys once a fortnight	Visible fat on meat (including crackling), belly pork, streaky bacon, salami, pâté, scotch eggs, duck, goose, pork pies, poultry skin. Sausages and luncheon meat, fried meats, rolled roasts, pressed meats
Eggs and dairy foods	Low fat (<1% fat) milk, skimmed milk, cottage cheese, low fat quarg, curd cheese, egg white, low fat yoghurt	Semi-skimmed 1.5 and 2% fat milk, medium fat cheeses, i.e. those with 24% total fat (45% fat content in dry matter) or less, e.g. Brie, Edam, Camembert, Mozarella, special processed and blue (12–13% fat) cheeses. 2–4 egg yolks per week including those in cooking and baking	Full cream milk, evaporated or condensed milk, cream, imitation cream. Full fat cheeses, e.g. stilton, cheddar, cheshire, cream cheeses, full fat yoghurt
Fish	All white fish, e.g. cod, sole, ling. Oily fish, e.g. herring, mackerel, salmon, sardines (if possible eat 200–400 g of oily fish twice per week)	Fish fried in suitable oil (oil should not be heated to smoke point or re-used) once per fortnight, avoid using fat in cooking if on a weight reducing diet. Mussels, oysters, scallops, clams	Fish roe, shrimps, squid
Fruit and vegetables	All fresh and plain frozen vegetables. Peas, beans of all kinds (e.g. haricot, red kidney, butter beans, lentils, chick peas) are particularly high in 'soluble fibre' and should be eaten regularly. Jacket or boiled potatoes, eat skins wherever possible. Fresh fruit, dried fruit, unsweetened tinned fruit	Chips and roast potatoes if cooked in suitable oil. Avocado pears, olives, fruit in syrup, crystallised fruit (restrict the latter two items if triglycerides raised) and avoid all of the above if following a weight reducing diet	Chips or roast potatoes cooked in unsuitable fat or oil. Oven chips, potato crisps
Cereals	Wholemeal flour, wholemeal and especially wholegrain bread, whole grain cereals, oatmeal, cornmeal, porridge oats, sweetcorn, whole grain rice and wholemeal pasta, crispbreads, oatcakes. Low fat crackers	White flour, white bread, sugary breakfast cereals, commercial muesli, white rice and pasta, plain semi-sweet biscuits, higher fat crackers	Fancy breads, croissants, brioches, savoury cheese biscuits, bought pastry. Egg noodles, pasta made with eggs

Table 41.13   *contd*

	Advisable	May be eaten in moderation	Should be avoided
Cakes and desserts	Low-fat puddings, e.g. jelly, sorbet, skimmed milk puddings, low-fat yoghurt, low-fat sauces	Cakes, pastry, puddings, biscuits and sauces made with suitable margarine or oil. Low-fat or soya-based ice cream. If triglycerides are raised or if following a weight-reducing diet, choose foods mainly from the 'Advisable' column	Cakes and pastry, puddings and biscuits made with saturated fats. Suet dumplings and puddings, butter and cream sauces. Deep fried snacks, dairy ice cream
Drinks	Tea, coffee, mineral water, slimline or sugar-free soft drinks, unsweetened fruit juice. Clear soups, homemade vegetable soup. Low alcohol beer	Sweet soft drinks, low-fat malted drinks or low-fat chocolate drinks occasionally. Meat soups, packet soups (avoid if on low salt diet). Alcohol (no more than 1–2 drinks for women, 2–3 drinks for men). Avoid alcohol and sugary drinks if triglycerides raised or if following a weight reducing diet	Irish coffee, Bailey's Irish Cream, full-fat malted milk drinks, e.g. Horlicks, Ovaltine, drinking chocolate, Cream soups
Sweets, preserves and spreads	Unless on a lower salt diet, clear pickles, Bovril, Marmite, Vegemite, Oxo. If on a weight-reducing diet, sugar-free sweeteners, e.g. saccharine tablets or liquid, aspartame sweetener, e.g. Nutrasweet tablets or powder, sucaryl liquid	Sweet pickles and chutney, jam, honey, marmalade, syrup, marzipan, lemon curd (made without eggs and butter), boiled sweets, pastilles, sugar, peppermints, wine gums. If triglycerides are raised or if following a weight-reducing diet choose foods mainly from the 'Advisable' column	Chocolate spreads, mincemeat containing suet, toffees, fudge, butterscotch, chocolate, coconut bars
Nuts and seeds	Linseed	Peanuts, walnuts, almonds, Brazil nuts, hazelnuts, cashew nuts, sunflower seeds, pumpkin seeds, sesame seeds	Coconut
Miscellaneous	Herbs, spices, mustard, pepper, vinegar, Worcester sauce, soy sauce, low-fat dressings, e.g. lemon or low-fat yoghurt	Meat and fish pastes, low calorie salad cream or low calorie mayonnaise bottled sauces, French dressing. If on a weight-reducing diet, choose foods mainly from the 'Advisable' column	Ordinary salad cream, mayonnaise, cream or cream cheese dressings

Table prepared by Alex Chisholm, Research Dietitian, Dept of Human Nutrition, University of Otago, Dunedin, New Zealand.

advantages to dietary change. However, the fact that there is no clear cut-off point for age, and that absence of clinical trial data reflects failure to include many elderly people in clinical trials rather than negative results, suggests that it is inappropriate to exclude all older people from relatively simple advice from which they may benefit. They should at least be given dietary advice which is compatible with the nutritional recommendations for high-risk populations described above. With regard to those who already have cardiovascular disease but no obvious risk factors, it should be appreciated that the existence of vascular disease is one of the major determinants of subsequent adverse events (Gofman et al 1966) and that what were previously regarded as relatively low levels of risk can be associated with unfavourable outcomes, especially when more than one factor is present in a susceptible individual. For these reasons they too should be given dietary advice.

OTHER NUTRITIONAL ISSUES RELEVANT TO DIET AND CHD

The importance of CHD as a major cause of premature morbidity and mortality has led to this disease becoming a highly emotive issue in many high-risk populations. Consequently the public is bombarded with an enormous amount of nutritional advice, some of which is valid, some of which is without any justification and some of which is confusingly based on half truths. Fad diets cause particular confusion. An example of the latter is the diet which is largely based on advice to increase oatbran and niacin. Oatbran may be rich in soluble forms of non-starch polysaccharides, which have some cholesterol-lowering properties, and nicotinic acid can certainly lower LDL and VLDL; however, pharmacological doses of nicotinic acid are required to produce an effect on lipoproteins, so that unless attention is paid to the other more important determinants of cardiovascular risk factors, this diet is likely to have a rather small overall beneficial effect. Similarly, n-3 polyunsaturated fatty acids (often referred to as omega-3 fatty acids and sold as concentrates in capsules) are sometimes advertised as a useful means of lowering cholesterol. Although these preparations can have a profound effect on thrombogenesis, VLDL, and may indeed reduce the risk of CHD, they do not have consistent effects on LDL and total cholesterol, except in pharmacological quantities. The safety of such preparations in large amounts has not been established, and whereas it seems reasonable to recommend an increased intake of fish, it is inappropriate to be advising large amounts of these fatty acids in concentrated form until requirements and safety have been established. On the other hand, garlic has been used for medicinal purposes since at least 1550 BC. It now seems that garlic can favourably influence a whole range of cardiovascular risk factors. Popular interest appears to be greatest in Germany, where garlic preparations have become the largest-selling over-the-counter 'drugs'. Much research is still required, and it seems clear that active ingredients may be lost in processing (Mansell & Reckless 1991).

From time to time there is a resurgence of interest in the association between coffee drinking, cholesterol levels and coronary heart disease. Relationships have not been consistent but evidence is emerging which suggests that the hypercholesterolaemic effect of coffee may be related to the method of preparation. Boiled coffee, which is most frequently drunk in the Nordic countries, may be more hypercholesterolaemic than coffee prepared in other ways, since this method of preparation requires more prolonged exposure of coffee and water at higher temperatures than is usual in other methods (Thelle et al 1987). These effects have not been sufficiently studied to justify the inclusion of advice concerning coffee drinking in dietary recommendations, though Thelle has suggested that the evidence may be strong enough to examine the coffee intake of people with high cholesterol levels and, where appropriate, recommend a switch in method of preparation.

Another highly controversial issue relates to the effects of alcohol on cardiovascular disease. There is now a considerable body of evidence to suggest that a modest intake of alcohol has a protective effect against CHD, perhaps via a beneficial effect on HDL, fibrinogen and platelet activity. However, the sharp increase in mortality from cerebrovascular disease, cancer, accidents and violence, as well as total mortality associated with more than two drinks per day, suggests that public health recommendations that emphasized the positive health effects of alcohol would be likely to do more harm than good (Marmot & Brunner 1991).

Given the complexity of the aetiology of CHD, it is quite conceivable that foods and nutrients other than those already extensively investigated will be found to have beneficial or deleterious effects. In view of the potentially powerful effects of advertising by those with vested interests, nutritionists have a critical role to play in the evaluation of, and public commentary on, new findings.

CEREBROVASCULAR DISEASE AND PERIPHERAL DISEASE

Despite the fact that atherosclerosis in the cerebral and femoral arteries resembles the equivalent pathological processes in the coronary arteries, the clinical syndromes of stroke and peripheral arterial disease are associated with a risk factor profile which is not identical to that of CHD. For stroke, systolic blood pressure, cigarette smoking and a heavy intake of alcohol are the most important potentially modifiable risk factors. Raised levels of fibrinogen also seem to confer risk (Shaper et al 1991, Qizilbash et al 1991). The lipoprotein-mediated risk seems to be of less importance, and consequently the dietary determinants of LDL, VLDL and HDL, so important in CHD, are likely to be of far less significance. The role of dietary factors in the aetiology, prevention and management of stroke has been little studied. An epidemiological study carried out several years ago suggested a protective effect of green vegetables and fruit (Acheson & Williams 1983) and in view of the importance of hypertension, dietary factors influencing this risk factor warrant attention. Obviously, patients found to have lipoprotein abnormalities should be advised accordingly and general dietary advice for the population at large seems appropriate. Diet-related factors may also be less important in the aetiology of peripheral vascular disease, for which smoking is unquestionably the most important risk factor (Hughson et al 1978), though once again individualized advice is appropriate for those with abnormalities.

CARDIOMYOPATHY AND CARDIAC FAILURE

Disorders of the heart and circulation are common in less affluent societies. Occasionally, cardiomyopathy and cardiac failure may occur as a result of specific nutrient deficiencies. The two classic examples are beriberi resulting from thiamin deficiency, which occurs in populations consuming highly milled rice, and Keshan disease, which has been reported in China and results from a deficiency of selenium. In both these conditions, replacing the nutrient will result in prevention as well as treatment of the clinical consequences of the deficiency. A much more common clinical situation is one where alcohol, in association with deficiencies of thiamin and other nutrients, results in a clinical syndrome sometimes labelled as cardiomyopathy and usually characterized by cardiac failure. There has been considerable controversy regarding the extent to which this condition results from nutrient deficiencies or alcohol excess, but clearly the management involves withdrawing or reducing alcohol and appropriate nutrient intakes. This clinical situation may occur in affluent societies, when it is invariably seen in those who have a long-standing excessive alcohol intake. Anaemia resulting from a range of nutrient deficiencies may also result in cardiac failure. This nutrition-related disorders of the heart and circulation remain a significant health issue in many developing countries, but it should be noted that, in many such societies, CHD is rapidly overtaking these conditions in terms of public health significance. Although it is clearly necessary to address the problems of undernutrition, nutritional recommendations in less affluent countries must also take cognisance of this fact in order to ensure that CHD does not reach the epidemic proportions it has achieved in so many westernized nations (Shaper et al 1974, Yang et al 1988).

REFERENCES

Acheson RM, Williams DRR 1983 Does consumption of fruit and vegetables protect against stroke? Lancet i: 1191–1193

Agner E 1984 Some cardiovascular risk markers are also important in old age. Acta Medica Scandinavia i (Suppl 696) : 1–50

Anderson JW, Deakins DA, Bridges SR 1990 Soluble fibre: hypocholesterolemic effects and proposed mechanisms. In: Kritchevsky D (ed) Dietary fiber – chemistry, physiology and health effects. Plenum Press, New York, pp 339–347

Armstrong BK, Mann JI, Adelstein AM, Eskin F 1975 Commodity consumption and ischaemic heart disease mortality with special reference to dietary practices. Journal of Chronic Diseases 28: 455–469

Ball M, Mann JI 1986 Apoproteins: predictors of coronary heart disease? British Medical Journal 293: 769–770

Banaona E, Lieber CS 1975 Effects of ethanol on lipid metabolism. Journal of Lipid Research 20: 289–315

Bang HO, Dyerberg J, Sinclair HM 1980 The composition of the Eskimo food in north western Greenland. American Journal of Clinical Nutrition 33: 2657–2661

Beaglehole R, Hay DR, Foster FH, Sharpe DN 1981 Trends in coronary heart disease mortality and associated risk factors in New Zealand. New Zealand Medical Journal 93: 371–375

Beilin LJ, Rouse IL, Armstrong BK et al 1988 Vegetarian diet and blood pressure levels: incidental or causal association? American Journal of Clinical Nutrition 48: 806–810

Bonanome A, Grundy SM 1988 Effect of dietary stearic acid on plasma cholesterol and lipoprotein levels. New England Journal of Medicine 318: 1244–1248

Broitman SA 1988 Dietary cholesterol, serum cholesterol and colon cancer: a review. Advances in Experimental Medical Biology 206: 137–152

Burr ML, Butland BK 1988 Heart disease in British vegetarians. American Journal of Clinical Nutrition 48 (Suppl): 830–832

Burr ML, Gilbert JF, Holliday RM et al 1989 Effects of changes in fat, fish and fibre intakes on death and myocardial reinfarction: Diet and Reinfarction Trial. Lancet ii: 757–761

Cappucio FP, MacGregor GA 1991 Does potassium supplementation lower blood pressure? A meta-analysis of published trials. Journal of Hypertension 9: 465–473

Castelli WP 1986 The triglyceride issue: a view from Framingham. American Heart Journal 112: 432–437

Cox KL, Puddley IB, Morton AR et al 1990 Controlled comparison of effects of exercise and alcohol on blood pressure and serum HDL cholesterol in sedentary men. Clinical and Experimental Pharmacology and Physiology 17: 251–255

Crawford MA 1987 The requirements of long-chain *n*-6 and *n*-3 fatty acids for the brain. In: Lands WEM (ed) Short course on polyunsaturated fatty acids and eicosanoids. American Oil Chemistry Society Biloxi, MI, pp. 270–295

Dayton S, Pearce ML, Hashimoto S et al 1969 A controlled trial of a diet high in unsaturated fat in preventing complications of atherosclerosis. Circulation 39/40 (Suppl II): 1–63

Department of Health 1984 Diet and Cardiovascular Disease. Report on health and social subjects, No 28. HMSO, London

Department of Health 1989 Dietary sugars and human disease. Reports on health and social subjects, No 37. HMSO, London

Department of Health 1991 Dietary reference values for food, energy and nutrients for the United Kingdom. Report on health and social subjects, No 41. HMSO, London

Descovich GC, Ceredi C, Gaddi A et al 1980 Multicentre study of soybean protein diet for outpatient hypercholesterolaemic patients. Lancet ii: 709–712

Duthie GG, Wahle KWJ, James WPT 1989 Oxidants, anti-oxidants and cardiovascular disease. Nutrition Research Review 2: 51–62

Dwyer T, Hetzel BS 1980 A comparison of trends of coronary heart disease mortality in Australia, USA and England and Wales with reference to three major risk factors – hypertension, cigarette smoking and diet. International Journal of Epidemiology 9: 65–71

Ederer F, Leren P, Turpeinen O, Frantz ID 1971 Cancer among men on cholesterol-lowering diets: experience from five clinical trials. Lancet ii: 203–206

Edington JD, Geekie M, Carter R et al 1987 Effect of dietary cholesterol concentration in subjects following reduced-fat high-fibre diet. British Medical Journal 294: 333–336

Edington JD, Geekie M, Carter R et al 1989 Serum lipid response to dietary cholesterol in subjects fed a low-fat high-fibre diet. American Journal of Clinical Nutrition 50: 58–62

Editorial 1988 Fish oil. Lancet i: 1081–1083

Elkan W, Buxton M, O'Brien B 1988 Coronary heart disease: Economic aspects of prevention. Lipid Review 2: 41–46

Farquhar JW, Maccaby N, Wood PD et al 1977 Community education for cardiovascular health. Lancet 1: 1192–1195

Fisher M, Devine PM, Weiner PH 1986 The potential clinical benefits of fish consumption. Archives of Internal Medicine 146: 2322–2333

Glieberman L 1973 Blood pressure and dietary salt in human populations. Ecology of Food and Nutrition 2: 143–156

Gofman JW, Young W, Tandy R 1966 Ischaemic heart disease, atherosclerosis and longevity. Circulation 34: 679–197

Gordon DJ, Prebstfield JL, Garison RJ et al 1989 High-density lipoprotein cholesterol and cardiovascular disease. Four prospective American studies. Circulation 79: 8–15

Gordon T, Kannel WB, Castelli WP, Dawber TR 1981 Lipoproteins, cardiovascular disease and death. The Framingham Study. Archives of Internal Medicine 141: 1128–1131

Grundy SM 1986 Comparison of monounsaturated fatty acids and carbohydrates for lowering plasma cholesterol. New England Journal of Medicine 314: 745–748

Haskell WL, Camargo C, Williams PT et al 1984 The effect of cessation and resumption of moderate alcohol intake on serum high-density lipoprotein subfractions. New England Journal of Medicine 310: 805–810

Hegsted DM, McGrandy RB, Myer ML et al 1965 Quantitative effects of dietary fat on serum cholesterol in man. American Journal of Clinical Nutrition 17: 281–295

Hjermann I, Byre K, Holme I et al 1981 Effect of diet and smoking intervention on the incidence of coronary heart disease. Lancet ii: 1303–1310

Hjermann I, Holme I, Leren P 1986 Oslo study diet and antismoking trial: results after 102 months. American Journal of Medicine 80 (Suppl 2A): 7–11

Holme 1990 An effect of randomised trials evaluating the effect of cholesterol reduction on total mortality and coronary heart disease incidence. Circulation 82: 1916–1924

Horlick K 1959 Studies on the regulation of serum cholesterol levels in man: the effects of corn oil, ethyl stearate, hydrogenated soybean oil and nicotinic acid when added to a very low-fat based diet. Laboratory Investigation 8: 723–735

Hornstra G 1989 Dietary lipids, platelet function and arterial thrombosis. Wiener Klinica Wochenschr 101: 272–277

Hornstra G, Lessenberg RN 1975 Relationship between the type of dietary fatty acid and the arterial thrombus tendency in rats. Atherosclerosis 22: 499–516

Hughson WG, Mann JI, Garrod A 1978 Intermittent claudication: prevalence and risk factors. British Medical Journal 1: 1379–1381

Intersalt Cooperative Research Group 1988 Intersalt: an international study of electrolyte excretion and blood pressure. Results for 24-hour urinary sodium and potassium excretion. British Medical Journal 297: 319–328

Isles CG, Hole JH, Gillis CR et al 1989 Plasma cholesterol, coronary heart disease and cancer in the Renfrew and Paisley survey. British Medical Journal 298: 920–924

Jenkins DJA, Rainey-Macdonald CG, Jenkins AL, Benn G 1986 Fibre in the treatment of hyperlipidemia. In: Spiller G (ed) CRC handbook of dietary fibre in human nutrition. CRC Press, Boca Raton, Florida, pp 327–344

Judd PA, Truswell AS 1985 Dietary fibre and blood lipids in man. In: Leeds A, Avenell A (eds) Dietary fibre perspectives: reviews and bibliography. John Libbey, London, pp 23–39

Junshi C, Campbell TC, Junyao L, Peto R 1990. Diet, life-style and mortality in China, a study of the characteristics of 65 Chinese counties. Oxford University Press, Oxford

Keys A 1980 Seven Countries: a multivariate analysis of death and coronary heart disease. Harvard University Press, Cambridge Massachusetts

Keys A, Anderson JT, Grande F 1965a Serum cholesterol response to changes in the diet I. Iodine value of dietary fat versus 2S-P. Metabolism 14: 747–758

Keys A, Anderson JT, Grande F 1965b Serum cholesterol response to changes in the diet. IV. Particularly saturated fatty acids in the diet. Metabolism 14: 776–787

Keys A, Anderson JT, Grande F 1977 Prediction of serum cholesterol responses of man to changes in fats in the diet. Lancet 2: 959–966

Keys A, Menotti A, Karvonen MJ et al 1986 The diet and 15-year death rate in the Seven Countries Study. American Journal of Epidemiology 124: 903–915

Klatsky AL, Armstrong MA, Friedman G et al 1988 The relations of alcoholic beverage use to colon and rectal cancer. American Journal of Epidemiology 128: 1007–1015

Kromhout D, Bosschieter EB, Coulander D 1985 The inverse relation between fish consumption and 20-year mortality from coronary heart disease. New England Journal of Medicine 312: 1205–1209

Lagarde M 1990 Metabolism of n-3/n-6 fatty acids in blood and vascular cells. Biochemical Society Transactions 18: 770–772

Lagarde M, Guichardant M, Dechavanne M 1981 Human platelet PGE, and dihomogammalinolenic acid. Comparison to PGE$_2$ and arachidonic acid. Progress in Lipid Research 20: 439–443

Law MR, Fost CD, Wald NJ 1991 By how much does dietary salt reduction lower blood pressure? British Medical Journal 302: 811–815, 815–818, 819–824

Leadbetter J, Ball MJ, Mann JI 1991 Effect of increasing quantities of oat bran in hypercholesterolaemic people. American Journal of Clinical Nutrition 54: 841–845

Lewis B 1987 Disorders of lipid transport. In: Weatherall DJ, Ledingham JGG, Warrel DA (eds) The Oxford textbook of medicine. Oxford University Press, Oxford

Lewis B 1991 Safety aspects of cholesterol lowering. Lipid Review 5: 45–47

Lewis B, Mann J, Mancini M 1986 Reducing the risks of coronary heart disease in individuals and in the population. Lancet 1: 956–959

McGregor L, Morazain R, Renaud S 1980 A comparison of the effects of dietary short- and long-chain saturated fatty acids on platelet functions, platelet phospholipids, and blood coagulation in rats. Laboratory Investigation 43: 438–442

MacIntyre DE, Hoover RL, Smith M et al 1984 Inhibition of platelet function by cis-unsaturated fatty acids. Blood 63: 848–857

Mann JI 1984 Lines to legumes: changing concepts of diabetic diets. Diabetes Medicine 1: 191–198

Mann JI, Lewis B, Shepherd J et al 1988 Blood lipid concentrations and other cardiovascular risk factors: distribution, prevalence and detection in Britain. British Medical Journal 296: 1702–1706

Mansell P, Reckless JPD 1991 Garlic: effects on serum lipids, blood pressure, coagulation, platelet aggregation and vasodilation. British Medical Journal 303: 379–380

Marmot M, Brunner E 1991 Alcohol and cardiovascular disease: the status of the U-shaped curve. British Medical Journal 303: 565–568

Martin MJ, Hulley SB, Browner WS et al 1986 Serum cholesterol, blood pressure and mortality: implications from a cohort of 361 662 men. Lancet 2: 933–936

Maserei JRC, Rouse IL, Lynch WJ et al 1984 Effects of a lacto-ovovegetarian diet on serum concentration of cholesterol, triglyceride, HDL-C, HDL$_2$-C, HDL$_3$-C, apoprotein-β and Lp(a). American Journal of Clinical Nutrition 40: 468–479

Mattson FH, Grundy SM 1985 Comparison of effects of saturated, monounsaturated and polyunsaturated fatty acids on plasma lipids and lipoproteins in man. Journal of Lipid Research 26: 194–202

Meade TW, North WRS 1977 Population based on distributions of haemostatic variables. British Medical Journal Bulletin 33: 283–288

Meade TW, North WRS, Chakrabarti R et al 1980 Haemostatic function and cardiovascular death. Lancet 1: 1050–1054

Meade TW, Vickers MV, Thompson SG et al 1985 The epidemiological characteristics of platelet aggregatibility. British Medical Journal 290: 428–432

Mensink RP, Katan MB 1990 Effects of dietary trans fatty acids on high-density and low-density lipoprotein cholesterol levels in healthy subjects. New England journal of Medicine 323: 439–445

Miettinen TA, Nakkarinen V, Huttunen JK et al 1982 Fatty acid composition of serum lipids predicts myocardial infarction. British Medical Journal 285: 993–996

Miller GV, Cruickshank JK, Ellis LJ et al 1989 Fat consumption and factor VII coagulant activity in middle aged men. An association between a dietary and thrombogenic risk factor. Atherosclerosis 78: 19–24

Morris JN, Marr JW, Clayton DG 1977 Diet and heart: a postcript. British Medical Journal 2: 1307–1314

Muldoon MF, Mannicle SB, Andrews KA 1990 Lowering cholesterol concentrations and mortality: a quantitative review of primary prevention trials. British Medical Journal 301: 309–314

Multiple Risk Factor Intervention Trial Research Group 1982 Multiple Risk Factor Intervention Trial: risk factor changes and mortality results. Journal of the American Medical Association 248: 1465–1477

Nutrition Task Force 1991 The report of the Nutrition Task Force to the Department of Health. Shortcut Publishing, Wellington, pp. 1–189

O'Dea K, Steel M, Naughton J 1988 Butter-enriched diets reduce arterial prostacyclin production in rats. Lipids 23: 234–241

Oliver MF 1991 Might treatment of hypercholesterolaemia increase non-cardiac mortality? Lancet 337: 1529–1531

Ornish D, Brown SE, Sherwitz LW et al 1990 Can lifestyle changes reverse coronary heart disease? Lancet 336: 129–133

Parthasarathy S, Kloo JC, Miller E et al 1990 Low-density lipoprotein rich in oleic acid is protected against oxidative modification: implications for dietary prevention in atherosclerosis. Proceedings of the National Acadamy of Science USA 87: 3894–3898

Peto R, Yusuf S, Collins R 1987 Cholesterol-lowering trial results in their epidemiologic context. Circulation 75 (Suppl 2): 451

Phillips RL, Kuzma JW, Beeson WL, Letz T 1980 Influence of selection versus lifestyle on risk of fatal cancer and cardiovascular disease among Seventh Day Adventists. American Journal of Epidemiology 112: 296–314

Qizilbash N, Jones L, Warlow C, Mann JI 1991 Fibrinogen and lipid concentrations as risk factors for transient ischaemic attacks and minor ischaemic strokes. British Medical Journal 303: 605–609

Rao GHR, Radha E, White JG 1983 Effect of docosahexaenoic acid on arachidonic acid metabolism and platelet function. Biochemical and Biophysical Research Communications 117: 549–555

Reisin E, Abel R, Madan M et al 1978 Effect of weight loss without salt restriction on the reduction of blood pressure in overweight hypertensive patients. New England Journal of Medicine 298: 1–6

Renaud S, Morazain R, Godsey F et al 1986 Nutrients,

platelet function and composition in nine groups of French and British farmers. Atherosclerosis 60: 37–48

Riemersma RA, Wood FA, Butler S et al 1986 Linoleic acid content in adipose tissue and platelet fatty acids and coronary heart disease. British Medical Journal 292: 1423–1427

Ritz E, Schnid M, Guo JZ et al 1988 Salt and the action of Ca antagonists. Journal of Cardiovascular Pharmacol 12 (Suppl. 6): 533–536

Rosengren A, Wilhelmsen L, Eriksson E et al 1990 Lipoprotein (a) and coronary heart disease: a prospective case control study in a general population sample of middle aged men. British Medical Journal 301: 1248–1251

Shaper AG, Hutt MSR et al (eds) 1974 Cardiovascular disease in the tropics. British Medical Association, London

Shaper AG, Phillips AN, Pocock SJ et al 1991 Risk factors for stroke in middle aged British men. British Medical Journal 302: 1111–1115

Shekelle RB et al 1981 Diet, serum cholesterol and death from coronary heart disease: the Western Electric Study. New England Journal of Medicine 304: 65–70

Shepherd J, Packard CJ, Patsch JR et al 1978 Effects of dietary polyunsaturated and saturated fat on the properties of high-density lipoproteins and the metabolism of apolipoprotein A-1. Journal of Clinical Investigation 61: 1582–1592

Sigfusson N, Sigvaldason H, Steingrimsdottir L et al 1991 Decline in ischaemic heart disease in Iceland and change in risk factor levels. British Medical Journal 302: 1371–1375

Sinclair HM 1984 Essential fatty acids in perspective. Human Nutrition. Clinical Nutrition 38C: 245–260

Stamler I 1979 Population studies. In: Levy RI, Rifkind BM, Dennis BH, Ernst N (eds) Nutrition, lipids and coronary heart disease. Raven Press, New York, pp 25–88

Swain JF, Rouse IL, Curley CB, Sacks FM 1990 Comparison of the effects of oat bran and low fibre wheat on serum lipoprotein levels and blood pressure. New England Journal of Medicine 322: 147–152

Swales JD 1991 Salt substitutes and potassium intake. British Medical Journal 303: 1084–1085

Sytkowski PA, Kannel WB, D'Agostino RB 1990 Changes in risk factors and the decline in mortality from cardiovascular disease. The Framingham heart study. New England Journal of Medicine 322: 1635–1641

Thelle DS, Heyden S, Foder JG 1987 Coffee and cholesterol in epidemiological and experimental studies. Atherosclerosis 67: 97–103

Thorogood M, Carter R, Benfield L et al 1987 Plasma lipids and lipoprotein cholesterol concentrations in people with different diets in Britain. British Medical Journal 295: 351–353

Thorogood M, Roe L, McPherson K, Mann J 1990 Dietary intake and plasma lipid levels: lessons from a study of the diet of health-conscious groups. British Medical Journal 300: 1297–1301

Tornberg SA, Holm LE, Cartensen JM et al 1986 Risks of cancer of the colon and rectum in relation to serum cholesterol and beta lipoprotein. New England Journal of Medicine 315: 1629–1633

Truswell AS, Mann JI 1972 Epidemiology of serum lipids in Southern Africa. Atherosclerosis 16: 15–19

Tuomilehto, Geboers J, Salonen T et al 1986 Decline in cardiovascular mortality in North Karelia and other parts of Finland. British Medical Journal 293: 1068–1071

Uemura K, Pisa Z 1988 Trends in cardiovascular disease mortality in industrialised countries since 1950. World Health Status Quo 41: 155–178

Ulbricht TLV, Southgate DAT 1991 Coronary heart disease: seven dietary factors. Lancet 338: 985–992

van Raaij JMA, Katan MB, West CE et al 1982 Influence of diets containing casein, soy isolate and soy concentrate on serum cholesterol and lipoproteins in middle-aged volunteers. American Journal of Clinical Nutrition 35: 925–934

Watts GF, Ahmed W, Quing J et al 1988 Effective lipid-lowering diets including lean meat. British Medical Journal 296: 235–237

Weatherall DJ, Warrell DA, Ledingham JGG 1987 (eds) Oxford Textbook of Medicine, 2nd edn, Vol II, Sections 13.138 and 13.167. Oxford University Press, Oxford

West KM, Ahuva MMS, Bennet PF 1983, The role of circulating glucose and triglyceride concentrations and their interactions with other 'risk factors' as determinants of arterial disease in nine diabetic population samples from the WHO multinational study. Diabetic Care 6: 361–369

WHO Expert Committee 1982 Prevention of coronary heart disease. Technical Report series. World Health Organization, Geneva

WHO Collaborative Group 1983 Multifactorial trial in the prevention of coronary heart disease :3. Incidence and mortality rates. European Heart Journal 4: 141–147.

Yang G, Chen J, Wen Z, Ge K, Khu L, Chen X, Chen X 1988 The role of selenium in Keshan disease. Advances in Nutritional Research 6: 203–231

42. Diet in relation to the nervous system

T. Westermarck and E. Antila

The purpose of this chapter is to provide general information concerning nutrients essential for the nervous system, and particularly its development and function. There is evidence that dietary elements or their absence influence the brain's neurochemistry, and even behaviour. Many questions remain on how diet influences the progress of neurological and neuropsychiatric disorders. Individual susceptibility to these effects also suggests that both genetic and environmental factors are involved in the aetiology and pathogenesis of neurological diseases.

DEVELOPMENT

Normal fetal development involves the production of a vast number of cells in the brain, and soon after birth this cell division stops. The brain continues to develop, however, as the cells migrate, organize and myelinate. The proliferation period of the neurons is complete by mid-pregnancy, while cell migration within the cerebral cortex is completed by the time an infant is 5 months of age. The neuronal organizational phase begins in mid-pregnancy and continues for several years postnatally.

The neurons produce cell extensions or neurites, which may be the principal component of the cell, i.e. as axons of great length. In addition, multiple small extensions or dendrites grow to interact with other neural cells. This dendritic development depends on the degree and nature of afferent stimulation of the brain and on the availability of nutrients to support the continued processing of dendritic development. The major period of intense neuronal development and interaction occurs from mid-gestation, when cell division stops, to about the age of 2 years. General brain maturation continues, however, until the age of 20 years in women and 25 years in men.

The adult brain has 100 billion neurons and an equal number of the supporting structural or glial cells. In the cortex alone there are 20 billion neurons and 40 billion glial cells. This minority of brain cells controls most of the function of the central nervous system. Each neuron develops 1000–10 000 connections – or synapses – with other cells, and receives input from about 1000 other neuronal synapses. Glial cells do not possess axons or synapses. They normally divide up to about 2 years of age, but retain the potential to divide throughout life. There are two groups of glial cells: the macroglia, which include the astrocytes and oligodendrocytes, and the smaller microglia, which act as macrophages in the brain (Davison 1981). The astrocytes are located close to the blood vessels and their projections surround the vessel, perhaps thereby controlling the nutrient supply to the brain. The oligodendrocytes synthesize and maintain the myelin sheath in the white matter of the brain, but serve as neuronal satellite cells within the grey matter of the brain. The myelin of the peripheral nerves is produced, however, by the Schwann cells.

The process of myelination involves the secretion of up to 40 layers of lipid-rich membrane, which surround each axon. This sheath is important for electrically insulating the axons and thereby allowing neuronal stimulus to pass down the axon. The myelin accounts for a high proportion of the white matter, and contains about 30% protein. The remainder consists of phospholipid, some cholesterol and glycolipids, e.g. galactocerebroside, which is a sphingoglycolipid important in myelin metabolism and found to be especially limited in immature brains. The n-3 and n-6 fatty acid content of both the myelin and the other membranes of the brain is high, and places unusual demands on the supply of these long-chain (C_{24} and C_{26}) polyunsaturated fatty acids during fetal life and in the first year or two of postnatal

651

development. The need for dihomo-γ-linolenic acid ($C_{20:3}$) and for arachidonic acid ($C_{20:4}$) derived from linoleic acid ($C_{18:2}$) is also important in the structure and function of cerebral membranes.

Myelin and the neuronal and glial cells are also rich in protein, so the demand for appropriate nutrients during fetal cell proliferation and postnatal brain maturation is relatively high. Thereafter, brain myelin, lipid and protein turnover require the provision of new substrates for maintaining brain structures. Nutrients are also required for the provision of energy for cellular metabolism and for the synthesis of a complex series of molecules which serve as neuro-transmitters in the interplay of neuronal activity throughout the brain. Understanding the effects of nutrition on brain development and function is therefore complex and a neglected area. In this chapter some attempt will be made to rationalize the numerous changes in brain function and behaviour in nutritional disorders, but our understanding remains primitive.

BRAIN METABOLISM

The brain is metabolically very active, accounting for about 20–30% of the body's resting metabolic rate. The brain's energy requirement varies from birth to old age, as does its blood flow. The newborn brain can withstand hypoxia for a longer time than in adulthood. The cerebral oxygen consumption, which is rather low at birth, rises during childhood and cerebral blood flow and oxygen uptake is highest at the age of 6 years, when the brain consumes over 60 ml O_2/min – more than 50% of total body basal oxygen consumption. In the adult brain of 1400 g, oxygen uptake is about 49 ml O_2/min.

The brain's high energy need is due to the mature neurons' requirement for a continuous supply of energy to maintain their function, with an appropriate transmembrane electrical potential in each of the huge number of extremely active cells. The neurons themselves have only a minimal substrate store of glycogen, which has in any case a rapid turnover. Glucose is the main energy substrate for both synthetic and functional activities of the central and peripheral nervous system. The glucose crosses the blood–brain barrier by facilitated transport involving a hexose-specific carrier. About one-fifth of the glucose in the arterial flow to the brain is taken up for metabolic purposes. Over 50% of the glucose meta-bolized by the brain during the first month of life passes via the hexose monophosphate shunt to supply both ribose molecules for nucleic acid synthesis and

NADPH (the reduced form of nicotinamide adenine dinucleotide phosphate) for lipid synthesis.

Glucose is the normal fuel for the brain at all ages. The newborn child may transiently be hypoglycaemic. They are not generally ketotic, but can produce ketones from their own body fat. Breast milk is high in fat, and is able to supply a substrate for ketogenesis. The developing brain has a great ability to take up and utilize ketones from the blood, and during the neonatal period these are an important source of energy for the brain. When weaned on to the normally relatively high-carbohydrate diet, cerebral ketone utilization disappears. Normally, aerobic respiration is dominant, with 90% of brain glucose being meta-bolized through the glycolytic pathway. Only a small part of pyruvate is then transferred to lactate. The principal part of glucose is converted to carbon dioxide and water in the citric acid cycle; the γ-aminobutyrate shunt bypasses the succinyl-CoA step in the Krebs cycle (see below and Chapter 8).

The catabolism of amino acids contributes less than 10% of the total energy supply of the brain. Most of the amino acids are required for the synthesis of proteins, peptides and certain neurotransmitters. Nervous tissue can synthesize some amino acids in situ, but all essential amino acids pass from the blood across the blood–brain barrier. The amino acids pass into nerve cells by diffusion and carrier-mediated transport, and nutritional factors can moderate this transfer and influence brain metabolism (see below).

The brain contains about 8% of its wet weight as protein, and the accumulation of protein is linear from 6 months of gestation until the second postnatal year, when it begins to slow. Biosynthesis of brain protein depends upon a continuous supply of amino acids. In the first few months of life the plasma concentrations of amino acids are to a great extent determined by the protein content of the feed. The amino acids of human milk protein are present in approximately the proportions necessary for tissue synthesis, but cysteine, taurine and tryptophan are present in higher levels. The level of free amino acids in brain is similar to that in plasma, with a few exceptions: there are much higher levels of glutamine, aspartate, N-acetylaspartate, and γ-butyric acid (GABA) in brain than plasma. The transmitters glutamate, GABA and glycine are released at approx-imately 90% of the synapses in the mammalian brain. The dominant excitatory neurotransmitter glutamate is of particular interest, when its post-synaptic recep-tors are implicated in pathways of memory and learning and mechanisms of ischaemic brain damage (Nicholls 1992).

NUTRITIONAL ABNORMALITIES AND BRAIN DEVELOPMENT

Given the fact that the brain has a critical period for its anatomical, biochemical and physiological development, it is not surprising that nutritional factors are increasingly recognized as important in determining brain function, particularly during fetal and early postnatal life. The vulnerable period extends throughout gestation and infancy. The effects of an extrinsic and harmful agent, such as a teratogenic drug, fetal hypoxia or malnutrition, depend largely on the timing of damage in relation to the stage of brain development. For example, there may be a vulnerable period for myelination, with the fetus showing sensitivity to external factors such as maternal malnutrition and placental insufficiency. However, in placental insufficiency associated with intrauterine growth retardation, the human brain is affected much less than other organs.

Developmental disturbances in the brain may result from many causes, including genetic factors and exposure to various teratogenic agents. Interference with any stage of brain development may then cause persisting intellectual and/or behavioural impairments. Nutritional deprivations seem to have particular effects on brain development from the last trimester of gestation until the second year of postnatal life. Subcortical functions are mature at birth, but higher cortical functions are present at birth only in immature form. Defective brain growth usually results in a reduced rate of growth of the head and, consequently, in a small head circumference. Microcephaly, i.e. a small head, resulting from a prenatal disorder is usually obvious at birth, but may sometimes only become evident later.

A prenatal developmental disorder of the brain may result in general functional defects of varying severity. The child may present with subnormal intelligence, but other specific cognitive deficits can occur with the preservation of normal general intelligence. Serious intellectual defects, such as mental deficiency, are usually obvious in the first year of life. Cognitive development depends on brain maturation, which continues until young adult life.

Specific nutrient deficiencies in the mother can also produce a variety of abnormalities in the development and function of the fetal brain. The early impact of a specific nutrient deficiency, e.g. folate, is seen with the development of neural tube defects (NTD) (Scott et al 1990). Included in the NTDs are spina bifida, where the neural tube fails to close at 4 weeks of fetal life, and anencephalus, where the forebrain fails to develop. There are also other conditions, such as encephalocele (hernial protrusion of the brain) and iniencephaly (brain matter protruding through a fissure in the occiput, generally associated with fissure of the vertebral column). Zinc deficiency may play a role in these conditions. These disorders seem to arise as a complex interplay between genetic and environmental factors. Thus female children are particularly affected in cases of anencephaly, for unknown reasons. The environmental influences are shown by the changing incidence of these problems, especially spina bifida and anencephaly, with variations being seen by season, year, region and decade of conception. Thus, in Britain and Ireland anencephalus and spina bifida show an excess incidence in babies conceived in the spring. Babies born with spina bifida show the highest rate of birth 2 months after babies having the maximum incidence of anencephalus. In populations with high NTD rates, the poorer classes have the highest incidence, but the prevalence rate of NTDs is falling worldwide, with new evidence suggesting that the availability of dietary folate plays a dominant role (see Chapters 14, 25 and 39).

Maternal illness also affects the incidence of NTD, thus diabetic mothers are particularly susceptible to NTD. One theory is that this is accounted for by a delayed switch from anaerobic to aerobic glucose metabolism in early uterine life because of the high prevailing glucose levels. This might then explain the failure of normal cell development and the induction of an NTD.

Experimental studies confirm the importance of an appropriate micronutrient intake. Rats fed folate-deficient diets supplemented with antifolates produce NTDs; vitamin B_{12} deficiency causes hydrocephalus, pyridoxal deficiency also causes NTD, as does pantothenic acid deficiency. Vitamin E deficiency may also cause NTDs in some species, and zinc deficiency has been found to increase the rate of hydrocephalus, but not NTDs (Scott et al 1990).

Vitamin A excess also leads to major abnormalities in fetal development. This teratogenic effect of excess vitamin A has led to advice for pregnant women in the UK to avoid eating liver which, under UK husbandry conditions, contains excess vitamin A derived from the animal feed.

The impact of iodine deficiency and the development of cretinism induced by the failure to produce the brain triiodothyroxine on which cellular development depends is set out in Chapter 36. The fetal alcohol syndrome is also described in Chapter 7. Mothers on phenytoin or phenobarbital may also produce babies with features similar to those with fetal alcohol syndrome, and drug-induced changes in folate absorption and metabolism have been suggested as an explanation (Yerby 1991). These possible anti-folate effects of drugs seem to occur later in fetal development than the more clearly defined effect of folate deficiency on the development of NTD (see Chapter 14).

The role of essential fatty acid deficiency in modulating brain development is receiving increasing attention (Neuringer et al 1988). Docosahexaenoic acid (22:6 n-3, or DHA) is produced by either the mother or the fetus from α-linolenic acid (18:3 n-3) by competing with the desaturase and elongation enzymes, which are also involved in the transformation of linoleic acid (18:2 n-6) to arachidonic acid, AA, (20:4 n-6). Both DHA and the other long-chain n-3 fatty acid, eicosapentaenoic acid (20:5 n-3, or EPA), are found in plentiful amounts in fish. Small amounts are obtained from leafy vegetables and some plant seeds, e.g. soy and rape seed. Increasing evidence suggests that the fetus in later pregnancy is dependent on the placental uptake of these long-chain n-3 fatty acids because of the limited capacity of the fetal liver or brain to produce enough DHA from α-linolenic acid. DHA and AA levels are higher in fetal blood than maternal blood, despite the fetus having lower plasma levels of α-linolenic and linoleic acids. Levels of DHA are so high in cerebral grey matter that DHA comprises up to a third of the total fatty acid content of ethanolamine and serine phospholipids. DHA is at its highest concentration in the synaptosomes and synaptic vesicles, and is also found in high concentrations in the retina. About half the adult DHA content of the brain and retina is deposited during fetal life. The DHA and arachidonate content of the cerebrum and cerebellum increase 3–5 times during the last trimester of pregnancy, with a similar increase in the first 3 months of infancy. Thus the provision of these fatty acids in the diet or from their precursors is crucial for both the fetus and infant.

After birth the milk of most mammals, including humans, provides a preformed source of DHA, but this is not present in current artificial milk formulae produced with bovine fat. Experimentally, diets deficient in EFAs tend to affect n-6 more than n-3 metabolism. In monkeys, n-3 deficiency in pregnancy leads to reduced visual acuity in the infants, and to abnormalities in the electroretinogram recordings of retinal activity. It is not surprising therefore that recent evidence suggests that prematurely born babies, who will have missed their late-pregnancy phase of DHA and other essential fatty acid accumulation in the brain, respond to feed supplements of fish oils rich in DHA.

They show changes in their electroretinograms, an enhanced growth in head circumference and accelerated functional development. These preliminary studies (Marabou Symposium 1992) are of great importance but need careful study. Studies with non-human primates show that DHA can rapidly be accumulated by the brain at 1–2 years of age in previously deficient young animals, but recovery does not occur in retinal function with this delayed therapy.

Effects of food deprivation and selective micronutrient deficiency on brain development and function in childhood

These issues have been dealt with in detail by Simeon and Grantham-McGregor (1990). Short-term food deprivation, e.g. missing breakfast, was considered in early US studies to lead to a deterioration in classroom behaviour (Tuttle et al 1946), but these well known studies were in practice poorly designed. More recent studies in the US and Jamaica suggest that for well nourished children, missing breakfast on a single occasion has only modest effects on school performance, although there are changes in the responses of both the central and autonomic nervous systems. In mildly malnourished children, however, the effects are more evident, with a deterioration in fluency and the efficiency of arithmetic problem-solving. When school feeding programmes are introduced for deprived groups there does seem to be some improvement in mental function, but the effects are subtle and surprisingly poorly documented.

In the acute phase of severe protein–energy malnutrition (PEM) mental changes are marked (see Chapter 30), with early changes in mood and responsiveness after the first few days of successful therapy. Nevertheless, malnourished children have very low development levels even after recovery and the long-term effects of PEM can be marked. Grantham-McGregor and colleagues (1991), however, in a series of major well controlled studies, showed that a substantial portion of the effect is also found in the children's siblings, who had not been severely malnourished. This suggests that familial or social factors are also very important, and distinguishing the specific effects of the illness from general social deprivation is not easy.

In mild to moderate cases of malnutrition there is a clear association between the degree of stunting in height and poor mental development by the time the child is of school age. By providing both nutritional supplements and training for mothers in simple play therapy as a social stimulus, Grantham-McGregor was able to show that interventions lasting a year produced substantial benefits. The food supplement improved locomotor development most, but both mental stimulation and food supplements were needed to produce the greatest benefit. Her recent follow-up studies suggest that this improvement may be sustained for many years after only 1–2 years' intervention and training. This suggests that brain function is still very plastic in early childhood, and that the critical period for brain development is not simply confined to fetal life and early infancy.

IRON DEFICIENCY

The severity and duration of iron deficiency influence brain development. The brain seems to be most sensitive to iron deficiency during the first 2 years of life, which produces long-term consequences. There is increasing evidence that children over 2 years of age with moderate iron deficiency in developing countries improve their mental function and school achievement if their anemia is corrected by iron supplementation. Detailed experiments with young children (Pollitt et al 1989) strongly support the view that prophylactic iron supplements in early infancy improve subsequent mental performance in children in developing countries. The effects are less striking in developed country studies. Nevertheless, these findings, together with animal experimental evidence showing the dependence of brain development and function on iron supply, strongly support the public health importance of ensuring an adequate iron status in both infancy and childhood (Simeon & Grantham-McGregor 1990).

AMINO ACID METABOLISM AND BRAIN FUNCTION

Table 42.1 lists some neurotransmitters and their precursor amino acids. Three features emphasize the significance of amino acids in determining brain function. Abnormalities of amino acid metabolism, with the accumulation of a specific amino acid or its catabolite, leads to brain damage and mental defects. By manipulating the diet to alter the transport of individual amino acids into the brain it is possible to alter both animal and human behaviour. This change in behaviour is preceded experimentally by altered synthesis rates of neurotransmitters from the precursor amino acids, so it has been inferred that the rate of

Table 42.1 Precursor amino acids for neurotransmitters

Precursor amino acids	Neurotransmitter
	Amino acids
As in transmitter	γ-amino butyrate (GABA)
	Glycine
	Aspartate
	Glutamate
	Acetylcholine
	Monoaminergic
Tyrosine	Dopamine
	Adrenaline
	Noradrenaline
Tryptophan	Serotonin
	Purinergic
	Adenosine
	ADP
	ATP
	AMP
Arginine	*Nitric oxide*
As in transmitter	*N-acetyl amino acids*
	N-acetyl peptides

cerebral amino acid uptake modulates neurotransmitter responses (Wurtman 1980). Uptake of tryptophan, phenylalanine and tyrosine occurs via a special transport system for the large neutral amino acids. Valine, leucine and isoleucine are transported by the same system. The ingestion of starch or sugar, which stimulates insulin secretion, will produce a selective fall in the plasma concentration of these branched-chain amino acids as they are transferred into muscle. This fall then allows the enhanced uptake of tryptophan and tyrosine into the brain. This mechanism, with the induced synthesis of 5-hydroxytryptamine (5HT) from tryptophan is proposed as an explanation for the increased drowsiness and mood changes after a carbohydrate-rich meal. 5HT is also now linked to the selective appetite drive for carbohydrate; drugs for appetite control, e.g. the fenfluramines and fluoxetines, have been developed to inhibit 5HT reuptake and therefore induce anorexia, particularly for carbohydrate-rich foods. Protein-rich meals paradoxically lower brain tryptophan levels, but brain tyrosine levels do rise and catecholamine formation may then also increase (Wurtman 1980). Patients with sleep disorders or depression have been treated with large doses of tryptophan to enhance serotonin but depress catecholamine synthesis. It is claimed that those patients with a low ratio of plasma tryptophan to large neutral amino acids benefit most from the treatment (Wurtman 1980), but many psychiatrists remain sceptical.

ABNORMALITIES OF AMINO ACID METABOLISM AND BRAIN FUNCTION

There is a series of amino acid metabolic disorders which lead to brain damage or mental disturbances. This is not surprising, given the importance of amino acid and protein metabolism in brain function. In utero the fetus normally has plasma concentrations 1.5–3 times those seen in the mother. The placenta has active transport systems for all the amino acids except cysteine, taurine, glutamic acid and aspartic acid. When the mother fasts the fetal concentrations change, with a fall in the essential amino acids and a rise in glycine concentrations. This has been likened to the pattern seen in kwashiorkor. Fetal tissues have not developed the capacity to metabolize amino acids well, because in utero the main route for use of fetal amino acids is in protein synthesis. The fetus is protected from high concentrations of an amino acid, e.g. phenylalanine, because any rise in amino acid concentrations will tend to be buffered by exchange of the amino acid across the placenta.

Phenylketonuria (see Chapter 47)

The microencephaly and mental retardation observed in phenylketonuria are well recognized but, with the now standard practice of screening newborns for this condition, it is possible to prevent mental retardation by maintaining babies and children on special diets with restricted phenylalanine intakes. Permanent damage may occur by 2–3 months of age without appropriate treatment. Blood levels should be maintained between 180 and 600 µmol/l (30–100 mg/l) for this, but care needs to be taken to ensure that phenylalanine deficiency is not induced. Phenylalanine deficiency is likely if plasma levels fall below 60 µmol/l, with the early clinical sign of reduced weight gain, feeding difficulties and nappy rash. Dystrophic changes in the skin, hair and nails then develop, with frequent infections, and if the condition is not treated, convulsions, mental retardation and death can occur. It is important therefore to maintain phenylalanine levels at the correct level to avoid mental deterioration. This control is crucial during infancy and childhood, but once brain development is complete dietary control is often considered less important (but see Chapter 47).

Adult women with phenylketonuria who conceive are very likely to have either spontaneous abortions, or babies with mental retardation, microencephaly, congenital heart disease and other organ defects. Both fetal and childhood brain development requires plasma and cerebral amino acids at their normal concentrations. Maternal plasma values have to be maintained below 250 µmol/l to prevent fetal values rising above 400 µmol/l (Krywawych et al 1991). If dietary restriction is reinstituted periconceptually, congenital heart disease is avoided but not if introduced at 2–3 months following conception, i.e. when the women recognizes she is pregnant. Head circumference and birthweight are related to the mother's phenylalanine concentration at conception, and good dietary control from the time of conception seems to allow normal fetal growth with little or no evidence of mental impairment in the offspring (Krywawych et al 1991).

Tyrosinemia (see Chapter 47)

In this inborn error there is a defect in tyrosine catabolism, with elevated tyrosine and sometimes phenylalanine concentrations. The babies fail to thrive and become mentally retarded, with behavioural abnormalities. Peripheral nerve abnormalities also develop. In the neonate dietary restriction and the use of ascorbic acid has been advocated.

Glycine, serine and threonine

Serine seems to be an important precursor for glycine in the brain, and rare conditions occur where glycine deficiency occurs. The babies become spastic but may respond to dietary glycine supplementation, which may affect the glycine-responsive receptors in the spinal cord. In patients with the adult progressive and fatal disease of amyotrophia lateral sclerosis, there is a reduced number of glycinergic receptors. Some improvement occurs with 2–4 g/day threonine; threonine experimentally increases the glycine content of the spinal cord (Roufs 1991).

Other amino acid abnormalities

Table 42.1 shows a range of amino acid precursors of neurotransmitters and there is increasing interest in manipulating the diet to assess their usefulness in a variety of brain disorders. Thus 60% of patients with epilepsy are found to have a reduced ability to synthesize γ-aminobutyric acid (GABA) in those regions of the brain responsible for the seizures. GABA is known to be an inhibitory neurotransmitter, but whether this reduced synthetic capacity is a primary phenomenon is not known.

MICRONUTRIENTS AND BRAIN FUNCTION

An adequate supply of both vitamins and minerals is essential for normal brain function. The clinical syndromes associated with the deficiency diseases are set out in Chapters 12, 13, 14 and 36, so only the behavioural aspects will be dealt with here. The brain requires micronutrients for their normal role as constituents of brain tissue and for normal metabolism, but some may be specifically needed for their free radical scavenging role in the brain, which is such a highly metabolically active organ. Thus vitamin C concentrations are 4–10 times higher in the brain than the plasma and may have an important antioxidative role in the retina and lens, preventing or delaying the development of age-related retinal atrophy and cataract. Other vitamins also play a crucial cofactor role in metabolic pathways of particular importance in the brain, e.g. in neurotransmitter synthesis. Vitamin C has also been described as being needed for the binding of serotonin to its receptors. Thus the micronutrients have many functions in the normal metabolism of the brain.

Thiamin

Thiamin deficiency interferes with the synthesis of the neurotransmitter amino acids glutamate and aspartate, as well as being crucially involved in the glucose metabolism on which the brain normally depends. The infantile form of beriberi seen in babies breastfeeding from mothers on a deficient diet may be acute, and occurs in association with cardiac failure. It may simulate meningitis because the baby becomes irritable, vomits, and may convulse, with a bulging fontanelle and nystagmus. A less severe form may simulate the Wernicke–Korsakoff syndrome (see Chapter 7). In developed countries this is rarely seen, and takes the form of a subacute encephalo-myelopathy (Haas 1988).

In older children and adults the progressive loss of the sense of vibration, with paraesthesia and a burning sensation in the feet, is the first symptom of peripheral neuritis. The motor paralysis and loss of tendon reflexes develop later.

Alcoholics often develop thiamin deficiency which, when severe, leads to the range of Wernicke–Korsakoff disorders (see Chapter 7). In epileptics treated long-term with phenytoin there is a substantial risk of thiamin deficiency developing unrelated to alcohol, and a prevalence of 25% has been reported (Keyser & De Brujin 1991). Thiamin therapy may also help alter the CNS signs in children with some forms of maple syrup urine disease; this implies that some of their metabolic features may be corrected by unusually high thiamin intakes.

Pyridoxine

Pyridoxine is essential for the synthesis or metabolism of almost all neurotransmitters. It is also critical in the synthesis of many hormones, e.g. insulin and growth hormone.

Pyridoxine deficiency disorders are characterized by fatigue, nervousness, irritability, depression, insomnia and walking difficulties. In adults dizziness, peripheral neuritis, neuralgia and carpal tunnel syndrome, induced by connective-tissue swelling at the wrist, can also appear.

Many years ago it was shown that infants fed milk substitutes which were pyridoxine-deficient developed irritability and convulsive seizures. The disorder was successfully treated with pyridoxine. This illustrates the need for dietary pyridoxine in early infancy.

Increased requirement for pyridoxine

A number of unusual genetic disorders seem to benefit from pharmacological doses of pyridoxine. Infantile spasms, or West's syndrome (sudden brief flexion of neck and trunk and raising of both arms), is a rare genetic disorder which leads to seizures and mental retardation in infancy, boys being more frequently affected than girls. A rapid therapeutic response to a high dose of 500 mg pyridoxine may be seen in these children. Testing the response of babies with neonatal seizures may, however, be dangerous, since this dose of pyridoxine may induce hypotonia, requiring assistance with ventilation. The dose is huge compared with a child's usual requirement of 0.3–0.9 mg/day. Abnormalities of pyridoxine and tryptophan metabolites have been reported in Down's syndrome, but pyridoxine therapy is of uncertain benefit. It has also been reported that long-term anticonvulsive therapy with phenytoin or succinimide has been associated with reduced plasma levels of pyridoxine, but in this case only modest supplements with pyridoxine seem to be needed.

Homocystinuria (see Chapter 47) is an inborn error of methionine catabolism involving cystathione synthase deficiency, which results in mental retardation. Convulsions have been reported in 10–15% of the cases. Marked biochemical and clinical improvement has been reported to occur in some patients after the administration of pyridoxine. The effective dose of vitamin B_6 has ranged from 50 to 500 mg/day. If the children fail to respond, a low-methionine diet is also of considerable value if started in the newborn period. The rise in homocystine generated from methionine catabolism may then be prevented, as homocystine oxidation matches methionine catabolism. Another form of homocystinuria involves a defect in the remethylation of homocysteine and a deficiency of the methyl groups for the formation of *S*-adenosylmethionine. The clinical presentation varies with the precise biochemical abnormality, but additional folic acid and vitamin B_{12}, in addition to pyridoxine and a low-methionine diet, may ensure that the plasma homocysteine levels do not rise, thrombosis is not accelerated and it is possible to prevent the clinical features of homocystinuria from developing (Brett & Smith 1991).

Pyridoxine deficiency induced by drugs

A number of hydrazine-derived drugs, when used long-term, induce even in adults pyridoxine deficiency symptoms such as irritability, peripheral neuropathy and convulsions. Examples include the antidepressant drugs iproniazid, nialamide and isocarboxazid; the monoamine oxidase (MAO) inhibitor phenalzine; the anticancer drug procarbazine; the antihypertensive drug hydralazine; and the antituberculosis drug isonicotinylhydrazine (INH). Penicillamine and cycloserine may also bind and inactivate pyridoxine. Patients taking these drugs and drinking excessive alcohol may also increase their need for vitamin B_6, a need which can be met effectively with pyridoxine supplementation.

Isoniazid treatment of tuberculous patients results in pyridoxine deficiency. Isoniazid pyridoxine hydrazone is excreted in the urine in amounts sufficient to deplete body stores of pyridoxal phosphate. The peripheral neuropathy that may occur in these patients responds to oral pyridoxine, and the vitamin supplement does not reduce the pharmaceutical effect of INH. Pyridoxine at 10 mg/day is recommended during long-term treatment with isoniazid.

Oral contraceptives with a high progesterone content may induce depression, as a side effect due to disturbed tryptophan metabolism. The excretion of tryptophan metabolites is normalized by an administration of 20 mg pyridoxine (Dickerson 1988). An induction of tryptophan pyrrolase is probably the explanation. This enzyme is the rate-limiting enzyme in the nicotinic acid pathway, and pyridoxine is utilized for the synthesis of nicotinic acid at the expense of the serotonin pathways, thus interfering

with the synthesis of this neurotransmitter. Only those women showing evidence of a disturbance in tryptophan metabolism respond to vitamin B_6 supplementation.

Corticosteroid treatment of long duration may also result in depression, and it has been suggested that this depression may be prevented by vitamin B_6 supplementation. Controlled trials to test these reports are not available, however.

Side effects of overdoses

It has been reported that a daily ingestion of 100–1000 mg pyridoxine may impair memory. Ingestion of large doses of pyridoxine also nullifies the beneficial effect of L-dopa in the control of Parkinson's disease. This effect seems to depend on pyridoxine accelerating the decarboxylation of L-dopa to dopamine in extracerebral tissues. This then reduces the amount of L-dopa entering the brain to replenish striatal dopamine, which is deficient in Parkinson's disease.

Vitamin B_{12} (see Chapter 14)

Vitamin B_{12} not only interacts with folate metabolism (see Chapter 14), but it is also required as a coenzyme for the conversion of methylmalonyl coenzyme A to succinyl coenzyme A in the citric acid cycle. Deoxyadenosyl vitamin B_{12} is essential for the last step. This reaction serves to reduce the plasma level of the potentially toxic methylmalonate. Vitamin B_{12} is needed for the maintenance of myelin in the nervous system, and inadequate myelin synthesis results in neurological damage, the metabolic basis of which is considered in Chapter 14, where the role of methionine is emphasized. It is recognized that decreased methylene tetrahydrofolate leads to depressed synthesis of DNA, and this could affect dividing cells in the growing brain. Deficient remethylation of homocysteine to methionine also leads to decreased availability of *S*-adenosylmethionine, and thus interferes with essential methylation reactions. A further component results from deficient methylmalonyl-CoA mutase. The content of odd fatty acids in myelin, 15- and 17-carbon fatty acids and branched fatty acids then increases in the nervous tissue (Kühne et al 1991). Whatever the mechanism, the consequences of vitamin B_{12} deficiency can be serious.

Breastfed infants of mothers consuming strict vegan diets are at high risk of serious infantile neurological disorders, which may even be irreversible. Brain atrophy, myoclonic seizures disorder, microcephaly and cortical blindness due to deficiency develop after birth; during pregnancy the placenta transports vitamin B_{12} actively to the growing fetus, and thereby protects it. The concentration of vitamin B_{12} in mothers' milk is similar to that in serum. Permanent brain damage due to vitamin B_{12} deficiency in vegan children is a real risk unless prophylactic vitamin B_{12} is given. More subtle effects of B_{12} deficiency are evident in patients with pernicious anaemia, who can develop a dementia. It is also possible that some of the decline in cognitive function associated with ageing is preventable or reversible with improved vitamin B_{12} and folate status (Rosenberg & Miller 1992). Decreased vitamin B_{12} status and specific malabsorption of vitamin B_{12} are reported in Down's patients (Cartilidge & Curnock 1986).

Nitrous oxide anaesthesia (see Chapter 14)

Nitrous oxide inactivates vitamin B_{12}, so postoperative B_{12} deficiency may develop. Non-toxic doses of N_2O can cause postoperative neurological deterioration due to myeloneuropathy; this is particularly likely in marginally B_{12}-deficient patients (Holloway & Alberico 1990). Increased plasma or urine methylmalonic acid and homocysteine are more sensitive indicators of vitamin B_{12} deficiency than haematological abnormalities. Treatment and full recovery depend on the severity of structural changes, and may take months.

Folic acid (see Chapters 14, 25 and 39)

The role of folic acid in precipitating neural tube defects, and its involvement in alcoholism and in patients treated with phenytoin and phenobarbital, has been considered earlier. Many psychiatric inpatients and psychogeriatric patients may develop folate deficiency due to selecting and eating a diet with a low folic acid content. Depression and even dementia may sometimes result (Dickerson 1988).

Niacin deficiency and pellagra (see Chapter 14)

Mild niacin deficiency may produce weakness, tremor, anxiety, depression and irritability. In more severe cases delirium may develop, but chronic severe deficiency may progress to dementia. The clinical picture is not pathognomic to pellagra, and patients may even be admitted to mental hospitals. The possibility of pellagra should be considered in any unexplained delirium or dementia in a person who has been taking a poor diet for a prolonged period. The condition may be accompanied by signs of

protein–energy malnutrition, by anaemia and by other deficiencies, e.g. of thiamin and other vitamins. Careful examination may reveal decreased sensation in the feet, and loss of vibration and position sense, which may be accompanied by hyperaesthesia. The loss of position sense may give rise to ataxia. Spasticity and exaggerated tendon reflexes are evidence of involvement of the pyramidal tracts. These features are those of subacute combined degeneration of the cord, and may be due to associated vitamin B_{12} deficiency. Alternatively, there may be footdrop and impairment of tendon reflexes, indicating peripheral nerve defects.

Pantothenic acid and biotin deficiency

These are considered in more detail in Chapter 14. Biotin may be decreased in patients receiving long-term treatment with anticonvulsant medication, and some physicians advocate the use of moderate amounts of biotin in long-term anticonvulsant therapy (Sweetman & Nyhan 1986).

Vitamin A (see Chapter 13)

The visual effects of deficiency are profound, but infants and children suffering from trisomy 21, prematurity and zinc deficiency, and those treated with anticonvulsants, are at risk of having a low serum vitamin A concentration.

Raised intracranial pressure, with infantile hydrocephalus and with headache and nausea in adults, has been reported in patients with vitamin A deficiency. These effects also occur paradoxically in patients suffering from hypervitaminosis A, who also complain of drowsiness, vertigo and vision problems. Children and adults who abuse alcohol are more sensitive to vitamin A overdose. Vitamin E supplementation induces a fall in plasma retinol-binding protein and retinol concentrations (Garrett-Laster et al 1981), and may limit vitamin A toxicity.

Vitamin E (see Chapter 13)

Attempts have been made to relate vitamin E to different neurological disorders such as epilepsy, intracranial haemorrhage, Parkinson's disease, Werdnig–Hoffman disease, neuronal ceroid lipofuscinoses, multiple sclerosis, myotonic dystrophy, Down's syndrome and Alzheimer's disease. It has also been suggested that oxygen-derived free radical species may be involved in neurological conditions such as cerebral ischaemia, tardive dyskinesia, Down's syndrome, Duchenne muscular dystrophy and mental retardation. Free radicals may be particularly induced by free transition metals, such as iron and copper. The decomposition of lipid hydroperoxides to form peroxyl and alkoxyl radicals may then occur in the nervous system. The neuronal ceroid lipofuscinoses, Hallervorden–Spatz syndrome, Parkinson's disease, Alzheimer's disease and Zellweger syndrome are conditions where some excess free radical activity may occur. These claims depend on clinical observations during supplementation with vitamin E, alone or in combination with other antioxidants (Gutteridge et al 1986, Sokol 1989, Muller 1990).

Vitamin E therapy

Vitamin E has been used to increase vitamin E stores and to prevent the complications of periventricular haemorrhage and retinopathy in premature babies, but the results are conflicting (Muller 1990).

In Down's syndrome the cytoplasmic Cu:Zn-superoxide dismutase activity is increased by 50%, but brain glutathione peroxidase remains normal. This means that the brain is likely to be more susceptible to oxygen free radical stress. Acceleration of oxidative processes in Down's syndrome might explain the clinical and biochemical signs of rapid ageing and the early occurrence of clinical dementia in these patients. A brain degeneration similar to that seen in Alzheimer's disease has been reported, and the increased amounts of ceroid lipofuscin pigments in the neurons are similar to those seen in the neuronal ceroid lipofuscinoses. A highly positive correlation has also been reported between erythrocyte glutathione peroxidase levels and the intelligence quotient in Down's children (Sinet et al 1979). Nevertheless, there is no evidence as yet of vitamin E depletion (Metcalfe et al 1989), nor that therapy with vitamin E will alter the accelerated ageing process in patients with this syndrome.

There is now increasing interest in considering the use of vitamin E to prevent the epilepsy induced after brain haemorrhage, when extravasated iron is likely to induce secondary tissue damage from free radical activity, and there are increasingly hopeful reports of the usefulness of vitamin E therapy in a number of rare brain disorders, such as the neuronal ceroid lipofuscinoses and Batten's disease.

In Finland selenium intakes were low for geophysical reasons, until the introduction of selenium-rich fertilizers. Selenium therapy, in conjunction with vitamin E, has therefore been a prominent feature of several studies on mentally retarded patients with a variety of disorders. The benefits in the rare group of patients with neuronal ceroid lipofuscinoses are promising. The best responders to antioxidant therapy show no neurological dysfunction, except deteriorated vision, even by the age of 20, so the expectancy of meaningful life in juvenile patients receiving antioxidants may be significantly prolonged in the future (Santavuori et al 1988, 1989, Rotteveel & Mullaart 1989).

MITOCHONDRIAL DISORDERS (see Chapter 47)

These include a group of patients with neuromuscular disorders and with a wide variety of clinical disorders. Combination vitamin therapy has been tried, but has not been clearly shown to be successful.

MULTIPLE SCLEROSIS

Multiple sclerosis is considered to result from a disorder involving the demyelination and scarring of the brain and spinal cord. This condition is a chronic disabling fluctuating neurological disease which has a peak onset between the ages of 25 and 35 years. There may be impairment of vision, coordination, sensation, intellect and sphincter control, and death may occur within a few years.

One of the most consistent epidemiological findings is the higher prevalence of the disease in populations living in countries with a cold climate and consuming diets rich in animal fats containing saturated fatty acids (Bates 1990). There is a high prevalence in many parts of the Nordic or Scandinavian countries. In 1972 Thompson found decreased levels of serum linoleate as well as unsaturated fatty acids of brain phospholipids in patients with multiple sclerosis. It has also been suggested that supplementation with essential fatty acids may improve the clinical status of young patients diagnosed early (Clausen et al 1988).

Vitamin E with selenium and vitamin C, and a balanced intake of ω-6 and ω-3 polyunsaturated fatty acids, has been tried in the treatment of multiple sclerosis because, as early as 1975, Mickel suggested that an increased peroxidation rate was a pathological factor in multiple sclerosis.

The problem with any nutritional study in such a distressing disease is that the episodic nature of multiple sclerosis requires that large numbers of patients should be studied by properly designed 'double-blind' trials conducted over many months, or even 1–2 years. This is difficult to organize, but it is all too easy to assume that a group of patients is improving and responding to treatment when in practice they are improving spontaneously. Multiple sclerosis is known to show a fluctuating and unpredictable clinical course.

PARKINSON'S DISEASE

Parkinson's disease is a degenerative neurological disease, with progressive degeneration of the pigmented nuclei in the brainstem and a loss of neurotransmitter dopamine in the basal ganglia. Clinical trials indicate that antioxidative treatment with vitamin E may postpone the need for L-dopa antiparkinson treatment (Parkinson Study Group 1989, Fahn 1991).

ALZHEIMER'S DISEASE

Alzheimer's disease is a frequent cause of dementia in the elderly. Lassen et al (1957) proposed that the decrease in cerebral blood flow, glucose utilization and oxygen consumption common to many dementias results from abnormalities of brain structure, with a high oxidative capacity. In dementia of the Alzheimer type, brain blood flow and oxidative metabolism are reduced. This situation may lead to loss of balance between pro-oxidants and antioxidants. More interest has been given to the possibility that aluminium toxicity may be one causal factor. Aluminium has been found in higher concentrations in the brains of some patients, and aluminium toxicity can lead to dementia similar to Alzheimer's disease. Aluminium is found as silicate in the cores of amyloid plaques. Simultaneous reductions in the cortical contents of selenium and zinc may indicate reduced antioxidant activity.

VITAMIN K (see Chapter 13)

Vitamin K is important for the function of a number of proteins, including plasma coagulation factors II, VII, IX and X, coagulation proteins C and S, and some other proteins less well investigated. The deficiency of vitamin K and the resulting coagulation defect is mostly a risk in newborns. There are three different types of haemorrhagic disease in newborns: the early haemorrhagic form, the classic type, and the late neonatal vitamin K deficiency.

The characteristic manifestations of the late neonatal haemorrhagic disease due to vitamin K deficiency are vomiting, lethargy, haemorrhage, convulsions, loss of appetite, unconsciousness, dyspnoea and intracranial bleeding. Vitamin K deficiency can occur in older infants for unknown reasons, or as a consequence of some other disorder. The incidence is higher among people in Asian countries than in the west.

Most infants suffering from late neonatal haemorrhagic disease have not had vitamin K prophylaxis at birth, and the mothers of these children have often been given drugs affecting vitamin K metabolism, such as anticonvulsants, isoniazid, rifampin and warfarin.

VITAMIN-LIKE SUBSTANCES

Choline and lecithin

Choline, a quaternary ammonium compound, is a component of phospholipids and has an important influence on the production of acetycholine, a neurotransmitter. Choline is not produced in the brain. Dietary intakes affect plasma and brain choline levels and alter acetycholine levels experimentally. Choline is consumed mostly as lecithin (95% of which is phosphatidylcholine). Oral doses of choline and phosphatidylcholine have been used as effective therapies for tardive dyskinesia, a disorder thought to involve disturbed cholinergic neurotransmission. This disorder is characterized by involuntary choreoathetotic movements of the face, extremities and trunk, and it is very frequently seen in patients treated with neuroleptics such as phenothiazines.

Chronic choline deficiency affects memory experimentally, and adult humans treated with anticholinergic drugs have developed memory deficits responsive to choline administration. There is no definite evidence that choline helps the memory of patients with Alzheimer's disease (Gelenberg 1981).

Carnitine

Carnitine (β-hydroxy-γ-N-trimethylammonium butyrate) is synthesized in the body from two essential amino acids, lysine and methionine. There may be a vitamin B_6 requirement for carnitine synthesis (Cho & Leklem 1990).

Carnitine is important in the transportation of long-chain fatty acids across the inner mitochondrial membranes. Carnitine also transports shortened acyl-CoA compounds from the peroxisomes to the mitochondria, and helps to deal with acyl-CoA compounds building up during anoxic or other abnormal metabolic conditions. In man, pure daily endogenous synthesis of carnitine may not be sufficient for needs, so some dietary carnitine is needed. Meat and dairy products are rich sources of carnitine.

Systemic carnitine deficiency results in recurrent attacks of acute encephalopathy characterized by vomiting, mental confusion and somnolence, followed by deepening stupor and coma. Decreased muscle strength is also commonly observed. Carnitine uptake in the brain is slow in vivo because it has to cross the blood–brain barrier. Carnitine may affect the activity of both GABA and acetylcholine. Carnitine deficiency is seen in patients with mitochondrial myopathies. Some antiepileptic drugs, e.g. valproic acid, sequestrate carnitine.

Winter et al (1987) reported that children with hypotonia, failure to thrive, recurrent infections, encephalopathy, non-ketotic hypoglycaemia and cardiomyopathy have a risk of carnitine deficiency. When the urine of these patients with encephalopathy were treated with 50–350 mg/kg/day of L-carnitine for 1–24 months, eight improved; patients with hypoglycaemic episodes had no further episodes once L-carnitine treatment had begun.

Taurine

Taurine, a β-aminosulfonic acid, is formed from methionine and cysteine, or is present in the food. It may be a cerebral osmoprotective molecule in chronic hypernatremic dehydration (Trachtman et al 1988).

Particularly high concentrations of taurine are found in the developing nervous and muscle systems. Oral taurine may induce a general depression of the central nervous system, and may inhibit short-term labile memory (Hayes & Sherman 1981, Hayes 1988). In the nervous system, the best-known experimental effect of taurine is as a generalized anticonvulsant.

Taurine membrane transport, e.g. of calcium and potassium, is considered to be a neurotransmitter and neuromodulator in the brain, in the olfactory bulbs and in the retina. Patients with small-intestinal bacterial overgrowth have shown abnormalities in retinal cone function as well as pigment epithelium defects, in association with significant decrease in plasma taurine, but the full physiological role of taurine is unclear.

MAGNESIUM AND TRACE ELEMENTS AND BRAIN FUNCTION

The importance of iron in brain development is covered in Chapter 12.

Magnesium

Magnesium is an activator of most of the enzymes involved in phosphorus metabolism and mitochondrial oxidative metabolism. Magnesium and calcium have complex interdependent influences on the excitability of neuromuscular activity. The blood–brain barrier limits the uptake of magnesium from blood into the central nervous system.

Tetany induced by hypomagnesaemia has been observed in newborns, and neonatal tetany due to magnesium deficit is often characterized by hypocalcaemia resistant to calcium therapy. Children suffering from magnesium deficit are restless, with psychomotor instability, but are not mentally retarded. Hypomagnesaemia in adults is characterized by nervousness, muscular twitchings, an unsteady gait, salivation and muscular tetany, which may progress to convulsions. Acute symptomatic hypomagnesaemia may sometimes be drastic, with carpopedal spasm, facial muscle twitching, apathy, anorexia, tremors, convulsive crises leading to tetanic crises, delirium and hallucinations, coma and then death.

Magnesium deficiency must also be considered in the following syndromes: organic brain syndrome, Alzheimer's disease, intestinal spasms, migraine, chronic fatigue syndrome, depression and panic attacks (Rogers 1992).

Treatment

Hypocalcaemia due to magnesium deficiency can be cured by giving magnesium (0.5–1.0 ml of 5% magnesium sulphate intramuscularly). Daily treatment with intramuscular magnesium (0.4–0.75 mmol/kg body weight) is needed for a full remission.

Manganese (see Chapter 12)

Manganese deficiency may rarely be a risk in institutionalized patients, but excessive intakes of Mn are documented as toxic. Miners of manganese ore in Chile develop a 'manganese madness' (locura manganica). Mn is deposited in the basal ganglia, and the disorder has some of the features of Parkinson's disease.

Copper (see Chapter 12)

Copper deficiency in experimental animals results in significant morphological and functional alternations in the brain, as well as in the pancreas, heart and adrenals. Major endocrine alternations in copper deficiency are characterized by changes in catecholamines, opiates and opiate receptors in the brain, and in the opiates and neuropeptides in the pituitary and hypothalamus. Decreases in noradrenaline and dopamine in discrete regions of the brain have been partly implicated in neurological disorders due to copper deficiency. It has also been demonstrated that feeding low-copper diets increases plasma β-endorphin and decreases plasma enkephalins in humans. Feeding fructose may produce a more severe copper deficiency in humans (Recant et al 1986, Bhathena et al 1991). Cerebellar ataxia occurs in humans with pure copper deficiency of nutritional origin.

Menkes' disease

In Menkes' disease, defective intestinal absorption leads to copper deficiency and extensive brain damage, convulsive seizures and mental retardation. The main clinical features are failure to thrive, poor psychomotor development, seizures, tendency to hypothermia, distinctive facial features, and very characteristic kinky or steel hair. It is a rare condition affecting one in 35 000 births, and death usually occurs in early childhood.

Treatment Copper supplements do not help. Parenteral copper-histidine supplemented by oral D-penicillamine (Nadal & Baerlocher 1988) was of benefit in one case, but further trials are necessary.

Wilson's disease

Wilson's disease (hepatolenticular degeneration) is a rare inherited defect, with excess copper accumulation leading to progressive fatal copper toxicity. Brain copper concentrations rise to 10 times the levels found in normal brain and cornea. Most patients with Wilson's disease present with liver disease or with neurological symptoms, but without mental retardation. Dysarthria and deterioration in coordination of voluntary movements are the most frequent neurological symptoms. Copper in the iris produces the Kayser–Fleischer ring, the most important sign of Wilson's disease. Its treatment is considered in Chapter 12.

Zinc (see Chapter 12)

A low cerebrospinal fluid zinc concentration has been found in patients with alcohol withdrawal seizures; increased values have been found in patients on oestrogen therapy. An expected increase in zinc levels in cerebrospinal fluid also occurs in patients with increased protein concentrations, or with sub-arachnoid haemorrhage (Palm 1982).

Deficiency

Acute severe zinc deficiency has been shown by Henkin et al (1975) to cause neurophysiological impairment in humans, particularly impairment of dark adaptation. In the central nervous system zinc influences appetite, taste, smell and vision. Zinc deficiency may also cause non-specific neuropsychiatric changes such as anorexia, apathy, irritability, jitteriness and mental lethargy. In cases of iatrogenically induced zinc deficiency, neurological features include jitteriness, impaired mental concentration, depression and mood lability. Zinc deficiency may also affect cone-mediated vision and may be associated with optic neuropathy (Dreosti 1983).

Acrodermatitis enteropathica

Only a few patients with acrodermatitis enteropathica are mentally handicapped. The misery of the condition responds rapidly to oral zinc.

Anorexia nervosa

It has been suggested that zinc deficiency may be involved in the aetiology of anorexia nervosa. Teenage girls who are restricting their food and mineral intake during the period of rapid body growth may develop a state of zinc deficiency and anorexia nervosa. Sauna users may also lose zinc by sweating, and starvation by itself is a catabolic state involving the release of tissue zinc into the plasma, and subsequent hyper-zincuria (Safai-Kutti 1990). A daily supplementation of 45 mg zinc, as zinc sulphate, has been reported to result in weight gain in 17 young female patients with long-standing anorexia nervosa (Safai-Kutti 1990). The weight gain continued over a 4-year follow-up period, and a multicentre clinical trial is now under way.

Selenium (see Chapter 12)

Attempts have been made to relate selenium to such different neurological disorders as epilepsy, phenyl-ketonuria and maple syrup urine disease, Parkinson's disease, amyotrophic lateral sclerosis, neuronal ceroid lipofuscinoses, myotonic dystrophy, multiple sclerosis, Down's syndrome, Alzheimer's disease and neuro-toxicity of mercury. The relevant connection between selenium and the majority of these disorders rests on clinical observations during selenium supplementation, alone or in combination with other antioxidants. The evidence so far is unimpressive.

Selenium food-borne toxicity

Genuine food-borne selenium toxicosis is rare: normal human diets seldom exceed the recommended safe level. Chronic dietary selenium intoxication has been reported from South America, where the consumption of coco de mono (*Lecythis ollaria*) nuts containing high levels of selenocystathione affects the gastro-intestinal tract, skin, hair and nails. Some intoxicated cases also suffer from lassitude. This effect on the brain was probably secondary to general malaise, since this form of selenium does not cross the blood–brain barrier.

Signs of selenosis in humans have also been reported from China. In the village with the most intense exposure, a toxic polyneuritis developed. The neurological symptoms were usually associated with disturbances in the digestive tract. Initially the patients could suffer from peripheral anaesthesia and pain in the extremities, with subsequent numbness, convulsions, paralysis, motor disturbance and hemiplegia. However, other factors, e.g. fluorosis and heavy metals, may also have contributed to the toxic effects. When residents were evacuated from affected areas they recovered as their diets changed.

NUTRIENTS AND MEMORY

Human and animal studies show that severe deficiencies of thiamin, niacin, pyridoxine, folic acid, or vitamin B_{12} result in impaired memory, which can be restored to normal by providing the deficient vitamin (Cherkin 1987).

NUTRIENTS AND PREGNANCY

Neonatal jaundice and kernicterus

Neonatal jaundice is a common disorder caused by bilirubin produced by the degradation of haemoglobin. It is important that this condition is diagnosed and treated early because free bilirubin is toxic to the brain. Jaundice in dark-skinned newborns is more difficult to detect, but may be seen by blanching the skin of the nasal bridge. Assessing the severity of the jaundice depends on measuring the level of total serum bilirubin. Any newborn infant whose serum bilirubin exceeds 175–210 µmol/1 by the third post-term day should be considered to have pathological jaundice.

Physiologically bilirubin production in the normal newborn infant is more than twice that of adults. The situation lasts about 1 week in Caucasian full-term infants. During this time the large mass and short lifespan of red cells, as well as the intestinal reabsorp-tion of bilirubin, lead to a rise in the concentration of serum bilirubin from 35 µmol/1 to 85–100 µmol/1 on the third post-term day. The higher concentration of bilirubin and its longer duration in normal full-term infants from China, Japan and Greece indicates the involvement of genetic and environmental factors. Several causes, such as blood group incompatibilities, sepsis and dehydration with the absence of appropriate intestinal flora, or the lack of mucosal β-glucuronidase to degrade bilirubin to urobilinogen, are accompanied by increased enterohepatic recirculation of bilirubin.

The routine use of 450–460 nm wave length phototherapy is recommended. Effective therapy needs a minimum irradiance of 1 mW/cm^2 of skin. Neonates in phototherapy require additional fluid, amounting to about 10–15% extra daily. Daily administration of riboflavin at doses of 0.5 mg/kg will shorten the need for phototherapy by stimulating the photolysis of bilirubin (Rivlin 1979). If the early diagnosis and treatment of pathological neonatal jaundice is missed, then bilirubin toxicity leads to brain damage. The affected infant becomes irritable or lethargic, sucks poorly, vomits its feed and develops later neurological signs pathognomic of kernicterus. These signs include hypertonia, paralysis of upward gaze, opisthotonus, a typical high-pitched cry, fever, apnoea and convulsions. Many babies survive with deafness, athetoid cerebral palsy and mental retardation (Chan 1991).

Favism

The most common cause of red-cell fragility is the inherited sex-linked recessive trait of favism. This is an expression of a mutation of the glucose-6-phosphate dehydrogenase (G6PD) gene, which has more than 300 variants. The gene for this trait is perpetuated in the tropics and in the Mediterranean area because heterozygotes suffer less from malarial infection by *Plasmodium falciparum*. Deficiency of the enzyme G6PD influences the first catalytic reaction in the pentose phosphate pathway which produces NADPH needed for glutathione reduction. Reduced glutathione protects red cells from oxidative stress, i.e. increased production of oxygen-derived free radicals, so that individuals with favism are liable to haemolysis because of their inability to regenerate glutathione.

Infants with G6PD deficiency should be protected from exposure to any haemolytic agents, such as naphthalene (inhalation of mothballs), oxidant drugs (see list below) and the faba (fava) bean. This exposure includes breastfeeding where the mother is eating the *Vicia faba* bean. Favism is an acute haemolytic anaemia caused either by the ingestion of faba beans or, by inhalation of pollen from the plant. The agents which inhibit G6PD are glycoside, vicinin and agglucon. Although herbal medicines may also have haemolytic properties, a versatile diet rich in antioxidant vitamins and minerals is recommended for mothers breastfeeding their babies. Any underfeeding or dehydration of the infant should be corrected by increasing the frequency of breastfeeding.

Drugs and chemicals to be avoided in favism are:

Antimalarials: primaquine, pamaquine, pentaquine
Sulphonamides
Sulphones
Nitrofurans
Nalidixic acid
Antihelminthics: niridazole, stibophan
Analgesics: acetophenetidin, acetosylic acid
Dimercaprol
Phenylhydrazine
Naphthalene
Probenecid
Vitamin K and water-soluble analogues
Methylene blue, toluidine blue
Faba bean

SPINAL ATAXIA

Spinal ataxia indicates a principal lesion in the dorsal column of the spinal cord. Loss of proprioceptive sensation makes the gait unsteady, and the patient sways when standing upright with the eyes closed (Rhomberg's test). Vibration sense in the legs is also often lost. Symptoms may occur in association with various nutritional conditions after long periods on unbalanced diets. This has been described as nutritional amblyopia in Malaysia, in strict vegetarians, and in the tropical ataxic neuropathy found in Africa.

The essential dietary abnormality is the lack of vitamin B_{12}, but in some forms of tropical ataxia vitamin B_{12} plays a secondary role. Epidemiologically this condition is found in people who regularly consume large amounts of cassava. Cassava contains the glyceride linamarin in its leaves and roots. Linamarin is cyanogenic, i.e. it can be broken down to yield free hydrogen cyanide by enzymes in the plant tissue itself if it is crushed or left standing in water. Hydrogen cyanide can be removed by soaking the roots and then drying them in the sun. If cyanide is ingested, however, it is detoxified by sulphur-containing amino acids, which convert it to thiocyanate, and by hydroxycobalamin, which forms cyanocobalamin. This then limits the availability of

B_{12} for normal neuronal function. Cyanogenic components may also be found in plants such as maize, millet, rice and sorghum, which are commonly used foods in many African countries. Thiocyanate overload resulting from consumption of this poorly detoxified cassava also worsens any iodine deficiency. Thiocyanate itself diminishes the secretory capacity of the thyroid gland, and cassava eaters are at increased risk of developing goitre.

Clinical features of tropical ataxia include tingling, coldness and numbness in the extremities due to peripheral neuropathy. Motor weakness and ataxia appear later, and become increasingly severe as the cord is involved. The physical signs depend on the relative involvement of the peripheral nerves and the dorsal and lateral columns of the cord. In severe cases ataxia is the outstanding feature, with loss of reflexes, especially in the lower limbs. Amblyopia and hearing disturbances may occur. If the brain is affected there may be an organic psychosis, which is occasionally the first sign of vitamin B_{12} deficiency.

Malabsorption of vitamins may be responsible in many of these cases, and deficiencies of the B group vitamins and of folic acid have been found in many cases. A causal link has been suggested with folic acid deficiency in Senegal, with vitamin B_1 and B_2 deficiency in Nigeria, and with vitamin B_{12} deficiency in Senegal and South Africa (Dumas et al 1990).

The toxic origin of African tropical myeloneuropathy has been demonstrated by many Nigerian investigators. The preparation of cassava's tuberous root leads to the release of cyanides. The toxicity of cyanide for the peripheral nerve and spinal cord is enhanced by low intakes of the sulphur-containing amino acids cysteine and methionine, which are involved in the uptake and detoxification of cyanides (Dumas et al 1990). This relates to modern concepts of B_{12} metabolism (see Chapter 14).

EXCITATORY AMINO ACIDS

Although in the industrialized countries excitatory amino acids have been suggested as being involved in the pathogenesis of such neurological disorders as Alzheimer's disease, Huntington's disease, epilepsy and Parkinson's disease, this is far from proven. However, there are two different tropical diseases where the role of excitatory amino acids has been established, namely in the amyotrophic lateral sclerosis found in Guam, and lathyrism.

The ingestion of the excitotoxin β-N-oxalylamino-L-alanine (BOAA), a compound of *Lathyrus sativus* peas, can result in lathyrism. These peas are often eaten in India and Ethiopia. This disease occurs in central India as an endemic, or sometimes as an epidemic, disorder. The symptoms of lathyrism include muscle cramps, weakness and stiffness, or it may present with an acute onset of paraplegia. This excitotoxin may be destroyed by boiling. A related compound to BOAA, namely β-*N*-methylamino-L-alanine, extracted from the *Cycas circinalis* palm, is linked to the Guamian amyotrophic lateral sclerosis, a particular form of amyotrophic lateral sclerosis present in various Pacific islands. BMAA has been shown in primate models to produce changes suggestive of pyramidal and extrapyramidal tract dysfunction (Dumas et al 1990).

REFERENCES

Bates D 1990 Dietary lipids and multiple sclerosis. Uppsala Journal of Medical Sciences 48 (Suppl): 173–187

Bhathena SJ, Recant L, Voyles NR, Fields M, Kennedy BW, Kim YC 1991 Interactions between dietary copper and carbohydrates on neuropeptides and neurotransmitters in CNS and adrenals. In: Momcilovic C (ed) Trace elements in man and animals 7. IMI, Zagreb, pp. 13–14

Brett EM, Smith I 1991 Phenylketonuria and its variants and some other amino acid disorders. In: Brett E (ed) Paediatric neurology, 2nd edn. Churchill Livingstone, Edinburgh, pp. 201–208

Cartilidge PHT, Curnock DA 1986 Specific malabsorption of vitamin B_{12} in Down's syndrome. Archives of Disease in Childhood 61: 514–515

Chan M 1991 Neonatal jaundice. In: Stanfield P, Brueton M, Chan M, Parkin M, Waterson TE (eds) Diseases of children in the subtropics and tropics, 4th edn. Edward Arnold, Sevenoaks

Cherkin A 1987 Interaction of nutritional factors with memory processing. In: Essman WB (ed) Nutrients and Brain Functions. Karger, Basel, pp. 72–94

Cho YK, Leklem JE 1990 In vivo evidence for a vitamin B_6 requirement in carnitine synthesis. Journal of Nutrition 120: 258–265

Clausen J, Jensen GE, Nielsen SA 1988 Selenium in chronic neurologic diseases. Biological Trace Element Research 15: 179–203

Davison AN 1981 Biochemistry of the nervous system. In: Davison AN, Thompson RHS (eds) The molecular basis of neuropathology. Edward Arnold, London, pp. 1–13

Dickerson JWT 1988 Nutrition and disorders of the nervous system. In: Dickerson JWT, Lee HA (eds) Nutrition in the clinical management of disease, 2nd edn. Edward Arnold, London, pp. 326–349

Dreosti IE 1983 Zinc and the central nervous system. In: Dreosti I, Smith RM (eds) Neurobiology of the trace elements, Vol 1. Humana Press, Clifton, NJ, pp. 135–162

Dumas M, Giordano C, Ndiaye IP 1990 African tropical myeloneuropathies. In: Chopra JS, Jagannathan K, Sawhney IMS (eds) Advances in neurology. Amsterdam, Elsevier Science Publications, pp. 343–352

Evans PH, Peterhans E, Burge T, Klinoswky J 1992 Aluminosilicate-induced free radical generation by murine brain glial cells in vitro: potential significance in aetiopathogenesis of Alzheimer's dementia. Dementia 3:1–6

Fahn S 1991 An open trial of high-dosage antioxidants in early Parkinson's disease. American Journal of Clinical Nutrition 53: 380S–382S

Garrett-Laster M, Oaks L, Russel RM, Oaks E 1981 A lowering effect of a pharmacological dose of vitamin E on serum vitamin A in normal adults. Nutrition Research 1: 559–564

Gelenberg AJ 1981 Use of choline, lecithin and individual amino acids in psychiatric and neurologic disease. In: Beers RF, Bassett EG (eds) Nutritional factors: modulating effects on metabolic processes. Raven Press, New York, pp. 239–254

Grantham-McGregor SM, Powell CA, Walker SP, Himes JH 1991 Nutritional supplementation, psychosocial stimulation, and mental development of stunted children: the Jamaican study. Lancet 338: 1–5

Gutteridge JMC, Westermarck T, Halliwell B 1986 Oxygen radical damage in biological systems. Modern Aging Research 8; 99–139

Haas RH 1988 Thiamin and the brain. Annual Review of Nutrition 8: 483–515

Hayes KC 1988 Taurine nutrition. Nutrition Research Reviews 1: 99–113

Hayes KC, Sherman JA 1981 Taurine in metabolism. Annual Review of Nutrition 1: 401–425

Henkin RI, Patten B, Re P, Bonzert DA 1975 A syndrome of acute zinc loss. Cerebellar dysfunction, metal changes, anorexia and taste and smell dysfunction. Archives of Neurology 32: 745–751

Holloway KL, Alberico AM 1990 Postoperative myeloneuropathy: a preventable complication in patients with B_{12} deficiency. Journal of Neurosurgery 72: 732–736

Keyser A, De Brujin SFTM 1991 Epileptic manifestations and vitamin B_1 deficiency. European Neurology 31: 121–125

Krywawych S, Haseler M, Brenton DP 1991 Theoretical and practical aspects of preventing fetal damage in women with phenylketonuria. In: Schamb J, Van Hoof F, Vis HL (eds) Inborn errors of metabolism. Nestlé Nutrition Workshop, Series Vol 24. Raven Press, New York, pp. 125–135

Kühne T, Bubl R, Baumgartner R 1991 Maternal vegan diet causing a serious infantile neurological disorder due to vitamin B_{12} deficiency. European Journal of Pediatrics 150: 205–208

Lassen NA, Munk O, Tottey ER 1957 Mental function and cerebral oxygen consumption in organic dementia. Archives of Neurology and Psychiatry 77: 126–133

Marabou Symposium 1992 The nutritional role of fat. Nutrition Reviews 50 Part II: 1–74

Metcalfe T, Bowen DM, Muller DPR 1989 Vitamin E concentrations in human brain of patients with Alzheimer's disease, fetuses with Down's syndrome, centenarians, and controls. Neurochemical Research 14: 12009–12012

Mickel HS 1975 Multiple sclerosis: a new hypothesis. Perspectives in Biological Medicine 18: 363–374

Muller DPR 1990 Antioxidant therapy in neurological disorders. Advances in Experimental Medicine and Biology 264: 475–484

Nadal D, Baerlocher K 1988 Menkes' disease: long-term treatment with copper and D-penicillamine. European Journal of Pediatrics 147: 621–625

Neuringer M, Anderson GJ, Connor WE 1988 The essentiality of n-3 fatty acids for the development and function of the retina and brain. Annual Review of Nutrition 8: 517–541

Nicholls D 1992 A bioenergetic approach to nerve terminal. Biochimica et Biophysica Acta 1101: 264–265

Palm R 1982 Zinc in cerebrospinal fluid and serum in some neurological diseases. In: Umeå University Medical Dissertations, New Series No 77

Parkinson Study Group 1989 DATATOP, deprenyl and tocopherol antioxidant therapy of Parkinsonism. Archives of Neurology 46: 1052–1060

Pollitt E, Haas J, Levitsky D 1989 International conference on iron deficiency and behavioural development. American Journal of Clinical Nutrition 50: 565–705

Recant L, Voyles NR, Timmers KI, Zalenski C, Fields M, Bhathena L 1986 Copper deficiency in rats increases pancreatic enkephalin containing peptides and insulin. Peptides 7: 1061–1069

Rivlin RS 1979 Hormones, drugs and riboflavin. Nutrition Reviews 37: 241–246

Rogers S 1992 Chemical sensitivity: breaking the paralyzing paradigm: how knowledge of chemical sensitivity enhances the treatment of chronic disease. Internal Medicine World Report 7: 13–41

Rosenberg IH, Miller JW 1992 Nutritional factors in physical and cognitive functions of elderly people. American Journal of Clinical Nutrition 55 (Suppl 6): 1237S–1243S

Rotteveel JJ, Mullaart RA 1989 Anti-oxydatieve therapie bij de ceroid lipofuscinoses. Tijdschrift Kindergeneeskunde 57: 181–186

Roufs JL 1991 L-threonine as a symptomatic treatment for amyotrophic lateral sclerosis (ALS). Hypotheses 34: 20–23

Safai-Kutti S 1990 Oral zinc supplementation in anorexia nervosa. Acta Psychiatrica Scandinavica Supplementum 361 82: 14–17

Santavuori P, Heiskala H, Westermarck T, Sainio K, Moren R 1988 Experience over 17 years with antioxidant treatment in Spielmeyer–Sjögren disease. American Journal of Medical Genetics 5(Suppl): 265–274

Santavuori P, Heiskala H, Autti T, Johansson E, Westermarck T 1989 Comparison of the clinical courses in patients with juvenile neuronal ceroid lipofuscinosis receiving antioxidant treatment and those without antioxidant treatment. Advances in Experimental Medicine and Biology 266: 273–282

Scott JM, Kirke PN, Weir DG 1990 The role of nutrition in neural tube defects. Annual Review of Nutrition 10: 277–295

Simeon DT, Grantham-McGregor SM 1990 Nutritional deficiencies and children's behaviour and mental development. Nutrition Research Reviews 3: 1–24

Sinet PM, Lejeune J, Jerome H 1979 Trisomy 21 (Down's syndrome), glutathione peroxidase, hexose monophosphate shunt and IQ. Life Science 24: 29–34

Sokol RJ 1989 Vitamin E and neurologic function in man. Free Radical Biology and Medicine 6: 189–207

Sweetman L, Nyhan WL 1986 Inheritable biotin-treatable disorders and associated phenomena. Annual Review of Nutrition 6: 317–343

Thompson RHS 1972 Fatty acid metabolism in multiple sclerosis. Biochemical Society Symposia 35: 103–111

Trachtman H, Del Rizzo R, Sturman JA, Huxtable RJ, Finberg L 1988 Taurine and osmoregulation. II. Administration of taurine analogues affords cerebral osmoprotection during chronic hypernatremic dehydration. American Journal of Diseases of Children 142: 1194–1198

Tuttle WW, Daum K, Larsen R, Salzano J, Roloff L 1946 Effect on schoolboys of omitting breakfast. Journal of the American Dietetic Association 30: 674–677

Winter SC, Szabo-Aczel S, Curry CJR, Hutchinson HT, Hogue R, Shug A 1987 Plasma carnitine deficiency. American Journal of Diseases of Children 141: 660–666

Wurtman RJ 1980 Nutritional control of brain tryptophan and serotonin. In: Hayaishi O, Ishimura Y, Kido R (eds) Biochemical and medical aspects of tryptophan metabolism. Elsevier Science Publications, Amsterdam, pp. 31–46

Yerby MS 1991 Pregnancy and teratogenesis. In: Trimble MR (ed) Women and epilepsy. Wiley, Chichester, pp. 167–192

43. Skin and hair

B. R. Allen

The skin, which is the largest single organ system in the body, provides an interface between an individual and the surroundings. The ability to survive in a climatically hostile world relies on its integrity and normal function. Both structurally and functionally it is divided into two interdependent but distinct layers (Figure 43.1). The outer epidermis of 0.04–1.5 mm thickness provides a flexible waterproof barrier between the internal and external environments, and is pigmented against damage from ultraviolet radiation. From it arise the skin appendages such as hair, nails, sebaceous glands and eccrine and apocrine sweat glands. Beneath it lies the inner dermis of 1.5–4 mm. Both rely heavily for their integrity and normal function on adequate and balanced nutrition. Dietary imbalance, whether in the form of overall deficiency, specific shortage, excess of one component or contamination of food, can disturb the equilibrium of the skin. Conversely, extensive skin disease can stress the body and cause or reveal relative nutritional deficiencies.

The barrier function of the epidermis is specifically localized to the stratum corneum, or horny layer. It is now recognized that the effectiveness of this barrier depends not only on normal keratinization but also on epidermal lipids, which constitute up to 10% of its dried weight. This lipid is derived from cell-wall phospholipid and is rich in essential fatty acids (EFAs). Deficiency of these EFAs results in a loss of the normal epidermal impermeability and an increase in epidermal water loss. Keratinization is influenced by nutrients such as vitamin A: the pilosebaceous opening becomes keratinized and is blocked in vitamin A deficiency. Dietary factors also affect the skin appendages, for example, there is lightening of the hair colour in kwashiorkor, copper deficiency, and sometimes in iron deficiency.

The underlying dermis allows nutrients to pass to the epidermis and also provides tough structural support which protects the body against mechanical injury. Deficiencies of vitamin C, copper or protein cause defects in collagen formation which render the skin more vulnerable to injury.

When, then, skin is stressed the demand for nutrients will alter and specific nutrients play an important role in countering disease, e.g. EFAs in eczema and psoriasis, and zinc in wound healing. Also the stimulus to sweat markedly increases the demand for water and electrolytes. The total mass of sweat glands in the skin approximates to that of one kidney, and 10 litres of sweat can be produced in 24 hours. Although there is normally considerable resorption of electrolytes in the eccrine duct, giving a very hypotonic secretion, at high sweating rates there is not time for this to occur and the sweat becomes almost isotonic, thus causing a substantial loss of body electrolytes, particularly sodium and chloride. Extensive inflammation of the skin (erythroderma) increases the requirements for energy and fluid as well as for specific nutrients such as folic acid and protein.

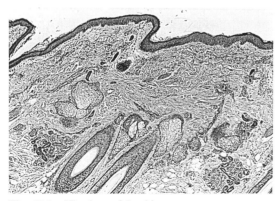

Fig. 43.1 Histology of the skin.

668

This chapter looks specifically at the interaction between diet and the skin; other aspects of the topics covered are considered elsewhere in this book.

VITAMIN A

Vitamin A is ingested either as the vitamin A alcohol or β-carotene, which can be split in the intestine to vitamin A (see Chapter 13). As well as its clearly defined role in vision and its effect on growth, reproduction and embryonic development, vitamin A is necessary for the maintenance of differentiated epithelia. The molecular mechanisms whereby this is achieved are not yet clear (Elias & Williams 1985), but the development of synthetic analogues of vitamin A (retinoids), which have reduced toxicity compared with the natural vitamin, has led to pharmacological doses of these derivatives being used to treat certain skin diseases. This was first achieved with all-*trans*-retinoic acid, which has been used both topically and systematically in acne, psoriasis, ichthyoses and actinic keratoses, but toxicity remained high. Newer derivatives which retain the beneficial effects of vitamin A but with much less toxicity, such as isotretinoin, etretinate and acetretin, have been developed and introduced into clinical practice (see Saurat 1991).

The effect of vitamin A on epithelial surfaces has generally been described as 'antikeratinizing'. In the absence of retinol, goblet mucous cells disappear from mucosal surfaces and are replaced by basal keratinocytes. These gradually convert the original epithelium into stratified keratinizing epithelium. As a result of the loss of the normal lubricating mucus, infection, irritation and sloughing of the surface occur. The skin itself shows an increase in keratinization: histologically this is seen as simple hyperplasia and hyperkeratosis, with a reduction in the number of sebaceous glands and blockage of sweat glands. A sign of vitamin A deficiency which has been claimed to be classic is plugging of the follicular openings with spiny horns (Frazier & Hu 1931) now known as phrynoderma. This has been the source of some dispute, since the histological changes in vitamin A deficiency do not show marked follicular plugging. The original patients in which this was described were treated successfully with cod-liver oil and this led Ramalingaswami & Sinclair (1953) to suggest that it is in fact due to essential fatty acid deficiency. During the second world war, conscientious objectors were recruited to a series of experiments, carried out in Sheffield, which included deprivation of vitamin A. Although follicular hyperkeratosis was seen as a clinical feature, it was not

possible to link it specifically to vitamin A intake (Hume & Krebs 1949).

β-Carotene

A variety of carotenoids are found in plants, of which β-carotene is the most abundant. It is contained in a number of green, yellow or orange fruits and vegetables, and the molecule can be split to provide vitamin A; approximately half of the vitamin in people on a mixed diet is supplied in this way. β-carotene appears to be non-toxic and when large amounts are taken it can be absorbed unchanged from the gut. As a result there is some carotene in normal skin, but excess amounts produce a yellow discoloration. In western countries it is occasionally seen in food faddists who eat excessive quantities of carrots, and in some parts of the world, e.g. West Africa, where red palm oil is used for cooking. An alteration in skin colour is first apparent when blood levels reach about four times normal, and can be distinguished from jaundice by its canary yellow appearance and the absence of staining of the sclera and mucous membranes. It is probable that carotenoids in plants have a dual role, playing a part in photosynthesis by absorbing wavelengths which are lower than those absorbed by chlorophyll, and also providing a photoprotective action against damage which might occur as a result of the plant's own chlorophyll. This has led to the investigation of its use as a photoprotective drug, but the only condition in which it has proved unequivocally effective is erythropoietic protoporphyria (Frain-Bell 1985).

Therapeutic aspects of vitamin A

A number of skin diseases show pathological changes in keratinization. These include congenital and inherited diseases, e.g. ichthyoses and Darier's disease, as well as common acquired conditions such as psoriasis, and also acne, where an alteration in follicular keratin is believed to be important. In the past there have been claims that some of them might be due to vitamin A deficiency (Peck et al 1941), but therapeutic trials were difficult because of the toxicity of high doses of vitamin A (Rapaport 1942, Straumfjiord 1943, Savitt & Obermayer 1950). Vitamin A may also prevent, or even reverse, the early changes of malignancy. Vitamin A influences cell differentiation and deficiency appears to enhance the effects of carcinogens (Bjelke 1975): the basal cells of many epithelia show decreased differentiation and enhanced DNA synthesis – changes which are reversed by giving vitamin A.

The administration of high doses of vitamin A is limited by its toxicity: 500 mg in an adult, 100 mg in a small child or 30 mg in an infant will result in an acute syndrome of raised intracranial pressure, followed after 24 hours by extensive peeling of the skin. Chronic administration of lesser amounts (doses over 7.5 mg per day are not recommended) may result in similar but milder cerebral symptoms, together with hepatosplenomegaly, pain and tenderness of the bones with, ultimately, bony overgrowth. The skin may become dry and pruritic, and desquamation, particularly of the palms and soles, may give rise to considerable tenderness. Hair growth is disturbed and the lips and nasal mucosa may become dry, cracked and irritable and may bleed.

Vitamin D

Dietary vitamin D_2 – calciferol – is originally formed by the solar irradiation of plant sterols, and in human skin vitamin D_3, cholecalciferol, is synthesized as a result of ultraviolet irradiation of 7-dehydrocholesterol (see Chapter 13). In northern Europe serum values of vitamin D are at their highest in the late summer and drop to a low in late winter, which suggests that irradiation of the skin might be an important source of the vitamin even when dietary intake appears adequate.

Deficiency is not associated with any cutaneous problems, but the recent discovery that vitamin D can interfere with keratinocyte proliferation has led to the development of synthetic derivatives, such as calcipotriol, which have only a slight influence on calcium metabolism but useful effects when applied topically in psoriasis (Kragballe 1991).

B COMPLEX VITAMINS

Niacin

Nicotinic acid (pyridine 2-carboxylic acid) and its derivatives, collectively known as niacin, are essential for the formation of nicotinamide adenine dinucleotide (NAD) and nicotinamide adenine dinucleotide phosphate (NADP), which are central to oxidation-reduction reactions in virtually all living cells. It is widely distributed in the diet and can also be formed from tryptophan, 60 mg of which will give 1 mg of niacin. Deficiencies should therefore be rare, but in maize, which is also low in tryptophan, the niacin is highly protein-bound and not readily available without roasting or alkali pretreatment. Deficiency, and the resulting disease of pellagra, can therefore occur in communities where bread made from maize is the staple food item.

Pellagra is often said to be the disease of the three Ds: diarrhoea, dementia and dermatitis. The gastrointestinal upset and the confusional state are not specific, may fluctuate and are not constant features, but the cutaneous eruption is consistent, typical and almost diagnostic. Usually the disease starts with a prodromal phase of mild gastrointestinal upset. At the same time, the patient might be aware of a reduction in mental acuity. The rash develops shortly afterwards and usually starts as a sensation of burning or irritation in light-exposed areas. Slight symmetrical oedema becomes apparent, followed by blistering or the development of thick brown scales. As the disease becomes more chronic the scaling increases and the skin begins to fissure, and haemorrhage may occur giving blackish crusts. The changes rarely extend beyond the hands, feet, face and neck, where a typical distribution known as 'Casal's necklace' may occur. On the limbs lesions are limited to the extremities, with a boot and gauntlet type of distribution which has a very clear line of demarcation. Facial lesions stop before the hairline and may have a butterfly type of distribution across the nose, in a manner reminiscent of lupus erythematosus. A distribution of this kind is highly suggestive of light sensitivity, but this has been difficult to show conclusively. Light testing has failed to demonstrate abnormal sensitivity (Smeenk & Hulsmans 1969). It is possible that skin which has sustained previous light damage might be more vulnerable to the deficiency. Blockage of sebaceous glands on the face with inspissated sebum (known as 'dyssebacea') has been described in adult males (Smith & Smith 1941). Histologically, early lesions show a chronic inflammatory infiltrate in the upper dermis. If vesicles and bullae are present they are situated subepidermally. In more chronic lesions there is hyperkeratosis, with patchy retention of the cell nuclei (parakeratosis) and some thickening of the epidermis. Consistent with the clinical appearance of darkening of the skin, the amount of melanin is increased. In cases which have become chronic there may be hyalinization of the dermal collagen followed by fibrosis and epidermal atrophy (Moore et al 1942).

Other causes of niacin deficiency

As the amino acid tryptophan can be converted into niacin, interference with its metabolism can result in a pellagra-like syndrome. In the rare autosomal recessive condition of Hartnup disease, the renal clearance of many amino acids, including tryptophan, is increased. The resulting loss can result in pellagra, and the same phenomenon may be seen in severe Crohn's disease, where uptake is impaired.

In the carcinoid syndrome the malignantly proliferating argentaffin cells avidly take up tryptophan, converting it to 5-hydroxytryptamine. Normally only about 1% of dietary tryptophan is metabolized in this way, but the increased excretion of 5-hydroxyindole acetic acid from a normal of 10 mg/day to over 500 mg/day indicates a major diversion of the metabolic pathway, with consequent depletion and the development of a pellagra-like rash. The antituberculous drug isoniazid was developed as a result of the observation that niacin had bacteriostatic properties against the tubercle bacillus, and the drug can interfere with the metabolism of the natural vitamin, with resulting pellagra (Cohen et al 1974).

Riboflavin

Riboflavin deficiency rarely occurs in isolation, but usually in association with other vitamin deficiencies. Studies on patients who were deficient in both niacin and riboflavin showed that the oral, flexural and genital lesions which were originally included in the clinical manifestations of pellagra were actually due to riboflavin deficiency (Sebrell & Butler 1938). Typically, after a period of 1–2 years on a deficient diet, a moist angular cheilitis develops, associated with a seborrhoeic dermatitis-like eruption in the nasolabial folds and eyelids, glossitis, and fissuring of the vermilion of the lips. There may also be maceration of the skin on the genitalia.

Pyridoxine

Pyridoxine deficiency produces symptoms and signs very much like those of riboflavin deficiency. These will appear within a few weeks if a diet poor in B vitamins is administered, together with the pyridoxine antagonist desoxypryridoxine. The lesions clear rapidly if pyridoxine is given, but are unresponsive to other B vitamins (Mueller & Vilter 1950). Isoniazid and penicillamine enhance the excretion of pyridoxine, and cycloserine and hydrallazine are antagonists of pyridoxine. Patients on these drugs should receive regular supplements of the vitamin.

Biotin

Raw egg white contains a glycoprotein known as avidin, which binds to biotin and prevents its absorp-

tion. It was discovered when experimental animals which were fed a diet containing raw egg white as the sole source of protein developed a severe exfoliative dermatitis. Biotin originally crystallized from egg yolk would protect against this injury. A similar but milder dermatitis has been produced in humans fed large amounts of egg white, and has been described in patients on total parenteral nutrition deficient in biotin (Innis & Allardyce 1983).

SCURVY

As humans lack the microsomal enzyme L-gulonolactone oxidase they are unable to synthesize vitamin C, which therefore needs to be obtained directly from fresh fruit and vegetables in the diet. The major metabolic defect which occurs in the deficiency state is impairment of the hydroxylation of proline and lysine in collagen formation. Collagen insufficiently hydroxylated in this way has a lower melting point and cannot form normal fibres, and this results in changes in structures with a high collagen content, such as bones, mucous membranes and the skin.

In studies of experimental deficiency carried out in Sheffield and Iowa (Bartley et al 1953, Hodges et al 1969) the first cutaneous changes seen were enlargement and keratosis of the hair follicles, especially on the upper arms. Plugging of the follicles was followed by coiling of the hairs into the typical corkscrews (Fig. 43.2). Although characteristic of scurvy, these hairs are often found in elderly patients who show no evidence of deficiency, and the sign cannot be regarded as diagnostic of vitamin C deficiency. The next change to occur was capillary dilatation followed by haemorrhage around the follicle, particularly on the lower limbs, no

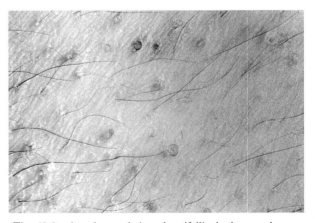

Fig. 43.2 A corkscrew hair and perifollicular haemorrhage in a patient with scurvy.

doubt as a result of high gravitational pressure in the defective capillaries. Histologically, (Figure 43.3) the capillaries around the follicles proliferate and show decreased amounts of collagen both within and around the vessel walls.

In naturally acquired scurvy, mood alterations such as apathy and depression, together with increasing bone pain, result in immobility and long hours of inactivity, with resulting high venous pressure and leakage through the weak capillary wall. The amount of haemorrhage in the lower limbs may then be extreme (Figure 43.4). The breakdown of old scars, as recorded in the early descriptions of scurvy, is a very late occurrence and rarely seen, but fresh wounds are slow to heal and haemorrhage into scars may result in their taking on a livid appearance. The classic gum changes of spongy swelling and haemorrhage are likely to occur soonest in patients with poor oral hygiene. In extreme cases the teeth become loose and are lost. Gum changes are not seen in edentulous patients.

The response of all symptoms to treatment with ascorbic acid is dramatic, with improvement being evident within hours.

In some experimental patients who were also suffering from acne, the lesions became more prominent and haemorrhagic but there is no evidence that giving high doses of vitamin C above those necessary to prevent deficiency has any therapeutic effect on otherwise healthy acne patients.

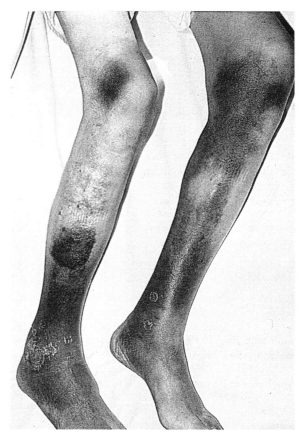

Fig. 43.4 Severe haemorrhage into the legs of a patient with scurvy.

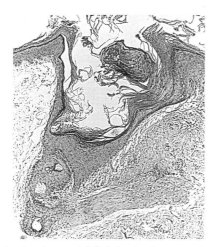

Fig. 43.3 An abnormal follicle in classic scurvy showing distension and plugging (courtesy of Dr A Stevens and Mr W Brackenberry)

METALS

Zinc

The first demonstration that zinc was an essential element in any biosystem was in 1869, when it was found necessary for the growth of *Aspergillus niger*. In 1926 it was shown to be a requirement of plants and has been known to be a vital component in the diets of rats since the early 1930s (Prasad 1988).

The total amount of zinc in the adult body has been estimated at between 1.4 and 2.3 g of which 20% is in the skin. The epidermis contains 70.5 µg/g dry weight and the dermis 12.6 µg/g. Scalp hair from school children contained 125–225 µg/g (Weismann 1980). Animals deficient in zinc show growth retardation and testicular atrophy, together with loss of hair and thickening and hyperkeratosis of the epidermis. The cutaneous manifestations of zinc deficiency which are

Table 43.1   Cutaneous manifestations of zinc deficiency

Skin Surface
Weeping dermatitis
    around the body orifices
    of the extremities
Secondary infection
Poor wound healing
'Eczéma craquelé'

Hair
Excessive fragility
Sparse scalp hair
Absent pubic hair

Nails
Paronychia
Nail deformities

now recognized are given in Table 43.1. In view of the ubiquity of zinc, deficiency might seem unlikely but it can occur in association with the conditions outlined in Table 43.2. The topic is considered in detail in Chapter 12.

For many years a link between zinc and human disease was missing, although a psoriasiform parakeratotic disease of pigs had been recognized as being due to a shortage of zinc (Tucker & Salmon 1955). Similarly adema disease (hereditary parakeratosis), which is an autosomal recessive disease of cattle, presents symptoms which are very like those found in affected pigs and it, too, is easily cured by supplements of zinc (Flagstad 1977). The parakeratotic, red, scaling, well-demarcated plaques which develop on the skin surface were thought to resemble psoriasis most closely, but zinc supple-

Table 43.2   Causes of zinc deficiency

Acrodermatitis enteropathica
Total parenteral nutrition
Intestinal disease
    Crohn's disease
    Jejunoileal bypass
    Steatorrhoea
    Chronic diarrhoea
Pancreatic disease
    Alcoholic pancreatitis
    Cystic fibrosis
Liver disease
    Alcoholic cirrhosis
    Primary biliary cirrhosis
Renal disease
    Chronic renal failure
Fetal alcohol syndrome
Penicillamine therapy
Phytate-rich diet

mentation to psoriatics was of no benefit. Studies carried out over 25 years ago (Greaves & Boyd 1967) showed decreased circulating levels of zinc in patients with extensive skin disease, but the changes were almost certainly secondary to the skin problem rather than the cause of it, since a similar reduction is seen following trauma and in almost any infection. The link with a specific human disease was missing until Moynahan & Barnes (1973) showed that dietary supplements of zinc could completely cure acrodermatitis enteropathica, an otherwise miserable and usually fatal skin disease.

Acrodermatitis enteropathica (AE)

This is a rare congenital disease characterized by alopecia, diarrhoea and an exudative dermatitis affecting the skin around body orifices and on the extremities. It carried a high mortality, with many children not surviving into adult life. In a typical case a breast-fed infant starts to develop symptoms shortly after weaning, usually at the age of about 6 months. Bottle-fed infants develop symptoms somewhat earlier, because the zinc in cow's milk is less easily available than in breast milk, even though the total amounts are similar. The difference might be due to the lower total protein in human (5.3 mg/ml) compared to bovine (29.0 mg/ml) milk (Cousins & Smith 1980). In mildly affected infants the reintroduction of breast milk has been found to improve the symptoms. The skin manifestations are the first signs of the disease to develop, with erythematous scaling and moist lesions appearing around the mouth, nose and anus. As the condition progresses the cutaneous lesions become more extensive and affect the flexures and extremities as well. Vesicobullous lesions have been described, but it is rare to see intact blisters although erosions are common. Sometimes a psoriasiform scaling occurs and, as with true psoriasis, the lesions are well demarcated. The histopathological changes in the skin are not specific. Secondary infections with candida and pyogenic organisms are also frequent, and when the lesions are extensive, give rise to an offensive odour.

Hair is lost diffusely and extensively, and the hairs themselves are hypopigmented and fragile. Consequently the alopecia is often apparent first on the occiput, as an exaggeration of the loss normally found in young infants, and is a result of excessive breakage of the weakened hairs due to friction. The analysis of hairs, which are normally rich in zinc, can provide a more accurate picture of the overall zinc status than the measurement of serum levels. After treatment the hair returns to normal.

If the extremities are involved the nails may be distorted owing to involvement of the nail matrix. Some of the damage is the result of secondary infection and can be permanent, with persisting deformity after otherwise successful treatment.

Diarrhoea is the second most common feature, but this is variable. Anorexia and general failure to thrive, together with impairment of growth, are usual features but they may not be marked and adults with the condition may have normal stature. Other features include hypogonadism and impaired wound healing, together with reduced senses of taste and smell.

In the 1950s the antifungal agent diodoquin was regularly and successfully used to treat AE. It is now known that this drug enhances intestinal zinc absorption (Cousins & Smith 1980), which accounts for its effectiveness. The response of the disease to the introduction of zinc supplements is rapid, even in adults where the condition has been present since infancy (Fig. 43.5a,b) (Gartside & Allen 1975).

It is now recognized that the manifestations of AE are due solely to a shortage of zinc, and that the features are simply those which would occur in any human deprived of the element. Before the report by Moynahan & Barnes, fluids prepared for total parenteral nutrition were lacking in zinc, and in young infants needing total parenteral nutrition, cutaneous signs identical to those of AE would occasionally develop (Fig. 43.6). The first published cases were described in adults in 1975 (Kay & Tasman-Jones) and in children in 1976 (Arawaka et al).

Even before the cause of AE was recognized, it was known to be an autosomal recessive condition. Following the discovery that the disease was due to zinc deficiency despite a normal dietary intake, the next challenge was to define the abnormality by delineating the pathway of zinc absorption from the gastrointestinal tract, it was obviously not just a passive process. This has led to a search for a species-specific ligand which binds zinc, and which is absent or reduced in patients with AE. This has not yet been discovered but it does appear that, once absorbed, zinc handling is normal. One suggestion is that prostaglandins of the 2 series are low in the guts of patients with AE, and that this impairs zinc absorption (Song & Adham 1979).

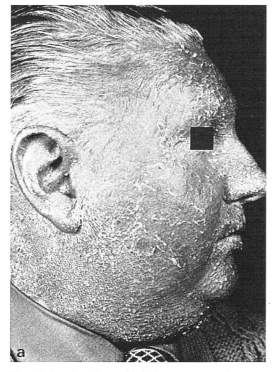 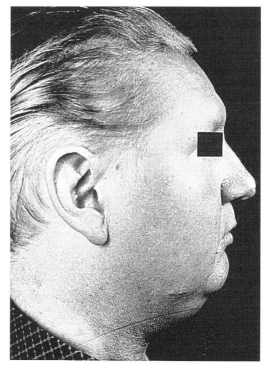

Fig. 43.5a   Acrodermatitis before treatment; **b** acrodermatitis after treatment with zinc sulphate 220 mg daily for 4 weeks.

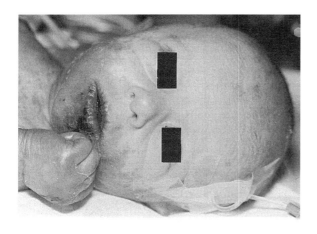

Fig. 43.6 Zinc deficiency due to total parenteral nutrition with zinc-deficient fluids.

Zinc depletion from other causes is unusual but it may arise in patients with chronic diarrhoea and other long-term gastrointestinal problems, alcoholism, and as a result of total parenteral nutrition where zinc supplementation is absent (Table 43.2). Under these circumstances the major symptoms are identical to those of AE. Milder cases associated with alcoholism may present with an eczéma craquelé type of appearance on the lower legs. It is not associated with itching and fails to respond to topical steroids, but improves with zinc supplements.

Treatment Colostrum has a high zinc, copper and iron content, and contains a ligand which enhances zinc absorption. This ligand declines as lactation is established and mature milk contains little. Whereas in normal adults a recommended intake of zinc may be 15 mg Zn per day, patients with AE can be relieved of their symptoms by receiving one 220 mg tablet of zinc sulphate per day, which provides 55 mg of Zn. The actual salt is not important and the acetate, chloride or gluconate salts of zinc are all equally effective. As high concentrations of oral zinc act as a local irritant on the stomach mucosa and may induce vomiting, capsules of zinc should be given with food.

Zinc in other diseases

In volunteers, zinc deficiency has been shown to worsen pre-existing facial acne (Baer et al 1978), but zinc supplements in ordinary acne vulgaris are not helpful (Wiesmann et al 1977). Zinc supplementation has also been recommended for the treatment of alopecia areata, but there is little evidence that either

condition is associated with defective zinc metabolism. Patients who are zinc-deficient have poor wound healing and, as a result, zinc supplements have been recommended in the management of chronic gravitational ulcers. Husain (1969) reported a healing time of 32 days in patients who were given zinc supplements, compared to a control time of 77 days. This degree of improvement has not been reproduced in venous ulcers (Phillips et al 1972) but some elderly patients with bed sores may be zinc-deficient (Thomas et al 1988).

Iron deficiency (see also Chapters 12 and 39)

The effects of iron deficiency on tissues other than the haemopoietic system are more difficult to clarify, but the element is essential for haem-containing cytochromes in many tissues, including epithelial cells. Depletion of these enzymes may be dissociated from clinically obvious anaemia and the haemoglobin is not necessarily low, although iron absorption is always increased in deficiency states. Chronic iron deficiency may result in spoon-shaped nails (koilonychia), hair loss, glossitis with loss of papillae, angular cheilitis and pruritus. The response of these features to iron replacement is often slow, or even non-existent, raising the possibility that they are secondary to other factors rather than a primary effect. This might explain their low overall prevalence in an iron-deficient population. Koilonychia is due to an unexplained disturbance in the growth of the nail. The nail itself may be thin and brittle as well as concave. Spoon-shaped nails are a normal finding in some young infants, and do not automatically indicate iron deficiency. They may also be found in adults as an idiopathic feature, and in nails damaged by chronic excessive exposure to detergents and other degreasing agents.

Although diffuse hair loss has been described in iron deficiency, an exact relationship between the two has yet to be proved. Any debilitating illness may cause diffuse hair loss, known as telogen effluvium, and it may be that in many cases of iron deficiency there is a common underlying cause for both conditions, rather than the shortage of iron itself resulting in the loss. The same can be said for pruritus. Itching is now accepted as a feature of iron deficiency and has been said to occur in 7–14% of patients. It may develop before the haemoglobin drops, and is believed by some to indicate an underlying malignancy. In a large Finnish study (Takkunen 1978) looking at 43 091 people, 0.7% of the men and 3.7% of the women were iron-deficient; 13.6% of the affected men complained of itching, compared with 3.7% of the controls, whereas in females the result was less pronounced, with 7.4% of those with anaemia complaining of itching compared with 5.1% of controls.

Angular cheilitis has also been attributed to iron deficiency (Dreizen & Levy 1981), but as with so many other putative causes of this condition it remains a possible although unproven factor (Darby 1946).

Iron overload

The commonest cause of iron overload is repeated blood transfusions. Iron from transfused cells is taken up into macrophages where, from the metabolic point of view, it is relatively harmless. Iron in cutaneous macrophages causes the skin to gradually take on a dusky grey colour. In idiopathic haemochromatosis a defect in the control of iron absorption from the gut leads to excess iron deposition in many tissues, especially the liver, resulting in serious dysfunction. Pancreatic damage and the skin changes lead to the clinical picture of 'bronze diabetes'. In haemochromatosis 82% of patients show skin pigmentation (Milder et al 1980) which is of a slightly different colour from that seen following multiple transfusions, since there is also increased melanin formation. Other cutaneous signs of haemochromatosis include the loss of body hair and gynaecomastia, both probably a consequence of testicular atrophy.

Cutaneous hepatic porphyria

Patients suffering from this disease present with photosensitivity and increased fragility of light-exposed skin, for example on the backs of the hands, where even the slightest trauma, such as rubbing against clothing, may be enough to damage the skin surface. As the condition becomes more severe, bullae develop after sun exposure and there may be scarring, hyperpigmentation and an increase in hair growth, evident in both sexes. The disorder is the result of a reduction in the activity of the hepatic enzyme uroporphyrinogen decarboxylase. In nearly every case there is evidence of a prolonged positive iron balance, with considerable hepatic siderosis and cirrhosis. Iron is obviously important in causing the disease but its role is not clear, since it does not directly inhibit uroporphyrinogen decarboxylase and patients with haemochromatosis do not develop porphyria cutanea tarda. Amongst the Bantus of South Africa, siderosis, which is a consequence of drinking beer with a low pH brewed in iron pots, is associated with a high frequency of the disease (Dean

1971). It is induced in the majority of patients in western countries by an alcohol intake which is high, although often much less than that seen in true alcoholics. In such patients it may be the alcohol itself which enhances iron absorption. Treatment by repeated venesection to remove iron and cause slight anaemia is usually curative. Many patients remain free of further trouble, even though abstension from alcohol may not be complete.

Copper

Human serum contains 100 μg copper per 100 ml, most of it tightly bound to caeruloplasmin and not exchangeable in vivo. Exchangeable copper is bound to albumin. The main importance of copper in the skin lies in its role in collagen and elastin synthesis. The enzyme lysyl oxidase requires copper as a cofactor. This enzyme is responsible for forming the cross-linkages in collagen which provide its tensile strength. In Menkes' disease (Menkes et al 1962) there is a deficiency in both caeruloplasmin and albumin-bound copper, due to a block in intestinal absorption (Lott et al 1975) and the manifestations of the disease are believed to be due to lack of the metal. The disease is a recessive disorder the gene for which has been firmly identified as situated on the long arm of the X chromosome (Xcen-q13)(Moss 1991). It has been postulated that these patients are deficient in lysyl oxidase, which is copper-dependent. Patients with Ehlers-Danloss syndrome type V have a different defect in the same enzyme.

Menkes' disease results in death from cerebral degeneration within a couple of years or so, and at postmortem the arteries are found to be tortuous, variable in calibre and with a fragmented internal elastic lamina. There are four cutaneous features: pallid skin,

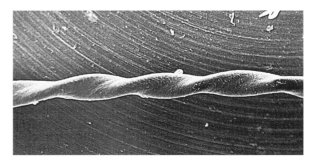

Fig. 43.7 Scanning electron micrograph of a hair in Menkes' disease (courtesy of Dr A Stevens).

horizontal tangled eyebrows, a change in the appearance of the upper lip to produce a Cupid's bow, and hypopigmented brittle and twisted hair. In affected children the hair is normal at birth but is gradually replaced with hair which is light in colour, brittle and breaks easily, and under the microscope shows twists similar to those found in the condition of pili torti (Fig. 43.7). The skin is paler than normal, a defect more readily seen in Negro children. The abnormal hair has been reported as showing a ninefold increase in free sulphydryl groups, a change which has also been shown in copper-deficient sheep (Gillespie 1964). A syndrome very similar to Menkes' disease has been described in infants fed for a prolonged period by total parenteral nutrition. It responded rapidly to the introduction of copper (Bennani-Smires et al 1980).

In Wilson's disease, where a metabolic abnormality results in a chronic positive copper balance, there are no skin abnormalities.

Selenium

Selenium is an essential constituent of the enzyme glutathione peroxidase which breaks down in the presence of reduced glutathione, potentially damaging reactive peroxides. In China, dietary deficiencies are endemic and may result in cardiomyopathy and inflammatory joint disease, but the only cutaneous symptom which has been described is whitening of the nails in a child on total parenteral nutrition. It was reversed by selenium administration (Kien & Ganther 1983).

Manganese

The human body contains about 15 mg of manganese, with high concentrations in the nuclei and mitochondria of liver cells. Whether naturally acquired deficiency ever occurs is doubtful due to the abundance of the element, but a case has been described in a volunteer being fed a purified diet to study the effects of vitamin K deficiency. The subject lost weight, developed dermatitis and hair and nail growth were slowed and his hair became reddened (Doisy 1972).

Toxic trace metals

Lead

Many trace metals may be inadvertently ingested with the diet as a result of environmental pollution. In no case is this more true than with lead, which has been used for plumbing purposes for 2000 years. A blue line on the gums is characteristic but not diagnostic, and may occur with other metallic poisons such as mercury, bismuth, iron, silver and thallium. This blue line is due to the interaction of hydrogen sulphide from anaerobic organisms and circulating lead compounds, and does not occur in babies before the teeth have appeared, people with good oral hygiene, or edentulous patients. Otherwise cutaneous involvement is not a recognized feature of chronic lead ingestion, despite the profound effect the metal has on porphyrin metabolism. Nevertheless, chronic lead ingestion has been reported as a possible cause of porphyria-like blistering of the skin (Allen et al 1974, 1975).

Mercury

Chronic mercury poisoning from environmental pollution may produce vague symptoms which are hard to diagnose (Gesterner & Huff 1977) but mercurous chloride (calomel) was formerly widely used in children's teething powder, and in 1948 Warkany and Hubbard first linked it with 'Pink disease' or acrodynia which continued to occur sporadically into the early 1960s. Typically, a child of 1–2 years would develop pink cheeks and pink desquamating extremities, together with joint pains and photophobia. Recovery occurred once the source of mercury was removed and cases ceased to occur once the mercury salt was removed from all teething powders. As it occurred in only a fraction of the infants exposed to mercury in this way, it is believed to have represented an allergy rather than a direct toxic effect (Matherson et al 1980).

Arsenic

Arsenic has been used as a therapeutic agent, and a poison, for over 2500 years. It was formerly a frequent ingredient of 'tonics' and was used therapeutically in the form of 'Fowler's solution', which contains inorganic trivalent arsenic to treat (with some success) inflammatory skin diseases such as psoriasis. High intakes may also result from contaminated drinking water and foods polluted with pesticides and herbicides. After prolonged exposure the skin may take on a pigmented appearance, with characteristic 'raindrop' hypopigmented macules on a diffusely bronzed background. The palms and soles often show punctate hyperkeratoses, and there is a very strong predisposition towards the development of basal and squamous-cell carcinomata, although this is not seen until a minimum of 13 years after exposure.

Thallium

Thallium-containing pesticides have been known to contaminate food. It is highly toxic, but if the patient survives the acute phase an extensive characteristic alopecia may develop about 2 weeks later.

Lithium

Lithium is abundant in some alkaline spring waters, but not in sufficient amounts to be toxic. Lithium salts used therapeutically to treat manic depressive illness frequently worsen psoriasis.

Nickel

Manufacturing has made nickel a ubiquitous element, so that we are daily exposed to it both in the diet, from the use of nickel-containing cooking utensils, and topically in coins used for currency and clips on clothing and in cheap jewellery. There is little evidence of any direct toxicity due to ingestion, but topical allergy in the form of allergic contact dermatitis is extremely frequent, especially in women, in whom the prevalence has been estimated as 10%. Some dermatologists believe that a low-nickel diet will help control the dermatitis, which may persist, particularly on the hands, long after exposure to topical nickel has ceased.

ESSENTIAL FATTY ACIDS

The epidermal barrier

During dietary studies carried out in the 19th century it was discovered that animals could convert carbohydrate into fat, and yet many animals fed on a fat-free diet died (Sinclair 1990). This was later found to be due to a deficiency of fat-soluble vitamin A, and it was not until the 1920s that fats themselves were found to be a necessary component of the diet. During the course of their research on vitamin E, George and Mildred Burr (1929, 1930) showed that if rats were reared on a fat-free diet, a deficiency disease developed which had not previously been described. It was not correctable by the addition of fat-soluble vitamins A and D. In addition to kidney failure, the animals had a high fluid intake not accountable for by increased urinary output. It was discovered that the animals had a high transepidermal water loss (TEWL) resulting from a defective epidermal barrier. The disorder was correctable by the addition of fat to the diet, and the unsaturated fraction was found to be responsible. The action of the unsaturated fraction was competitively inhibited by saturated fat. The name 'essential fatty

acid' (EFA) has superseded the original one of 'vitamin F' and all EFAs are now known to be polyunsaturated fatty acids (PUFA), although not all PUFAs are essential. There are two groups of EFAs, ω-3 derived from α-linolenic acid, and ω-6 derived from linoleic acid (18:2ω-6). The former are formed in marine plankton and reach the diet through fish or the flesh of marine mammals. The ω-6 EFAs are found in vegetables and red meat (see Chapter 6). The two groups are entirely separate and cannot be metabolized one from the other (see Figs 6.5 and 41.9).

Basnayake & Sinclair (1956) found that if, immediately after weaning, rats were placed on a diet lacking in EFA, the first cutaneous change, evident after 1 week, was a rapid reduction in linoleic and arachidonic acids. After 5 weeks skin scaliness would develop and the animals drank more. By 10 weeks on the diet TEWL was about 10 times normal. As the available linoleic acid falls, the enzymes which normally convert linoleic acid into arachidonic acid act on oleic acid to form Δ5,8,11-eicosatrienoic acid (ω-9). This abnormal fatty acid is detectable only in trivial amounts in normal skin, and is a marker for fatty acid deficiency. Table 43.3 summarizes the effects of experimentally produced fatty acid deficiency in a growing rat.

The essentiality of the ω-3 group is still a subject of debate. In experimental EFA deficiency the cutaneous changes are reversible either by the ω-3 or the ω-6 group, but are more sensitive to the ω-6 group (Ziboh & Chapkin 1987).

The cutaneous barrier

Dried epidermis contains approximately 10% lipid by weight. It is now known that its structural integrity and barrier function depend on both the 'bricks' provided by the stratum corneum cells and the 'mortar' provided by the lipid between the cells. In EFA deficiency there are two problems. Structural failure results from the incorporation of more saturated – or monounsaturated – fats into the phospholipid of cell walls, which results

Table 43.3   Features of essential fatty acid deficiency

Hair loss
Scaling dermatitis
Sebaceous-gland hyperplasia
Increased transepidermal water loss
Poor wound healing
Stunted growth
Renal failure
Atrophy of exocrine glands
Fatty atrophy of the liver
Reproductive failure

in a loss in fluidity. Also, defective intercellular lipid results in the increased water loss (Landmann 1975). This lipid is itself originally derived from the metabolism of intracellular phospholipid extruded by the exocytosis of lamellar granules evident in the upper layers of the epidermis. Lamellar granules disappear in EFA deficiency, and are also absent in epithelium such as oral mucosa, which has no water-barrier properties. Because linoleic acid (18:2 ω-6) is absent in EFA deficiency, oleic acid (18:1 ω-9) is incorporated into ceramides in its place. This results in a failure to form normal lamellar granules, and the water barrier becomes defective (Elias & Brown 1978).

The histological changes which occur in EFA-deficient skin have been reviewed by Prottey (1976). The epidermis thickens, with the development of a well developed granular layer but without the parakeratosis which is such a marked feature of certain scaling diseases of the skin such as psoriasis.

EFA deficiency in man

It is difficult to demonstrate EFA deficiency in any adult animal because body stores are usually too great. Most experimental work has been carried out in animals, but there have been occasional cases of deficiency reported in humans.

In otherwise healthy humans, naturally acquired EFA deficiency of a purely dietary origin does not occur, and would in any case be masked by a fat-soluble vitamin deficiency. Nevertheless, the fact that eicosatrienoic acid (ω-9) is a marker for EFA deficiency has led to the detection of some cases in patients following extensive bowel resection (Prottey et al 1975). Interestingly, although there was scaling of the skin there did not appear to be an increase in transepidermal water loss, unlike the situation in rats. In the 1950s the addition of inadequate amounts of EFAs to artificial milk preparations resulted in a dry scaling rash and increased appetite, corrected by the addition of EFA (Hansen 1957, Hansen et al 1958)

EFA deficiency can be corrected by the topical application of linoleic acid, and also by using derivatives of EFAs such as prostaglandin E_2 (Ziboh & Hsia 1972). Fatty acids of the ω-3 series are much less potent at reversing the cutaneous changes than those of the ω-6 series (Ziboh & Chapkin 1987).

Manipulation of dietary EFAs in the treatment of skin disease

PUFAs are important in maintaining the fluidity of cell membranes. Following trauma they are released again from cell-wall phospholipid and are then the precursors of prostaglandins, leukotrienes and other proinflammatory eicosanoids, the properties of which vary according to the EFA from which they are derived. Thus, for example leukotriene B_5 (LTB$_5$), derived from the major ω-3 EFA eicosapentaenoic acid, is a far less potent chemoattractant than LTB$_4$, its ω-6 equivalent derived from linoleic acid (Terano et al 1986), and indeed may even inhibit its release (Prescott 1984). This, together with the increasing recognition of the interrelationship between the lipid-derived proinflammatory mediators and the cytokine network in cell-to-cell signalling in general, has prompted the study of the manipulation of EFA intake as a means of modulating inflammation in certain inflammatory skin diseases.

Atopic eczema

The eczema which so often occurs as part of the atopic state usually has its onset between the ages of 4 and 24 months. Thus it is probable that environmental factors play a part in causing it and it is understandable that dietary factors should come under scrutiny, although it is clear that they are not the fundamental cause of the problem. If diet is significant, there are two mechanisms by which it could exert an influence: there may be a dietary deficiency or the eczema could constitute an adverse reaction to something eaten. With regard to both these aspects it is easy to argue that breastfeeding should be of benefit, but the proposal was first put forward over 50 years ago (Grulee & Sanford 1936) and there is still no persuasive evidence that it is correct, with many trials producing contrary evidence (Bonfazi et al 1980, van Asperen et al 1984). At about the same time, Hansen (1933) claimed that infantile eczema was associated with a deficiency of the newly discovered EFAs. This hypothesis has not stood the test of time, although the interest in the contribution that might be made by EFAs has been revived by suggestions that the lamellar granules in atopic skin may be abnormal (Werner et al 1987), and that sufferers may be deficient in Δ-6 desaturase (Manku et al 1984). This enzyme converts linoleic acid into γ-linolenic acid, allowing its further metabolism to dihomogammalinolenic acid and arachidonic acid, both of which can be incorporated into cell-wall phospholipid. Gammalinolenic acid itself is not plentiful in a normal diet, but it is found in breast milk (Gibson & Kneebone 1981) and oil from the seeds of the evening primrose (*Oenothera biennis*) (Hudson 1984). Trials using the oil as a dietary supplement in atopic eczema have yielded conflicting results (Wright & Burton 1982, Bamford et al 1985) but an analysis of all published work has indicated a modest beneficial effect (Morse et al 1989).

In an attempt to modulate the inflammatory component of atopic eczema dietary supplements of fish oil have also been used, but here again the results have not been clear-cut (Bjørneboe et al 1987, Kunz et al 1989).

Psoriasis

There seems little doubt that eicosanoid metabolism is disturbed in psoriasis, with high levels of leukotrienes B$_4$ and C$_4$ (LTB$_4$, LTC$_4$), 12-hydroxy eicosatetraenoic acid (12 HETE) and free arachidonic acid all being described in the skin. For a review see Camp (1988). Similar changes are not seen in other inflammatory skin diseases such as eczema. It is not clear whether the disturbances are primary or the consequence of other preceding phenomena, but research into the possibility that dietary supplements of fish oil might be beneficial in psoriasis was stimulated by the observation that the prevalence of psoriasis was low in Eskimos (Kromann & Green 1980) whose natural diet is rich in ω-3 EFAs. Thus preliminary studies describing benefit from fish oils in rheumatoid arthritis (Kremer et al 1985) and ulcerative colitis (McCall et al 1986) might extend to psoriasis, although the low frequency of psoriasis in Mongoloid races generally has to be taken into account.

Theoretically, increasing the amount of eicosapentaenoic acid in the diet might be beneficial. LTB$_5$ has only about 10% of the activity of LTB$_4$ in causing aggregation, degranulation and chemokinesis of polymorphonuclear neutrophilic leucocytes (Prescott 1984, Terano et al 1984, Lee et al 1985), and is only weakly agonistic in potentiating bradykinin-induced plasma exudation in rabbit skin (Terano et al 1986). Polymorphonuclear leucocytes are prominent in psoriatic lesions, and reducing the availability of potent chemoattractants, especially LTB$_4$, by the dietary substitution of ω-3 EFAs for ω-6 EFAs might influence psoriasis by the mechanisms outlined above.

There have now been a number of trials of dietary supplements with fish oil in the treatment of psoriasis. Ziboh et al (1986) and Maurice et al (1986) found that daily therapy with, for example, 50 ml fish oil to provide about 9 g EPA led to clinical improvement in over half the patients treated. These studies have been confirmed by Bittiner et al (1988), who conducted a double-blind trial. After 8 weeks' treatment there was a significant reduction in the itching, erythema and scaling of the active group, with a decrease in the area of skin affected by the psoriasis. Not all studies have been so successful (Bjørneboe et al 1988).

Other skin diseases

There is little firm evidence that manipulation of dietary EFAs in other skin conditions is beneficial, but low levels of linoleic acid have been found in the ducts of the sebaceous glands in acne (Downing et al 1986). It has been suggested that this is the cause of the abnormal keratinization which occurs, but there is little evidence to support dietary supplementation with EFAs (Allen 1990).

URICARIA AND THE CUTANEOUS ASPECTS OF FOOD ALLERGY (see also Chapter 44)

The lesions of urticaria consist of pruritic areas of redness and dermal swelling, which are variable in size, shape and distribution and transient in nature. When they affect deeper tissues they give rise to angio-oedema. They are caused by the local release of histamine from mast cells. The most clearly defined mechanism by which mast cells are induced to degranulate is through the binding of IgE to the cell surface. This has resulted in the assumption that there is an immunological cause in all cases of urticaria and, in the absence of any other obvious provoking factor, food is usually blamed. In the majority of cases no immunological cause is detectable. Nevertheless, when it does occur an IgE-mediated reaction to food will produce an urticarial reaction. Milk, egg, fish and nuts are the most likely foods to cause the problem (Lessof et al 1980). Usually the symptoms develop rapidly, 10 min–2 h after challenge, but sometimes an attack once triggered may persist for several days. Food allergies of this type are acquired early in childhood, and are rarely seen arising for the first time in adults. In children it has commonly been held that breastfeeding will prevent the development of true food allergy, but this is not the case, as has been clearly shown in a 7-year follow-up study of 1753 children initially fed on breast, soya or cow's milk: the occurrence of allergy was similar in each group (Halpern et al 1973). There is a tendency for an allergy to lessen over the years, and adults who have suffered an allergic response in childhood may later be able to tolerate the offending foods. Urticaria may also be triggered pharmacologically by agents in the diet, of which salicylates, yeast products, benzoate preservatives and the dye tartrazine have been most frequently implicated. These substances lower the threshold at which mast cells are triggered to release histamine. Certain foods, such as shellfish and straw-berries, may similarly act in a pharmocological way to produce urticaria, although the clinical picture is identical to one of an IgE-mediated food allergy.

Atopic children show a high incidence of true food allergy of this type, and may have eczema (Lessof et al 1980) but the two problems are separate and it is increasingly accepted that there is little evidence that food allergy plays a direct part in causing eczema (Allen 1988), although this is not universally accepted (Atherton 1983, 1988). In an investigation of 541 patients with atopic dermatitis, 84 gave histories of cutaneous symptoms related to food but, whereas in a group with urticaria there was a good correlation between the history, RAST (radioallergosorbent) tests and the results of a challenge, there was no such correlation in those who believed that their eczema was made worse (Bonfazi et al 1980). Unfortunately, most studies of diet in eczema rely heavily on apparent improvement following exclusion of an item, whereas the true test of an adverse reaction is the development of an exacerbation on double-blind challenge (Pearson 1985).

It is the assumption of many people, both lay and medical, who advocate dietary manipulation in skin disease, particularly eczema, that the condition is being caused by a food 'allergy'. Unfortunately, the subject of food-associated disease is one which is bedevilled by unsubstantiated claims and often a complete mis-use of the word 'allergy', which should be restricted to describing only those reactions in which an immune response can be demonstrated. Otherwise the terms 'adverse reaction' or 'intolerance' should be used (Pearson 1985 and Chapter 44). The only immuno-logical reaction which has been shown unequivocally to occur from food is a Type I IgE-mediated reaginic response. Its characteristics are immediate onset, angio-oedema-like swelling around the lips, burning of the mouth and throat, widespread urticaria, and an immediate recurrence on challenge with the offending substance.

Food additives generally have also been blamed for causing eczema but, as Lessof (1987) has pointed out, there is no logic in considering additives as a unified group because they are such a wide range of chemicals. The yellow food dye tartrazine is a histamine-release agent and will cause deterioration in urticaria, but a survey of the prevalence of reactions to food additives in 18 582 people failed to identify one in whom challenge produced eczema (Young et al 1987).

Dermatitis herpetiformis

Dermatitis herpetiformis is a relatively uncommon skin condition characterized by the development of intensely itchy blisters, particularly over the knees, elbows and sacral area. Sufferers are nearly always well nourished and show no symptoms of malabsorp-tion, but it has nevertheless been shown that they have subtotal villous atrophy in the small intestine of the type seen in coeliac disease (Shuster et al 1968). Despite the lack of symptoms, patients often show slight folate and iron deficiency and impaired D-xylose absorption, and the difference seems to be one of degree. As with coeliac disease the gastrointestinal changes respond to the exclusion of gluten from the diet, but the skin lesions rarely show a complete response. Dermatitis herpetiformis responds drama-tically to treatment with dapsone, but the drug needs to be continued indefinitely. It is usual to find that, after gluten has been excluded from the diet, the dosage of dapsone can be reduced.

REFERENCES

Allen BR 1988 Role of diet in treating atopic eczema: dietary manipulation has no value. British Medical Journal 297: 1459–1460

Allen BR 1990 Essential fatty acids of the *n*-6 series in acne and psoriasis. In: Horrobin D (ed) Omega-6 essential fatty acids: pathophysiology and roles in clinical medicine. Wiley-Liss, New York

Allen BR, Hunter JAA, Beattie AD, Moore MR 1974 Lead poisoning and blistering. Scottish Medical Journal 19: 3–6

Allen BR, Moore MR, Hunter JAA 1975 Lead and the skin. British Journal of Dermatology 92: 715–719

Arawaka T, Tamara T, Igrashi Y et al 1976 Zinc deficiency in two infants during total parenteral alimentation for diarrhea. American Journal of Clinical Nutrition 29: 197–204

Atherton DJ 1983 The role of foods in atopic eczema. Clinical and Experimental Dermatology 8: 227–232

Atherton DJ 1988 Role of diet in treating atopic eczema: elimination diets can be beneficial. British Medical Journal 297: 1458–1460

Baer MT, King JC, Tamura T, Margen S 1978 Acne in zinc deficiency. Archives of Dermatology 114: 1093

Bamford JTM, Gibson RW, Renier CM 1985 Atopic eczema unresponsive to evening primrose oil. Journal of the American Academy of Dermatology 13: 959–965

Bartley WH, Krebs A, O'Brien JRP 1953 Medical Research Council Special Report Series N°280. HMSO, London

Basnayake V, Sinclair HM 1956 The effect of deficiency of essential fatty acids upon the skin. In: Popjak G, LeBreton E (eds) Biochemical problems of lipids. Butterworths, London

Bennani-Smires C, Medina J, Young LW 1980 Infantile nutritional copper deficiency. American Journal of Diseases of Childhood 134: 1155–1156

Bittiner SB, Tucker WFG, Cartwright I et al 1988 A double-blind, randomised, placebo-controlled trial of fish oil in psoriasis. Lancet 1: 378–380

Bjelke E 1975 Dietary vitamin A and human lung cancer. International Journal of Cancer 15: 561–565

Bjørneboe A, Soyland E, Bjørneboe GEA et al 1987 Effect of dietary supplementation with eicosapentaenoic acid on the treatment of atopic dermatitis. British Journal of Dermatology 117: 463–469

Bjørneboe A, Kleymeyer-Smith A, Bjørneboe G-E 1988 Effect of dietary supplementation with n-3 fatty acids on clinical manifestations of psoriasis. British Journal of Dermatology 118: 77–83

Bonifazi E, Garofalo L, Monterisi A, Meneghini CL 1980 History of food allergy, RAST and challenge tests in atopic dermatitis. Acta Dermatologica Venereologica 92: 91–93

Burr GO, Burr MM 1929 A new deficiency disease produced by rigid exclusion of fat from the diet. Journal of Biological Chemistry 82: 345–367

Burr GO, Burr MM 1930 On the nature and role of the fatty acids essential in nutrition. Journal of Biological Chemistry 86: 587–621

Camp RDR 1988 Role of arachidonic acid metabolites in psoriasis and other skin diseases. In: Lewis A, Ackerman N, Otternes I (eds) New perspectives in anti-inflammatory therapies. Advances in Inflammation Research Vol 12, Raven Press, New York, 163–172

Cohen LK, George W, Smith R 1974 Isoniazid-induced acne and pellagra. Archives of Dermatology 109: 377–381

Cousins RJ, Smith KT 1980 Zinc-binding properties of bovine and human milk in vitro: influence of changes in zinc content. American Journal of Clinical Nutrition 33: 1083–1087

Darby WJ 1946 The oral manifestations of iron deficiency. Journal of the American Medical Association 130: 830–835

Dean G 1971 The porphyrias: a study of inheritance and environment, 2nd edn. Pitman Medical, London

Doisy EA 1972 (quoted by Korc M) Manganese homeostasis in humans and its role in disease states. In: Prasad AS (ed) 1988 Essential and toxic trace elements in human health and disease. Alan R. Liss, New York, 253–273

Downing DT, Stewart ME, Wertz PW, Strauss JS 1986 Essential fatty acids and acne. Journal of the American Academy of Dermatology 14: 221–225

Dreizen S, Levy BM 1981 Handbook of experimental stomatology. CRC Press Boca Raton, Florida

Elias PM, Brown BE 1978 The mammalian cutaneous permeability barrier:defective barrier function in essential fatty acid deficiency correlates with the abnormal intercellular lipid deposition. Laboratory Investigation 39: 574–583

Elias PM, Williams ML 1985 Retinoid effects on epidermal differentiation. In: Saurat J-H (ed) Retinoids: new trends in research and therapy. Karger, Basel, 138–158

Flagstad T 1977 Intestinal absorption of ^{65}Zn in A46 (adema disease) after treatment with oxychinolones. Nordisk Veterinaer-Medecin 29: 96–100

Frain-Bell W 1985 Cutaneous photobiology. Oxford Medical Publications, Oxford University Press, Oxford

Frazier CN, Hu CK, 1931 Cutaneous lesions associated with deficiency of vitamin A in man. Archives of Internal Medicine 48: 507–514

Gartside JM, Allen BR 1975 Treatment of acrodermatitis with zinc sulphate. British Medical Journal 3: 521–522

Gesterner H, Huff J 1977 Clinical toxicology of mercury. Journal of Toxicology and Environmental Health 2: 491–526

Gibson RA, Kneebone GM 1981 Fatty acid composition of human colostrum and mature breast milk. American Journal of Clinical Nutrition 34: 252–257

Gillespie JM 1964 The isolation and properties of some soluble proteins from wool. VIII The proteins of copper-deficient wool. Australian Journal of Biological Sciences 17: 282–300

Greaves M, Boyd TRC 1967 Plasma zinc concentrations in patients with psoriasis, other dermatoses and venous leg ulceration. Lancet ii: 1019–1020

Grulee CG, Sanford HN 1936 The influence of breast and artificial feeding on infantile eczema. Journal of Pediatrics 9: 223–225

Halpern SR, Sellars WA, Johnson RB et al 1973 Development of childhood allergy in infants fed breast, soy or cow's milk. Journal of Allergy and Clinical Immunology 51: 139–151

Hansen AE 1933 Essential fatty acid deficiency in atopic eczema. Proceedings of the Society for Experimental Biology and Medicine 31: 160–161

Hansen AE 1957 Role of unsaturated dietary fat in infant nutrition. American Journal of Public Health 47: 1367–1370

Hansen E, Hagard ME, Boelsche AN et al 1958 Essential fatty acids in human nutrition. Journal of Nutrition 60: 565–576

Hodges RE, Baker EM, Hood J et al 1969 Experimental scurvy in man. American Journal of Nutrition 22: 535–548

Hudson BJF 1984 Evening primrose oil and seeds. Journal of the American Oil Chemists Society 61: 540–543

Hume EM, Krebs HA 1949 Vitamin A requirements of human adults: experimental study of vitamin A deprivation in man. Report of vitamin A Subcommittee of Accessory Food Factors Committee MRC Special Report N° 264. HMSO, London

Husain SL 1969 Oral zinc sulphate in leg ulcers. Lancet 2: 1069–1071

Innis SM, Allardyce DB 1983 Possible biotin deficiency in adults receiving long-term parenteral nutrition. American Journal of Clinical Nutrition 37: 185–187

Kay RG, Tasman-Jones C 1975 Zinc deficiency and intravenous feeding. Lancet 2: 605–606

Kien CL, Ganther HE 1983 Manifestations of chronic selenium deficiency in a child receiving total parenteral nutrition. American Journal of Clinical Nutrition 37: 319–328

Kragballe K, Gjertsen BT, de Hoop G et al 1991 Double-blind, right/left comparison of calcipotriol and betamethasone valerate in treatment of psoriasis vulgaris. Lancet 337: 193–196

Kremer JM, Bigauoette J, Michalek AV et al 1985 Effects of manipulation of dietary fatty acids on clinical manifestations of rheumatoid arthritis. Lancet 1: 184–187

Kromann N, Green A 1980 Epidemiological studies in the Uppernarvik district of Greenland. Acta Medica Scandinavica 200: 401–406

Kunz B, Ring J, Braun-Falco O 1989 Eicosapentaenoic acid (EPA) treatment in atopic eczema: a prospective double-blind trial. Journal of Allergy and Clinical Immunology 83: 196

Landmann L 1975 The epidermal permeability barrier. Anatomy and Embryology 178: 1–13

Lee TH, Hoover RL, Williams JD et al 1985 Effect of dietary enrichment with eicosapentaenoic and docosaenoic acids on in-vitro neutrophil and monocyte leukotriene generation and neutrophil function. New England Journal of Medicine 312: 1217–1224

Lessof MH 1987 Adverse reactions to food additives. Journal of the Royal College of Physicians of London 21: 237–240

Lessof MH, Wraith DG, Merrett TG et al 1980 Food allergy and intolerance in 100 patients - local and systemic effects. Quarterly Journal of Medicine 195: 259–271

Lott IT, Di Paolo R, Schwartz D et al 1975 Copper metabolism and steely hair syndrome. New England Journal of Medicine 292: 197–199

McCall T, O'Leary D, Bloomfield J et al 1986 The effect of eicosapentaenoic acid in treatment and neutrophil function of patients with ulcerative colitis. 6th International Conference on Prostaglandins and Related Compounds, Florence, Italy

Manku MS, Horrobin DF, Morse N et al 1984 Essential fatty acids in the plasma phospholipids of patients with atopic eczema. British Journal of Dermatology 110: 643–648

Matherson DS, Clarkson TW, Gelfand EW 1980 Mercury toxicity induced by long-term injection of gammaglobulin. Journal of Pediatrics 97: 153–155

Maurice PD, Bather PC, Allen BR 1986 Arachidonic acid metabolism by polymorphonuclear leukocytes in psoriasis. British Journal of Dermatology 114: 57–64

Menkes JH, Alter M, Steigleder GK et al 1962 A sex–linked recessive disorder with retardation of growth, peculiar hair and focal and cerebral and cerebellar degeneration. Pediatrics 29: 764–799

Milder MS, Cook JD, Stray S, Finch CA 1980 Idiopathic hemochromatosis, an interim report. Medicine 59: 34–49

Moore RA, Spies TD, Cooper ZK 1942 Histopathology of the skin in pellagra. Archives of Dermatology and Syphilology 46: 100–104

Morse PF, Horrobin DF, Manku MS et al 1989 Meta-analysis of placebo-controlled studies of the efficacy of Epogam® in the treatment of atopic eczema. Relationship between plasma essential fatty acid changes and clinical response. British Journal of Dermatology 121: 75–90

Moss C 1991 Dermatology and the human gene map. British Journal of Dermatology 124: 3–9

Moynahan EJ, Barnes PM 1973 Zinc deficiency and a synthetic diet for lactose intolerance. Lancet i: 676–677

Mueller JF, Vilter RW 1950 Pyridoxine deficiency in human beings induced with desoxypyridoxine. Journal of Clinical Investigation 29: 193–201

Pearson DJ 1985 Food allergy, hypersensitivity and intolerance. Journal of the Royal College of Physicians of London 19: 154–162

Peck SM, Chargin L, Sobotaka H 1941 Keratosis follicularis (Darier's disease) a vitamin A deficiency disease. Archives of Dermatology and Syphilology 43: 223–229

Phillips A, Davidson M, Greaves MW 1972 Venous leg ulceration: evaluation of zinc treatment, serum zinc and rate of healing. Clinical and Experimental Dermatology 2: 395–399

Prasad AS 1988 Clinical spectrum and diagnostic aspects of human zinc deficiency. In: Prasad AS (ed) Essential and toxic trace elements in human health and disease. Alan R. Liss, New York, 3–53

Prescott SM 1984a The effect of eicosapentaenoic acid on leukotriene generation and neutrophil function. Journal of Biological Chemistry 258: 7615–7621

Prescott SM 1984b The effect of eicosapentaenoic on leukotriene B formation by human neutrophils. Journal of Biological Chemistry 259: 7615–7621

Prottey C 1976 Essential fatty acids and the skin. British Journal of Dermatology 94: 579–587

Prottey C, Hartop PJ, Press M 1975 Correction of the cutaneous manifestations of essential fatty acid deficiency in man by the application of sunflower seed oil to the skin. Journal of Investigative Dermatology 64: 228–234

Ramalingaswami V, Sinclair HM 1953 The relation of deficiencies of vitamin A and of essential fatty acids to follicular hyperkeratosis in the rat. British Journal of Dermatology 65: 1–21

Rapaport HG 1942 The treatment of ichthyoses with vitamin A. Journal of Pediatrics 21: 733–746

Saurat J-H (ed) 1991 Retinoids 10 Years on. Karger, Basel

Savitt LE, Obermayer ME 1950 Treatment of acne vulgaris and senile keratoses with vitamin A, results of a clinical experiment. Journal of Investigative Dermatology 14: 282

Sebrell WH, Butler RE 1938 Riboflavin deficiency in man: preliminary note. Public Health Report 53: 2282

Shuster S, Watson AJ, Marks J 1968 Coeliac syndrome in dermatitis herpetiformis. Lancet i: 1101–1106

Sinclair HM 1990 History of essential fatty acids. In: Horrobin DF (ed) Omega-6 essential fatty acids: Pathophysiology and roles in clinical medicine. Wiley Liss, New York, 1–20

Smeenk G, Hulsmans HAM 1969 Dermatological and biochemical anomalies in two patients with pellagroid syndrome. Dermatologica 138: 295–302

Smith SG, Smith DT 1941 Journal of Investigative Dermatology 4: 23

Song MK, Adham NF 1979 Evidence for an important role of prostaglandin E_2 and F_2 in the regulation of zinc transport in the rat. Journal of Nutrition 109: 2152–2159

Straumfjiord JV 1943 Vitamin A: its effects on acne. Northwestern Medicine 42: 219

Takkunen H 1978 Iron deficiency pruritus. Journal of the American Medical Association 239: 1394

Terano T, Salmon JA, Moncada S 1984 Biosynthesis and biological activity of leukotriene B_5. Prostaglandins 27: 217–232

Terano T, Salmon JA, Higgs GA, Moncada S 1986 Eicosapentaenoic acid as a modulator of inflammation. Biochemical Pharmacology 35: 779–785

Thomas AJ, Bunker VW, Hinks LJ et al 1988 Energy, protein, zinc and copper status of 21 elderly inpatients: analysed dietary intake and biochemical indices. British Journal of Nutrition 59: 181–191

Tucker HF, Salmon WD 1955 Parakeratosis or zinc deficiency disease in the pig. Proceedings of the Society of Experimental Biology and Medicine 88: 613–616

Van Asperen PP, Kemp AS, Mellis CM 1984 Relationship of diet in the development of atopy in infants. Clinical Allergy 14: 525–532

Warkany J, Hubbard DM 1948 Mercury in the urine of children. Lancet i: 829–830

Weismann K 1980 Zinc metabolism and the skin. In: Rook A, Savin J (eds) Recent advances in dermatology (5).

Churchill Livingstone, Edinburgh, pp. 109–129

Weismann K, Knudson L 1978 Effects of penicillamine and hydroxychloroquine on absorption of orally ingested ^{65}Zn in the rat. Journal of Investigative Dermatology 71: 242–244

Wiesmann K, Wadskov S, Søndergaard J 1977 Oral zinc sulphate therapy in acne vulgaris. Acta Dermatovenereologica 57: 357–360

Werner Y, Lindberg M, Forslind B 1987 Membrane-coating granules in 'dry' non-eczematous skin of patients with atopic dermatitis. Acta Dermatovenereologica (Stockholm) 67: 385–388

Wright S, Burton JL 1982 Oral evening primrose oil improves atopic eczema. Lancet i 19: 1120–1122

Young E, Patel S, Stoneham M et al 1986 The prevalence of reaction to food additives in a survey population. Journal of the Royal College of Physicians of London 21: 241–247

Ziboh VA, Chapkin RS 1987 Biologic significance of polyunsaturated fatty acids in the skin. Archives of Dermatology 123: 1686–1690

Ziboh VA, Hsia SL 1972 Effects of prostaglandin E$_2$ on rat skin: inhibition of sterol ester biosynthesis and clearing of scaly lesions in essential fatty acid deficiency. Journal of Lipid Research 13: 458–467

Ziboh VA, Cohen KA, Ellis CN et al 1986 Effects of dietary supplementation with fish oil on neutrophil and epidermal fatty acids. Archives of Dermatology 122: 1277–1282

44. Nutrition and the immune system

A. Ferguson

GENERAL STRUCTURE AND FUNCTIONS OF THE IMMUNE SYSTEM

The science of immunology arose from the study of man's resistance to infection. It was appreciated that, after recovery from a particular infectious disease, the same disease rarely occurred again. This altered reactivity is what we now call specific immunity, and is mediated by T- and B-lymphocytes and antibodies. Immunology also encompasses a number of entirely non-specific antimicrobial protective mechanisms, both molecular and cellular. These are innate, in that they are not affected by prior contact with the infectious agent, although their activity can be regulated by a number of factors. Roitt (1988) and Male et al (1987) are recommended as source material for a general account of the immune system.

Cells and tissues involved in immunity comprise about 2% of the body's weight. Cells which participate in immune responses are collected together in the lymphoid organs – thymus, spleen, lymph nodes and Peyer's patches. In this environment they can perform their functions very effectively, and they also disseminate immunity by migrating throughout the body. There are many other sites, particularly the mucosae, where cells of the immune system are dispersed between other cells, for example within the gut epithelium and lamina propria.

Cells involved in immunity

A wide range of cells participate in non-specific and specific immunity, and many of these fulfil several different functions.

T- (thymus-dependent) cells perform important immunoregulatory functions via their secreted products, and also act as effector cells, being capable of killing other cells. Many immunological diseases, both immunodeficiency and abnormally enhanced reactivity, can ultimately be attributed to defects of T-cell regulatory function. In terms of protective immunity, T-cells are particularly important in defence against intracellular bacterial and protozoal pathogens, viruses and fungi.

B-lymphocytes are independent of the thymus and, in man, probably complete their early maturation within the bone marrow. They are called B-cells because they mature within the Bursa of Fabricius in birds. When appropriately stimulated, B-lymphocytes undergo proliferation, maturation and differentiation to form plasma cells. Eventually there are many identical daughters derived from a single B-cell, forming a clone. The enormous diversity of antibodies an individual can produce is explained partly by rearrangements of nucleic acid within precursor B-cells, and partly by random mutation.

Other cells, found mainly in the lymphoid organs and the skin, have as their main role the presentation of antigen in a particular way to lymphocytes to start the immune responses specific to that antigen.

Molecules of the immune system

Immunoglobulins

Immunoglobulin (Ig) molecules are the effector products of B-cells, and although they all have a broadly similar structure, minor differences within the main immunological classes (IgG, IgM, IgA, IgD and IgE) are associated with a range of important biological properties. Molecules almost identical to secreted immunoglobulins are incorporated in the cell membranes of B-cells (surface Ig), and there are many related molecules concerned with antigen recognition and cell–cell communication.

In healthy adults, IgG accounts for more than 70% of the immunoglobulins in normal serum, and is distributed equally between the blood and extracellular fluids. About a quarter of all the body's IgG passes out of the bloodstream each day, and the same amount returns via the thoracic duct.

The macromolecular IgM is predominantly intravascular. IgM is especially effective in activating complement to produce immune lysis of foreign cells. IgM antibodies are also much more efficient than IgG antibodies in linking particulate antigens together for agglutination and phagocytosis, and seem to be specially adapted for dealing with cell debris or bacteria in the bloodstream.

IgA accounts for about 20% of the total serum immunoglobulins. However, its function, if any, within the bloodstream and tissues is thought to be much less important than its role as a secretory antibody. The major sites of IgA synthesis are the laminae propriae underlying the respiratory tract, the gut and other mucosae. Secretory IgA confers immunity to infection by enteric bacterial and viral pathogens, and may also be involved in the regulation of the commensal gut flora. Oral immunization is now being used to try to induce protective immunity to intestinal infections such as cholera and rotavirus.

IgE concentration in serum is very low. This is partly because it has a considerable affinity for cell surfaces and binds firmly to mast cells and basophils. IgE antibodies are necessary for immediate hypersensitivity reactions, such as occur in atopic individuals, for example in hay fever. The physiological function of IgE antibodies is obscure, but appears to be important in defence against helminth parasites (worms).

Cytokines

Some of these are often still called lymphokines; others are being renamed as interleukins. The most important are interleukin 1 (IL1) made by macrophages; IL2 and γ-interferon, made by the T-cells responsible for delayed hypersensitivity, and IL4, IL5 and IL6, involved in the regulation of B-cell function.

Induction and expression of immunity

A distinction must be made between the *induction* phase of immunity in which, at the first encounter with antigen, a pattern of altered reactivity is established, and *expression* of one or more types of immune response upon subsequent re-encounter with the same antigen. Expression of specific immunity is usually beneficial, for example by neutralizing toxins and killing bacteria. However, expression of immunity sometimes produces hypersensitivity reactions, tissue damage resulting from what may be a necessary protective immune response, or an inappropriate reaction, e.g. to a self-antigen or a food. There are

also circumstances where antigen encounter leads to down-regulation of specific reactivity. This is called tolerance, and is discussed below.

Patterns of immune responses to fed antigen

The immune system of the gastrointestinal tract (gut-associated lymphoreticular tissue, GALT) has a number of different roles (Gastroenterology Clinics of North America 1991). When the route of entry is through the follicle-associated epithelium of Peyer's patches of immunologically normal and mature mammals, the general trend is towards suppression of immunity – in other words, *oral tolerance*. However, active immunization may also follow the feeding of antigen, and this is typically in the form of harmless secretory IgA antibody. In some circumstances there is, however, induction of potentially immunopathogenic immune reactions when antigen is fed, for example IgE, IgG antibody or T-cell-mediated immunity. Thus there may be either induction or suppression of a particular immune response, whether antibody or T-cell-mediated, when antigen is encountered via the gut.

Regulation of immunity

It is inappropriate for a specific immune response to progress and expand indefinitely, and so there have evolved several factors which inhibit rather than potentiate specific immunity.

As the concentration of antigen in the body drops, so the intensity of the immune response falls off. Antibody itself exerts negative feedback control, partly by neutralizing the available antigen.

There are suppressor-inducer and suppressor-effector subgroups of T-cells, which down-regulate immunity. Some antigenic determinants much more readily evoke suppressor T-cell responses than active immunity. If such determinants could be identified (for example, in relation to allergic and hypersensitivity diseases), such diseases could be cured by the deliberate evoking of suppressive responses. Another practical issue is that deficiency of T-cell function, as may occur in some forms of malnutrition, can result in overall loss of suppression and thus lead to hypersensitivity damage or autoimmunity, in addition to the more readily recognized problems of susceptibility to infection.

Regulation of gut immunity

There are many T-lymphocytes dispersed in the mucosa as well as in the organized lymphoid tissues of the GALT, and, just as in the systemic immune system, gut T-lymphocytes have two types of function – immunoregulatory and effector. There appears to be dual activation of the T-cells which regulate B-lymphocytes: of helper cells for the IgA system and suppressor cells for IgM and IgG synthesis. At the same time there is induction of T_S cells which suppress cell-mediated immune responses. Experiments with protein antigens have shown that there is subtle alteration – 'processing' – of antigen as it crosses the gut epithelium, and such material is tolerogenic for cell-mediated immunity, rather than immunogenic.

Gut lymphoid cells generate protective immunity to infectious microorganisms and parasites. However, immune responses may disrupt intestinal anatomy and function by the 'innocent bystander' phenomenon. This occurs when substantial tissue damage occurs as an unavoidable by-product of a specific immune response to an infectious agent. The classic example of this is tuberculosis or leprosy. Inappropriate immune responses developing in response to harmless antigens such as foods are well recognized as ancillary manifestations of disease, as well as sometimes being primarily responsible for the disease. Immune responses exert important influences on the absorptive capacity of the gut, and thereby on the body's utilization of ingested nutrients.

Protein malnutrition has significant effects on the structure and integrity of the gut epithelium. Since the nature and quantity of circulating antigen, passing across a 'leaky' epithelium, may determine the pattern of induction of immunity to fed antigen, malnutrition may influence the pattern of protective immunity and hypersensitivity to gut antigens.

Immunological tolerance

The clinical relevance of regulation of immunity is enormous. The phenomenon of tolerance, i.e. the specific down-regulation of the capacity to amount an immune response to a particular antigen, has been well recognized for years. For example, potential antigens which reach the lymphoid cells of the fetus during their immunological development specifically suppress any future response to that antigen when the individual is immunologically mature. This is how unresponsiveness develops to the body's own constituents, i.e. 'self'; this then enables the lymphoid cells to distinguish potentially harmful antigens as 'non-self'. Immunological tolerance therefore protects us against overwhelming auto-(antiself) immunity.

A state of tolerance can sometimes be induced in adult life by giving particularly large or extremely small doses of antigen, or chemically modified antigen. Additionally, antigens which are normally encountered via the gut usually induce a state of oral tolerance. Thus food-allergic diseases such as coeliac disease can be envisaged as being due to a breakdown in the usual physiological down-regulation of immunity to dietary and other gut antigens.

Aberrant immunity, malabsorption and infection

A variety of dietary antigens eaten every day reach the organized lymphoid tissues in sufficient amounts to induce a variety of humoral and cellular immune responses. If an active immune response is induced, then the entry of that same antigen in a further meal may result in a local immune reaction which causes tissue damage – this is immunological hypersensitivity.

A deficient immunological response in the gut is in itself unlikely to affect nutritional status. However, the infections which occur in immunodeficient hosts often themselves cause severe diarrhoea and malabsorption, so this is a secondary intestinal consequence of immunological changes.

To evaluate the links between immunological reactivity and nutritional status it is important to have a clearly defined programme of testing.

AN APPROACH TO CLINICAL INVESTIGATION OF THE IMMUNE SYSTEM

Systemic immunity

Protocols for the clinical evaluation of systemic immunity are widely used by clinical and laboratory immunologists for the investigation and management of patients with primary, acquired and iatrogenic immunodeficiency syndromes. Patients can normally be classified by the type of effector mechanism involved, for example T-cell-mediated immunity, immunoglobulin isotype, polymorphonuclear function or reticuloendothelial system.

History and clinical examination

Important features to be elicited include a family history of parental consanguinity as well as of immunodeficiency states, autoimmune disease and atopy. Evidence of a previous but normal recovery from bacterial or viral infections is important. The history of the responses to immunization, particularly with live vaccines (smallpox, BCG) is valuable and can indicate earlier normal cell-mediated immunity.

An aberrant immune status can usually be deduced from a history of atopy, e.g. rhinitis, eczema and asthma. Important features to note on general clinical examination include the presence of palpable lymph nodes, size of the tonsils, splenomegaly, and thymic shadow on the chest X-ray of an infant.

Cellular basis of immunity

Examination of blood films should be the first investigation, with total white cell count, an accurately performed differential and inspection of cell morphology. The absolute lymphocyte count in peripheral blood is a simple but often neglected test. There is now, of course, a range of techniques for defining lymphocyte subsets in blood. The minimum should now involve counts of CD4, CD8 and B-cells in the peripheral blood.

Lymphocytes and specific cell-mediated immunity

Evidence of the existence of specific cell-mediated immunity (implying both normal afferent and efferent limbs) can be obtained by in-vivo tests of delayed-type hypersensitivity using a range of antigens to which the body will usually have been exposed. These 'recall' antigens include tuberculin, mumps antigen, streptokinase–streptodornase and candida.

Many in-vitro tests of antigen-reactive T-cell function are available, ranging from antigen-driven blast transformation to the secretion of cytokines in culture with antigen. Usually these tests are carried out using peripheral blood lymphocytes.

Immunoglobulins and antibodies

Assays of total immunoglobulins can be readily carried out on serum by a variety of techniques in which polyclonal anti-heavy chain antisera are used. Immediate skin-prick tests are used for the in-vivo detection of IgE class antibodies. There are also many tests for assessing the presence of serum antibodies and their titres and avidities, e.g. to antigens of commensal bacteria, vaccines and blood-group substances.

More precise information on the induction and expression of humoral immunity is obtained by studying the primary and secondary immune responses to defined antigens not previously encountered, if these preparations of antigens can be made. The induction of antibody-producing B-cells can also be measured, by using plaque or enzyme immunoassay techniques on suspensions of peripheral blood lymphocytes.

Polymorphonuclear leucocyte and other non-antigen specific functions

The techniques of assessment include basal and stimulated peripheral blood polymorph counts, studies of chemotaxis, phagocytic function and intracellular bacterial killing capacity. A wide range of other cellular and humoral components may be aberrant and a full immune status evaluation should include an appraisal of eosinophils, mast cells, basophils, complement and reticuloendothelial function.

Gastrointestinal mucosal immunity

It is difficult to study the immune system of the gastrointestinal tract in detail, and clinical tests of gastrointestinal immune function have been slow to develop. General guidelines for the investigation of an individual patient or of a group of patients in whom intestinal mucosal immunodeficiency or hypersensitivity state may be present, are given below.

History and clinical examination

Attention must be paid to the potential roles of non-immunological digestive factors. These may not only act as alternative mechanisms of disease, mimicking immunological disorders (e.g. certain infections), but also as factors which will alter immunity in general (e.g. malnutrition) or change intestinal antigen patterns (e.g. pancreatic insufficiency).

Cellular basis of mucosal immunity

Cells serving effector functions are present in mucosal biopsies taken from any level of the gastrointestinal tract. Both histological and in-vitro techniques can be applied. Immunofluorescence or immunoenzyme techniques using polyclonal or monoclonal antibodies targeted to either membrane or cytoplasmic antigens, have greatly expanded the information which can be accrued from mucosal biopsy histopathology.

Lymphocytes and specific cell-mediated immunity

These are used only in research studies. In general, methods available concern non-antigen specific functions such as helper activity, suppressor inducer, suppressor cytotoxic and natural killer-cell functions.

Currently there are no standard methods for detecting the presence of antigen-specific T-effector cells in the mucosae. The existence of an ongoing delayed-type hypersensitivity (DTH) reaction in the small-intestinal and/or the colonic mucosa can be inferred by a cluster of features defined on the basis of work on experimental animals. These include villous atrophy, crypt hyperplasia and a high intraepithelial lymphocyte count.

Immunoglobulins and antibodies

Numbers and immunoglobulin class distribution of plasma cells within the lamina propria of the human gastrointestinal tract can be assessed by using appropriately stained mucosal biopsies.

Immunoglobulins and antibodies can be studied by using ELISA techniques and various intestinal secretions (with appropriate processing to inactivate proteases). Such materials include pure parotid saliva, upper small-intestinal fluid (for example obtained by jejunal intubation), gut perfusates obtained by perfusion of a defined segment of the small intestine with occluding balloons above and below, and fluid obtained from whole-gut lavage, used to cleanse the gastrointestinal tract prior to colonoscopy, barium enema examination or colonic surgery.

Antigens which are used to evaluate intestinal mucosal secretory function include those of gut microorganisms, vaccines and dietary proteins. Just as with the systemic immune apparatus, the generation of a primary antibody response to a new antigen such as cholera vaccine should be incorporated in any full protocol of evaluation of immune status.

Mucosal hypersensitivity reactions

Normally, it appears that antigen-specific immunity of T-cell origin does not develop in the intestine to enterically encountered antigens such as foods. Whether this is true tolerance, antigen-specific suppression, or whether it is merely the absence of this limb of the immune response at gut level, is unknown.

The three jejunal mucosal histopathological features of villous atrophy, crypt hyperplasia and high intraepithelial lymphocyte count, may imply the existence of a cell-mediated immune reaction within the mucosa. In antibody-mediated hypersensitivity, proof of an IgE-mediated immune response requires first, the demonstration of mucosal mast cells; secondly, if possible, evidence from in-vivo skin tests or RASTs on serum, that the patient has IgE antibodies to the antigen concerned, and finally, evidence that mucosal mast-cell degranulation occurs on antigen re-encounter from the gut lumen or bloodstream. An eosinophil infiltrate is also suggestive (Ferguson 1987).

A key factor in immune-mediated tissue damage is the capacity of the tissue to respond to stimuli such as cytokines. In the malnourished state the capacity to mount non-specific inflammation is impaired, and this may partly protect the gut epithelium from some of the potentially adverse effects of mucosal immune reactions.

NUTRITION AND IMMUNODEFICIENCY DISORDERS

Virtually any component of the immune system, specific or non-specific, can be absent or abnormal; the consequent immunodeficiency states vary in severity from trivial to fatal. There are many genetically determined conditions, but immunodeficiency can also result from acquired disease. This is well illustrated in severe form in the acquired immunodeficiency syndrome (AIDS), but it is also common in many infections including influenza, infectious mononucleosis and measles. Acquired immunodeficiency may also be iatrogenic, for example as a result of corticosteroid treatment. In addition to causing susceptibility to infection, immunodeficiency may be associated with abnormally regulated immune reactions, as in allergy or autoimmunity.

In general, immunodeficiency itself has no effect on nutrition but secondary effects occur with diarrhoea, malabsorption and gut losses of blood and protein when immunodeficiency is complicated by chronic bacterial, viral and protozoal infections in immunodeficient animals and humans.

Primary immunodeficiencies

Abnormalities of polymorph function, and deficiencies of complement components or antibodies, all result in susceptibility to bacterial infection. Deficiencies of the humoral and cellular components of the specific immunological system may occur separately or together.

A severe combined immunodeficiency syndrome can be caused by several different gene defects, which are autosomal or X-linked. It is characterized by a defect of stem-cells that leads to deficiency in both the T- and B-lymphocyte systems, and therefore to impairment of cell-mediated immunity and of humoral antibody synthesis. Failure of early stem-cell development has the additional feature of agranulocytosis, with normal red-cell and platelet production. The affected infants are susceptible to even the most benign viral infections, and may die from generalized chicken pox, measles, cytomegalovirus or other viral infections.

Selective deficiency of the B-lymphocyte system occurs in X-linked recessive hypo- or agammaglobulinaemia. The lack of immunoglobulins is not absolute, but the patient fails to respond to antigenic stimuli. However, cell-mediated immunity is normal. This disorder is compatible with survival for many years, though the patient is very susceptible to bacterial infections.

Most patients with immunoglobulin deficiency have 'acquired' or 'late-onset' hypogammaglobulinaemia, known as 'common, variable immunodeficiency'. This is associated with an unusually high incidence of autoimmune disease, such as pernicious anaemia and haemolytic anaemia. An occasional complication is a malabsorption syndrome which may be due to *Giardia lamblia* infection.

Isolated IgM deficiency renders the patient susceptible to blood-borne infection such as that due to meningococcus. Lack of IgA may be associated with gastrointestinal or respiratory tract infections.

In the inherited complement deficiencies there is usually a total absence of the complement protein, and this implies the lack of a functional gene. The association of C1, 4 and 2 deficiencies with immune complex-like or lupus-like disorders is probably due to the failure to eliminate immune complexes.

Secondary immune deficiencies

Immunoglobulin deficiency may result from abnormal losses of serum proteins, for example in lymphangiectasia. Drugs may also depress the immune system; for example, phenytoin or penicillamine may induce IgA deficiency.

Secondary T-cell defects may occur in Hodgkin's disease or sarcoidosis, and following infections such as leprosy, miliary tuberculosis or measles. It may also result from loss of lymphocytes from the gut in protein-losing enteropathy, or due to thoracic duct fistula, and may be caused by treatment with cytotoxic drugs.

HIV-associated intestinal disease and malabsorption

Diarrhoea, malabsorption and weight loss are important clinical features of AIDS. Lesions of the gut may be produced by Kaposi's sarcoma, by opportunistic bacterial, viral, protozoal or fungal infection, or by other sexually transmitted diseases. Even in the absence of intestinal infection, abnormalities of small-bowel histology and function may occur, perhaps due to direct HIV infection of epithelial cells.

There is a reduction in villus length, and in the absence of other infections crypts are short, with a low mitotic activity; when there is associated opportunistic infection, the findings are of short villi with slightly longer crypts, although these have inappropriately low mitotic activity in relation to the villus damage present. Studies of mucosal lymphocytes in duodenal biopsies from HIV-infected patients have revealed low counts of mucosal T-cells, and markers of activated T-cells, such as IL2 receptor expression, are absent. The enterocytes which cover the shortened villi are abnormal, usually with no detectable lactase activity in the duodenal brush border. The prevalence of clinical lactose intolerance in AIDS patients is uncertain, and the classic chronic diarrhoea is probably multifactorial.

There has been considerable attention paid to the dietary treatment of gross undernutrition in AIDS. A pragmatic approach should be taken; if possible, treat infection aggressively, recognize and treat, with appropriate changes in the balance of the diet, pancreatic insufficiency and disaccharidase intolerance; consider the relevance of ileal dysfunction, which might be treated symptomatically with cholestyramine. The appropriateness of a regimen of assisted nutrition, enteral or parenteral, will depend on the patient's general prognosis and the importance of malnutrition in the context of the overall disability (Kotler 1991).

EFFECTS OF MALNUTRITION ON IMMUNITY

Poor nutrition compromises immune function, not only in individuals with generalized protein–energy malnutrition in developing countries, but also in undernourished persons in developed nations – hospitalized patients, alcoholics, the elderly and food faddists (Chandra 1989, 1990). In fact, tests of immunocompetence are included in protocols for the assessment of nutritional status (see Chapter 30).

The majority of studies investigating the relationship between nutrition and immune factors have focused on protein–energy malnutrition (PEM) in children in developing countries, and on debilitated hospitalized patients in industrialized nations. Since, in these groups, there are often multiple deficiencies of protein, energy, vitamins and minerals of variable degrees, interpretation of the data is difficult. Furthermore, associated infection will in turn have profound effects on both the host's immune response and nutritional status.

Investigations of the effects of deficiency of single nutrients on immunity have generally been performed in experimental animals, since single-nutrient imbalances are relatively rare in humans. The results of such experimental studies may have little relevance to complex human conditions.

Protein–energy malnutrition

PEM influences specific immunological functions to different degrees. Humoral immunity is largely spared. Circulating B-lymphocytes are relatively unaffected by nutritional stresses; serum levels of IgG and IgM are usually normal; serum IgA may be modestly elevated; secretory IgA in nasopharyngeal and other external secretions is reduced in malnutrition. Almost all studies of severe malnutrition in humans and experimental animals show reductions in many complement components.

The most consistent and profound effect of PEM is on the cellular immune system. In malnourished children, there is atrophy of the thymus, lymph nodes, tonsils and spleen. The absolute number and functions of circulating T-lymphocytes are reduced. Impaired cellular immunity in the malnourished individual is clinically apparent by a decrease in delayed cutaneous hypersensitivity reactions to a battery of recall antigens.

In terms of phagocytosis, there is evidence that whereas total leucocyte count is normal, bactericidal activity (i.e. intracellular ability to kill bacteria and fungi) is reduced.

The extent of immunological impairment depends not only on the severity of malnutrition, but also on the presence of infection and/or other metabolic stresses, and the age of onset of nutritional deprivation. Malnutrition is one of several factors, along with infection, trauma, surgery, neoplastic disease and metabolic disorders, which contributes to a decrease in immune function in hospitalized patients. In fact, suppression of the immune system by malnutrition has been implicated as one of the major causes of complications in hospitalized patients. Nutritional repletion of many patients improves their immunocompetence and decreases their risk of infection.

Essential fatty acid deficiency

Essential fatty acid deficiencies result in lymphoid atrophy and depressed antibody responses both to T-cell dependent and T-cell independent antigens in experimental animals. Similar findings have not been reported in humans, in whom essential fatty acid deficiency is rare.

Single vitamins

Under normal social conditions, deficiencies or excesses of single vitamins are rarely encountered in humans in developed countries. Consequently, most of the data concerning the role of individual vitamins in immunity have been obtained from experimental animal studies. As reviewed by several authors, single vitamins exert unique effects on the immune system.

Of the fat-soluble vitamins, vitamins A and E have been shown to influence the immune response, whereas there is little evidence for a role for vitamins D and K. Vitamin A deficiency, a frequent complication of PEM, is associated with an increased incidence of infection, both in humans and experimental animals. This may be due to epithelial changes and/or decreased cell-mediated and humoral immunity. In experimental animals, vitamin A deficiency causes a decrease in immunocompetence, evidenced by a reduction in the number and function of T-cells and suppressed production of antibodies by B-cells. The addition of vitamin A to the deficient diet restores immunocompetence. In experimental animals, deficiency of vitamin E decreases humoral and cellular responses.

Among the water-soluble vitamins, deficiencies of pyridoxine (vitamin B_6), pantothenic acid, and folic acid cause impairments in both cell-mediated and humoral immunity in many animal species. In contrast, most of the other B-group vitamins have only a minimal influence on the immune response. Vitamin C enhances bacterial phagocytosis by macrophages, but there is no evidence that it has a role in specific immunity.

Minerals and trace elements

Many minerals and trace elements are required for adequate immune responsiveness. Deficiencies of iron, calcium, magnesium, manganese, copper, selenium, cadmium, chromium and iodine depress immunocompetence in experimental animals. Immune functions also are compromised by an excess of toxic heavy metals, such as lead, mercury and cadmium. The mechanisms by which these nutrient imbalances influence immunocompetence is unknown. Of the various minerals and trace elements examined, considerably more information has accumulated on the role of iron and zinc in immune function.

Both iron deficiency and iron excess are associated with increased susceptibility to infection in experimental animals and humans. Iron deficiency, with or without anaemia, results in a wide range of defects in immune function. While iron is obviously necessary for optimum immune function in the host, it is also essential for the multiplication and growth of bacteria. Thus, theoretically, an increase in iron intake may activate latent bacterial or parasitic infections by providing free iron to support bacterial multiplication. This is the basis of the recommendation that treatment of iron deficiency be carried out cautiously in severely malnourished or infected patients. In healthy individuals, there is little evidence that physiological or moderate increases in iron intake compromise immune responses or increase the occurrence of infectious illness.

Zinc has a critical role in immunocompetence. Zinc deficiency in experimental animals and humans is associated with multiple immunological defects, including atrophy of lymphoid tissue and abnormalities in both cellular and humoral components. Furthermore, zinc deprivation during the fetal or early postnatal periods delays normal development of the immune system. In humans, zinc deficiency occurs in many children with PEM, in hospitalized patients receiving total parenteral nutrition, and in individuals with acrodermatitis enteropathica, a hereditary disorder of zinc absorption. These individuals have an increased incidence of infectious diseases and altered immune responses. Adequate zinc in the diet restores immunocompetence to normal in many zinc-deficient animals and humans.

FOOD INTOLERANCE AND FOOD ALLERGY

The increased public awareness of the relevance of diet to health has also enhanced the idea that 'allergy' to foods, food additives, beverages and even water, causes a wide range of distressing physical and psychological problems and chronic, disabling diseases. However, despite many claims for effective in vitro diagnostic tests for food sensitivity, the precise diagnosis of either food intolerance or allergy generally relies on clinical methodology. Recent advances in understanding the immunological and pharmacological mechanisms of food intolerance help distinguish these from psychologically based reactions to foods. Several authoritative monographs and books provide excellent sources of further information. The EC Scientific Committee for Food (1982) deals with the problem of sensitivity to food additives, provides a useful list of definitions, recommends appropriate labelling of foods and identifies the need to develop better tests of the allergenic potential of dietary substances. The Royal College of Physicians and the British Nutrition Foundation (1984) expanded the definitions of food-related diseases to include the important group of patients without evidence of organic disease but with psychologically based food intolerance. A monograph from the American Academy of Allergy and Immunology and National Institute of Allergy and Infectious Diseases (1984) gives excellent coverage of truly allergic phenomena. An appendix lists and classifies almost 400 diseases transmitted by foods. For excellent, comprehensive and up-to-date coverage of specific diseases see Metcalf et al (1992). The general principles of food intolerance are discussed here; lactase deficiency and milk allergy are considered in greater detail.

SCOPE AND DEFINITIONS

Adverse reactions to ingested food cause a wide variety of symptoms, syndromes and diseases for which the general descriptive terms 'sensitivity' and 'intolerance' are useful. These terms do not imply specific mechanisms for their pathogenesis and can be applied to a reaction with an unknown mechanism as well as to a clearly defined metabolic, pharmacologic or immunopathologic process. The provoking agent may be a single food or ingredient, but sometimes – particularly in IgE-mediated food allergy – many different foods are involved.

Recommended definitions

Food intolerance or *food sensitivity* is a reproducible, unpleasant (i.e. adverse) reaction to a specific food or food ingredient, which is not psychologically based. This occurs even when the affected person cannot identify the type of food which has been given. Mechanisms responsible include enzyme deficiency (e.g. lactase deficiency), pharmacological effects (e.g. due to caffeine), non-immunological histamine-releasing effects (e.g. by certain shellfish), and direct irritation (e.g. by gastric acid in oesophagitis or colonic wind in carbohydrate intolerance).

Food allergy is a form of food intolerance where there is both a reproducible food intolerance and evidence of an abnormal immunological reaction to the food.

Psychologically based food reactions (food aversions) comprise both psychological avoidance – when the subject avoids food for psychological reasons – and psychological intolerance, which is an unpleasant bodily reaction caused by emotions associated with the food rather than the food itself, and which does not occur when the food is given in an unrecognizable form.

DIAGNOSTIC APPROACHES

Elimination diet and challenge

Even the most experienced clinician may have difficulty in elucidating the exact relationship between dietary constituents and the clinical phenomena observed in an individual patient or a specific disease. It has therefore become established practice to use, as diagnostic criteria, the objectively monitored effects of exclusion diets and provocation tests. Some ingenuity may be required to define the objective measures, which may include serial recordings of forced expiratory volume or of nasal airflow, mapping of the extent and severity of skin rashes, daily aphthous ulcer counts, measurements of faecal characteristics, intestinal permeability tests, morphometry of mucosal biopsies, and so on.

For example, in children with atopic eczema appropriate elimination and challenge protocols have clearly shown that around 60% respond positively to specific food challenges, with dermal, gastrointestinal and respiratory reactions. Many different foodstuffs can be implicated and the mechanism of food intolerance is allergic, involving IgE and mast cells. Coeliac disease is currently defined by a different approach, i.e. the effects on small-bowel histology of a gluten-free diet and then a gluten challenge. The intestinal damage is probably induced by activated T-cells. On the other hand, the common condition of lactose intolerance is highly dose-dependent and due to deficiency of the intestinal brush border enzyme, lactase.

Problems with placebo responses

Experience of elimination diet and challenge protocols has revealed that patients' perceptions and doctors' diagnoses of food intolerance are not invariably accurate or correct. In patients with clear and convincing histories of adverse reactions, less than half can normally be confirmed as intolerant on objective testing. Furthermore, double-blind protocols reveal a high rate of symptomatic responses to placebo in some groups of adults; this placebo effect is rare in children.

Clinical ecology

Some health professionals and many members of the public have become convinced that adverse reactions to foods and other environmental agents are extremely common. It is suggested that food sensitivity is a common cause of distressing symptoms such as headache, insomnia, tinnitus, palpitations, breathlessness, ankle swelling, abdominal bloating and fatigue; and in children, of bad behaviour, bed-wetting, poor school performance and hyperactivity. Practitioners may diagnose food intolerance by bizarre laboratory and clinical investigation techniques, such as hair analysis, cytotoxic blood tests, iridology, sublingual and injection provocation tests. These doctors often use highly unconventional treatments, but are genuinely convinced of the accuracy and value of their work, despite many criticisms of their concepts by the 'medical establishment' on both sides of the Atlantic.

SYMPTOMS, SYNDROMES AND DISEASES OF FOOD INTOLERANCE

Food aversion, intolerance and allergy are very difficult to distinguish from one another. Whether objective changes are present or not, the diagnosis of food intolerance can only be established if the symptoms disappear with an elimination diet and if a controlled challenge then leads either to a recurrence of symptoms or to some other clearly identified change – for example, in a jejunal biopsy.

Food intolerance in children

In childhood, a wide range of conditions have been associated with food intolerance and these include eczema, wheeze, urticaria, mood alterations, angio-oedema, epilepsy, failure to thrive, diarrhoea, vomiting and gastrointestinal blood loss. The evidence linking hyperactivity to food intolerance is poor, despite some claims to the contrary.

Milk-induced colitis differs from ulcerative colitis in many clinical and pathological features. Small-intestinal mucosal damage with malabsorption is best documented for cow's milk protein intolerance, but can also occur with soy, chicken, rice, fish and egg intolerance. Coeliac disease and lactose intolerance are described in detail elsewhere.

It seems likely that the symptoms, signs or disease have an immune basis in a higher proportion of children than adults with food intolerance. However, interpreting food antibody tests in infants is difficult because many normal infants have quite high titres of circulating antibody to dietary proteins in the absence of disease.

Food intolerance in adults

In adults the classic allergic symptoms of urticaria, asthma or anaphylaxis may be found, but urticaria in response to food additives can develop from prostaglandin release rather than from an allergy mechanism. The relationship between food sensitivity and migraine is complex; when present, this is likely to have a pharmacological rather than an allergic basis, i.e. is produced by a direct effect of chemical substances on the blood vessel walls. The threshold for the development of a food-induced migraine is altered by many other factors, such as fatigue, smoking and the menstrual cycle.

There are anecdotal claims for an association between food allergy and arthritis, but there is little evidence which can withstand critical examination. Psychiatric symptoms such as irritability and depression may accompany other manifestations of food intolerance, but it remains to be established whether foods can provoke psychiatric disease directly.

Other food-provoked symptoms are gastrointestinal and include nausea, bloating, abdominal pain, constipation and diarrhoea. These features are those of the irritable bowel syndrome. The symptoms may arise either because of abnormal motility or because an individual is unduly aware of sensations accompanying normal contraction or distention of the gut. Not surprisingly, these symptoms are often closely related to foods. Many people who avoid specific foods and have an unsubstantiated self-diagnosis of food allergy suffer from the irritable bowel syndrome. Their self-imposed alterations in diet will influence gut motility, the composition of the stools and the production of gas, and in an introspective individual such physiological changes greatly reinforce the patient's concern.

Despite many erroneous diagnoses of food allergy, there is plenty of evidence that local immunological reactions can influence gastrointestinal motility. Local reactions of immediate hypersensitivity can produce prepyloric or pyloric spasm, hypermotility of the small and large intestines, and oedema with increased secretion of mucus and rectal spasm. The clinical effects include nausea, vomiting, abdominal pain and diarrhoea, but in such patients the basis for the symptoms is truly allergic.

Psychological food intolerance

The psychological aspects of food intolerance are fascinating. There is no doubt that attitudes to food vary widely. Dieting, overeating and food fads are extremely common. Intolerance of food by proxy has been described, whereby in a patient with an eating disorder such as anorexia nervosa the suggestion that the problem could be 'allergic' is seized upon to avoid the stigma of a primarily psychiatric diagnosis. Among those patients complaining of food intolerance, there are significant numbers who are psychiatrically ill and may respond to psychiatric treatment. The mistaken idea that food allergy or intolerance is the cause of their condition appeals to several different types of patient. Some have vague, relatively harmless symptoms such as those of the irritable bowel syndrome. Others suffer from serious allergic disease (e.g. atopic eczema), or progressive diseases with a poor prognosis (e.g. multiple sclerosis, rheumatoid arthritis, schizophrenia). These people may then embark on a radical elimination diet without any proper medical or dietary advice. Since dramatic cure is rare, they eventually present to a hospital specialist asking for an identification of those substances in foods or in the environment which are responsible for their symptoms or disease. Such patients may have already embarked on costly and highly unorthodox investigations and treatments. They will often have experience of alternative medicine, including homeopathy, osteopathy, iridology, medical herbalism and acupuncture. Current conventional medical opinion is that there is no truth in their claim that food intolerance is widespread, unrecognized and a danger to society.

Prevalence of food intolerance

The incidence and prevalence of food intolerance are unknown. Informed medical opinion is that when lactose intolerance is excluded, the prevalence of other conditions is probably less than 1%, with a relatively higher proportion of allergic food intolerance in infants.

APPROACHES TO DIETARY TREATMENT

There are two patterns. The symptoms and clinical features may conform to well recognized phenomena, or to a disease associated with a specific food. This will be suspected from the history and confirmed by a small number of tests. Examples include asthma, rhinitis and eosinophilia associated with salicylate intolerance; flatus and diarrhoea induced by sorbitol from diabetic foods; an increase in milk consumption unmasking a previously asymptomatic lactose intolerance; coeliac disease presenting in an anaemic child with failure to thrive and a positive family history.

In other patients, food intolerance will be included in a wider differential diagnosis. When symptoms are mild, simple symptomatic treatment such as antihistamines for nasal stuffiness, antidiarrhoeals for diarrhoea and analgesics for headache may be more appropriate initially than diagnostic and therapeutic diets, which tend to be time-consuming and difficult. If food intolerance is to be pursued, a baseline elimination diet is taken for some weeks; if symptoms and signs disappear, relevant foods are identified during a planned period of reintroduction, and confirmed by placebo-controlled challenges if feasible.

RELEVANCE OF ALLERGY IN DISEASE – THE EXAMPLE OF MILK

Antigens in cow's milk

Whole cow's milk contains some 3.3 g protein per ml, 80% of which is casein and 20% whey. β-Lactoglobulin (BLG) is the major whey protein, composed of two identical polypeptide chains each having a molecular weight of around 18 000 D. Antigens of cow's milk which induce hypersensitivity reactions are confined to the protein components. Neither milk fat nor lactose is antigenic. On the other hand, digestion of milk proteins may reveal new immunogenic structures which are not present on the intact molecule. In clinical studies, particular attention has been paid to BLG, but reactions to all of the milk proteins may occur. There is considerable antigenic similarity between the proteins of cow's milk and the proteins in milk of other related species, such as goats and sheep.

Patterns of antibody responses to cow's milk protein in man

There have been many reports, using a wide range of techniques, of the titres and patterns of antibodies to cow's milk proteins in the serum of human infants and children. Antibodies are present in the serum of most children, and also 10–20% of healthy adults. Patients with diffuse small-bowel disease and enhanced intestinal permeability from whatever cause, tend to have high titres of serum antibody to many foods. IgE responses to food proteins are of greater relevance than other immunoglobulin responses as the mechanisms of food allergic disease. Transient IgE antibodies to food proteins also occur in some healthy children and may be present in high titre in some individuals. IgE antibodies to food antigens are evidence of an atopic state in general (i.e. a predisposition to become allergic), rather than being of direct diagnostic use in a particular situation.

Allergy as a mechanism within the spectrum of food intolerance and disease

It is very important to define the relevance of immunological mechanisms, and of each particular foodstuff, as the cause of a symptom or disease. In relation to milk allergy, three different groups of patients may be found:

1. All cases of the disease are caused by milk allergy (for example cow's milk sensitive enteropathy). However, usually there are other single foods which can produce an identical condition, such as soya.
2. Several substances – milk, other foods and other allergens, particularly inhalants, are implicated in the pathogenesis of the disease (for example atopic eczema).
3. Allergy (including food allergy) is only one of several possible causes of a symptom or disease (for example diarrhoea, wheeze).

Goldman originally diagnosed milk allergy if the symptoms subsided after dietary elimination of milk and recurred within 48 hours after milk challenge. Reactions to three such challenges had to be positive, with a similar onset, duration and clinical features before a diagnosis could be made. Now, however, such challenge is recognized as too dangerous for some atopic infants, so clinical improvement on an elimination diet should be the main criterion of diagnosis. The increasing use of double-blind testing of foods and placebo in older children and adults, and the use of objective indices of change, such as pathological changes in a jejunal biopsy, greatly strengthen the clinical information to be obtained from a challenge test.

DISEASES CAUSED BY MILK ALLERGY IN SOME PATIENTS

Atopic eczema

The incidence of atopic eczema is rising in Britain and foods are among the many environmental factors which contribute to making this distressing skin disease worse. The strongest evidence of a role for food in the pathogenesis of atopic eczema comes from studies in which children with atopic eczema have responded well to exclusion diets in double-blind controlled crossover trials. Eczema can occur in exclusively breastfed infants, but this can be due to the transfer of absorbed food antigens from the mother's diet to her milk. Food intolerance and enhanced immune responsiveness to foods are also features of atopic eczema in adults. The antigens concerned are usually fish, shellfish, eggs and nuts, and milk sensitivity does not seem to be important.

Asthma

Clinical observations suggest that milk intolerance is not an important factor in asthma.

Malabsorption syndrome with cow's milk intolerance

The classic description is of infants with diarrhoea and a failure to thrive; vomiting is also a feature and some patients have atopic eczema and recurrent respiratory infections. Gastrointestinal investigations show malabsorption, and jejunal biopsy reveals abnormalities of the jejunal mucosa, ranging from moderate villus atrophy to a pathology indistinguishable from coeliac disease. Treatment with a cow's milk-free diet (e.g. banked human milk, elemental diet) induces rapid remission. Once clinical recovery is complete, it may be appropriate to confirm the diagnosis by an in-hospital milk provocation test. Most of these children will be clinically tolerant of cow's milk by the age of 1 year, although the proximal jejunal mucosa often shows persistent but minor abnormalities.

Lactose intolerance overlaps with the syndrome of cow's milk protein-sensitive enteropathy. Where there is extensive villus atrophy, loss of disaccharidase-containing mature enterocytes leads to a relative reduction in the disaccharidase activity of the small-bowel mucosa. Hence there may be a reversible lactose intolerance induced by the intestinal damage, which itself has been caused by cow's milk protein intolerance. The most important practical aspect of this is that lactose intolerance should not be accepted as a primary explanation of malabsorption, failure to thrive, etc. Lactose intolerance can accompany a number of other more serious enteropathies. When a milk challenge is to be given, it is often advisable first to carry out a lactose challenge in the healthy infant on a milk-free diet. When this produces no clinically adverse effect, then a subsequent reaction to a challenge with whole cow's milk can be attributed to the protein constituents, rather than to the lactose.

Cow's milk-sensitive colitis

Many years ago, rectal bleeding was described as a feature of cow's milk allergy in infants. However, when studies of the age distribution of children with colitis were performed, an excess of infants emerged, producing a bimodal distribution, and this suggested that there might be different aetiologies in infants and at other ages. From careful clinical descriptions the specific entity of allergic infantile colitis was recognized and formally documented. Typically, an infant with food-sensitive colitis presents before the age of 1 year, with loose stools containing mucus and blood. An elimination diet and clinical monitoring with rectal biopsy shows a pattern of improvement similar to that seen clinically and with jejunal biopsy in cow's milk-sensitive malabsorption syndrome. The pathology of the rectum differs from classic ulcerative colitis in that there is preservation of the architecture of the mucosal crypts, with no crypt abscess formation and no depletion of goblet cell mucus. Additionally, there are substantial numbers of eosinophils and plasma cells in the infiltrate of the lamina propria. These infants respond well to elimination of the cow's milk from their diet, or from the mother's diet if they are still breastfed. Severe clinical colitis may be induced by a milk challenge, and it is recommended that the rectal pathology, and clinical and pathological improvement on an elimination diet, should be used to diagnose food-sensitive colitis. As is the case in food-sensitive enteropathy, most children can tolerate cow's milk by the age of 2.

Principles of management

The problem lies in the patient's immune system, not in the nature of the food. Young infants are particularly at risk of developing a food allergy because of the immaturity of their immunoregulatory mechanisms. The incriminating foodstuff is usually cow's milk, occasionally soya or egg, because of the limited repertoire of food antigens encountered by human infants. If an individual becomes actively immunized to a food and expresses the immune response as a hypersensitivity reaction, either in the gut or in the skin, then the best treatment is by an elimination diet. This is not too difficult to achieve when the sensitivity is to cow's milk protein. Since mast cells and IgE antibodies are involved, drugs which modify mast-cell functions, such as sodium cromoglycate, may also have a role in suppressing the child's responsiveness to the allergen. T-cell-mediated immunity is probably the underlying mechanism of enteropathy and colitis in the majority of infants with these rare syndromes. New developments, with immune manipulation of the T-cells with either monoclonal antibodies or drugs, are becoming possible. Ultimately one would hope to develop treatment regimens which recreate the normal, healthy state where there is immunological tolerance (specific down-regulation of immunity) to the whole array of antigens which are normally found in the diet.

LACTOSE INTOLERANCE

Patterns of lactase activity in the small intestine

Lactase is one of several disaccharidases contained within the brush border of the small intestine's epithelial cells (enterocytes). In the human, lactase activity is detectable in the fetal gut as early as 8 weeks' gestation. In most mammals lactase activity drops sharply after weaning, and this maturation phenomenon is biologically appropriate since mammalian milk is the only known source of lactose. The human species is unusual in that, in some races, e.g. western European Caucasians, intestinal lactase persists into adult life, probably as a result of selective pressures which allowed persistence of a mutant gene in certain ethnic groups.

Family studies suggest that the ability to express lactase in adult life is inherited at a single gene locus. Thus, within a family the dual inheritance of the gene for lactase absence leads to very low lactase activity in homozygotes; intermediate values are found when one gene for lactase persistence is inherited; and high intestinal lactase activities occur when the individual has both genes for lactase persistence.

Studies of the quantitative distribution of enterocyte enzymes along the villi and crypts of the intestine have shown quite different distribution patterns. In the case of lactase, there is virtually no enzyme activity in crypt enterocytes. Enzyme activity increases sharply in the mid-part of the villi and maximal enzyme activity per enterocyte is reached at the apex. Thus enzyme activity may be reduced when there is disease of the small intestine with villus damage, even in those with a homozygous inheritance for lactase persistence. Transient lactase deficiency and lactose intolerance are extremely important in diarrhoeal diseases and infections of infants. However, because the adult intestine is relatively resistant to extensive epithelial damage, lactose intolerance secondary to infection, or in association with coeliac disease, is very rarely seen in the adult.

Lactose absorption, lactase activity, lactose intolerance

In a healthy individual without small-bowel disease, a randomly taken mucosal biopsy is, in general, representative of the whole of the intestine, and lactase activity in such a specimen gives a good index of the lactase status and lactose absorptive capacity of that individual. The capacity for lactose absorption can also be evaluated by a number of relatively non-invasive blood or breath tests (Chapter 33).

Lactose intolerance is a clinical phenomenon, usually associated with lactose malabsorption and delivery of unabsorbed carbohydrate into the colon. However, lactose intolerance may occasionally be due to the osmotic effects of a carbohydrate load in the upper small intestine, even in a lactose absorber. For example, after peptic ulcer surgery, rapid stomach emptying presents a concentrated load to the upper gut; there is then a shift of fluid from the bloodstream into the gut and accelerated passage down the intestine.

Diagnostic tests

Jejunal biopsy Tissue lactase activity in a jejunal biopsy is the critical investigation, but the result must be interpreted in the context of the histopathology of the jejunum. If this is absolutely normal and there is no evidence of other gastrointestinal disease, such as coeliac disease, parasite infection, Crohn's disease etc., then a low tissue lactase activity usually indicates a state of lactose malabsorption. Obtaining a biopsy from the correct site is important because the normal values for tissue lactase activity in the first and second parts of the duodenum are substantially lower than the normal reference values for the jejunum.

Lactose absorption: lactose tolerance test This is the method which was used in the classic early epidemiological studies in North America, Europe and Africa. The profile of blood glucose after an oral loading dose of glucose is compared with the profile of blood glucose after a similar loading dose of lactose. If there are striking differences between the two curves, then lactose malabsorption can be inferred. Alternatively, a blood glucose rise of less than 20 mg/100 ml after a 50 g lactose load is taken as diagnostic.

Lactose malabsorption: reducing substances in stools In infants with diarrhoea, unabsorbed lactose in the diarrhoea stools can be clearly identified by paper chromatography, and a simple test for faecal reducing substances, using Clinitest tablets, is very useful as a screening test to detect unabsorbed lactose in a child with diarrhoea.

Lactose malabsorption: breath tests These non-invasive tests are extremely valuable for population screening and for other clinical investigations of carbohydrate digestion. The principle of the test is as follows: normal mammalian cells do not produce hydrogen metabolically; however, many bacteria, including the normal gut flora of virtually all humans, generate hydrogen if a suitable energy source is presented. Usually, when lactose or other sugars are eaten, their absorption is complete in the jejunum so no sugar enters the colon, and no extra hydrogen is produced by the colonic bacteria. If unabsorbed carbohydrate such as lactose is presented to the colonic flora, then there is a sudden burst of metabolic activity by these bacteria, with the production of hydrogen. This gas is absorbed into the blood and can therefore be detected and measured as it is excreted in the breath. An increase in fasting hydrogen levels of more than 20 ppm after a 50 g lactose oral load indicates lactose intolerance.

Clinical lactose intolerance When an oral dose of lactose causes the production of flatus, abdominal discomfort or diarrhoea *and* the ingestion of a similar dose of another carbohydrate does not produce these effects, it can be concluded that lactose malabsorption is likely to be present. However, some 10% of healthy individuals will develop gastrointestinal symptoms, dizziness, nausea and palpitation after eating 50 g of any carbohydrate, and so it is essential to be cautious in the interpretation of these clinical features.

Clinical features of lactose intolerance

Adverse reactions which may develop when a lactase-deficient individual ingests lactose in food include nausea, bloating, abdominal pain and diarrhoea. The clinical effects of lactose ingestion are closely related to dose, and there is a wide variation among individuals in the dose–response phenomenon. The conventional lactose load, 50 g, used in tolerance tests, produces symptoms in 70–80% of malabsorbers, whereas 10–15 g of lactose, equivalent to half a pint of milk, will produce abdominal symptoms in only 30–60%.

For reasons that are poorly understood, lactose presented in a food is less likely to induce symptoms than an identical load of lactose presented in solution. One relevant factor may be the rate of gastric emptying, so the fat content of the food or drink consumed may slow the entrance of lactose into the small intestine.

Clinical syndromes of lactose intolerance

Modification of milk-drinking habits

Individuals who are aware of the clinical effects of milk or lactose ingestion modify their dietary habits accordingly. Milk avoidance is significantly commoner in lactose-intolerant than tolerant patients.

Irritable bowel syndrome

Since the clinical effects of lactose intolerance are produced by altered gastrointestinal motility, the symptoms produced in some people will suggest a diagnosis of irritable bowel syndrome. In the early literature, lactose intolerance as a cause of irritable bowel syndrome was overemphasized; unrecognized lactose intolerance is not a common cause of irritable bowel syndrome. Even when lactase deficiency is present in a patient with irritable bowel syndrome, the two diseases often coexist and it is appropriate to treat the primary motility disorder by pharmacological or other dietary means (e.g. by an increase in dietary fibre).

The flatus production associated with lactose malabsorption may cause distress to patients, and there are extremely colourful case reports in the literature.

Abdominal pain in children

Recurrent abdominal pain in children is almost as common as irritable bowel syndrome. The post-weaning drop in intestinal lactase activity may occur as early as 2 years in some races – 5 years in Caucasians – so that schoolchildren may be intolerant of lactose. Studies of recurrent abdominal pain in children in the USA have shown malabsorption of lactose and clinical lactose intolerance in a substantial proportion, and particularly so in black children. Lactose intolerance associated with abdominal pain is mainly relevant in children of ethnic groups with a high prevalence of lactose malabsorption, in whom clinical symptoms may be precipitated by a scheme to provide free school milk or other measures aimed at encouraging high milk consumption.

Diarrhoea after gastric surgery

Gastric surgery and surgery of the small intestine radically alters the physiology of the upper gastrointestinal tract. As noted above, the rate of gastric emptying may affect the tolerance to lactose in a susceptible individual; with lactose feeding after surgery, a lactase-deficient person may develop bloating, faintness and discomfort known as 'dumping', and diarrhoea.

Multiple pathology

Since lactose malabsorption may be the norm in some racial groups, lactose malabsorption and even lactose intolerance will often coexist with other diseases. Since coincident lactose intolerance may modify the pattern of clinical presentation, a period on a lactose-free diet may be of diagnostic value in patients with a puzzling combination of symptoms. For example, lactose malabsorption will clearly affect faecal volume and gastrointestinal symptoms in patients with Crohn's disease or ulcerative colitis, and it is sensible to establish the absorptive capacity for lactose in these patients. If appropriate, dietary lactose can be restricted so that changes in abdominal symptoms can be correlated with disease activity, rather than confused by variations in the lactose content of the diet.

Secondary, reversible lactose intolerance

Disaccharide intolerance may occur as a transient phenomenon associated with a wide variety of diseases (see Chapter 33). Currently World Health Organization recommendations for the management of children recovering from acute diarrhoea are that nutrition, including breastfeeding, should, in general, be introduced within 24 hours. Although many low-lactose and modified milk preparations are now available for patients with acute and chronic diarrhoeas, these are likely to be more relevant in the management of immunologically based milk protein intolerance, or in chronic diarrhoeal disease, than during acute gastroenteritis.

Treatment of lactose intolerance

As with other states of food intolerance, the strict diagnosis of lactose intolerance relies on objective measurements of the clinical effects of the withdrawal and reintroduction of lactose. Milk is such an important nutrient that, before recommending a low-lactose diet with the avoidance of milk, milk intolerance should be formally confirmed by one of the techniques described above. The only satisfactory treatment of lactose intolerance is a diet with a low lactose content. The strictness of the diet depends on the clinical susceptibility of the individual. Patients should be reassured that the symptoms are not due to any disease and can readily be prevented by diet modification. Milk and milk products can be used conveniently for their laxative effect in these patients. Foodstuffs high in lactose, such as fresh milk, powdered milk and milk puddings, should be avoided but most lactose-intolerant patients can tolerate fermented milk products.

Lactose-reduced milk and milk products are available. They can be prepared in various ways, either by removing the lactose or by its hydrolysis, using solid-phase bacterial lactases in the manufacturing process. There are now commercially available lactase preparations which can be used in the home for hydrolysing the lactose in milk and milk products.

FOOD INTOLERANCE AND THE DOCTOR–PATIENT RELATIONSHIP

Many patients with diseases and syndromes of food intolerance are unaware of the relevance of food to their symptoms, and will present to many different specialists concerned with diseases of various systems, general physicians or paediatricians. All specialists need educating on the subject of food intolerance, the diagnostic approaches and the management of the many clinical forms of intolerance. Many patients complaining of food intolerance in fact have psychologically based symptoms without organic disease, and this should be recognized early. Management is often difficult, because many refuse to accept the opinion of a conventional physician or allergist. Such patients may then revise their diagnosis to the 'chronic fatigue syndrome' or to 'chronic candidiasis', and although greatly disabled, refuse to accept the possibility of a psychiatric diagnosis. Physicians and dietitians must give them a sympathetic hearing, with both clinical examination and general support. Patients need gentle persuading that their problem will not be helped by odd diagnostic procedures, which are widely available from sources ranging from witch doctors in the developing world to unscientific practitioners in the affluent world. The latter are good at marketing their theories, often with considerable commercial success.

CONCLUSION

Aspects of nutritional status, host resistance, infection and tissue healing are covered in several other chapters in this book, reflecting the complexity of interactions between the immune system and nutritional status. Research targeted on specific nutrients and specific types of immunity is difficult, and requires an interdisciplinary approach. The protocol described above for clinical assessment of systemic and gut immunity in man, should have many applications.

REFERENCES

American Academy of Allergy and Immunology and National Institute of Allergy and Infectious Diseases 1984 Adverse reactions to foods. NIH Publication No 84–2442, July

Chandra RK 1989 Nutritional regulation of immunity and risk of infection in old age. Immunology 67: 141–147

Chandra RK 1990 Nutrition and immunity. American Journal of Clinical Nutrition 53: 1087–1101

Commission of the European Communities 1982 Food – science and techniques. Sensitivity of individuals to food components and food additives. Reports of the Scientific Committee for Food (Twelfth series) EUR 7823

Ferguson A 1987 Models of immunologically driven small-intestinal damage. In: Marsh MN (ed) Immunopathology of the small intestine. John Wiley & Sons Ltd, Chichester, pp. 225–252

Gastroenterology Clinics of North America 1991 Mucosal immunology: basic principles, Vol 20 no 3

Kotler DP (ed) 1991 Gastrointestinal and nutritional manifestations of the acquired immunodeficiency syndrome. Raven Press, New York

Male DK, Champion B, Cooke A (eds) 1987 Advanced immunology. J B Lippincott, Philadelphia

Metcalf D, Simon R, Sampson HA (eds) 1992 Adverse reactions to foods and food additives. Blackwell, Cambridge, Mass

Roitt IM (ed) 1988 Essential immunology. Blackwell Scientific Publications, Oxford

Royal College of Physicians and The British Nutrition Foundation (Joint Report) 1984 Food intolerance and food aversion. Journal of the Royal College of Physicians of London 18: 83–123

45. Nutritional factors and cancer

P. Boyle

Food production, processing and distribution have been transformed this century, as highlighted in Chapter 21. This and changes in economic and social organization has revolutionized patterns of eating (Trowell 1976). In the developed world greater affluence has led to falling levels of physical activity, both at work and during leisuretime. The pace of change is astonishing with Marcel Pagnol's father telling his class of amazed schoolchildren in 1900 that the developments of the 20th century would lead, among others, to a reduction in the working day to 10 hours (M. Pagnol *'La Gloire de mon Pere'*).

The widespread use of tobacco, alcohol and other addictive substances and recent major changes in sexual habits, modern contraception and family size have all contributed to great changes in western lifestyle. Diet and health must be viewed within this wider context (Hetzel & McMichael 1987).

With the many benefits have come changes in the risk of several diseases, including cancer. For nearly 40 years there has been conclusive proof of an association between cigarette smoking and increased levels of different forms of cancer (IARC 1985). Alcohol drinking is now established as a factor that increases the risk of several forms of cancer (IARC 1988), and coffee consumption has been associated with increased risks of bladder cancer (IARC 1991). Evidence is accumulating that dietary practices may also be associated with changes in the risk of various forms of cancer (Doll & Peto 1981, Armstrong et al 1982, National Academy of Science 1982, Willett & MacMahon 1984, United States Surgeon General 1988). This chapter concentrates on the link between diet and cancer risk, although other lifestyle factors must not be ignored.

THE NATURE OF THE EVIDENCE

During the first half of this century several classic experiments in animals demonstrated the potential impact of diet on carcinogenesis (Tannenbaum 1940). Attention then focused on identifying preformed carcinogens and assessing their role. More recently attention has shifted to the concept that metabolic changes induced by diet may influence indirectly the risk of cancer and that carcinogens may themselves be produced from dietary substrates (Armstrong et al 1982).

'Cancer' is a term greatly feared by the general population. It more correctly refers to a disease process ('carcinogenesis' (Sporn 1992)) whose development is thought to be multistep, with both reversible and irreversible steps. The steps are characterized by the appearance of new types of cells thought to represent stages in the transformation from normal to malignant cells (Hetzel & McMichael 1987); some of the reversible steps may be influenced by dietary factors which can also limit the multistep process from progressing and thereby protect against the development of clinical cancer.

Evidence of the association between cancer risk and dietary factors comes from a number of different study designs. The most widely used initially was the *correlation* study (now more commonly referred to as an *'ecological'* study), where national cancer mortality rates were plotted against national food disappearance data and the correlation coefficient was calculated. This is a useful technique for generating hypotheses and can be used also for testing whether any observed dietary associations obtained from other studies are in broad agreement with morbidity or mortality rate differences or changes found in the correlation studies. Correlation studies are, however, a poor way of establishing that a dietary factor causes, promotes or protects against cancer. It is also a poor way of estimating the magnitude of the dietary link. There are some major drawbacks to using international data which rely on estimates of per capita food consumption. These figures are calculated from complex data on food supplies, imports and exports, etc., provided to the UN Food and Agriculture

Organization by the Ministries of Agriculture. Thus national fat consumption is calculated by adding together the fat contents of all imported food and all local production and subtracting that which is exported. Importantly, no account is taken of food wasted for various reasons and, therefore, not consumed by the population: the consequences of this are outlined by Willett (1990). The total food available for consumption is then divided by the total number of men, women and children in the population. Thus, national rates for breast cancer have been correlated with fat consumption but the quantities involved are different. Thus, cancer usually occurs in women over the age of 60 and fat intake is taken as an average percentage of energy for both sexes and all ages (Baghurst & Baghurst 1982).

It is always advisable to examine the aetiological role of diet by comparing the dietary exposure of persons with the disease under study with comparable individuals without that disease. The most frequently used study design in epidemiology is the *case-control* study. This involves identifying cases and choosing appropriate controls to compare their dietary experience. Questionnaires are used to build up a picture of the lifetime history of exposure to different dietary components and then seeing whether consistent differences emerge. This study is one form of *retrospective* study. Great care is needed when conducting retrospective analyses of lifetime habits, particularly diet, because an ill person tends to highlight for themselves factors that they may believe precipitated their disease. Bias is therefore a potential problem with cases having a 'better' recall than controls. Great care must be taken to minimize these distortions. A more useful study design is the *cohort* (or *prospective*) study where disease-free individuals are identified and the exposure information collected; these individuals are then followed prospectively until groups of cases are identified which can be compared directly to groups without the disease. This study design has the advantage that the exposure information is unbiased. The disadvantage is that large numbers of subjects with lengthy follow-up are needed so these studies are very expensive.

The ideal scientific study design is the *randomized clinical trial* of diet as a preventive measure. This is not a feasible alternative in epidemiological studies on diet and cancer, particularly when the problem is first to identify the dietary risk factors.

THE CURRENT EVIDENCE

Different populations throughout the world experience different rates of different forms of cancer.

These rates also change with time. Groups of migrants acquire the cancer pattern of their new country or region (Haenszel 1981) and this may happen within decades (as found in migrants to Australia) or may take generations, as in the case of breast cancer in Japanese migrants to the United States (Boyle & La Vecchia 1993). Groups of individuals within a community with different characteristics (such as Seventh Day Adventists, Mormons or US blacks) have markedly different cancer patterns. From evidence such as this the environmental theory of carcinogenesis was developed (Higginson & Muir 1979, Doll & Peto 1981) and it is widely held that upwards of 80%, and perhaps 90%, of human cancer may be attributable to environmental factors. 'Environment' is defined broadly to include a wide range of lifestyle factors, including diet, social and cultural practices, with some of these being poorly specified.

It is widely accepted that one-third of human cancer could relate directly to some dietary component (Doll & Peto 1981): in the European Community, this would mean that 400 000 new cases of cancer each year have a major dietary basis (Jensen et al 1990). Furthermore, it seems plausible (but not yet proven) that nutrition plays a permissive role in enhancing the development of many other cancers. Up to 80% of all cancers may have some link with nutrition. The importance of the topic is therefore huge, since within the European Community this represents nearly 1 million new cases per year. Since, theoretically, changes in nutritional intake could induce major changes in cancer rates, it is little surprise that this field is emerging as a topic for intense research.

Research in this area is difficult but much progress has been made in the past decade (Willett 1990). Dietary intakes in terms both of food items and nutrients can now be assessed in the 'usual diet' of very large numbers of individuals. Statistical analytical techniques are also improving as epidemiologists attempt to separate the effects of specific nutrients, e.g. fat, from the possible effect of their contribution to total energy intake (Willett 1990). In these nutritional studies, analysis is more difficult because one is attempting to identify individuals at different levels of dietary exposure, whereas in 'classic' epidemiology there may often be an unexposed group, e.g. of lifetime non-smokers, to compare with cigarette smokers. This need to look at graded effects has important implications for study design and data analysis. To detect trends in the effect of different levels of nutrient intake requires many more subjects than in the much simpler comparison of 'exposed' and 'unexposed' groups (Lubin et al 1988).

Four simple criteria allow the quality of a study to be assessed. First, a validated method of estimating dietary and total energy intakes must be used; secondly, in the analysis the effect of each nutrient should be adjusted to take account of the energy intake; thirdly, the study must be of sufficient size to detect the risk envisaged; and fourthly, the range of dietary intakes in the population must be sufficiently large to allow the graded effects of dietary components or nutrients to be assessed. Few studies as yet fulfil these criteria, so it is no surprise that early epidemiological studies proved inconclusive. In this chapter what evidence there is has been summarized and related to individual cancers in the order specified by the 'International Statistical Classification of Diseases, Injuries and Causes of Death' (WHO 1975).

Tongue, mouth and pharyngeal cancer

These cancers have been combined in the majority of analytical studies and it is difficult to discuss them separately. Their incidence and mortality rates are rising among younger persons in many parts of the world. Cigarette smoking and alcohol consumption are independent risk factors for oral cancer, but their combined effects are usually multiplicative rather than simply additive. After stopping smoking for 10 years the risk among ex-smokers falls to a level similar to that of lifelong non-smokers (Boyle et al 1992). Oral snuff (Winn et al 1981) and fine homeground tobacco powder (Sankaranarayanan et al 1989) are linked to an increased risk of oral cancer. Betel nut chewing is also a risk for inducing oral cancer in many parts of the world, e.g. the Indian sub-continent (IARC 1985). Poor dental hygiene seems to be an independent risk factor (Zheng et al 1990), but the risk of cancer of these sites is reduced by the frequent consumption of fruits and vegetables (McLaughlin et al 1988, Steinmetz & Potter 1991a).

Nasopharyngeal cancer

This shows a different pattern from oral tumours. Epstein-Barr virus (EBV) infections seem to be involved. There is also a very substantial risk of nasopharyngeal cancer among those Chinese weaned on to salted fish, preserved foods and fermented foods, and also among those who consume these foods during childhood (Yu et al 1989). This association is biologically plausible since these foods are sources of volatile nitrosamines, some of which have been shown to be capable of inducing nasal cavity tumours in experimental animals (Delemarre & Themans 1971). Rats fed these salty foods also produce urine containing mutagens (Fong et al 1979).

Cancer of the oesophagus

The most important risk factors for cancer of the oesophagus in developed countries are cigarette smoking (IARC 1986) and alcohol intake (IARC 1988). The highest rates of oesophageal cancer in Europe are found in France (Levi et al 1990); in north-west France, 85% of all oesophageal cancers are attributable to the joint effects of cigarette smoking and alcohol consumption, which are difficult to separate because the two behaviours are closely linked. Nevertheless, other studies show that the risk of oesophageal cancer is increased among non-cigarette smokers who drink alcohol, and among non-drinkers who smoke (La Vecchia & Negri 1989).

Patients with oesophageal cancer have a high prevalence of alcoholism and from the early 19th century the disease was noted to occur in workers involved in the production and distribution of alcoholic beverages (Clemmesen 1965). A prospective study of Danish brewery workers also showed a two-fold increased risk of oesophageal cancer (Jensen 1980), and the more alcohol consumed among men in the French department of Ille-et-Villaine the greater the progressive risk of cancer (Tuyns 1977).

Neither alcohol nor tobacco are substantially involved in the high incidence areas of several developing countries such as Iran (Cook-Mozaffari et al 1979) and China. Drinking very hot drinks (Victora et al 1987) or contaminated foods have been suggested as risk factors but generalized dietary deficiencies are probably major contributing factors to the carcinogenic process (Franceschi et al 1990). The diet in these high-risk areas is poor in vitamins A and C and several other micronutrients as a result of a low intake of fruits and vegetables (Iran–IARC Study Group 1977). These deficiencies and dietary patterns may also be related to oesophageal cancer risk in developed countries (Decarli et al 1987). Recently, estimates suggest that 90% of oesophageal cancer in males in northern Italy is attributable to cigarette smoking, high alcohol use and low β-carotene intake; the corresponding proportion of risk explained by these factors in females was 58% (Negri et al 1992). In areas where the 'diet' is poor, consumption of meat and fish has been shown to reduce the risk of oesophageal cancer, but African and northern Italian studies have also suggested an association between oesophageal cancer risk and maize consumption (Franceschi et al 1990). A monotonous maize-based diet can induce deficiencies of several micronutrients (thiamin, riboflavin and particularly niacin) and, in severe cases, pellagra, a disease which leads to widespread inflammation of the upper digestive tract mucosa (see Chapter 14).

Cancer of the stomach

This was the leading cause of mortality from cancer on a global scale up until the early 1980s, and only recently has been overtaken by the 'epidemic' of lung cancer. There are still areas of the world, notably China and Japan, but also Eastern European countries and northern Italy, where gastric cancer rates are very high. The incidence of stomach cancer in Western countries in declining for reasons that remain unclear. However, there is now consistent evidence from descriptive and analytical epidemiology suggesting that a more affluent diet, and improved methods of food preservation, especially refrigeration, are to some extent linked to these favourable trends. There is, however, a considerable time lag, and migrants show changes in stomach cancer mortality later than they do changes in mortality in colorectal or breast cancer. These studies suggest that diet in early life may be important in altering gastric carcinogenesis.

Diets rich in fresh fruit and vegetables (Risch et al 1985) and, specifically, garlic (allium) (Buiatti et al 1989, Yu et al 1989) are protective against stomach cancer, whereas diets rich in traditional starchy foods tend to be positively associated with risk, although this may simply be an index of a poor diet. If the risks and benefits of high- and low-risk foods are combined in a model, it is possible to envisage a 5–10 fold variation in risk, which could account for much of the observed geographical variation (Trichopoulos et al 1984, La Vecchia et al 1987). The proposed links with dietary salt and with salt nitrates or nitrites are less clear, as are the supposed protective effects of specific micronutrients, such as the antioxidants, β-carotene or ascorbic acid (Buiatti et al 1990).

Colorectal cancer

Colorectal cancer is the third commonest form of cancer and occurs worldwide with an estimated 570 000 new cases diagnosed in 1980 (Parkin et al 1988) and 166 000 new cases each year in the European Community alone (Jensen et al 1990). High incidence rates are found in western Europe and North America, intermediate rates in Eastern Europe and the lowest rates in sub-Saharal Africa (Boyle et al 1985). Few specific risk factors of a non-dietary origin have been established for colorectal cancer.

Energy intakes seem to be consistently higher in cases of colorectal cancer than in comparison groups but any proposed mechanism reflecting this is complex (Willett 1989). Physically active individuals tend to consume more energy but physical activity seems to reduce colorectal cancer risk (Vena 1987, Slattery et al 1988, Whittemore et al 1990). There is no consistent association between obesity and colorectal cancer risk but retrospective studies have to cope with the problems of weight loss from the disease. This positive effect of energy does not appear to be merely the result of overeating, therefore, and may reflect differences in metabolic efficiency or body composition.

Epidemiological studies consistently show that fat intake is positively related to colorectal cancer risk: this evidence is obtained from ecological studies, animal experiments, case–control and cohort studies. However, there have been few methodologically sound analytical studies performed in humans. Many fail to show an energy-independent effect of fat intake. Willett et al (1990) assessed prospectively the health of nurses in the United States: 88 571 women aged 34–59 years, who were without cancer or inflammatory bowel diseases at recruitment, were assessed over many years. After adjustment for total energy intake, consumption of animal fat was found to be associated with increased colon cancer risk. The trend in risk was highly significant ($p=0.01$) when the relative risk of different quintiles of fat intake was related to the risk of cancer. The relative risk in the highest compared with the lowest quintile of fat intake was 1.89 (95% confidence limits of 1.13 and 3.15). This means that with such a large group a graded effect of up to nearly double the lowest risk was discerned and that there was only a 5% chance that the true observed risk fell outside the limits given. (This way of expressing the data is now common in modern studies of this nature.) Curiously, Willett et al found no association with vegetable fat but the relative risk of colon cancer in women who ate beef, pork of lamb as a main dish every day was 2.49 (95% CL 1.24–5.03) compared with those women reporting their consumption as less than once per month. The authors interpreted their data as providing evidence for the hypothesis that a high intake of animal fat increases the risk of colon cancer, and they support existing recommendations to substitute fish and chicken for meats with a high fat content (Willett et al 1990).

This study provides the best epidemiological evidence to date identifying increased meat consumption as a risk factor for colon cancer independently of its contribution to fat or to total energy intake.

Laboratory evidence strongly suggests that cooked meats may be carcinogenic because aminoimidazoazarenes (AIAs) are produced when meats are cooked (Sugimura 1986, Felton et al 1986). These compounds are highly mutagenic in bacterial assays, but there is now evidence that AIAs are mammalian carcinogens – feeding experiments with mice have produced tumours in various anatomic sites (Schiffman & Felton 1990). However, the situation is not entirely straightforward: fried ground beef can also produce anticarcinogenic compounds (Ha et al 1987), so you have a food that has the potential to produce mixtures of potentially carcinogenic and anticarcinogenic substances.

Whittemore et al (1990) performed a case–control study of Chinese in both North America and China, thus ingeniously utilizing the large difference in risk of colorectal cancer which exists between the two continents. Colorectal cancer risk in both continents was increased with increasing total energy intake and specifically from saturated fat: however, no relationship was found with other sources of energy in the diet. Colon cancer risk was elevated among men employed in sedentary occupations. In both continents and both sexes the risks for cancer of the colon and rectum increased with the time spent sitting: the association between colorectal cancer risk and saturated fat was stronger among the sedentary than the active. The risk among sedentary Chinese Americans of either sex increased more than four-fold from the lowest to the highest category of saturated fat intake. Among migrants to North America, risk increased with increasing years spent in North America. Attributable risk calculations suggest that, if these associations are causal, saturated fat intakes exceeding 10 g/day, particularly in combination with physical inactivity, could account for 60% of colorectal cancer incidence among Chinese–American men and 40% among Chinese–American women.

The specific fatty acids in the diet may also be important: animal experiments suggest that linoleic acid (an n-6 polyunsaturated fatty acid) promotes colorectal carcinogenesis (Zaridze 1983, Sakaguchi et al 1984) and that a low-fat diet rich in eicopentaenoic acid (an n-3 polyunsaturated fatty acid) has an inhibitory effect on colon cancer (Minoura et al 1988). However, there have been no epidemiological studies conducted to date regarding n-3 and n-6 fatty acids and colorectal cancer risk.

The original hypothesis of the protective effect of dietary fibre was based on a clinical/pathological observation and a hypothesis that proposed that increasing intakes of dietary fibre increased fecal bulk and reduced transit time. More recent thinking suggests that this mechanism may not be as relevant to colorectal carcinogenesis as previously thought (Kritchevsky 1986). The term 'fibre' encompasses many components, each of which has specific physiological functions (see Chapter 4). The commonest classification is into the insoluble, non-degradable constituents (mainly present in cereal fibre) and into soluble, degradable constituents like pectin and plant gums, which are present mainly in fruits and vegetables. Epidemiological studies have reported differences in the effect of these components. For example, Tuyns et al (1987) and Kune & Kune (1987) found a protective effect for total dietary fibre intake in case–control studies and the same was found in one prospective study (Heilbrun et al 1986). However, a large number of studies could find no such protective effect (see Willett 1989 for review). The large majority of studies in humans have found no protective effect of fibre from cereals but have found a protective effect of fibre from vegetable and, perhaps, fruit sources (Willett 1989). This could conceivably reflect an association with other components of fruits and vegetables, with 'fibre' intake acting merely as an indicator of consumption.

Although calcium was proposed as capable of modifying colorectal carcinogenesis (Newmark et al 1984), there is little supporting evidence (Sorenson et al 1988), although the study was of questionable design and diet was estimated inadequately. A number of studies have reported positive associations with alcohol consumption (Longnecker et al 1990), but it remains to be proven whether the putative association is with alcohol per se and not with some energetic effect of the alcohol. There is some experimental evidence that vitamin E and selenium may be protective against colon tumours (Zaridze 1983) and that vitamin A and/or its precursor β-carotene protects also (Willett 1989). Lactobacilli, found in some dairy products, may have a favourable effect on the intestine (Goldin & Gorbach 1984). Twelve case–control studies of acceptable quality have addressed the issue of coffee consumption and the risk of colorectal cancer, and 11 of these have found an inverse relationship, i.e. suggesting that coffee drinking may be protective (IARC 1991). No association has been found with tea drinking or caffeine intake from all sources considered.

Therefore, dietary factors seem to be important determinants of colorectal cancer risk, but methodological problems remain. An effect of saturated fat appears to exist independently of energy intake and meat intake may also increase risk. Whether this is independent of its fat content or its contribution to energy intake is currently unclear: if the risk is independent, then it may relate to the mutagenic products formed in the cooking process. Vegetable fibre, directly or indirectly, appears to be protective, as does coffee consumption. Associations with other dietary factors, including cereal fibre consumption, are still open questions.

Liver cancer

An increased frequency of *primary* liver cancer has been observed among individuals with a high alcohol intake in a number of studies, although this is not a universal finding (IARC 1988). Of four cohort studies, two found an increased risk with increasing alcohol consumption, while a third study showed an elevated risk in only a sub-group. Alcoholics have a 50% excess of liver cancer compared with non-alcoholics. This risk may well be underestimated, however, because the liver damage induced by alcohol may lead people to stop drinking before the diagnosis of liver cancer becomes apparent in a patient.

Part of the excess liver cancer risk in alcoholics can be attributed to dietary deficiencies, since it has been shown that a diet poor in vitamin A and other micronutrients increases the risk of hepatocellular carcinoma (La Vecchia et al 1988). In tropical areas of Africa and Asia, aflatoxin – a metabolite of *Aspergillus flavus*, contaminates foods, particularly cereals, and increases the risk of primary liver cancer, especially in those who have had hepatitis B virus and consume alcohol. The risk of primary liver cancer has been found to be greatly elevated among subjects exposed to more than one factor (Bulatao-Jayme et al 1982). Animal experiments suggest that very early exposure to hepatitis B virus is particularly conducive to hepatonic development.

Pancreatic cancer

This is consistently reported to occur more frequently in men than in women, in blacks than in whites and in urban compared with rural population groups. In some countries, mortality rates continue to rise, whereas in others declining levels of disease can be seen among members of younger birth cohorts (Boyle et al 1989). Although some of the patterns observed can be explained by variation in pancreas cancer risk factors, many cannot.

Analytical studies based on patients with pancreatic cancer consistently demonstrate that cigarette smok-

ing increases the risk (IARC 1986, Boyle et al 1989).

Speculation of a link with coffee consumption (MacMahon et al 1981) has not been sustained (IARC 1991), and there is no convincing link with alcohol intake either (Velema 1986). Beer consumption was suggested as a risk (Cuzick & Babiker 1989), but three other case–control studies do not support this (Bouchardy et al 1990).

Specific dietary factors are likely to emerge as important in determining pancreatic cancer risk (Bueno de Mesquita et al 1990, Howe et al 1990a, b, Ghadirian et al 1991, Baghurst et al 1991, Zatonski et al 1991). The SEARCH study (Howe et al 1991) found positive associations between carbohydrate and cholesterol intake and an inverse relationship with dietary fibre and vitamin C intakes. The consistency, strength and specificity of these associations among the five centres involved suggest underlying causal relationships (Howe et al 1990b).

Laryngeal cancer

Tobacco smoking (IARC 1986) and alcohol consumption (IARC 1988) are the major established risk factors for laryngeal cancer. Different types of alcohol seem unimportant (Rothman et al 1989). Pipe and cigar smoking are strongly related to laryngeal cancer, with a lower risk for filter, low-tar cigarettes. Dietary factors are implicated by the strong and inverse relationship of the cancer with social class, with diet being one of the biggest distinctions between classes of relevance to carcinogenesis. A few case–control studies show that a poor diet (Zatonski et al 1991), especially one limited in fresh fruit, vegetables and therefore also in the availability of vitamin A and C, is associated with the risk of laryngeal cancer (Graham et al 1981, De Stefani et al 1987, La Vecchia et al 1990).

Lung cancer

Although cigarette smoking (La Vecchia et al 1990) is the overwhelming cause of lung cancer in humans, there is now a considerable body of evidence of dietary associations. Eight case–control studies examined the effects of fruit and vegetables and all found lower risks associated with the regular consumption of one or more fruits and vegetables. Steinmetz & Potter (1991a), in reviewing the results, observed that each study found a lower risk with intakes of at least one vegetable high in β-carotene. In four of these eight studies, the lower risk was more evident in smokers than in non-smokers.

Breast cancer

Despite many detailed epidemiological studies, including a large number with biological measurements, the aetiology of breast cancer remains unclear (Boyle 1988). There are over half a million new breast cancers diagnosed worldwide each year (Parkin et al 1988).

The risk of breast cancer appears to increase with increasing body mass index among postmenopausal women (de Waard et al 1964) and a number of studies have suggested that the same risk factor reduces the risk of breast cancer at premenopausal ages, although a number of biases, including the increased likelihood of finding a lump in thinner women, complicate the interpretation of these findings (Swanson et al 1988). Former college athletes have been found to have a reduced risk of breast cancer compared with non-athletes (Frisch et al 1985), as have ballet dancers (Warren 1980). This may be associated with physical activity or reduced body weight around menarche, early adolescence or throughout lifetime.

The association with diet, particularly dietary fat intake, was originally suggested by cross-cultural ecological studies and by some animal experiments, but the subject is very controversial (Willett 1989). Theoretical considerations of biological processes lead to the conclusion that an increased risk of breast cancer with increasing saturated fat intake in postmenopausal women was plausible (Boyle & Leake 1988). However, the evidence from detailed analytical studies in humans with breast cancer is unclear. Case–control studies provide minimum support for this association (Howe et al 1990) and no association can be found in the prospective studies reported to date (Willett et al 1987a, Jones et al 1988). The most recent analysis of the United States Nurses Health Study found no association between fat intake and intake of fibre and breast cancer risk in either pre- or post-menopause women (Willett et al 1992). There is little consistent evidence in humans of a fat–breast cancer association.

Studies from Greece (Katsouyanni et al 1986) and Italy (La Vecchia et al 1987) have suggested that green vegetable consumption is an indicator of a low risk dietary pattern. This may simply reflect low intake of fat or calories, or suggest that some constituent of green vegetables may be protective (Michnovicz & Bradlow 1990). If such an association exists, current evidence suggest it is weak (Steinmetz & Potter 1991a, b).

A modest increase in risk of breast cancer has been observed consistently with increased alcohol intake from a large number of studies (Willett et al 1987b, Longnecker et al 1988), although no satisfactory biological explanation has been proposed. The overview conducted by Longnecker et al (1988) resulted in four conclusions: (1) at intakes of 24 g alcohol/day (two drinks/day), there is a strong association between alcohol consumption and an increased risk of breast cancer; (2) at lower levels of intake, weaker or modest associations are found, although the 95% statistical confidence limits usually include 1.0, i.e. that there is no relative risk within the range of risk which could have occurred by chance; (3) evidence in favour of a dose–response relationship between alcohol intake and risk of breast cancer is strong; and (4) the very small relative risk of 1.1 obtained by pooling a large number of studies that compare those who have drunk some alcohol with those who have never drunk, does not alter the conclusions since most women are light or moderate drinkers so their impact on the analysis will diminish the association. There is therefore no proof that alcohol causes breast cancer, but the evidence does support an association between breast cancer risk and alcohol consumption.

Cervical cancer

Cervical cancer resembles in several ways a sexually transmitted disease (Brinton & Fraumeni 1986). The younger the age at first intercourse, and the greater the number of sexual partners (Brinton et al 1987), the greater the risk, which is also increased in proportion to the number of pregnancies (Brinton et al 1989). The risk is greater in the lower social classes in long-term users of oral contraceptives and in cigarette smokers (IARC 1986). Pre-vitamin A (carotenoids) and vitamin E (Cuzick et al 1989), or other aspects of a vegetable-rich diet, seem to be protective, but this association may simply reflect one index of a more health-conscious lifestyle (La Vecchia et al 1988), the key factor being sexual behaviour.

Endometrial cancer

Endometrial cancer is the gynaecological malignancy that most readily correlates with hormonal changes. It is strongly related to increased oestrogen levels and to oestrogen drug use and to low levels of progestogens. It therefore relates to states of non-ovulation in many women, to oestrogen replacement treatment in the menopause and to obesity, which increases endogenous oestrogen levels. The risks of long-term hormonal replacement therapy (HRT) use and of severe obesity are 5–10 times greater than normal (Lew & Garfinkel 1979). Menopausal treatment with hormones was the major determinant of the epidemic of endometrial cancer observed in the United States during the 1970s (Ziel & Finkle 1975), whereas obesity is the major established risk determinant of endometrial cancer in Europe (Parazzini et al 1989) where HRT has not been so widely used.

There is some suggestion that both nutritional status and diet are related to endometrial cancer. Ecological studies show positive correlations with meat, eggs and milk consumption and with protein, fat and total energy intakes. The few analytical studies available suggest positive associations with total energy intake and with dietary carbohydrates, fats and oils, but protective effects of green vegetables (La Vecchia 1989).

Ovarian cancer

Epithelial ovarian cancer is the commonest type of ovarian neoplasm and the leading cause of death from gynaecological cancer in most Western countries. The role of nutrition and diet are the major issues in ovarian cancer epidemiology. The American Cancer Society One Million Study showed an elevated risk of ovarian cancer among obese women (Lew & Garfinkel 1979), but the evidence from case–control studies is largely null. Loss of weight secondary to the cancer may complicate the analysis. Ecological studies show positive correlations with fats, proteins and energy intakes, but these are less strong than for endometrial cancer. Case–control studies show a possible association with total fat intake and some protective effect from green vegetables (La Vecchia 1989).

Recently, there has been debate on the possible role of milk fat (Mettlin & Piver 1990) and lactose (Cramer et al 1989, Cramer 1989, Harlow et al 1991) in increasing the risk of ovarian cancer. According to Cramer's model (1989), galactose is considered toxic for the oocytes. Laboratory evidence has been supported by ecological and case–control studies but others claim that the real mechanism involves animal fats rather than milk sugars (Mettlin 1991, Cramer & Harlow 1991).

Prostatic cancer

In 1980 it was estimated that prostatic cancer was the fifth most frequent cancer in men, with an estimated 235 000 cases occurring annually worldwide (Parkin et al 1988). Its cause is poorly understood. Sex hormones have been implicated simply because the growth and development of this organ requires the presence of androgens. The hormonal promotion theory has received little support from epidemiological studies and clinical observations (Griffiths et al 1990).

International analyses relate prostatic cancer rates to per capita fat intake (Zaridze & Boyle 1987), but recent interest has focused on three aspects of diet: animal fat, β-carotene and milk intakes. Fat probably does increase the risk of prostatic cancer but milk consumption does not appear to be related other than through its effects on fat intake. The association with vegetable intake is very confusing: some studies are positive, some negative and a smaller number show no association. The precise nature of the dietary involvement in prostatic cancer remains to be identified.

Bladder cancer

Here the link with cigarette smoking is overwhelming (IARC 1986, La Vecchia et al 1991): the only remaining question is the strength of the association. A number of studies have also reported increased risks of bladder cancer with coffee consumption; an IARC Working Group considered that there was some evidence that coffee may be carcinogenic for the human bladder (IARC 1991). Another widely used potential risk factor is saccharine, but the results of extensive investigation is largely reassuring (IARC 1987). There is some evidence that a diet rich in fresh fruit and vegetables and, possibly in vitamin A, is protective.

Kidney cancer

This occurs more frequently in men than women with a ratio of 2:1. Renal cell adenocarcinoma accounts for about 85% of all kidney cancers. Very little, however, is known about their causes. The single established risk factor is cigarette smoking, but the relative risk is about 2 for current versus never smokers, i.e. lower than for bladder and most other tobacco-related neoplasms (IARC 1986). A few case–control studies have shown a positive association with obesity (Maclure & Willett 1990), but the evidence is not totally consistent (Talamini et al 1990). There is no consistent evidence regarding the role of alcohol (IARC 1988) or methylxanthine-containing beverages (IARC 1991) on the risk of renal cell cancer.

Maclure & Willett (1990) reported that cases ate more meat than controls in a study from Massachusetts. They also reported significant trends in risk with increasing intake of animal protein, animal fat and saturated fat; there were negative trends with markers of vegetable intake (Maclure & Willett 1990). The association seen for meat intake was confirmed by McLaughlin et al (1984), but not by McCredie et al (1988). The link with protein intake is supported by the increased death rates seen among meat cutters and fishermen (Petersen & Milham 1980), ranchers and creamery workers (Milham 1976) who usually have access to cheaper meat fats and milk. The risk has also been found to be increased by kidney stones (McLaughlin et al 1984, Maclure & Willett 1990).

Thyroid cancer

This is a rare form of cancer in general; it is also unusual in being more common in women, with various histological types showing a wide range of malignancy from the relatively benign to the rapidly fatal (Franceschi et al 1991). The influence of iodine deficiency, suspected for a long time as a major influence on this disease, is not totally understood. Scanty data suggest that a poorer diet, particularly if containing natural goitrogens, is related to an increased risk (Franceschi et al 1991, 1993).

MECHANISMS FOR DIETARY EFFECTS ON CANCER

Diet may influence human carcinogenesis in six general ways (Armstrong et al 1982, Hetzel & McMichael 1987):

1. Diet provides the carcinogens or their immediate precursors;
2. Diet facilitates or inhibits the endogenous production of carcinogens;
3. The modification of carcinogens by metabolic activation or inactivation could be affected by other dietary components;
4. Increasing or impeding the delivery of carcinogens to their site of action may be influenced by dietary changes;
5. Diet may alter the susceptibility of tissues to cancer induction or growth by dietary effects or tissue metabolism;
6. Diet may alter the body's capacity to eliminate transformed cells.

The existence of each of these mechanisms in studies from humans can be demonstrated to some degree or another and no unifying theory can be proposed as yet.

PROSPECTS FOR PREVENTION

Identifying the risk factors for cancer is not an end in itself: it is merely a first step in the process of cancer prevention. Prevention can be started even though the underlying mechanism is poorly understood. Thus, lung cancer was linked to cigarette smoking and preventive policies started years before any mechanism of action was identified.

It seems clear that there is a link between fat and particularly saturated fat intake and colon cancer. This is a consistent finding and it could be reasonably concluded that if a population were to reduce its intake of fat, then a reduction in the incidence of colon cancer can be expected. However, the magnitude of the effect is unclear and it is uncertain whether the effects of fat are mediated through some precise biochemical mechanism which would allow another specific prevention strategy.

At the beginning of the chapter the reversible nature of the multi-step process of carcinogenesis was noted. If agents responsible for reversing these processes could be found, then this would be important for prevention. The most likely prevention measure lies in fruits and vegetables and their constituents (Steinmetz & Potter 1991a, b). Up until early 1991, a total of 13 ecological studies, nine cohort studies and 115 case–control studies could be used to conclude that consumption of higher levels of vegetables and fruits is associated consistently, although not universally, with a reduced risk of cancer at most sites. The association is most marked for epithelial cancers (particularly those in the intestinal and respiratory tracts). These links are, however, weak or non-existent for hormone-related cancers (Steinmetz & Potter 1991a). A wide variety of vegetables and fruits seem to be involved, with some suggestion that raw forms are associated most consistently with a lower risk.

Possible mechanisms for these associations have also been considered (Steinmetz & Potter 1991b). A large number of potentially anti-carcinogenic agents are found in these food sources, including carotenoids, vitamins C and E, selenium, dietary fibre, dithiolthiones, glucosinolates and indoles, isothiocyanates, flavenoids, phenols, protease inhibitors, plant sterols, allium compounds and limonene. These agents have a number of distinct complementary and overlapping mechanisms of action. It is therefore considered unlikely that any one substance in the fruit and vegetables is responsible.

The next step is to identify the precise nutrients or non-nutrients responsible for these protective effects, but it is still premature to estimate the level of intake of these foods, nutrients or non-nutrients needed to confer protection. Nevertheless, a WHO group proposed that intakes of 400 g/day for fruit and vegetables (excluding potatoes) was a reasonable goal since this corresponded to intakes in general Mediterranean areas where cancer rates are lower than in North America or Northern Europe.

PROSPECTS FOR INTERVENTION

Several studies are underway with randomized trials of vitamin supplementation to see whether a decrease in cancer rates is achieved. Trials such as these are important in evaluating the possible impact of dietary changes which are more difficult to use as the basis of intervention trials. There is an excellent discussion of many issues related to changing individual and population diets in Hetzel & McMichael (1987).

REFERENCES

Armstrong BK, McMichael AJ, McLennan R 1982 Diet. In: Schottenfeld D, Fraumeni J (eds) Cancer epidemiology and prevention. WB Saunders, Philadelphia

Baghurst KI, Baghurst PA 1982 Public perceptions of the role of dietary and other environmental factors in cancer causation or prevention. Journal of Epidemiology and Community Health 46: 120–126

Baghurst PA, McMichael AJ, Slavolinek AH, Baghurst KI, Boyle P, Walker AM 1991 A case-control study of diet and cancer of the pancreas. American Journal of Epidemiology 134: 167–179

Bouchardy C, Clavel F, La Vecchia C, Raymond L, Boyle P 1990 Alcohol, beer and cancer of the pancreas. International Journal of Cancer 45: 842–846

Boyle P 1988 Epidemiology of breast cancer. In: Bailliere's Clinical Oncology 2: 1–57

Boyle P, Leake RE 1988 Progress in understanding breast cancer: epidemiologic and biological interactions. Breast Cancer Research and Treatment 11: 91–112

Boyle P, La Vecchia 1993 Cancer aetiology. In: Peckman MJ, Pinedo R, Veronesi U. Oxford Textbook of Oncology. Oxford University Press, Oxford

Boyle P, Hsieh CC, Maisonneuve P et al 1989 Epidemiology of pancreas cancer. International Journal of Pancreatology 5: 327–346

Boyle P, Zaridze DG, Smans M 1985 Descriptive epidemiology of colorectal cancer. International Journal of Cancer 36: 9–18

Boyle P, Macfarlane GJ, Zheng T, Maisonneuve P, Evstifeeva T, Scully C 1992 Recent advances in epidemiology of head and neck cancer. Current Opinion in Oncology 4: 471–477

Brinton LA, Fraumeni JF 1986 Epidemiology of uterine cervical cancer. Journal of Chronic Diseases 39: 1051–1065

Brinton LA, Hamman RF, Huggins GR et al 1987 Sexual and reproductive risk factors for invasive squamous cell cervical cancer. Journal of the National Cancer Institute 79: 23–30

Brinton LA, Reeves WC, Brenes MM et al 1989 Parity as a risk factor for cervical cancer. American Journal of Epidemiology 130: 486–496

Bueno de Mesquita HB, Moerman CJ, Runia S, Maisonneuve P 1990 Are energy and energy-providing nutrients related to carcinoma of the exocrine pancreas? International Journal of Cancer 46: 435–444

Buiatti E, Palli D, Decarli A et al 1989 A case-control study of gastric cancer and diet in Italy. International Journal of Cancer 44: 611–616

Buiatti E, Palli D, Decarli et al 1990 A case-control study of gastric cancer and diet in Italy. II. Association with nutrients. International Journal of Cancer 45: 896–901

Bulatao-Jayme J, Almero EM, Castro CA, Jardeleza TR, Salamat LA 1982 A case-control dietary study of primary liver cancer risk from aflatoxin exposure. International Journal of Epidemiology 11: 112–119

Clemmesen J 1965 Statistical studies in the aetiology of malignant neoplasms. I. Copenhagen Danish Cancer Registry

Cook-Mozaffari P, Azordegan F, Day NE, Ressicaud A, Sabai C, Armesh B 1979 Esophageal cancer studies in the Caspian Littoral of Iran: results of a case-control study. British Journal of Cancer 39: 293–309

Cramer DW 1989 Lactase persistence and milk consumption as determinants of ovarian cancer risk. American Journal of Epidemiology 130: 904–910

Cramer DW, Harlow BC, Willett WC et al 1989 Galactose consumption and metabolism in relation to the risk of ovarian cancer. Lancet 2: 66–71

Cramer DW, Harlow BL 1991 A case-control study of milk drinking and ovarian cancer risk. American Journal of Epidemiology 134: 454–456

Cuzick J, Babiker AG 1989 Pancreatic cancer, alcohol, diabetes mellitus and gall bladder disease. International Journal of Cancer 43: 415–421

Cuzick J, De Stavolo B, McCance D 1989 A case-control study of cervix cancer in Singapore. British Journal of Cancer 60: 238–243

De Stefani E, Correa P, Oreggia F et al 1987 Risk factors for laryngeal cancer. Cancer 60: 3087–3091

de Waard F, Baanders-van Halewijin EA, Huizinga J 1964 The bimodal age distribution of patients with mammary carcinoma. Cancer 17: 141–151

Decarli A, Liati P, Negri E, Franceschi S, La Vecchia C 1987 Vitamin A and other dietary factors in the aetiology of esophageal cancer. Nutrition and Cancer 10: 29–37

Delemarre JF, Themans HH 1971 Adenocarcinoma of the nasal cavities. Nederlands Tijdschrift voor Geneeskunde 115: 688–690

Doll R, Peto R 1981 The causes of cancer: quantitative estimates of avoidable risks of cancer in the United States today. Journal of the National Cancer Institute 66: 1191–1308

Felton JS, Knize MG, Shen NH et al 1986 Identification of the mutagens in cooked beef. Environmental Health Perspective 67: 17–24

Fong LY, Ho JH, Huang DP 1979 Preserved foods as possible cancer hazards. WA rats fed salted fish have mutagenic urine. International Journal of Cancer 23: 342–346

Franceschi S, Bidoli E, Baron AE, La Vecchia C 1990 Maize and risk of cancers of the oral cavity, pharynx and oesophagus in north-eastern Italy. Journal of the National Cancer Institute 82: 1407–1411

Franceschi S, Levi F, Negri E, Fassina A, La Vecchia C 1991 Diet and thyroid cancer: a pooled analysis of four European case-control studies. International Journal of Cancer 48: 395–398

Franceschi S, Boyle P, Maisonneuve P et al 1993 The epidemiology of thyroid cancer. Critical Reviews in Oncogenesis (in press)

Frisch RE, Wyshak G, Albright NL et al 1985 Lower prevalence of breast cancers and cancers of the reproductive system among former college athletes compared to non athletes. British Journal of Cancer 52: 885–891

Ghadirian P, Simard A, Baillargeon J, Maisonneuve P, Boyle P 1991 Nutrition and pancreatic cancer in the Francophone community in Montreal, Canada. International Journal of Cancer 47: 1–6

Goldin BR, Gorbach SL 1984 The effect of milk and lactobacillus feeding on human intestinal bacterial enzyme activity. American Journal of Clinical Nutrition 39: 756–761

Graham S, Mettlin C, Marshall JR, Priore R, Rzepka T, Shedd D 1981 Dietary factors in the epidemiology of cancer of the larynx. American Journal of Epidemiology 113: 675–680

Griffiths K, Eaton CL, Davies P 1990 Prostatic cancer: aetiology and endocrinology. Hormone Research 32 (Suppl 1): 38–43

Ha YL, Grimm NK, Pariza MW 1987 Anticarcinogens from fried beef: heat altered derivatives of linoleic acid. Carcinogenesis 8: 1881–1887

Haenszel W 1981 Migrant studies. In: Schottenfield, Fraumei JF (eds) Cancer epidemiology and prevention. WB Saunders, Philadelphia

Harlow BL, Cramer DL, Geller J, Willett WC, Bell DA, Welch WR 1991 The influence of lactose consumption on the association of oral contraceptive use and ovarian cancer risk. American Journal of Epidemiology 134: 445–453

Heilbrun LK, Hankin JH, Nomura A et al 1986 Colon cancer and dietary fat, phosphorous and calcium in Hawaiian-Japanese men. American Journal of Clinical Nutrition 43: 306–309

Hetzel B, McMichael AJ 1987 The LS factor: lifestyle and health. Penguin Books, Australia

Higginson J, Muir C 1979 Environmental carcinogenesis: misconceptions and limitations to cancer control. Journal of the National Cancer Institute 63: 1291–1298

Howe GR, Hirohata T, Hislop TG et al 1990a Dietary factors and risk of breast cancer: combined analysis of 12 case-control studies. Journal of the National Cancer Institute 82: 561–569

Howe GR, Jain M, Miller AB 1990b Dietary factors and risk of pancreatic cancer: results of a Canadian population-based case-control study. International Journal of Cancer 45: 604–608

IARC 1985 Monographs on the evaluation of carcinogenic risk of chemicals to humans. Tobacco habits other than smoking; betel-quid and areca-nut chewing; and some related nitrosamines, no. 37 IARC, Lyon

IARC 1986 Monographs on the evaluation of the carcinogenic risk of chemicals to humans, tobacco smoking, no. 38: IARC, Lyon, pp. 279–284

IARC 1987 Overall evaluations of carcinogenicity: an updating of IARC Monographs volumes 1–42. IARC Monographs (Suppl. 7). IARC, Lyon

IARC 1988 Monograph on the evaluation of carcinogenic risks to humans, alcohol drinking, no. 44. IARC, Lyon, pp. 215–222

IARC 1991 Monographs on the evaluation of carcinogenic risk to humans, coffee, tea, maté, methylxanthines (caffeine, theophylline, throbromine) and methylglyoxal, no. 51. IARC, Lyon

Iran-IARC Study Group 1977 Esophageal cancer studies in the Caspian Littoral of Iran: results of population studies. A prodrome. Journal of the National Cancer Institute 59: 1127–1128

Jensen OM 1980 Cancer morbidity and causes of death among Danish brewery workers. IARC Non-serial publication. IARC, Lyon

Jensen OM, Esteve J, Moller H, Renard H 1990 Cancer in the European Community and its member states. European Journal of Cancer 26: 1167–1256

Jones DY, Schatzkin A, Green SB et al 1988 Dietary fat and breast cancer in the National Health and Nutrition Survey 1 (NHANES 1). Epidemiologic follow-up study. Journal of the National Cancer Institute 79: 465–471

Katsouyanni K, Trichopoulos D, Boyle D et al 1986 Diet and breast cancer: a case-control study in Greece. International Journal of Cancer 38: 815–820

Kritchevsky D 1986 Diet, nutrition and cancer. The role of fiber. Cancer 58 (Suppl 8): 1830–1836

Kune S, Kune GA, Watson LF 1987 Case-control study of dietary aetiological factors: the Melbourne colorectal cancer study. Nutrition and Cancer 9: 21–42

La Vecchia C 1989 Nutritional factors and cancers of the breast, endometrium and ovary. European Journal of Cancer and Clinical Oncology 25: 1945–1951

La Vecchia C, Negri E 1989 The role of alcohol in oesophageal cancer in non-smokers and of tobacco in non-drinkers. International Journal of Cancer 43: 784–785

La Vecchia C, Bidoli E, Barra S et al 1990 Type of cigarettes and cancers of the upper digestive and respiratory tract. Cancer Causes Control 1: 69–74

La Vecchia C, Boyle P, Franceschi S et al 1991 Smoking and cancer with emphasis on Europe. European Journal of Cancer 27: 94–104

La Vecchia C, Decarli A, Fasoli M et al 1988 Dietary vitamin A and the risk of intra-epithelial and invasive cervical neoplasia. Gynecologic Oncology 30: 187–195

La Vecchia C, Decarli A, Franceschi S, Gentile A, Negri E, Parazzini F 1987 Dietary factors and the risk of breast cancer. Nutrition and Cancer 10: 205–214

Levi F, Ollyo JB, La Vecchia C, Boyle P, Monnier P, Savary M 1990 The consumption of tobacco, alcohol and the risk of adeno-carcinoma in Barrett's oesophagus. International Journal of Cancer 45: 852–854

Lew EA, Garfinkel L 1979 Variations in mortality by weight among 750,000 men and women. Journal of Chronic Diseases 32: 563

Longnecker MP, Berlin JA, Orza MJ, Chalmers TC 1988 A meta-analysis of alcohol consumption in relation to the risk of breast cancer. Journal of American Medical Association 260: 652–656

Longnecker MP, Orza MJ, Adams ME, Vioque J, Chalmers TC 1990 A meta-analysis of alcoholic beverage consumption in relation to risk of colorectal cancer. Cancer Causes Control 1: 59–68

Lubin JH, Gail MH, Ershaw AG 1988 Sample size and power for case-control studies when exposures are continuous. Statistics in Medicine 7: 363–376

McCredie M, Ford JM, Stewart JH 1988 Risk factors for cancer of the renal parenchyma. International Journal of Cancer 42: 13–16

Maclure M, Willett W 1990 A case-control study of diet and risk of renal adenocarcinoma. Epidemiology 1: 430–440

MacMahon B, Yen S, Trichopoulos D, Warren K, Nardi G 1981 Coffee and cancer of the pancreas. New England Journal of Medicine 304: 630–633

McLaughlin JK, Gridley G, Block G et al 1988 Dietary factors in oral and pharyngeal cancer. Journal of the National Cancer Institute 80: 1237–1243

McLaughlin JK, Mandel JS, Blot WJ, Schuman LM, Mehl ES, Fraumeni JF 1984 A population-based case-control study of renal cell carcinoma. Journal of the National Cancer Institute 72: 275–284

Mettlin CJ 1991 Progress in the nutritional epidemiology of ovary cancer. American Journal of Epidemiology 134: 457–459

Mettlin CJ, Piver MS 1990 A case-control study of milk-drinking and ovarian cancer. American Journal of Epidemiology 132: 871–876

Milham S 1976 Occupational mortality in Washington State, 1950–1971, Vol. 1. US Government Printing Office, Washington, DC

Michnovicz JJ, Bradlow HL 1990 Induction of estradiol metabolism by dietary indole-3-carbinol in humans. Journal of the National Cancer Institute 82: 947–949

Minoura T, Takata T, Sakaguchi M et al 1988 Effect of dietary eicosapentaenoic acid on azoxymethane-induced colon carcinogenesis in rats. Cancer Research 48: 4790–4794

National Academy of Science Committee on Diet, Nutrition and Cancer 1982 Diet, nutrition and cancer. National Academic Press, Washington DC

Negri E, La Vecchia C, Franceschi S, Decarli A, Bruzzi P 1992 Attributable risk for oesophageal cancer in northern Italy. European Journal of Cancer 28A: 1167–1171

Newmark HL, Wargovich MJ, Bruce WR 1984 Colon cancer and dietary fat, phosphate and calcium: a hypothesis. Journal of the National Cancer Institute 72: 1323–1325

Parazzini F, Negri E, La Vecchia C, Bruzzi P, Decarli A 1989 Population attributable risk for endometrial cancer in northern Italy. European Journal of Cancer and Clinical Oncology 25: 1451–1456

Parkin DM, Laara E, Muir C 1988 Estimates of the worldwide frequency of twelve common cancers in 1980. International Journal of Cancer 41: 184–197

Petersen GR, Milham S 1980 Occupational mortality in the State of California, 1959–1961. US Government Printing Office (US DHEW-NIOSH pub. no. 80–104), Washington, DC

Risch HA, Jain M, Choi NW 1985 Dietary factors and the incidence of cancer of the stomach. American Journal of Epidemiology 122: 949–959

Rothman KJ, Cann CI, Fried MP 1989 Carcinogenicity of dark liquor. American Journal of Public Health 79: 1516–1520

Sakaguchi M, Hiramatzu Y, Takada H 1984 Effect of dietary unsaturated and saturated fats on azoxy-methane-induced colon carcinogenesis in rats. Cancer Research 44: 1472–1477

Sankaranarayanan R, Duffy SW, Padmakumary G, Day NE, Padmanabhan TK 1989 Tobacco chewing, alcohol and

nasal snuff in cancer of the gingiva in Kerala, India. British Journal of Cancer 60: 638–643

Schiffman MH, Felton JS 1990 Fried foods and the risk of colon cancer. American Journal of Epidemiology 131: 376–378 (Comment on American Journal of Epidemiology 128: 1000–1006)

Slattery ML, Shumacher MC, Smith WR, West DW, Abd-Elghany N 1988 Physical activity, diet and risk of colon cancer. American Journal of Epidemiology 128: 989–999

Sorenson AW, Slattery ML, Ford MH 1988 Calcium and colon cancer: a review. Nutrition and Cancer 11: 135–145

Sporn MB 1992 Carcinogenesis and cancer. Different perspectives of the same disease. Cancer Research 51: 6215–6218

Steinmetz KA, Potter JD 1991a Vegetables, fruit and cancer. I. Epidemiology. Cancer Causes Control 2: 325–357

Steinmetz KA, Potter JD 1991b Vegetables, fruit and cancer. II. Mechanisms. Cancer Causes Control 2: 427–442

Sugimura T 1986 Past, present, and future mutagens in cooked foods. Environmental Health Perspectives 67: 5–10

Swanson CA, Jones DY, Schatzkin A, Brinton LA, Zeigler RG 1988 Breast cancer risk assessed by anthropometry in the NHANES I epidemiological follow-up study. Cancer Research 48: 5363–5367

Talamini R, Baron AE, Barra S 1990 A case-control study of risk factor for renal cell cancer in northern Italy. Cancer Causes Control 1: 125–131

Tannenbaum A 1940 Relationship of body weight to cancer incidence. Archives of Pathology 30: 509–517

Trichopoulos D, Yen S, Brown J, Cole P, Macmahon B 1984 The effect of westernization on urine estrogens, frequency of ovulation and breast cancer risk. A study of ethnic Chinese women in the Orient and the USA. Cancer 53: 187–192

Trowell H 1976 Definition of dietary fiber and hypotheses that it is a protective factor in certain diseases. American Journal of Clinical Nutrition 29: 417–427

Tuyns A 1977 Cancer of the oesophagus in Ille-et-Vilaine in relation to levels of consumption of alcohol and tobacco. Bulletin du Cancer 64: 45–60

Tuyns AJ, Haelterman M, Kaaks R 1987 Colorectal cancer and the intake of nutrients: oligosaccharides are a risk factor, fats are not: a case-control study in Belgium. Nutrition and Cancer 10: 181–196

United States Surgeon General 1988 Report on nutrition and health. US DHH Public Health Service Publication No. 88–5021O

Velema JP, Walker AM, Gold EB 1986 Alcohol and pancreatic cancer. Insufficient epidemiological evidence for a causal relationship. Epidemiologic Reviews 8: 28–31

Vena JE, Graham S, Zielezny M, Brasure J, Swanson MK 1987 Occupational exercise and risk of cancer. American Journal of Clinical Nutrition 45: 318–327

Victora CG, Munoz N, Day NE, Barcelos LB, Peccin DA, Braga NM 1987 Hot beverages and oesophageal cancer in Southern Brazil: a case-control study. International Journal of Cancer 39: 710–716

Warren MP 1980 The effects of exercise on pubertal progression and reproduction function in girls. Journal of Clinical Endocrinology and Metabolism 51: 1150–1157

Whittemore AF, Wu-Williams AH, Lee M et al 1990 Diet, physical activity and colorectal cancer among Chinese in North America and China. Journal of National Cancer Institute 82: 915–926

Willett W 1989 The search for causes of breast and colon cancer. Nature 338: 389–394

Willett W 1990 Nutritional epidemiology. Monographs in epidemiology and biostatistics 15. Oxford University Press, New York

Willett W, MacMahon B 1984 Diet and cancer – an overview. New England Journal of Medicine 310: 633–638, 697–703

Willett WC, Hunter DJ, Stampfer MJ et al 1992 Dietary fat and fibre in relation to role of breast cancer. Journal of the American Medical Association 268: 2037–2044

Willett WC, Stampfer MJ, Colditz GA, Rosner BA, Hennekens CH, Speizer FE 1987a Dietary fat and the risk of breast cancer. New England Journal of Medicine 316: 22–28

Willett WC, Stampfer MJ, Colditz GA, Rosner BA, Hennekens C H, Speizer F E 1987b Moderate alcohol consumption and risk of breast cancer. New England Journal of Medicine 316: 1174–1180

Willett WC, Stampfer MJ, Colditz GA, Rosner BA, Speizer FE 1990 Relation of meat, fat, and fiber intake to the risk of colon cancer in a prospective study among women. New England Journal of Medicine 323: 1664–1672

Winn DM, Blot WJ, Shy CM, Pickle LW, Toledo A, Fraumeni JF 1981 Snuff dipping and oral cancer among women in the Southern United States. New England Journal of Medicine 304: 745–749

World Health Organization 1975 International statistical classification of diseases, injuries and causes of death, 9th revision. WHO, Geneva

Yu MC, Huang TB, Henderson BE 1989 Diet and nasopharyngeal carcinoma: a case-control study in Guangzhou, China. International Journal of Cancer 43: 1177–1182

Zaridze DG 1983 Environmental etiology of large-bowel cancer. Journal of National Cancer Institute 70: 389–399

Zaridze DG, Boyle P 1987 Cancer of the prostate: epidemiology and aetiology. British Journal of Urology 59: 493–502

Zatonski W, Przewozniak K, Howe GR, Maisonneuve P, Walker AM, Boyle P 1991 Nutritional factors and pancreatic cancer: a case-control study from south-west Poland. International Journal of Cancer 48: 390–394

Zheng TZ, Boyle P, Hu HF et al 1990 Dentition, oral hygiene, and risk of oral cancer: a case-control study in Beijing, China. Cancer Causes Control 1: 235–241

Ziel HK, Finkle WD 1975 Increased risk of endometrial carcinoma among users of conjugated estrogens. New England Journal of Medicine 293: 1167–1170

46. The low-birthweight infant

P. J. Aggett

There are three categories of underweight babies at birth: low-birthweight (LBW) weighing less than 2.5 kg; very low-birthweight (VLBW) below 1.5 kg; and extremely low-birthweight (ELBW) weighing less than 1.0 kg. LBW infants can be small because they have been born preterm (before 37 completed weeks of gestation); their weight may then be appropriate for gestational age (AGA). If, however, they have not grown in utero they show intrauterine growth retardation and are small for dates (SFD). A baby is classified as SFD if its birthweight is below the 10th centile of expected weight for its gestational age: 2.5 kg is the 10th weight centile for a fetus of about 31 weeks' gestation.

About 16% of the world's live births are of LBW; 90% of them are born in developing countries and of these about 75% are SFD. The proportion of SFD infants amongst babies weighing less than 1.5 kg is much smaller. As a generalization, SFD babies are relatively mature, having been delivered late in pregnancy. They do not then experience the difficulties arising from the loss of intrauterine development of their metabolic functions. Immaturity is the characteristic problem, however, for the AGA infants of similar weights. AGA infants are also vulnerable to cardiopulmonary problems and other stresses which disrupt their metabolism. They are therefore more vulnerable than SFD babies of equivalent weight. Advances in the care of these problems have improved the survival of LBW AGA infants, but meeting their nutritional needs has emerged as a major challenge.

The AGA infant will have been deprived of many of the phases of development during the last 3 months of gestation. Between 24 and 36 weeks post-conceptional age, the fetus trebles its body weight at a rate of 15–20 g/kg/day. The only comparable weight gain is seen in children recovering from severe malnutrition, and LBW AGA infants have similar problems with protein, energy and mineral supply. They are also susceptible to infections and to metabolic disturbances arising from stress such as surgery.

During the last trimester of gestation the fetus accumulates 550 g of fat, and the proportion by weight of fat in the body increases from 1% to 16%. This is an important energy reserve: whereas a starved term infant weighing 3.5 kg would survive for 30 days, LBW infants weighing 1.0 kg and 2.0 kg survive for only 4 and 12 days respectively (Heird et al 1972). LBW infants, both of the AGA and SFD types, are particularly vulnerable to hypoglycaemia. This is because they have limited glycogen and fat stores, and because VLBW infants have impaired gluco-neogenesis and limited fat oxidation. At term, the surge in the capacity for gluconeogenesis and fatty acid oxidation appears to match the loss from trans-placental supply of glucose, amino acids and other nutrients. This switch allows the full-term newborn child to metabolize a lipid-rich diet. Fatty acid oxidation inhibits glucose oxidation and stimulates the formation of gluconeogenic substrates (lactate, pyruvate and alanine). These adjustments at birth are slower to develop in the preterm infant (Girard 1990), so LBW infants require a nutrient inflow to match their specific needs, and their capacity to adapt without harm resulting may be very limited. Thus these LBW infants need glucose as the main oxidative substrate for brain. Their overall glucose consumption (5–6 mg/kg/min) is higher than that of the term infant (3–5 mg/kg/min) (Kalhan et al 1980). Even moderate hypoglycaemia (plasma glucose <2.6 mmol/l) can be associated with subsequent impaired neuro-development (Lucas et al 1988). During fetal and postnatal life there is a progressive series of changes in brain-cell division, migration and organization that requires a whole range of appropriate nutrients (see Chapter 42).

Table 46.1 Current recommended nutrient intakes for the oral feeding of low-birthweight infants

	American Academy of Pediatrics (1985)	ESPGAN (1987)
Protein (g 100/kcal)	2.25–4.5	2.25–3.1
Total energy	≈ 120	≈ 130
Fat (% total energy)	40–50	30–50
Linoleic acid (% total energy)	3	4.5–12.6[a]
Carbohydrate (% total energy)		30–60
Minerals		
Sodium (mmol/100 kcal)	2.1–6.7	1.0–2.3
Potassium (mmol/100 kcal)	1.7–2.5	1.8–3.8
Chloride (mmol/100 kcal)		1.3–2.5
Calcium (mmol/100 kcal)	4.2–5.2	1.8–3.5
Phosphorus (mmol/100 kcal)	3.0–3.4	1.6–2.9
Calcium: Phosphorus	1.1–2.0	1.4–2.0
Magnesium (mmol/100 kcal)	0.25	0.25–0.5
Iron (μmol/100 kcal)		≈ 23
Zinc (μmol/100 kcal)	7.7	8.5–16.9
Copper (μmol/100 kcal)	1.4	1.4–1.9
Iodine (μmol/100 kcal)	0.04	0.08–0.35
Fat-soluble vitamins		
A (μg/100 kcal)	75–150	90–150
D (μg/100 kcal)	27	≤ 3[b]
E (IU/100 kcal)	0.7	>0.6
(mg/g linoleic acid)	1.0	≥0.9
(IU/day)		5(+above)
K (μg/100 kcal)		4.15
Water–soluble vitamins		
Thiamin B$_1$ (μg/100 kcal)		20
Riboflavin B$_2$ (μg/100 kcal)		60
Niacin B$_3$ (μg/100 kcal)		>800
Pyridoxine B$_6$ (μg/100 kcal)		35–250
Pantothenic acid (μg/100 kcal)		≥300
Biotin (μg/100 kcal)		≥1.5
B$_{12}$ (μg/100 kcal)		≥0.15
Folic acid (μg/100 kcal)	50 μg/day	≥60
C (mg/100 kcal)		7.5–40
Inositol[c] (mg/kg/day)	80	

[a] ESPGAN (1991) suggest that 0.5% of total fatty acids should be as ω-3 (*n*–3) fatty acids.
[b] Extra vitamin D may be needed
[c] Recently proposed by Hallman et al (1992)

NUTRITIONAL MANAGEMENT

The nutritional management of the LBW infant is set out in detail elsewhere, and this chapter summarizes the current policy (American Academy of Pediatrics 1985, ESPGAN 1987, Shaw 1988, Cowett 1991).

The ideal criteria for evaluating the nutritional management of LBW babies have not been established. LBW infants can be very different from normal babies, so their problems are unique and not part of normal physiology. Preterm infants, rapidly lose extracellular fluid after delivery, with an 8–10% weight loss. Metabolic demands ex utero differ from those in utero.

The adequacy of supplying 'idealized' nutrient intakes is being increasingly evaluated, not just by short-term systematic biochemical, anthropometric and metabolic studies, but also by long-term studies of the development and performance of the children at school and later in life. This involves sufficiently large cohorts of ex-preterm infants to ensure adequate statistical analysis. Thus the recommended intakes listed in Table 46.1 should not be confused with the potential requirements for LBW infants; the table simply provides a basis for current feeding systems until more refined recommendations can be made. For some nutrients recommended intakes have been derived empirically from calculating the amount that would be supplied by human breast milk, but this is unsuitable for some nutrients such as energy, protein, calcium and sodium.

ENERGY (Table 46.2)

LBW infants have higher energy requirements than heavier or term infants because they have higher resting metabolic rates, inefficient intestinal absorption, less efficient thermal regulation and increased growth rates. The RMR (resting metabolic rate) increases during the neonatal period, and is related directly to energy intake and the rate of weight gain. It is therefore highest in babies who are growing fast or recovering from starvation; the RMR of SFD babies is usually higher than in AGA infants, who are not simply malnourished and need to have nutrients to support their developmental changes.

Table 46.2 Estimated energy requirements of LBW neonates

Component	kcal/kg body weight/day
Resting metabolic rate	30–60
Energy cost of growth (3.0–5.7 kcal/g/ new tissue) assuming a weight gain of 15 g/kg	
cost of tissue synthesis	10–25
energy deposited in tissue	20–30
Spontaneous activity and crying	5–10
Thermoregulation	7–10
Theoretical total estimated requirement	72–135
Intake needed assuming 80% absorptive efficiency	90–170
Recommended intake in practice	120–130

The cost of tissue synthesis depends on the composition and hydration of the newly forming tissue, on the rates of growth of the child, and on the supply of all the nutrients needed for efficient growth and lean tissue synthesis (e.g. indispensable amino acids and intracellular cations Mg and Zn) (Sinclair 1978, Reichman et al 1982, ESPGAN 1987).

The energy intake lost in faeces varies with the amount of feed and on its composition, and the efficiency of intestinal absorption. Optimum energy absorption can be achieved by selecting the quality and quantity of both the fat (see below) and the carbohydrate. An absorptive efficiency of 80% or more can be expected in the stable LBW infant; this would amount to a daily faecal loss of 10–30 kcal/kg (Reichman et al 1982).

Evaporative water loss increases energy requirements, but these can be reduced by measures which minimize insensible water loss (IWL). The energy required for thermoregulation can be minimized by scrupulous attention to nursing the child in a thermoneutral environment and by avoiding cooling during nursing procedures. Infants nursed just below their thermoneutral environment use 7–8 kcal/kg/day in supporting the evaporation of water and body temperature. Thus it seems wise to allow up to 10 kcal/kg/day for thermoregulatory activity.

The upper energy figure (170 kcal/24 h) in Table 46.2 is probably an overestimate. Current recommendations suggest an intake of 120–130 kcal/kg/day, but sometimes infants need more than this to achieve weight gain. Since human breast milk has an energy density of 65–70 kcal/day, this energy requirement could be met with a volume of 180–200 ml/kg/day. There is no clear evidence that the energy density of milk from mothers who deliver preterm is higher than that from mothers delivering at term, but the mothers should be encouraged to provide the milk anyway. Proprietary formulae with an energy density of 65–85 kcal/day will meet these requirements at volumes of 200–150 ml/kg/day. Pasteurized human milk does not support growth as well as raw human breast milk because of enzyme denaturation (see below). There is probably no benefit in providing higher energy intakes. Although SFD infants grow faster than AGA ones, they do this with a low energy deposition (i.e. predominantly protein and water deposition) (Chessex et al 1984) and do not necessarily benefit from increased energy intakes; the AGA baby simply becomes fat on higher intakes.

Infants with bronchopulmonary problems because of immature lungs, i.e. dysplasia, and growth failure have increased resting metabolic rates and decreased prealbumin values. This suggests a degree of malnutrition and indicates the increased and possibly long-standing metabolic demands of sick infants (Kurzner et al 1988).

FAT

Fat provides 50% of the energy in breast milk and is the main energy source for the neonate. The digestion and absorption of lipid depends on infant pancreatic, gastric and lingual lipases and on bile salts. In LBW babies, especially preterm, lipase activity is low but this is compensated for by lipase activity in breast milk, and by the type of milk-fat globule in human breast milk. The efficiency of fat absorption by breastfed LBW infants is about 80%. It is lower in babies born more prematurely, lower with formula feeds and also in infants fed pasteurized human milk in which the lipases have been denatured.

Human breast milk contains large amounts of long-chain unsaturated fatty acids (linoleic (C18:2 ω–6), linolenic (C18:3 ω–3), arachidonic (C20:4 ω–6) and docosahexanoic (C22:6 ω–3)). Unsaturated fatty acids are more efficiently absorbed than are saturated fatty acids of the same chain length, and in human milk 60–70% of the long-chain fatty acids are unsaturated, whereas approximately 60% of those in cow's milk are saturated.

LBW infants have clinical, biochemical and histological evidence of essential fatty acid deficiency if their linoleic acid intake comprises less than 1% energy intake. It has been suggested that formula-fed LBW babies should receive at least 4.5% and 0.5% of their energy intake as linoleic and linolenic acids respectively.

Many proprietary formulae already contain vegetable oils as sources of unsaturated fatty acids, but marine fish oils are better sources of the longer-chain polyenoic acids. The importance of the latter in human milk is becoming apparent. They accumulate rapidly in the fetal brain during the last trimester of pregnancy when the brain is growing fast (Clandinin et al 1982). Many LBW infants miss this crucial phase but it has been shown that VLBW infants fed a formula with a fatty acid content simulating that of human milk achieve retinal function similar to that of infants fed breast milk (Uauy et al 1990, Koletzko 1992) (see Chapter 6).

Medium-chain fatty acids (MCFA; C8–12) are more easily absorbed than long-chain fatty acids and can enter the mitochondria for oxidation without the carnitine transfer system. However, although medium-chain triglycerides (MCT) are absorbed 20% more efficiently, there is no evidence that they produce energy balances or weight gains better than with long-chain triglycerides (LCT).

Some LBW babies may not be able to synthesize carnitine from lysine. However, no deficiency syndrome has been reported as yet, and carnitine supplementation seems only to improve fatty acid oxidation transiently (Larsson et al 1990). There is, however, recent evidence of the vital importance of inositol as a new addition needed in LBW infant feeds. Inositol has a fundamental role not only in phospholipid metabolism and intracellular signalling, but also in stimulating the normal development of the child. Inositol supplementation in preterm infants reduces the incidence of pulmonary and retinal damage. Table 46.1 includes the new proposal that a LBW infant should receive an intake equivalent to that of breast milk (Hallman et al 1992).

CARBOHYDRATE

Carbohydrate provides some 40% of the energy of breast milk. Although lactose is the predominant carbohydrate in milk, the LBW infant can assimilate other dissacharides and polysaccharide sources because by mid-gestation the activities of intestinal lactase, sucrase, isomaltase and maltase are 50–70% of those at term. There is also some α-amylase activity and this has led to the use in synthetic formulae of polysaccharides and glucose polymers as carbohydrate sources; these polymers are used as a device to reduce the osmolality of the feeds and to minimize the risk of osmotic diarrhoea in some immature neonates who cannot hydrolyse lactose.

Lactose is considered not to be essential because it is its constituent galactose which is needed for cerebroside and glycosaminoglycan synthesis. Galactose can, in theory, be made from glucose in the liver. However, the assumption that the LBW child has the capacity to produce enough galactose is unclear, and galactose is also an important precursor for glycogen synthesis. Thus, the inclusion of lactose or galactose in a feed is wise. Further benefits arising from providing LBW infants with lactose depend on the sugar's ability to increase the absorption of minerals and promote the growth of intestinal lactobacilli, which tend to minimize intestinal infection.

The hydrolysis of polysaccharides in breast milk is helped by breast milk α-amylase, but the under-development of endogenous α-amylase in LBW infants may limit the use in formulae of glucose polymers and partially hydrolysed starch (e.g. corn-syrup solids and maltodextrins) as energy sources.

PROTEIN

The nitrogen content of the fetus rises from 14.6 g/kg to 18.6 g/kg between 24 and 36 weeks of gestation; this corresponds to a daily net protein accumulation of from 1.6 g to 2.0 g/kg. Protein is digested and absorbed efficiently and about 90% of absorbed dietary protein nitrogen is incorporated into the infant's tissues. Protein should comprise about 10% of the energy intake. The overall efficiency of this incorporation and the tolerance of dietary protein depends on the supply of the indispensable amino acids, energy and of other nutrients (e.g. Mg, Zn, P) needed for the synthesis of lean tissue. The maturity of the metabolism of amino acids and the ability of the kidney to handle any metabolite of unused amino acids present considerable problems in specifying the mixture of amino acids needed by LBW infants. There is also a specific need for some amino acids, glycine, cysteine and taurine (Jackson et al 1981, Chesney 1988) which are not thought to be indispensable for adults. These amino acids are needed for tissue synthesis and cannot be formed in sufficient amounts by the immature metabolic pathways of the child.

Inadequate protein intakes cause poor growth, hypoalbuminaemia and oedema. Protein intakes greater than 4 g/kg/day (3.1 g/100 kcal) may not be used effectively (Kashyap et al 1988). At intakes above this, neonates may develop acidosis, high blood ammonia concentrations and increased plasma levels of phenylalanine, tyrosine and methionine, because the liver enzymes for their catabolism have not developed properly. Other amino acids can be catabolized, however, so urea is produced but accumulates as the kidney tries to excrete it. The increased renal solute load then leads to dehydration. These problems are exacerbated if the metabolism of amino acids is disrupted by deficiencies of nutrients essential for their optimum use, and by stress and intercurrent infections.

Human breast milk may not supply all the estimated needs of the LBW infant even at daily intakes of 180–200 ml/kg, especially if the infant is gaining weight rapidly. Supplementing the feed with other protein sources, such as whey-based formula, hydrolysed casein or human milk protein, may then be beneficial (Jackson et al 1981, Ronholm et al 1986, Putet et al 1987).

WATER

Water comprises 50–70% of the weight gain of the growing, well-fed LBW infant. Thus, with a weight gain of 20 g, about 12 g (ml) is water. This volume is, however, relatively small compared with the need to replace water losses.

Water loss occurs via the kidney, skin, lungs and gut. Extrarenal or insensible water loss (IWL) via the skin (transepidermal water loss, TEWL) and lungs amounts to 30–60 ml daily. IWL is increased by activity, respiratory stress (including high ventilator rates), low humidity and a high temperature in the infant's environment. In an infant of 32 weeks' gestation, TEWL in the first 3 days of life is 2–6 ml/kg/h. It is higher in infants of shorter gestations (Rutter 1988), but the skin keratinizes rapidly postnatally and by 1–2 weeks of age TEWL has become similar to that of term infants. Phototherapy to reduce bilirubin levels and nursing under radiant heaters can increase TEWL two- to threefold. IWL loss can be reduced by nursing LBW infants in an air humidity of 80% or more, or under heat shields to increase local humidity. Faecal water loss is 5–20 ml/kg body weight daily.

The urinary volume depends on the osmotic load to be excreted. Even the normal neonate, born at 40 weeks' gestation, cannot achieve a urinary osmolality greater than 500 mmol/kg, even with maximum production of the antidiuretic hormone, arginine-vasopressin (AVP). VLBW infants usually have a urine osmolality of 60–200 mmol/kg (Coulthard & Hey 1985). Most LBW infants can achieve a urinary osmolality of only 170 mmol/kg, so this means that they will excrete more water with any solutes or osmolar loads than usual. If the customary renal solute load amounts to 14–15 mmol/kg body weight daily, then their load needs to be excreted in 90 ml/kg/day.

When these losses are all added, the daily water requirement amounts to 150–200 ml/kg body weight. Some of this water is produced endogenously by nutrient oxidation (approximately 12 ml/100 kcal), so on a daily energy intake of 120–130 kcal/kg, 15 ml of water per kg will be produced. The adequacy of an infant's water intake has to be monitored by clinical evaluation, regular weighing, by measuring changes in plasma sodium, and by measuring urine specific gravity or osmolality.

Water excretion may be limited inappropriately by the secretion of AVP induced by stress, such as asphyxia or respiratory distress (Rees et al 1984). This will then lead to water overload. Water intake may need to be restricted, but there is then the risk of restricting the intakes of the other nutrients.

SODIUM AND POTASSIUM

The 25-week fetus contains 94 mmol of sodium per kg body weight; by term this has fallen to 74 mmol/kg. The daily accumulation of sodium in the second half of gestation is 0.5–1.1 mmol/kg.

In the first 4–5 days of life, the LBW infant loses about 12% of body weight and 6–16 mmol of sodium per kg. This represents the loss of extracellular fluid and the acquisition of body water compartmentation similar to full-term infants (Bauer et al 1991). Most LBW infants achieve positive sodium balance during the second week of life; intakes of 1.6 mmol sodium/kg/day can achieve this, but do not necessarily prevent a low plasma sodium, specified as that below 130 mmol Na/l. The sodium intake then needs to be adjusted to maintain normal plasma sodium concentrations (130–135 mmol/l). Since LBW infants may not be able to excrete high sodium loads it is usually prudent to supply low amounts which can be supplemented when necessary. Infants, especially those under 30 weeks' gestation, with immature renal tubular sodium reabsorption, may need as much as 8–12 mmol/kg/day. After 32–34 weeks' gestational age, most LBW infants are able to maintain normal plasma sodium concentrations irrespective of whether they are fed a full-term formula providing 1.2 mmol/kg/day or a preterm formula providing 3.9 mmol/kg/day.

Potassium deficiency is rare, even during rapid growth when it is essential for new tissue, and daily intakes of 2.0–3.5 mmol/kg which would be provided by mature breast milk (10–17.5 mmol/l) should meet the needs of most LBW neonates.

MINERALS

Between 26 and 36 weeks' gestation the normal fetus accumulates 120–150 mg (3–3.25 mmol) of calcium/kg/day and 60–75 mg (1.94–2.42 mmol) phosphorus/kg/day; 99% of the calcium and 80% of the phosphorus are deposited in bone. Neither human breast milk nor proprietary formulae can match the calculated fetal accretion rates of these minerals.

Early neonatal calcium deficiency may cause an asymptomatic hypocalcaemia which stimulates a release of parathormone and the mobilization of skeletal calcium. Early introduction of feeds, or of calcium with parenteral nutrition, reduces the incidence of this problem. Late neonatal hypocalcaemia (3–15 days of age), unless it is detected biochemically, can present initially with convulsions.

After birth, extensive bone turnover and remodelling combined with continued bone growth leads to bone changes, varying between a barely discernible radiological hypomineralization ('physiological osteoporosis') and severe rachitic changes with fractures. Nearly all infants <1.5 kg will develop reduced bone mineralization and as many as 57% of ELBW infants develop severe changes (Koo & Tsang 1991). Adequate deposition of skeletal calcium depends on the supply of phosphorus, and without enough phosphorus metabolic bone disease occurs even when infants are given sufficient intakes of vitamin D to produce normal or raised plasma concentrations of vitamin D metabolites (Koo et al 1989). Metabolic bone disease and hypomineralization are more prevalent in infants fed human milk (Gross 1987, Abrams et al 1988). Silent early bone disease retards subsequent linear growth, and this emphasizes the importance of solving the problem of optimizing the provision of calcium and phosphorus to preterm infants, especially those fed human milk (Lucas et al 1989).

The requirements for phosphorus retention can be calculated from the following formula:

P retention (mg) =
calcium retention/2 + nitrogen retention/17.4

which makes specific allowance for the requirements of bone and soft tissue for phosphorus. If these demands of about 0.6 mmol/kg/day are not met by diet, plasma inorganic phosphate falls below 1.5 mmol/l and calcium incorporation into bone slows. LBW infants fed breast milk are vulnerable to this phosphorus depletion syndrome, which is associated with elevated plasma calcium concentrations. These rise not only because of impaired deposition of calcium in bone but because of increased bone resorption. A high urinary calcium is observed (>0.4 mmol/kg/day) and urinary phosphorus falls below 0.1 mmol/kg/day and the plasma alkaline phosphatase activity often increases to above 1000 IU/l. Phosphate supplements (0.3 mmol/kg/day) improve calcium retention and eliminate the hypercalcuria (Senterre et al 1983), but the response to extra phosphorus must be monitored carefully because excessive supplements may cause phosphaturia and loss of further calcium in the urine, with a fall in plasma calcium (Carey et al 1985). Growth is improved but hypomineralization is not prevented. The phosphate depletion syndrome is rare in LBW formula-fed infants because their phosphorus intake is higher than that of those fed breast milk.

Thus calcium and phosphorus supplies should be carefully balanced. Calcium cannot be utilized effectively for bone formation in the absence of phosphorus. The use of large calcium intakes (>140 mg/kg/day) is ineffective in improving bone mineralization when the problem is one of phosphorus supply. Indeed, such intakes may be detrimental because they may lead to impaired absorption of fat, intraluminal precipitation of calcium, hypercalcaemia, metabolic acidosis and phosphorus depletion.

Magnesium

A 1 kg fetus contains 0.2 g of magnesium. Body Mg increases to 0.8 g in the term infant weighing 3.5 kg, and 65% of this is in the skeleton. The LBW infant weighing 1 kg would accumulate 10 mg of Mg/kg/day whilst at 1.5 kg the rate is 8.5 mg/kg/day. However, 10 mg/kg/day may be inadequate for VLBW infants who are receiving sufficient calcium and phosphorus to approximate fetal accretion rates, and as much as 20 mg/kg/day may be required (Giles et al 1990). Human breast milk only provides 3.0 mg/day.

A low plasma magnesium concentration in preterm infants may result from the incorporation of magnesium into tissues during rapid weight gain; the problem may present clinically with convulsions and a persistent low plasma calcium.

Iron

At 1 kg the fetus contains 65 mg of iron, but it gains 1.8 mg/kg/day during the last trimester. The iron stores of infants weighing less than 1.4 kg is exhausted after 6–8 weeks of postnatal life without iron intakes, whereas those in heavier LBW infants would probably last until about 12 weeks' postnatal age. Frequent blood sampling also depletes the infant of iron (1 g of haemoglobin contains 3.4 mg of iron). Iron supplements, if used, are probably best delayed until 4–8 weeks' postnatal age. It is not certain if extra iron introduced during the neonatal period is used efficiently. A total iron intake, including that supplied by feeds, of 2–2.5 mg/kg/day is adequate for most LBW infants. Some proprietary formulae contain sufficient iron to achieve this intake without any supplement. Excessive iron supplements may theoretically cause increased lipid peroxidation and haemolytic anaemia, alter intestinal flora and increase the risk of Gram-negative septicaemia, but these problems are not often linked to excess iron supply. Since blood transfusions supply significant amounts of iron, infants who are having their haemoglobin concentrations maintained in this way have no need for additional iron supplements.

Copper

The fetus accumulates copper at the rate of 51 µg/kg/day, and at term the infant contains 14 mg of the element. Since half of this is accumulated in the liver during the last trimester, it is not surprising that sporadic copper deficiency occurs in artificially fed, low-birthweight infants (see Chapter 12). Copper deficiency has not been described in infants fed breast milk.

Zinc

The zinc content of the fetus is about 19.5 mg/kg fat-free tissue; approximately 25% of this is in the liver and 40% is in the skeleton. A dietary supply of Zn and the release of zinc from these pools usually meets the demands of newly synthesized lean tissue, but symptomatic zinc deficiency occasionally occurs at 2.5–4.5 months' postnatal age in LBW infants receiving breast milk (see Chapter 12).

VITAMINS

Deficiencies of vitamins are rare, but there are circumstances when such possibilities need to be remembered. LBW infants are at risk of inadequate intake of all the fat-soluble vitamins. Low plasma levels of retinol are often found, with metabolic evidence of vitamin A deficiency (Woodruff et al 1987). Overt deficiency is rare, however. The turnover of vitamin A is increased in babies who are being ventilated (Shenai et al 1985) and it has been proposed, but not proven, that vitamin A depletion may predispose infants to chronic lung disease. Similarly, vitamin E might reduce the risk of pulmonary damage, but neither this nor possible benefits in preventing retinal damage and brain haemorrhages have yet been clearly demonstrated.

The independence of metabolic bone disease from vitamin D supply has been described above. However, before 32 weeks' gestation the intestinal response to 1,25-dihydroxycholecalciferol is poor, and such preterm babies may need extra vitamin D to optimize calcium and phosphorus metabolism.

LBW infants have a need for vitamin K supplements because of their rapid systemic utilization of vitamin K, their low dietary intake, and the limited intestinal production of the vitamin. The standard practice is to give all infants 0.5–1 mg of vitamin K intramuscularly on the first day of life. This can be repeated at weekly intervals until the child is on adequate oral feeding, which should provide 2–3 µg/kg/day.

WATER-SOLUBLE VITAMINS

Deficiencies of water-soluble vitamins are rare. Thiamin, ascorbic acid and folic acid are heat-sensitive, and their loss from heat-treated formulae or from pasteurized breast milk is high. As much as 90% of breast-milk vitamin C can be lost as a result of pasteurization. Thiamin deficiency may occur in LBW infants fed soya milk, or who have been breastfed by thiamin-deficient mothers.

Ascorbic acid (vitamin C) is important in influencing iron absorption and, possibly, reducing the transient hypertyrosinaemia and hyperphenylalaninaemia seen in LBW infants.

Riboflavin is photosensitive and exposure of human milk to light degrades it, resulting in a variable loss of vitamin activity. Additionally, phototherapy may cause a transient biochemical riboflavin deficiency in breastfed babies.

Pyridoxine (vitamin B_6) deficiency occasionally presents in LBW infants. Biotin deficiency has only been recognized in infants fed intravenously. Vitamin B_{12} deficiency has only been seen in infants being breastfed by vitamin B_{12}-deficient mothers.

FEEDING TECHNIQUES

When possible, enteral feeds are prepared but in ELBW babies, i.e. <1.0 kg, it is difficult to provide for the full nutritional needs of the child. Therefore, supplementation with intravenous feeding is needed. The management of feeding is thus very complicated and is best done in specialized units.

Several concerns about feeding LBW infants arise because of their gut and other organ immaturity, which leads to cardiopulmonary and other systemic disorders. The fetus can swallow at 16 weeks and gut motility appears at 28 weeks' gestation. However, effective sucking, intestinal motility and protection of the airways is not present until 34 weeks (Milla & Bisset 1988). Before this time gastric emptying is impaired, and since gastric capacity is small, there is a danger of stomach contents refluxing into the airways. Furthermore, gastric distension may interfere with inflation of the lungs.

Enteral feeding of critically ill LBW babies may not be possible or easy, and many neonatologists prefer to use intravenous feeding routinely. Even small amounts of enteral feeds are beneficial, however, because they stimulate a more physiological hormonal surge, stimulate bile flow and help to induce maturation of the intestinal mucosa.

When enteral feeds are given, large volumes should be avoided because they predispose to apnoea, ileus and necrotizing enterocolitis. Very rapid advancement of enteral feeding and excessive fluid volumes predispose premature infants to the development of necrotizing enterocolitis (Anderson & Kliegman 1991).

Enteral feeds are often given via naso- or orogastric tubes. The distal end can be placed either in the stomach, jejunum or, more commonly, the duodenum.

The use of intermittent boluses rather than continuous infusions of feeds is controversial. The former is more physiological, and recent studies indicate that adverse metabolic effects and altered body composition may arise from continuous feeding.

The practice has evolved of gradually increasing the volumes fed to infants during the first week of life, even though they can tolerate intakes of 90–260 ml/kg/day from 3 days of age (Coulthard & Hey 1985). The immediate introduction of large-volume feeds predisposes the babies to intestinal damage and necrotizing enterocolitis (Lucas & Cole 1990).

Although human milk may not provide some preterm LBW infants with enough nutrients such as protein, energy, calcium, phosphorus, iron, sodium, vitamin C and folic acid, breast milk confers improved immune function and protection (Lucas & Cole 1990), a better lipid profile and better developmental progress (Lucas et al 1992). For SFD infants breast milk is clearly the best food source. This applies therefore to the vast majority of LBW infants. However, if they cannot be breastfed, LBW babies progress better on specific formulae designed for preterm LBW infants than on conventional term formulae.

During later infancy it may well be important to consider the baby's post-conceptional age rather than postnatal age in assessing nutrient requirements and metabolism. Many ex-preterm babies have the formula feed used for normal babies introduced inappropriately early (Ernst et al 1990). Introducing cow's milk and weaning cereals should also be delayed to a time appropriate for the full post-conceptional age of the child.

REFERENCES

Abrams SA, Schanler RJ, Garza C 1988 Bone mineralization in former very low birthweight infants fed either human milk or commercial formula. Journal of Pediatrics 112: 956–960

American Academy of Pediatrics: Committee on Nutrition 1985 Nutritional needs of low birthweight infants. Pediatrics 75: 976–986

Anderson DM, Kliegman RM 1991 The relationship of neonatal alimentation practices to the occurrence of endemic necrotizing enterocolitis. American Journal of Perinatology 8: 62–67

Bauer K, Bovermann G, Roithmaier A et al 1991 Body composition, nutrition, and fluid balance during the first two weeks of life in preterm neonates weighing less than 1500 grams. Journal of Pediatrics 118: 615–620

Carey DE, Goetz CA, Horak E, Rowe JC 1985 Phosphorus wasting during phosphorus supplementation of human milk feedings in preterm infants. Journal of Pediatrics 107: 790–794

Chesney RW 1988 Taurine: is it required for infant nutrition? Journal of Nutrition 118: 6–10

Chessex P, Reichman B, Verellen G et al 1984 Metabolic consequences of intrauterine growth retardation in very low-birthweight infants. Pediatric Research 18: 709–713

Clandinin MT, Chappell JE, Heim T 1982 Do low-birthweight infants require nutrition with chain elongation desaturation products of essential fatty acids? Progress in Lipid Research 10: 901–904

Coulthard M, Hey EN 1985 Effect of varying water intake on renal functions in healthy preterm babies. Archives of Diseases of Childhood 65: 614–620

Cowett RM (ed) 1991 Principles of perinatal–neonatal metabolism. Springer-Verlag, London

Ernst JA, Bull MJ, Rickard KA et al 1990 Growth outcome and feeding practices of the very low-birthweight infant (less than 1500 grams) within the first year of life. Journal of Pediatrics 177: S156–S166

ESPGAN Committee on the Nutrition of the Preterm Infant 1987 In: Wharton B (ed) Nutrition and feeding of preterm infants. Blackwell Scientific Publications, Oxford

ESPGAN Committee on Nutrition 1991 Comment on the content and composition of lipids in infant formulas. Acta Paediatrica Scandinavica 80: 887–896

Giles MM, Laing IA, Elton RA et al 1990 Magnesium metabolism in preterm infants: effects of calcium, magnesium, and phosphorus, and of postnatal and gestational age. Journal of Pediatrics 117: 147–154

Girard J 1990 Metabolic adaptations to change of nutrition at birth. Biology of the Neonate 58 (Suppl 1): 3–15

Gross SJ 1987 bone mineralization in preterm infants fed human milk with and without mineral supplementation. Journal of Pediatrics 111: 450–458

Hallman M, Bry K, Hoppu K et al 1992 Inositol supplementation in premature infants with respiratory distress syndrome. New England Journal of Medicine 326: 1233–1239

Heird WC, Driscoll JM, Schullinger JN et al 1972 Intravenous alimentation in pediatric patients. Journal of Pediatrics 80: 351–372

Jackson AA, Shaw JCL, Barber A, Golden MHN 1981 Nitrogen metabolism in preterm infants fed human donor breast milk: the possible essentiality of glycine. Pediatric

Research 15: 1454–1461

Kalhan S, Bier D, Savins et al 1980 Estimation of glucose turnover and 13C recycling in the human newborn by simultaneous [1–13C] glucose and [6,62H2] glucose tracers. Journal of Clinical Endocrinology and Metabolism 50: 456–460

Kashyap S, Schulze KF, Forsyth M et al 1988 Growth, nutrient retention, metabolic response in low-birthweight infants fed varying intakes of protein and energy. Journal of Pediatrics 113: 713–721

Koletzko B 1992 Fats for brains. European Journal of Clinical Nutrition 46: S51–S62

Koo WW, Sherman R, Succop P et al 1989 Serum vitamin D metabolites in very low-birthweight infants with and without rickets and fractures. Journal of Pediatrics 114: 1017–1022

Koo WW, Tsang RC 1991 Mineral requirements of low-birthweight infants. Journal of the American College of Nutrition 10: 474–486

Kurzner SI, Garg M, Bautista DB et al 1988 Growth failure in infants with bronchopulmonary dysplasia: nutrition and elevated resting metabolic expenditure. Pediatrics 81: 379–384

Larsson LE, Olegard R, Ljung BM et al 1990 Parenteral nutrition in preterm neonates with and without carnitine supplementation. Acta Anaesthesiologica Scandinavica 34: 501–505

Lucas A, Cole, TJ 1990 Breast milk and neonatal necrotising enterocolitis. Lancet 336: 1519–1523

Lucas A, Morley R, Cole TJ 1988 Adverse neurodevelopmental outcome of moderate neonatal hypoglycaemia. British Medical Journal 297: 1304–1308

Lucas A, Brooke OG, Baker BA et al 1989 High alkaline phosphatase activity and growth in preterm neonates. Archives of Diseases of Childhood 64: 902–909

Lucas A, Morley R, Cole TJ et al 1992 Breast milk and subsequent intelligence in children born preterm. Lancet

339: 261–264

Milla PJ, Bisset WM 1988 The gastrointestinal tract. British Medical Bulletin 44: 1010–1024

Putet G, Rigo J, Salle B, Senterre J 1987 Supplementation of pooled human milk with casein hydrolysate: energy and nitrogen balance and weight gain composition in very low-birthweight infants. Pediatric Research 21: 458–461

Rees L et al 1984 Hyponatraemia in the first week of life in preterm infants. 1. Arginine-vasopressin secretion. Archives of Disease of Childhood 59: 414–422

Reichman BL, Chessex P, Putet G et al 1982 Partition of energy metabolism and energy cost of growth in the very low-birthweight infant. Pediatrics 69: 446–451

Ronholm KA, Perheentupa J, Siimes MA 1986 Supplementation with human milk protein improves growth of small premature infants fed human milk. Pediatrics 77: 649–653

Rutter N 1988 The immature skin. British Medical Bulletin 44: 957–970

Senterre J, Putet G, Rigo J 1983 Effects of vitamin D and phosphorus supplementation on calcium retention in preterm infants fed banked human milk. Journal of Pediatrics 103: 305–307

Shaw JCL 1988 Growth and nutrition of the very preterm infant. British Medical Bulletin 44: 984–1009

Shenai JP, Chytil F, Stahlman MT 1985 Vitamin A status of neonates with chronic lung disease. Pediatric Research 19: 185–189

Sinclair JC (ed) 1978 Temperature regulation and energy metabolism in the newborn. Grune & Stratton, New York

Uauy RD, Birch DG, Birch EE et al 1990 Effect of dietary omega-3 fatty acids on retinal function of very low-birthweight neonates. Pediatric Research 28: 485–492

Woodruff CW, Latham CB, Mactier H, Hewett JC 1987 Vitamin A status of preterm infants: correlation between plasma retinol concentration and retinol dose response. American Journal of Clinical Nutrition 46: 985–988

47. Dietetic treatment of inherited metabolic disease

B. Clayton

More than 3000 disorders displaying Mendelian patterns of inheritance and caused primarily by a single mutant gene have been described. Many of them are very rare, but as they are so numerous they make a significant contribution to morbidity and mortality, especially in childhood (McKusick 1988, Scriver et al 1989). A few of them can be treated with therapeutic diets with varying degrees of success. Such treatment may:

1. prevent the accumulation of a substrate and its derivatives, e.g. such as in a low-phenylalanine controlled diet for phenylketonuria;
2. provide a metabolite which becomes rate-limiting as a result of a metabolic block, e.g. the administration of arginine in children with argininosuccinase deficiency;
3. provide a metabolite, deficiency of which is dangerous, e.g. a diet to prevent hypoglycaemia in glycogen-storage disease;
4. provide a cofactor or precursor, e.g. large doses of pyridoxine for a variant of homocystinuria.

The close cooperation of the dietitian, hospital doctor, laboratory staff, nurse and general practitioner is very important, and the education of the patient and/or parents is essential. The support of industry so that suitable synthetic foods are available commercially is also essential. Within the UK the Advisory Committee on Borderline Substances advises on those conditions where 'foods' may be classified as NHS drugs and be prescribable as such. The products and the indications for their use are listed in each edition of the British National Formulary and also in the Monthly Index of Medical Specialities, MIMS.

A diet may be scientifically excellent but it is useless if the patient will not eat it – and most of the patients are young. In many diets, everyday items of food cannot be used and the presentation of their substitutes may tax the ingenuity of the dietitian to the full.

The composition of proprietary dietetic products may change from time to time and this occurs too with many normal commercial foodstuffs, such as tinned soups, biscuits and so on. For this reason, lists of commercial preparations have not been included in this chapter as they soon go out of date. It is essential that the doctor and dietitian work with up-to-date information, which is readily available from the manufacturers, and information is also given in the British National Formulary.

Many of the diets are very complicated and have to be modified to suit each patient. For this reason, only a few diet sheets are included in this chapter. A dietitian who does not normally treat a rare inborn error would be well advised to consult a colleague in a centre specializing in the particular disorder, in order to obtain detailed and up-to-date advice.

In some metabolic disorders, the patient may respond to the administration of a particular cofactor, which should be administered on a trial basis. If the patient is very ill, both cofactor and a diet may be given, and whether or not the diet is essential can be sorted out later. The diagnosis of an inborn error can be very difficult to make in some cases. Opinions differ on whether or not to try a cocktail of cofactors before an accurate diagnosis has been made.

The treatment of phenylketonuria (PKU) is described in some detail, as it illustrates the principles and problems of providing a diet for an inherited metabolic disorder. The major textbook by Scriver et al (1989) is an excellent source of advice on inherited metabolic disorders. Major textbooks on paediatric nutrition have been written by Francis (1986, 1987) and Bentley & Lawson (1988).

AMINO ACID DISORDERS

Phenylketonuria

This heterogenous disorder (Cotton 1990) is one of the few causes of mental handicap for which

723

reasonably effective treatment is available. In the UK neonates are screened between the 6th and 14th days after birth. Definitive diagnosis and the commencement of treatment where it is indicated must be pursued with urgency. Different populations tend to carry different alleles for hyperphenylalaninaemia. Smith et al (1991), in a review of the UK screening programme during 1984–1988, found that about 1 in 10 000 neonates (445 subjects) had levels of blood phenylalanine persistently above 240 μmol/l. In the majority of cases this resulted from mutations in the gene for phenylalanine hydroxylase, and 273 had classic phenylketonuria. Three had defects in the metabolism of the cofactor. In the classic form of the disease, the blood phenylalanine concentration exceeds 1200 μmol/l. In addition, tyrosine levels in plasma are low or low normal, and large amounts of abnormal metabolites appear in the urine (see Fig. 47.1).

Hyperphenylalaninaemia in classic PKU is due to <1% of normal activity of the enzyme phenylalanine hydroxylase, which is present in liver and converts phenylalanine to tyrosine (Fig. 47.1). If the enzyme activity is 1–5% of normal, it produces a milder form of the condition (sometimes referred to as variant or atypical PKU). If the activity is reduced but nevertheless >5% of normal, this causes mild hyperphenylalaninaemia. In 1–3% of patients with defective hydoxylation of the phenylalanine, there is a deficiency of the cofactor tetrahydrobiopterin, and brain damage in this rare condition is not prevented by dietary treatment.

In hyperphenylalaninaemia responsive to diet, it has been customary to treat the infant if the plasma level is above 600 μmol/l, and those with levels of 240–600 μmol/l are followed up by the paediatrician. It is generally customary to try and maintain blood levels of phenylalanine between 180 and 480 μmol/l during treatment. However, in a recent study of a large number of patients (Smith et al 1990) it was shown that although treated children with PKU appear to have 'normal' IQs, they do have cognitive deficits, educational problems and an increased incidence of behavioural disorders, especially hyperactivity. Smith and her colleagues concluded that this policy may require revision, so that levels are maintained between 120 and 300 μmol/l.

The practical and social difficulties for achieving such tight control must not be underestimated. A complicating factor is that failure to provide the essential requirement for phenylalanine can itself lead to brain damage. The policy of not usually treating children with untreated levels between 240 and 600 μmol/l may also require revision.

High levels of phenylalanine lead to changes in the metabolism of myelin and amines. This is likely to interfere with the integrity of the nervous system throughout life, and there is now evidence that lifelong

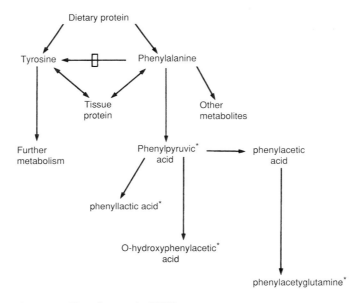

Fig. 47.1 Phenylketonuria (PKU)
÷ Impairment of phenylalanine hydroxylase activity in PKU
⋆ Major urinary metabolites in untreated PKU

treatment will probably be required (Thompson et al 1990). A recent confusing observation is that magnetic resonance imaging shows distinct abnormalities in the brain, but they do not appear to correlate with the clinical severity.

Treatment is by a low-phenylalanine controlled diet and regular monitoring of the blood phenylalanine concentrations is essential. Although the recommended intake of nutrients, apart from the phenylalanine and tyrosine, is similar to that for a normal infant (see DHSS 1988 (Department of Health 1991)) the restricted use of protein-containing conventional foods requires that supplements of amino acids (except phenylalanine), protein-free energy and a comprehensive range of vitamins, macro and trace elements be given. Phenylalanine is an essential amino acid (1 g natural protein contains approximately 50 mg). Its complete exclusion from the diet is incompatible with life, and if the amount in the diet is insufficient brain damage will be caused. The essential requirement must be ingested each day, an aliquot of the total daily requirement being given with each meal. In order to restrict the phenylalanine levels within the range of 180–480 μmol/l plasma, only one-third to one-tenth of the normal protein intake is required, and therefore a synthetic protein substitute is necessary. The synthetic protein substitute for PKU must contain the essential amino acids leucine, valine, isoleucine, threonine, methionine, lysine and tryptophan. For infants and young children, cystine, histidine, arginine and probably proline are also essential. In addition, tyrosine becomes essential owing to the metabolic block. The substitute may be a mixture of amino acids from which phenylalanine is excluded, an enzymic hydrolysate of protein which still contains some phenylalanine, or an acid hydrolysate of protein which is phenylalanine-free. The synthetic preparations contain added tyrosine. The protein substitutes must be given in divided portions at meals during the day, so far as is practicable. This is especially important in infants and young children. Affected infants usually tolerate 70–90 mg phenylalanine per kg body weight per 24 h. In the first month of life and during periods of rapid growth the patient may tolerate 110 mg/kg/ 24 h. Frequent monitoring of blood levels is essential, as there is considerable variation between patients and from time to time in any individual patient. In addition to the protein substitute, the commercial preparations vary in their content of other nutrients and it is essential to study the literature on a particular product. 'Complete' products which are made up like conventional dried milks for infants, have advantages for the mother, who then only has to supplement with

the essential requirement for phenylalanine (as infant formula or cow's milk) at each feed. The degree of 'completeness' varies – therefore consult the label! Preparations of amino acids without fat but including carbohydrate are recommended for older children and adults, as they are more palatable and allow the diet to be more varied and include more natural foodstuffs.

The essential requirement for the macro elements calcium, magnesium, phosphorus, potassium and sodium, and for the trace elements iron, zinc, copper, manganese, chromium, molybdenum, iodine, cobalt, nickel and selenium, should be provided. These elements may be given as separate supplements or may be included in the commercial protein substitute.

A complete vitamin supplement should be provided, either separately or as part of the manufacturer's formulation of a low-phenylalanine protein substitute. The vitamins required are A and D, α-tocopherol, vitamin K, ascorbic acid, thiamin, riboflavin, niacin, pyridoxine, vitamin B_{12}, folic acid, biotin and pantothenic acid; choline and inositol are also in some preparations.

The practical management of the diet is very important. Blood levels of phenylalanine should be monitored on non-fasting specimens taken 3.5–4 h after a feed or main meal, and the laboratory should employ a micromethod so that a capillary sample can be used. If spots of blood are collected onto a Guthrie card, the parent or child can take the specimen. The card is then posted to the laboratory and this freedom is much appreciated. The recommended frequency of monitoring is weekly in infants during the first months of life; every 2 weeks after weaning and during the toddler age after adjusting the diet; every 3–4 weeks in the preschool child; and 4-weekly thereafter until the teens, when the frequency may be only every 2 or 3 months or even less. If the stricter limits suggested by Smith et al (1990) are adopted, more frequent monitoring and a chemical method for measuring phenylalanine will be needed. In addition, the levels should be checked in younger children following infections or after pilfering food.

Examples of a low-phenylalanine infant feeding plan, of a weaning menu and of the diet for a schoolchild are shown in Tables 47.1–47.3.

If the patient has an infection and will not eat, a high-energy drink is recommended in order to prevent catabolism, with a rise in phenylalanine. Details of such a regimen are given in Table 47.3.

Breastfeeding of a newly diagnosed infant may be continued if the mother wishes. Close cooperation between the parents and the caring team is particularly important in this situation. Human milk is lower in phenylalanine per unit of nitrogen than cow's milk, and breast milk can be combined with the use of a protein substitute (see Table 47.1). Frequent monitoring of blood levels is essential. The intake of breast milk must be varied in response to the blood levels by adjusting the length of time for which the infant is at the breast, and varying the amount of protein substitute which is given. If the infant's tolerance for phenylalanine is very low, larger amounts of the substitute should be given so that the infant will not suckle for so long and the flow of milk will be reduced.

Not only must the dietitian educate and encourage the patient and the parents, but she must also provide adequate interpretation of how a diet which is scientifically correct is to be made into one which the patient is willing to eat and which is socially acceptable. She needs to provide low-phenylalanine cooking hints and numerous recipes for suitable ice-cream, gravy, apple cake and so on, how to make a low-phenylalanine birthday cake that the rest of the family can enjoy too, and how to cope with school meals. She needs to provide lists of the phenylalanine content of many manufactured foods, the composition of which changes quite frequently. Useful leaflets and booklets are published regularly by the National Society for Phenylketonuria and Allied Disorders, 26 Towngate Grove, Mirfield, West Yorkshire. The use of any item listed must be checked by the patient's dietitian or doctor before including it in the diet.

If a child has an intercurrent infection he frequently loses his appetite. No attempt should be made to force-feed the low-phenylalanine protein substitute, which can be stopped for a few days if necessary. The patient should be given fluids containing carbohydrates, such as fruit juices with sugar or glucose polymer, and encouraged to take whichever foods containing phenylalanine exchanges he particularly fancies. The protein substitute should not be recommended until he is taking phenylalanine exchanges.

It should be noted that the sweetener aspartame (such as Canderel and Nutrasweet) contains phenylalanine and should not be given to phenylketonuric patients of any age. These sweeteners are put in a wide variety of manufactured foods and the labels should be checked. Saccharine is suitable for use.

If a mother who has phenylketonuria consumes a normal diet during pregnancy, her offspring have a

Table 47.1 Example of a low-phenylalanine infant feeding plan

Bottle-feeding regimen

Daily
1. —— ml milk (infant formula or cow's). The amount of milk (phenylalanine source) is adjusted according to blood levels.
2. —— g low phenylalanine milk substitute, e.g. Analog XP, Lofenalac, Minafen, plus boiled water to give a 15% w/v concentration.

The average total volume of feed (i.e. 1. + 2.) is 150–200 ml/kg. The total amount should be divided equally between 5 feeds. The milk providing the phenylalanine should be given BEFORE the low-phenylalanine milk substitute.

Aminogran Mineral Mixture and a comprehensive vitamin supplement, such as 3 Ketovite Tablets plus 5 ml Ketovite Liquid, may be required, depending on the type of milk substitute and the amount used. Manufacturer's data should be checked to assess nutritional adequacy.

Feeding pattern
—— ml milk (phenylalanine source). Replace if rejected or vomited.
—— ml milk substitute (low phenylalanine), plus vitamins and minerals if necessary.

Breast feeding regimen

The amount of low-phenylalanine milk substitute required varies depending upon blood phenylalanine levels and growth. The total volume is divided into 5 feeds and given BEFORE demand breastfeeds.

Feeding pattern
—— ml milk substitute (low phenylalanine) plus vitamins and minerals if necessary.
Breastfeeds (phenylalanine source), on demand

Table 47.2 Example of a weaning diet for a bottle-fed infant with phenylketonuria

Daily	1. — g Analog XP, diluted to produce a 15% w/v concentration. 2. — 50 mg phenylalanine exchanges – divide between meals as advised.
Morning meal:	— 50 mg phenylalanine exchanges e.g. rusk/cereal + milk Analog XP Low-protein bread/toast, butter or margarine, jam, honey, marmalade
Midday meal:	— 50 mg phenylalanine exchanges, e.g. milk, potato, cereal Analog XP Pureed or mashed low-protein vegetables Pureed or mashed fruit
Snack:	Diluted fruit juice Low-protein biscuit or piece of fruit, e.g. apple, to chew
Evening meal:	— 50 mg phenylalanine exchanges, e.g. milk, cereal, ordinary custard, yoghurt* Analog XP Pureed or mashed fruit
Bedtime:	— 50 mg phenylalanine exchanges as milk Analog XP

In this example Analogue XP is used; however, other suitable products are available. It is important to check manufacturer's data to assess the need for vitamin and mineral supplementation.

Lists of 50 mg phenylalanine exchanges are available; contact the dietitian.

* Food or drink containing aspartame ('Nutrasweet') is unsuitable for patients with phenylketonuria

very high chance of having a number of severe congenital abnormalities, particularly microcephaly, mental subnormality and heart defects. The infant will not have PKU unless the father is a carrier or has the condition.

If a woman with PKU wishes to have a child and is not already receiving a low-phenylalanine controlled diet, such treatment should be commenced some weeks before contraception is stopped, and the diet must be continued throughout pregnancy. The diet must be strict and the aim should be to control blood levels between 60 and 180 μmol/l. Frequent monitoring of blood levels is essential. Mild forms of the disease with untreated levels above 300 μmol/l should also be treated. The results of such a regimen are encouraging, but ideal levels of phenylalanine are

difficult to attain (Smith et al 1990). During pregnancy, adequate amounts of a low-phenylalanine protein substitute must be provided, together with additional tyrosine (4–8 g) in order to maintain the plasma tyrosine levels within the range of 30–80 μmol/l. Careful monitoring of the plasma levels of phenylalanine is important, as after about the 20th week of pregnancy the requirement for this amino acid increases rapidly. At the end of pregnancy the diet will contain about three times the amount of phenylalanine given in the early part of the pregnancy. The energy intake should be sufficient for the pregnant woman to gain weight at the appropriate level. If the patient is overweight when she decides to have a baby, she should be encouraged to reduce her weight while she is still practising contraception. It is very difficult indeed to maintain satisfactory phenylalanine levels while losing weight, and it would therefore be likely to harm the fetus if she slimmed during the pregnancy.

Homocystinuria

Classic homocystinuria is due to deficient activity of cystathionine synthetase (see Fig. 47.2). The impaired conversion of homocystine to cystathionine results in the accumulation of homocystine, methionine and other sulphur-containing metabolites, and a low level of plasma cystine. The classic description of the condition includes mental subnormality (usually not severe), lens displacement, skeletal abnormalities and thrombotic episodes. There is considerable variation in the presentation and course of the disease. Although there is some evidence that

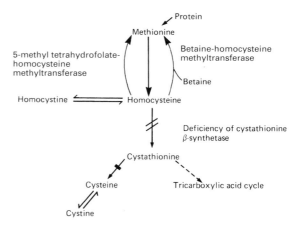

Fig. 47.2 Homocystinuria

Table 47.3 A temporary high-energy protein-free regimen (adapted from Francis 1987), for use during the initial diagnostic period and subsequent metabolic relapses in a variety of conditions

	0–6 months	6–12 months	Teenage
Optimal energy/kg actual weight per 24 h	kJ 525–540 kcal 125–150	420–525 100–125	330–190 70–45
Fluid (ml/kg)	160–200	130–160	60–40*
Carbohydrate (g/100 ml) as glucose polymer	15	15	20*
Optional 50% fat emulsion (g/100 ml)	2	2	4

Notes
1. The osmolality should not exceed 500 mosmol/kg
2. Monitoring of blood gases and electrolytes is required in very ill patients and the doctor may wish to prescribe sodium and potassium
3. The minimum energy provided from carbohydrate should be 168 kJ/kg per 24 h
4. The fat emulsion should not be used in disorders of fat metabolism and during severe relapse in organic acidaemias
5. Only use this regimen for up to 3 days maximum

*Older children may prefer Lucozade, Coke etc. plus glucose polymer. (Do not give drinks containing aspartame to a patient with PKU)

dietary treatment is of value, the variable course of the condition, even amongst siblings, makes assessment difficult. In some families there is a clear biochemical response to large doses of pyridoxine, and some evidence that it is clinically beneficial.

The diet prescribed for patients who do not respond to pyridoxine, or show only a partial biochemical response, is one which is low in methionine and supplemented with cystine. The diet follows the same principles as that described for phenylketonuria. Several commercial protein substitutes low in, or free of, methionine are available. Pulses, soya, lentils and gelatine, which are relatively low in methionine, can be incorporated into the diet. Lists of foods providing 25 mg methionine exchanges are available.

Cystine is not synthesized properly and a supplement of 150–200 mg/kg body weight per 24 h is required for infants, increasing to 1–2 g/24 h in children and adults, unless it is already incorporated in the proprietary protein substitute. The cystine will provide at least some cysteine, which is probably an essential amino acid in this condition.

The administration of choline, which is the precursor of the methyl donor betaine, or of betaine itself, will reduce the plasma levels of homocysteine, although it also increases the level of methionine. It is believed that the rate of homocysteine methylation is increased through betaine–homocysteine methyl transferase. If betaine is prescribed, the accumulation of methionine must not be allowed to become too large. This aspect of treatment requires further study and it is too early to know whether betaine is really helpful. Some patients with homocystinuria require folic acid, but this too may lead to the accumulation of methionine and the levels must be monitored.

Hereditary tyrosinaemia type I

This rare condition arises from a deficiency of fumarylacetoacetate hydrolase, which catalyses the final step in the breakdown of tyrosine (Kvittingen 1991). It presents in early life with progressive liver failure. Even if diagnosed and treated early, it carries a poor prognosis. Most patients die of liver failure and

Table 47.4   Sample menu for a schoolchild with phenylketonuria

Daily:	— g, (—- scoops), Maxamaid XP Mix with water to a paste or drink. If unflavoured, suitable flavourings are available. Divide into 3 portions and give with meals. Always offer an accompanying drink. — 50 mg phenylalanine exchanges – divide between meals as advised.
Breakfast:	Maxamaid XP Fruit juice, tea or coffee with no-protein 'milk'* — 50 mg phenylalanine exchanges, e.g. cereal and/or milk Sugar (optional) Low-protein bread or toast, butter or margarine, jam, honey, marmalade
Mid-morning (between-meal snack):	Suitable fruit squash/cordial** Low-protein biscuits Fruit
Snack meal/ packed lunch:	Maxamaid XP Suitable fruit squash/cordial** — 50 mg phenylalanine exchanges, e.g. chips/crisps Low-phenylalanine vegetables or salad Low-protein bread, butter or margarine Fruit Low-protein biscuits Permitted sweets, e.g. protein-free chocolate or boiled sweets
Main meal:	Maxamaid XP Suitable fruit squash/cordial**, tea or coffee with no-protein 'milk'* — 50 mg phenylalanine exchanges, e.g. potato, rice Low-phenylalanine vegetables or salad — 50 mg phenylalanine exchanges, e.g. as ordinary custard or yoghurt or ice cream** Fruit, fresh, stewed or tinned and/or no-protein 'milk' puddings Low-protein bread, butter or margarine, jam or honey Low-protein biscuits
Bedtime:	Suitable fruit squash/cordial** or tea with no-protein 'milk'* Fruit

In this example Maxamaid XP is used; however, other suitable products are available. It is important to check manufacturer's data to assess the need for vitamin and mineral supplementation.
Lists of 50 mg phenylalanine exchanges are available; contact the dietitian.
*   No-protein 'milk': 240 ml water + 60 ml Calogen + 2 tsps sugar
** Food or drink containing aspartame (Nutrasweet), is unsuitable for patients with phenylketonuria

those who do survive have a high risk of developing a hepatoma. Clinical presentation is highly variable and the acute form in infancy usually causes death in the first year of life. Some of the more chronic forms respond to a diet low in phenylalanine and tyrosine, and often methionine. Vitamin D supplementation may be required; frequently a liver transplant is the only successful treatment.

Branched-chain amino acid disorders

Many inborn errors of branched-chain amino acid metabolism have been described, and these are shown in Fig. 47.3. In some instances the condition may be vitamin-responsive, e.g. a rare form of maple syrup urine disease (MSUD) responsive to thiamin, or some forms of propionic acidaemia responsive to biotin. Some paediatricians will prescribe an empirical trial of large doses of vitamins. Many of the conditions are very rare and often go unrecognized as the true cause of death in infancy.

Generally these disorders present as emergencies in infancy, with relatively non-specific symptoms and signs which include lethargy or irritability, hypotonia, failure to feed, acidosis (which may not be present), hypoglycaemia, convulsions, vomiting and diarrhoea. The diagnosis is often difficult, and sepsis in infancy may cause similar clinical features. The biochemical studies required to make a definitive diagnosis may take several days, and in the meantime the infant has to be fed. The urgent requirement is to stop catabolism and promote anabolism by giving a high-energy protein-free supplement. This may be administered as a continuous nasogastric feed, or as frequent feeds. A suitable composition is shown in Table 47.3. Gradually a very low-protein diet should be introduced to provide 0.5 g protein per kg body weight per 24 h, plus a comprehensive vitamin supplement to provide the recommended intake for any infant (DHSS 1988, Collins & Leonard 1985).

For those patients who do not respond to treatment with a cofactor vitamin, or who respond only partially, a permanent protein-restricted diet will be required, with the aim of preventing the accumulation of metabolites. The amount of protein which can be tolerated will have to be determined by trial and error, but will be in the region of 0.75–1.5 g/kg body weight per 24 h, the higher amount being required by younger patients and during periods of growth. If the amount of protein which can be tolerated is so low that growth is inhibited, supplementary amino acids appropriate for the particular metabolic block should be given.

It is essential to avoid sodium overload and hypoglycaemia. To correct acidosis the following therapies may assist: methylmalonate excretion is increased if the urine is kept alkaline; glycine may reduce the accumulation of some organic acids such as isovaleric acid; carnitine may prevent the accumulation of propionyl-CoA.

This group of disorders is very difficult to manage and the prognosis is generally poor (unless of course the patient is responsive to a cofactor vitamin and the diagnosis has been made early in life). The patients are particularly vulnerable during early life and at times of intercurrent infections thereafter. Many do not survive and those that do are all too frequently handicapped. Nevertheless, some patients do well. While using the high-energy low-protein regimen for feeding, the infant should be transferred to a centre with special expertise in managing this type of problem (Leonard et al 1984).

Maple syrup urine disease (MSUD)

In the classic form of this disorder there is a failure of oxidative decarboxylation of the α-ketoacids derived from the branched-chain amino acids (see Fig. 47.3). These amino acids and their α-ketoacids increase in the blood, cerebrospinal fluid and urine. Dietary treatment is monitored by measuring the branched-chain amino acids in the plasma.

The condition is named after the odour of the urine. Classically it presents acutely in an apparently normal

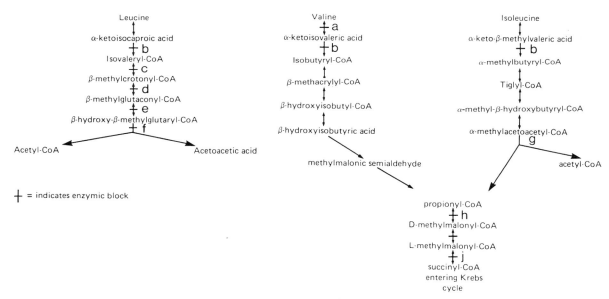

Fig. 47.3   Inherited disorders of branched chain amino acid metabolism
a. hypervalinaemia
b. maple syrup urine disease
c. isovaleric acidaemia
d. β-methylcrotonyl glycinuria
e. 3-methylglutaconic aciduria
f. β-hydroxy-β-methylglutaric aciduria
g. α-methylacetoacetyl-CoA thiolase deficiency
h. propionic acidaemia
j. methylmalonic aciduria (methylmalonic-CoA-mutase)

infant in the neonatal period, with feeding difficulties, vomiting, irregular respiration and severe neurological degeneration. Untreated, the infant usually dies; in the rare survivor there will be brain damage. Prompt treatment is therefore essential. Milder variant forms of the condition are occasionally seen.

The initial emergency treatment (to be used during intercurrent infections) has been described above. The dietary treatment consists of restricting the intake of leucine, valine and isoleucine; this requires severe restriction of natural protein and supplementation with an amino acid mixture free of the three branched-chain amino acids (about 2–3 g amino acid mixture per kg body weight per 24 h). Appropriate vitamins and macro and micro elements must be provided (see the treatment of phenylketonuria), as well as adequate energy from carbohydrate and fat. During the early stages of the introduction of the branched-chain synthetic amino acids, it is necessary to monitor the plasma levels daily and a prompt laboratory service is essential. It is desirable to introduce natural protein (by means of modified milk formulae) to replace the synthetic leucine, valine, and isoleucine once the blood levels have become more stable. Food tables are available so that weaning onto restricted quantities of some normal foods is possible. The principles are similar to those for PKU, but since three amino acids have to be titrated regularly and acute metabolic episodes easily occur, particularly in infants, the management of this diet is far more difficult. Early diagnosis and treatment in the neonate is vital, but even so, if the infant survives the prognosis for normal neurological development is poor.

Urea cycle disorders

Although these disorders (Fig. 47.4) may present at any age, the neonatal period is most likely. Any patient, even with milder forms, may have acute episodes of hyperammonaemia, which is largely responsible for the clinical features of vomiting, focal neurological signs, convulsions and coma, which may be fatal. Older patients may complain of headaches and ataxia, and become confused. The onset of coma carries a poor prognosis. The ammonia levels in neonates may rise to >400 μmol/l plasma, and in acute encephalopathy in older children levels will usually be above 250 μmol/l.

In severe ammonia intoxication haemodialysis or peritoneal dialysis is necessary. Dietary treatment aims to limit the total nitrogen intake by giving a low-protein diet of 0.7 g/kg body weight per 24 h and a

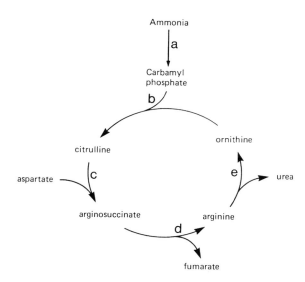

Fig. 47.4 Disorders of the urea cycle
a. Carbamylphosphate synthetase deficiency
b. Ornithine transcarbamylase deficiency
c. Argininosuccinic acid synthetase (citrullinaemia)
d. Argininosuccinic acid lyase (argininosuccinic aciduria)
e. Arginase deficiency (argininaemia)

supplement of 0.7 g/kg body weight of essential amino acids. In the urea cycle defects, specific supplementation with L-arginine or L-citrulline is used for relative insufficiency of these amino acids. Drugs may be used to increase the renal excretion of nitrogen, which is the precursor of ammonia. For example, sodium benzoate will conjugate with glycine to form hippuric acid, which is then excreted in the urine. The efficiency of the diet is determined by monitoring growth and plasma levels of ammonia and essential amino acids. It is not easy to obtain adequate growth in these children, as they have poor appetites and may refuse food. A high-energy protein-free regimen is necessary during periods of food refusal and when ammonia levels are raised, as catabolism worsens the clinical state.

CARBOHYDRATE DISORDERS

Glycogen storage disease

There are a number of inherited disorders which affect glycogen metabolism, and those which require dietary therapy are discussed here (Fig. 47.5).

Glucose-6-phosphatase deficiency

(Also referred to as Type 1a glycogen storage disease or Von Gierke disease.)

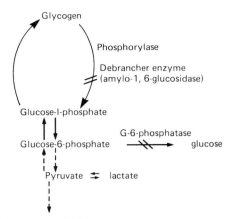

Fig. 47.5   Glycogen metabolism

This enzyme is normally present in liver, renal tubular cells and enterocytes. Endogenous glucose, which is formed by glycogenolysis or gluconeogenesis, cannot be released by the liver (see Fig. 47.5). Severe hypoglycaemia, hyperlacticacidaemia, hyperuricaemia, hyperlipidaemia and hepatomegaly are the main features of the condition. Patients may tolerate the low blood sugar, but all of them fail to grow and develop normally. During childhood dietary therapy has to be intensive, but after growth has ceased the patient becomes more tolerant.

Oral supplements of glucose and/or glucose polymers should be given to the infant to provide 0.5 g carbohydrate per kg bodyweight per hour. The concentration should not be stronger than 15–20%, as it may cause diarrhoea. As the child grows the necessary glucose drinks can be reduced in amount (though not necessarily in frequency), so that by adolescence 0.1 g carbohydrate/kg/h will be sufficient, and the concentration of the solution may be increased to 25%. At night it is more practical to use a continuous nasogastric feed in prepubertal patients with severe disease, and parents and child cope well with this regimen. It should be noted that patients who are being well treated become very vulnerable indeed to falls in blood glucose levels.

For older patients uncooked corn starch should be prescribed: about 2 g/kg body weight made up 1:3 with water at room temperature and given every 4–6 h in addition to normal meals. Such a regimen must be adjusted to suit the individual patient.

Lactose and fructose should be avoided as galactose and fructose are converted to lactate. In infants a lactose (and therefore galactose) + sucrose + fructose-free milk substitute should be prescribed. Older children and adults should avoid drinking ordinary milk, avoid cane sugar, and eat fruit in small quantities sweetened with glucose.

Similar treatment is required for Type 1b, in which there is defective transport of glucose-6-phosphate across the microsomal membrane of hepatocytes and leucocytes.

Deficiency of the debranching enzyme (amylo-1, 6-glucosidase) and of the hepatic phosphorylase complex

Patients with the debrancher enzyme deficiency have hepatomegaly and fasting hypoglycaemia which may be asymptomatic. They often improve considerably at puberty and the condition carries a better prognosis than glucose-6-phosphatase deficiency. Patients with the phosphorylase defect also have hepatomegaly, but

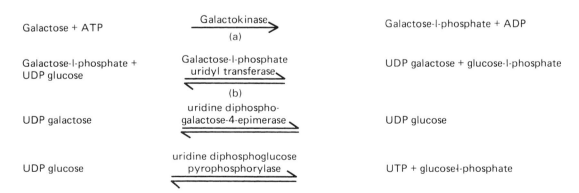

Fig. 47.6   Metabolism of galactose
(a)   Galactokinase deficiency (cataracts)
(b)   Galactosaemia (severe disorder)

growth retardation is slight and their symptoms are mild. Both groups should be treated with a diet in which the protein intake is twice that of normal for age, with frequent meals and snacks. At bedtime a high-protein snack containing some starch is normally sufficient, but with the debrancher deficiency another snack during the night, or even a nocturnal drip feed, may be required. Retarded growth, adenomas and hyperlipidaemia are long-term complications in most patients (Smit et al 1990).

Galactosaemia

Galactosaemia is due to a deficiency of galactose-1-phosphate uridyl transferase (Fig. 47.6), which metabolizes galactose to glucose. This produces an accumulation of galactose-1-phosphate in tissues and erythrocytes. The condition usually presents when the infant begins to receive milk, but there is considerable variation in the rate at which symptoms and signs develop. It can be an acute fulminating disorder associated with an infective agent such as *Escherichia coli*, and death can occur within 24 hours without a diagnosis being made. More usually there is failure to thrive, with vomiting, diarrhoea, jaundice and hepatomegaly. If the infant should survive without treatment, and this is very unusual, the child will be mentally retarded and have cirrhosis of the liver and cataracts.

It is important to exclude the diagnosis in a jaundiced infant and, if the condition is suspected, it is wise to treat empirically for a day or two until the diagnosis is confirmed or excluded by the laboratory. Lactose-free milk will not harm a sick infant who does not have galactosaemia. Early dietary management prevents renal and hepatic damage and cataracts. Unfortunately, although severe mental retardation is usually prevented, these patients often only achieve intelligence in the low normal range and have visual problems and ovarian dysfunction. It seems likely that the prenatal accumulation of galactose-1-phosphate and galactitol leads to some brain damage and eye changes in utero, but further biochemical studies are required. The diet should exclude galactose and therefore lactose. Whether or not it can be relaxed a little at adolescence remains a matter for debate, but there is no biochemical reason for relaxing it.

The infant should receive a galactose–lactose free milk substitute and this should be used to replace normal milk thereafter. All foods containing lactose should be excluded from the diet. Milk is added to many manufactured foods, lactose is used in tablets and lists of suitable foods must be available from the dietitian. She will require up-to-date lists from manufacturers, who are helpful in such matters. It used to be thought that α-galactosides, as found in beans and offal, were harmful, but this now seems unlikely. A suitable diet is shown in Table 47.5. The diet is monitored by the determination of galactose-1-phosphate in erythrocytes. It is impossible to reduce the level to zero.

Hereditary fructose intolerance

This serious condition is due to a deficiency of fructose-1-phosphate aldolase B (Fig. 47.7). The condition will only manifest itself in the infant when

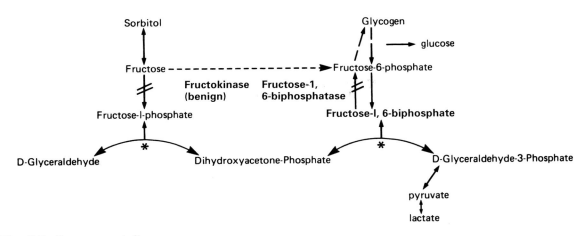

Fig. 47.7 Fructose metabolism
* Fructose-1-phosphate aldolase B deficiency

fructose (or sucrose) is given as cane sugar or in fruit juice. It is potentially fatal, as liver failure may develop if the condition is not recognized and treated. The infant fails to thrive, feeds badly, is lethargic after meals and develops hepatomegaly, or possibly

Table 47.5 Example of a minimal-galactose diet for children (also suitable in lactose intolerance)

Breakfast:	Fruit juice
	Breakfast cereal without milk solids
	Sugar (optional)
	Milk substitute
	Egg, bacon (optional)
	Milk-free bread or toast
	Milk-free margarine e.g. Tomor, some low-fat spreads
	Jam, honey, marmalade, peanut butter
	Tea or coffee and milk substitute
Mid-morning:	Milk substitute or fruit juice
	Milk-free biscuit
Snack meal/ packed lunch:	Milk-free meat, chicken, fish or egg
	Salad/vegetables without milk products or butter
	Plain crisps (check label), chips, jacket potato or milk-free pasta
	Milk-free bread or roll
	Milk-free margarine
	Jam, honey, peanut butter
	Milk-free biscuit or cake
	Fruit
Main meal:	Milk-free meat, chicken, fish or egg
	Rice or potato, prepared without milk/butter
	Vegetables/salad without milk products or butter
	Gravy
	Fruit, fresh, stewed or tinned
	Fruit jelly
	Puddings made with milk substitute and/or milk-free margarine
Bedtime:	Milk substitute or fruit juice
	Milk-free biscuit or cake or sandwich with suitable margarine and filling or fruit

To be used in addition to a suitable milk substitute e.g. Nutrilon Soya (Cow & Gate), Wysoy (Wyeth Nutrition), Prosobee, Pregestimil (Mead Johnson), Ostersoy (Farley Health).
Fortified infant formula soya milks are recommended for children under 5 years of age. For children over 5 and adults, alternative milk substitutes may be used; however, vitamin and mineral (particularly calcium), intakes may need to be supplemented.
Check all ingredients of manufactured products to exclude lactose, milk, whey etc.

jaundice. Treatment is by the removal of all fructose, sucrose and sorbitol from the diet. These patients dislike anything sweet, but even very small amounts of fructose are harmful and lead to hypoglycaemia and liver disease.

Fructose-1, 6-biphosphatase deficiency

This condition (Fig. 47.7) which affects gluco-neogenesis, presents in infancy with hypoglycaemia and with signs and symptoms of acidosis due to the accumulation of acetate and ketones. These patients do not dislike sweet foods. They should receive regular feeds or meals, preferably using glucose or glucose polymers, especially during infections. Although the diet does not have to be too strict and small amounts of fruit are allowed, added cane sugar, fructose and honey should be avoided.

Favism

This condition, which is well recognized in southern Italy and Greece, and is now seen in ethnic groups in the UK, is associated with a deficiency of the B variant of erythrocyte glucose-6-phosphatase. Acute haemolytic anaemia follows the ingestion of broad beans, which should therefore be excluded from the diet. It has been reported even in breastfed infants whose mothers have eaten the beans (see Chapter 42).

Malabsorption of carbohydrates

Lactose intolerance without lactase deficiency

Although these patients do not lack intestinal lactase activity, lactose is absorbed and marked lactosuria, together with aminoaciduria, proteinuria and renal tubular acidosis is found. The infant develops severe diarrhoea, vomiting and acidosis within the first few days of life, and it is a life-threatening condition. Treatment is with a lactose-free diet, to which the response is excellent. It should be noted that even a very small amount of lactose can precipitate the symptoms, but it is a transient disorder from which the child recovers between 12 and 18 months of age.

Congenital lactase deficiency

Many healthy older children and adults have intestinal hypolactasia and, indeed, the low incidence of this finding within Scandinavia and northern Europe is exceptional compared with most parts of the world. Normally infants of all races are born with intestinal lactase. The congenital deficiency presents during the first few days of life as profuse watery diarrhoea and severe failure to thrive. The stool may be acid and may contain lactose, and there may be some lactosuria. Intestinal lactase deficiency is often detected with the hydrogen breath test, but in some instances the enzyme deficiency may be confirmed by a jejunal biopsy. Treatment is with a lactose-free proprietary milk and then weaning onto a lactose-free diet. Care should be taken to make sure that additional vitamins, macro and micro nutrients are given as appropriate, depending upon the composition of the proprietary preparations which are being used.

Congenital sucrose–isomaltase deficiency

This condition is rare in the UK as an inherited disorder. It may cause severe diarrhoea in infancy or occasional bouts in older children. A definitive diagnosis is made by determining enzyme activities on a jejunal biopsy. Treatment is the removal of sucrose from the diet. The condition usually improves with age.

Glucose–galactose malabsorption

This condition is due to the absence of an intestinal transport system shared by glucose and galactose. About 10% of glucose can be absorbed, perhaps due to the presence of another transport system. Profuse, watery diarrhoea appears soon after the infant receives the first feed, whether breast milk, cow's milk or an artificial milk, and severe dehydration and acidosis develop. The infant may be hungry and continue to feed.

Fructose absorption has a separate carrier mechanism. Treatment therefore involves the removal of all glucose and galactose (and therefore sucrose and lactose) from the diet and replacement of these sugars by fructose. Since the fructose molecule is small, preparations containing this sugar have a high osmolality and should be introduced gradually whilst the infant is still on an intravenous drip. A proprietary infant feed with fructose as the sole carbohydrate may be given, or a feed based on a protein module such as comminuted chicken can be made. At the time of weaning, the variety of foodstuffs allowed will be very limited indeed. Gradually the patient may be able to tolerate a little glucose and later may be able to eat small amounts of starchy foods such as potatoes. With such a restricted diet supplements of vitamins and macro and micro nutrients will require careful consideration.

CYSTIC FIBROSIS

Cystic fibrosis is a hereditary disease affecting exocrine glands and characterized by abnormal composition of the exocrine secretions. The disease is the commonest cause of pancreatic insufficiency in childhood. The energy requirements of patients with cystic fibrosis may be 20–50% or even more above normal requirements, but this remains an area under discussion. There are repeated respiratory infections and varying degrees of steatorrhoea. The emphasis therefore is on foods which are high in energy. Fat intake should not be limited (contrary to earlier practice), and meals containing whole milk, full-fat cheese, full-cream yoghurt, butter and margarine, crisps, chips, cream, fried foods and chocolate should be encouraged. For a patient on the old-style low-fat diet, transfer to the new diet should be gradual. Other high-energy foods include sugar, sweets, jam and honey. Glucose polymers can be added to savoury as well as sweet foods, as they do not taste sweet, and concentrated glucose drinks and supplemented flavoured milk shakes are also useful.

Breastfeeding is acceptable but must be combined with a pancreatic supplement. Bottle-fed infants should receive a standard formula supplemented with additional energy. In order to boost energy intake, weaning should be commenced if possible at about 3 months of age.

Pancreatic enzymes should be taken during every meal and snack unless the latter just consists of items such as squash, fruit or boiled sweets. The more recent preparations of pancreatic enzymes in the form of enteric-coated pH-sensitive microspheres are a major advance. Pancreatic powder is required in infants.

The diet should include at least two good portions of protein as well as fruit and vegetables. A daily supplement of 8000 IU vitamin A, 800 IU vitamin D and 100–200 mg of vitamin E should be given. If the appetite is very poor, a comprehensive vitamin supplement and possibly trace elements will be necessary.

INBORN ERRORS OF CELLULAR ORGANELLES

There are three well defined groups of genetic disorders in which the functions of an intracellular organelle are impaired: lysosomal storage disorders, mitochondrial disorders and peroxisomal disorders. These conditions arise both from mutations in the structural genes for the proteins in an organelle, and from mutations in the gene coding for components necessary for the transport of the proteins and their incorporation into the organelles. No dietary treatment is available for lysosomal storage disorders.

Mitochondrial disorders and fat oxidation defects

These result from defects of a) transport (carnitine deficiency is included in this group); b) substrate utilization of the Krebs cycle; c) oxidation–phosphorylation coupling; and d) the respiratory chain. They may present as a myopathy or an encephalomyopathy with episodic hypoglycaemia. Their diagnosis is highly complex, requires extensive biochemical facilities and such patients are likely to be investigated fully in a teaching hospital (Pollit 1989). Treatment is still very experimental and its long-term effect on prognosis requires further experience.

Przyrembel (1987) has summarized dietary treatments as follows:

Defect	*Diet*
Carnitine deficiency	Low fat, high carbohydrate
Carnitine deficiency Carnitine palmitoyl transferase	MCT fat, high carbohydrate
Pyruvate carboxylase?	High protein, high carbohydrate
Acyl-CoA dehydrogenases Phosphoenolpyruvate carboxykinase	High carbohydrate – frequent meals
Pyruvate dehydrogenase	High fat, low carbohydrate

Periods of fasting should be avoided. Such diets may include trials of megadoses of a variety of vitamins and/or carnitine 50–200 mg/kg body weight per 24 h.

Peroxisomal disorders

Important peroxisomal functions include the catabolism of very long-chain fatty acids and phytanic acid and the synthesis of bile acids (for a review see Monnens & Heymans 1987). There are two diseases in which peroxisomal function is impaired and which respond to dietary therapy.

Refsum disease – adult type

In this disorder oxidation of phytanic acid (PA) which is a 20-carbon acid is impaired due to deficient activity of phytanic acid α-hydrolase. In man, PA is derived from food and also from the conversion of free phytol in food. Normally only a trace of PA is present in serum, but it is greatly increased in amount in Refsum disease. The condition is characterized by a number of features, which include cerebellar ataxia, peripheral neuropathy, retinitis pigmentosa with night blindness and cardiomyopathy. The onset of signs and symptoms is variable, but usually before the age of 20 years. Dietary treatment aimed at maintaining the plasma PA levels below 10 mg/100 ml has given encouraging results. The main sources of PA are dairy produce and fats and meat from ruminants, but also other fats too. Phytol occurs in various foods including corn oil, nuts and spices. There is uncertainty about whether or not chlorophyll-bound phytol should be restricted.

A practical diet is one with severe restrictions of fat, and no ruminant meat, but fruit, skimmed milk and perhaps vegetables may be allowed. Plasma exchanges in the early stages of treatment may be indicated and during periods of loss of appetite a high carbohydrate intake should be administered (Dickson et al 1989).

Adrenoleukodystrophy

This is a group of degenerative neurological disorders in which there is demyelination and an accumulation of saturated, very long-chain fatty acids in body fluids and tissues. Using a diet in which these acids are restricted, together with a supplement of oleic acid, may produce a reduction in, and be of value in, X-linked leukodystrophy, which presents at about 8 years of age. Whether this is clinically beneficial remains to be established. Inherited disorders of lipid metabolism are discussed in Chapter 41.

A review of peroxismal disorders is given by Moser et al (1991).

Acknowledgement

I am very grateful to Mrs Hilary Warwick SRD, District Dietitian, Southampton and South West Hampshire Health Authority for providing the diet sheets and reading the manuscript. During the writing of this chapter I held an Emeritus Leverhulme Fellowship.

REFERENCES

Advisory Committee on Borderline Substances Recommendations published in British National Formulary. Publ. British Medical Association and the Pharmaceutical Society of Great Britain. New editions twice yearly

Bentley D, Lawson M 1988 Clinical nutrition in paediatric disorders. Baillière Tindall, London

Collins JE, Leonard JV 1985 The dietary management of inborn errors of metabolism. Human Nutrition: Applied Nutrition 39A: 255–272

Cotton RG 1990 Heterogeneity of phenylketonuria at the clinical, protein and DNA levels. Journal of Inherited Metabolic Disease 13: 739–750

Department of Health 1991 Dietary reference values for food energy and nutrients for the United Kingdom. Report on Health and Social Subjects 41, HMSO, London

Department of Health and Social Security 1988 Present-day practice in infant feeding: third report. Report on Health and Social Subjects 32, HMSO, London

Dickson N, Mortimer JG, Faed JM et al 1989 A child with Refsum's disease: successful treatment with diet and plasma exchange. Developmental Medicine and Child Neurology 31: 81–87

Francis D 1986 Nutrition for children. Blackwell Scientific Publications, Oxford

Francis D 1987 Diets for sick children. Blackwell Scientific Publications, Oxford

Kvittingen EA 1991 Tyrosinaemia type 1 – an update. Journal of Inherited Metabolic Disease 7: 13–17

Leonard JV, Daish PD, Naughten ER, Bartlett K 1984 The management of longterm outcome of organic acidaemias. Journal of Inherited Metabolic Disease 7: 13–17

McKusick VA 1988 Mendelian inheritance in man, 8th edn. Johns Hopkins University Press, Baltimore

MIMS Monthly Index of Medical Specialities, 30 Lancaster Gate, London W2 3LP

Monnens L, Heymans H 1987 Peroxisomal disorders: clinical characterisation. Journal of Inherited Metabolic Disease 10 (Suppl 1): 23–32

Moser HW, Bergin A, Cornblath D 1991 Peroxisomal disorders. Biochem Cell Biology 69: 463–474

Pollitt RJ 1989 Disorders of mitochondrial β-oxidation: prenatal and early postnatal diagnosis and their relevance to Reye's syndrome and sudden infant death. Journal of Inherited Metabolic Disease 12 (Suppl 1): 215–230

Przyrembel H 1987 Therapy of mitochondrial disorders. Journal of Inherited Metabolic Disease 10: 129–146

Scriver CR, Beaudet AL, Sly WS, Valle D (eds) 1989 The metabolic basis of inherited disease, 6th edn. McGraw-Hill, New York

Smit GPA, Fernandes J, Leonard JV et al 1990 The long-term outcome of patients with glycogen storage diseases. Journal of Inherited Metabolic Disease 13: 411–418

Smith I, Beasley MG, Ades AE 1990 Intelligence and quality of dietary treatment in phenylketonuria. Archives of Diseases of Childhood 65: 472–478

Smith I, Cook B, Beasley M 1991 Review of neonatal screening programme for phenylketonuria. British Medical Journal 303: 333–335

Smith I, Glossop J, Beasley M 1990 Fetal damage due to maternal phenylketonuria: effects of dietary treatment and maternal phenylalanine concentrations around the time of conception. (An interim report from the UK Phenylketonuria register). Journal of Inherited Metabolic Disease 13: 651–657

Thompson AJ, Smith I, Brenton D et al 1990 Neurological deterioration in young adults with phenylketonuria. Lancet 336: 602–605

PRODUCTS NAMED IN THE TABLES

The following products are mentioned in the tables but, in addition, many other suitable preparations are available.

Analog XP	Scientific Hospital Supplies Group UK 100 Wavertree Boulevard Wavertree Technology Pk Liverpool L7 9PT
Aminogran Food Supplement Aminogran Mineral Mixture	UCB (PHARMA) Limited Star House 69 Clarendon Road, Watford Herts WD1 1DJ
Calogen	Scientific Hospital Supplies Ltd
Nutrilon Soya	Cow & Gate Ltd Cow & Gate House, Trowbridge Wilts BA14 OXQ
Ketovite tablets and liquid	Paines and Byrne Limited Pabyrn Laboratories 177 Bilton Road, Perivale Greenford, Middlesex UB6 7HG
Maxamaid XP	Scientific Hospital Supplies Ltd
Minafen	Cow & Gate Ltd
Ostersoy	Farley Health Products Nottingham NG2 3AA
Pregestimil	Mead Johnson Nutritionals Division of Bristol Myers Co Ltd Station Road, Langley Slough SL3 6ED
Tomor margarine	Van den Bergh Sussex House, Burgess Hill West Sussex RH15 9AW
Wysoy	Wyeth Nutrition Huntercombe Lane South Taplow, Maidenhead Berks SC6 OPH

48. Nutritional management of alcohol-related disease

L. M. Blendis

Alcoholism has been suggested as a major cause of malnutrition in the developed world, but in practice malnutrition is only found in ill patients with cirrhosis and pancreatitis. Alcoholics without medical complications have no evidence of malnutrition: 88% of US alcoholics admitted for treatment had ideal or excess body weight (Hurt et al 1981). Patients on adequate energy intakes but with 30% energy from alcohol may still eat enough protein and other nutrients to satisfy their needs (Neville et al 1968).

Alcohol normally accounts for >5% of energy in half of North American business executives, and a quarter take more than 10% of energy in this form (Bebb et al 1971). Alcohol intakes of 11–12% of energy are not unusual in general medical studies, e.g. of hyperlipidaemic men (Dennis et al 1985). Chapter 7 sets out the variable impact of alcohol as an energy source depending on the level and chronicity of intake.

ALCOHOLIC LIVER DISEASE: GENERAL CONSIDERATIONS

In the majority of nutritional studies in alcoholic liver disease one or a number of tests are performed (Table 48.1) and these may be used as a more sensitive index of malnutrition than body weight. An apparently overweight 'healthy'-looking chronic drinker may still be suffering from underlying nutritional deficiencies. For example, in a study of 100 consecutive chronic alcoholic patients without obvious liver disease, nearly two-thirds had abnormal liver biopsies but normal anthropometric measurements (Bunout et al 1983). By the time patients have developed clinical liver disease they often have haematological, biochemical and immunological indicators of protein–energy malnutrition (PEM) (O'Keefe et al 1980). However, many of the blood tests, e.g. albumin and transferrin, are affected by liver damage itself as well as malnutrition and

Table 48.1 Nutritional assessment in liver disease

Assessment of dietary intake
Anthropometric measurements
    Arm muscle circumference – skeletal muscle
    Skinfold thickness – fat stores
Biochemistry
    Creatinine/height index – lean body mass
Intradermal skin testing for anergy – generalized malnutrition
Tests for specific deficiencies
    RBC folate
    Serum vitamin levels
    Assessment of trace mineral deficiency
Energy balance – indirect calorimetry compared to dietary caloric intake
Studies of nitrogen status and metabolism
    Serum amino acid levels
    Ratio of branched-chain to aromatic amino acids (BCAA/AAA)
    Nitrogen balance
    Total body nitrogen – capture of neutron activation
    Nitrogen index
    Labelled amino acid kinetic studies – ^{13}C, ^{14}C leucine

therefore have to be interpreted with caution (Merli et al 1987). Older patients may exhibit more evidence of PEM in the absence of clinical liver disease (Mendenhall et al 1984), but alcoholic hepatitis is particularly likely to be linked to the presence of adult kwashiorkor or marasmus. In a more recent study the percentage of total calories derived from protein in cirrhotics was 12%, compared to 17% in normal controls (Schneeweiss et al 1990). The severity of PEM may correlate with the degree of liver damage and predict 6-month mortality (Mendenhall et al 1986), although this clear link is not always found (Mills et al 1983). Patients with significant alcoholic liver disease tend to have a lower protein intake than usual but still remains above the minimum requirement in health (Gabuzda & Shear 1970).

ACUTE ALCOHOLIC HEPATITIS (AAH)

Patients with AAH are often anorexic and wasted and their nitrogen balance is often negative (Soberon et al 1987). They are unable to tolerate oral food and their condition is frequently complicated by the presence of encephalopathy, necessitating protein restriction, and a tendency to maldigestion or malabsorption of protein and fat (Soberon et al 1987). This problem led to trials of the value of enteral feeding in patients with AAH. Early trials with well tolerated polyurethane feeding tubes showed that protein intakes of more than 80 g/day could be tolerated and positive nitrogen balances achieved without exacerbating the encephalopathy (Smith et al 1982). Table 48.2 shows, however, that two randomized controlled trials of enteral feeding have not demonstrated a clear benefit for enteral nutrition rather than a routine hospital diet with abstinence from alcohol. However, positive nitrogen balances may not be consistently achieved without the enteral use of energy-dense diets, with 9.4 g N/l given as a continuous infusion (Rees et al 1989).

A review of trials using corticosteroid treatment, and the possible protection by propylthiouracil in patients with severe AAH, is given by Blendis (1992).

Parenteral nutrition (PN) in acute alcoholic hepatitis

PN has been restricted by the fear that infused amino acids, especially the aromatic amino acids (AAA), and methionine will cause portosystemic encephalopathy (PSE) (see below). However, in an initial observation, Galambos et al (1979) showed that Travasol infused via a peripheral vein did not induce PSE in patients with AAH, even when up to 2 l/day were infused to provide 50–77 g of protein. Albumin concentrations increased and liver enzyme levels fell, while urinary urea excretion rose. Even patients with fulminant hepatic failure have been shown to tolerate PN well (Forbes et al 1987). These findings led to five randomized control trials of intravenous amino acid therapy in patients with AAH (Table 48.2), but the majority have found no significant improvement in

Table 48.2   Controlled trials in the nutritional treatment of alcoholic hepatitis

Reference	Number of patients	Study	Length of study (days)	Outcome
Enteral				
Mendenhall et al (1985)	67	Routine 2500 kcal hospital diet vs. hospital diet + 2240 kcal/day high in BCAA		PSE decreased in both. Little advantage.
Calvey (1985)	64	Hospital diet vs. supplement with 200 kcal + 10 g N	18	No effect on mortality.
Parenteral				
Nasrallah & Galambos (1980)	35	70–80 g Aminosyn or 8.5% Travasol	28	Increase in serum albumin. Decrease in mortality.
Diehl et al (1985)	15	AA/glucose vs. glucose	28	No change in nutrition or histology. No difference in mortality.
Achord (1987)	28	Conventional diet vs. 2L AA/glucose	21	Increase in serum albumin. No difference in mortality.
Simon & Galambos (1988)	34	Peripheral PN vs. standard diet	28	No difference in mortality. Improved morbidity in severe AH.
Mezey et al (1991)	54	Dextrose + Freamine III (350 kcal) vs. Dextrose	28	No difference in mortality. Improved biochemical, metabolic and nutritional parameters.

mortality. Thus enteral feeding and PN in AAH may promote an improvement in both nutrition and liver function, but studies remain inconclusive in terms of an improvement in mortality.

CIRRHOSIS

In patients with cirrhosis but without alcoholic hepatitis, analyses of the plasma amino acids have shown a generalized elevation of plasma AAA, but a decrease in the branched chains (BCAA) (Blendis & Jenkins 1988). However, an analysis of skeletal muscle biopsies show that only valine is depleted (Montanari et al 1988). Thus the problem of the ideal intake for maintenance and repair remains. In an earlier metabolic study, Gabuzda & Shear (1970) showed that with an intake of at least 1500–3500 kcal/day, nitrogen balance was maintained on only 35–50 g protein daily, i.e. 0.6–0.7 g/kg body weight/day. Cirrhotic patients had an average minimum protein requirement of 0.74 g/kg/day, whether natural or BCAA-enriched protein was used. At 0.93 g/kg/day, positive nitrogen balance was achieved with an average gain of 1.2 g/N/day (Swart et al 1988).

Whole-body protein synthesis rates in cirrhosis may be unchanged, increased (Swart et al 1988) or decreased (Morrison et al 1990) depending on the severity of the liver disease (Schneeweiss et al 1990) or the presence of glucose intolerance and insulin resistance (Petrides et al 1991). Malnourished patients, however, show greater nitrogen retention on the same nitrogen intake (Golden et al 1977), and the organ basis for changes in protein synthesis or breakdown is uncertain. In answer to the question 'Are patients with chronic liver disease hypermetabolic?' (Heymsfield et al 1990), Wagner et al (1991) suggest there are about 20% who metabolically mimic acute starvation (McClain et al 1991b). The cirrhotic patient seems to maintain a positive nitrogen balance on only modest increases in protein intake equivalent to the RNI of protein, i.e. 0.75 g/kg/day.

Enteral and parenteral nutrition

The difficulty in assessing studies on enteral feeding is that they are often very short-term studies performed on small numbers of patients, whose disease lasts for many years. Only long-term studies on large groups of patients are likely to provide the essential information as to whether improved nutrition will affect liver function and the lifespan of cirrhotic patients. For example, 9 out of 10 patients with cirrhosis, most of whom were malnourished, tolerated a high-energy (2000 kcal), low-protein (40 g), low-salt (1 g Na)

formula, with significant increases in albumin and transferrin levels as well as increases in their creatinine/height ratio and in mid-arm muscle and fat areas (Smith et al 1982), but these biochemical and anthropometric improvements were all short-term. Cabre et al (1990) in a similar, larger study also showed reduced hospital mortality. Cirrhotic patients have consistently been shown to have low plasma levels of BCAA associated with decreased appearance rates (Marchesini et al 1987). Supplementation with branched-chain amino acids (BCAA) has also been tested, with satisfactory early responses over a 5-week period (Okita et al 1984).

However, the role of parenteral nutrition (PN) in a chronic disease such as cirrhosis remains problematical (Silk 1988). For example, supplementation of an oral diet of 40 kcal/kg/day with parenteral nutrition of 200 mg nitrogen/kg/day resulted in a significant decrease in serum bilirubin (Naveau et al 1986). However, short-term metabolic studies have provided important information about the disturbances in amino acid metabolism in these patients. Using intravenous amino acids in patients with malabsorption syndrome allows them to go into positive nitrogen balance, but some may fail to respond because of selective needs for specific amino acids, e.g. cystine and tyrosine. With oral supplementation of these amino acids patients then go into positive nitrogen balance, with improvement in their nutritional and hepatic function tests (Rudman et al 1981). In another acute metabolic study the effect of intravenous amino acid, together with infusions of glucose and insulin, was assessed in patients with decompensated chronic liver disease (O'Keefe et al 1988). The infusion of the mixture reduced body protein breakdown so that there was a progressive positive N balance without a rise in plasma amino acids. As liver function decreases, the ability of the liver to clear amino acids such as proline, lysine, threonine and arginine may become increasingly impaired as the capacity to synthesize urea declines (Vilstrup et al 1982). Recently the failure of intravenous BCAA-enriched solutions to effect nitrogen balance was confirmed (Weber et al 1990), but they did result in a fall in plasma ammonia levels, indicating a possible therapeutic role in the management of encephalopathy.

Portal systemic encephalopathy (PSE)

This is a brain abnormality with disturbances in mental function and changes in neuromuscular movement. Acutely it occurs after fulminant liver failure, but it may be episodic in cirrhotics before becoming a chronic condition. It is associated with the shunting of blood from the portal system directly into the systemic circulation, thereby bypassing the liver. Patients at first show subtle changes in mood or sleep rhythm and may become apathetic or irritable. Progression to drowsiness precedes semi-stupor and coma. Simple tests to draw a five-point star and to link consecutive numbers on a page by straight lines – the number connection test – reveal the early mental abnormalities. A 'flapping' tremor can be shown by having the patient stretch their arms, hands and fingers out: the hands suddenly flex or extend at the wrist and then resume their position. The central role of nitrogenous material in the gastrointestinal tract in the pathogenesis of PSE is undisputed (Conn & Lieberthal 1984), although clearly there are other precipitating factors such as infection, electrolyte disturbances, intravascular volume depletion and increased sensitivity to CNS depressants such as the benzodiazepines. Several nitrogen-containing materials have been implicated, including ammonia (Kirk 1936, Walshe 1951), methionine (Phear et al 1956) and its metabolites, the mercaptans (Chen et al 1970), disturbances in serum amino acid metabolism (Walshe 1953) and in the metabolism of CNS-depressant gamma-aminobutyric acid (GABA) (Schafer & Jones 1982).

Amino acid metabolism and the false neurotransmitters

One theory that has received a great deal of attention has been that of the false neurotransmitters. The aromatic amino acids, phenylalanine and tyrosine, rise markedly in severe liver disease. These amino acids compete for the transport carrier process across the blood–brain barrier which also transfers the branched-chain amino acids. An excess phenylalanine concentration in the brain will saturate the phenylalanine–catecholamine pathway (Fischer & Baldessarini 1971). This in turn leads to an excessive production of the sympathomimetic amines, tyramine and octopamine, which by combining with the amino receptors on neuronal membranes as weak neuro-transmitters could in theory interfere with normal neurotransmission. Therefore, despite much conflicting evidence, amino acid solutions rich in BCAA, in addition to protein restriction, were proposed as a treatment for both acute and chronic PSE (Fischer et al 1976). After the initial uncontrolled observations which suggested that BCAA infusions improved acute PSE, several randomized controlled trials have been published (Table 48.3). The trials differ in many aspects, including the proportion of men, the percentages of alcoholics, the proportions of different grades of PSE and the length of follow-up. The trials all used different nutrient regimens, so it is difficult to assess any synergistic or antagonistic effects between the other nutrients used and the action of the BCAA. Mortality rates varied from 25% to 50% in the control groups and it was not clear whether the variety of causes of PSE producing equivalent grades of encephalopathy had the same prognosis. PSE linked to gastrointestinal bleeding and to sepsis, for example, are known to carry a worse prognosis than excessive

Table 48.3 Effects of intravenous BCAA on the management of PSE: a summary of 6 clinical trials

Study	Number of patients	BCAA additional treatment	Control 'treatment'	Mortality (%)		Improved mental state (%)	
				BCAA	Controls	BCAA	Controls
Rossi-Fanelli et al (1982)	34	20% glucose	20% glucose lactulose	24	41	70	47
Wahren et al (1983)	50	30 kcal/kg/day 50% glucose + 20% intralipid	50% glucose	40	20	56	48
Cerra et al (1985)	75	25% glucose *Oral nutrition as tolerated <1500 kcal/day	25% glucose neomycin	17	55	77	45
Fiaccadori et al (1984)	48	30% glucose *With or without lactulose	30% glucose lactulose	0	0	94	62
Michel et al (1985)	70	*Lipids (100 g)	Conventional AA solution Lipids	20	20.9	33	29
Gluud et al (1983)	20	50% glucose	50% glucose	20	10	70	60

* All groups received a modified AA solution enriched with BCAA + glucose

protein ingestion or constipation, with greater colonic absorption of microbial metabolites. The weight of evidence indicates that intravenous BCAA solutions may result in a more rapid improvement in PSE, but no change in mortality compared to conventional therapy (Eriksson & Conn 1989, Vilstrup et al 1990). Naylor et al (1989) showed reduction in mortality; the different results depend on which studies are included in the analysis, so the situation remains unresolved.

Oral BCAA

The enrichment of oral feeds with BCAA mixtures is even more difficult to assess. Ten trials, often with small groups of patients, have been performed (Table 48.4). Only two of the trials showed a distinct improvement with BCAA compared to the control diet. Thus it is still difficult to support the recommendation of oral BCAA solutions for the treatment of chronic PSE at the present time.

Amino acid analogues

With the confusing results of BCAA supplementation, an alternative approach has been the use of amino acids as the α-ketoanalogues. The administration of five essential amino acids – valine, leucine, isoleucine, methionine and phenylalanine – as the calcium salts in gelatin capsules significantly improves the behaviour of patients on clinical and psychological testing (Maddrey et al 1976). Finally, when oral ornithine salts of branched-chain ketoacids (34 mmol/day) were compared with the effects of BCAA (68 mmol/day) in a double-blind crossover study, the ornithine salts produced a significant improvement (Herlong et al 1980), but calcium salts of branched-chain ketoacids (34 mmol/day) had little effect; ornithine α-keto-glutarate induced mental deterioration. Ornithine itself might effect some change in ammonia metabolism because it is part of the hepatic urea cycle, with two amino groups being added to form urea.

Table 48.4 Effects of oral BCAA on the management of PSE: a summary of 10 clinical trials

| Study | Number of patients | Treatment | | Duration of treatment | Type of study | Outcome |
		BCAA	Controls			
McGhee et al (1983)	4	'Hepataid' Casein 20 g	Casein 50 g	11	Crossover	No change None developed PSE
Horst et al (1984)	37	20 g 'Hepataid' 20 g protein diet	20 g protein oral diet+ glucose solution	30	Prophylaxis controlled randomized	BCAA better PSE became more severe in controls with increasing protein intake
Eriksson et al (1982)	7	30 g BCAA + sucrose 40–100 g protein diet lactulose	Sucrose/ maltodextrin	14	Crossover	No difference
Egberts et al (1984)	22	BCAA 0.25 g/kg l g protein/kg/day, 35 kcal	Casein 0.25 g/kg	7	Prophylaxis crossover	BCAA better improved psychometrics only
Riggio et al (1984)	28	BCAA 0.5 g protein/kg/day	Lactulose	60	Controlled randomized	No difference
Simko (1983)	15	'Hepataid' 20-60 g standard unrestricted diet	Placebo	90	Controlled randomized	No change
Sieg et al (1983)	14	BCAA carbohydrates 40 g protein diet lactulose	Placebo isocaloric carbohydrate intake	90	Crossover	No change
Von Schafer et al (1981)	8	45 g BCAA enriched protein & usual diet	45 g milk protein	30–60	Crossover	No difference Milk protein not tolerated
Swart et al (1981)	8	Up to 80 g BCAA enriched protein (35% BCAA)	Up to 80 g mixed protein (20% BCAA)	30 Alternating five day regimes	Prophylaxis controlled randomized	No difference
Guarnieri et al (1984)	8	30 g amino acid Basic diet		100–200	Controlled randomized	No difference

Oral therapy with lactulose and neomycin

Lactulose is a synthetic non-absorbable disaccharide which is now widely used in managing some forms of constipation. It is particularly valuable in PSE because it provides substrates for colonic microflora to grow; this then diverts N-containing compounds from ammonia and other metabolites to providing the substrate for bacterial protein synthesis. Faecal N therefore rises. A reduction in colonic pH as lactulose ferments may also alter the colonic absorption of ammonia or aromatic amino acids. This therapy, if introduced rapidly, can lead to cramps and flatulence. It is often combined with oral neomycin, which is a non-absorbed antibiotic which tends to reduce small-intestinal fermentation. Their combined use is considered by some to be controversial but by others particularly valuable.

Use of vegetable protein in portosystemic encephalopathy

Whatever the cause of PSE, dietary protein intake has been uniformly implicated in its pathophysiology and protein restriction is a standard part of therapy. Sir Andrew Aguecheek in Shakespeare's *Twelfth Night* considered meat was harmful: '. . . but I am a great eater of beef and I believe that does harm to my wit', but it was Pavlov who first pointed out that meat protein induced mental changes in dogs with Eck-fistulae, whereas milk protein did not. Later, blood was shown to produce more ammonia than either fish or milk protein (Bessman & Minck 1958). This prompted the use of a milk and cheese diet in the treatment of PSE, with some success (Fenton et al 1966). Another rationale for this diet was the possible change in colonic bacterial flora, from urease-containing bacteria on a meat diet (with ammonia produced from urea) to predominantly lactobacilli on a milk-rich diet.

With the advent of highly successful oral therapy for PSE, such as lactulose and neomycin, the need for special diets has diminished. However, the fact remains that these patients need protein and yet are being treated by protein restriction. Intakes of 40 g of protein daily or less may be below requirements, since nitrogen balance studies have shown that in some patients protein requirements may vary from 0.7 to 1.0 g/kg body weight. Greenberger et al (1977) first suggested that vegetable protein might be beneficial and the results of four studies comparing animal and vegetable protein are shown in Table 48.5. The vegetable protein produced no deleterious effects and had some possible benefits. This is a considerable reversal of the old advice to use animal protein for its superior biological value in patients with hepatic encephalopathy.

What are the possible mechanisms by which the benefits of vegetable protein might occur? There is little or no difference in the aromatic or branched-chain amino acid content of the meat and vegetable diets, so the false neurotransmitter explanation seems hard to sustain. Vegetable protein diets are richer in arginine. Both of the basic amino acids, arginine and ornithine, however, are involved as intermediates in the hepatic urea cycle. Thus they induce an increase in uptake of blood ammonia, so that blood ammonia levels fall in both normal and cirrhotic subjects as urea production rises (Najarian & Harper 1956, Bessman & Minck 1958). However, one controlled trial of oral arginine alone (Reynolds et al 1958) failed to show benefit.

Other factors also may explain differences in the response to animal and vegetable protein diets. Animal protein diets contain significantly more methionine and this could be detrimental due to the formation of mercaptans. Vegetable protein diets may also reduce the net absorption of nitrogen because the increased fibre content of the diet leads to enhanced

Table 48.5 PSE animal or vegetable protein?

Reference	Number of patients	Type of study	Anti-PSE therapy	Results
Greenberger et al (1977)	3	Crossover	Yes	Improvement with vegetarian
Uribe et al (1982)	10	Crossover with 80 g protein	No	Improvement with vegetarian
DeBruijn et al (1983)	8	Crossover < 45 g protein	No	Improvement with vegetarian
Shaw et al 1983	5	Crossover with 50 g protein	Yes	No difference

bacterial synthesis in the colon, with greater endogenous protein losses and an increase in faecal nitrogen excretion on vegetable diets (Stephen & Cummings 1980, Weber et al 1985). There is then a significant reduction in urinary urea (Weber et al 1985) and total nitrogen excretion (deBruijn et al 1983). Thus the mechanisms for any beneficial effect of vegetable protein are many.

SALT AND WATER RETENTION

Another common complication of portal hypertension is that of salt and water retention, leading to the development of massive ascites with or without peripheral oedema. Even cirrhotics without ascites appear to have a problem with sodium handling and compensate with an increase in levels of atrial natriuretic peptide (ANP). With increasing dietary sodium intake, plasma ANP levels rise further (Warner et al 1990). However, in cirrhotic patients with ascites plasma ANP levels can no longer compensate for increased dietary sodium intake, which therefore has to be restricted (Warner et al 1990), together with fluid intake, and diuretic therapy is needed. Patients with only a moderate amount of ascites require a 'no-added salt diet', in which salt is neither added to the food nor to cooking. This may restrict sodium intake to 2 g or 100 meq daily, but much depends on the amount of salty foods eaten (Shepherd & Farleigh 1987). In addition they usually require 'potassium-sparing' diuretics, which act at the distal nephron site. However, as the patients become more resistant to these drugs and require additional 'loop' diuretics, such as furosemide, sodium intake must be restricted further to 1 g of sodium, or 50 meq per day. The more 'refractory' patients, i.e. those that do not respond to such a regimen, will require hospitalization with bedrest and restriction of sodium intake to the lowest palatable level – 20 meq per day – together with 1 litre of fluid. These patients usually excrete less than 3 meq sodium per day in the urine. The diets can be made more palatable with salt substitutes such as potassium chloride, but care must be taken in patients on 'potassium-sparing' diuretics, that they do not develop hyperkalaemia.

The small group of patients who become virtually refractory to all diuretic regimens may be managed by removing large volumes of fluid from the abdominal cavity by paracentesis (Gines et al 1987). If this treatment fails or is impractical, a peritoneovenous shunt (PVS) may result in an impressive diuretic response (Blendis et al 1979). In the longer term,

ascites either disappears or is easily controlled with a no-added salt diet with or without small doses of diuretics (Greig et al 1981).

One of the complications associated with massive ascites is the loss of muscle mass from the limbs and trunk, resulting in a cachetic appearance. In a recent study of body composition in seven patients undergoing PVS, the initial diuresis was associated with a mean loss of 9 kg in weight. The urinary loss of sodium and potassium was associated with a decrease in total body potassium (TBK) but not in total body nitrogen (TBN), resulting in a significant decrease in the body's TBK/TBN ratio from 2.12 to 1.66 ($p<0.01$). This signifies a state of potassium depletion rather than a reduction in potassium capacity. After more than a year there were significant increases in TBN (Harrison et al 1984). These improvements were associated with the use of extra non-alcohol calories but not dietary protein (Blendis et al 1986). These studies therefore indicate the usefulness of assessing TBN as a measure of lean body mass. It is also possible that the state of ascites affects nitrogen metabolism in the liver as well as elsewhere, in addition to its effect in diminishing food intake.

IMPAIRED CARBOHYDRATE METABOLISM AND DIABETES

It has long been recognized that there is an association between cirrhosis and an increased incidence of diabetes: up to 70% of cirrhotic patients have an

Table 48.6 Factors involved in the reduced carbohydrate tolerance in patients with chronic alcoholism

Liver disease causing:
    Hyperinsulinaemia from diminished hepatic uptake of insulin
    Hypokalaemia from aldosteronism
    Diminished total body potassium
    Hyperglucagonaemia from reduced hepatic hormonal uptake
    Increased hepatic gluconeogenesis
    Diminished hepatic uptake of glucose from:
        decreased liver cell mass and decreased hepatic insulin action due to blood shunting past the liver by portal systemic anastomoses developing naturally or induced surgically
    Down regulation of peripheral insulin receptors induced by hyperinsulinaemia
    Post-insulin receptor defect for reasons unknown

Pancreatic disease inducing relative insulin deficiency for the prevailing state of insulin resistance
Causes:
    Chronic pancreatitis
    Secondary haemachromatosis

impaired carbohydrate tolerance, and up to 30% are clinically diabetic. Hyperglucagonism and glucagon resistance appear to be early findings associated with normal glucose and insulin levels (Silva et al 1988). The high fasting and postprandial serum insulin levels (Table 48.6) and down-regulated insulin receptors mimic overweight patients with non-insulin dependent diabetes (Blei et al 1982). The hyperinsulinaemic response to oral glucose only partially compensates for peripheral tissue insensitivity, resulting in glucose intolerance in some patients (Kruszynska et al 1991).

The principles of dietary management currently being applied to non-cirrhotic diabetics should apply equally well to cirrhotic patients with diabetes. The recommended increase in the intake of carbohydrate to 50% of dietary calories in the form of high-fibre foods may have definite advantages for the diabetic cirrhotic. Legume – as opposed to bread-based, meals induce lower postprandial glucose, insulin and gastric inhibitory peptide (GIP) responses. This may be due to a slower absorption of these foods, as indicated by higher enteroglucagon and neurotensin levels or smaller increases in amino acid levels (Jenkins et al 1987). When 40 g of vegetable protein, in the form of legumes, is included in the diets of insulin-dependent diabetic cirrhotic patients, they show a reduction in their insulin requirements and increasing episodes of hypoglycaemia (Uribe et al 1982). In a follow-up crossover study in patients with chronic encephalopathy and diabetes, equicaloric diets of vegetable and animal protein were supplemented with 35 g of fibre daily. Significant reductions in fasting blood glucose levels were found on the vegetable protein diets (Uribe et al 1985). At present it is therefore appropriate to treat cirrhotic patients with 'hepatogenous diabetes' with more slowly digested carbohydrate, high-fibre and vegetable protein-rich diets. This should improve carbohydrate tolerance and reduce insulin requirements.

FAT MALABSORPTION

The contribution of fat to the total metabolic requirement is increased in cirrhosis, associated with a great turnover of free fatty acids (FFA) (Owen et al 1983), with increased splanchnic production of ketone bodies (Merli et al 1986). Impaired fat absorption has been noted in patients with alcoholic cirrhosis, particularly in the presence of chronic pancreatitis or, as expected, in response to neomycin therapy. Small-intestinal morphology on light microscopy is unchanged, but small-intestinal damage

is seen on electron microscopy. A reduced bile-salt pool size in cirrhosis will also affect fat absorption but the effect is, as expected, small. Of possibly greater nutritional significance is that the lower concentration of luminal bile salts will impair the absorption of fat-soluble vitamins (Jenkins et al 1976). One therapy with bile acids, such as ursodiol, reduced faecal fat excretion from 14 to 10 g per day (Salvioli et al 1990). When skin irritation (pruritus) occurs from accumulating bile acids in skin, as in primary biliary cirrhosis, then treatment with the bile salt binding agent cholestyramine will also induce modest fat malabsorption. Should oral lipid supplementation be necessary, medium-chain triglycerides can be given in doses of 5 ml, 3–4 times daily, providing 350–450 kcal, emulsified in milk shakes (Munoz 1991).

ALCOHOLIC PANCREATITIS

Alcohol is responsible for two syndromes affecting the pancreatic gland. These syndromes develop on a background of diminished protein, carbohydrate and fat intake (Mezey et al 1988). In acute pancreatitis the patient presents with acute abdominal pain, characterized by the development of small-intestinal paralysis (ileus) and an acute elevation of serum levels of the pancreatic enzymes amylase and lipase. The illness is usually short-lasting (5–10 days). A minority of patients develop haemorrhagic pancreatitis with a bloody peritoneal exudate. Local complications include the development of a pancreatic pseudocyst, abscess or fistula formation; prolonged morbidity may result for weeks or months. The patient may also develop life-threatening complications, including hypocalcaemia, hyperglycaemia and hypoxia.

The management of these patients requires fasting to induce bowel rest and, if the disorder lasts for more than a few days, parenteral nutrition. For hypocalcaemia, additional intravenous calcium is required and insulin may be needed for persistent hyperglycaemia.

Chronic pancreatitis

The mechanism by which alcohol results in pancreatic inflammation is unknown. One of the earliest lesions is the formation of plugs in the small pancreatic ducts formed by protein precipitates of glycoproteins and calcium (Nakamura et al 1972). Alcohol has been shown to alter pancreatic secretion in both animals (Tiscornia et al 1973) and man (Mott et al 1972), but the results differ between the species and in the response to different stimuli of secretion. Alcohol may act indirectly via the autonomic nervous system or by stimulating gastrointestinal hormones; pancreatic metabolism of alcohol with an altered redox state or acetaldehyde production may also be involved.

The geographic distribution of chronic calcific pancreatitis shows a strong correlation with alcoholism and the western diets high in protein and fat, but there is also a form of chronic alcoholism which has been linked to malnutrition (Sarles 1973).

Once pancreatic secretion and enzyme output fall below 10% of normal, patients with chronic pancreatitis suffer principally from fat malabsorption with steatorrhea (DiMagno et al 1973, 1975); N malabsorption is much less severe and vitamin deficiencies are uncommon (Toskes et al 1979). Treatment requires a low-fat diet, e.g. 25 g fat daily, together with pancreatic enzyme replacement. Since 8000 units of lipase per hour needs to be delivered to the duodenum for efficient lipolysis, this means that about the equivalent has to be given as pancreatic enzyme capsules every 4 hours. Maximizing the enzymes' activity by creating an alkaline duodenal pH normally depends on pancreatic bicarbonate secretion. In its absence, gastric acidity can be reduced, e.g. by using an H_2 blocker such as cimetidine 800 mg daily, ranitidine 300 mg daily, or omeprazole 20 mg daily. This significantly reduces the steatorrhea (DiMagno et al 1977, Regan et al 1977). Should parenteral lipid replacement therapy be required for any reason, despite theoretical objections,

there is no practical contraindication (Rossner et al 1979).

Alcoholic cardiomyopathy and myopathy

Classically the alcoholic cirrhotic has a hyperkinetic circulation with a high cardiac output (Kowalski & Abelmann 1953). Occasionally a patient will present with the extreme of this picture, in high-output heart failure. Although the clinical picture is typical of beriberi cardiomyopathy, only a minority of patients will respond to thiamin supplementation with 50 mg thiamin daily (Ikram et al 1981). Although thiamin deficiency has been claimed to be common in chronic alcoholics, the assessment usually depends on measurements of transketolase activity in vitro, which exaggerate the incidence of deficiency. The more sensitive measurement of thiamin phosphate ester concentrations (Dancy et al 1985) shows that only about 8% of patients with alcoholic liver disease have thiamin deficiency. The cardiomyopathy and the proximal myopathy of chronic alcoholism are more the result of chronic muscular damage from alcohol than an acute vitamin deficiency (Urbano-Marquez et al 1989).

VITAMINS AND MINERALS

Deficiencies of all four fat-soluble vitamins occur in patients with chronic liver disease (Leevy & Baker

Table 48.7 Nutritional deficiency in liver disease: fat-soluble vitamins

Vitamin	Source	Mechanism	Diagnosis	Clinical	Reference	Recommended
A	Apricots Peaches Carrots Green veg	Fat malabsorption Hepatic synthesis	Carotene Plasma retinol Hepatic A levels	Defective sepermatogenesis Defective night vision Defective dark adaptation Xerophthalmia (± zinc deficiency)	Van Thiel & Lester (1976) Herlong et al (1981)	Vit A, 5000 U daily
D	Dairy foods Sunlight	Intake Malabsorption Def. 25-OH of D Environment Cholestyramine	Serum 25-OH D Skeletal X-ray Bone biopsy	Osteopenia	Reed et al (1980) Long et al (1978)	Vit D, 50 000 U weekly
E	Nuts Seeds Meat Fish Green veg Cereal	Malabsorption	Plasma-tocopherol	Neuropathic ataxia syndrome Haemolytic anaemia with acanthocytosis	Rosenblum et al (1981) Sokol et al (1983)	α-Tocopherol Acetate 30–100 mg
K	Gut bacteria Hepatic synthesis	Malabsorption Liver failure	Prothrombin time	Bleeding diathasis	Blanchard et al (1981)	Vitamin K, 10 mg

Table 48.8   Nutritional deficiency in liver disease: water-soluble vitamins and minerals

Vitamins	Source	Diagnosis	Clinical syndromes	Prevention treatment
B_1 Thiamin	Unpolished rice, bran wheat, meat fish, peas	RBC transketolase activity	High output cardiac failure Wernicke-Korsakoff Peripheral neuropathy	5–10 mg daily
Riboflavin	Meat, dairy, cereals, pulses	RBC glutathione reductase activity ± holoenzyme		5 mg daily
B_6 Pyridoxine	Egg yolk, meat, fish, dairy	RBC transaminase activity ± pyridoxal phosphate	Peripheral neuropathy	10 mg daily
Folic acid	Green veg	RBC folate	Megaloblastic anaemia	5 mg weekly
B_{12} Cyanocobalamin	Most foods	Serum B_{12}	Megaloblastic anaemia	
Iron	Red meat, green veg	Serum Fe/MBC serum ferritin	Microcytic hypochromic anaemia	50 mg daily
Zinc	Meat	Serum, hair or total body zinc	Deficient retinol protein–dark adaptation Hypogonadism	10 mg daily

1968) (Table 48.7). The commonest is vitamin K deficiency, found both in patients with chronic obstructive jaundice and in hepatic insufficiency. In obstructive liver disease an abnormal prothrombin time is corrected by vitamin K injections. In other liver diseases a pure fat-soluble vitamin deficiency is unusual. For example, the ophthalmic complications associated with vitamin A deficiency may not be reversed without adding a zinc supplement; osteomalacia from vitamin D deficiency is less common than osteoporosis in patients with primary biliary cirrhosis (Eastell et al 1991) and in primary sclerosing cholangitis (Hay et al 1991), whereas clinical vitamin E deficiency may only be found in patients with biliary atresia and, rarely, in primary biliary cirrhosis.

Similarly, significant deficiencies of water-soluble vitamins (Table 48.8) are usually confined to thiamin and folate deficiency. Once again, folate deficiency is an infrequent cause of macrocytic anaemia associated with liver disease, and Wernicke's encephalopathy is the only neurological disorder clearly corrected by thiamin therapy (Diamond 1989).

As far as the metals are concerned, iron deficiency is common but usually related to chronic blood loss rather than deficient intake, whereas zinc deficiency is rarely a clinical problem. Although thought to be a factor in the pathogenesis of PSE, retinal dysfunction and anorexia, there is no firm evidence that dietary zinc supplementation results in significant improvements (McClain et al 1991a).

REFERENCES

Achord JL 1987 A prospective randomized clinical trial of peripheral amino acid glucose supplementation in acute alcoholic hepatitis. Americal Journal of Gastroenterology 82: 871–875

Bebb HT, Houser HB, Witschi MS et al 1971 Calorie and nutrient contribution of alcoholic beverages to the usual diets of 155 adults. American Journal of Clinical Nutrition 24: 1042–1052

Bessman AN, Minck G S 1958 Blood ammonia levels following the ingestion of casein and whole blood. Journal of Clinical Investigation 37: 990–998

Blanchard RA, Furie B C, Jorgensen M et al 1981 Acquired vitamin K-dependent carboxylation deficiency in the liver. New England Journal of Medicine 305: 242–248

Blei AJ, Robbins D C, Drobney E et al 1982 Insulin resistance and insulin receptors in hepatic cirrhosis. Gastroenterology 83: 1191–1199

Blendis LM 1992 Review article: the treatment of alcoholic liver disease. Alimentary Pharmacology and Therapeutics 6: 541–548

Blendis LM, Jenkins DJA 1988 Nutrition and diet in management of diseases of the gastrointestinal tract; nutritional support in liver disease. In: Shils ME, Young V (eds) Modern nutrition in health and disease, 7th edn. Lea & Febiger, Philadelphia, 1182–1200

Blendis LM, Greig PD, Langer B et al 1979 The renal and hemodynamic effects of the peritoneovenous shunt for intractable hepatic ascites. Gastroenterology 77: 250–256

Blendis LM, Harrison JE, Russell D et al 1986 The effects of peritoneovenous shunting on body composition. Gastroenterology 90: 127–134

Bunout D, Gattas V, Iturriaga H et al 1983 Nutritional status of alcoholic patients: its possible relationship to alcoholic liver damage. American Journal of Clinical Nutrition 38: 469–473

Cabre E, Gonzalez-Hvix F, Abad-Lacruz A et al 1990 Effect of total enteral nutrition on the short-term outcome of severely malnourished cirrhotics. Gastroenterology 98: 715–721

Calvey H, Davis M, Williams R 1985 Controlled trial of nutritional supplementation with and without branched-chain amino acid enrichment in the treatment of acute alcoholic hepatitis. Journal of Hepatology 1: 141–151

Cerra FB, Cheung NK, Fischer JE et al 1985 Disease-specific amino acid infusion (F080) in hepatic encephalopathy: a prospective randomised, double-blind controlled trial. Journal of Parenteral and Enteral Nutrition 9: 288–295

Chen S, Zieve L, Mahadevan V 1970 Mercaptans and demethyl sulfide in the breath of patients with cirrhosis of the liver. Journal of Laboratory and Clinical Medicine 75: 628–635

Conn HO, Lieberthal MM 1984 The hepatic coma syndromes and lactulose. Williams and Williams, Baltimore, 46

Dancy M, Bland JM, Leech G et al 1985 Preclinical left ventricular abnormalities in alcoholics. Lancet i: 1122–1125

DeBruijn KM, Blendis LM, Zilm DH et al 1983 The effect of dietary protein manipulations in subclinical portal systemic encephalopathy. Gut 24: 53–60

Dennis BH, Haynes SG, Anderson JJ et al 1985 Nutrient intakes among selected North American populations in the lipid research clinics prevalence study. American Journal of Clinical Nutrition 41: 312–329

Diamond I 1989 Alcoholic myopathy and cardiomyopathy. New England Journal of Medicine 320: 458–459

Diehl AM, Boitnott JK, Herlong H F et al 1985 Effect of parenteral amino acid supplementation in alcoholic hepatitis. Hepatology 5: 57–63

DiMagno EP, Go VLW, Summerskill WHJ 1973 Relations between pancreatic enzyme outputs and malabsorption in severe pancreatic insufficiency. New England Journal of Medicine 288: 813–815

DiMagno EP, Malagelado JR, Go VLW 1975 Relationship between alcoholism and pancreatic insufficiency. Annals of the New York Academy of Sciences 252: 200–207

DiMagno EP, Malagelado JR, Taylor WF et al 1977 Fate of orally ingested enzymes in pancreatic insufficiency: comparison of two dosage schedules. New England Journal of Medicine 297: 737–742

Eastell R, Dickson ER, Hodgson SF et al 1991 Rates of vertebral bone loss before and after liver transplantation in women with primary biliary cirrhosis. Hepatology 14: 296–300

Egberts EH, Schomerus H, Hamster W, Jurgens P 1984 Effective treatment of latent portosystemic encephalopathy with oral branched-chain amino acids. In: Capocaccia L, Fischer JE, Rossi-Fanelli F (eds) Hepatic encephalopathy in chronic liver failure. Plenum Press, New York, 351–357

Eriksson LS, Persson A, Wahren J 1982 Branched-chain amino acids in the treatment of chronic hepatic encephalopathy. Gut 23: 801–806

Eriksson LS, Conn HO 1989 Branched-chain amino acids in the management of hepatic encephalopathy: an analysis of variants. Hepatology 10: 228–246

Fenton JCB, Knight EJ, Humpherson PL 1966 Milk and cheese diet in portosystemic encephalopathy. Lancet i: 164–165

Fiaccadori F, Ghinelli F, Pedretti G et al 1984 Branched-chain amino acid-enriched solutions in the treatment of hepatic encephalopathy: a controlled trial. In: Capocaccia L, Fischer JE, Rossi-Fanelli F (eds) Hepatic encephalopathy in chronic liver failure. Plenum Press, New York, 323–333

Fischer JE, Baldessarini RJ 1971 False neurotransmitters and hepatic failure. Lancet ii: 75–80

Fischer JE, Rosen HM, Ebeid AM et al 1976 The effect of normalization of plasma amino acids on hepatic encephalopathy in man. Surgery 80: 77–91

Forbes A, Wicks C, Marshall W et al 1987 Nutritional support in fulminant hepatic failure: the safety of lipid solutions. Gut 28: 1347–1349

Gabuzda GJ, Shear L 1970 Metabolism of dietary protein in hepatic cirrhosis. Nutritional and clinical considerations. American Journal of Clinical Nutrition 23: 479–487

Galambos JT, Hersh T, Fulenwider T 1979 Hyperalimentation in alcoholic hepatitis. American Journal of Gastroenterology 72: 535–541

Gines P, Arroyo V, Quintero E et al 1987 Comparison of paracentesis and diuretics in the treatment of cirrhotics with tense ascites. Gastroenterology 93: 234–241

Gluud C, Deigaard A, Hardt F 1983 Preliminary treatment results with balanced amino-acid infusion to patients with hepatic encephalopathy. Scandinavian Journal of Gastroenterology 18 (Suppl 86): 19

Golden MHN, Waterlow JC, Picou D 1977 Protein turnover, synthesis and breakdown before and after recovery from protein energy malnutrition. Clinical Science and Molecular Medicine 53: 473–477

Greenberger NJ, Carley JE, Schenkers S et al 1977 Effect of vegetable and animal protein diets in chronic hepatic encephalopathy. American Journal of Digestive Diseases 22: 845–855

Greig PD, Blendis LM, Langer BR et al 1981 The renal and hemodynamic effects of the peritoneovenous shunt. Long-term effect. Gastroenterology 80: 119–125

Guarnieri GF, Toigo G, Situlin R et al 1984 Muscle biopsy studies on malnutrition in patients with liver cirrhosis. In: Capocaccia L, Fischer JE, Rossi-Fanelli F (eds) Hepatic encephalopathy in chronic liver failure. Plenum Press, New York, 193–208

Harrison JE, McNeil KG, Strauss AL 1984 A nitrogen index – total body protein normalized for body size for diagnosis of protein status in health and disease. Nutrition Research 4: 209–224

Hay JE, Lindor KD, Wiesner RH et al 1991 The metabolic bone disease of primary sclerosing cholangitis. Hepatology 14: 257–261

Herlong HF, Maddrey WC, Walser M 1980 The use of ornithine salts of branched-chain ketoacids in portal systemic encephalopathy. Annals of Internal Medicine 93: 545–550

Herlong HF, Russell RM, Maddrey WC 1981 Vitamin A and zinc therapy in primary biliary cirrhosis. Hepatology 1: 348–351

Heymsfield SB, Waki M, Reinus J 1990 Are patients with chronic liver disease hypermetabolic? Hepatology 11: 502–505

Horst D, Grace ND, Conn HO et al 1984 Comparison of dietary protein with an oral branched-chain enriched amino acid supplement in chronic portal systemic encephalopathy: a randomized controlled trial. Hepatology 4: 279–287

Hurt RD, Higgins JA, Nelson RA et al 1981 Nutritional status of alcoholics before and after admission to an alcoholism treatment unit. American Journal of Clinical Nutrition 34: 386–392

Ikram H, Maslowski AH, Smith BL et al 1981 The haemodynamic histopathological and hormonal features of alcoholic cardiac beriberi. Quarterly Journal of Medicine NS 50: 359–375

Jenkins DJA, Gassull MA, Leeds AR et al 1976 The relation of impaired vitamin A and E tolerance to fat absorption in biliary diversion. International Journal of Vitamin and Nutrition Research 2: 226–230

Jenkins DJA, Thorne MJ, Taylor RH et al 1987 Effect of modifying the rate of digestion of a food on the blood glucose, amino acid and endocrine responses in patients with cirrhosis. American Journal of Gastroenterology 3: 223–230

Kirk E 1936 Amino acid and ammonia metabolism in liver diseases. Acta Medica Scandinavica 77 (Suppl 1): 1–147

Kowalski HJ, Abelmann WK 1953 Cardiac output at rest in Laennec's cirrhosis. Journal of Clinical Investigation 32: 1025–1033

Kruszynska YT, Home PD, McIntyre N 1991 Relationship between insulin sensitivity, insulin secretion and glucose intolerance in cirrhosis. Hepatology 14: 103–111

Leevy CM, Baker H 1968 Introduction: vitamins and alcoholism. American Journal of Clinical Nutrition 21: 1325–1328

Long RG, Meinhard E, Skinner RK et al 1978 Clinical, biochemical and histological studies of osteomalacia, osteoporosis and parathyroid function in chronic liver disease. Gut 19: 85–90

McClain CJ, Marsano L, Burk RF, Bacon B 1991a Trace metals in liver disease. In: McCullough AJ, Tavill AG (eds) Nutrition and the liver. Seminars in liver disease, Vol 11, no 4. Thieme Medical Publishers, New York, 321–329

McClain CJ, McCullough AJ, Tavill AS 1991b Disordered energy and protein metabolism in liver disease. In: McCullough AJ, Tavill AS (eds), Nutrition and the liver. Seminars in liver disease, Vol 11, no 4. Thieme Medical Publishers, New York, 265–277

McGhee A, Henderson JM, Millikan WJ et al 1983 Comparison of the effects of hepatic aid and casein modular diet on encephalopathy, plasma amino acids and nitrogen balance in cirrhotic patients. Annals of Surgery 197: 288–293

Maddrey WC, Weber FL, Coulter AW et al 1976 Effects of keto analogues of essential amino acids in portosystemic encephalopathy. Gastroenterology 71: 190–195

Marchesini G, Branchi GP, Vilstrup H et al 1987 Plasma clearances of branched-chain amino acids in control subjects and in patients with cirrhosis. Journal of Hepatology 4: 108–117

Mendenhall CL, Anderson S, Weesner RE et al 1984 Protein-calorie malnutrition associated with alcoholic hepatitis. American Journal of Medicine 76: 211–222

Mendenhall CL, Bongiovanni G, Goldberg S et al 1985 VA cooperative study group on alcoholic hepatitis. III Changes in protein-calorie malnutrition associated with 30 days of hospitalization with and without enteral nutrition. Journal of Parenteral and Enteral Nutrition 9: 590–599

Mendenhall CL, Tosch T, Weesner RE et al 1986 VA cooperative study on alcoholic hepatitis. II Prognosis significance of protein-calorie malnutrition. American Journal of Clinical Nutrition 43: 213–218

Merli M, Eriksson LS, Hagenfeldt L, Wahren J 1986 Splanchnic and leg exchange of free fatty acids in patients with liver cirrhosis. Journal of Hepatology 3: 348–355

Merli M, Romiti A, Riggio O, Capocaccia L 1987 Optimal nutritional indexes in chronic liver disease. Journal of Parenteral and Enteral Nutrition 11 (Suppl): 130S–134S

Mezey E, Kolmari CJ, Dietzl AM et al 1988 Alcohol and dietary intake in the development of chronic pancreatitis and liver disease in alcoholism. American Journal of Clinical Nutrition 48: 148–151

Mezey E, Caballeria J, Mitchell MC et al 1991 Effect of parenteral amino acid supplementation on short-term and long-term outcomes in severe alcoholic hepatitis: a randomized controlled trial. Hepatology 14: 1090–1096

Michel H, Bories P, Aubin JP et al 1985 Treatment of acute hepatic encephalopathy in cirrhotics with a branched-chain amino acids enriched versus a conventional amino acid mixture. Liver 5: 282–289

Mills PR, Shenkin A, Anthony RS et al 1983 Assessment of nutritional status and in vivo immune responses in alcoholic liver disease. American Journal of Clinical Nutrition 38: 849–859

Montanari A, Simoni I, Vallisa D et al 1988 Free amino acids in plasma and skeletal muscle of patients with liver cirrhosis. Hepatology 8: 1034–1039

Morrison WL, Bouchier IAD, Gibson JNA et al 1990 Skeletal muscle and whole-body protein turnover in cirrhosis. Clinical Science 78: 613–619

Mott C, Sarles H, Tiscornia O et al 1972 Inhibitory action of alcohol on human exocrine pancreatic secretion. American Journal of Digestive Disease 17: 902–910

Munoz SJ 1991 Nutritional therapies in liver disease. In: McCullough AJ, Tavill AS (eds) Nutrition and the liver. Seminars in liver disease, Vol 11, no 4. Thieme Medical Publishers, New York, 278–291

Najarian JS, Harper HA 1956 A clinical study of the effect of arginine on blood ammonia. American Journal of Medicine 21: 832–842

Nakamura K, Sarles H, Payan H 1972 Three-dimensional reconstruction of the pancreatic ducts in chronic pancreatitis. Gastroenterology 62: 942–949

Nasrallah SM, Galambos JT 1980 Amino acid therapy of alcoholic hepatitis. Lancet ii: 1276–1277

Naveau S, Pelletier G, Poynard T et al 1986 A randomized clinical trial of supplementary parenteral nutrition in jaundiced alcoholic cirrhotic patients. Hepatology 6: 270–274

Naylor CD, O'Rourke K, Detsky AS et al 1989 Parenteral nutrition with branched-chain amino acids in hepatic encephalopathy. A meta-analysis. Gastroenterology 97: 1033–1042

Neville JN, Eagles JA, Samason G et al 1968 Nutritional status of alcoholics. American Journal of Clinical Nutrition 21: 1329–1340

O'Keefe SJD, El Zayadi A, Carrahet T et al 1980 Malnutrition and immune competence in patients with liver disease. Lancet ii: 615–617

O'Keefe SJD, Ogden J, Ramjee G, Moldawer LL 1988 Short-term effects of an intravenous infusion of a nutrient solution containing amino acids, glucose and insulin on leucine turnover and amino acid metabolism in patients with liver failure. Journal of Hepatology 6: 101–108

Okita M, Watanabe A, Nagashima H 1984 A branched-chain amino acid supplemented diet in the treatment of liver cirrhosis. Current Therapeutic Research 35: 83–87

Owen OE, Trapp VE, Reichard GA et al 1983 Nature and quantity of fuels consumed in patients with alcoholic cirrhosis. Journal of Clinical Investigation 72: 1821–1832

Petrides AS, Luzi L, Reuben A et al 1991 Effect of insulin and plasma amino acid concentration on leucine metabolism in cirrhosis. Hepatology 14: 432–441

Phear EA, Ruebner B, Sherlock S et al 1956 Methionine toxicity in liver disease and its prevention by chlortetracycline. Clinical Science 15: 93–117

Reed JS, Meredith SC, Nemchausky BA 1980 Bone disease in primary biliary cirrhosis: reversal of osteomalacia with oral 25-hydroxy vitamin D. Gastroenterology 78: 513–517

Rees RGP, Cooper TM, Beetham R et al 1989 Influence of energy and nitrogen contents of enteral diets on nitrogen balance. Gut 30: 123–129

Regan PJ, Malagelada JR, DiMagno EP et al 1977 Comparative effects of antacids, cimetidine and enteric coating on the therapeutic response to oral enzymes in severe pancreatic insufficiency. New England Journal of Medicine 297: 854–857

Reynolds TB, Redeker AG, Davis P 1958 A controlled study of the effects of L-arginine on hepatic encephalopathy. American Journal of Medicine 25: 359–367

Riggio O, Cangiano C, Cascino A et al 1984 Long-term dietary supplement with branched-chain amino acids, a new approach in the prevention of hepatic encephalopathy: results of a controlled study in cirrhotics with portocaval anastomosis. In: Capocaccia L, Fischer JE, Rossi-Fanelli F (eds) Hepatic encephalopathy in chronic liver failure. Plenum Press, New York, 183–192

Rosenblum JL, Keating JP, Prensky AL 1981 A progressive neurologic syndrome in children with chronic liver disease. New England Journal of Medicine 304: 503–508

Rossi-Fanelli F, Riggio O, Cangiano C et al 1982 Branched-chain amino acid vs lactulose in the treatment of hepatic coma. A controlled study. Digestive Disease and Sciences 27: 929–935

Rossner S, Johansson C, Walldivs G et al 1979 Intralipid clearance and lipoprotein pattern in men with advanced alcoholic liver cirrhosis. American Journal of Clinical Nutrition 32: 2022–2026

Rudman D, Kutner M, Ansley J 1981 Hypotyrosinemia hypocystinemia and failure to retain nitrogen during total parenteral nutrition of cirrhotic patients. Gastroenterology 81: 1025–1036

Salvioli G, Carati L, Lugli R 1990 Steatorrhoea in cirrhosis: effect of ursodeoxycholic acid administration. Journal of International Medical Research 18: 289–294

Sarles H 1973 An international survey on nutrition and pancreatitis. Digestion 9: 389–403

Schafer DF, Jones EA 1982 Hepatic encephalopathy and the gamma-aminobutyric acid neutotransmitter system. Lancet i: 18–20

Schneeweiss B, Graninger W, Ferenci P et al 1990 Energy metabolism in patients with acute and chronic liver disease. Hepatology 11: 387–393

Shaw S, Worner TM, Lieber CS 1983 Comparison of animal and vegetable protein sources in the dietary management of hepatic encephalopathy. American Journal of Clinical Nutrition 38: 59–62

Shepherd R, Farleigh CA 1987 Salt intake assessment by questionnaire and urinary sodium excretion. Nutrition Research 7: 557–565

Sieg A, Walker S, Czygan P et al 1983 Branched-chain amino acid enriched elemental diet in patients with cirrhosis of the liver. A double-blind crossover trial. Zeitschrift für Gastroenterologie 21: 644–650

Silk DBA 1988 Parenteral nutrition in patients with liver disease. Journal of Hepatology 7: 269–277

Silva G, Gomis R, Bosctz J et al 1988 Hyperglucagonism and glucagon resistance in cirrhosis. Journal of Hepatology 6: 325–331

Simko V 1983 Long-term tolerance to a special amino acid oral formula in patients with advanced liver disease. Nutrition Reports International 27: 765–773

Simon D, Galambos JT 1988 A randomized controlled study of peripheral parenteral nutrition in moderate and severe alcoholic hepatitis. Journal of Hepatology 7: 200–207

Smith J, Horowitz J, Henderson JM 1982 Enteral hyperalimentation in undernourished patients with cirrhosis and ascites. American Journal of Clinical Nutrition 35: 56–73

Soberon S, Pauley MP, Duplantier R et al 1987 Metabolic effects of enteral formula feeding in alcoholic hepatitis. Hepatology 7: 1204–1209

Sokol RJ, Heubi JE, Iannaccone S, Bave KE, Balisteri F 1983 Mechanism causing vitamin E deficiency during chronic childhood cholestasis. Gastroenterology 85: 1172–1182

Stephen AM, Cummings JH 1980 Mechanism of action of dietary fibre in the human colon. Nature 284: 283–284

Swart GR, Frenkel M, van den Berg JWO 1981 Minimum protein requirements in patients with advanced liver. In: Walser M, Williamson JR (eds) Metabolic and clinical implications of branched-chain amino and ketoacids. Elsevier, North Holland, 427–432

Swart GR, van den Berg JWO, Wattimena JLD et al 1988 Elevated protein requirements in cirrhosis of the liver investigated by whole-body protein turnover studies. Clinical Science 75: 101–107

Tiscornia OM, Gullo L, Sarles H 1973 The inhibition of canine exocrine pancreatic secretion by intravenous ethanol. Digestion 9: 231–240

Toskes PP, Dawson W, Curington C et al 1979 Non-diabetic retinal abnormalities in chronic pancreatitis. New England Journal of Medicine 300: 942–946

Urbano-Marquez A, Estruch R, Navarro-Lopez F et al 1989 The effect of alcoholism on skeletal and cardiac muscle. New England Journal of Medicine 320: 409–415

Uribe M, Marquez MA, Ramos GG et al 1982 Treatment of chronic portal systemic encephalopathy with vegetable and animal protein diets. A controlled crossover study. Digestive Disease and Science 27: 1109–1116

Uribe M, Debilodox M, Malpica G et al 1985 Beneficial effect of vegetable protein diet supplemented with psyllum plantago in patients with hepatic encephalopathy and diabetes mellitus. Gastroenterology 88: 901–907

Van Theil DH, Lester R 1976 Alcoholism: its effect on hypothalamic pituitary gonadal function. Gastroenterology 71: 318–327

Vilstrup H, Bucher D, Krog B, Damgard SE 1982 Amino acid clearance in cirrhosis. European Journal of Clinical Investigation 65: 197–202

Vilstrup H, Gluud C, Hardt F et al 1990 Branched-chain enriched amino acid versus glucose treatment of hepatic encephalopathy. A double-blind study of 65 patients with cirrhosis. Journal of Hepatology 10: 291–296

Von Schafer K, Winther MG, Ukida M et al 1981 Influence of an orally administered protein mixture enriched in branched-chain amino acids on chronic hepatic encephalopathy (CHE) of patients with liver cirrhosis.

Zeitschrift für Gastroenterologie 19: 356–362

Wagner S, Lautz HU, Muller MJ, Schmidt FW 1991 Pathophysiology and clinical basis of prevention and treatment of complications of chronic liver disease. Klinischer Wochenschrift 69: 112–120

Wahren J, Denis J, Desurmont P et al 1983 Is intravenous administration of branched-chain amino acid effective in the treatment of hepatic encephalopathy? A multicentre study. Hepatology 13: 475–480

Walshe JM 1951 Observations on the symptomatology and pathogenesis of hepatic coma. Quarterly Journal of Medicine 20: 421–438

Walshe JM 1953 Disturbances of amino acid metabolism following liver injury: study by means of paper chromatography. Quarterly Journal of Medicine 22: 483–505

Warner LC, Campbell PJ, Morali GA et al 1990 The response of atrial natriuretic factor and sodium excretion to dietary sodium challenges in patients with chronic liver disease. Hepatology 12: 460–466

Weber FL, Minco D, Fresard KM, Banwell JG 1985 Effects of vegetable diets on nitrogen metabolism in cirrhotic subjects. Gastroenterology 89: 538–544

Weber FL, Bagby BS, Licate L, Kelson SG 1990 Effects of branched-chain amino acids on nitrogen metabolism in patients with cirrhosis. Hepatology 11: 942–950

49. Eating disorders

S. Gilbert

Interest in the eating disorders has expanded greatly since 1979, when Professor Russell, known for his work with anorexia nervosa, first noted a similar form of disorder in young women who were not underweight (Russell 1979). At about the same time, workers in other centres were also collating data on the phenomenon of binge-eating in women of normal weight, and the disorder known as 'bulimia nervosa' became widely studied.

The advent of bulimia nervosa cast a new perspective on the relative importance of the physical versus the psychological aspects of shape and weight, and brought into sharp focus the eating behaviour both of obese people and of anorexics, in that it now became apparent that both groups can be divided into two – those who are able successfully to curb their eating, and those who overeat in an uncontrolled way.

ANOREXIA NERVOSA

Anorexia nervosa is a state in which the sufferer, usually female, refuses to eat enough to maintain normal body weight for her height. Usually she claims to want to lose weight to be slimmer; sometimes she says that she does not feel hungry or that it is uncomfortable to eat. It is important not to confuse the disorder with undereating for other reasons: for example, undereating may be present in depression, a phobia of eating (perhaps for fear of eating in public or because of an irrational fear of choking), where there is underlying disease such as cancer, and in old age for a variety of reasons, both physical and psychological.

The currently accepted definition of anorexia nervosa is given in the American Psychiatric Association's Diagnostic and Statistical Manual (DSM-IIIR 1987) and has four criteria:

1. Refusal to maintain body weight over a minimal normal weight for age and height.

2. An intense fear of gaining weight or becoming fat, even though underweight.
3. A disturbance in the way one's body weight, size or shape is experienced.
4. In females, absence of at least three consecutive menstrual cycles when otherwise expected to occur.

All anorexics refuse food and count calories, and many eat as little as 200–300 calories per day. They may also take strenuous exercise, and often appear 'faddy' with their food. They may take an immense interest in cookery and in cooking for other people, although they will avoid eating the food they cook themselves. Anorexics are also thought to have a distorted body image, in that they grossly overestimate their own size or weight. This is in common, however, with many other people with abnormal eating habits.

About one-half of anorexics also binge-eat, or binge-eat and purge themselves by means of vomiting or taking laxatives or diuretics, and are called 'bulimic'. The bulimics are usually older when they present for treatment than are the 'restrictors', and have been ill for longer. More of the bulimics appear to seek help for themselves, while the restrictors often deny that they have a problem at all. Researchers are not very clear as to whether the binge-eating is a progression of the disorder or whether those people who binge and vomit are an entirely different group of people from the restrictors.

Anorexia nervosa appears in less than 0.5% of women. It is said to be increasing in prevalence, but it is not known how far this is because there really are larger numbers of anorexics than in previous years, or because people in general – and doctors in particular - are more likely to recognize it than before.

Between 1 in 16 and 1 in 19 anorexics is male. Sufferers are usually in their adolescence, but the disorder can appear at any time between 12 and 44 years and there are recent reports of its appearance in young prepubescent girls (see Lask & Bryant-Waugh 1986 for a review). It is said to be over-represented in the upper social classes, and traditionally was thought to be confined to white people, both in the USA and in the UK. However, the disorder is reported increasingly in women of all classes, and in Asian and Afro-Caribbean women, which suggests that eating disorder is linked rather to the cultural and family difficulties engendered by change than to social class or culture per se.

The disorder takes a physical toll on sufferers in that they may have dry skin; excessive growth of dry brittle hair over the nape of the neck, cheeks, forearms and thighs, called 'lanugo' hair; they often have cold hands and feet, and peripheral oedema. They can develop cardiac abnormalities and arrhythmias, and suffer from constipation. Long-term amenorrhoea may lead to premature bone loss and place sufferers at risk of osteoporosis in later life.

Outcome of anorexia nervosa

Most anorexics have just one episode of the disorder and eventually return to a normal weight. Of those who are treated in clinics and survive, between 40% and 80% have been reported to achieve normal weight by between 2 and 10 years after they are first seen. However, many continue to have abnormal attitudes to food and weight for a very long time, and about half of previous sufferers do not return to eating normally. Between 13% and 50% do not recommence menstruating. About 60% of those who continue to maintain a low weight and have problems with eating manage to live apparently normal lives, and hold down jobs. On the other hand, however, between 2% and 16% of anorexics will eventually starve themselves to death. Poor outcome has been associated with a later age of onset of the disorder, a longer duration, and poor family relationships (Ratnasuriya et al 1991).

BULIMIA NERVOSA

Bulimia nervosa was first described by Gerald Russell in 1979 in a series of 30 patients, most of whom had a history of anorexia nervosa but whose weight was currently normal. These young women had powerful urges to overeat, which they alternated with periods of starving themselves. Like anorexics, they had a 'morbid fear' of fatness and had developed the habit of vomiting or purging in order to control their weight.

There has been some controversy in the scientific literature about the nature of this disorder. A part of

the problem relates to the definition of what is a binge: this is normally accepted as being 'eating in an uncontrolled way', past any feeling of hunger, eating more than the person 'needs', and implies the existence of a feeling of guilt about the eating. Given, however, that there is no generally accepted definition of what is meant by hunger and of what is meant by 'controlled' eating, the term is still problematic. Also, many normal people binge occasionally, and there is the problem of defining what exactly or how much food constitutes a binge. One person's 'binge' may be defined as a sole chocolate bar in the context of an otherwise healthy, low-fat and stringent diet. On the other hand, another person may eat several chocolate bars per day without feeling that their behaviour was particularly excessive. For that person, a 'binge' might constitute several small meals followed by a whole cake, a large restaurant meal or several packets of biscuits.

In addition, the definition of the disorder itself has been the subject of some controversy, as until 1987 the US and UK definitions differed, making direct comparison between studies difficult. In the USA, it was known as 'bulimia' and did not necessarily encompass purging behaviour (American Psychiatric Association 1980), while in the UK Professor Russell's definition, which necessitated purging, was used. Since 1987, purging behaviour has been included in the American Psychiatric Association's definition, although it is still not a necessary precondition of having the disorder (American Psychiatric Association 1987). There are five main criteria:

1. Recurrent episodes of binge eating
2. Experience of lack of control over the binges
3. Attempts to prevent weight gain by the regular use of self-induced vomiting, laxatives, diuretics, or strict dieting or fasting, or by vigorous exercise
4. A minimum average of two binge-eating episodes per week for at least 3 months
5. Persistent concern over body shape and weight.

Typically, bulimics start the day by eating nothing or very little, then possibly are 'good' at lunchtime with a yoghurt or an apple; then eating may escalate to include several meals or several items of food, typically high in calories, fat and carbohydrates: packets of biscuits, confectionery, cereals, etc.

Bulimics usually eat in private, hiding the problem from other people. Often they do not eat normal meals, and have difficulty in experiencing hunger or knowing when they have reached 'fullness' at the end of a meal. They may stop eating only when uncomfortably full, or if interrupted. After an eating binge they will experience extreme guilt and dysphoria. Days of binge-eating may alternate with several days of strict dieting or starving.

Sufferers are usually women between the ages of 18 and 34, with an average age of 24 years. The disorder has its onset on average between ages 16–18, usually after a period of extreme dieting and loss of weight. People present themselves for treatment between 1 and 5 years after the disorder has started. Estimates of the prevalence of the disorder have varied as widely as between 1% and 20%, largely because of the wide variations in definition. However, when studies using comparable strict criteria are examined, prevalence appears to be about 1% of young adolescent and adult women (Fairburn & Beglin 1990). Little has been said about males with bulimia nervosa, but Carlat & Camargo (1991) have reviewed the literature between 1966 and 1990 and have concluded that it affects approximately 0.2% of adolescent boys and young adult men, and that 10–15% of all bulimics identified in community-based studies are male.

A survey of the relevant literature suggests that the disorder is not just a progression of anorexia nervosa, as only about one-quarter of sufferers may have been anorexic in the past, and between 30% and 40% of sufferers have previously been overweight. Some bulimia sufferers also have problems with controlling their alcohol consumption; many steal, initially food but sometimes also other items; some demonstrate impulsive self-destructive behaviour such as cutting themselves with knives, or attempting suicide. This group of sufferers has been called 'multi-impulsive' as they appear in addition – or perhaps as the main characteristic of their problem – to be suffering from a personality disorder focusing around self-destructive, out-of-control behaviour. These people are notoriously more difficult to treat than are those for whom the eating disorder is the primary problem. Some people have suggested an association between eating disorder and major personality disturbance (for example, see Lacey & Evans 1986). However, this association has been found in only a small proportion of patients in other studies.

Like anorexia nervosa, bulimia nervosa can take its toll physically on the health of sufferers. Some bulimics experience amenorrhoea, some experience oedema and possible kidney dysfunctions. The vomiting itself causes potassium, chloride and hydrogen ions to be lost in the vomitus, resulting in symptoms of muscle weakness, constipation and headache. Sufferers also experience palpitations, abdominal pain, easy fatiguability, sore throat and swollen salivary glands. The disorder leads to a predisposition to cardiac arrhythmias. Many bulimics have dental problems, and indeed may first be picked up by their dentists, as the continual presence of vomitus in the mouth can cause tooth enamel to dissolve. For an excellent explanation of some of these problems, in a form suitable also for patients to read, see French (1987).

CAUSES OF THE EATING DISORDERS

Many causes have been posited for these eating disorders, but given their complex nature and the very different ways in which they present in individual patients, it is likely that different causal factors will influence their development in each person. Thus, many workers now accept the notion that the disorders are multidetermined in nature. (For a detailed review of the aetiology of eating disorders see Gilbert 1986.)

Early medical sources looked for a physical cause for anorexia nervosa. The idea of a hypothalamic disturbance was posited, given that the hypothalamus is the part of the brain thought to control appetite. Indeed, hypothalamic changes could be seen in anorexics but these changes revert to normal as sufferers are cured of their disorder, and it is likely that the physical changes are a consequence of rather than a cause of the disorder in the first place.

Psychodynamic views

One of the earliest psychological explanations was couched in psychodynamic terms. Psychoanalytic psychology emphasizes past and early experience as an important causal factor influencing psychopathology, and uses as its method of discovery series of sessions with individual patients in which they recall and explore issues to do with their early upbringing, and relationships with parents and other important people in their lives. Using her psychiatric work as a basis for her conclusions, Bruch (1974) concluded that anorexia nervosa was a disorder which was secondary to an underlying disturbance of personality, which arose from the child having a faulty relationship with a mother who consistently misinterpreted her child's signals of hunger, distress, or other needs at an early age. Hence the child does not learn to know when he/she is upset and what he/she really wants or needs by way of comfort, and comes to use food as a cure for all ills. Such a child typically would be seen as a 'good' child, anxious to please, and would rarely make its needs or wants heard, but as a result would experience a paralysing sense of ineffectiveness. Bruch suggested that such a child may be triggered into dieting when faced by new and stressful experiences, such as going to a new school or away from home to summer camp. The child may be vulnerable to criticism and may diet as a way of being liked by her peers.

Crisp (1980) has conceptualized anorexia nervosa more specifically as a disorder of adolescence, triggered by the onset of puberty and representing a fear of growing up and the responsibilities of adulthood in general, and a fear of sexuality in particular.

The family as a source of eating disorder

Clinical observations of families with an anorexic or bulimic member have led to many attempts to identify common characteristics. Some workers have suggested that such families are characterized by disturbed relationships, for example where a marriage is good on the surface but where the couple is masking a high degree of dissatisfaction. Minuchin and his colleagues (1978) have identified a number of characteristics which they believe are typical of anorexic families: overprotectiveness, rigidity, lack of conflict resolution, and an atmosphere which allows for little privacy so that the anorexic child is involved in unresolved marital or family conflicts.

Other family-related stress factors which have been implicated in the development of anorexia nervosa and bulimia nervosa include a tendency by the parents to avoid social activities; a family with an unusual interest in weight, food or shape; one or other parent working in the food or fashion industry; a family history of anorexia nervosa or obesity, and the implication that the eating disorder might be carried through families. In addition, recent authors have pointed to the possibility that child sexual abuse is more prevalent in the families of women with eating disorders than in the families of normal women. (For example, see Sloan & Leichner 1986 and Palmer et al 1990.) Whether or not this is the case, clinical observation often suggests that the sufferer has been exposed to abuse of either a physical or an emotional nature, and that the eating disorder serves as a focus for her attempt to bring control into an otherwise chaotic life.

Eating disorder and other psychiatric diagnoses

Some workers have suggested that anorexia nervosa and bulimia are really forms of affective disorder, akin to major depression; in other words, sufferers and their families have a predisposition to general neurotic morbidity which may be genetic. In support of this idea, they note that many anorexics and bulimics describe themselves as depressed. Also, several studies have suggested a high prevalence of affective disorder, anxiety disorders and alcoholism, both in patients with eating disorders and their first-degree relatives (Halmi et al 1991). However, if indeed eating disorder in these people is an expression of affective disorder, it is not clear why the individuals concerned should develop an eating disorder in particular. Also, it is possible that the depression is secondary to eating disorder, as the depressive symptoms often appear after the eating disorder and usually improve with improvement in the eating disorder.

Anorexia and bulimia as sociocultural disorders

An alternative explanation is that anorexia nervosa and bulimia nervosa are both diseases of our modern society, which idolizes slimness and health and denigrates fatness. (For a review of attitudes to fat people see Gilbert 1989.) In this context, very many adolescent and preadolescent girls are self-conscious and very sensitive to fatness and changes in body shape, and it is an easy thing for dieting to be triggered by a chance remark, or by contact with other dieters; indeed several recent surveys have suggested that up to 70% of adolescent girls have tried dieting (Hill et al 1992).

Several surveys have been carried out to explore the prevalence of dieting and attitudes to weight among men and women of all ages. Estimates have varied widely, but even the most conservative suggest that dieting and negative attitudes to current weight in people of normal weight are fairly common. At least 50% of women would like to be slimmer, and as many as 50–75% have tried dieting, with a current prevalence of dieting of up to 50% for men and 70% for women. Estimates of admitted binge eating in females have ranged from 20% in a community survey of women of reproductive age, to 90% in a sample of college students.

Of course, dieting, while clearly a risk factor for eating disorder, is not necessarily the sole prerequisite. Ballet dancers and athletes who need to maintain a low maximum body weight are known to be at higher risk than are other people of becoming anorexic or bulimic, but in general are more amenable to cure with simple advice and counselling than are other people with eating disorders. There is a difference between a normal dieter who simply wishes to be more physically attractive and more socially acceptable, and the young woman who may also have problems with low self-esteem and is struggling with wider issues to do with control over her life, and for whom an interest in dieting may predispose her to eating disorder.

Eating disorder as learned behaviour

This idea has led to the notion put forward by Slade (1982), among others, that eating disorder might become rewarding to some young women, not in the sense of being pleasant, but as a way – albeit destructive – out of an impossible emotional turmoil. He suggested that the behaviour of non-eating, started as a means of avoiding obesity, may take over as the sufferer begins to feel satisfaction about being in control. Binging, if it occurs, has a negative reinforcement value in that it makes the person feel bloated, uncomfortable and out of control, and the consequent dieting, starving or purging behaviour becomes extremely rewarding as a consequence. Hence the sufferer is in a vicious circle from which she cannot escape.

Eating disorder as a corollary to dieting and food-deprivation

This latter idea is given added strength by the notion that dieting itself, or at least starvation, may render some people more vulnerable to binging behaviour. Evidence from studies of starvation suggests that normal-weight people who have been underfed for a considerable period of time will demonstrate symptoms akin to those of anorexics, such as talking constantly about food and hoarding food, and that even after a period of refeeding they may continue to eat when full, and alternately diet and binge-eat in an uncontrolled way. It is not clear how far this effect may have a physical rather than a psychological basis. It is possible that the mere thought of having to control their eating can act as a stress on some individuals, as evidenced by the suggestion that the prevalence of eating disorder in diabetics, who need to control their intake of certain foods, is greater than in the normal population (Rodin et al 1986).

In addition, it has been suggested that people who diet may find it increasingly difficult subsequently to lose the same amount of weight on successive occasions. Research with animals has suggested that there may be an underlying metabolic basis for this, in that rats fed on exactly the same reducing diet on two subsequent occasions took longer to reach their target weight on the second occasion than on the first (Brownell et al 1986). Athletes needing to achieve competition weight find this increasingly difficult to achieve from year to year, and a similar effect has been claimed in obese dieters on closely supervised reducing diets followed by refeeding and further dieting (Blackburn et al 1989). Hence, dieters who frequently fail to achieve their targets, overeat, gain weight and then diet again ('weight cyclers'), may unwittingly compromise their ability to diet successfully and render themselves vulnerable to cyclical binging and dieting behaviour.

IS OBESITY AN EATING DISORDER?

Obesity results from an excess of energy intake over expenditure. However, as obese people have been found to expend more energy on average than normal-weight people, they must on average take in more food in order to remain obese (see Garrow 1988). Nevertheless, much research time and effort has gone into asking the question of whether obese people do indeed eat more, with inconclusive results. The question then arises as to how far the cause of this increased intake has to do with the extremes of lack of control over eating behaviour found in people with eating disorders. The existence of bulimia has not been widely studied in relation to obesity, but certainly there is some evidence, both from clinical observation and from research, that perhaps 50% of obese people binge-eat, and that at least a small proportion meet the DSM-III (1980) criteria for bulimia. In addition, some workers have found a higher incidence of depression in obese people seeking treatment than in the normal-weight population. This raises the question of whether obese people eat more as a consequence of depression or whether they are depressed simply because they have a chronic untreatable condition. (For a more detailed review of the incidence of depression and eating disorder in obese people, see Gilbert 1990.)

Thus, it is not possible to generalize about the existence of eating disorder in obesity, except perhaps to conclude that while some obese people simply eat more than they need, it is feasible that there is a small group who experience an eating disorder.

TREATMENT OF EATING DISORDERS

Hospitalization

Most medical treatments for anorexia nervosa advocate bedrest in hospital, although the weight level at which this is considered essential varies between treatment centres. Patients are encouraged to take in between 1600 and 5500 calories per day, and in some units are offered increasing degrees of freedom in return for weight gain. Occasionally patients are fed by a tube or through hyperalimentation, but although these treatments can produce weight gains of 5–12 kg fairly quickly, they carry certain medical complications, such as sepsis, deep-vein thrombosis, water overload and liver toxicity, and are now avoided as far as possible in favour of dietary counselling alone (for an excellent description of the role of the dietitian in eating disorders see Bowyer 1988).

Where bulimia nervosa is concerned, few centres routinely admit patients for treatment, given that the disorder appears often to be determined by the person's situation and appears rapidly to normalize while she is in the safety of the hospital ward and spared the need to control her own eating behaviour. Where inpatient admission is used to stabilize a chaotic eating pattern, outpatient follow-up is invariably needed in order to ensure that the sufferer is able to continue with her new-found control in her home environment.

Behaviour modification

Given that it is extremely difficult to persuade a determined anorexic to put on weight in hospital, many programmes have adopted a so-called behaviour modification approach. Behaviour modification is essentially the use of principles of learning to teach people new behaviours or to modify maladaptive behaviours. Patients on behavioural programmes are rewarded either for weight gain or for eating more. Results are similar to those of pure medical treatments, but there are several problems associated with this kind of approach. First, the treatment is not purely 'behavioural', as it does not usually include a means of ensuring that the newly learned behaviour will continue after the end of treatment; secondly, the patient could be gaining weight merely in order to avoid being in hospital, and not to acquire privileges such as visitors, telephone calls, etc. In fact, behavioural treatments of this type have no advantage over medical treatments alone, and it is possible that patients simply gain weight so as to get out of hospital as quickly as possible.

Pharmacological treatments

Drug treatments for anorexia nervosa have fallen into three categories: drugs to promote food intake and weight gain, drugs to treat the associated psychiatric symptoms, and drugs to treat the physical complications of starvation. (For a detailed review of drug treatments in anorexia nervosa and bulimia nervosa see Kennedy & Goldbloom 1991.) In the 1960s, chlorpromazine became popular in the treatment of anorexia nervosa. However, this lowers blood pressure and reduces body temperature and is no longer widely used.

Some authorities favour the use of the minor tranquillizers to reduce anxiety about eating, and this can certainly be helpful as a short-term measure. More recently, in the USA in particular, others have advocated the use of antidepressant drugs, based on the hypothesis that anorexic and bulimic patients are in fact suffering from forms of affective disorder akin to depression.

There have been few controlled trials of the use of antidepressants in anorexia nervosa, with no significant response. However, several trials have shown a clear advantage of antidepressant medication over placebo in the treatment of bulimia, whether or not the patients are depressed (Walsh 1991). The side effects caused by monoamine oxidase inhibitors (MAOIs) render these drugs inappropriate in the case of people with no control over their eating behaviour, but several trials have demonstrated the efficacy of tricyclic antidepressants such as imipramine and desipramine, and fluoxetine. On average, patients receiving active medication achieve a decline in binge frequency of about 50%, but only about 20% of the patients stop binge-eating altogether, and in many trials patients have been able to maintain their improvement only through continued use of the antidepressant drugs. Also, there is no evidence that drug treatment has any effect on the patients' attitudes to weight and shape.

Psychological treatments

Most units provide some form of psychotherapeutic intervention as an adjunct to medical treatment, or as a means of treatment in itself. Until recently, this has largely been psychoanalytic in nature, or at least with some psychodynamic focus. This means that the patient's problems and history are couched in terms of links with their past relationships and developmental history, and the implication is that they can be cured as a result of having explored and understood the nature of these links. In addition, patients are given information about their disorder based on the idiosyncratic view of the unit, all in a setting where skilled nursing care and a relationship of trust are considered important. For a review of the full range of psychological treatments, see Garner & Garfinkel (1985).

Family therapy

Given the evidence that people with eating disorders often have difficulties with family relationships, family therapy has seemed to be the treatment of choice for many young women with anorexia nervosa or bulimia nervosa. The methods of either Selvini-Palazzoli, known as the 'Milan method', or of Salvador Minuchin, have been widely adopted.

Selvini-Palazzoli sees the anorexic as having become part of a dirty 'game' in a family where the channels of communication have gone very wrong. Her therapy involves the whole family in a short series of no more than 20 sessions, where the main aim is to help the family to redefine their relationships with the help of a non-confrontative therapist, using as his or her main tools a method of circular questioning in order to clarify the relationships between and the needs of individual family members, and prescription of the symptom – a method which involves describing symptomatic behaviour in a positive, uncritical light, so that the participants have the opportunity to accept and hence to discard it.

Minuchin's therapy is based on the 'systems theory' approach. His therapy aims to create a change in a malfunctioning 'system' by challenging four basic family characteristics: enmeshment, or overinvolvement of family members with each other; overprotectiveness; rigidity, or a strong desire to maintain the status quo; and an inability to resolve conflict. These methods were largely untested in any controlled way until a recent study at the Institute of Psychiatry in London randomly allocated 57 discharged anorexic and bulimic patients either to family therapy or to individual therapy. Their findings, based on the small group of patients who remained in therapy, were that family therapy was more effective than individual therapy in anorexic patients whose illness was not chronic and had begun before the age of 19 years, but that older patients and bulimics appeared to do better with individual therapy (Russell et al 1987).

Behaviour therapy aimed at attitude change

Behaviour modification for anorexia nervosa is enhanced where the therapist takes account of the patient's thoughts and feelings about food and eating. To this end, certain traditional behavioural techniques have been found useful. One of these is 'self-monitoring', where the patient is asked to keep a record of her eating and possibly the thoughts and feelings around it, so that the therapist can help her move towards further change. Some therapists will help their patients with 'graded exposure' to previously 'forbidden' foods – in other words, helping their patients to contemplate eating successively more 'fattening' foods. In addition, exposure together with 'response prevention' may be used in order to help people who purge to interrupt the binge–purge cycle at successively earlier points.

Behaviour therapy has proved particularly useful in modifying eating habits in the treatment of overeating. The treatment works by helping the person to reduce eating in response to environmental and social cues (stimulus control). It has produced improved long-term maintenance of weight loss in comparison with other treatments, largely through recent attempts to continue treatment for longer and build in means of helping patients to handle relapse (for a detailed review see Brownell & Kramer 1989).

In relation to eating disorder, the thoughts and feelings of patients about weight and shape are of primary importance, and treatments which can focus on attitude change and help to reduce restraint rather than increase it are essential. To this end, a recent addition to the behavioural repertoire, cognitive therapy, has proved useful. This is a therapy initially worked out by Meichenbaum (1977) in the USA for helping people to cope with anxiety through practice at changing the way they think about anxiety-provoking situations. A form of cognitive therapy has been devised by Beck in Philadelphia for the treatment of depression, and extended also for the treatment of anxiety, personality difficulties and many other disorders (Beck et al 1979, Beck & Emery 1985). This short-term therapy aims to produce attitude change through helping patients to modify negative ways of thinking about their situations and dysfunctional basic assumptions about life and experience.

Fairburn in the UK and Garner and Bemis in the USA have tested cognitive behavioural programmes for the treatment respectively of bulimia nervosa and to a lesser extent anorexia nervosa (Fairburn & Cooper 1989, Garner & Bemis 1985). Fairburn's treatment is in three phases: in phase one, the emphasis is on improving self-control over eating, and the methods used include self-monitoring, the prescription of a pattern of regular eating, and stimulus-control measures. In addition, patients are given information about body-weight regulation, dieting, and the effects of starving or using self-induced vomiting or purging as a means of controlling their weight. In the second phase, designed to modify disturbed attitudes to weight and shape, patients are taught to modify negative self-statements and to expose themselves to increasing amounts of 'forbidden' foods. The third stage consists of measures designed to reduce the risk of relapse.

The cognitive therapy process, with its emphasis on collaboration in a joint venture between patient and therapist, makes sense as a treatment for anorexia nervosa, a disorder in which the motivation of the patient is the greatest barrier to change (Hollin & Lewis 1988). However, cognitive therapy has as yet shown no clear advantage over other therapies in relation to the treatment of this disorder. In one of the few controlled studies to date (Channon et al 1989), there did appear to be a slight effect in terms of better compliance in relation to attendance at therapy sessions.

In relation to bulimia nervosa, on the other hand, cognitive therapy has shown itself to be effective in the short term for many sufferers. It also appears to have had an advantage in terms of better outcome at long-term follow-up in several research studies when compared with drug therapy (Mitchell 1991). Cognitive behaviour therapy has proved equally effective to other short-term psychological treatments in reducing the symptoms of binging and purging behaviour, but it may have an advantage in terms of its ability to modify the disturbed attitudes to shape and weight and extreme dieting which appear to maintain eating disorders (Fairburn et al 1991).

Studies which have attempted to predict the outcome of therapy for bulimia nervosa have concluded that poor outcome relates to a high degree of personality disturbance, alcohol abuse, high impulsivity (including suicidal behaviour), and low self-esteem (Herzog et al 1991). These conclusions appear to support the notion of the utility of pursuing effective long-term psychological treatments for the eating disorders.

REFERENCES

American Psychiatric Association 1980 Diagnostic and statistical manual of mental disorders (DSM-III), 3rd edn. American Psychiatric Association, Washington DC

American Psychiatric Association 1987 Diagnostic and statistical manual of mental disorders (DSM-III-R), 3rd edn, revised. American Psychiatric Association, Washington DC

Beck AT, Emery G 1985 Anxiety disorders and phobias: a cognitive perspective. Basic Books, New York

Beck AT, Rush AJ, Shaw BF, Emery G 1979 Cognitive therapy of depression. John Wiley & Sons, Chichester

Blackburn GL, Wilson GT, Kanders BS et al 1989 Weight cycling: the experience of human dieters. American Journal of Human Nutrition 49: 1105–1109

Bowyer C 1988 Dietary factors in eating disorders. In: Scott D (ed) Anorexia and bulimia nervosa: practical approaches. Croom Helm, London

Brownell KD, Kramer FM 1989 Behavioural management of obesity. Medical Clinics of North America 73(1): 185–201

Brownell KD, Greenwood MRC, Stellar E, Shrager EE 1986 The effect of repeated cycles of weight loss and regain in rats. Physiology and Behaviour 38: 459–464

Bruch H 1974 Eating disorders: anorexia, obesity and the person within. Routledge and Kegan Paul, London

Carlat DJ, Camargo CA 1991 Review of bulimia nervosa in males. American Journal of Psychiatry 148: 831–843

Channon S, de Silva P, Helmsley D, Perkins R 1989 A controlled trial of cognitive behavioural and behavioural treatment of anorexia nervosa. Behaviour Research and Therapy 27(5): 529–536

Crisp AH 1980 Anorexia nervosa: let me be. Academic Press, London

Fairburn CG, Beglin SJ 1990 Studies of the epidemiology of bulimia nervosa. American Journal of Psychiatry 147: 401–408

Fairburn CG, Cooper PJ 1985 Eating disorders. In: Hawton

K, Salkovskis PM, Kirk J, Clark DM (eds) Cognitive behaviour therapy for psychiatric problems: a practical guide. Oxford Medical Publications, Oxford

Fairburn CG, Jones R, Peveler RC et al 1991 Three psychological treatments for bulimia nervosa: a comparative trial. Archives of General Psychiatry 48: 463–469

French B 1987 Coping with bulimia: the binge–purge syndrome. Thorsons, Wellingborough

Garner DM, Bemis KM 1985 Cognitive therapy for anorexia nervosa. In: Garner DM, Garfinkel PE (eds) Handbook of psychotherapy for anorexia nervosa and bulimia. Guilford, New York

Garner DM, Garfinkel PE (eds) 1985 Handbook of psychotherapy for anorexia nervosa and bulimia. Guilford, New York

Garrow JS 1988 Is obesity an eating disorder? Journal of Psychosomatic Research 12(6): 585–590

Gilbert S 1986 Pathology of eating: psychology and treatment. Routledge and Kegan Paul, London

Gilbert S 1989 Tomorrow I'll be slim: the psychology of dieting. Routledge, London

Gilbert S 1990 Psychological aspects of obesity and its treatment. In: Shepherd R (ed) Handbook of the psychophysiology of human eating. Wiley, Chichester

Halmi KA, Eckert E, Marchi P, Sampugnaro V, Apple R, Cohen J 1991 Comorbidity of psychiatric diagnoses in anorexia nervosa. Archives of General Psychiatry 48: 712–718

Herzog T, Hartmann A, Sandholz A, Stammer H 1991 Prognostic factors in outpatient psychotherapy of bulimia. Psychotherapy and Psychosomatics 56: 48–55

Hill AJ, Oliver S, Rogers PJ 1992 Eating in the adult world: the rise of dieting in childhood and adolescence. British Journal of Clinical Psychology 31: 95–105

Hollin C, Lewis V 1988 Cognitive–behavioural approaches to anorexia and bulimia. In: Scott D (ed) Anorexia and bulimia nervosa: practical approaches. Croom Helm, London

Kennedy SH, Goldbloom DS 1991 Current perspectives on drug therapies for anorexia nervosa and bulimia nervosa. Drugs 41(3): 367–377

Lacey JH, Evans CDH 1986 The impulsivist: a multi-impulsive personality disorder. British Journal of Addiction 81: 715–723

Lask B, Bryant-Waugh R 1986 Childhood-onset anorexia nervosa. In: Meadow R (ed) Recent advances in paediatrics Vol. 8 Churchill Livingstone, Edinburgh, 21–31

Meichenbaum D 1977 Cognitive behaviour modification: an integrative approach. Plenum Press, New York

Minuchin S, Rosman BL, Baker L 1978 Psychosomatic families: anorexia nervosa in context. Harvard, Cambridge, Massachusetts

Mitchell JE 1991 A review of the controlled trials of psychotherapy for bulimia nervosa. Journal of Psychosomatic Research 35 (Suppl 1): 23–32

Palmer RL, Oppenheimer R, Dignon A, Chaloner DA, Howells K 1990 Childhood sexual experiences with adults reported by women with eating disorders: an extended series. British Journal of Psychiatry 156: 699–703

Ratnasuriya RH, Eisler I, Szmukler GI, Russell GFM 1991 Anorexia nervosa: outcome and prognostic factors after 20 years. British Journal of Psychiatry 158: 495–502

Rodin GM, Johnson LE, Garfinkel P, Daneman D, Kenshole A B 1986 Eating disorders in female adolescents with insulin-dependent diabetes mellitus. International Journal of Psychiatry in Medicine 16: 49–57

Russell GFM 1979 Bulimia nervosa: an ominous variant of anorexia nervosa. Psychological Medicine 9: 429–488

Russell GFM, Szmukler GI, Dare C, Eisler I 1987 An evaluation of family therapy in anorexia nervosa and bulimia nervosa. Archives of General Psychiatry 44: 1047–1056

Slade PD 1982 Towards a functional analysis of anorexia nervosa and bulimia nervosa. British Journal of Clinical Psychology 21(3): 167–179

Sloan G, Leichner P 1986 Is there a relationship between sexual abuse or incest and eating disorders? Canadian Journal of Psychiatry 31: 656–660

Walsh BT 1991 Fluoxetine treatment of bulimia nervosa. Journal of Psychosomatic Research 35 (Suppl 1):33–40

50. Drug–nutrient interactions

D. A. Roe

Drug–nutrient interactions consist of the physico-chemical, physiological and pathophysiological processes that may alter the disposition, intended function or toxicity of food components or foreign compounds. The outcomes of drug and nutrient interactions may be beneficial or adverse (Table 50.1). An example of a beneficial outcome is the ability to reduce the risk of convulsions from an overdose of the antituberculosis drug, isoniazid, if vitamin B_6 is administered promptly. This is explained by the formation of a drug–vitamin complex which is excreted and thereby reduces the neurotoxic potential of the drug. Adverse interactions include the acute hypertension occurring when an individual receives a drug with a monoamine oxidase activity inhibitor, and then eats foods high in tyramine. The inhibition of catecholamine metabolism and the acute effects of tyramine in increasing plasma and tissue noradrenaline levels can then have serious effects. Another example is the megaloblastic anaemia which can develop when a drug antagonizes the effects of folic acid.

MALABSORPTION DUE TO DRUGS

Some drugs cause direct damage to the intestine and thereby induce malabsorption. Table 50.2 provides some examples. The commonest drug with direct intestinal effects is ethyl alcohol which can cause inflammatory changes in the oesophagus and stomach of heavy drinkers (see Chapter 7). Its small intestinal effects include folate malabsorption (see Chapter 14). In alcoholics, pancreatic damage and liver changes can limit the input of pancreatic enzymes and bile salts; folate deficiency itself contributes to the malabsorption and neomycin, when given to combat hepatic encephalopathy, may enhance the malabsorption. Thus alcoholics can be found to have malabsorption of fat and fat-soluble vitamins, carbohydrate and the vitamins B_1, B_{12} and folic acid.

Neomycin is a poorly absorbed antibiotic widely used to reduce the bacterial production of amines and other bacterial metabolites in hepatic encephalopathy (see Chapter 34). It produces a reversible malabsorption of fat, protein and carbohydrates, as well as of carotene, iron and vitamin B_{12}. It acts not only by a direct effect on the intestine but by binding bile salts and limiting the micelle formation needed for long-chain fat absorption. Neomycin can also induce the malabsorption of other drugs. Kanamycin, an alternative drug used to reduce the intestinal flora, can have similar effects which are dose-dependent.

Colchicine also tends to induce fat malabsorption by a direct intestinal effect if used long term in doses of 2 g or more per day. Para-aminosalicylic acid also

Table 50.1 Beneficial and adverse drug–nutrient interactions

Beneficial	Harmful
Drug absorption enhanced by foods	Impaired drug absorption by foods
Appetite stimulation	Altered drug metabolism with toxicity in
Improved nutrition with antibiotics in infection	malnutrition
Drug prevention of disease by antinutritional effects	Drug-induced nutrition deficiencies
Anticancer effects based on changed nutrient metabolism	Hyperphagic side-effects of some drugs
Vitamin use as drug toxicity antidotes	

Table 50.2 Drug–nutrient interactions in the intestine

Direct mucosal damage
  Ethyl alcohol; oral antidiabetic biguanides
  Neomycin, kanamycin, colchicine
  Methotrexate and other antimitotic drugs used in cancer
  chemotherapy
  Chronic purgative abuse (colonic effects predominate)

Bile salt precipitation/sequestration
  Neomycin, kanamycin
  Cholestyramine

Drug-induced malabsorption
  Folate: by sodium bicarbonate, cholestyramine,
  sulphasalazine
  B_{12}: by gastric hydrogen ion inhibitors of secretion, e.g.
  cimetidine
  Vitamins A, D and K: by mineral oil and bile salt
  sequesters
  Calcium: by phenolphthalein laxatives
  Phosphate: by aluminium hydroxide

Drug-induced changes in appetite
  Reduced: amphetamines and other catecholaminergic
  agonists, serotonin uptake inhibitors, e.g. fenfluramine,
  fluoxitine
  Increased: some antidepressants, antibiotics in infected
  patients

induces malabsorption of a variety of nutrients, so this common antituberculous drug may exacerbate the poor nutritional state of tuberculous patients.

Cholestyramine, the quarternary ammonium resin which exchanges with anions such as bile acids, is used deliberately for its capacity to induce bile salt malabsorption. It is commonly used in patients with intolerable itching from the bile acid accumulation in the skin of patients with obstructive jaundice. Patients with diarrhoea following a modest resection of the ileum, e.g. <100 cm, improve once sequestration of the bile salts limits colonic water loss. These two clinical problems are the principal gastrointestinal conditions where the drug is used in sufficient amounts to enhance the malabsorption of fat and fat-soluble vitamins. Cholestyramine is also increasingly used in high doses to enhance cholesterol excretion and catabolism in hypercholesterolaemia (see Chapter 41), so again the likelihood of vitamin malabsorption needs to be recognized.

The drug effects on nutrient absorption (Table 50.2) include chelation, e.g. between calcium and tetracycline; ionic binding such as between folate and cholestyramine; precipitation, e.g. between phosphate and aluminium hydroxide; solubilization, e.g. of β-carotene within malabsorbed mineral oil; and changes in pH, e.g. where sodium bicarbonate reduces folate absorption.

EFFECTS OF FOOD ON DRUG ABSORPTION AND METABOLISM

The interactions with food can have profound effects on the availability and effectiveness of drug therapy. Table 50.3 provides examples where drug absorption or catabolism is altered. The important impairment in the absorption of penicillins and tetracyclines by food is often neglected but these drugs are much more efficiently absorbed in the fasting state. Penicillins affect the absorption of many foods and the absorption of tetracyclines is selectively inhibited by dairy products high in calcium or other foods rich in magnesium or iron. Tetracyclines form chelates with divalent ions, e.g. calcium, magnesium, zinc and iron. Harju's (1989) review suggests that an interaction between iron and tetracycline preparations will always occur but, if the iron is given 2–3 hours after the tetracycline, the tendency for the drug and the iron mutually to inhibit the absorption of each is no longer of clinical importance. However, Harju also notes that interactions between doxycycline and iron not only decrease the absorption of the drug and the nutrient but also enhance the body's metabolism and excretion of both the drug and the iron. Therefore, tetracyclines

Table 50.3 Effects of food on drug therapy

Effect	Example	Response time
Food-induced drug malabsorption	Tetracycline–milk	
		1–3 h ↓ absorption
	Methyldopa–amino acids	
Food-enhanced drug metabolism	Phenytoin–indole-induced oxidases	Days
	Theophylline–protein	≥ 5 days
Nutrient modulated responsiveness to drugs	Iron–doxycycline	1–3 h ↓ absorption
		Drug ↑ catabolism

are best taken at least 2 hours before or after the intake of milk, other dairy products or protein foods. In hospital this demands proper organization in the ward to standardize nursing regimens for drug dispensing with meal times.

Drug formulation also affects the rate and amount of drug absorbed. Suspensions or solutions of drugs are not always better absorbed than solid drug products when given with food. The nutritionist or dietitian therefore needs to check the industry's evidence on dietary interactions with the specific drug being used, because often there is evidence available on the timing of meals in relation to the particular form of the drug, but is poorly publicized.

Drug catabolism may be enhanced by food components. For example, smoked foods contain substances that induce intestinal and hepatic mixed function oxidases (MFO), which are involved in drug metabolism. Indoles present in cabbage and Brussels sprouts also induce these oxidases, which therefore enhance the catabolism of the antiepileptic drug phenytoin, of anticoagulants such as the coumarins and barbiturate catabolism. A high protein diet promotes the catabolism of theophylline, so this can reduce the time during which an asthmatic attack can be controlled by a single dose of theophylline. The chelation of isoniazid by pyridoxine is an example of a direct interaction of a drug with a nutrient that can be used advantageously if too much isoniazid has been given. However, a high pyridoxine intake, e.g. in patients treating themselves with vitamin supplements in an effort to improve their health when they have tuberculosis, will also reduce the effectiveness of the isoniazid therapy.

PHYSIOLOGICAL INTERACTIONS

Physiological interactions between drugs and nutrients induce a variety of effects which include drug-induced disturbances in the rate of absorption of nutrients, and nutrient-induced changes in gastric emptying which affect the rate of drug absorption. The latter may affect the development of clinically obvious side-effects. For example, when the calcium channel blocking agent, nifedipine, is given fasting or, curiously, with a high fat breakfast meal, the drug is absorbed faster and is more likely to cause headache and flushing than when it is given with a low fat breakfast meal (Reitberg et al 1987). These interactions may be only of relevance in particular disease states. For example, a diabetic taking long-acting antidiabetic oral drugs in a fasting rather than a fed state shows different effects on blood glucose, but the postprandial glucose response is reduced if a drug that slows gastric emptying time, e.g. propantheline bromide, is also taken. Another functional side-effect of chlorpropamide, which occurs in a subgroup of non-insulin dependent diabetics, is the chlorpropamide–alcohol flush, which is induced by ingestion of a modest intake of an alcoholic beverage, such as a glass of sherry. This flush reaction can be suppressed if aspirin is given with the sherry, because the aspirin suppresses the prostaglandin release which causes the flush reaction (Chapter 7).

PATHOPHYSIOLOGICAL INTERACTIONS

Interactions between drugs and nutrients can have toxic effects. The severity of the outcome may relate to the immediate interference with essential metabolic functions or reflect the effect of progressive cell injury with functional loss. Pathophysiological effects attributable to drug–nutrient interactions include acute and chronic malabsorption states induced by drugs such as methotrexate and colchicine, some drug–induced hepatotoxicities, e.g. those due to ethanol, and the effects of isoniazid, potent folate antagonists and drugs which induce neuropathies by producing vitamin B_6 deficiency. Examples of pathophysiological drug–nutrient interactions are listed in Table 50.4. Important factors to be considered in the prognosis of these reactions are the reversibility of tissue damage, the complexity of multiple drug effects on cell damage, and the nature of a patient's disease and their diet. An example of the difficulty in risk assessment is provided by the evidence of methotrexate-induced hepatotoxicity in which the effect of this cytotoxic folate antagonist on liver pathology and

Table 50.4 Pathophysiological drug–nutrient interactions

Drug	Nutrient	Effect	Risk
Methotrexate	Folic acid	Villous atrophy	Multiple nutrient deficiencies due to malabsorption
Alcohol	Vitamin K	Toxic hepatitis	Vitamin K deficiency + haemorrhage

function are related to prior toxic and adverse nutritional effects of alcohol abuse (Newman et al 1989).

Outcomes of drug and nutrient interactions which impose the risk of tissue damage also vary in that the prognosis may be worse in the elderly, who are more likely to have structural and functional deficits of the liver and kidneys due to chronic disease or prior drug use (Roe 1989).

THERAPEUTIC INTERACTIONS

Beneficial effects of drug–nutrient interactions need to be emphasized because the interactions can be used therapeutically. For example, a diabetic regimen with a short-acting oral sulphonylurea drug, such as glipizide, and caloric restriction, improve the early management of non-insulin dependent diabetics (NIDDM). The glipizide controls the early postprandial hyperglycaemia and the diet controls the later postprandial phase of blood glucose elevation (Melander et al 1989). Bile acid sequestrants, together with niacin and a diet low in cholesterol and in saturated fatty acids, can also be used as a combination therapy in the management of hypercholesterolaemic states.

EFFECTS OF NUTRITIONAL STATE ON DRUG METABOLISM

Protein–energy malnutrition (PEM) in children in the Third World can have profound effects on drug metabolism. Malnourished children have a reduction in organ size and this may affect drug disposal. Differences can also be expected between marasmic children and those with kwashiorkor because the total amount of body fat may be remarkably different. Thus fat-soluble drugs will have a very different uptake and distribution in the two forms of malnutrition. Malnourished children may also have selective nutritional deficiencies that make them more susceptible to the effects of drugs. To these effects of organ size and specific nutritional deficiencies must be added the effects of a persistently low intake of food and of specific nutrients, all of which will affect drug uptake and metabolism. The child with kwashiorkor may have a particularly damaged small intestine, but drug uptake may also be impaired by the common bacterial overgrowth in the small intestine (see Chapter 30).

Drug conjugation may come to be dependent on the availability of glycine, sulphate, glutathione or other metabolites, e.g. for acetylation. The capacity to respond to drugs, e.g. by inducing enzyme activity, is also likely to be impaired in malnutrition. So it is not surprising if experimental animal and clinical studies demonstrate the unusual sensitivity of the malnourished child, adult or elderly patient to drug toxicity.

Children with kwashiorkor excrete a higher ratio of the antimalarial, chloroquine, as hepatic metabolites. Another antimalarial, pyrimethamine, inhibits dihydrofolate reductase, so this can exacerbate folate deficiency. The same enzyme is also inhibited by trimethoprin which usually exerts a more profound effect on folate metabolism in bacteria than man. Nevertheless, a marginally folate-deficient child or adult can be expected to have their nutritional problem amplified by the use of this antibacterial drug. Chloramphenicol, still used for treating children and adults with typhoid, is cleared much more slowly in the malnourished patient, e.g. 30 hours compared with a plasma clearance time of 12 hours in well-nourished children. This probably reflects the dominant glucuronide pathway for its normal excretion: 35–55% of the drug is excreted in this form in malnutrition compared with a normal percentage of 75–85% (Mehta et al 1975). The slow excretion of penicillin in children with kwashiorkor seems, however, to depend on the inadequate renal function in these children during the acute phase of their illness (Buchanan & Hansen 1976). Thus several commonly used antibiotics have very different effects in malnourished patients.

Another common drug, tetrachloroethylene, used in the treatment of hookworm infestations, seems, however, to be less toxic than expected in malnourished children, presumably because of the impaired metabolic capacity for producing toxic metabolites.

DRUG–NUTRIENT INTERACTIONS IN THE ELDERLY

The effectiveness of drugs is influenced by both the physiological and pathological changes which occur with ageing and the problems may be particularly difficult because the elderly often have multiple abnormalities and receive several drugs for different conditions simultaneously and over a prolonged period of time. The elderly seem at particular risk of drug-induced nutritional deficiencies but this may simply reflect the fact that older people eat much less because of their reduced physical activity and much smaller lean tissue mass. With nutrient intakes close to the requirement levels because of the reduced appetite for energy, then any effect of drugs on the absorption or metabolism of nutrients is likely to have a great impact. The propensity for the elderly to develop mild forms of malnutrition also means that these changes of malnutrition will affect drug metabolism. Drugs for combating cardiovascular problems are widely used in older people, as are those for psychiatric and gastrointestinal problems. Older people also take laxatives for their constipation and analgesics for pain from, for example, the musculoskeletal system. The majority of the elderly in the developed world therefore take 2–5 different drugs daily and have 2–3 times the rate of drug complications seen in younger age groups. Cardiovascular and psychotropic drugs are a particular problem.

Drug malabsorption is not a special problem of the elderly but plasma binding is often reduced and the lower lean body mass reduces tissue uptake unless the drug is lipid-soluble and therefore readily taken up by the relatively large fat mass in the elderly. However, changes in drug distribution rarely affect peak concentrations of the drug.

Given the frequent initial oxidative step in drug metabolism via the hepatic cytochrome P-450 dependent enzyme system and the recognized changes with age in this system, it is not surprising that drug metabolism is altered in the elderly. Usually drug oxidation rates are reduced in the elderly, but the activity of the hepatic conjugative pathway, e.g. for glucuronidation, sulphation or linkage with glutathione, seems to be preserved in older humans but not in aged animals. Reduced hepatic blood flow which can occur in older patients also reduces the hepatic clearance of some drugs, e.g. of the β-adrenergic blocker, propranolol.

Reduced renal function is the main contributor to drug sensitivity in the elderly. This affects, for example, the excretion of digoxin, propranolol, cimetidine and procainamide, as well as the excretion of most antimicrobial drugs. Clearance is proportional to endogenous creatinine clearance, so dosage adjustments can be made by assessing the clearance rate.

Changes in tissue sensitivity may also contribute. For example, the elderly's brain proves to be more sensitive to benzodiazepines. Coumarin anticoagulants and adrenergic agonists and antagonists are also more effective in the elderly.

All these effects explain the undue sensitivity of the elderly to drug therapy. Given this sensitivity, additional nutritional effects on drug absorption or metabolism can produce marked effects because of the sensitivity. Thus the non-cardiac effects of digoxin can be severe in the elderly, with 50–90% of patients complaining of both fatigue and anorexia which can lead to substantial weight loss. This response can then be misinterpreted as a further clinical problem. Hypokalaemia from diuretics is also more likely because of the reduced potassium intake in older people on a smaller total food intake, so particular care with potassium therapy is needed given the changes in renal function.

Similarly muscle wasting and bone loss may be especially important in elderly patients treated with steroids which will accentuate any nutritional limitation, e.g. in calcium uptake or vitamin D metabolism. Long-term ascorbate deficiency may also alter drug metabolism. The normal induction of cytochrome P-450 by cabbage, Brussels sprouts and charcoal-cooked meat may be less in the elderly simply because the intake of these foods is reduced.

Given this complexity of effects, it is best to assume that when old people are being treated for cardiovascular, psychiatric, gastrointestinal and infective conditions, then they are likely to exhibit undue sensitivity to drugs and the chronic use of these drugs is likely to induce or accentuate nutritional problems, which might best be combated by ensuring a very high-quality diet, i.e. rich in nutrients, and with relatively small amounts of fat, sugar and alcohol.

PRACTICAL ASPECTS OF DRUG–NUTRIENT INTERACTIONS

Physicians, nurses, pharmacists and clinical nutritionists need to be able to predict the risk of drug–nutrient interactions from their knowledge of the medication list, the patient's diet and nutritional status and the timing of medications in relation to meals. It is also their responsibility to identify when unwanted outcomes of drug and nutrient interactions occur by recognizing the clinical signs and applying the appropriate laboratory tests. They should also know what appropriate interventions are required both to reduce the risk of problems and to handle the effects of these drug interactions.

Such interventions can make a great difference to the clinical condition of the patient. Clinical experience with new drugs has to be carefully collected and dietary changes kept in mind if the drug–nutrient interaction is to be identified quickly and effectively. The probability of reaching the correct diagnosis usually depends on recognizing a cluster of symptoms and signs present and on the results of laboratory tests (Albert et al 1988).

For nutritionists, one issue is whether the effect of a drug is likely to be sufficient to alter the nutritional state of the child or adult. Conversely, if the absorption of a drug is of special interest to the physician or the pharmacist, then the effect of taking the drug with or without meals and with or without particular foods is of particular concern. The effects of drugs on the usefulness of therapeutic iron preparations are a particular example where both the drug and the nutritional effects become important. It needs to be clearly understood whether these effects apply only at high levels of iron intake or simply when ordinary levels of food iron are being considered.

There are simple preventive strategies to reduce the risk of serious effects from the physicochemical interactions between dietary factors and drug therapy. Giving a drug several times a day reduces the risk that meal components are present in the same part of the gut lumen as the drug. In hospital, patients, nursing staff and those providing food need to cooperate to adjust the times for giving drugs and meals to meet the needs of patients rather than adjusting therapy to their own hours of duty. In patients fed by nasogastric tube, care has to be taken with some drugs that interact with the enteral feed and block the tube (Cutie et al 1983). Drug suspensions of low pH are a particular problem, but if the formula feeding is stopped and the tube flushed with water before and after drug delivery, then the feed can be recommenced 1 or more hours later, once the drug has been allowed to pass down into the small intestine for absorption.

Any simple assumption that a particular drug does or does not interact with food is unwise unless the form of the drug and the nature of the meal is specified. For example, when the anticonvulsant phenytoin is given as a suspension to neurosurgical patients with epilepsy who are being fed by continuous nasogastric feeding, seizures may not be controlled because therapeutic blood levels of phenytoin are not attained (Bauer 1982). However, it is recognized that phenytoin, given to healthy adults as a single dose in capsule form, is well absorbed even if enteral formula feedings are used (Nishimura et al 1988). Thus identifying whether the capsular or suspension form of phenytoin is to be used becomes important in management. Furthermore, normal subjects given phenytoin in a solution form with a formula containing a hemicellulose fibre source show an enhanced absorption of phenytoin when the fibre is included in the feeding system. These different outcomes are related to the magnitude of the physicochemical interactions between the drug in its particular form and food components. The effects of the formula ingredients (e.g. a fibre source) on, for example, gastric emptying time, may itself alter the rate or amount of the phenytoin reaching the systemic circulation. Conversely, a drug can have a profound impact on nutrient availability and therefore on nutritional status by virtue of its effects on nutrient absorption. Thus laxative abusers may take a mineral oil in the form of liquid paraffin and develop fat-soluble vitamin deficiency because the laxative oil also solubilizes and traps β-carotene, as well as reducing the absorption of other fat-soluble vitamins, probably through effects on micelle formation (Curtis & Ballmer 1939, Roe 1985).

It is clear therefore that as advances in nutrition are made the doctor, nutritionist and dietitian need to be aware of the latest evidence on the absorptive and metabolic interactions of new drugs and the effect of their formulation.

REFERENCES

Albert DA, Munson R, Resnik MD 1988 Reasoning in medicine. Johns Hopkins University Press, Baltimore, pp. 216–217

Bauer LA 1982 Interference of oral phenytoin absorption by continuous nasogastric feedings. Neurology 32: 570–572

Buchanan N, Hansen JDL 1976 Chloramphenicol metabolism in children with PCM. American Journal of Clinical Nutrition 29: 327–330

Curtis AC, Ballmer RS 1939 The prevention of carotene absorption by liquid petrolatum. Journal of American Medical Association 113: 1785–1788

Cutie AJ, Altman E, Lenkel L 1983 Compatibility of enteral products with commonly employed drug additives. Journal of Parenteral and Enteral Nutrition 7: 186–191

Harju E 1989 Clinical pharmacokinetics of iron preparations. Clinical Pharmacokinetics 17: 69–89

Mehta S, Kalsi, HK, Jayaraman S, Mathur VS 1975 Chloroamphenicol metabolism in children with protein–calorie malnutrition. American Journal of Clinical Nutrition 28: 977–981

Melander A, Bitzen P-O, Schersten B 1989 Food cultures and NIDDM therapeutics: the Western community model. In: McLean AJ, Wahlqvist ML (eds) Current problems in nutrition, pharmacology and toxicology. John Libbey, London, pp. 19–25

Newman M, Auerbach R, Feiner H et al 1989 The role of liver biopsies in psoriatic patients receiving long-term methotrexate treatment. Archives of Dermatology 125: 1218–1224

Nishimura LY, Armstrong EP, Plezia PM, Iacono RP 1988 Influence of enteral feedings on phenytoin sodium absorption from capsules. Drug Intell Clinical Pharmacology 22: 130–133

Reitberg DP, Love SJ, Quercia GT, Zinny MA 1987 Effect of food on nifedipine pharmacokinetics. Clinical Pharmacokinetics 42: 72–75

Roe DA 1985 Drug-induced nutritional deficiencies, 2nd edn. AVI Publishing Company, Westport, CT, pp. 113–114

Roe DA 1989 Drug–nutrient interactions in the elderly. In: Munro HN, Danford DE (eds) Nutrition, aging, and the elderly. Plenum Press, New York, pp. 363–384

51. Policy and a prudent diet

W. P. T. James

The historical account of changes in food supply, disease patterns and attitudes to food, health and nutrition research given in Chapter 1 illustrates the complex factors that affect nutrition policy in different parts of the world. International committees have been able to draw together evidence from all over the world on what constitutes a healthy diet and these now provide recommendations of the optimum range of intake of those nutrients needed to sustain the health of individuals of all ages. The development of these recommendations has been slow and modern approaches that specify nutrient goals to limit the development of the chronic diseases of adult life, rather than the avoidance of deficiency diseases, have only emerged since the early 1960s.

DEVELOPMENT OF MODERN CONCEPTS OF HEALTHY NUTRITION

By the end of World War II, Keys and his colleagues (1950) had completed their classic studies on the effects of semi-starvation. Keys then embarked on a new endeavour to explain the extraordinary differences in the disease patterns in reasonably affluent societies. His 'Seven Country Study' (Keys 1980) led to the first major example of 'metabolic epidemiology' and a preliminary understanding of the nutritional basis for coronary heart disease (CHD) (see Chapter 41). While these collaborative studies were in progress, Keys demonstrated in volunteer medical students that standard amounts of a specific type of saturated fatty acid increased total blood cholesterol to a varying degree in different individuals and that switching to diets rich in polyunsaturated fatty acids lowered blood cholesterol concentrations.

Keys and his colleagues in public health were soon advocating major changes in the eating pattern of Americans. So successful was their campaign that the American Heart Association, formed to combat the increasing problem of heart disease, in 1963 advocated a new diet based on reducing total fat and saturated fatty acid intakes and increasing polyunsaturated fatty acid intake. It is noteworthy that this was an action plan by a voluntary organization for the benefit of the public. Advice was given but any dietary change depended on personal decision-making in a society with no national health service and a growing public awareness that American doctors were business men as well as carers of patients. An American had to decide the choice of doctor and medical specialists he consulted and he paid the bills for any care given. This led to intense personal interest in health and a fear that illness in middle and old age could become financially crippling.

American government also had a tradition of ensuring freedom of choice with minimal government interference, so government responded on the one hand to public pressure to increase research into the causes of heart disease and cancer but remained extremely reluctant to engage in economic measures to improve public health, e.g. to tax tobacco or subsidize 'healthy' foods. Whereas Europe was still recovering from the devastation and hardship of the post-war period, America had enjoyed no food deprivation during World War II, and its agriculture was varied, successful and highly productive. Support for the American tobacco industry and farmers was, and continues to be, based on economic and political rather than on health grounds (Taylor 1984). Thus, in the USA and indeed in Canada, public health was not seen in coherent public policy terms as requiring governmental action. Governments were therefore there to help individuals to respond to health messages. On this basis it is little wonder that Americans are far more responsive to new ideas on the promotion of healthy living than Europeans who have a much greater sense of being passive with government taking responsibility for policy-making, for providing health care and for protecting the consumer.

767

Cannon (1992) collected and reviewed the 100 different reports published on diet in relation to the chronic diseases of affluent societies. The first country to establish such a national policy was Norway which, like its Scandinavian neighbours, sees it as natural that the government takes steps through its many departments to promote all measures necessary to encourage its population to eat a healthy diet. Thus, the Norwegians decided in 1974 to change agriculture, retail, tax and food policies in a coherent way to reduce the prevalence of CHD. Since then other governments have introduced schemes that in part attempt to rectify many of their original policies, which, after the World War II, were geared to the promotion of animal products. This led eventually to the subsidizing of structural changes in society that encouraged the consumption of an unhealthy diet. Cannon's review shows that the many committee reports are surprisingly consistent and distinguish between advice suitable for individuals and policies suitable for implementation at a population level. The new reports also specify the ideal amounts of nutrients in quantitative terms rather than simply advising people to eat less or more of a particular food. The last decade has also seen an integration of preventive programmes aimed at a range of diseases, e.g. obesity and cancer as well as heart disease.

These developments still confuse doctors, policy-makers and government officials who have been educated, until recently, in the concepts of healthy nutrition developed in the 1940s.

Table 51.1 Trends in life expectancy at birth, for different regions (both sexes combined)

Region	1950–1955	1980–1985	2020–2025 (projected)
Northern America	69.0	74.6	79.7
Europe	65.3	73.2	79.1
Oceania	60.8	68.0	75.6
The former USSR	64.1	67.9	76.7
Latin America	51.2	64.5	72.8
Asia	41.1	59.3	72.8
Africa	38.0	49.9	65.2
Developed countries	65.7	72.3	78.7
Developing countries	41.0	57.6	70.4
World total	45.9	59.6	71.3

Source: WHO 1990

Table 51.2 Causes of death in 1980 in developed and developing countries, and world total

Causes of death	Developed countries (%)	Developing countries (%)	World total (%)
Diseases of the circulatory system	54	19	26
Neoplasms	19	5	8
Infectious and parasitic diseases	8	40	33
Injury and poisoning	6	5	5
Perinatal mortality	2	8	6
All other causes	12	23	21

Source: WHO 1990

CHANGING DISEASE PATTERNS IN DEVELOPING COUNTRIES

While some developing countries remain concerned with the problems of hunger, malnutrition and communicable diseases, in others there are rapid increases in obesity, heart disease and cancers. Many countries also now have to deal with the dual problems of malnutrition in the rural areas and the chronic diseases of cardiovascular disease and cancer in the urban centres. Table 51.1 shows the estimated life expectancies of individuals from the different regions of the world in the 1950s and 1980s, and the projected changes by the years 2020–2025. Every region has seen an increase in life expectancy over the last 30 years, and this is expected to increase markedly in Africa and Asia over the next 30 years.

As infant and childhood mortality declines, the proportion and total numbers of people living into old age can be expected to increase rapidly. Thus, it can be predicted that there will be many millions of elderly in all regions of the world who, having acquired immunity to the many prevalent infections, will become susceptible to cardiovascular diseases and cancers if their dietary patterns are inappropriate. This change is already evident: if infant mortality is excluded, then cardiovascular disease and cancers already account for a very high proportion of deaths in the developing world (Table 51.2).

The stage at which cardiovascular disease 'actively emerges' as a significant cause of death corresponds to a national life-expectancy level between 50 and 60 years; cardiovascular mortality then accounts for 15–25% of all deaths. Cardiovascular diseases emerged in developing countries between 1970 and 1975, and on current projections these diseases will be established as a substantial health problem in virtually every country in the world by the year 2000.

NUTRIENT GOALS AND DIETARY GUIDELINES

Nutrient goals are the average values for a particular nutrient intake that may be considered appropriate

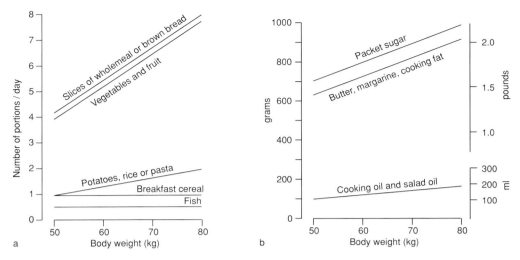

Fig. 51.1   a, Minimum recommended daily intake which should be built up to limit hunger and reduce intake of fatty foods, b, maximum recommended monthly purchases of restricted foods.

for ensuring the optimum health of a population. Alternatively, intermediate targets may be set in preference to the optimum nutrient goals; a government committee may consider the optimum to be so far removed from the prevailing intake in a society that to advocate such drastic change would appear unproductive. This pragmatic policy was developed by several Scandinavian countries, the UK and the Netherlands and was recognized by the WHO European Region as appropriate for northern Europe and perhaps now for eastern Europe.

The difference between a nutrient and a dietary goal is important. If it is considered appropriate to have, for example, an intake of complex carbohydrates corresponding to 50% of total energy intake, then this can be achieved by consuming starchy foods of a wide variety, these foods varying dramatically from one country to another. Thus in one country potatoes may make a major contribution, whereas elsewhere it may be bread, pasta, rice or a variety of other cereals. It is usual to set nutrient goals on a scientific basis but to specify dietary guidelines rather than goals so that individuals recognize that there are many culinary ways of achieving a nutrient goal; when the range of food patterns is considered that can achieve the nutrient goals, this need not be restrictive. A scheme for converting goals to guidelines for consumption and purchase of specific foods is shown in Fig. 51.1a and b (James & Ralph 1990).

The 1982 WHO committee (WHO 1982) specified that total fat intake should be 20–30% of energy, with saturated fatty acid intakes below 10%. This means that although the average national intake should com-

ply with these values, individuals' intake will vary. This distinction is important because it distinguishes between a population strategy and the prescribing of diets for individuals. This public health emphasis leads to a very different approach to policy-making because populations at risk can be specified. This means that the average level of weight, blood pressure, serum cholesterol, faecal weight or alcohol intake in a population may be seen as inappropriate because there is a very clear relationship between the mean body mass index (BMI) (weight in kg/(height in m)^2) and the proportion of the population that is obese. Similarly, as the average alcohol intake of a population increases, so does the proportion of people who may be classified as alcoholics. If this simply reflects the emergence of a distinct group of obese or alcoholic patients, then it is possible to argue that the average BMI or alcohol intake is bound to increase since there are more people with an extreme problem. In practice, a group of individuals responds to a change in any nutrient in a variable way but this response varies in a statistically normal or lognormal way. This reflects the impact of the polygenic control of the metabolic pathways involved in these responses to changes in nutrients. Only occasionally is there a distinct genetically determined subgroup of people with a very unusual response to food, e.g. gluten sensitivity, or familial hypercholesterolaemia. Thus for most conditions of public health importance the whole population tends to shift up or down as behavioural, eating and drinking patterns change. This implies that government strategies need to consider the lifestyle of the whole population and not just the high-risk groups who present themselves to their doctors with a particular condition such as diabetes or hypertension.

A further reason for considering population strategies comes from considering the attributable risk for a population. This was dealt with in Chapter 41 in relation to cardiovascular diseases but the concept applies elsewhere. Thus more lives may be saved by tackling the modest risk that applies to a very large number of people with a blood pressure or serum cholesterol that is the average for the population rather than by treating the small number of people at very high personal risk. Thus the interests of the individual and of government in a society may be very different. An individual will be happy to take a small risk of being overweight, mildly hypertensive or having a total blood cholesterol level of 5.5 mmol/1, but it is not in any government's interest to have to provide huge resources for coronary care units, stroke rehabilitation services or for all those developing type II diabetes in old age as a result of their life-long overweight.

The average individual may be content with his nutrient intake and dietary pattern but from a national perspective the distribution of intakes is too high and everybody, including this individual, needs to be encouraged to change their diet. Thus it is also a common mistake to consider people in a northern European country as having 'normal' levels of serum cholesterol. It is only when an international perspective is taken that the value of reducing the whole population's saturated fatty acid intake from 14% to, perhaps, 9% or less becomes clear.

WHO has taken a global view of diet in relation to health and produced a lower and an upper nutrient goal (Table 51.3). This is to take account of, for example, Chinese, Indonesian or southern Indian diets where fat intake is low and there is no perceived benefit from an intake as high as 30%. Therefore, lower values for these populations seem reasonable, there being either no or only modest evidence of harm when populations change between the lower and upper values. Table 51.4 includes an intermediate goal deemed by the WHO European Office (James 1988) to signify that the UK and Scandinavian countries would find a large-scale change in fat intake too daunting for immediate policy development.

Validity of nutrient goals

Inevitably there is much debate about the scientific basis for nutrient goals. Although many scientists and doctors consider that the nutrients chosen and the levels set are based on crude epidemiological analyses,

this is quite wrong. In practice committees attach far greater importance to the biological plausibility of links between nutrient intakes and disease and are often more impressed by animal experiments, clinical studies, metabolic and physiological analyses of nutrient responses and the effects of short-term clinical trials than by crude cross-cultural associations. One example relates to the level of serum cholesterol and the development of coronary heart disease. There continues to be intense debate about whether cholesterol levels are important in the development of CHD but this neglects the vital importance of the natural experiment of the homozygous hypercholesterolaemic child who dies in childhood from CHD. Studies on these children and those with the heterozygous disease clearly show that a single base change in the DNA controlling the amino acid sequence for the hepatic receptors for low density lipoprotein (LDL) can completely alter LDL uptake with a marked rise in plasma levels and fulminating heart disease. When different saturated and polyunsaturated fatty acids are then shown to modulate the activity of LDL binding and plasma levels the issue becomes one of trying to link this evidence with the severe familial form of hypercholesterolaemia. Again clinical dietary trials demonstrate the ability to slow or even reverse the narrowing of the coronary vessels but epidemiological trials are needed to see the progressive increase in risk of increasing LDL cholesterol levels. Epidemiology also highlights the presence of other factors that interact with this process and shows the overall development of CHD to be multifactorial. This, however, does not deny the role of elevated LDL cholesterol levels in promoting coronary atherosclerosis. It is now recognized that half the variation in risk is unexplained by smoking, hypertension and elevated LDL levels with support growing for the role of antioxidants. In practice, committees have to work on the basis of recognized risk factors that are biologically plausible and involved mechanistically in the disease process.

Where epidemiological analyses come into their own is when it is necessary to establish the likelihood within a population of there being people with a particular diet or disease. Rarely is it possible to have dietary intervention trials to prove that people will definitely benefit from a change in diet, although this has been attempted for CHD.

The lower fat goal of 15% was developed because of concern that too low a fat content usually signifies a bulky diet with inadequate energy intakes for young children in Africa and for very active adults, e.g. cane cutters of Central America. The goal was chosen on a judgemental basis without any detailed evaluation of

Table 51.3   Population nutrient goals

| | Limits for population average intakes | |
	Lower	Upper
Total energy	See[1]	
Total fat (% total energy)	15	30[2]
Saturated fatty acids (% total energy)	0	10
Polyunsaturated fatty acids (% total energy)	3	7
Dietary cholesterol (mg/day)	0	300
Total carbohydrate (% total energy)	55	75
Complex carbohydrate[3] (% total energy)	50	70
Dietary fibre[4] (g/day):		
As non-starch polysaccharides	16	24
As total dietary fibre	27	40
Free sugars[5] (% total energy)	0	10
Protein (% total energy)	10	15
Salt (g/day)	–[6]	6

[1]Energy intake needs to be sufficient to allow for normal childhood growth, for the needs of pregnancy and lactation, and for work and desirable physical activities, and to maintain appropriate body reserves of energy in children and adults. Adult populations on average should have a body mass index (BMI) of 20–22 (BMI = weight in kg/(height in m)^2).

[2]An interim goal for nations with high fat intakes; further benefits would be expected by reducing fat intake towards 15% of total energy.

[3]A daily minimum intake of 400 g of vegetables and fruits, including at least 30 g of pulses, nuts, and seeds, should contribute to this component.

[4]Dietary fibre includes the non-starch polysaccharides (NSP), the goals for which are based on NSP obtained from mixed food sources. Since the definition and measurement of dietary fibre remain uncertain, the goals for total dietary fibre have been estimated from the NSP values.

[5]These sugars include monosaccharides, disaccharides, and other short-chain sugars produced by refining carbohydrates.

[6]Not defined.

Source: WHO 1990

Table 51.4   Intermediate and ultimate nutrient goals for Europe

| | Intermediate goals | | Ultimate goals |
	General population	Cardiovascular high-risk group	
Energy (%)[1] derived from:			
Complex carbohydrates[2]	>40	>45	45–55
Protein	12–13	12–13	12–13
Sugar	10	10	10
Total fat	35	30	20–30
Saturated fat	15	10	10
P:S ratio[3]	≤0.5	≤1.0	≤1.0
Dietary fibre (g/day)[4]	30	>30	>30
Salt (g/day)	7–8	5	5
Cholesterol (mg/4.18 MJ)	—	<100	<100
Water fluoride (mg/l)	0.7–1.2	0.7–1.2	0.7–1.2

[1]All the values given refer to alcohol-free total energy intakes.

[2]The complex carbohydrate figures are implications of the other recommendations.

[3]This is the ratio of polyunsaturated to saturated fatty acids.

[4]Dietary fibre values are based on analytical methods that measure non-starch polysaccharide and the enzyme-resistant starch produced by food processing or cooking methods.

Alcohol intake should be limited. Iodine prophylaxis should be applied when necessary and nutrient density should be increased. A BMI of 20–25 is both an intermediate and an ultimate goal, although this value is not necessarily appropriate for the developing world, in which the average BMI may be 18 (James 1988).

fat intakes worldwide. Now it is recognized that the average fat intake in China is about 14% with only about 13% of the population having even the first degree of chronic energy deficiency, i.e. with a BMI between 17.0 and 18.4. On these fat intakes a very small proportion of the population is obese so the 15% goal may prove to be well chosen.

The upper fat goal was originally chosen on a pragmatic basis to combat CHD even though it was recognized by Keys and his colleagues that total fat intakes in Greece and Crete were about 40%, there being a substantial number of obese people but a very low rate of CHD. Whereas Keys showed neither total fat intake nor obesity as necessarily conducive to the development of CHD, elsewhere it was considered that in practice lowering the total fat intake could also reduce saturated fatty acid consumption. Alternatively, an upper fat goal was specified in an attempt to reduce the prevalence of obesity with its many complications in addition to any effect of CHD.

The upper goal for total fat intake was also established because of concerns about the prevalence of cancers in many societies with high fat diets. Since animal experiments suggested that fat intake promotes carcinogenesis (Chapter 45), cancer epidemiologists are anxious to advocate a lowering of fat intakes, perhaps even below 30%. This level is not, however, based on detailed assessment in case-control, prospective or metabolic studies of the graded effects of fat on the risk of carcinogenesis. The level must therefore be seen as one chosen pragmatically.

The proposed levels for saturated fatty acids, i.e. with an upper limit of 10% of energy intake, is recognized as arbitrary. There is a gradient of risk from levels of 1–2% in rural China to those of 20% or more in Scotland in the 1970s and in eastern Europe now. For this reason the latest WHO group specified 0% as the lower limit, recognizing that this simply signified that there was no lower limit below which there was no further reduction in risk.

The proposed goals for polyunsaturated fatty acid (PUFA) intakes are more difficult to justify. A minimum intake of essential fatty acids is considered to be about 1% of energy so the 3% value, shown in Table 51.3, is in keeping with this. Originally an upper limit of 10% was chosen but concern for the possible free radical inducing effect of high PUFA intakes has led to a moderation of this goal even though high PUFA intakes are usually accompanied by higher intakes of antioxidants such as α-tocopherol. No longer is the P:S ratio considered a suitable index because the primary benefit is thought to come from a lower saturated fatty acid intake.

Carbohydrate goals

Sugar

The goals chosen for sugar are based on the recognition that animal, clinical and epidemiological evidence all support the importance of free refined sugar in inducing dental caries, even though some scientists as well as the sugar industry are anxious to emphasize the importance of other factors of the diet. As there is no need for refined sugar in the diet, the WHO 1990 committee set the lower goal at 0% of energy intake (WHO 1990). The upper goal was chosen from epidemiological studies with a variety of other authorities suggesting goals corresponding to 7.5%–15% of energy. There has been much contention about this because claims were originally made for the role of sucrose in inducing hypertriglyceridaemia, CHD and diabetes. No recent committee has proposed these reasons for limiting sugar intakes and to do so would be unscientific on the basis of current understanding.

Non-starch polysaccharides

Only recently have attempts been made to establish goals for intakes of 'dietary fibre'. Unfortunately there is continuing controversy about what constitutes dietary fibre, the original definition being based on supposed physiological criteria, i.e. those fractions of the plant that remain undigested in the small intestine and therefore pass into the colon. This definition is difficult to use because only now are those components of the diet that do pass into the colon being identified. These include starches which traditionally were thought to be digested and absorbed in the small bowel. A new chemical and enzymatic approach has therefore been devised for measuring the total carbohydrate fraction of the plant cell wall that resists digestion by α-amylases in the intestine. These non-starch fractions of the dietary polysaccharides are found in the plant cell wall and their intake has profound effects on both the small and large intestine. There is therefore an increasing tendency to formulate studies and analyse epidemiological and physiological data in relation to non-starch polysaccharide (NSP) intakes.

A further complication comes from the widespread adoption of the Association of Official Analytical Chemists (AOAC) method for analysing dietary fibre. This relies on weighing the residue of the diet after chemical and enzymatic treatment and ashing of the diet rather than measuring the carbohydrate fraction directly. Values vary depending on food processing and the extent to which the structure of starch alters during heating and cooling. For these reasons WHO related the physiological effects of dietary fibre to the NSP content of the food.

The approach used for deciding the goals for NSP intakes are instructive. There has been great interest in the role of dietary fibre in the prevention of colonic diverticular disease and large bowel cancer but the best coherent evidence stems from the effects of NSP in preventing constipation by increasing faecal bulking. Fig. 33.3 shows the combination of a large number of physiological feeding studies in which mean daily faecal weight was the measured effect. Since constipation occurs at faecal weights below 100 g and transit times lengthen at faecal weights below 150 g, a goal of 150 g daily was used, while recognizing that because of individual variability a proportion of the population might still have constipation if the average faecal output for adults was 150 g/day. From Fig. 33.3 this corresponds to an NSP intake of about 22 g /day. The upper value of 32 g of NSP was chosen as the upper limit beyond which no further benefit had been shown. These figures of 22 and 32 g NSP obtained on northern European and American adults had to be modified to take account of the shorter, lighter populations of the world with a high proportion of children. By relating intakes to energy requirements, the lower and upper values of 16 g and 24 g of NSP were obtained, as shown in Table 52.3. This approach chose nutrient goals based on physiological and clinical criteria but took account of population analyses of energy requirements.

Complex carbohydrates

Currently these values are obtained by subtracting the specified fat and protein values from the total energy intake, because there are few criteria for specifying how much starch is required for health. Starchy foods are usually rich in micronutrients and have other effects in terms of bulking the food and slowing the passage and diffusion of nutrients, which may prove to be important. The evidence is too weak as yet, however, to allow direct development of nutrient goals.

Protein goals

These goals have often been established pragmatically on the grounds that it is unusual to find societies with protein intakes that are not between 10 and 15% of the energy intake. Recently, however, a controversy has emerged over essential amino acid requirements, which are higher in adults than previously thought. This is not an unimportant issue because the latest proposal that adults should have the same amino acid ratios as children at the minimum protein intake, triggers the need for a profound change in agricultural production to ensure that enough animal protein is eaten. Young et al (1989) believe that the FAO/WHO/UNU values for the essential amino acids are too low and they have revised them, with tacit support from FAO (1990) and WHO (1990), and the original approach was sustained by the UK COMA Panel in 1991 and by the European Community's group of nutritionists meeting in late 1992. New nutrient goals for protein may in due course emerge from detailed physiological and nutritional studies.

The WHO committee broke new ground in suggesting that a dietary as well as a nutrient goal could be developed with a healthy population eating on average 400 g of vegetables (excluding potatoes) plus fruit daily and 30 g of pulses. These values were taken from data on Mediterranean food patterns and were developed because the protective role of vegetables and fruit in relation to many diseases is difficult to assign to any specific nutrient. The choice of quantitative goals is relatively new in some countries, but is much more useful than the often meaningless suggestion that 'moderation in everything' or 'choosing a varied diet' is the key to health. These old concepts are based on folklore or ideas developed in the 1940s.

DIETARY GUIDELINES

Once nutrient goals are set, it is then the responsibility of nutritionists and dietitians to interpret these in relation to prevailing nutrient intakes and dietary patterns. Migrant studies suggest that the response to diet is surprisingly uniform in different racial and cultural groups who may have very different ways of achieving a set of nutrient goals. These goals do not therefore specify the dietary changes that are needed; dietary guidelines are, however, appropriate and can be developed as general national targets or as individual guidelines.

NATIONAL STRATEGIES FOR IMPLEMENTING CHANGES IN DIETARY PATTERNS

Governments have many responsibilities that affect the dietary patterns of the population and extend far beyond the instant assumption that health education

Table 51.5 UK government departments with responsibility for nutrition and health

Agriculture, Fisheries, Food	Education and Science
Employment	Energy
Environment	Finance
Foreign Affairs	Health
Health and Safety Commission	Home Office
Information	Social Security
Trade and Industry	Transport

is the only, or even the main, method of instituting change (Table 51.5). Social policy will affect the purchasing power of the poor and differential tax rates on food may make some items more expensive. Import/export regulations limit or extend the variety of foods available for purchase. Within the Ministries of Health and Agriculture a range of unseen policies affect the production, processing, distribution and retailing of food in ways that are rarely considered. The promotion of water fluoridation can have a marked influence on dental caries but this requires rather complex technical support and monitoring. Policies on prevention in the dental services will also influence caries rates as well as the care being provided through maternal and child health clinics. Industrial policies are also important. In western societies, for example, dairy farming has been steadily built up by government subsidy and support into a huge industry with vested interests now capable of influencing government policy on food regulation and marketing. Some industries also manipulate public perceptions through advertising and subtle promotion. Past policies based on post-war food policies have distorted the marketplace by allowing food marketing monopolies and cooperatives to develop. These vested interests frequently promote the philosophy of individual food choice rather than government policy initiatives as the appropriate mechanism for influencing dietary patterns. However, the advertising of food and drink often exceeds government health education funding by 100-fold. On this basis it is surprising that the public can discern the unbiased information of doctors and dietitians from the huge amount of other confusing and sometimes banal information on diet and health.

Government can also influence food patterns by establishing standards for catering in official institutions, such as government offices, schools, hospitals, prisons and the armed forces. Institutional caterers can also be influenced in a coordinated campaign. The Health Service also has a major responsibility for providing information, advice and practical help in changing diets since in the UK 75% of the population attends a primary health care unit each year. The opportunity for promoting appropriate eating habits is therefore substantial. It is, however, often limited by the ignorance of doctors, nurses and other health workers who do not know what constitutes a healthy diet nor how to help individuals to change their eating habits. Dietitians have a particular responsibility for educating their colleagues but traditionally they have had little involvement in evaluating the most effective ways of influencing eating behaviour and have not seen themselves as educators of their fellow professionals.

Experience worldwide has shown that very few changes occur if civil servants and politicians are left to implement policy. Traditionally, civil servants are well able to plan, analyse and respond to crises by limiting damage and protecting the status quo. Given the dominance of economics in almost all government policy-making, Departments of Health are readily overwhelmed by Ministries of Finance, Trade, Foreign Affairs and Agriculture, all of which have a profound effect on food prices and policies. Although health promotion includes the development of institutional change, Departments of Health usually end up promoting health education alone. Political pressure from voluntary or non-governmental organizations then becomes essential to ensure not only effective community involvement through the use of preexisting networks but to force Members of Parliament and Ministers to recognize their responsibility for promoting change within their own sphere. The active involvement of non-governmental organizations by Ministers of Health was therefore proposed by WHO in its analysis of the most effective ways of stimulating effective government action (WHO 1990).

Effective action is now being stimulated by government policies which set targets for changes in dietary behaviour and for achieving reductions in illnesses, e.g. obesity and premature deaths from heart disease and some cancers. This is a new strategy of the UK government, which in 1991 revolutionized its approach to nutrition policy-making by accepting that many government departments were involved. Its Cabinet-approved White Paper (Health of the Nation 1992) adjusted and even extended these targets, which requires new analyses of how public health policies can be changed. The next decade will provide many comparisons between Britain's astonishing societal change in food patterns during war-time and those developed from a different philosophy 50 years later.

REFERENCES

Cannon G 1992 Food and health: the experts agree. Consumers' Association, London

Food and Agriculture Organization 1990 Report of the Joint FAO/WHO Expert Consultation on Protein Quality Evaluation, Bethesda 1989. FAO, Rome

Health of the Nation 1992 A strategy for health in England. HMSO, London

James WPT 1988 Healthy nutrition. WHO European Series No 24. WHO, Copenhagen

James WPT, Ralph A 1990 What is a healthy diet? Medicine International 82: 3364–3368

Keys A 1980 Seven countries: a multivariate analysis of death and coronary heart disease. Harvard University Press, Harvard

Keys A, Brozek J, Henschel A, Mickelson O, Taylor HL 1950 The biology of human starvation. University of Minnesota Press, Minnesota

Taylor R 1984 The smoke ring. The politics of tobacco. Bodley Head, London

WHO 1982 Prevention of coronary heart disease. Technical Report Series No 678. WHO, Geneva

WHO 1990 Diet, nutrition and the prevention of chronic diseases. WHO Technical Report No 797. WHO, Geneva

Young VR, Bier DM, Pellet PL 1989 A theoretical basis for increasing current estimates of the amino acid requirements in adult man with experimental support. American Journal of Clinical Nutrition 50: 80–92

Appendix 1: Methods for dietary assesssment

A. Ralph

A variety of methods for assessing dietary intake of individuals or population groups is given below. (The list was prepared for a British Nutritional Epidemiology Group.) Each method has its advantages and limitations. It is important that published work giving the results of dietary assessment should include an adequate description of the technique used, so the reader can make a judgement about the reliability of the data.

DEFINITIONS OF DIETARY ASSESSMENT METHODS

Dietary assessment: A blanket term for any method. Past intake may be assessed by interview or questionnaire and present intake by records at the time of eating. Either approach may be qualitative or quantitative.

Interview techniques

Dietary questionnaire: This phrase has no precise meaning. It is not an adequate description.

1. *Diet recall*. The respondent is asked to recall the actual food and drink consumed on specific days, usually the immediate past 24 hours (24-hour recall) but sometimes for longer periods.
2. *Diet history*. The respondent is questioned about 'typical' or 'usual' food intake in a 1–2 hour interview. The aim is to construct a typical 7 days' eating pattern. The interview may discuss each meal and inter-meal period in turn or each day of the week in turn. Questions are usually open-ended, although a fully structured interview may be used. The diet history may be preceded by a 24-hour recall and/or supplemented with a check list of foods usually consumed.
3. *Food frequency (and amount) questionnaires (FFQ)*. The respondent is presented with a list of foods and is required to say how often each is eaten per day/per week/per month, etc. Food lists are usually chosen because they are important sources of the

particular nutrient under study, and may not assess total diet. The FFQ may be interviewer-administered or self-completed. Assessment of the quantities of food consumed on each eating occasion/day may also be included.

4. *Study-specific dietary questionnaire*. A term covering all dietary assessments using a set of pre-determined questions but not conforming to any of the classic techniques defined above. The method is defined only by the questionnaire itself. The questionnaire may be interviewer-administered or self-completed.

Record techniques

Diet record is a blanket term for all record methods. In American literature the term is often used without qualification but with 'quantified in household measures' understood. Since there are other forms of records, it is an inadequate description. A record is of actual food and drink consumed on specified days after the first contact by the investigator. The usual number of days recorded is 7 but may be fewer or more.

1. *Menu record (or food frequency record)* (the first term is preferable to avoid confusion with FFQ). Record obtained without quantifying the portions. It may be subsequently analysed in terms of frequencies of consumption, or the investigator may assign 'average' weights to portions. Because the respondent does not indicate quantity, there can be no attempt to identify the true weight of individual portions (cf estimated record).
2. *Estimated record*. A record with portions described in household measures (cups, spoons, etc.) with/without the aid of diagrams or photographs. This method aims to estimate the actual quantity eaten.
3. *Weighed record (weighed inventory technique)*. Record with weights of portions as served and the plate

waste. (Weighed records are rarely fully weighed; estimated portions are usual for food eaten away from home.)

4. *Precise weighed record.* A record kept by the respondent of all ingredients used in the preparation of meals, also inedible waste, total cooked weight of meal items, cooked weight of individual portions and plate waste.

5. *Cardiff photographic record.* Respondents photograph food on the plate at the time of consumption. Portions are quantified by comparison with reference photographs of portions of known weight projected alongside the survey photographs (Elwood & Bird 1983).

6. *Semi-weighed method for measuring family food intake.* Method of Nelson & Nettleton (1980). Total quantity of food served to a family is weighed and quantities served to individuals are given in household measures. The term is sometimes mistakenly used for a weighed diet record where the authors acknowledge that not all food is in fact weighed.

Techniques of direct analysis

1. *Duplicate diets.* Respondents keep a weighed record and also weigh out and put aside a duplicate portion of each food as consumed for later analysis by the investigator.

2. *Aliquot sampling technique.* Respondent keeps a weighed record and puts aside aliquot samples of food as consumed for later analysis.

3. *Equivalent composite technique.* Respondent keeps a weighed record. Subsequently a combined sample of raw foods, equivalent to the mean daily amounts of foods eaten, is made up by the investigator for analysis.

It should be noted that in some situations the foods need to be described in some detail bcause the preparation or cooking method or variety may be relevant to the study.

A checklist of information which should be provided when writing a report or publishing work on dietary assessment is shown in Table A1.1. These points also should be noted when reading such a study.

Table A1.1   Checklist of information required for dietary surveys

Sample characteristics	
Sample (and control) recruitment	How subjects were recruited Sampling framework Numbers contacted, recruited and completing study Reasons for non-completion Use of incentives
Sample (and Control) characteristics	Age, sex, height, weight, social class Other demographic/clinical information Whether sample represents the population studied Geographic coverage
Other information relevant to response or interpretation of results	Timing in relation to disease processes Timing in relation to interventions Timing in relation to season
Method of dietary assessment	
Information required for all methods	
Method of dietary assessment	See definitions above
Validity of the method	Rationale for choice of method Have techniques used been pre-tested on a similar population? Has method been validated against another dietary method or external markers of intake? Has the repeatability been assessed?
Methods used for quantifying portions	See definitions below Specify: Source of 'average' portions Details of aids used to help quantifying portions Scales used for weighing Method for quantifying unweighed foods in a weighed record

Table A1.1   Checklist of information required for dietary surveys – *contd*

Method of dietary assessment

Information required for all methods

Food composition database used for the anlysis	Which database was used? How foods were dealt with which were not in the database Any supplementary analytical work
Interviewers or field workers	Whether qualified (dietitians/nutritionists) Training given to unqualified field workers Have the same workers both collected data and coded it for analysis?
Data collection procedures	Where and how data were collected (home/clinic/by interview —face to face or telephone/self-completed—by post or by computer) Number of interviews per subject Duration of interviews
Checking procedures	When and how often were records checked over with respondents Any checks for coding errors Any checks on the consistency of field workers

Information required specific to different methods

Recall method	How many and which days recalled Were all days of the week included? If not, were results weighted?
Diet history	Attempted time scale (current/recent distant past/past/season/whole year) Open-ended questions or fully structured interview Structure of interview (Did it start with a 24-hour recall? Did it take each meal or each day of the week in turn to build up a picture of the diet? Did it include any cross checks for types or frequency of foods consumed? Were the subjects given any prompt lists?)
Food frequency (and amount) questionnaires	Whether interviewer-administered or self-completed Rationale for the choice of foods Was the technique pre-tested in a similar population? Foods covered and options for frequency
Study-specific questionnaires	Was it interviewer-administered or self-completed? Rationale for the form of the questionnaire Was the technique pre-tested in a similar population? Include the questionnaire as an appendix
All record methods	How many and which days were studied Were all days of the week included? (If not, was any adjusment or weighting used?) How food eaten away from home was quantified What instructions and equipment were given to the respondent

GENERAL NOTE ON QUESTIONNAIRES

It is desirable for the questionnaire to be included as an appendix even if much reduced in size. This best describes the methods since it shows the questions asked and the foods and frequencies chosen. For the instrument to be 'available from the authors' is unsatisfactory, since it does not permit immediate evaluation of the study and in later years is unobtainable. At the very least a copy of the questionnaire must be made available for review purposes.

Definitions: quantifying portions

Qualitative (or unquantified) assessment: An assessment made only in terms of foods eaten, usually by counting the frequency of consumption.

Quantitative assessment: A dietary assessment that quantifies the portions of foods eaten in order to calculate nutrient consumption.

A. *Average portions.* The investigator assigns 'average' portion weights derived from previous studies, experience or publications, e.g. Crawley (1988). 'Small', 'medium' or 'large' may also be used to indicate portion size in relation to the 'average'.
B. *Household measures.* The respondent describes portions in terms of household measures, e.g. cups, spoons, etc. 'Standard' weights are assigned to the descriptions.

Photographic measures. Respondent is shown photographs of portions of known weight and asked how their own portion relates to the pictured portion. (Not to be confused with the Cardiff Photographic Record, see above.)

Food models/replicas. Respondent is shown three-dimensional models representing foods and asked how their own portion relates to the models. Models may be realistic replica foods or a variety of neutral shapes and sizes.

Weighed. The subject weighs and records each food item as it is consumed.

COMPUTERIZED ASSESSMENTS

The phrase 'computer assessment' does not define a method. Assessments conducted by computer should be described in the terms defined above.

Computer-conducted assessments differ from person-conducted assessments in the mechanics used. The computer may substitute for the paper and pencil of a self-completion questionnaire or it may substitute for the interviewer in a diet history by fully-structured interview.

Computerized interviewing may be combined with nutrient analysis to provide 'instant' information on nutrient intake. Here the assumptions necessary to code foods and quantify portions are built into the programme. The computer substitutes for the investigator in performing the post-interview coding tasks.

COMPARISON OF METHODS AND USE OF DATA

A detailed and extensive account of the methodology of food consumption studies is given in Cameron & Van Staveren (1988). The book was produced by the International Union of Nutritional Sciences (IUNS) and EURO-NUT, the Concerted Action Programme on Diet and Health of the Commission of European Communities. One chapter is devoted to the coding of foods and the conversion to nutrients using different analyses, food tables and databases. Further reviews and recommendations on methods of collection of dietary intake data are given by Bingham (1987, 1991), who places particular emphasis on the importance of the validity and precision of methods. Possible sources of error are shown in Table A1.2.

Analysis of coefficient of variation within individuals, between individuals and between methods shows that some of these errors are random, and precision can be improved by increasing the number of observations on each individual, or the numbers in a group. A more serious potential source of error is a systematic bias, due either to different methods of dietary assessment or from consistent over- or under-reporting by the subjects. Independent methods for validating dietary assessments, such as the 24-hour urine nitrogen output or the doubly-labelled water technique (see Chapter 3), should be included in any study of the free-living individual.

Table A1.2   Sources of error in dietary surveys

Source of error	Records with weight	Records with estimated weights	Daily recalls	Dietary histories and questionnaires
Food tables	+	+	+	+
Coding errors	+	+	+	+
Wrong weights of food	−	+	+	+
Reporting error	−	−	+	+
Variation with time	+	+	+	−
Wrong frequency of consumption	−	−	−	+
Change in diet	±	±	−	−
Response bias	±	±	±	±
Sampling bias	+	+	+	+

+ = Error known to be present; − = error not present; ± = error may be present.
From Bingham (1991)

Accuracy requires freedom from both random error and bias.

Dietary intake may be used, along with health data, in policy making. Per capita food consumptions estimated from national food balance sheets, or from institutions or households give no indication of individual variation. A critical assessment of how different sources of data may be used, and their limitations, is given in a book produced by the World Health Organization (WHO 1991).

REFERENCES

Bingham SA 1987 The dietary assessment of individuals; methods, accuracy, new techniques and recommendations. Nutrition Abstracts and Reviews (Series A) 57: 705–742

Bingham SA 1991 Limitations of the various methods for collecting dietary intake data. Annals of Nutrition and Metabolism 35: 117–127

Cameron ME, Van Staveren WA 1988 Manual on methodology for food consumption studies. Oxford University Press, Oxford

Crawley H 1988 Food portion sizes. Ministry of Agriculture, Fisheries and Food, HMSO, London

Elwood PC, Bird G 1983 A photographic method of diet evaluation. Human Nutrition: Applied Nutrition 37A: 474–477

Nelson M, Nettelton PA 1980 Dietary survey methods. 1. A semi-weighed technique for measuring dietary intake within families. Journal of Human Nutrition 34: 325–348

World Health Organization 1991 Food and health data. Their use in nutrition policy-making. WHO Regional Publications, European Series No 34, Copenhagen

Appendix 2: Dietary reference values

A. Ralph

Tables of dietary reference values:

TERMINOLOGY

United Kingdom (Department of Health 1991)

Dietary reference values (DRVs), revised in 1991, were previously known as recommended daily amounts (RDAs). The term applies to the range of intakes based on an assessment of the distribution of requirements for each nutrient. DRVs apply to groups of healthy people and are not appropriate for those with disease or metabolic abnormalities. The DRVs for one nutrient presuppose that requirements for energy and all other nutrients are met. For most nutrients, three values are given:

LRNI	Lower reference nutrient intake, 2 SD below EAR.
EAR	Estimated average requirement which assumes normal distribution of variability.
RNI	Reference Nutrient Intake, 2 SD above EAR. Where only one value is given in summary tables, this is the value chosen.
Safe intakes	Some nutrients are known to be important but there is insufficient data on human requirements to set any DRVs. A safe intake was judged to be a level or range of intakes above which there is no risk of deficiency and below a level where there is a risk of undesirable effects.
Individual minimum Individual maximum Population averages	Used for specifying carbohydrates (fibre) and fat needs

United States of America (National Research Council 1989)

The RDAs were revised in 1989 and are jointly produced by the Food and Nutrition Board, the National Academy of Sciences and the National Research Council. They are designed for the maintenance of good nutrition of practically all healthy people in the USA.

782

RDA — This is the average daily intake over time; it provides for individual variations among most normal persons living in the USA under the usual environmental stresses.

Safe intake — Estimated safe intakes and adequate daily dietary intakes are given for some vitamins and minerals where there is less information on which to base allowances, and figures are provided in the form of ranges of recommended intakes. Since the toxic levels for many trace elements may not be much greater than the safe intakes, e.g. for copper, these safe levels should not be habitually exceeded.

Europe, EC

European values are currently (1992) being revised and the values given here were provided prior to final publication of the report. Carbohydrate, fat and non-starch polysaccharide population goals are from James (1988).

LTI — Lowest threshold intake.
ARI — Average requirement intake.
PRI — Population reference intake: mean requirement +2 SD. This is the value chosen for most of the tables in this Appendix.
Acceptable range — Range of safe values given where insufficient information is available to be more specific.

World Health Organization (WHO 1974, 1988, 1990, 1992, FAO/WHO 1988, FAO/WHO/UNU 1985)

The WHO requirements have been revised for groups of nutrients at different times. The dates of the revisions are therefore given in the appropriate table. The trace elements are the most recent revision (1992); carbohydrate, fat, non-starch polysaccharides (1990); vitamin A, iron, folate and vitamin B_{12} (FAO/WHO 1988); energy and protein (FAO/WHO/UNU 1985); other nutrients (1974).

Population requirement safe ranges (1992)
Basal — Lower limit of safe ranges of population mean intakes.
Normative — Population mean intake sufficient to meet normative requirements. This value is used in most of the tables in the Appendix.

Maximum — Upper limit of safe ranges of population mean intakes.

Recommended intakes (1974)
Average requirement augmented by a factor that takes into account inter-individual variability. The amounts are considered sufficient for the maintenance of health in nearly all people.

UNITS

These vary for different nutrients

Energy (kcal/day, kJ/day or MJ/day)

All energy values are based on the Schofield equations (FAO/WHO/UNU 1985) and so should be similar for each source. Any variation occurs because the equations are based on weight and activity within broad age bands. The mean weight and activity level used for each age band is not the same in each source. Details of this are given in Chapter 3.

Carbohydrate and fat

These are expressed as a percentage of total energy intake, including 5% alcohol, or as a percentage of food energy, excluding alcohol.

Protein (g/day or g/kg/day)

Protein requirements are all based on the FAO/WHO/UNU 1985 Report and, like energy, should be similar from various sources, the only difference being the average weight chosen for each age group. Requirements for specific amino acids are discussed in Chapter 5.

Most nutrients (g/day, mg/day or μg/day)

Some nutrient interactions:

Niacin: mg/1000 kcal or mg/MJ
Vitamin B_6: μg/g protein
Vitamin E: mg/g polyunsaturated fatty acids

Iron, zinc

Requirements depend on the bioavailability of the diet, which may be low, moderate or high (Chapter 12). In this Appendix levels were chosen for medium availability from WHO values. The UK and the USA values assume western diets of high availability.

AGE BANDS

The different national and international sources of data have used slightly different age bands in some instances. Where necessary these have been adjusted to correspond as closely as possible with the most frequently used age bands.

REFERENCES

Department of Health 1991 Report on Health and Social Subjects, 41. Dietary reference values for food energy and nutrients for the United Kingdom. Committee on Medical Aspects of Food Policy. HMSO, London

EEC Scientific Committee for Food 1992 Reference nutrient intakes for the European Community. EC, Brussels (in press)

FAO/WHO 1988 Requirements for vitamin A, iron, folate and vitamin B_{12}. Report of a joint FAO/WHO expert consultation. Food and Nutrition Series. FAO, Rome

FAO/WHO/UNU 1985 Energy and protein requirements. Report of a joint FAO/WHO/UNU expert consultation. Technical Report Series, 724. WHO, Geneva

James WPT 1988 Healthy nutrition. Preventing nutrition-related diseases in Europe. WHO Regional Publications, European Series No 24. WHO, Copenhagen

National Research Council, Food and Nutrition Board, Commission on Life Sciences 1989 Recommended dietary allowances, 10th edn. National Academy Press, Washington, DC

WHO 1974 Handbook on human nutritional requirements. Monograph Series No 61. WHO, Geneva

WHO 1990 Diet, nutrition, and the prevention of chronic diseases. Technical Report Series 797. WHO, Geneva

WHO 1992 Trace elements in human nutrition. WHO, Geneva (in press)

Table A2.1a   Dietary reference values for energy for males

| Age | UK and WHO EAR | | USA AER[1] | | European | |
	(MJ/day)	(kcal/day)	(MJ/day)	(kcal/day)	Lower[2,4] (MJ/day)	Higher[3] (MJ/day)
0–3 months	2.28	545	2.7	650	2.3	
4–6 months	2.89	690	2.7	650	3.0	
7–9 months	3.44	825	3.5	850	3.5	
10–12 months	3.85	920	3.5	850	3.9	
1–3 years	5.15	1230	5.4	1300	5.3	
4–6 years	7.16	1715	7.5	1800	7.2	
7–10 years	8.24	1970	8.3	2000	8.2	
11–14 years	9.27	2220	10.4	2500	9.4	
15–18 years	11.51	2755	12.5	3000	11.6	
19–50 years	10.60	2550	12.1	2900	11.3	12.0
51–59 years	10.60	2550	9.6	2300	11.3	12.0
60–64 years	9.93	2380	9.6	2300	8.5	9.2
65–74 years	9.71	2330	9.6	2300	8.5	9.2
75+years	8.77	2100	9.6	2300	7.5	8.5

[1]Average Energy Allowance
[2]No physical activity
[3]Desirable physical activity } + desirable body weight for adults
[4]Children's values are Estimated Average Requirement

Table A2.1b   Dietary reference values for energy for females

| Age | UK and WHO EAR | | USA AER[1] | | European | |
	(MJ/day)	(kcal/day)	(MJ/day)	(kcal/day)	Lower[2,4] (MJ/day)	Higher[3] (MJ/day)
0–3 months	2.16	515	2.7	650	2.1	
4–6 months	2.69	645	2.7	650	2.8	
7–9 months	3.20	765	3.5	850	3.3	
10–12 months	3.61	865	3.5	850	3.7	
1–3 years	4.86	1165	5.4	1300	5.0	
4–6 years	6.46	1545	7.5	1800	6.6	
7–10 years	7.28	1740	8.3	2000	7.4	
11–14 years	7.92	1845	9.2	2200	8.0	
15–18 years	8.83	2110	9.2	2200	8.8	
19–50 years	8.10	1940	9.2	2200	8.4	9.0
51–59 years	8.00	1900	9.2	2200	8.4	9.0
60–64 years	7.99	1900	9.2	2200	7.0	7.7
65–74 years	7.96	1900	9.2	2200	7.0	7.7
75+ years	7.61	1810	9.2	2200	6.7	7.6
Pregnancy	+0.80[5]	+200[5]	+1.2	+300		
Lactation	+1.9–2.0	+450–480	+2.1	+500	+1.5–1.7	

[1]Average Energy Allowance
[2]No physical activity
[3]Desirable physical activity } + desirable body weight for adults
[4]Children's values are Estimated Average Requirement
[5]Last trimester

Table A2.2   Dietary reference values for protein (g/day)

Age	UK and WHO EAR[1]	UK and WHO RNI[1]	USA RDA	European PRI[3]
0–3 months	—[2]	12.5[2]	13.0	
4–6 months	10.6	12.7	13.0	14.0
7–9 months	11.0	13.7	14.0	14.5
10–12 months	11.2	14.9	14.0	14.5
1–3 years	11.7	14.5	16.0	14.7
4–6 years	14.8	19.7	24.0	19.0
7–10 years	22.8	28.3	28.0	27.3
Males				
11–14 years	33.8	42.1	45.0	42.0
15–18 years	46.1	55.2	59.0	48.5
19–50 years	44.4	55.5	60.0	55.0
50+ years	42.6	53.3	63.0	55.0
Females				
11–14 years	33.1	41.2	46.0	39.7
15–18 years	37.1	45.0	44.0	51.4
19–50+ years	36.0	45.0	46.0	47.0
50+ years	37.2	46.5	50.0	47.0
Pregnancy		+6	60.0	48–60
Lactation		+11	65.0	63.0

[1]Based on egg and milk protein, assume complete digestibility
[2]No WHO value
[3]Children's values are safe levels

Table A2.3   Dietary reference values for fat and carbohydrate for adults as a percentage of daily total energy intake (percentage food energy[1])

	UK Individual minimum	UK Population average[1]	UK Individual maximum	USA RDA	WHO (1990) Lower[2]	WHO (1990) Upper[2]	European PRI[3] or goal[4]
Saturated fatty acids		10(11)		<10	0	10	10[4]
Cis-polyunsaturated fatty acids		6(6.5)	10	7	3	7	
	n-3 0.2						0.5[3]
	n-6 1.0						2.0[3]
Cis-monounsaturated fatty acids		12(13)					
Trans-fatty acids		2(2)					
Total fatty acids		30(32.5)					
Total fat		33(35)		<30	15	30	20–30[4]
Non-milk extrinsic sugars	0	10(11)			0	10	10[4]
Intrinsic milk sugars and starch		37(39)					
Total carbohydrate		47(50)		>50	55	75	55–65[4]
Non-starch polysaccharide (g/day)	12	18	24		16	24	30[4]

[1]Total energy intake assumes 5% alcohol; food energy (in parenthesis) excludes alcohol
[2]Population nutrient goal
[3]Population Reference Intake
[4]Ultimate goal

Table A2.4   Dietary reference values for vitamin A (µg retinol equivalent/day)

Age	UK			USA RDA	WHO (1988) safe level[1]	European PRI
	LNRI	EAR	RNI			
0–12 months	150	250	350	375	350	350
1–3 years	200	300	400	400	400	400
4–6 years	200	300	400	500	400	400
7–10 years	250	350	500	700	400	500
Males						
11–14 years	250	400	600	1000	550	600
15–50+ years	300	500	700	1000	600	700
Females						
11–50+ years	250	400	600	800	500	600
Pregnancy			+100	⋆	600	⋆
Lactation			+350	1300	850	⋆

⋆No increment
[1]Safe level = upper end of normative storage requirement

Table A2.5   Dietary reference values for vitamin D (µg/day)

Age	UK RNI	USA RDA	WHO RNI (1970)	European safe range
Males and females				
0–6 months	8.5	7.5	10	10–25
7 months–3 years	7.0	10	10	10–25
4–6 years	0[1]	10	10	5–15
7–10 years	0[1]	10	2.5	5–15
11–24 years	0[1]	10	2.5	10–15
25–50+ years	0[1]	5	2.5	0–15
65+ years	10	5	2.5	10–15
Pregnancy and lactation	10	10	10	10–15

[1]If exposed to the sun

Table A2.6   Dietary reference values for vitamin E (mg/day α-tocopherol) (No WHO values available)

Age	UK safe intake	USA RDA	European PRI
0–6 months	0.4 mg/g PUFA[1]	3	0.4 mg/g PUFA[1]
7–12 months	0.4 mg/g PUFA[1]	4	0.4 mg/g PUFA[1]
1–3 years	0.4 mg/g PUFA[1]	6	0.4 mg/g PUFA[1]
4–10 years		7	
Males			
11–50+ years	> 4	10	> 4
Females			
11–50+ years	> 3	8	> 3
Pregnancy		10	
Lactation		12	

[1]PUFA = polyunsaturated fatty acid

Table A2.7   Dietary reference values for vitamin K (µg/day) (No WHO or European values available)

Age	UK safe intake	USA RDA
0–6 months	10	5
7–12 months	10	10
1–3 years		15
4–10 years		20
7–10 years		30
Males		
11–14 years	1 µg/kg body weight	45
15–18 years	1 µg/kg body weight	65
19–24 years	1 µg/kg body weight	75
25+ years	1 µg/kg body weight	80
Females		
11–14 years	1 µg/kg body weight	45
15–18 years	1 µg/kg body weight	55
19–24 years	1 µg/kg body weight	60
25+ years	1 µg/kg body weight	65
Pregnancy	1 µg/kg body weight	65
Lactation	1 µg/kg body weight	65

Table A2.8 Dietary reference values for vitamin C (mg/day)

Age	UK			USA RDA	WHO RNI (1970)	European PRI
	LNRI	EAR	RNI			
0–6 months	6	15	25	30	20	
7–12 months	6	15	25	35	20	20
1–3 years	8	20	30	40	20	25
4–6 years	8	20	30	45	20	25
7–10 years	8	20	30	45	20	30
Males						
11–14 years	9	22	35	50	30	35
15–50+ years	10	25	40	60	30	45
Females						
11–14 years	9	22	35	50	30	35
15–50+ years	10	25	40	60	30	40
Pregnancy			+10	70	50	50
Lactation			+30	95	50	65

Table A2.9 Dietary reference values for thiamin

Age	UK			UK RNI (mg/day)	USA RDA (mg/day)	WHO RNI (1970) (mg/day)	European PRI (mg/day)
	LNRI (mg/1000 kcal)	EAR (mg/1000 kcal)	RNI (mg/1000 kcal)				
0–6 months	0.2	0.23	0.3	0.2	0.3	0.3	
7–12 months	0.2	0.23	0.3	0.3	0.4	0.3	0.3
1–3 years	0.23	0.3	0.4	0.5	0.7	0.5	0.5
4–6 years	0.23	0.3	0.4	0.7	0.9	0.7	0.7
7–10 years	0.23	0.3	0.4	0.7	1.0	0.9	0.8
Males							
11–14 years	0.23	0.3	0.4	0.9	1.3	1.2	1.0
15–50+ years	0.23	0.3	0.4	0.9	1.2	1.2	1.1
Females							
11–14 years	0.23	0.3	0.4	0.7	1.1	1.0	0.8
15–50+ years	0.23	0.3	0.4	0.8	1.0	0.9	0.9
Pregnancy	0.23	0.3	0.4	+0.1[1]	1.5	+0.1	1.0
Lactation	0.23	0.3	0.4	+0.2	1.6	+0.2	1.1

[1]For last trimester only

Table A2.10 Dietary reference values for riboflavin (mg/day)

Age	UK			USA RDA	WHO RNI (1965)	European PRI
	LNRI	EAR	RNI			
0–6 months	0.2	0.3	0.4	0.4	0.5	
7–12 months	0.2	0.3	0.4	0.5	0.5	0.4
1–3 years	0.3	0.5	0.6	0.8	0.8	0.7
4–6 years	0.4	0.6	0.8	1.1	1.1	1.0
7–10 years	0.5	0.8	1.0	1.2	1.3	1.1
Males						
11–14 years	0.8	1.0	1.2	1.5	1.7	1.3
15–18 years	0.8	1.0	1.3	1.8	1.8	1.6
19–50 years	0.8	1.0	1.3	1.7	1.8	1.6
50+ years	0.8	1.0	1.3	1.4	1.8	1.6
Females						
11–14 years	0.8	0.9	1.1	1.3	1.5	1.0
15–50+ years	0.8	0.9	1.1	1.2	1.3	1.4
Pregnancy			+0.3	1.6	+0.2	1.7
Lactation			+0.5	1.8	+0.4	1.7

Table A2.11 Dietary reference values for niacin (nicotinic acid equivalent)

Age	UK			UK	USA	WHO	European
	LNRI (mg/1000 kcal)	EAR (mg/1000 kcal)	RNI (mg/1000 kcal)	RNI (mg/day)	RDA (mg/day)	RNI (1970) (mg/day)	PRI[1] (mg/day)
0–6 months	4.4	5.5	6.6	3	5	5.4	
7–12 months	4.4	5.5	6.6	5	6	5.4	5
1–3 years	4.4	5.5	6.6	8	9	9.0	8
4–6 years	4.4	5.5	6.6	11	12	12.1	11
7–10 years	4.4	5.5	6.6	12	13	14.5	12
Males							
11–14 years	4.4	5.5	6.6	15	17	19.1	18
15–18 years	4.4	5.5	6.6	18	20	20.3	18
19–50 years	4.4	5.5	6.6	17	19	18.8	18
50+ years	4.4	5.5	6.6	16	15	19.8	18
Females							
11–14 years	4.4	5.5	6.6	12	15	16.4	14
15–18 years	4.4	5.5	6.6	14	15	15.2	14
19–50 years	4.4	5.5	6.6	13	15	14.5	14
50+ years	4.4	5.5	6.6	12	13	14.5	14
Pregnancy	★	★	★	★	17	+2.3	★
Lactation	★	★	+2.3 mg/day	+2	20	+3.7	+2

★No increment
[1]1.6 mg/MJ

Table A2.12 Dietary reference values for vitamin B$_6$ (No WHO values available)

Age	UK			UK	USA	European
	LNRI (µg/g protein)	EAR (µg/g protein)	RNI (µg/g protein)	RNI (mg/day)	RDA (mg/day)	PRI[1] (mg/day)
0–6 months	3.5	6	8	0.2	0.3	
7–9 months	6	8	10	0.3	0.6	0.4
10–12 months	8	10	13	0.4	0.6	0.4
1–3 years	8	10	13	0.7	1.0	0.7
4–6 years	8	10	13	0.9	1.1	0.9
7–10 years	8	10	13	1.0	1.4	1.0
Males						
11–14 years	11	13	15	1.2	1.7	1.3
15–18 years	11	13	15	1.5	2.0	1.5
19–50+ years	11	13	15	1.4	2.0	1.5
Females						
11–14 years	11	13	15	1.0	1.4	1.1
15–18 years	11	13	15	1.2	1.5	1.1
19–50+ years	11	13	15	1.2	1.6	1.1
Pregnancy	★	★	★	★	2.2	1.3
Lactation	★	★	★	★	2.1	1.3

★No increment
[1]15 µg/g protein

Table A2.13   Dietary reference values for folate (µg/day)

Age	UK			USA RDA	WHO (1988) safe level[1]	European PRI
	LNRI	EAR	RNI			
0–3 months	30	40	50	25	16	50
4–6 months	30	40	50	25	24	50
7–12 months	30	40	50	35	32	50
1–3 years	35	50	70	50	50	90
4–6 years	50	75	100	75	50	120
7–10 years	75	110	150	100	102	140
Males						
11–14 years	100	150	200	150	170	160
15–50+ years	100	150	200	200	200	200
Females						
11–14 years	100	150	200	150	170	160
15–50+ years	100	150	200	180	170	200
Pregnancy			+100	400	370–470	400
Lactation			+60	280	270	350

[1]Based on normative storage requirement with 15% coefficient of variation

Table A2.14   Dietary reference values for vitamin B_{12} (µg/day)

Age	UK			USA RDA	WHO (1988) safe level	European PRI
	LNRI	EAR	RNI			
0–6 months	0.1	0.25	0.3	0.3	0.1	
7–12 months	0.25	0.35	0.4	0.5	0.1	0.5
1–3 years	0.3	0.4	0.5	0.7	0.5	0.6
4–6 years	0.5	0.7	0.8	1.0	0.8	0.9
7–10 years	0.6	0.8	1.0	1.4	1.0	1.0
Males						
11–14 years	0.8	1.0	1.2	1.7	1.0	1.2
15–50+ years	1.0	1.25	1.5	2.0	1.0	1.4
Females						
11–14 years	0.8	1.0	1.2	1.4	1.0	1.2
15–50+ years	1.0	1.25	1.5	1.5	1.0	1.4
Pregnancy			★	2.2	1.4	1.6
Lactation			+0.5	2.6	1.3	1.9

★No increment

Table A2.15   Dietary reference values for biotin (µg/day) (No WHO values available)

Age	UK safe intake	USA RDA	European acceptable range
0–6 months		10	
7–12 months		15	
1–3 years		20	
4–10 years		25–30	
Males and females			
11–50+ years	10–20	30–100	15–70

Table A2.16   Dietary reference values for pantothenic acid (mg/day) (No WHO values available)

Age	UK safe intake	USA RDA	European acceptable range
0–6 months	1.7	2.0	
7–12 months	1.7	3.0	
1–3 years	1.7	3.0	
4–10 years	3–7	3–5	
Males and females			
11–50+ years	3–7	4–7	3–12

Table A2.17   Dietary reference values for calcium (mg/day)

Age	UK			USA RDA	WHO RNI (1961)	European PRI
	LNRI	EAR	RNI			
0–6 months	240	400	525	400	500	
7–12 months	240	400	525	600	600	400
1–3 years	200	275	350	800	400	400
4–6 years	275	350	450	800	450	450
7–10 years	325	425	550	800	500	550
Males						
11–14 years	450	750	1000	1200	600–700	1000
15–18 years	450	750	1000	1200	500–600	1000
19–24 years	400	525	700	1200	400–500	700
25–50 years	400	525	700	800	400–500	700
15–50+ years	400	525	700	800	400–500	700
Females						
11–14 years	480	625	800	1200	600–700	800
15–18 years	480	625	800	1200	500–600	800
19–24 years	400	525	700	1200	400–500	700
25–50 years	400	525	700	800	400–500	700
50+ years	400	525	700	800	400–500	700
Pregnancy	★	★	★	1200	1000–1200	★
Lactation			+550	1200	1000–1200	+500

★ No increment

Table A2.18   Dietary reference values for phosphorus (mg/day) (No WHO values available)

Age	UK RNI[1]	USA RDA	European PRI
0–6 months	400	300	
7–12 months	400	500	310
1–3 years	270	800	310
4–10 years	350	800	350–450
Males			
11–18 years	775	1200	775
19–24 years	550	1200	540
25–50 years	550	800	540
50+ years	550	800	540
Females			
11–18 years	625	1200	625
19–24 years	550	1200	540
25–50+ years	550	800	540
Pregnancy	★	1200	540
Lactation	+440	1200	+400

★No increment
[1]Phosphorus RNI is set equal to calcium in molar terms

Table A2.19   Dietary reference values for magnesium (mg/day)

Age	UK			USA RDA	WHO (1974) RNI	European acceptable range
	LNRI	EAR	RNI			
0–3 months	30	40	55	40		
4–6 months	40	50	60	40		
7–9 months	45	60	75	60		
10–12 months	45	60	80	60		
1–3 years	50	65	85	80		
4–6 years	70	90	120	120		
7–10 years	115	150	200	170		
Males						
11–14 years	180	230	280	270		
15–18 years	190	250	280	400		
19–50+ years	190	250	300	350	200–300	150–500
Females						
11–14 years	180	230	280	280		
15–18 years	190	250	300	300		
19–50 years	190	250	300	280	200–300	150–500
50+ years	150	200	270	280		
Pregnancy	★	★	★	320		
Lactation			+50	355		

★No increment

Table A2.20   Dietary reference values for sodium (mg/day[1])

Age	UK		USA minimum requirement[2]	WHO population average[3]	European acceptable range
	LNRI	RNI			
0–3 months	140	210	120		
4–6 months	140	280	120		
7–9 months	200	320	200		
10–12 months	200	350	200		
1–3 years	200	500	225		
4–6 years	280	700	300		575–3500
7–10 years	350	1200	400		575–3500
Males and females					
11–14 years	460	1600	500		575–3500
15–50+ years	575	1600	500	3900	575–3500
Pregnancy	★	★			★
Lactation	★	★			★

★   No increment
[1]1 mmol sodium = 23 mg
[2]No allowance for large losses, from the skin through sweat
[3]Upper limit

Table A2.21   Dietary reference values for potassium (mg/day[1]) (No WHO values available)

Age	UK		USA minimum requirement[2]	European PRI
	LNRI	RNI		
0–3 months	400	800	500	
4–6 months	400	850	500	
7–9 months	400	700	700	800
10–12 months	450	700	700	800
1–3 years	450	800	1000	800
4–6 years	600	1100	1400	1100
7–10 years	950	2200	1600	2000
Males and females				
11–14 years	1600	3100	2000	3100
15–50+ years	2000	3500	2000	3100
Pregnancy	★	★	★	★
Lactation	★	★	★	★

★No increment
[1] 1 mmol potassium = 39 mg
[2] Desirable intakes may exceed these values (3500 mg for adults)

Table A2.22   Dietary reference values for chloride (mg/day) (No WHO values available)

Age	UK RNI[1]	USA minimum requirement[2]	European acceptable range[1]
0–3 months	320	180	
4–6 months	400	300	
7–9 months	500	300	
10–12 months	500	300	
1–3 years	800	350	
4–6 years	1100	500	
7–10 years	1100	600	
Males and females			
11–50+ years	2500	750	Should match sodium intake
Pregnancy	★	★	★
Lactation	★	★	★

★No increment
[1] Corresponds to sodium. 1 mmol = 35.5 mg
[2] No allowance for large losses from the skin through sweat

Table A2.23 Dietary reference values for iron[1] (mg/day)

Age	UK			USA RDA	WHO[2]	Europe[3]
	LNRI	EAR	RNI			
0–3 months	0.9	1.3	1.7	6	—	
4–6 months	2.3	3.3	4.3	6	8.5	
7–12 months	4.2	6.0	7.8	10	8.5	6
1–3 years	3.7	5.3	6.9	10	5.0	4
4–6 years	3.3	4.7	6.1	10	5.5	4
7–10 years	4.7	6.7	8.7	10	9.5	6
Males						
11–14 years	6.1	8.7	11.3	12	15.0	10
15–18 years	6.1	8.7	11.3	12	9.0	13
19–50+ years	4.7	6.7	8.7	10	9.0	9
Females						
11–14 years	8.0	11.4	14.8[4]	15	16.0	18–22[5]
15–50 years	8.0	11.4	14.8[4]	15	12.5	17–21[5]
50+ years	4.7	6.7	8.7	10	9.5	8
Pregnancy	★	★	★	30	★	★
Lactation	★	★	★	15	10.5	10

★No increment
[1] 1 μmol iron = 55.9 μg
[2] Median basal requirement on intermediate bioavailability diet
[3] Bioavailability 15%
[4] Insufficient for women with high menstrual losses who may need iron supplements
[5] Lower value for 90% of population, upper value for 95% of population

Table A2.24 Dietary reference values for zinc (mg/day)

Age	UK			USA RDA	WHO (1992)[1]	European PRI
	LNRI	EAR	RNI			
0–3 months	2.6	3.3	4.0	5.0		
4–6 months	2.6	3.3	4.0	5.0		
7–12 months	3.0	3.8	5.0	5.0	5.6	4.0
1–3 years	3.0	3.8	5.0	10.0	5.5	4.0
4–6 years	4.0	5.0	6.5	10.0	6.5	6.0
7–10 years	4.0	5.4	7.0	10.0	7.5	7.0
Males						
11–14 years	5.3	7.0	9.0	15.0	12.1	9.0
15–18 years	5.5	7.3	9.5	15.0	13.1	9.5
19–50+ years	5.5	7.3	9.5	15.0	9.4	9.5
Females						
11–14 years	5.3	7.0	9.0	12.0	10.3	9.0
15–18 years	4.0	5.5	7.0	12.0	10.2	7.0
19–50+ years	4.0	5.5	7.0	12.0	6.5	7.1
Pregnancy	★	★	★	15.0	7.3–13.3	★
Lactation						
0–4 months			+6.0	19.0	12.7	+5.0
4+ months			+2.5	16	11.7	+5.0

★No increment
[1] Normative requirement on diet of moderate zinc availability

Table A2.25   Dietary reference values for copper[1] (mg/day)

Age	UK RNI	USA safe intake[2]	WHO (1992)[3]	European PRI
0–3 months	0.3	0.4–0.6	0.33–0.55	
4–6 months	0.3	0.4–0.6	0.37–0.62	
7–12 months	0.3	0.6–0.7	0.60	0.3
1–3 years	0.4	0.7–1.0	0.56	0.4
4–6 years	0.6	1.0–1.5	0.57	0.6
7–10 years	0.7	1.0–2.0	0.75	0.7
Males				
11–14 years	0.8	1.5–2.5	1.00	0.8
15–18 years	1.0	1.5–3.0	1.33	1.0
19–50+ years	1.2	1.5–3.0	1.35	1.1
Females				
11–14 years	0.8	1.5–2.5	1.00	0.8
15–18 years	1.0	1.5–3.0	1.15	1.0
19–50+ years	1.2	1.5–3.0	1.15	1.1
Pregnancy	★	★	★	★
Lactation	+0.3	★	1.25	+0.25

★No increment
[1] 1 µmol = 63.5 µg
[2] Upper levels should not be habitually exceeded because of toxicity
[3] Normative requirement

Table A2.26   Dietary reference values for selenium[1] (µg/day)

Age	UK LNRI	UK RNI	USA RDA	WHO (1992)[2]	European PRI
0–3 months	4	10	10	6	
4–6 months	5	13	10	9	
7–9 months	5	10	15	12	15
10–12 months	6	10	15	12	15
1–3 years	7	15	20	20	15
4–6 years	10	20	20	24	20
7–10 years	16	30	30	25	30
Males					
11–14 years	25	45	40	36	45
15–18 years	40	70	50	40	70
19–50+ years	40	75	70	40	55
Females					
11–14 years	25	45	45	30	45
15–18 years	40	60	50	30	60
19–50+ years	40	60	55	30	55
Pregnancy	★	★	65	39	★
Lactation	+15	+15	75	42–46	+12

★No increment
[1] 1 µmol selenium = 79 µg
[2] Normative requirement

Table A2.27   Dietary reference values for iodine (µg/day)

Age	UK		USA RDA	WHO (1992) RNI	European PRI
	LNRI	RNI			
0–3 months	40	50	40	40	
4–6 months	40	60	40	40	
7–12 months	40	60	50	50	70
1–3 years	40	70	70	70–120	70
4–6 years	50	100	90	70–120	100
7–10 years	55	110	120	70–120	110
Males and females					
11–14 years	65	130	150	120–150	130
15–18 years	70	140	150	120–150	140
19–50+ years	70	140	150	120–150	130
Pregnancy	⋆	⋆	175	175	⋆
Lactation	⋆	⋆	200	175	⋆

⋆No increment

Index